The Kidney and Hypertension in Diabetes Mellitus

This book is dedicated to the memory of Knud Lundbæk (1912–1995), distinguished diabetologist, my friend and mentor, and a great inspiration for all of us. He also became strongly engaged in exciting and penetrating new studies in the field of sinology, his second science.

CEM

The Kidney and Hypertension in Diabetes Mellitus

Sixth edition

Edited by

Carl Erik Mogensen MD
Professor of Medicine
Medical Department M
Aarhus University Hospital
Aarhus
Denmark

Editorial Secretary
Anna Honoré

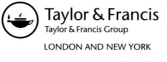

Taylor & Francis
Taylor & Francis Group
LONDON AND NEW YORK
A MARTIN DUNITZ BOOK

© 2004 Taylor & Francis, an imprint of the Taylor & Francis Group

First published in 1988 by Martinus Nijhoff Publishing, Boston (MA), USA

Sixth edition published in the UK in 2004 by
Taylor & Francis, an imprint of the Taylor & Francis Group, 11 New Fetter Lane,
London EC4P 4EE

Tel.: +44 (0) 20 7583 9855
Fax: +44 (0) 20 7842 2298
E-mail: info@dunitz.co.uk
Website: http://www.dunitz.co.uk

A CIP record for this book is available from the British Library.

Library of Congress Cataloging-in-Publication Data

Data available on application

ISBN 1-84184-433-0

Distributed in North and South America by

Taylor & Francis
2000 NW Corporate Blvd
Boca Raton, FL 33431, USA

Within Continental USA
Tel.: 800 272 7737; Fax: 800 374 3401
Outside Continental USA
Tel.: 561 994 0555; Fax: 561 361 6018
E-mail: orders@crcpress.com

Distributed in the rest of the world by
Thomson Publishing Services
Cheriton House
North Way
Andover, Hampshire SP10 5BE, UK
Tel.: +44 (0)1264 332424
E-mail: salesorder.tandf@thomsonpublishingservices.co.uk

Printed and bound in Great Britain by TJ International Ltd, Padstow, Cornwall

CONTENTS

Contents

PREFACE to the first edition

The first sporadic observations describing renal abnormalities in diabetes were published late in the 19th century, but systematic studies of the kidney in diabetes started only half a century ago after the paper by Cambier in 1934 and the much more famous study by Kimmelstiel and Wilson in 1936. These authors described two distinct features of renal involvement in diabetes: early hyperfiltration and late nephropathy. Diabetic nephropathy is, despite half a century of studies, still a very pertinent problem, renal disease in diabetes now being a very common cause of end-stage renal failure in Europe and North America and probably throughout the world. It is a very important part of the generalized vascular disease found in long-term diabetes as described by Knud Lundbæk in his monograph *Long-term Diabetes* in 1953, published by Munksgaard, Copenhagen.

Surprisingly, there has not been a comprehensive volume describing all aspects of renal involvement in diabetes, and the time is now ripe for such a volume summarizing the very considerable research activity within this field during the last decade and especially during the last few years.

This book attempts to cover practically all aspects of renal involvement in diabetes. It is written by colleagues who are themselves active in the many fields of medical research covered in this volume: epidemiology, physiology and pathophysiology, laboratory methodology, and renal pathology. New studies deal with the diagnosis and treatment of both incipient and overt nephropathy by metabolic, antihypertensive, and dietary invention.

Considerable progress has been made in the management of end-stage renal failure and also in the management and treatment of nephropathy in the pregnant diabetic woman. Diabetic nephropathy is a world-wide problem, but it is more clearly defined in Europe and North America where facilities for the diagnosis and treatment of diabetes and its complications are readily available. Much more work needs to be done in other parts of the world, as it appears from this book.

It is hoped that we now have a handbook for the kidney and hypertension in diabetes and that further progress can be made in clinical work in diagnosing and treating diabetic patients. Much more work still needs to be done regarding patient education with respect to complications. Many diabetics have now been trained to take part in the management of their metabolic control; they should also be trained to take part in the follow-up and treatment of complications.

This volume also underlines the considerable need for future research. So far, research in this field has been carried out in relatively few countries and centres in the world. The editor is sure that this volume will also stimulate further advancement in clinical science within the field of diabetic renal disease.

In 1952, the book *Diabetic Glomerulosclerosis, The Specific Renal Disease in Diabetes Mellitus*, by Harold Rifkin and co-workers, published by Charles C. Thomas, Springfield, Illinois, USA, summarized all current knowledge on the diabetic kidney in about 100 short pages, including many case histories. Much more space is needed now and the many disciplines involved will undoubtedly attract many readers.

Carl Erik Mogensen

PREFACE to the second edition

The sum of clinical problems caused by diabetic renal disease has been steadily increasing since the first edition of this book was published in 1988. Indeed, it is now estimated that throughout the world about 100,000 diabetic individuals are receiving treatment for end-stage renal failure. Obviously, this means a burden with respect to human suffering, disease and premature mortality, but additionally these treatment programmes are extremely costly, so costly that in many areas resources are not available for this kind of care. It is therefore clear, that every efforts should be made to prevent or postpone the development of end-stage disease.

The years since the first edition appeared we have seen a tremendous progress in research activities. Importantly, this also includes improvement in the treatment programmes to prevent end-stage renal failure. Thus it has become clear that the diabetic kidney is extremely pressure-sensitive, responding to effective antihypertensive treatment by retarded progression of disease. Some agents may be more beneficial in this respect than other, although the effective blood pressure reduction per se is crucial throughout the stages of diabetic renal disease. However, the prime cause of diabetic renal disease is related to poor metabolic control and it is now documented beyond doubt that good metabolic control is able to postpone or perhaps even prevent the development of renal disease. However, in many individuals we are not able to provide such a quality of control that will prevent complications, and therefore non-glycaemic intervention remains important. Maybe in the future non-glycaemic intervention will become the most important research area in diabetic nephropathy.

With respect to the exact mechanisms behind poor metabolic control and development of renal disease, much information is now being gained. It is likely that a combination of genetic predisposition and metabolic and haemodynamic abnormalities explain the progression to renal disease, seen in about 30% of the diabetic individuals. Much of this development probably relates to modifiable genetic factors, such as blood pressure elevation or haemodynamic aberrations. However, mechanisms related to the response to hyperglycaemia are also of clear importance as is the possibility that these metabolic or haemodynamic pathway may be inhibited.

This volume reviews older data as well as the progress seen within the research of diabetic nephropathy over the last five years and provides a state of the art of the development. However, we are still far from the main goal, which is the abolition of end-stage renal disease in diabetic individuals. Obviously, much work still needs to be done and one of the intentions of this book is to stimulate further research in this area where so many sub-disciplines of medical science are involved from the extremes of genetic and molecular biology to clinical and pharmacological research trials.

Carl Erik Mogensen
January 1994

PREFACE to the third edition

Many new dimensions have been added to the concepts regarding diabetic renal disease in the past few years. In addition some considerably amounts of new studies have been published since the second edition of this book. Therefore, there is a clear need to update the issue on diabetic renal disease. Ever more focus is placed on pressure-induced and metabolic related aberration, in relation to genetic abnormalities and also changes developing in foetal life. New chapters also include exercise, lipidemia and retinopathy in diabetic renal disease. New data are also included regarding structural changes in NIDDM-patients. Much of the development in diabetic renal disease is also relevant to non-diabetic renal disease, and therefore chapters comparing diabetic and non-diabetic renal disease have been included. As a result of the studies on pathogenesis of treatment of diabetic renal disease, new guidelines have been published as recently reviewed in the *Lancet* 1995. These guidelines are also included in this new edition, where the editor has tried to focus on all major issues relevant to diabetic renal disease. Many groups are working within this field, but the most cited authors are the following as recently reviewed by JDF (for the years 1981-95).

Measure Diabetes Research 1981-95 - Hypertension, Nephropathy (T-10)

		<u>Cites</u>	<u>Papers</u>	<u>C/P</u>
USA	Brenner B	2499	33	76
DK	*Christiansen JS*	2659	115	23
DK	*Deckert T*	4229	157	27
USA	Knowler WC	2975	127	23
USA	Krolewski AS	2220	74	30
USA	Mauer SM	2307	101	23
DK	*Mogensen CE*	3456	146	24
DK	*Parving HH*	4702	216	22
F	*Passa P*	1570	196	8
UK	*Viberti GC*	2820	119	24

Carl Erik Mogensen
August 1996

PREFACE to the fourth edition

We have witnessed a rapid development within the field of the kidney and hypertension in diabetes mellitus. A lot of work within the traditional areas has been published, and several new dimensions are now being developed, mostly in the experimental setting as discussed in several chapters. Therefore, there is now a need for an updated edition of this volume. A clear policy has been to have completely updated versions of the book, at disposal for the clinicians and the scientists in the area.

New guidelines are being developed within the field of hypertension and also in the field of diabetes mellitus, where new definitions are being introduced, mainly relevant for type 2 diabetes. The number of patients entering end-stage renal failure programmes are still increasing, underscoring the need for better management of these patients. The number of patients with diabetes is predicted to increased over the next decade, mainly due to changing patterns of life-style and an older population. Therefore, we need to be even more prepared to look after these patients, also with respect to renal, hypertensive and cardiovascular complications.

Since diabetic nephropathy is in most cases associated with heart disease and with retinopathy, new chapters on these aspects have been added. Very importantly, there is now more and more scientific support for early treatment in normotensive patients with microalbuminuria with ACE-inhibitors. This treatment seems beneficial also for diabetic heart disease and diabetic retinopathy according to new studies, also discussed in the book. The maxim is that diabetic nephropathy, retinopathy and heart disease often go together. The same seems to be the case regarding treatment and prevention.

Carl Erik Mogensen
January 1998

PREFACE to the fifth edition

Over the years this volume may have developed as the OPUS MAGNUM within in diabetic renal disease and hypertension. This is a rapidly expanding area as will be seen from all the new references, which have been included since the fourth edition.

Also knowledge within the field of hypertension in type 2 diabetes has developed very rapidly with the publication of many new trials, including the UKPDS. This study and other studies really emphasise the importance of good glycemic control and especially control of hypertension in these patients. Effective treatment would greatly minimise all vascular complications.

It is likely that the number of patients entering renal end-stage programs is still increasing but we can expect that this is due to better survival and postponement of the disease and also to better acceptance of patients that were earlier not allowed into this treatment programme.

The number of publications regarding microalbuminuria is continuously increasing, not only regarding diabetic nephropathy in its early phase, but also as a marker for cardiovascular disease, both in hypertension and in the general background population.

The maxim is still true that diabetic nephropathy, retinopathy, heart disease and vascular disease all go together often with neuropathy. This is also apparent in this volume, with focus on good glycemic control and the best possible antihypertensive treatment program to be implemented early.

Carl Erik Mogensen
March 2000

PREFACE to the sixth edition

The main subjects of this book, hypertension and renal disease in diabetes, are areas where developments rapidly occur all the time, and therefore there is a clear need for a new edition – also even though it is only three years after the latest volume. During these three years, there have been many important new publications and numerous new trials have been conducted.

Increasing emphasis is now put on screening meaning identifying patients early on by measuring microalbuminuria. Microalbuminuria is a unique predictor of worsening of renal disease, cardiovascular disease and also early mortality. An increasing number of studies documents that treatment improve prognosis.

Unfortunately, the number of end-stage renal disease related to type 2 diabetes is increasing but there seems to be a decline, at least in some countries of patients with type 1 diabetes – and it seems that also the age where patients enter advanced renal disease programmes has increased, probably related to greatly improved medical care in general.

With this new edition it is my hope that the number of diabetic patients entering ESRD finally will start to decrease.

Carl Erik Mogensen
January 2004

Contributors

Amanda Adler, MD, PhD, FRCP
Radcliffe Infirmary
Oxford Diabetes Research Laboratories
Woodstock Road
Oxford OX2 6HE, UK
Tel: +44 1865 2245 25
Fax: +44 1865 723884
E-mail: amanda.adler@dtu.ox.ac.uk

Niels Holmark Andersen
Medical Dept. M
Aarhus Kommunehospital
Aarhus University Hospital
DK-8000 Aarhus, Denmark
Fax: +45 8949 2010
E-mail: nielsholmark@dadlnet.dk

Sharon Anderson, M.D.
Division of Nephrology and Hypertension
Oregon Health and Science University
Portland, OR 97201, USA
Tel: +1-503-494-8490
Fax: +1-503-721-7810
E-mail: anderssh@ohsu.edu

George L. Bakris, MD, F.A.C.P
Rush University Hypertension Center
Rush-Presbyterian-St. Luke's Medical Center
1700 W. Van Buren
Suite #470
Chicago, IL 60612-3833, USA
Tel: +1 312 563 2195
Fax: +1 312 942 4464
E-mail: gbakris@rush.edu

Hans-Jacob Bangstad, M.D.
Unit of Nephrology
Pediatric Department
Aker Diabetes Research Center
Ullevål University Hospital
0407 Oslo, Norway
Tel: +47 2211 7954
Fax: +47 2211 8663
E-mail: hans-jacob.bangstad@uus.no

Rudy W. Bilous, MD, FRCP
Professor of Clinical Medicine
Audrey Collins Teaching Unit
Education Centre
James Cook University Hospital
Marton Road, Middlesbrough TS4 3BW, UK
Tel: +44 1 642 854 145
Fax: +44 1 642 854 148
E-mail: r.w.bilous@ncl.ac.uk

Geoffrey Boner, M.B.B.Ch.
Diabetic Complications Group
Baker Heart Res. Institute
Commercial Rd
Prahran 3181, VIV, Australia
E-mail: geoff.boner@baker.edu.aul

Knut Borch-Johnsen, M.D.
Steno Diabetes Center
Niels Steensens Vej 2
2820 Gentofte, Denmark
Tel: +45 4443 9415
Fax: +45 4443 8233
E-mail: kbjo@novo.dk

Vito M. Campese, M.D.
LAC/USC Medical Center
1200 North State St.
Los Angeles, CA 90033, USA
Tel: +1 213 226 7307
Fax: +1 213 226 5390
E-mail: campese@hsc.usc.edu

Professor John Chalmers
Institute for International Health
University of Sydney
PO Box 576 Newtown
NSW 2042, Australia
Tel: +61 2 9351 0063
Fax: +61 2 9352 0064
E-mail: chalmers@iih.usyd.edu.au

Per K. Christensen
Steno Diabetes Center
Niels Steensens Vej 2
2820 Gentofte, Denmark
tel: +45 3968 0800
fax: +45 3968 1048
E-mail:pkc@novonordisk.com

Mark Cooper, M.D.
Diabetes Complications Group
Baker Medical Research Institute
PO Box 6492
Melbourne 8008 VIC, Australia
Tel: +613 8532 1362
Fax: +613 8532 1480
E-mail: mark.cooper@baker.edu.au

Pedro Cortes, M.D., Director
Henry Ford Hospital & Medical Centers
Nephrology and Hypertension
2799 West Grand Boulevard
Detroit, Michigan 48202-2689, USA
Tel: +1 313 876 2711/2702
Fax: +1 313 876 2554
E-mail: cortes.pedro@usa.net

Dr. Ralf Dikow
Department of Internal medicine
Ruperto Carola University
Heidelberg, Germany
E-mail: ralf.dikow@med.uni-heidelberg.de

Bo Feldt-Rasmussen, M.D.
Medical Department P 2132
Rigshospitalet
DK-2100 Copenhagen Ø, Denmark
Tel: +45 3545 2135
Fax: +45 3545 2240
E-mail: bfr@rh.dk

Ele Ferrannini, M.D.
Istituto di Fisiologia Clinica del CNR
CNR Institute of Clinical Physiology
Consiglio Nazionale delle Ricerche - C.N.R.
c/o Università di Pisa
Via Savi, 8
I-56100 Pisa, Italy
Tel: +39 50 500087
Fax: +39 50 553235
E-mail: ferranni@ifc.pi.cnr.it

Paola Fioretto, M.D.
Istituto di Medicina Interna
Università di Padova
Via Giustiniani, 2
I-35128 Padova, Italy
Tel: +39 49 821 2150
Fax: +39 49 821 2151
E-mail: paola.fioretto@unipd.it

G. Alexander Fleming, MD
President and CEO
Kinexum LLP
550 Ridge St
Harper's Ferry, WV 25425
PO Box 1476, USA
E-mail: zanfleming@kinexum.com

Allan Flyvbjerg, MD. D.Sc.
Ass. Professor
Medical Department M
Diabetes & Endocrinology
Aarhus Kommunehospital
Aarhus University Hospital
DK-8000 Aarhus C, Denmark
Fax: +458949 2010/86 56 00 87
E-mail: allan.flyvbjerg@dadlnet.dk

Amy L. Friedman
Department of Surgery, Yale University School of
Medicine,
New Haven, Connecticut, USA
E-mail: amy.friedman@yale.edu

Eli A. Friedman, M.D.
Division of Renal Disease
Department of Medicine
State University of New York Health Science
Center at Brooklyn
450 Clarkson Avenue, Box 52
Brooklyn, NY 11203, USA
Tel: +1 718 270 1584
Fax: +1 718 270 3327
E-mail: elifriedmn@aol.com

Giovanni Gambaro
Division of Nephrology,
Dept. of Medical and Surgical Sciences
School of Medicine
Università di Padova
I-35128 Padova, Italy
E-mail: giga@unipd.it

Andy IM Hoepelman
University Medical Centre Utrecht
Dept. of Medicine,
3508 GA Utrecht, The Netherlands
Tel: +31 30 2506288
Fax: +31 302523741
e-mail: i.m.hoepelman@digd.azu.nl

Henrik Post Hansen
Steno Diabetes Center
Copenhagen, Denmark
e-mail: posthansen@dadlnet.dk

Klavs Würgler Hansen, M.D.
Medical Department
Silkeborg Centralsygehus
Falkevej 1-3
DK-8600 Silkeborg, Denmark
E-mail: kwh@dadlnet.dk

Tom Hostetter, Director
National Kidney Disease Education Program
Senior Scientific Advisor
National Instutes of Health
National Institutes of Diabetes, Digestive and
Kidney Diseases,
6707 Democracy Blvd., Room 625
Bethesda, Maryland 20892, USA.
Tel: 301 594 8864
Fax: 301 480 3510
E-mail: HostetterT@extra.niddk.nih.gov

Dr. Giuseppina Imperatore
Division of Diabetes Translation
Centers for Disease Control and Prevention
Atlanta, Georgia, USA
E-mail: gai5@cdc.gov

George Jerums, M.D.
Endocrine Unit
Austin Hospital
Burgundy Street
Heidelberg Victoria 3084, Australia
Tel: +61-39-496-5489
Fax: +61-39-496-3365
E-mail: endo@austin.unimelb.edu.au

Dr. Susan E. Jones
Department of medicine
The Medical school
Framlington Place
Newcastle Upon Tyne NE2 4HH, UK
Tel: +44 (0) 191 2227 019
Fax: +44 (0) 191 2220 723
E-mail: susan.jones@ncl.ac.uk

Professor William F. Keane, M.D.
Merck & Co. Inc
One Walnut Grove, HM 215
Horsham PA 19044, USA
E-mail: williamf_keane@merck.com

George L. King, M.D.
Vascular Cell Biology and Complications
Joslin Diabetes Center
One Joslin Place 02215
Boston, MA, USA
Tel: +1-617-732-2660
Fax: +1-617-732-2637
E-mail: george.king@joslin.harvard.edu

John L. Kitzmiller, M.D.
Chief, Maternal Fetal Medicine
Good Samaritan Health System
Perinatal Associates of Santa Clara Valley
2425 Samaritan Drive
San Jose, California 95124, USA
Tel: +1 408 559 2258
Fax: +1 408 559 2658
E-mail: kitz@batnet.com

William C. Knowler, M.D., Dr.P.H.
Chief, Diabetes and Arthritis Epidemiology
Section
National Institute of Diabetes and Digestive and
Kidney Diseases
1550 East Indian School Road
Phoenix, Arizona 85014, USA
Tel: +1 602 200-5206
Fax: +1 602 200-5225
E-mail: wknowler@phx.niddk.nih.gov

Gozewijn D. Laverman
Department of Internal Medicine, Division of
nephrology, University Hospital Groningen,
Groningen, The Netherlands
E-mail: gd_laverman@hotmail.com

Paulette Lyle
Merck & Co. Inc
One Walnut Grove, HM 215
Horsham PA 19044, USA
E-mail: paulette_lyle@merck.com

Professor Carl Erik Mogensen, M.D.
Medical Department M
Aarhus Kommunehospital
Aarhus University Hospital
DK-8000 Aarhus C, Denmark
Tel: +45 8949 2011
Fax: +45 8613 7825/8949 2010
E-mail: carl.erik.mogensen@afdm.au.dk

Henrik Bindesbøl Mortensen, M.D.
Pediatric Department L
Amtssygehuset i Glostrup
Ndr. Ringvej
DK-2600 Glostrup, Denmark
E-mail: HBMO@glolstruphosp.kbhamt.dk

Gerjan J. Navis, M.D.
Department of Internal Medicine
Division of Nephrology
University Hospital
Hanzeplein 1
9700 RB Groningen, The Netherlands
Fax: +31 50 3169310
E-mail: g.j.navis@int.azg.nl

Steen Olsen, M.D.
Professor Emeritus
Department of Pathology
Herlev Hospital
DK-2730 Herlev, Denmark
Tel: (home: 45 3976 2520)
E-mail: steeno@dadlnet.dk

Hans-Henrik Parving, M.D.
Steno Diabetes Center
Niels Steensens Vej 2
2820 Gentofte, Denmark
Tel: 44 43 90 53
Fax: 44 43 82 32
E-mail: HHParving@dadlnet.dk

Dr. Margrethe Mau Pedersen
Department of Internal Medicine
and Cardiology,
Aarhus University Hospital
DK-8000 Aarhus, Denmark
E-mail: mmp@hi.au.dk

David J. Pettitt, M.D.
Sansum Medical Research Foundation
2219 Bath Street
Santa Barbara, CA 93105, USA
Tel: +1 805 682 7640
Fax: +1 805 682 3332
E-mail: dpettitt@sansum.org

Per Løgstrup Poulsen, M.D.
Medical Department M
Aarhus Kommunehospital
Aarhus University Hospital
DK-8000 Aarhus C, Denmark
Tel: +45 8949 2019
Fax: +45 8949 2010
E-mail: logstrup@dadlnet.dk

Eberhard Ritz, M.D.
Sektion Nephrologie
Klinikum der Universität Heidelberg
Medizinische Klinik
Bergheimer Strasse 56a
D-69115 Heidelberg, Germany
Tel: +49 6221 91120
Fax: +49 6221 162476
E-mail: Prof.E.Ritz@T-online.de

Peter Rossing, M.D.
Steno Diabetes Center
Niels Steensensvej 2
DK-2820 Gentofte, Denmark
Fax: +45 4443 8232
E-mail: prossing@dadlnet.dk

Dr. Piero Ruggenenti
Mario Negri Institute for Pharmacological
Research
Via Gavazzeni 11
24125 Bergamo, Italy
Tel: +39 035 319 888
Fax: +39 035 319 331
E-mail: ruggenenti@irfmn.mnegri.it

Erwin Schleicher, M.D.
Institute of Internal Medicine
Dep. Of Endocrinology, Metabolism and
Pathobiochemistry
University of Tübingen
Otfried-Müller-Str. 10
D-72076 Tübingen, Germany
Tel: +49 7071 29 87599
Fax: +49 7071 29 5974
e-mail: enschlei@med.uni-tuebingen.de

Dr. Neil Sheerin
Department of Nephrology and Transplantation
Guy's King's and St Thomas' School of Medicine
King's College London
London SE1 9RT, UK
Tel: +44 (0) 7955 2117
Fax: +44 (0) 7955 4303
E-mail: neil.sheerin@kcl.ac.uk

Coen D.A. Stehouwer, M.D.
Department of Internal Medicine
VU University Medical Centre
De Boelelaan 1117
1081 HV Amsterdam, The Netherlands
Tel: +31 20 444 309
Fax: +31 20 444 313
E-mail: cda.stehouwer@vumc.nl

Lise Tarnow, M.D.
Steno Diabetes Center
Niels Steensensvej 2
2820 Gentofte, Denmark
Fax: +45 4443 8232
E-mail: LTAR@steno.dk

Merlin C Thomas
Danielle Alberti Memorial Centre for Diabetes
Complications
Baker Heart Research Institute
Melbourne 8008, Victoria, Australia
E-mail;: merlin.thomas@baker.edu.a

Dr. Stephen .M. Thomas
King's Diabetes Centre
Kings College Hospital
London, UK
Tel: +44 (0) 207 737 1737
Fax: +44 (0) 207 737 -
E-mail: Stephen.Thomas@kingsch.nhs.uk

GianCarlo Viberti, M.D.
Division of Medicine
Guy's and St Thomas's Medical and
Dental School
Unit for Metabolic Medicine
Diabetes, Endocrinology, Metabolism
Floor 5 Hunt's House, Guy's Hospital
London Bridge, London SE1 9RT, UK
Tel: +44 1 71 955 4826
Fax: +44 1 71 955 2985
E-mail: giancarlo.viberti@kcl.ac.uk

Dr. Cora Weigert
Department of medicine
Div. of Endocrinology, Metabolism and
Pathobiochemistry
University of Tübingen, Germany
E-mail: caweiger@med.uni-tuebingen.de

Contributors

Fuad N. Ziyadeh, M.D.
Renal-Electrolyte and Hypertension Division
700 Clinical Research Building
University of Pennsylvania Medical Center
415 Curie Boulevard
Philadelphia, PA 19104-6144, USA
Tel: +1 215 573 1837
Fax: +1 215 898 0189
E-mail: ziyadeh@mail.med.upenn.edu

Giulio Zuanetti, M.D.
Department of Cardiovascular Research
Istituto Mario Negri
via Eritrea 62
I-20157 Milan, Italy
Tel: +39 2 3901 4454
Fax: +39 2 3320 004
E-mail: zuanetti@irfmn.mnegri.it

1

RATIONALE FOR EARLY SCREENING FOR DIABETIC KIDNEY DISEASE

Thomas H Hostetter

University of Minnesota, Director, National Kidney Disease Education Program, Senior Scientific Advisor, National Institutes of Health, National Institute of Diabetes, Digestive, and Kidney Diseases, 6707 Democracy Blvd, Room 625, Bethesda, MD 20892, fax +1 301-480-3510

Primary prevention of diabetic nephropathy is probably possible with rigorous glucose and blood pressure control [1-3]. Indeed, many people at risk for type 2 diabetes could even prevent the development of diabetes [4, 5]. However, screening for diabetic renal disease falls within the scope of secondary prevention. The goal of such screening is not to prevent the appearance of renal damage but to detect it early enough that its course can be favorably deflected. Thus, at first approximation such screening has the same general goals as mammography for breast cancer or fecal occult blood detection for colon cancer.

Several principles guide the decision for any screening of this type [6]. First, the disease should be serious but also be predictably indolent in its course so that interventions can be applied before the most serious outcomes transpire. It should also be relatively common. The screening test must be specific and sensitive but also it must identify the disease early in its course. Next, therapy that improves outcome when given early must exist. Finally, the costs of screening and therapy must be acceptable. Evidence for the currently recommended screening and consequent treatments for diabetic nephropathy approach but do not completely satisfy all these criteria.

GOALS OF SCREENING

Before assessing the degree to which screening for kidney damage meets the above principles, the goals of screening for this condition should be considered in some more detail. They are wider than for cancer screening wherein the only purpose is to prevent or perhaps delay cancer related death. To be sure, the major goal of screening for early diabetic nephropathy is to delay the course of progressive loss of renal function and the need for dialysis or transplantation. Although preventing the occurrence of ESRD is not predictably possible after evidence of the disease appears, the rate may be slowed sufficiently in some patients so as to avoid ESRD. Furthermore, with the links between renal injury and wider cardiovascular risk, the implications of screening have wider and more difficult to delimit implications than testing for a cancer.

Other benefits, which are harder to measure, also accrue to a positive screening test.

The specific therapeutic consequences of a positive result are actually only a very modest adjustment to the ongoing guidelines for care of people with diabetes without nephropathy, principally addition of an angiotensin converting enzyme inhibitor (ACEI) or angiotensin receptor blocker (ARB) [7]. However, these drugs may have special benefits for non-renal complications especially cardiovascular ones, although debate still exists on this point [8-10]. In any case, the presence of renal damage predicts cardiovascular risk and should be an occasion to redouble the search for classic risk factors for heart and vascular disease. This added scrutiny is especially desirable as cardiovascular death supervenes before ESRD in most patients with diabetic renal disease. (See Chapter 39). Perhaps the psychological impact, for both patient and provider, is as important as the specific recognition of kidney dysfunction. The solid identification of a very serious diabetic complication could intensify adherence to the overall guidelines of glycemic control, blood pressure control, retinal screening, lipid monitoring, etc. Some of these will dampen kidney injury but they will also have more general benefits. A final potential merit of screening for kidney function is preparation of the patient for ESRD. Secondary prevention of nephropathy is imperfect and patients can develop ESRD despite adequate care. Preparation for uremia –vascular access placement, attention to mineral metabolism, planning for transplantation, anemia management, etc, - has value and tardy recognition of impending renal failure carries a large cost [11].

Given the nexus between renal disease and the wide range of diabetic complication especially cardiovascular one, screening for nephropathy should not be seen as purely isolated to ESRD outcomes.

MAGNITUDE OF DIABETIC NEPHROPATHY

In 2000 in the United States, 42,000 people developed end stage renal disease due to diabetic nephropathy for an incidence rate of 146 per million population [12]. This leads to a prevalence of 131,000 people receiving ESRD care due to diabetes. All of these numbers had more than doubled over the prior ten years [12]. Diabetes was the leading cause of ESRD accounting for about 43% of prevalent cases. These trends have begun to be recognized worldwide [13]. With an annual mortality of 23% during renal replacement therapy in the United States, 31,000 people with diabetic nephropathy and ESRD died in 2000 despite dialysis or transplantation [12]. These data compare with the death rates for the third and fourth leading causes of cancer death in the United States, breast and prostate, which accounted for 42,000 and 31,000 deaths respectively. Unlike ESRD due to diabetes, the death rates for these two cancers have been essentially stable for more than a decade [14]. Thus, the disease burden diabetic nephropathy is large and increasing.

The cost of caring for patients with diabetes and ESRD is also large and growing. All ESRD care is costly but people with diabetes incur greater expenses than others. Approximately $19 billion (US) was expended for all of ESRD care in 2000 in the United States and at least half of that went to treat diabetic ESRD[14]. Hence, in economic as well human terms diabetic nephropathy represents a substantial societal cost.

TEMPO OF THE DISEASE

Diabetic nephropathy can be envisioned as proceeding through some initial period of diabetes usually exceeding 10 years in type 1 diabetes and a less clearly defined interval in type 2 in which the presence of injury is currently undetectable by laboratory tests [1, 15-18]. Then, in some patients abnormal amounts of urinary albumin become detectable. This low-grade albuminuria is termed microalbuminuria, usually defined as more than 30 mg per day. (Definitions and further details of microalbuminuria are contained in Chapters 6, 26 and 47). At the onset of this second step of microalbuminuria, variable amounts of histologic injury may be present but glomerular filtration rate (GFR) is within the normal range. Higher rates of albuminuria, usually defined as greater than 300mg per day and called macroalbuminuria or dipstick positive proteinuria, are associated with declining GFR. This phase is often styled overt diabetic nephropathy. Patients with microalbuminuria develop overt nephropathy at variable and unpredictable rates but these average 5% per year [15, 19]. Hence, upward of 10 years may be spent in this microalbuminuric phase. With overt nephropathy, decay in GFR also shows wide individual variability but averages a loss of approximately 12ml/min per year [1, 15, 16]. If such a rate of decline began at a GFR of 100 ml/min then about seven years would elapse before ESRD care would be required. A major shortcoming in our present knowledge is the lack of predictability of rate of progression for individual patients as the above averages lie within vary wide ranges. However, at not only the microalbuminuric phase but also with overt nephropathy, relatively long, if highly variable, periods of time are available for effective therapy.

STRENGTH OF SCREENING TESTS FOR DIABETIC NEPHROPATHY

At present only two general classes of tests are used to detect diabetic nephropathy. First, GFR can be assessed. This is done most conveniently by measuring serum creatinine and entering that value in an estimating equation. Current equations have been incompletely validated for patients with diabetes and serum creatinine measurements are not so true as desirable especially in the near normal range [20, 21]. However, these deficiencies are not the major reason that GFR based screening has not been favored as a screening tool. Indeed, despite these weaknesses estimation of GFR is still a useful and needed adjunct to usual screening. As described above, when GFR has descended into the clearly abnormal range, much of the course of nephropathy has been run and the opportunity for intervention has diminished. Thus, GFR decline is a late index of kidney damage

Albuminuria precedes the decline in GFR and testing for microalbuminuria is the commonly recommended screening test for diabetic nephropathy and the stage of disease has been called incipient nephropathy [1, 15, 18, 22]. Microalbuminuria is not specific to diabetic nephropathy. Other renal diseases can provoke it and transient and presumably trivial transient conditions such as fever or exertion can as well. For this reason the test should not be done under such conditions and at least two out of three samples obtained within in a six month period should be positive before designating a patient as microalbuminuric is made. Although structural changes in the glomerulus are said to be uniformly present in microalbuminuric patients, not all patients who have persistent microalbuminuria progress to overt nephropathy and then to ESRD [1, 19, 23]. Some of them will die prematurely of cardiovascular disease since microalbuminuria predicts cardiovascular as well as renal risk (See Chapter 4). Initial reports held that approximately 80 % of microalbuminuric patients with type 1 diabetes progressed to overt proteinuria [1, 18, 19]. Some have contended that a lower fraction progress and the portion ultimately reaching ESRD is less clear [24]. At present there is simply insufficient data to state with precision what percentage of diabetics with microalbuminuria progress to ESRD, die of cardiovascular disease, or remain alive with only age attributable change in renal function. Indeed, given the current guidelines to test for microalbuminuria and treat if present, a true sensitivity in a natural history sense will never be obtainable.

The sensitivity of microalbuminuria seems less problematic but no more subject to thorough analysis than its specifity. At any rate, to the author's knowledge no reports exist of a patient who developed ESRD due to proven diabetic nephropathy but without antecedent microalbuminuria despite annual surveillance. The test is likely to be highly sensitive.

VALUE OF EARLY THERAPY

The treatment of hypertension has long been recognized as a means for attenuating the course of overt nephropathy [18] (See Chapters 31 and 33). In recent years the particular value of ACEI or ARBs in such treatment has been established [1, 25-28]. When applied at a GFR of approximately 40 ml/min, ARBs delays ESRD by about two years compared to other antihypertensives. Probably another two years reprieve would occur for every 30 ml/min higher level of initiation [1, 25]. That is, four years would likely be gained if the drugs were started with overt proteinuria but a GFR of 70 ml/min. The earlier the treatment of overt nephropathy, the more time free of ESRD is gained.

For some observers, the major remaining point of uncertainty is the advantage of applying these drugs during the microalbumiuric phase and particularly in those who remain normotensive at that phase. Most patients with type 2 diabetes and microalbuminuria have hypertension especially if current JNC 7,

ADA, and NKF guidelines for target blood pressure of less than 130/80 are used [7, 29-32]. However, many type 1 diabetics with microalbuminuria may remain within these bounds [33]

The result of treatment with ACEIs or ARBs during microalbuminuria has been established by in randomized controlled trials and is similar in both types of diabetes though more extensive with type 2 disease. Such treatment clearly delays the appearance of overt nephropathy [1, 33, 34]. However, studies demonstrating delay to ESRD are lacking. Nevertheless, the continuous nature of albuminuria- the division between micro and overt is largely arbitrary- coupled with the clear diminution in deterioration in GFR by ACEI and ARB in the overt stage, both argue for a benefit in the earlier phase. The micro HOPE trial provides some additional support for these drugs at this phase [8]. In the final analysis though it must be admitted that formal evidence of prevention or delay of ESRD from a randomized clinical trial has not been adduced for treatment during microalbuminuria.

Current therapy applied at the stage of microalbuminuria cannot promise complete interdiction of progressive renal injury. Retrospectively identified subsets of patients do show stabilization or at least the slow declines comparable to aging alone [35]. Still, the follow-ups are not long enough to confidently consider these in remission. Thus, cure in the sense that successful surgery for cancer can cure, is not yet predictable in even early diabetic nephropathy. Substantial delay in ESRD is predictable and the earlier the application the longer the respite.

COSTS OF SCREENING AND TREATMENT

Economic analyses have generally suggested that screening followed by therapy with an ACEI reduces costs or results in acceptable expenditure for each quality adjusted life year gained [1, 36-39]. However, some have been more skeptical [40, 41]. Critique of the more detailed modeling required for these projections is beyond the scope of this chapter. However, such exercises can depend critically on input variables some of which are either uncertain or changing. For example, the cost of drugs generally declines as their patent lives expire. As noted above, the specificity of urinary albumin testing in predicting ESRD may be unknowable since guidelines dictate treatment when microalbuminuria is detected. Also benefits to cardiovascular outcomes and the potential for a positive test for nephropathy to inspire better observance of all facets of care have not been included in these computations. Finally, overall costs to society are of paramount concern but these may vary somewhat depending on the health care system even within the developed countries and the specific economic implications can differ greatly within components of a heterogeneous system of payers as seen in the United States.

CURRENT STATUS

Multiple health providers and groups such as the American Diabetes Association have promulgated guidelines for screening for nephropathy and they are generally similar [15]. As can be gleaned from the above discussion all criteria for screening are not perfectly satisfied but in this author's judgment the available data support it. One major issue raised in critical analyses is that a prospective randomized trial of screening has not been performed. This is true. However, the duration of such a trial from normoalbuminuria to ESRD or death would be so long, more than 2 decades that it will never occur. Moreover, equipoise on the usefulness of screening clearly does not exist. The current scheme proposed by the American Diabetes Association shown in Figure 1 is sound.

ALTERNATIVE VIEWS AND FUTURE DIRECTIONS

Current guidelines for the general care of patients with diabetes emphasize lower than usual blood pressure goals (typically 130/80 mm Hg), smoking cessation, and the best possible glycemic control [7]. Hence, within the armamentarium for treating early renal disease, the finding of microalbuminuria leads only to the addition of an ACEI or ARB to the recommended regimen. (Other issues such as low protein diets, phosphate control, and anemia management are in the province of more established renal insufficiency) Furthermore, since these drugs are generally well tolerated, some have proposed treating all diabetics, or at least those at higher risk, with an ACEI and forgoing screening for albuminuria altogether. One economic analysis concluded that for type 2 diabetics over 50 years, this was a cost saving strategy [42]. Another model also held that such an approach for high-risk patients with type 1 diabetes was cheaper [43]. Of course, identification of the higher risk subgroup is at present weak. As the authors note, these analyses are sensitive to either poorly defined or changing assumptions. Nevertheless, the idea has appeal not only because of the drugs' tolerability but also because in United States screening is done for only a small minority who should receive it and even when done and positive patient or provider does not begin therapy.

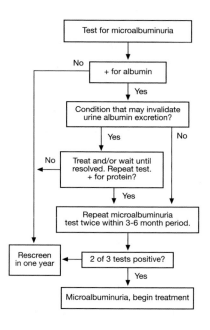

Figure 1. A suggested path for screening for diabetic nephropathy. From the American Diabetes Association reference 15.

Data bearing on the usefulness of universal, preemptive treatment with ACEI or ARB should be forthcoming. Mauer and his colleagues are conducting a study in type 1 diabetes to assess largely by morphometry the value of ACI and ARB in normoalbuminuric type 1 patients [44]. If proven effective, these results would influence the debate on screening versus treating all and screening none.

Other trials of this approach with an endpoint of development of microalbuminuria and economic analyses would be of interest. They should also consider not only fixed annual screening versus prophylactic treatment but also the third issue of whether patients are actually screened and treated in current practice.

No strong rationale exists for continued annual testing for albuminuria once it has been detected and ACEI or ARB begun. Some have argued for titration of blood pressure downward or ACEI ARB upward dependent upon albuminuria. Continued monitoring of albuminuria for this purpose does not now have a strong evidence base. Here too trials would be useful.

Finally, better markers of renal damage and better tools for identifying patients at high risk would greatly advance this area. The desirability of better therapies is almost self-evident. Such progress could improve screening or better yet abolish its need.

REFERENCES

1. Retinopathy and nephropathy in patients with type 1 diabetes four years after a trial of intensive therapy. The Diabetes Control and Complications Trial/Epidemiology of Diabetes Interventions and Complications Research Group. N Engl J Med, 2000. 342(6): p. 381-9.
2. Intensive blood-glucose control with sulphonylureas or insulin compared with conventional treatment and risk of complications in patients with type 2 diabetes (UKPDS 33). UK Prospective Diabetes Study (UKPDS) Group. Lancet, 1998. 352(9131): p. 837-53.
3. Tight blood pressure control and risk of macrovascular and microvascular complications in type 2 diabetes: UKPDS 38. UK Prospective Diabetes Study Group. BMJ, 1998. 317(7160): p. 703-13.
4. Knowler, W.C., et al., Reduction in the incidence of type 2 diabetes with lifestyle intervention or metformin. N Engl J Med, 2002. 346(6): p. 393-403.
5. Tuomilehto, J., et al., Prevention of type 2 diabetes mellitus by changes in lifestyle among subjects with impaired glucose tolerance. N Engl J Med, 2001. 344(18): p. 1343-50.
6. M T Connelly, T.S.I., Principles of Disease Prevention, in Harrison's Principles of Internal Medicine, E.B. A S Fauci, K J Isselbacher, et al, Editor. 1998, Mcgraw-Hill: New york. p. 46-48.
7. Standards of medical care for patients with diabetes mellitus. Diabetes Care, 2003. 26(Supplement 1): p. 1- 156.
8. Effects of ramipril on cardiovascular and microvascular outcomes in people with diabetes mellitus: results of the HOPE study and MICRO-HOPE substudy. Heart Outcomes Prevention Evaluation Study Investigators. Lancet, 2000. 355(9200): p. 253-9.

9. Wing, L.M.H., et al., A Comparison of Outcomes with Angiotensin-Converting-Enzyme Inhibitors and Diuretics for Hypertension in the Elderly. N Engl J Med, 2003. 348(7): p. 583-592.

10. Major outcomes in high-risk hypertensive patients randomized to angiotensin-converting enzyme inhibitor or calcium channel blocker vs diuretic: The Antihypertensive and Lipid-Lowering Treatment to Prevent Heart Attack Trial (ALLHAT). Jama, 2002. 288(23): p. 2981-97.

11. Kinchen, K.S., et al., The timing of specialist evaluation in chronic kidney disease and mortality. Ann Intern Med, 2002. 137(6): p. 479-86.

12. U.S. renal Data System, USRDS 2002 Annual Data Report: Atlas of End-stage Renal Disease in the United States. 2002, National Institutes of Health, National Institute of Diabetes and Digestive and Kideny Diseases.

13. Ritz, E., et al., End-stage renal failure in type 2 diabetes: A medical catastrophe of worldwide dimensions. Am J Kidney Dis, 1999. 34(5): p. 795-808.

14. SEER: Surveillance , Epidemiology and End Results, National Cancer Institute.

15. Diabetic Nephropathy. Diabetes Care, 2003. 26(90001): p. 94S-98.

16. Remuzzi, G., A. Schieppati, and P. Ruggenenti, Nephropathy in Patients with Type 2 Diabetes. N Engl J Med, 2002. 346(15): p. 1145-1151.

17. Ritz, E. and S.R. Orth, Nephropathy in patients with type 2 diabetes mellitus. N Engl J Med, 1999. 341(15): p. 1127-33.

18. Parving, H.H., Osterby R, Anderson P W, Hsueh W A, Diabetic Nephropathy, in The Kidney, B.M. Brenner, Editor. 1996, W. B. Saundesr: Philadelphia. p. 1864-1892.

19. Parving, H.H., et al., Does microalbuminuria predict diabetic nephropathy? Diabetes Care, 2002. 25(2): p. 406-7.

20. Coresh, J., et al., Calibration and random variation of the serum creatinine assay as critical elements of using equations to estimate glomerular filtration rate. Am J Kidney Dis, 2002. 39(5): p. 920-9.

21. Manjunath, G., M.J. Sarnak, and A.S. Levey, Prediction equations to estimate glomerular filtration rate: an update. Curr Opin Nephrol Hypertens, 2001. 10(6): p. 785-92.

22. Kasiske, B.L., Keane WF, Laboratory Assessment of Renal Disease, in The Kidney, B.M. Brenner, Editor. 1996, W. B. Saunders: Philadelphia. p. 1137-1174.

23. Caramori, M.L., P. Fioretto, and M. Mauer, The need for early predictors of diabetic nephropathy risk: is albumin excretion rate sufficient? Diabetes, 2000. 49(9): p. 1399-408.

24. Tabaei, B.P., et al., Does microalbuminuria predict diabetic nephropathy? Diabetes Care, 2001. 24(9): p. 1560-6.

25. Brenner, B.M., et al., Effects of losartan on renal and cardiovascular outcomes in patients with type 2 diabetes and nephropathy. N Engl J Med, 2001. 345(12): p. 861-9.

26. Hostetter, T.H., Prevention of end-stage renal disease due to type 2 diabetes. N Engl J Med, 2001. 345(12): p. 910-2.

27. Lewis, E.J., et al., The effect of angiotensin-converting-enzyme inhibition on diabetic nephropathy. The Collaborative Study Group. N Engl J Med, 1993. 329(20): p. 1456-62.

28. Lewis, E.J., et al., Renoprotective effect of the angiotensin-receptor antagonist irbesartan in patients with nephropathy due to type 2 diabetes. N Engl J Med, 2001. 345(12): p. 851-60.

29. The Seventh Report of the Joint National Commission on Prevention, Detection, Evaluation and Treatment of High Blood Pressure. 2003, National Heart, Lung, and Blood Institute.

30. Levey, A.S., et al., National Kidney Foundation Practice Guidelines for Chronic Kidney Disease: evaluation, classification and stratification. Ann Inter Med, 2003. 139: p.137–41.

31. Olivarius Nde, F., et al., Epidemiology of renal involvement in newly-diagnosed middle-aged and elderly diabetic patients. Cross-sectional data from the population-based study "Diabetes Care in General Practice", Denmark. Diabetologia, 1993. 36(10): p. 1007-16.

32. Gall, M.A., et al., Prevalence of micro- and macroalbuminuria, arterial hypertension, retinopathy and large vessel disease in European type 2 (non-insulin-dependent) diabetic patients. Diabetologia, 1991. 34(9): p. 655-61.

33. Mathiesen, E.R., et al., Efficacy of captopril in postponing nephropathy in normotensive insulin dependent diabetic patients with microalbuminuria. Bmj, 1991. 303(6794): p.81-7.

34. Parving, H.H., et al., The effect of irbesartan on the development of diabetic nephropathy in patients with type 2 diabetes. N Engl J Med, 2001. 345(12): p. 870-8.

35. Hovind, P., et al., Remission and regression in the nephropathy of type 1 diabetes when blood pressure is controlled aggressively. Kidney Int, 2001. 60(1): p. 277-83.

36. Borch-Johnsen, K., et al., Is screening and intervention for microalbuminuria worthwhile in patients with insulin dependent diabetes? Bmj, 1993. 306(6894): p. 1722-5.

37. Klonoff, D.C. and D.M. Schwartz, An economic analysis of interventions for diabetes. Diabetes Care, 2000. 23(3): p. 390-404.

38. Palmer, A.J., et al., The cost-effectiveness of different management strategies for type I diabetes: a Swiss perspective. Diabetologia, 2000. 43(1): p. 13-26.

39. Siegel, J.E., et al., Cost-effectiveness of screening and early treatment of nephropathy in patients with insulin-dependent diabetes mellitus. J Am Soc Nephrol, 1992. 3(4 Suppl): p. S111-9.

40. Scheid, D.C., et al., Screening for microalbuminuria to prevent nephropathy in patients with diabetes: a systematic review of the evidence. J Fam Pract, 2001. 50(8): p. 661-8.

41. Kiberd, B.A. and K.K. Jindal, Screening to prevent renal failure in insulin dependent diabetic patients: an economic evaluation. Bmj, 1995. 311(7020): p. 1595-9.

42. Golan, L., J.D. Birkmeyer, and H.G. Welch, The cost-effectiveness of treating all patients with type 2 diabetes with angiotensin-converting enzyme inhibitors. Ann Intern Med, 1999. 131(9): p. 660-7.

43. Kiberd, B.A. and K.K. Jindal, Routine treatment of insulin-dependent diabetic patients with ACE inhibitors to prevent renal failure: an economic evaluation. Am J Kidney Dis, 1998. 31(1): p. 49-54.

44. Mauer, S. Zinman B, Gardiner R, Drummond KN, Suissa S, Donnelly SM, Strand TD, Kramer MS, Klein R, Sinaiko AR. ACE-I and ARBs in early diabetic nephropathy. JRAAS 2003. 3(4): 262-9.

2

PRESSURE-INDUCED AND METABOLIC ALTERATIONS IN THE GLOMERULUS: CYTOSKELETAL CHANGES

Pedro Cortes and Jerry Yee
Henry Ford Hospital, Detroit, Michigan USA

INTRODUCTION

One renal alteration that appears to be common to type 1 and type 2 diabetes is an early period of glomerular hyperfiltration [1-4]. Increased glomerular filtration rate (GFR) and renal plasma flow have been extensively documented in type 1 diabetes presage the onset of nephropathy [5]. Studies in experimental, insulin-deficient diabetes have shown that this hyperfunction is mainly due to glomerular hypertrophy and increased glomerular capillary pressure that are widely recognized as important factors in the genesis of glomerular injury [6-8]. Numerous studies have repeatedly shown an improvement or prevention of experimental diabetic glomerulosclerosis by normalizing intraglomerular pressure.

Thus, agents that limit the formation or action of angiotensin II whose receptor distribution in the renal arteriolar circulation is preponderant on the efferent arteriole may slow the progression of glomerulosclerosis in type 1 and type 2 diabetic patients, independently of changes in systemic pressure, presumably by inducing vasorelaxation of the efferent arteriole with consequent reduction of intraglomerular pressure and filtration [9-13]. However, it is less abundantly clear how this glomerular hypertension occurs and by which mechanism the

Mogensen CE (ed.) THE KIDNEY AND HYPERTENSION IN DIABETES MELLITUS. Copyright©
2004 by Martin Dunitz, a member of the Taylor & Francis Group, plc. All rights reserved.

increased intraglomerular pressure translates into metabolic alterations that lead to glomerular extracellular matrix accumulation.

AFFERENT ARTERIOLAR HYPOCONTRACTILITY

Glomeruli are normally subjected to minimal variations in internal pressure due to the precise afferent arteriolar autoregulatory control of glomerular pressure [14, 15]. Importantly, early in the course of glomerular sclerosis, such as in the remnant kidney and in insulin-deficient diabetes, there is a characteristic afferent arteriolar vasodilation and impairment of pressure-induced vasoconstriction [16-18]. This lack of afferent arteriolar autoregulation permits the free intraglomerular transmission of systemic arterial pressure and its variations and fosters hemodynamic strain [19, 20]. Therefore, restoring the functionality of the afferent arteriole appears as the logic target for therapeutic intervention. However, the pathobiology that underlies this arteriolar hypocontractiliy remains elusive.

Increased capillary wall tension is, obviously, the force causing distention of the elastic glomerulus. This wall tension depends on the level of intraluminal hydrostatic pressure and the diameter of the vessel, as defined by the LaPlace's principle. Thus, for any given pressure, glomerular expansion will be greater in large glomeruli containing capillaries with increased vessel radius than in smaller glomeruli formed by capillaries of smaller radius. However, independently of the prevalent stiffness and capillary diameter, it is the wide oscillation in intraglomerular pressure the force which ultimately may cause the repeating glomerular expansion/contraction that causes mesangial mechanical stretch.

Numerous studies have implicated abnormal renal eicosanoid metabolism as the cause for diabetic renal vasodilation and hyperfiltration. A preferential increase in vasodilatory prostaglandins associated with overexpression of cyclooxygenase-2, and reduced glomerular thromboxane receptors have been described in experimental diabetes [16, 21-23]. Other evidence has suggested an important role of an overactive kallikrein-kinin system as mediator of hyperfiltration in human and experimental diabetes [24-26]. More recently, the role of nitric oxide has been extensively studied with sharply conflicting results [27-29]. Finally, a defective contractility of the afferent arteriole has been related to a basal activation of its K_{ATP} channels induced by diabetes, however, chronic blocking of these channels does not result in amelioration of hyperfiltration [30, 31]. Therefore, it remains uncertain if any of the mechanisms proposed, or their combination, may be responsible for the abnormal arteriolar contractility.

GLOMERULAR DISTENSIBILITY

How intraglomerular hypertension may induce hemodynamic strain and trigger a cascade of metabolic events has been clarified following the demonstration of the unique elastic properties of the glomerular structure and the response of mesangial cells when subjected to mechanical stretch in tissue culture. Conclusive evidence of glomerular elasticity has been provided by studies in isolated microperfused glomeruli *ex vivo* [20]. As the intraglomerular pressure is increased from zero to levels approximating those observed in the diabetic and in the remnant kidney, glomerular volume increases by about 30% [32]. In addition, due to the high elasticity of the glomerular structure, volume changes reach their maximum within 3-4 seconds following alteration in intraglomerular pressure [19]. This elasticity, therefore, allows the occurrence of significant volume changes even with the most transient variations in intraglomerular pressure. Further, for the same increase in internal pressure, the degree of distention of the hypertrophied diabetic glomeruli is significantly greater than that in normal sized ones [33].

Glomerular expansion is, obviously, associated with the stretching of its structural components, including the extracellular matrix and the cellular constituents. Because both capillary lumina and mesangial regions equally participate in the overall increase in glomerular volume [19], endothelial, mesangial and epithelial cells will all be subjected to stretch as intraglomerular pressure increases. Due to the central location of the mesangial regions within the glomerular lobule, mesangial cells (MC), in particular, experience substantial mechanical strain. Detailed morphological studies have demonstrated how numerous cytoplasmic projections emerging from the MC body extend between adjacent capillaries and firmly attach to the perimesangeal regions of the glomerular basement membrane [34]. Therefore, the centrifugal displacement of these regions during glomerular expansion is expected to result in marked tridimensional MC stretch.

In addition to MC, podocytes are also expected to be subjected to intense mechanical strain during glomerular distention. Since these cells are commonly attached to several capillaries via their extended foot processes, capillary dilation will result in their bi-dimensional stretch extending over a wide surface [35].

REGULATION OF GLOMERULAR EXPANSION

Cellular mechanical strain is derived from the repetitive stretching and contracting of the cell body as the consequence of cyclic variations in glomerular volume. Therefore the elements opposing distention, i.e., overall glomerular stiffness are important modulators of mechanical strain. The degree of glomerular stiffness is primarily determined by the rigidity of the glomerular scaffold, i.e., peripheral basement membrane and mesangial matrix [19, 36] and by the cellular component. The composition and distribution of the extracellular matrix is probably an important determinant of the glomerular mechanical properties because, contrary to what might have been predicted, the rigidity of the passive component of glomerular stiffness is diminished in conditions of incipient glomerulosclerosis [19].

The contribution of the cellular component depends on cytoskeletal elements of MC and podocytes, particularly the actin cytoskeleton. The actin cytoskeleton and its cell membrane attachments are highly dynamic structures responsible for the maintenance of cell shape and contractility, polarity, migration, cytokinesis, and matrix assembly, which are all influenced by the activity of GTP-binding Rho proteins [37-40]. Intuitively, mechanical stretch should be limited by the main fibrillar actin (F-actin) cytoskeletal structure in MC, i.e., stress fibers. Stress fibers are temporary contractile bundles formed by F-actin and myosin II. At one end, these fibers insert into the intracellular side of the focal adhesion plaques where the external face of the cell is firmly attached to the extracellular matrix. At the other end, they insert into a second focal adhesion or in the perinuclear actin cytoskeleton [40]. Stress fibers appear as tensional cables prominent in cells that are exposed to high mechanical forces or shear stress, including MC [41] suggesting their prominent role in opposing cellular deformation.

GLOMERULAR CELL RESPONSE TO MECHANICAL STRAIN AND HIGH GLUCOSE: SIGNALING EVENTS

Our knowledge of the cellular events triggered by mechanical strain has been greatly advanced by the capability of stimulating cells in culture by controlled stretch. This is achieved by culturing cells on elastic surfaces, coated with extracellular matrix components that can be cyclically stretched at specific frequencies and amplitudes [42]. In MC subjected to cyclic stretch in tissue culture, recent evidence points to the early and transient activation of specific pathways that may act as triggering mechanisms for later events. Stretch-induced activation of extracellular signal-regulated kinase (ERK) and stress-activated protein kinase/Jun terminal kinase (SAPK/JNK) has been observed early after mechanical stimulation, and DNA-binding activity of AP-1 transiently enhanced at 60 min [43-46]. These early changes are apparently independent of PKC activation. However, the induction of c-*fos,* the increase in cytosolic S6 kinase and p38 mitogen activated protein kinase, described by others is dependent on PKC activity [47-49]. Interestingly, the activation of some of these signaling pathways has been shown to be greatly enhanced in the presence of high glucose concentrations [45, 46].

In summary, even though the data is fragmentary, the overall evidence is that transient activation of mitogen-activated protein kinases is an early event in the response to stretch by MC which is magnified in the presence of high glucose.

GLOMERULAR CELL RESPONSE TO MECHANICAL STRAIN AND HIGH GLUCOSE: GROWTH FACTORS AND EXTRACELLULAR MATRIX

Particularly important among stretch-induced metabolic changes is the stimulation of extracellular matrix formation. Cyclic stretch of MC in culture stimulates the synthesis and deposition of collagen and other extracellular matrix constituents [20, 49-51]. This stimulation is proportional to the intensity of cellular stretch and its deposition strongly influenced by the extracellular glucose concentration. While cyclic stretch of mesangial cells in culture stimulates collagen synthesis at all glucose concentrations, at high levels of the sugar net collagen accumulation is augmented as the result of catabolic rates insufficient to match the increased synthesis [33]. This extracellular matrix deposition may be, at least in part, the result of growth factor hyperactivity.

A number of studies have now conclusively shown that stimulated growth factor expression is an important pathogenetic component in the excessive matrix deposition occurring in the diabetic glomerulus [52-56]. Abundant evidence indicates that the autocrine activation of TGF-β is part of the mechanism translating the stimulus of cellular stretch into alterations in extracellular matrix synthesis in MC in tissue culture. Thus, it has been shown that cyclic stretch of MC specifically upregulates the expression, secretion and activation of TGF-β1 [49, 57]. Since exposure of MC to high levels of glucose also increases the secretion of TGF-β1, a further elevation in the expression of this growth factor occurs when these two stimuli are combined [57, 58]. Consequently, the potentiating effect of high glucose concentration on the stretch-induced enhancement of collagen formation is likely to be mediated via this enhanced growth factor expression [58]. However, the increased TGF-β1 action induced by stretch is not just due to this increased expression. Exposure to cyclic stretch also significantly augments the overall number of TGF-β receptors as well as the ligand associated with TGF-β receptors (βR)) I, II and III [59]. Therefore, the modulation of TGF-β receptors may be an additional control point in the mechanism of mechanical force-induced increase in ECM deposition by MC.

Another molecule that may play a role in the response of MC to mechanical strain is vascular endothelial growth factor (VEGF). A promoter of vascular permeability, VEGF is induced in MC by both TGF-β and stretching [60]. Interestingly, stretch-induced VEGF production is unaffected by the addition of TGF-β neutralizing antibody. Finally, there is a significant additive effect on VEGF production when MC are pre-exposed to stretch and then treated with angiotensin II suggesting possible *in vivo* interaction between hemodynamic changes and proteinuria in the mechanically stressed glomerulus [61].

Connective tissue growth factor (CTGF) has also been investigated as a possible component in the response of MC to mechanical stretch. The potential importance of this growth factor was originally suggested by studies demonstrating, in other cell types, its induction by TGF-β and the ability to stimulate fibrosis in the skin [62]. CTGF is overexpressed in the interstitium and glomeruli in a variety of sclerosing renal diseases and, specifically in diabetes, its activity has been considered responsible for the progression of tubulointerstitial injury [63]. In addition, the relevance of a glucose-stimulated CTGF in the pathogenesis of diabetic glomerulosclerosis has been shown in the diabetic db/db mouse. After 3.5 months of diabetes, when mesangial expansion is mild and interstitial disease absent CTGF mRNA levels in whole kidney and microdissected glomeruli are markedly increased [64]. Further, although MC express CTGF mRNA and secreted the protein in relatively low levels, these are markedly stimulated by both TGF-β and high glucose concentrations. This overexpression of CTGF closely correlated with increased levels of fibronectin mRNA expression.

Cyclic stretching of cultured MC upregulates CTGF expression in a rapid and sustained manner [64]. This induction precedes that of TGF-β, suggesting that the stretch-induced CTGF expression may occur independently of TGF-β action. These results suggest the CTGF upregulation may be an important factor in the pathogenesis of diabetic glomerulosclerosis, acting both downstream of TGF-β stimulated by high glucose levels and stretch, but also independently of TGF-β early during mechanical strain.

GLOMERULAR CELL RESPONSE TO MECHANICAL STRAIN AND HIGH GLUCOSE: CYTOSKELETAL CHANGES

Cells respond to changes in the mechanical environment by directionally reorienting their cytoskeleton and modifying their shape, presumably to adapt to a more favorable conformation for structural stability and function. Repetitive mechanical changes of opposing sign (stretch/relaxation) demand drastic cytoskeletal and ECM remodeling activity. In these circumstances, there is a change in cell orientation that seems to be universal to all adherent cells. Cyclic stretching of osteoblasts, fibroblasts, and vascular endothelial and smooth muscle cells, uniformly results in cell elongation with perpendicular alignment of the long cell axis to the direction of the stretching force [65-67]. In addition, actin filaments are reorganized, changing from a random network distribution to one of dense bundles of stress fibers arranged in the direction of the long cellular axis. Similarly, shear stress, a different form of mechanical strain, induces the realignment of endothelial cells and their intracellular stress fibers, in this case in parallel with the direction of flow, again minimizing cellular mechanical strain [68]. MC are not an exception to this morphologic change. MC *in vivo* and in tissue culture demonstrate a rich F-actin cytoskeleton mainly arranged in the form of contractile stress fibers which realigns during stretch perpendicularly to the distending force [50] (Fig. 1).

Exposure to an environment of high glucose concentration induces the disassembly of the contractile stress fibers in MC in tissue culture and in glomeruli of diabetic animals *in vivo* via a mechanism involving the activation of protein kinase C (PKC) [69, 70-73]. This disassembly of F-actin is associated with MC hypocontractility. Thus, the weakening of this important structural component will be associated with a diminished force opposing glomerular distention and impediment to cell realignment in response to mechanical strain.

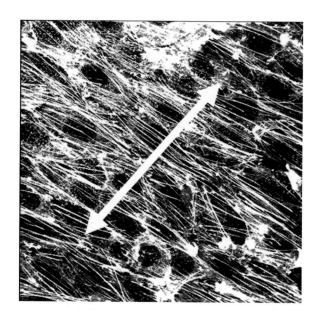

Figure 1. Alignment of stress fibers in cyclically stretched MC. A confluent culture of MC was stretched for 24 h at 3 cycles/min and 20% elongation. The cell layer was fixed and the F actin-containing stress fibers visualized with Alexa Fluor-488 phalloidin. The image is a reconstruction of confocal, 0.3 μm-thick images. The arrow indicates the direction of stretching force. Original magnification 63x.

CONCLUSION

The hemodynamic glomerular injury of diabetes is closely related to the loss of afferent arteriole autoregulation of pressure, the presence of glomerular hypertrophy and the occurrence of large moment-to-moment oscillations in capillary wall tension. This mechanical injury is possible due to the elasticity of the glomerular structure permitting the repeated stretch/relaxation of the cellular component. The cellular response to this mechanical stimulus is one leading to the enhanced activity of signaling cascades and overexpression of growth factors and the accumulation of extracellular matrix. These processes are further aggravated by an environment of high glucose concentration which, in turn, also induces the disassembly of the F-actin cytoskeleton, weakening of the structure-stabilizing forces and further amplification of mechanical strain (Fig. 2).

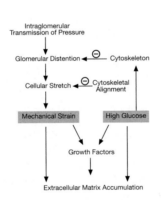

Figure 2. Schematic representation of the relationship between mechanical strain and high glucose concentration, and the role of the cytoskeleton as factors promoting glomerular extracellular matrix accumulation in diabetes.

REFERENCES

1. Ritz E, Stefanski A. Diabetic nephropathy in type II diabetes. Am J Kidney Dis 1996; 27: 167–194.
2. Nowack R, Raum E, Blum W, E. Ritz E. Renal hemodynamics in recent-onset type II diabetes. Am J Kidney Dis 1992; 20: 342–347.
3. Vora JP, Dolben J, Dean JD, Thomas D, Williams JD, Owens DR, Peters JR. Renal hemodynamics in newly presenting non-insulin dependent diabetes mellitus. Kidney Int 1992; 41: 829–835.
4. Bank N. Mechanisms of diabetic hyperfiltration. Kidney Int 1991; 40: 792–807.
5. Rudberg S, Persson B, Dahlquist G. Increased glomerular filtration rate as a predictor of diabetic nephropathy. An 8-year prospective study. Kidney Int 1992; 41: 822–828.
6. Anderson S, Meyer TW, Rennke HG, Brenner BM. 1985. Control of glomerular hypertension limits glomerular injury in rats with reduced renal mass. J Clin Invest 1985; 76: 612–619.
7. Anderson S, Rennke HG, Garcia DL, Brenner BM. Short and long term effects of antihypertensive therapy in the diabetic rat. Kidney Int 1989; 36: 526–536.
8. Zatz R, Dunn BR, Meyer TW, Anderson S, Rennke HG, Brenner BM. Prevention of diabetic glomerulopathy by pharmacological amelioration of glomerular capillary hypertension. J Clin Invest 1986; 77: 1925–1930.
9. Lewis EJ, Hunsicker LG, Bain RP, Rohde RD. 1993. The effect of angiotensin-converting-enzyme inhibition on diabetic nephropathy. The Collaborative Study Group. New Engl. J. Med. 1993; 329: 1456–1462.
10. Rudberg S, Aperia A, Freyschuss U, Persson B. Enalapril reduces microalbuminuria in young normotensive type 1 (insulin-dependent) diabetic patients irrespective of its hypotensive effect. Diabetologia 1990; 33: 470–476.
11. Mulec H, Johnsen SA, Björck S. 1994. Long-term enalapril treatment in diabetic nephropathy. Kidney Int. 1994; 45, Suppl. 45: S-141–S-144.
12. Ravid M, Savin H, Jutrin I, Bental T, Lang R, Lishner M. Long-term effect of ACE inhibition on development of nephropathy in diabetes mellitus type II. Kidney Int. 1994; 45, Suppl. 45: S-161–S-164.
13. Parving H-H, Hommel E, Jensen BR, Hansen HP. Long-term beneficial effect of ACE inhibition on diabetic nephropathy in normotensive type 1 diabetic patients. Kidney Int 2001; 60: 228–234.
14. Takenaka T, Harrison-Bernard LM, Inscho EW, Carmines PK, Navar LG. Autoregulation of afferent arteriolar blood flow in juxtamedullary nephrons. Am J Physiol 1994; 267 (Renal Fluid Electrolyte Physiol 36): F879–F887.
15. Casellas D, Moore LC. Autoregulation of intravascular pressure in preglomerular juxtamedullary vessels. Am J Physiol 1993; 264 (Renal Fluid Electrolyte Physiol 33): F315–F321.
16. Hayashi K, Epstein M, Loutzenhiser R, Forster H. Impaired myogenic responsiveness of the afferent arteriole in streptozotocin-induced diabetic rats: role of eicosanoids. J Am Soc Nephrol 1992; 2: 1578–1586.
17. Pelayo JC., Westcott JY. Impaired autoregulation of glomerular capillary hydrostatic pressure in the rat remnant nephron. J Clin Invest 1991; 88: 101–105.

18. Ohishi K, Okwueze MI, Vari RC, Carmines PK. Juxtamedullary microvascular dysfunction during the hyperfiltration stage of diabetes mellitus. Am J Physiol 1989; 267 (Renal Fluid Electrolyte Physiol. 36): F99–F105.

19. Cortes P, Zhao X, Riser BR, Narins RG. Regulation of glomerular volume in normal and partially nephrectomized rats. Am J Physiol 1996; 270 (Renal Fluid Electrolyte Physiol 39): F356–F370.

20. Riser BL, Cortes P, Zhao X, Bernstein J, Dumler F, Narins RG. Intraglomerular pressure and mesangial stretching stimulate extracellular matrix formation in the rat. J Clin Invest 1992; 90: 1932–1943.

21. DeRubertis FR, Craven PA. Eicosanoids in the pathogenesis of the functional and structural alterations of the kidney in diabetes. Am J Kindey Dis 1993; 22: 727–735.

22. Komers R, Lindsley JN, Oyama TT, Schutzer WE, Reed JF, Mader SL, Anderson S. Immunohistochemical and functional correlations of renal cyclooxygenase-2 in experimental diabetes. J Clin Invest 2001; 107: 889–898.

23. Wilkes BM, Kaplan R, Mento PF, Aynedjian HS, Macica CM, Schlondorff D, Bank N. Reduced glomerular thromboxane receptor sites and vasoconstrictor responses in diabetic rats. Kidney Int 1992; 41: 992–999.

24. Jaffa AA, Silva RH, Kim B, Mayfield RK. Modulation of renal kallikrein production by dietary protein in streptozotocin –induced diabetic rats. J Am Soc Nephrol 1996; 7: 721–727.

25. Harvey JN, Edmunson AW, Jaffa AA, Martin LL, Mayfield RK. Renal excretion of kallikrein and eicosanoids in patients with type 1 (insulin-dependent) diabetes mellitus. Relationship to glomerular and tubular function. Diabetologia 1992; 35: 857–862.

26. Jaffa AA, Rust PF, Mayfield RK. Kinin, a mediator of diabetes-induced glomerular hyperfiltration. Diabetes 1995; 44: 156–160.

27. Veelken R, Hilgers KF, Hartner A, Haas A, Böhmer KP, Sterzel RB. Nitric oxide synthase isoforms and glomerular hyperfiltration in early diabetic nephropathy. J Am Soc Nephrol 2000; 11: 71–79.

28. Schwartz D, Schwartz IF, Blantz RC. An analysis of renal nitric oxide contribution to hyperfiltration in diabetic rats. J Lab Clin Med 2001; 137:107–114.

29. Ito, A, Uriu K, Inada Y, Qie Y-L, Takagi I, Ikeda M, Hashimoto O, Suzuka K, Eto S, Tanaka Y, Kaizu K. Inhibition of neuronal nitric oxide synthase ameliorates renal hyperfiltration in streptozotocin-induced diabetic rat. J Lab Clin Med 2001; 138: 177–185.

30. Ikenaga H, Bast JP, Fallet RW, Carmines PK. Exaggerated impact of ATP-sensitive K^+ channels on afferent arteriolar diameter in diabetes mellitus. J Am Soc Nephrol 2000; 11: 1199–1207.

31. Biederman J, Cortes P, Giannico G, Hasset C, Yee J. Effect of sulfonylurea receptor (SUR) agonists on the hyperfiltration (HF) of diabetes mellitus (DM). J Am Soc Nephrol 2002: 13: 320A.

32. Cortes P, Riser BL, Zhao X, Narins RG. Glomerular volume expansion and mesangial cell mechanical strain: mediators of glomerular pressure injury. Kidney Int 1994; 45 (Suppl 45): S11-S16.

33. Cortes P, Zhao X, Riser BL, Narins RG. Role of glomerular mechanical strain in the pathogenesis of diabetic nephropathy. Kidney Int 1997; 51: 57–68.

34. Kriz W, Elger M, Lemley K, Sakai T. Structure of the glomerular mesangium: A biomechanical interpretation. Kidney Int 1990; 38 (Suppl 30): S2-S9.

35. Kritz W, Elger M, Mundel P, Lemley KV. Structure-stabilizing forces in the glomerular tuft. J Am Soc Nephrol 1995; 5: 1731–1739.

36. Welling LW, Grantham JJ. Physical properties of isolated perfused renal tubules and tubular basement membranes. J Clin Invest 1972; 51: 1063-1075.

37. Burridge K, Chrzanowska-Wodnicka M. Focal adhesions, contractility, and signaling. Annu Rev Cell Dev Biol 1996; 12: 463–519.

38. Aelst LV, D'Souza-Schorey C. Rho GTPases and signaling networks. Genes Develop 1997; 11: 2295–2322.

39. Zhong C, Chrzanowska-Wodnicka M, Brown J, Brown, Shaub A, Belkin AM, Burridge K. Rho-mediated contractility exposes a cryptic site in fibronectin and induces fibronectin matrix assembly. J Cell Biol 1998; 141:539–551.

40. Hall A. Small GTP-binding proteins and the regulation of the actin cytoskeleton. Annu Rev Cell Biol 1994; 10: 31–54.

41. Kreisberg JI, Ghosh-Choudhury N, Radnick RA, Schwartz MA. Role of Rho and myosin phosphorylation in actin stress fiber asembly in mesangial cells. Am J Physiol 1997; 273 (Renal Physiol 42): F283–F288, 1997.

42. Banes AJ, Gilbert J, Taylor D, Monbureau O. A new vacuum-operated stress-providing instrument that applies static or variable duration cyclic tension or compression to cells in vitro. J Cell Sci 1985; 75: 35–42.

43. Ishida T, Haneda M, Maeda S, Koya D, Kikkawa R. Stretch-induced overproduction of fibronectin in mesangial cells is mediated by the activation of mitogen-activated protein kinase. Diabetes 1999; 48: 595–602.

44. Ingram AJ, Ly H, Thai K, Kang M, Scholey JW. Activation of mesangial cell signaling cascades in response to mechanical strain. Kidney Int 1999; 55: 476–485.

45. Ingram AJ, Ly H, Thai K, Kang M-J, Scholey JW. Mesangial cell signaling cascades in response to mechanical strain and glucose. Kidney Int 1999; 56:1721–1728.

46. Dlugosz JA, Munk S, Kapor-Drezgic J, Goldberg HJ, Fantus IG, Scholey JW, Whiteside CI. Stretch-induced mesangial cell ERK1/ERK2 activation is enhanced in high glucose by decreased dephosphorylation. Am J Physiol Renal Physiol 2000; 279: F688–F697.

47. Akai Y, Homma T, Burns KD, Yasuda T, Badr KF, Harris RC. Mechanical stretch/relaxation of cultured rat mesangial cells induces protooncogenes and cyclooxygenase. Am J Physiol 1994; 267 (Cell Physiol. 36): C482–C490.

48. Homma T, Akai Y, Burns D, Harris RC. Activation of S6 kinase by repeated cycles of stretching and relaxation in rat glomerular mesangial cells. J Biol Chem 1992; 267: 23129–23135.

49. Grunden G, Zonca S, Hayward A, Thomas S, Maestrini S, Gnudi L, Viberti GC. Mechanical stretch-induced fibrinectin and transforming growth factor-$\beta 1$ production in human mesangial cells is p38 mitogen-activated protein kinase-dependent. Diabetes 2000; 49: 655–661.

50. Harris RC, Haralson MA, Badr KF. Continuous stretch-relaxation in culture alters rat mesangial cell morphology, growth characteristics, and metabolic activity. Lab Invest 1992; 66: 548-554.

51. Yasuda T, Kondo S, Homma T, Harris RC. Regulation of extracellular matrix by mechanical stress in rat glomerular mesangial cells. J Clin Invest 1996; 98: 1991–2000.

52. Nakamura T, Fukui M, Ebihara I, Osada S. Nagakoa I, Tomino Y, Koide H. mRNA expression of growth factors in glomeruli from diabetic rats. Diabetes 1993; 42: 450-456.

53. Sharma K, Ziyadeh FN. Hyperglycemia and diabetic kidney disease. The case for transforming growth factor-ß as a key mediator. Diabetes 1995; 44: 1139-1146.

54. Young BA, Johnson RJ, Alpers CE, Eng E, Gordon C, Floege J, Couser WG. Cellular events in the evolution of experimental diabetic nephropathy. Kidney Int 1995; 47: 935-944.

55. Ziyadeh FN, Sharma K, Ericksen M, Wolf G. Stimulation of collagen gene expression and protein synthesis in murine mesangial cells by high glucose is mediated by autocrine activation of transforming growth factor-ß. J Clin Invest 1994; 93: 536-542.

56. Yamamoto T, Nakamura T, Noble NA, Ruoslahti E, Border WA. Expression of transforming growth factor ß is elevated in human and experimental diabetic nephropathy. Proc Natl Acad Sci USA 1993; 90: 1814-1818.

57. Riser BL, Cortes P, Heilig C, Grondin J, Ladson-Wofford S, Patterson D, Narins RG. Cyclic stretching force selectively up-regulates transforming growth factor-beta isoforms in cultured rat mesangial cells. American Journal of Pathology 1996; 148: 1915-23.

58. Riser BL, Cortes P, Yee J, Sharba AK, Asano K, Rodriguez-Barbero A, Narins RG. Mechanical strain- and high glucose-induced alterations in mesangial cell collagen metabolism: Role of TGF-β. J Am Soc Nephrol 1998; 9: 827-36.

59. Riser B, Ladson-Wofford S, Sharba A, Cortes P, Drake K, Guerin C, Yee J, Choi ME, Segarini PR, Narins RG. TGF-β receptor expression and binding in rat mesangial cells: Modulation by glucose and cyclic mechanical strain. Kidney Int 1999; 56: 428–39.

60. Gruden G, Thomas S, Burt D, Lane S, Chusney G, Sacks S, Viberti GC. Mechanical stretch induces vascular permeability factor in human mesangial cells: mechanisms of signal transduction. Proc. Natl. Acad. Sci. USA 1997; 94: 12112-1216.

61. Gruden G, Thomas S, Burt D, Zhou W, Chusney G, Gnudi L, Viberti GC. Interaction of angiotensin II and mechanical stretch on vascular endothelial growth factor production by human mesangial cells. J Am Soc Nephrol 1999; 10: 730–737.

62. Grotendorst GR, Okochi H, Hayashi N. A novel transforming growth factor beta response element controls the expression of the connective tissue growth factor gene. Cell Growth Diff 1996; 7: 469–80.

63. Wang S, deNichilo M, Brubaker C, Hirschberg R. Connective tissue growth factor in tubulointerstitial injury of diabetic nephropathy. Kidney Int 2001; 60: 96–105.

64. Riser B, DeNichilo M, Cortes P, Baker C, Grondin J, Yee J, Narins RG. Regulation of connective tissue growth factor activity in cultured rat mesangial cells and its expression in experimental diabetic glomerulosclerosis. J Am Soc Nephrol 2000; 11: 25–38.

65. Buckley MJ, Banes JA, Levin LG, Sumpio BE, Sato M, Jordan R, Gilbert G, Link GW, Tay RTS. Osteoblasts increase their rate of division and align in response to cyclic, mechanical tension *in vitro*. Bone Mineral 1998; 4: 225–236.

66. Darsch PC, Betz E. Response of cultured endothelial cells to mechanical stimulation. Basic Res Cardiol 1989; 84: 268–281.

67. Darsch PP, Hämerle H. Orientation response of arterial smooth muscle cells to mechanical stimulation. Eur J Cell Biol 1986; 41: 339–346.

68. Davies PF, Robotewskyj A, Griem ML. Quantitative studies of endothelial cell adhesion. Directional remodeling of focal adhesion sites in response to flow forces. J Clin Invest 1994; 93: 2031–2038.

69.   Cortes P, Mendez M, Riser BL, Guérin CJ, Rodríguez-Barbero A, Hasset C, Yee J. F-Actin fiber distribution in glomerular cells structural and functional implications. Kidney Int 2000; 58: 2452–2461.

70.   Zhou X, Hurst RD, Templenton D, Whiteside CI. High glucose alters actin assembly in glomerular mesangial and epithelial cells. Lab Invest 1995; 73: 372–383.

71.   Zhou X, Li C, Dlugosz J, Kapor-Drezgic J, Munk S, Whiteside CI. Mesangial cell actin dissasembly in high glucose mediated by protein kinase C and the polyol pathway. Kidney Int 1997; 51 :1797–1808.

72.   Duglosz JA, Munk S, Ispanovic E, Goldberg HJ, Whiteside CI. Mesangial cell filamentous actin dissasembly and hypocontractility in high glucose are mediated by PKC-β. Am J Physiol Renal Physiol 2002; 282: F151–F163.

73.   Cevallos M, Hasset C, Giannico G, Biederman J, Yee J, Cortes P. Mesangial cell (MC) cytoskeletal effects of high glucose (HG) concentration: role of TGF-β1. J Am Soc Nephrol 2002; 13: 316A.

3

THE STENO HYPOTHESIS FOR CARDIOVASCULAR AND RENAL DISEASE REVISITED

Giovanni Gambaro, Monica Ceol, and Augusto Antonello
Division of Nephrology, Dept. of Medical and Surgical Sciences, School of Medicine, University of Padova, Padova, Italy

It is well known that diabetic patients are at increased risk of vascular disease, and that atherosclerosis is their main cause of death. Also, patients with diabetic nephropathy have an even higher risk of cardiovascular mortality. In a 10 year follow-up study, 15% of IDDM patients with normoalbuminuria, 25% with microalbuminuria and 44% with overt nephropathy died due to cardiovascular causes [1]. Indeed, several retrospective and prospective studies have demonstrated that micro- and macroalbuminuria predict cardiovascular morbidity and mortality in diabetes mellitus [2].

How albuminuria and proteinuria are linked with macroangiopathy is poorly understood. In this respect it is worth noting that patients with diabetic nephropathy suffer not only from increased macromolecolar permeability within the glomeruli, but also from an increased extrarenal capillary permeability as indicated by a 50% increase of the transcapillary escape rate of albumin and other plasma proteins [3]. It has been suggested that this increased permeability has some relevance to the augmented cardio-vascular morbidity and mortality seen in diabetic patients with nephropathy [4]. The increased extrarenal capillary permeability is not only related to augmented capillary pressure, but also to structural alterations of the macromolecular pathway, i.e. the extracellular matrix (ECM) between the endothelial cell and the limphatic capillaries [5]. The nature of these alterations is unknown, but as in the kidney they might be related to a loss of the compounds supplying the ECM with negative charges, and in particular a loss of the glycosaminoglycans (GAG) heparan sulfate (HS) [5]. Indeed, in accordance with studies performed on glomerular basement membranes (GBM) from kidney biopsies [6,7] it has been demonstrated that the content of the basement membrane HS in muscle capillaries is negatively correlated with the degree of tissue albumin clearance in the streptozotocin diabetic rat [8], and with the degree of albuminuria in diabetic patients with nephropathy [9]. Thus, albuminuria in insulin-dependent diabetic patients might reflect a universal alteration of the ECM [10].

THE CENTRAL ROLE OF THE HEPARAN SULFATE PROTEOGLYCAN AND THE STENO HYPOTHESIS OF DIABETIC MICRO AND MACROANGIOPATHY

It has been suggested that the first change in the extracellular matrix in diabetes might be an undersulphation of HS- proteoglycans (PGs) [10], followed by an absolute decrease of HS [11]. These alterations in HS-PG metabolism have been identified as the possible molecular basis for the abnormal permselectivity of glomerular and extrarenal capillaries in diabetes mellitus.

HS-PGs consist of a central core protein to which HS-GAG side chains are linked. These HS-GAG side chains are formed by repeating disaccharide units consisting of hexuronate and hexosamine. Sulfate groups covalently linked to the repeating units and carboxyl groups give the HS-GAG its highly negative charge. The biochemical processing of HS-GAG is extremely complex and involves a variety of enzymes required for the sulfation of the disaccharide unit [12]. A key actor in this process is the N-deacetylase/N-sulfotransferase enzyme, which substitutes the N-acetyl group of the glucosamine for a sulfate group.

The *Steno hypothesis* was put forward by Torsten Deckert and his group almost 15 years ago [10] and aimed at answering a number of clinical and patho-physiological observations gained in type 1 diabetic patients with nephropathy:

1. the high cardiovascular mortality;
2. the co-existence of a systemic derangement in vessel permeability;

3. the very selective proteinuria in the early stages of diabetic nephropathy in type 1 diabetes suggesting a pure abnormality in charge selectivity of the glomerular barrier;
4. the familial clustering of diabetics with nephropathy and the fact that only a subset of 20-40% of type 1 diabetic patients develops diabetic nephropathy.

According to this hypothesis a genetic defect in the regulation of HS synthesis by endothelial, myomedial, and mesangial cells determines the susceptibility of diabetic patients to develop proteinuria and angiopathy with its associated cardiovascular risk; the sulfation pattern of the GAG side chains of HS-PGs plays a pivotal role in this hypothesis. The central idea is that type 1 diabetic patients susceptible to nephropathy and macroangiopathy have a genetic trait that, under the diabetic milieu, leads to a lower activity of the enzymes (namely, the N-deacetylase/N-sulfotransferase) responsible for GAG sulfation. The resulting undersulfated GAG chains would then play a crucial role in the pathogenesis of proteinuria (due to the loss of anionic charges in the glomerular basement membrane), and diabetic nephropathy, as well as in the pathogenesis of diabetic micro- and macroangiopathy. Although genes have been cloned for N-deacetylase/N-sulfotransferase, 3-O-sulfotransferase and 6-O-sulfotransferase enzymes [13], it is still unclear whether different polymorphisms of these enzymes with a different susceptibility to high glucose concentrations really exist.

Thus, the Steno hypothesis embraces four different assumptions:

1. an altered sulfation of GAG, and namely of HS exists in diabetic nephropathy, and this might be the primary derangement.
2. this abnormality depends on the defective activity of the enzyme N-deacetylase/N-sulfotransferase.
3. it is a systemic abnormality, i.e. it is not a disorder occurring at the renal level only.
4. it is a genetically determined disturbance.

What are the data in favor of the Steno hypothesis? Does this hypothesis apply to type 2 diabetes as well? To answer these questions we have reviewed what is known about HS-PG metabolism in diabetes.

ABNORMAL HS-PG METABOLISM IN DIABETES

GAG abnormalities in diabetic nephropathy were originally investigated on the bases that albuminuria implies abnormal GBM permselectivity, and that GAGs, namely HS, were thought to be important determinants of GBM permeability. Indeed, a decreased ^{35}S sulfate incorporation in the GBM of diabetic glomeruli has been observed [14-16]. In experimental animal models of diabetes, a reduced synthesis of glomerular PGs and basement membrane HS-PG was also found [17-19]. However, the finding of the reduced sulfate incorporation is not without controversy, and a marked increase in ^{35}S sulfate incorporation in proteoglycans in diabetic tissues has also been observed [20]. Studies using biochemical techniques to measure the GAG content of kidneys obtained at autopsy demonstrated that the GBM of patients with diabetic nephropathy (it was not specified whether type 1 or type 2 diabetes) contained less GAGs than kidneys of non-diabetic controls [21,22]. That the synthesis of carbohydrate side chains of HS-PGs can be altered in type 1 diabetes mellitus was also shown by a ultrastructural investigation by Vernier et al [23] who described a negative correlation between GBM HS-PG deposition and mesangial expansion in diabetic nephropathy.

This was confirmed by a study using of JM-403, a monoclonal antibody that reacts with HS-GAG side chains, mainly staining the GBM in normal kidneys: in a mixed group of type 1 and type 2 patients with diabetic nephropathy it showed a decreased intensity of GBM staining correlated with proteinuria [7]. In the same subjects no statistically significant change in HS-PG core protein staining was observed. The effects of the diabetic milieu on glomerular HS-PG synthesis have been studied *in vitro* by different groups using glomerular cell cultures [24]. When human podocytes and mesangial cells were cultured under high glucose conditions, and stained with the monoclonal antibody JM-403, a decreased staining in the extracellular matrix was observed [25]. By metabolic labeling an altered GAG production under high glucose conditions was shown, with predominantly a decrease in HS, compared with dermatan or chondroitin sulfate [26].

A study carried out using two different antibodies raised against different epitopes of the HS-GAG side chain has shown a decreased HS N sulfation of urinary GAGs in type 2 diabetic patients possibly pointing to a reduced sulfation of HS within the GBM in diabetic patients [27]. However, whether the patients with diabetic nephropathy had a more severe disturbance was not evident from that study since normoalbuminuric patients and patients with incipient nephropathy had similar urinary levels of N sulfated HS.

The first major GBM HS-PG to be identified was perlecan [20]; this molecule is also a normal constituent of the basement membrane of vessels [28]. Therefore, it was an appealing candidate as a target for the deranged metabolism of diabetes in micro- and macroangiopathy and for explaining the reduced HS synthesis in diabetes mellitus and namely in diabetic nephropathy. However, immunohistochemistry with antibodies against perlecan HS-PG core proteins did not reveal any significant change in diabetic nephropathy in IDDM patients [7,29].

Thus, taken together the above mentioned findings suggested a vulnerability in the metabolism of the negatively charged side chain of HS-PG in diabetic nephropathy rather than a decreased synthesis of the whole HS-PG.

Nevertheless perlecan has a glomerular localization that does not resemble the distribution of HS-PG using antibodies directed against HS-PG isolated from the GBM [30-32]. Indeed, two other HS-PG core proteins have been identified in the GBM: agrin [33] and collagen XVIII [34]. Agrin, which has been demonstrated to be present only in the kidney [33], the retina [35] and the nervous system [33], seems to be the major HS-PG present in the GBM [33]; thus, it is reasonable to hypothesize that agrin contributes to the GBM charge permselectivity and, by interacting with laminin, to the GBM architecture. Yard et al [36] have recently discovered a reduction in both the agrin (core protein) and JM-403 (HS side chains) staining in renal biopsies from type 2 diabetic patients. Furthermore, a reduction in the agrin synthesis by podocytes in high glucose cultures was also revealed [36]. These recent findings in type 2 diabetic patients with diabetic nephropathy challenge the idea that a selective dysregulation of HS-PG sulfation occurs, rather than a reduction in the synthesis of HS-PG as a whole molecule.

ABNORMAL ACTIVITY OF THE ENZYMES RESPONSIBLE FOR GAG SULFATION IN DIABETES

To date three different forms of N-deacetylase/N-sulfotransferase have been cloned [37,38]. The activity of N-deacetylase/N-sulfotransferase is approximately 40% lower in hepatocytes from streptozotocin diabetic rats as compared with control cells [39]. Furthermore, Kofoed-Enevoldsen et al [40-42] found a reduction in N-deacetylase/N-sulfotransferase activity in streptozotocin diabetic rats. In humans, the activity or gene expression of N-deacetylase/N-sulfotransferase has been evaluated in cell cultures of skin fibroblasts obtained from diabetic patients with/without diabetic nephropathy. Neither the activity of N-deacetylase/N-sulfotransferase in type 1 diabetics [43] nor mRNA levels of N-deacetylase/N-sulfotransferase 1 and 2, in type 2 diabetic patients [44] levels were altered. Interestingly, only the N-deacetylase/N-sulfotransferase 2 gene expression was down-regulated by diabetes, but this was only in skin fibroblasts, not in mesangial cells [44].

It should be recognized that N-deacetylase/N-sulfotransferase 1 and 2 enzymes are not the only enzymes involved in HS-PG sulfation. Indeed, N-deacetylase/N-sulfotransferase 3, epimerase and the 3-O-sulfotransferases may also substantially contribute to HS-PG sulfation. Interestingly, while there is no data in the literature on the effect of the diabetic milieu on the activity of the two former, quite recently Edge and Spiro [45] have obtained findings suggesting an abnormal activity of isoforms of 3-O-sulfotransferase. Indeed, a highly specific reduction in the disaccharide unit IdUA(2S)α1$\rightarrow$4GlcN(3S) was observed in the GBM from kidneys of patients (not reported whether type 1 or 2 diabetics) with diabetic nephropathy. This disaccharide unit has so far been found only in the HS from GBM in substantial quantities representing approximately 20% of all HS disaccharide units.

DISTRIBUTION OF THE HS-PG METABOLISM ABNORMALITY IN DIABETES

The available data are contradictory. Studies using biochemical techniques to measure GAG content in the intima of the aorta of patients with type 2 diabetes mellitus have observed a reduction of HS [46], suggesting that the abnormalities in HS metabolism are not necessarily restricted to the kidney, although there has not been any examination of any possible relationship with coexistent diabetic nephropathy. The staining of skin basement membranes by JM-403, the monoclonal antibody that reacts with HS-GAG side chains, was significantly reduced in type 1 diabetic patients with diabetic nephropathy, as compared to patients with long-standing diabetes without nephropathy [47]. However, similar findings were observed also in patients with ESRD of non-diabetic origin [47]. The more recently discovered anomalies in HS-PG seem to be restricted, at least in type 2 diabetes, to the kidney taking into account the observation of the tissue distribution of agrin [36], of the finding that increased microvascular permeability in human diabetic retinopathy is not associated with changes in expression of agrin and perlecan [35], and the HS disaccharide unit IdUA(2S)α1→4GlcN(3S) [45]. Moreover, findings on the expression and regulation of N-deacetylase/N-sulfotransferase enzymes [44] at least demonstrate that alterations in HS-PG metabolism in type 2 diabetic patients with nephropathy are not generalized.

GENETICS OF HS-PG ABNORMALITIES IN DIABETES

The existence of genetic polymorphisms in the N-deacetylase/N-sulfotransferase enzymes has thus far not been reported. Animal experiments performed by Kofoed-Enevoldsen et al [40-42] support the influence of genetic factors in modulating the vulnerability of the N-deacetylase/N-sulfotransferase enzyme towards diabetes-induced inhibition, as evident from studies involving different rat strains.

Recently, a BamHI restriction fragment length polymorphism in the perlecan gene was found to be associated with diabetic nephropathy in Caucasian insulin-dependent diabetes mellitus [48]. However, in type 2 Japanese diabetic patients the BamHI HSPG2 genotype and allele frequencies were not significantly different between the patients with nephropathy and the patients without nephropathy [49]. No data are available on the role of variants of agrin in diabetes complications.

ALTERNATIVE HYPOTHESIS FOR THE HS-PG ALTERATIONS FINDINGS FROM THE ATHEROSCLEROSIS PROSPECT

The role of PGs in atherosclerosis has been the subject of intense investigations largely owing to the observation that chondroitin sulfate (CS) and dermatan sulfate (DS) PGs (manly versican and decorin) associate with apoB-containing lipoproteins [50], which are major components of the atherosclerotic plaque. The increase in CS/DS-PGs in the intima of atherosclerotic vessels might therefore explain an increased retention of lipoprotein. On the other hand, HS-PGs (mainly perlecan) are reduced in the vessel intima during atherosclerosis and diabetes, thus leading to an increased permeability to lipoproteins contributing to the increased vessel content of lipoproteins in these pathological conditions [51]. Indeed, the amount of cholesterol accumulated in atherosclerotic lesions is inversely proportional to the concentration of HS in the aorta [52].

However, matrix HS-PGs not only provide a physical barrier to the movement of large molecules such as lipoproteins into tissues, but the HS side chains bind and sequester a variety of bioactive proteins, including growth factors, cytokines, chemokines and enzymes [53] and in such a way modulate a number of events relevant to atherosclerosis: cell proliferation, matrix synthesis, monocyte recruitment, macrophage differentiation, etc. Moreover, the perlecan core protein, the major HS-PG in the subendothelial matrix, has a complex functional organization that can also influence events related to atherosclerosis, i.e. interaction between matrix proteins, integrin mediated cell attachment, matrix assembly, cell proliferation, lipoprotein binding [51].

Elevated levels of non-esterified fatty acids (NEFA) have been shown in smooth muscle cells (SMC) in culture to cause a substantial increase in the CS/DS-PGs versican and decorin [54]. Furthermore, in endothelial cell basement membranes NEFA exposure altered the matrix composition, and in particular reduced the sulfation of HS-PG [55] and the production of perlecan [56] making these membranes more permeable to macromolecules. Thus NEFA have the potential to induce those extracellular matrix alterations of the intima typical of atherosclerosis and diabetes.

NEFA may come into contact with vascular cells in different ways. They are one of the main products of phospholipases and other lipases on lipids of apoB-lipoproteins entrapped in the intima. In addition, in the dyslipidemia associated with insulin resistance and type 2 diabetes the vasculature is permanently exposed to a high influx of albumin-bound NEFA originating from the hydrolysis of post-prandial lipoproteins and from increased lypolysis of adipose tissue triglycerides. How NEFA alter the structure and production of matrix PGs is still a subject of investigation. However, it is known that NEFA impair the use of fructose-6-phosphate in the glycolytic pathway, thus increasing its availability for the hexosamine pathway and consequently for the synthesis of glucosamine that may stimolate GAG synthesis. Alternatively, the overdriven hexosamine pathway may lead to the up-regulation of the synthesis of transforming growth factor-β1 (TGF-β1), one of the leading stimulus to extracellular matrix production in SMC and, interestingly in mesangial cells.

Oxidized LDL and lysolecithin, a product of LDL oxidation, also modify the extracellular matrix composition of the intima. Specifically they decrease subendothelial HS-PGs [57]. This decrease is associated with both decreased core protein expression and increased HS degradation by heparanase [58].

May these findings be extrapolated to the kidney? We are not aware of studies examining the effect of increased NEFA on the extracellular matrix of glomerular cells, although lipoproteins and oxidized LDL affect the synthesis of α1(I), α1(III), and α1(IV) collagen and proteoglycan in mesangial cell cultures [59,60]. Moreover, it should be remembered that microalbuminuria is a very early marker of the insulin resistance that precedes type 2 diabetes; and, that dyslipidemia, characterized by elevated levels of triglyceride-rich particles and NEFA, is an early disturbance in insulin resistance that similarly precedes type 2 diabetes and is frequently associated with microalbuminuria [61,62]. Again, an increased heparanase activity has been discovered in the urine of diabetic patients that was associated with a poorer glycemic control [63]. In addition, the reduced HS N sulfation of urinary GAGs in type 2 diabetic patients might also be compatible with an increased degradation of HS within the GBM [27].

Thus, it is possible to speculate that, based on the effects of NEFA and oxidized LDL on endothelial cells and of oxidized LDL on mesangial cells, the dyslipidemia of insulin resistance may also contribute to the alterations in the glomerular matrix, namely in HS-PGs, observed in diabetic nephropathy at least in type 2 diabetics.

Alternative mechanisms can be put forward. There is growing evidence, that an imbalance in prooxidant and antioxidant activity and subsequent oxidative stress significantly contribute to the development and progression of renal disease. However, an oxidative imbalance is also a major actor of the endothelial dysfunction and enhanced vascular permeability in diabetes mellitus, a condition predisposing to atherosclerosis. Thus, the link between cardiovascular mortality and nephropathy in diabetes mellitus might well be related to the associated oxidative stress.

These considerations would suggest that the molecular basis for severe atherosclerosis (responsible for increased cardiovascular mortality) occurring simultaneously with diabetic nephropathy does not arise from a primary defect of the N-deacetylase/N-sulfotransferase enzymes, i.e. its special susceptibility to the diabetic milieu. The familial clustering and the fact that only a subset of diabetic patients develops the so-called "malignant angiopathy" might well be associated with polymorphisms of other genes, for instance

1. genes of the renin-angiotensin system whose polymorphisms have been found to be associated with both cardiovascular diseases and renal failure progression; or
2. the TGF-β1 gene, one of the more important stimuli to matrix synthesis in SMC and mesangial cells, that is triggered by many stimuli active in diabetes mellitus, and particularly by both high glucose levels and NEFA; or
3. genes involved in the oxidative stress, i.e. in the AGE metabolism and turnover, or in the antioxidant defense systems.

HEPARIN AND GAGs RENOPROTECTION IN DIABETIC NEPHROPATHY: DOES IT SUPPORT THE STENO HYPOTHESIS?

A number of reports showed that heparin and more generally GAGs prevent and cure experimental diabetic nephropathy [16,64-67] and decrease albuminuria in type 1 and 2 diabetic patients [68,69]. Because defects in HS-GAG synthesis are believed to be so striking in diabetic nephropathy, the treatment of diabetic nephropathy with HS-GAG like substances can be viewed as an experiment to test the Steno hypothesis. However, the activity of these drugs cannot be explained, by the Steno hypothesis, only in terms of recovery of the diabetes-induced abnormalities in HS-PG metabolism, restoration of anionic-HS charges in glomerular and other basement membranes, and recovery of derangement in basement membrane permeability. Indeed, Oturai [70] has shown that heparin treatment does not correct the diabetes-induced vascular hyperpermeability although heparin and GAGs are known to be curative in arteriosclerosis [71,72].

As a matter of fact the favorable remodeling effect of HS-GAG-like substances at the renal level may be explained by different mechanisms, i.e. down-regulation of proteases, modulation of extracellular mesangial matrix synthesis, all possibly reliant on the inhibition of the over-expression of TGF-β1 gene in diabetes mellitus [73-74].

It is true that heparin and GAGs improve glomerular permselectivity to proteins; this was clearly demonstrated by evaluating the fractional clearances of neutral and anionic dextrans in long-term streptozotocin diabetes in rats treated with a modified heparin [16], and indirectly confirmed by a number of studies demonstrating a reduction in the albumin excretion rate after heparin treatment in diabetic patients [68,69].

However, this effect on permselectivity depends on the complex activity of heparin on mesangial matrix and GBM protein synthesis, rather than on the selective effect on HS-PG synthesis (indeed, the opposite might be true, since heparin treatment induced the down-regulation of the perlecan gene in control and diabetic rats) [16], or on the trivial adhering of heparin to the GBM thereby correcting the charge deficiency. Indeed, the activity of heparin at the renal level on the sulfation and synthesis of proteoglycans, on the collagen IV/perlecan ratio, on collagen III synthesis and PAS positive matrix deposition appears to be relevant in maintaining the authentic architecture and permeability characteristics of the glomerulus and the GBM [16,75,76]. According to our data, the renoprotective effect of heparin and GAGs in diabetic nephropathy most likely depends on the modulation of the overactivated TGF-β1 gene cascade [75]. Although TGF-β1 was shown to increase HS-PG synthesis [77], a potentially favorable effect according to the Steno hypothesis, as a whole it has a more prominent and pivotal role in the pathogenesis of glomerulosclerosis as shown by the useful impact in the evolution of diabetic nephropathy of its long-term inhibition.

CONCLUSION

In summary, the Steno hypothesis has received very little scientific support in the 15 years since its proposal. Available data from the literature are fragmentary and contradictory; unfortunately many findings nee to be re-evaluated taking into account the new knowledge on the extracellular matrix composition and HS-PG biochemistry and molecular biology; and, most importantly, type 1 and 2 diabetes should be clearly separated in the hypothesis because it is likely that findings in one might not be extrapolated to the other.

However, alternative hypotheses - which do not assign to N-deacetylase/N-sulfotransferase enzymes a primary role - may be put forward which would explain both the association between severe atherosclerosis, cardiovascular mortality and diabetic nephropathy, as well as the genetical background.

From the point of view of the advancement of science in the field of diabetes complications the Steno hypothesis was an important step forward because, at least, it focussed the attention of researchers on the role of abnormalities of proteoglycans in the pathogenesis of diabetic microangiopathy.

ACKNOWLEDGEMENTS

This work was supported by the program MURST Cofin 40%, No. 2002062217_005, year 2002.

REFERENCES

1. Rossing P, Hougaard P, Borch-Johnsen K, Parving HH. Predictors of mortality in insulin dependent diabetes: 10 year observational follow up study. BMJ 1996; 313:779-784.
2. Parving HH, Osterby R, Anderson PW, Hsueh W. Diabetic nephropathy. In: Brenner BM (ed). The kidney. 5th ed. W.B.Saunders; Philadelphia; 1996; pp 1864-1892.
3. Feldt-Rasmussen B. Increased transcapillary escape rate of albumin in type 1 (insulin-dependent) diabetic patients with microalbuminuria. Diabetologia 1986; 29: 282-286.
4. Borch-Johnsen K, Kreiner S. Proteinuria: values as predictor of cardiovascular mortality in insulin dependent diabetes mellitus. BMJ 1987; 312: 1651-1654.
5. Bent-Hansen L, Feldt-Rasmussen B, Kverneland A, Deckert T. Plasma disappearance of glycated and non-glycated albumin in type 1 (insulin-dependent) diabetes mellitus: evidence for charge dependent alterations of the plasma to lymph pathway. Diabetologia 1993; 36: 361-363.
6. Makino H, Ikeda S, Haramoto T, Ota Z. Heparan sulfate proteoglycans are lost in patients with diabetic nephropathy. Nephron 1992; 61: 415-421.
7. Tamsma JT, van den Born J, Bruijn JA, Assmann KJM, Weening JJ, Berden JHM, Wieslander J, Schrama E, Hermans J, Veerkamp JH, Lemkes HHPJ, van der Woude FJ. Expression of glomerular extracellular matrix components in human diabetic nephropathy: Decrease of heparan sulphate in the glomerular basement membrane. Diabetologia 1994; 37: 313-320.
8. van der Born J, van Kraats AA, Hill S, Bakker MAH, Berden JHM. Vessel wall heparan-sulfate and transcapillary passage of albumin in experimental diabetes in the rat. Nephrol Dial Transplant 1997; 12: 27-31.
9. Yokoyama H, Høier PE, Hansen PM, van den Born J, Jensen T, Berden J, Deckert T, Garbarsch C. Immunohistochemical quantification of heparan sulfate proteoglycan and

collagen IV in skeletal muscle capillary basement membranes of patients with diabetic nephropathy. Diabetes. 1997; 46:1875-1880.

10. Deckert T, Feldt-Rasmussen B, Borch-Johnsen K, Kofoed-Enevoldsen A. Albuminuria reflects widespread vascular damage. The Steno hypothesis. Diabetologia 32:219-226,1989

11. van den Born J, Berden JHM. Is microalbuminuria in diabetes due to changes in glomerular heparan sulphate? Nephrol Dial Transplant 1995; 10: 1277-1296.

12. Kusche M, Lindahl U. Biosynthesis of heparin. O-sulfation of D-glucuronic acid units. J Biol Chem 1990; 265: 15403-15409.

13. Rosenberg RD, Shworak NW, Liu J, Schwartz JJ, Zhang L. Heparan sulfate proteoglycans of the cardiovascular system. Specific structures emerge but how is synthesis regulated? J Clin Invest 1997; 100, S67-S75.

14. Cohen MP, Surma ML. 35S sulfate incorporation into glomerular basement membrane glycosaminoglycans is decreased in experimental diabetes. J Lab Clin Med 1981; 98: 715-722.

15. Brown DM, Klein DJ, Michael AF, Oegema TR. 35S-glycosaminoglycan and 35S glycopeptide metabolism by diabetic glomeruli and aorta. Diabetes 1995; 31:418-425.

16. Gambaro G, Venturini AP, Noonan DM, Fries W, Re G, Garbisa S, Milanesi C, Pesarini A, Borsatti A, Marchi E, Baggio B. Treatment with a glycosaminoglycan formulation ameliorates experimental diabetic nephropathy. Kidney Int 1994; 46: 797-806.

17. Kanwar YS, Rosenzweig LJ, Linker A, Jakubowski ML.: Decreased de novo synthesis of glomerular proteoglycans in diabetes: Biochemical and autoradiographic evidence. Proc Natl Acad Sci USA 1983; 80: 2272-2275.

18. Rohrbach DH, Hassel JR, Kleinman HK, Martin GR. Alterations in the basement membrane (heparan sulfate) proteoglycan in diabetic mice. Diabetes 1982; 31: 185-188.

19. Rohrbach DH, Wagner CW, Star VL, Martin GR, Brown KS, Yoon JW. Reduced synthesis of basement membrane heparan sulfate proteoglycan in streptozotocin-induced diabetic mice. J Biol Chem 1983; 258: 11672-11677.

20. Iozzo RV, Cohen IR, Grässel S, Murdoch AD. The biology of perlecan: the multifaceted heparan sulphate proteoglycan of basement membranes and pericellular matrices. Biochem J 1994; 302: 625-639.

21. Parthasarathy N, Spiro R. Effect of diabetes on the glycosaminoglycan component of the human glomerular basement membrane. Diabetes 1982; 31: 738-741.

22. Shimomura H, Spiro R. Studies on macromolecular components of human glomerular basement membrane and alterations in diabetes: Decreased levels of heparan sulfate proteoglycans and laminin. Diabetes 1987; 36: 374-381.

23. Vernier RL, Steffes MW, Sissons-Ross S, Mauer M. Heparan sulfate proteoglycan in the glomerular basement membrane in type I diabetes mellitus. Kidney Int 1992; 41: 1070-1080.

24. Van der Woude FJ, van Det NF. Heparan sulphate proteoglycans and diabetic nephropathy. Exp Nephrol 1997; 5: 180-188.

25. Van Det NF, van den Born J, Tamsma JT, Verhagen NAM, Berden JHM, Bruijn JA, Daha MR, van der Woude FJ. Effects of high glucose on the production of heparan sulfate proteoglycan by human mesangial and glomerular visceral epithelial cells in vitro. Kidney Int 1996; 49: 1079-1089.

26. Gambaro G, Baggio B. Role of glycosaminoglycans in diabetic nephropathy. Acta Diabetol 1992; 29: 149-155.

27. Yokoyama H, Sato K, Okudaira M, Morita C, Takahashi C, Suzuki D, Sakai H, Iwamoto Y. Serum and urinary concentrations of heparan sulfate in patients with diabetic nephropathy. Kidney Int 1999; 56: 650-658.

28. Camejo G, Olsson U, Hurt-Camejo E, Baharamian N, Bondjers G. The extracellular matrix on atherogenesis and diabetes-associated vascular disease. Atherosclerosis Supplements 2002; 3: 3-9.

29. Van den Born J, van den Heuvel LPWJ, Bakker MAH, Veerkamp JH, Assman KJM, Weening JJ, Berden JHM. Distribution of GBM heparan sulfate proteoglycan core protein and side chains in human glomerular diseases. Kidney Int 1993; 43: 454-463.

30. van den Born J, van den Heuvel LP, Bakker MA, Veerkamp JH, Assman KJ, Berden JH. Monoclonal antibodies against the protein core and glycosaminoglycans side chain of glomerular basement membrane heparan sulfate proteoglycan: characterization and immunohistochemical application in human tissues. J Histochem Cytochem 1994; 42: 89-102.

31. van den Heuvel LP, Westenend PJ, van den Born J, Assman KJ, Knoers N, Monnens LA. Aberrant proteoglycan composition of the glomerular basement membrane in a patient with Denys-Drash syndrome. Nephrol Dial Transplant 1995; 10: 2205-2211.

32. Couchman JR, Ljubimov AV, Sthanam M, Horchar T, Hassel JR. Antibody mapping and tissue localization of globular and cysteine-rich regions of perlecan domain III. J Histochem Cytochem 1995; 43: 955-963.

33. Groffen AJ, Ruegg MA, Dijkman H, van de Velden TJ, Buskens CA, van den Born J, Assmann KJ, Monnens LA, Veerkamp JH, van den Heuvel LP. Agrin is a major heparan sulfate proteoglycan in the human glomerular basement membrane. J Histochem Cytochem 1998; 46: 19-27.

34. Halfter W, Dong S, Schurer B, Cole GJ. Collagen XVIII is a basement membrane heparan sulfate proteoglycan. J Biol Chem 1998; 273: 25404-25412.

35. Witmer AN, van den Born J, Vrensen GF, Schlingemann RO. Vascular localization of heparan sulfate proteoglycans in retinas of patients with diabetes mellitus and in VEGF-induced retinopathy using domain-specific antibodies. Curr Eye Res 2001; 22: 190-197.

36. Yard BA, Kahlert S, Engelleiter R, Resch S, Waldherr R, Groffen AJ, van den Heuvel LPWJ, van der Born J, Berden JHM, Kroger S, Hafner M, van der Woude FJ. Decreased glomerular expression of agrin in diabetic nephropathy and podocytes, cultured in high glucose medium. Exp Nephrol 2001; 9: 214-222.

37. Kusche-Gullberg M, Erikson I, Pikas DS, Kjellen L. Identification and expression of two heparan sulfate glucosaminyl N-deacetylase/N-sulfotransferase genes. J Biol Chem 1998; 273: 11902-11907.

38. Aikawa JI, Esko JD. Molecular clining and expression of a third member of the heparan sulfate/heparin GlcNAc N-deacetylase/N-sulfotransferase family. J Biol Chem 1999; 274: 2690-2695.

39. Unger E, Pettersson I, Eriksson UJ, Lindahl U, Kjellen L. Decreased activity of the heparan sulfate-modifying enzyme glucosaminyl N-deacetylase in hepatocytes from streptozotocin-diabetic rats. J Bio, Chem 1991; 266: 8671-8674.

40. Kofoed-Enevoldsen A, Eriksson UJ. Inhibition of N-acetylheparosan deacetylase in diabetic rats. Diabetes 1991; 40: 1449-1452.

41. Kofoed-Enevoldsen A. Inhibition of glomerular glucosaminyl N-deacetylase in diabetic rats. Kidney Int 1992; 41: 763-767.

42. Kofoed-Enevoldsen A, Noonan D, Deckert T. Diabetes mellitus induced inhibition of glucosaminyl N-deacetylase: effect of short term blood glucose control in diabetic rats. Diabetologia 1993; 36: 310-315.

43. Kofoed-Enevoldsen A, Petersen JS, Deckert T. Glucosaminyl N-deacetylase in cultured fibroblasts: comparison of patients with and without diabetic nephropathy, and identification of a possible mechanism for diabetes-induced N-deacetylase inhibition. Diabetologia 1993; 36: 536-540.

44. Yard B, Feng X, Keller H, Mall C, van der Woude F. Influence of high glucose concentrations on the expression of glycosaminoglycans and N-deacetylase/N-sulfotransferase mRNA in cultured skin fibroblasts from diabetic patients with or without nephropathy. Nephrol Dial Transplant 2002; 17: 386-391.

45. Edge ASB, Spiro RG. A specific structural alteration in the heparan sulphate of human glomerular basement membrane in diabetes. Diabetologia 2000; 43: 1056-1059.

46. Wasty F, Alavi MZ, Moore S. Distribution of glycosaminoglycans in the intima of human aortas: Changes in atherosclerosis and diabetes mellitus. Diabetologia 1993; 36: 316-322.

47. Van der Pijl JW, Daha MR, Van den Born J, Verhagen NA, Lemkes HH, Bucala R, Berden JH, Zwinderman AH, Bruijn JA, van Es LA, van der Woude FJ. Extracellular matrix in human diabetic nephropathy: reduced expression of heparan sulphate in skin basement membrane. Diabetologia 1998; 41:791-798.

48. Hansen PM, Chowdhury T, Deckert T, Hellgren A, Bain SC, Pociot F. Genetic variation of the heparan sulfate proteoglycan gene (perlecan gene). Association with urinary albumin excretion in IDDM patients. Diabetes 1997; 46:1658-1659.

49. Fujita H, Narita T, Meguro H, Ishii T, Hanyu O, Suzuki K, Ito S. Lack of association between the heparan sulfate proteoglycan gene polymorphism and diabetic nephropathy in Japanese NIDDM with proliferative diabetic retinopathy. Ren Fail 1999; 21: 659-664.

50. Hurt-Camejo E, Olsson U, Wiklund O, Bondjers G, Camejo G. Cellular consequences of the association of apoB lipoproteins with proteoglycans. Arterioscler Thromb Vasc Biol 1997; 17: 1011-1017.

51. Pillarisetti S. Lipoprotein modulation of subendothelial heparan sulfate proteoglycans (perlecan) and atherogenicity. Trends Cardiovasc Med 2000; 10: 60-65.

52. Hollmann J, Schmidt A, von Bassewitz D. Relationship of sulfated glycosaminoglycans and cholesterol content in normal and atherosclerotic human aorta. Arteriosclerosis 1989; 9: 154-158.

53. Lindahl U, Lidholt K, Spillmann D, Kjellen L. More to heparin than anticoagulation. Thrombosis Res 1994; 75: 1-32.

54. Olsson U, Bondjers G, Camejo G. Fatty acids modulate the composition of extracellular matrix in cultured smooth muscle cells by altering the expression of genes for proteoglycan core proteins. Diabetes 1999; 48: 616-622.

55. Ramasamy S, Boissoneault GA, Lipke DW, Hennig B. Proteoglycans and endothelial barrier function: effect of linoleic acid exposure to porcine pulmonary artery endothelial cells. Atherosclerosis 1993; 103: 279-290.

56. Ramasamy S, Lipke DW, Boissonneault GA, Guo H, Hennig B. Oxidized lipid-mediated alterations in proteoglycan metabolism in cultured pulmonary endothelial cells. Atherosclerosis 1996; 120; 199-208

57. Pillarisetti S, Obunike JC, Goldberg IJ. Lysolecithin induced alterations of subendothelial heparan sulfate proteoglycans increases monocyte binding to matrix. J Biol Chem 1995; 270: 760-765.

58.   Pillarisetti S, Paka L, Obunike JC, Berglund L, Goldberg IJ. Subendothelial retention of lipoprotein (a). Evidence that reduced heparan sulfate promotes lipoprotein (a) retention by subendothelial matrix. J Clin Invest 1997; 100: 867-874.

59.   Lee HS. Oxidized LDL, glomerular mesangial cells and collagen. Diabetes Res Clin Pract 1999; 45:117-122.

60.   Chana RS, Wheeler DC, Thomas GJ, Williams JD, Davies M. Low-density lipoprotein stimulates mesangial cell proteoglycan and hyaluronan synthesis. Nephrol Dial Transplant 2000;15:167-172.

61.   Mattock M, Barnes D, Viberti G, Keen H, Burt D, Hughes J, Fitzgerald A, Sanddhu B, Jackson P. Microalbuminuria and coronary heart disease in NIDDM. Diabetes 1998: 47: 1786-1792.

62.   Mykkänen L, Zaccaro D, Wagen Knecht L, Robbins D, Gabriel M, Haffner S. Microalbuminuria is associated with insulin resistance in non-diabetic subjects: the insulin resistance atherosclerosis studi. Diabetes 1988; 47: 793-800.

63.   Katz A, Van-Dijk DJ, Aingorn H, Erman A, Davies M, Darmon D, Hurvitz H, Vlodavsky I. Involvement of human heparanase in the pathogenesis of diabetic nephropathy. Isr Med Assoc J 2002; 4: 996-1002.

64.   Gambaro G, Cavazzana AO, Luzi P, Piccoli A, Borsatti A, Crepaldi G, Marchi E, Venturini AP, Baggio B. Glycosaminoglycans prevent morphological renal alterations and albuminuria in diabetic rats. Kidney Int 1992; 42: 285-291.

65.   Ceol M, Nerlich A, Baggio B, Anglani F, Sauer U, Schleicher E ,Gambaro G. Increased glomerular α1(IV) collagen expression and deposition in long-term diabetic rats is prevented by chronic glycosaminoglycan treatment. Lab Invest 1996; 74: 484-495.

66.   Oshima Y, Isogai S, Mogama K, Ohuchi H, Ohe K. Protective effect of heparin on renal glomerular anionic sites of streptozotocin-injected rats. Diab Res Clin Pract 1995 ; 25: 83-89.

67.   Oturai PS, Rasch R, Hasseleger E, Johansen PB, Yokoyama H, Thomsen MK, Myrup B, Kofoed-Enevoldsen A, Deckert T. Effects of heparin and aminoguanidine on glomerular basement membrane thickening in diabetic rats. APMIS 1996 ; 104: 259-264.

68.   Gambaro G, van der Woude FJ. Glycosaminoglycans: use in treatment of diabetic nephropathy. J Am Soc Nephrol. 2000; 11: 359-368.

69.   Gambaro G, Kinalska I, Oksa A, Pont'uch P, Hertlova M, Olsovsky J, Manitius J, Fedele D, Czekalski S, Perusicova J, Skrha J, Taton J, Grzeszczak W, Crepaldi G. Oral sulodexide reduces albuminuria in microalbuminuric and macroalbuminuric type 1 and type 2 diabetic patients: the Di.N.A.S. randomized trial. J Am Soc Nephrol. 2002;13:1615-1625.

70.   Oturai PS. Effects of heparin on vascular dysfunction in diabetic rats. Clin Exp Pharmacol Physiol 1999 ; 26: 411-414.

71.   Striker GE, Lupia E, Elliot S, Zheng F, McQuinn C, Blagg C, Selim S, Vilar J, Striker LJ. Glomerulosclerosis, arteriosclerosis, and vascular graft stenosis: treatment with oral heparinoids. Kidney Int Suppl 1997; 63: S120-123.

72.   Engelberg H. Actions of heparin in the atherosclerotic process. Pharmacol Rev 1996; 48:327–352.

73.   Gambaro G, Baggio B. Glycosaminoglycans: a new paradigm in the prevention of proteinuria and progression of glomerular disease. Nephrol. Dial. Transplant 1996; 11: 762-764.

74. Gambaro G, Barbanti M, Marchi E, Baggio B. Therapy with glycosaminoglycans in nephrology. In: Harenberg J, Casu B (eds). Nonanticoagulant actions of glycosaminoglycans, Plenum Press, New York; 1996; pp 281-286.

75. Ceol M, Gambaro G, Sauer U, Baggio B, Anglani F, Forino M, Facchin S, Bordin L, Weigert C, Nerlich A, Schleicher ED. Glycosaminoglycan therapy prevents TGF-beta1 overexpression and pathologic changes in renal tissue of long-term diabetic rats. J Am Soc Nephrol. 2000; 11: 2324-2336.

76. Caenazzo C, Garbisa S, Ceol M, Baggio B, Borsatti A, Marchi E, Gambaro G. Heparin modulates proliferation and proteoglycan biosynthesis in murine mesangial cells: molecular clues for its activity in nephropathy. Nephrol Dial Transplant 1995; 10: 175-184.

77. van Det NF, Tamsma JT, van den Born J, Verhagen NAM, van den Heuvel LPWJ, Lowik CWGM, Berden JHM, Bruijn JA, Daha MR, van der Woude FJ. Differential effects of angiotensin II and transforming growth factor β on the production of heparin sulfate proteoglycan by mesangial cells in vitro. J Am Soc Nephrol 1996; 7: 1015-1023.

4

MICROALBUMINURIA AND CARDIOVASCULAR DISEASE

S.M. Thomas[1], G.C. Viberti[2].
[1]King's Diabetes Centre, King's College Hospital, London
[2]Department of Endocrinology, Diabetes & Internal Medicine, Division of Medicine, GKT School of Medicine, Guy's Hospital Campus, KCL

INTRODUCTION

The term microalbuminuria was first coined in 1969 by Keen *et al* in Guy's Hospital Reports [1]. They described raised urinary albumin excretion rate (AER) in patients with type 2 diabetes. The authors noted that the AER correlated with the systolic blood pressure and made the prescient speculation that "the results of hypertension and hyperglycaemia combine to increase the degree of albuminuria". In 1974 Parving *et al* described that microalbuminuria was also present in non-diabetic populations with essential hypertension [2]. Over the last twenty years there has been increasing interest in the importance of microalbuminuria as a marker of not only renal disease but cardiovascular disease in populations both with and without diabetes.

MICROALBUMINURIA AND CARDIOVASCULAR DISEASE IN DIABETES

Type 2 Diabetes

In type 2 diabetes microalbuminuria is a stronger predictor of cardiovascular disease than it is of the risk of end-stage renal failure.

The association between microalbuminuria and CVD in type 2 diabetes has been shown in several cross-sectional and retrospective studies (Table 1). In Europid patients with Type 2 diabetes, the presence of an elevated UAE increases the relative risk of all cause mortality to between 1.6 and 2.7-fold.

Table 1. Microalbuminuria as a predictor of mortality in Type 2 Diabetes

Study	Follow up (years)	Outcome Relative risk of death (95% Confidence Interval)
Mattock *et al* [9]	7	2.73** (1.3 - 5.7)
Damsgaard *et al* [4]	8	1.57* (1.2 - 2.1)
Macleod *et al* [7]	9	1.7* (1.3 - 2.2)
Neil *et al* [9]	6	2.2** (1.3 - 3.7)

Prospective studies indicating risk of microalbuminuria for cardiovascular mortality in type 2 diabetes

Several prospective studies have shown microalbuminuria to be an independent predictor of mortality [3-9]. In 1988 in a 10-year follow up study of ~ 500 patients with type 2 diabetes, microalbuminuria was associated with CVD mortality [6]. Damsgaard *et al* found microalbuminuria to be the best predictor of long term mortality in type 2 diabetes in a 8 – 9 year follow-up of 228 patients with type 2 diabetes [4].

Macleod *et al* in a 8 year prospective follow up study compared 153 UK patients with type 2 diabetes with abnormal AER and 153 with AER in the normal range. Subjects with an abnormal AER had a higher all cause mortality (Odds Ratio (OR) 1.47). The increase in all-cause mortality was detectable at an AER over 10.6 μg/min in particular the risk of vascular deaths was also higher at these levels of AER (OR 1.7) [5]. This has led to the suggestion that in type 2 diabetes microalbuminuria should be defined as an AER > 10 μg/min. Similarly, in a recent 7 year prospective study of a hospital-based cohort, coronary heart disease (CHD) was the cause of death in 72% of patients with microalbuminuria as compared with 39% of patients with normoalbuminuria.

In a 9-year follow up of 134 patients with type 2 diabetes in Finland, thirty-eight patients died, 68% from CVD. The baseline predictors of death were a higher HBA1c, higher LDL and triglycerides, lower HDL-cholesterol, higher non –esterified fatty acid concentrations and AER. 45% of the patients who died had microalbuminuria as opposed to 6% of the survivors [6].

Whether under all circumstances microalbuminuria is an independent predictor of CHD has however been questioned. In a prospective ten-year study of patients with newly diagnosed type 2 diabetes, urinary AER measured at 5 years predicted independently of serum lipid abnormalities 10 year CVD mortality but was not an independent predictor when adjusted for plasma glucose [10]. At least in part the cardiovascular risk associated with microalbuminuria is related to disadvantageous alterations in conventional cardiovascular risk factors (Table 2) [9].

Table 2. Multivariate risk factors associated with the development of microalbuminuria in Caucasian patients with type 2 diabetes

	All Subjects
N	100
Fasting plasma glucose (mmol/l)	2.27 (1.33-3.88)
Log_{10} UAER (μg/min)	1.84 (1.09-3.11)
Current smoker (yes/no)	3.72 (1.23-11.3)
Pre-existing CHD (yes/no)	3.61 (1.09-11.9)
Data are OR (95% C.I.)	

Cardiovascular risk factors that also predict the risk of microalbuminuria in type 2 diabetes (modified from Mattock et al [9])

There are ethnic differences in the relationship between diabetes and microalbuminuria. In South Asian populations microalbuminuria is more common than in Europid patients [11] and is associated with more ischaemic heart disease in these populations but maybe less retinopathy, neuropathy [12] and peripheral vascular disease [13]. In a study of patients with diabetes in India microalbuminuria was associated with higher carotid intimal-media thickness and more coronary artery disease.

In Japanese populations however the relationship between microalbuminuria and cardiovascular disease appears weaker. In a six-year follow up of 297

Japanese patients with type 2 diabetes, 96 of whom had microalbuminuria, the all cause mortality was higher in those with microalbuminuria but there was no difference in cardiovascular death [14]. Similar results were seen in a ten-year follow up study of 47 Japanese patients ~ 60% of whom had microalbuminuria at baseline [15].

Overall however in type 2 diabetes in most populations microalbuminuria is associated with higher cardiovascular mortality with a pooled odds ratio of ~ 2.5 (95% Confidence Interval 1.8 - 3.60) for total mortality from a combined analysis using all available studies in 1995 [16].

MICROALBUMINURIA AND CARDIOVASCULAR DISEASE IN TYPE 1 DIABETES.

Microalbuminuria is strongly predictive of the development of overt diabetic nephropathy and its associated excess of coronary, cerebrovascular and peripheral arterial disease in type 1 diabetes [17]. In prospective studies those with microalbuminuria have a significantly higher risk of dying from a cardiovascular cause. In a twenty three year follow up study of patients with type 1 diabetes and microalbuminuria those with microalbuminuria had a significantly higher mortality from a cardiovascular cause (Relative Risk 2.94 95% Confidence Interval 1.18 - 7.34) [18]. Rossing *et al* confirmed this in a ten-year observational follow up of 939 patients with type 1 diabetes, 593 with normal AER, 181 with microalbuminuria and 165 with overt nephropathy [19]. Age, smoking, microalbuminuria and overt nephropathy were significant predictors of cardiovascular mortality. Myocardial involvement may even be present at the stage of microalbuminuria, aerobic work capacity is reduced in patients with microalbuminuria [20] and significant coronary lesions may be present [21]. In type 1 diabetes as in type 2 diabetes microalbuminuria may be associated with adverse cardiovascular risk factors In the EURODIAB IDDM study, AER was positively related to fibrinogen and Von Willebrand factor in those with concomitant retinopathy and also with increased fasting plasma triglycerides [22].

Microalbuminuria is associated with LVH in type 1 diabetes [23] and this effect seems independent of clinic measured blood pressure [24] although may be explained by higher 24-hour blood pressures and in particular by lack of a nocturnal dip in blood pressure even when clinic blood pressures seem similar [23]. Indeed higher nocturnal systolic pressures may precede the development of microalbuminuria and the presence of a nocturnal dip in systolic pressure is associated with a lower risk of progression to microalbuminuria in type 1 diabetes [25].

Microalbuminuria may be associated with salt-sensitivity in type 1 diabetes. In a study of 15 patients with type 1 diabetes a high salt diet increased mean BP only in those with microalbuminuria. In those with microalbuminuria high salt also, as may be expected, increased the pressor effect of Angiotensin II [26]. Salt sensitivity may mark derangements of capillary haemodynamics where in response to salt intake intracapillary pressure rises [27], possibly leading in the glomerulus leads to microalbuminuria and in other capillary beds may lead to other target organ damage [28].

MICROALBUMINURIA IN THE NON DIABETIC POPULATION

Several population based studies have suggested a link between microalbuminuria , blood pressure and cardiovascular disease [29, 30]. In the Islington heart study an elevated AER was found in 9% of non - diabetic patients over 40 years of age. Those with an elevated AER had more coronary disease (OR 5.7), more peripheral vascular disease (OR 7.45) and an increased mortality after 3.6 years (OR 24.3) [31]. Microalbuminuria is associated with rising blood pressure particularly systolic BP and increased pulse pressure in non-diabetic populations [32].

Essential Hypertension
Microalbuminuria is attracting increasing interest in essential hypertension. The quoted prevalence of microalbuminuria varies between 5 and 25% in treated hypertension and up to 40% in untreated hypertension [32-35] although some estimates are even higher [33].

Several observations indicate that those with microalbuminuria represent a distinct subpopulation amongst those with essential hypertension who may be at highest risk.

Those with microalbuminuria have more activation of the renin angiotensin system with higher peripheral renin activity [34] which some believe may drive the increased urinary albumin excretion. In addition those with essential hypertension and microalbuminuria have other distinguishing features.

Nocturnal blood pressure and microalbuminuria
Patients with microalbuminuria have higher 24 hour mean blood pressure levels, with an altered circadian rhythm with [35] less nocturnal blood pressure dip and greater variability of pressure readings [36].

There seems to be a circadian rhythm but also in urinary albumin excretion. In patients on a high sodium diet, nocturnal falls in both urinary sodium excretion and AER were observed in those with a nocturnal blood pressure dip but not in non-dippers [37].

Salt Sensitivity and Microalbuminuria
Microalbuminuria in essential hypertension is related to higher salt intakes and to salt-sensitive hypertension. In one study of 839 patients either "normotensive" or with untreated essential hypertension systolic blood pressure and urinary sodium excretion were both independent predictors of urinary albumin excretion. Furthermore sodium restriction may modify circadian rhythms both in BP and in AER [37].

Microalbuminuria as a marker of target organ damage
Patients with essential hypertension and microalbuminuria show more evidence of target organ damage. In a cross-sectional study of 333 treated hypertensive men aged 50 –72 years 47.6% of those with microalbuminuria had organ damage, as evidenced by a cardiovascular event or ECG changes as compared with 30.9% of those with a normal AER [38]. Patients with essential hypertension and microalbuminuria are more prone to retinopathy [39] and left ventricular hypertrophy [40-42]. The relationship between increasing left ventricular mass and AER is not confined to those with microalbuminuria but there is a continuous relationship into the normoalbuminuric range [43].

In several cross-sectional studies the prevalence of coronary artery disease and cardiovascular disease in general is significantly higher in patients with microalbuminuria [44-46]. One population based study of around 2000 patients followed for nearly ten years found that raised urinary albumin excretion was the strongest predictor of coronary artery disease implying a three to four fold risk over the duration of the study [47, 48]. Similarly in The Heart Outcomes Prevention Evaluation study, the presence of microalbuminuria was associated with around a two fold increase in the risk of cardiovascular events be it death or hospitalisation. In that study every 0.4mg/mmol increase in ACR level, increased the risk of a cardiovascular event by around 6% [49].

Microalbuminuria is also associated with cerebrovascular disease with increased carotid intimal-medial thickness and with a higher prevalence of cerebral ischaemic lacunae than normoalbuminuric patients although in this study not with left ventricular mass [50,51].

The significance of microalbuminuria for renal disease in essential hypertension is less clear. There have been few histological studies performed, and no specific renal lesion has been seen in patients with essential hypertension and microalbuminuria as compared with those with normoalbuminuria [52]

Functionally small retrospective and prospective studies suggest a faster rate of decline of creatinine clearance in patients with microalbuminuria [39, 48]. Overall however there is a paucity of data to confirm that microalbuminuria indicates a poor renal prognosis in essential hypertension in contrast to the data in diabetes.

Elderly
Microalbuminuria is a marker of increased mortality in the elderly [53] and of the subsequent development of coronary heart disease (CHD) especially in those with high circulating insulin levels [54]. Increasing age may be a particular risk factor for microalbuminuria in men In one study of 31 elderly patients with systolic hypertension 12 had microalbuminuria which was reversible by antihypertensive therapy but responded better to inhibition of the renin-angiotensin system [55].

CARDIOVASCULAR RISK FACTORS IN MICROALBUMINURIA

Familial Predisposition
Positive family histories of hypertension or CVD in the non-diabetic parents are related to the development of albuminuria in the diabetic proband emphasising the shared predisposition to these two conditions. These associations hold true for both Type 1 and Type 2 diabetes after adjustment for age, sex and duration of diabetes [56, 57]. There is also some evidence for a familial predisposition to develop microalbuminuria in association with essential hypertension. Children with one hypertensive parent have a higher AER than children of a normotensive parent while normotensive adults with at least one hypertensive parent have elevated AER compared to normotensive adults with a negative family history for arterial hypertension [58].

Smoking
In both Type 1 and Type 2 diabetes and in those without diabetes smoking is an independent risk factor for the development of microalbuminuria [59, 60]. The association between smoking and microalbuminuria is not strong however and it seems unlikely that smoking explains much of the excess cardiovascular risk.

Lipid Abnormalities
In both Type 1 and Type 2 diabetes, an unfavourable lipid profile is present at a very early stage of albuminuria. The concentrations of total cholesterol, VLDL cholesterol LDL cholesterol, triglycerides and fibrinogen rise with increasing AER in patients with Type 1 diabetes, 11 - 14 % higher in microalbuminuria and 26 - 87% higher in macroalbuminuria [61]. In addition, there is an increase in LDL mass and atherogenic small dense LDL particles, which correlates with the plasma triglyceride concentrations. HDL levels also tend to be reduced with a disadvantageous alteration in their composition [10, 62, 63].

Similarly in the non -diabetic population, those with elevated UAE have increased Lipoprotein (a), LDL: HDL cholesterol ratios and lower Apolipoprotein A-1 and HDL cholesterol levels [64, 65].

Insulin Resistance
In both Type 1 and Type 2 diabetes and non-diabetics, persistent microalbuminuria is associated with insulin resistance [66 –68]. In addition insulin resistance may be related to salt sensitivity [69, 70].

Endothelial dysfunction and Haemostatic abnormalities

Levels of Von Willebrand factor (vWF), PAI1, Factor VII and fibrinogen are higher in patients with microalbuminuria as compared with controls suggesting an association with endothelial activation and a hypofibrinolytic, hypercoagulable state [71, 72]. Recent evidence suggests that the increase in vWF may precede the onset of microalbuminuria in type 1 diabetes [73]. In addition there is a generalised increase in vascular permeability in both the non – diabetic and diabetic population indicated by an increased transcapillary escape of albumin [74, 75]. Other markers of vascular risk are also elevated in patients with microalbuminuria e.g. c-reactive protein , homocysteine and sialic acid suggesting low grade immune activation [76;77].

INTERVENTION

Glycaemic Control

The question of whether improved glycaemic control is of benefit in preventing CVD in either Type 1 Diabetes or Type 2 diabetes remains unresolved.

In the Diabetes Control and Complications Trial intensive insulin therapy significantly reduced development of hypercholesterolaemia with a 41% reduction in the risk of macrovascular disease although the number of outcome events was small [78]. The UKPDS in type 2 diabetes showed that intensive glycaemic control reduced the risk of myocardial infarction by 16% over a ten-year follow up although this failed to reach statistical significance [79].

In an open, parallel trial for ~8 years at the Steno centre 160 patients with type 2 diabetes and microalbuminuria were allocated to either standard treatment based on current guidelines or intensive treatment – a programme of behaviour modification and pharmacological therapy targeting hyperglycaemia, hypertension, dyslipidaemia.[80] The intensified treatment resulted in a fall in HbA1c of ~0.5% and around 50% less cardiovascular end-points (table 3).

Lipid lowering therapy.

There is from a number of studies evidence of the beneficial effects of lipid lowering therapy in diabetes in general. In the Heart Protection Study, which included 3982 people with diabetes mellitus, there was around a 25% reduction in the risk of a cardiovascular event in those with diabetes randomised to receive high dose statins irrespective of whether or not they had a previous cardiovascular event [81]. In the Steno study lipid lowering therapy aimed at those with type 2 diabetes and microalbuminuria aiming for a total cholesterol < 4.5 mmol/L and achieving a mean cholesterol of around 3.8mmol/L resulted in around a 50% reduction in the risk of cardiovascular disease [80].

In addition, there is some evidence that statin therapy in type 2 diabetes can also reduce microalbuminuria [82].

Table 3. Multifactorial intervention study to reduce complications in patients with type 2 diabetes and microalbuminuria

	Intensive	Conventional
Systolic blood pressure (mmHg)	-14	-3
Diastolic blood pressure (mmHg)	-12	-8
Total cholesterol (mmol/L)	-1.3	=
LDL cholesterol (mmol/L)	-1.2	0.3
HbA1c	-0.5	0.2
Urinary albumin (mg/24 hrs)	-20	30

Changes in cardiovascular risk factors targeted ion an eight year multifactorial intervention study resulting in a 50% reduction in the risk of a cardiovascular end-point in patiens with type 2 diabetes and microalbuminuria. (Modified from Gaede et al [80]).

Blood Pressure Reduction

The Hypertension in Diabetes study within the UKPDS showed that intensive therapy (144/82 c.f. 154/87) using primarily either an ACE inhibitor or a β-blocker resulted in significantly less strokes, heart failure and diabetes related deaths although not less myocardial infarctions [83].

The Appropriateness of Blood pressure Control in Diabetes trial (ABCD) addressed the benefits of intensive blood pressure control (mean 128/75 mmHg) compared with conventional blood pressure control over around 5 years demonstrated that those with more intensive control had less progression of the AER and less strokes [84].

There is also evidence in diabetes of the beneficial effects of renin angiotensin system inhibition in microalbuminuria in addition to the blood pressure lowering effect.

The MICRO-HOPE sub study of the Heart Outcomes Prevention Evaluation Study (HOPE) has published the benefits of treatment with an ACE inhibitor in patients with type 2 diabetes and microalbuminuria. 3577 patients aged 55 years or older with a history of diabetes and at least one other cardiovascular risk factor were enrolled in the HOPE study. At baseline ~ 30% of patients had microalbuminuria The study was terminated early as ACE inhibitor treatment lowered the risk of a primary combined end-point of myocardial infarction, stroke or CVD death by 25 % and total mortality by 24%. The presence of microalbuminuria and pre-existing cardiac disease were both baseline predictors of a beneficial effect of ACE inhibition [85]. Recent data suggest that initial therapy with a combination of an ACE inhibitior with a diuretic may be particularly beneficial as initial therapy result in lower BP and lower AER in patients with type 2 diabetes and microalbuminuria (Mogensen *et al* Hypertension in press).

Similarly an interim analysis of the ABCD study described that patients treated first-line with enalapril group had fewer myocardial infarctions (Risk ratio 7) as compared to those treated first-line with nisoldipine [86].

Studies in non – diabetic people also show a benefit of antihypertensive treatment in reducing microalbuminuria and suggested that inhibition of the renin – angiotensin system may again have specific benefits in renal protection [87, 88]. However there are no specific studies with CVD mortality end points available.

SUMMARY

Microalbuminuria is associated with excess all cause and cardiovascular mortality in both diabetic and non-diabetic people. Identification of microalbuminuria allows the physician to more accurately risk assess the cardiovascular risk of the individual and plan their treatment strategy accordingly. An intensive strategy of risk factor reduction is necessary to tackle this problem and does result in a significant benefit in cardiovascular outcomes.

REFERENCES

1   Keen H, Chlouverakis C, Fuller J, Jarrett RJ. The concomitants of raised blood sugar: studies in newly- detected hyperglycaemics. II. Urinary albumin excretion, blood pressure and their relation to blood sugar levels. Guys Hospital Reports 1969; 118(2):247-254.

2   Parving HH, Mogensen CE, Jensen HA, Evrin PE. Increased urinary albumin-excretion rate in benign essential hypertension. Lancet 1974; 1(7868):1190-1192.

3   Schmitz A, Vaeth M. Microalbuminuria: a major risk factor in non-insulin-dependent diabetes. A 10-year follow-up study of 503 patients. Diabet Med 1988; 5(2):126-134.

4   Damsgaard EM, Froland A, Jorgensen OD, Mogensen CE. Eight to nine year mortality in known non-insulin dependent diabetics and controls. Kidney Int 1992; 41(4):731-735.

5   Macleod JM, Lutale J, Marshall SM. Albumin excretion and vascular deaths in NIDDM. Diabetologia 1995; 38(5):610-616.

6   Forsblom CM, Sane T, Groop PH, Totterman KJ, Kallio M, Saloranta C et al. Risk factors for mortality in Type II (non-insulin-dependent) diabetes: evidence of a role for neuropathy and a protective effect of HLA-DR4. Diabetologia 1998; 41 (11):1253-1262.

7   Neil A, Hawkins M, Potok M, Thorogood M, Cohen D, Mann J. A prospective population-based study of microalbuminuria as a predictor of mortality in NIDDM. Diabetes Care 1993; 16(7):996-1003.

8   Gall MA, Borch-Johnsen K, Hougaard P, Nielsen FS, Parving HH. Albuminuria and poor glycemic control predict mortality in NIDDM. Diabetes 1995; 44(11):1303-1309.

9   Mattock MB, Barnes DJ, Viberti G, Keen H , Burt D, Hughes JM et al. Microalbuminuria and coronary heart disease in NIDDM: an incidence study. Diabetes 1998; 47 (11):1786-1792.

10   Uusitupa MI, Niskanen LK, Siitonen O, Voutilainen E, Pyorala K. Ten-year cardiovascular mortality in relation to risk factors and abnormalities in lipoprotein composition in type 2 (non- insulin-dependent) diabetic and non-diabetic subjects. Diabetologia 1993; 36 (11):1175-1184.

11   Mather HM, Chaturvedi N, Kehely AM. Comparison of prevalence and risk factors for microalbuminuria in South Asians and Europeans with type 2 diabetes mellitus. Diabet Med 1998; 15(8):672-677.

12   Tindall H, Martin P, Nagi D, Pinnock S, Stickland M, Davies JA. Higher levels of microproteinuria in Asian compared with European patients with diabetes mellitus and their relationship to dietary protein intake and diabetic complications. Diabet Med 1994; 11(1):37-41.

13   Abuaisha B, Kumar S, Malik R, Boulton AJ. Relationship of elevated urinary albumin excretion to components of the metabolic syndrome in non-insulin-dependent diabetes mellitus. Diabetes Research & Clinical Practice 1998; 39(2):93-99.

14   Araki S, Haneda M, Togawa M, Sugimoto T, Shikano T, Nakagawa T et al. Microalbuminuria is not associated with cardiovascular death in Japanese NIDDM. Diabetes Research & Clinical Practice 1997; 35(1):35-40.

15   Araki S, Kikkawa R, Haneda M, Koya D, Togawa M, Liang PM et al. Microalbuminuria cannot predict cardiovascular death in Japanese subjects with non-insulin-dependent diabetes mellitus. J Diabetes Complications 1995; 9(4):323-325.

16   Dinneen SF, Gerstein HC. The association of microalbuminuria and mortality in non-insulin- dependent diabetes mellitus. A systematic overview of the literature. Arch Intern Med 1997; 157(13):1413-1418.

17   Viberti GC, Hill RD, Jarrett RJ, Argyropoulos A, Mahmud U, Keen H. Microalbuminuria as a predictor of clinical nephropathy in insulin- dependent diabetes mellitus. Lancet 1982; 1(8287):1430-1432.

18   Messent JW, Elliott TG, Hill RD, Jarrett RJ, Keen H, Viberti GC. Prognostic significance of microalbuminuria in insulin-dependent diabetes mellitus: a twenty-three year follow-up study. Kidney Int 1992; 41(4):836-839.

19   Rossing P, Hougaard P, Borch-Johnsen K, Parving HH. Predictors of mortality in insulin dependent diabetes: 10 year observational follow up study. BMJ 1996; 313(7060):779-784.

20   Kelbaek H, Jensen T, Feldt-Rasmussen B, Christensen NJ, Richter EA, Deckert T et al. Impaired left-ventricular function in insulin-dependent diabetic patients with increased urinary albumin excretion. Scand J Clin Lab Invest 1991; 51(5):467-473.

21   Earle KA, Mishra M, Morocutti A, Barnes D, Stephens E, Chambers J et al. Microalbuminuria as a marker of silent myocardial ischaemia in IDDM patients. Diabetologia 1996; 39(7):854-856.

22   Mattock MB, Cronin N, Cavallo-Perin P, Idzior-Walus B, Penno G, Bandinelli S et al. Plasma lipids and urinary albumin excretion rate in Type 1 diabetes mellitus: the EURODIAB IDDM Complications Study. Diabet Med 2001; 18(1):59-67.

23   Sato A, Tarnow L, Parving HH. Prevalence of left ventricular hypertrophy in Type I diabetic patients with diabetic nephropathy. Diabetologia 1999; 42 (1):76-80.

24   Spring MW, Raptis AE, Chambers J, Viberti GC. Left ventricular structure and function are associated with microalbuminuria independently of blood pressure in type 2 diabetes [Abstract] Diabetes 1997, 46, 109A, 0426.

25   Lurbe E, Redon J, Kesani A, Pascual JM, Tacons J, Alvarez V et al. Increase in nocturnal blood pressure and progression to microalbuminuria in type 1 diabetes. N Engl J Med 2002; 347(11):797-805.

26   Trevisan R, Bruttomesso D, Vedovato M, Brocco S, Pianta A, Mazzon C et al. Enhanced responsiveness of blood pressure to sodium intake and to angiotensin II is associated with insulin resistance in IDDM patients with microalbuminuria. Diabetes 1998; 47(8):1347-1353.

27   Bigazzi R, Bianchi S, Baldari D, Sgherri G, Baldari G, Campese VM. Microalbuminuria in salt-sensitive patients. A marker for renal and cardiovascular risk factors. Hypertension 1994; 23(2):195-199.

28   Morimoto A, Uzu T, Fujii T, Nishimura M , Kuroda S, Nakamura S et al. Sodium sensitivity and cardiovascular events in patients with essential hypertension. Lancet 1997; 350(9093):1734-1737.

29   Jensen JS, Feldt-Rasmussen B, Borch-Johnsen K, Clausen P, Appleyard M, Jensen G. Microalbuminuria and its relation to cardiovascular disease and risk factors. A population-based study of 1254 hypertensive individuals. J Hum Hypertens 1997; 11(11):727-732.

30   Jensen JS, Borch-Johnsen K, Feldt-Rasmussen B, Appleyard M, Jensen G. Urinary albumin excretion and history of acute myocardial infarction in a cross-sectional population study of 2,613 individuals. J Cardiovasc Risk 1997; 4(2):121-125.

31   Yudkin JS, Forrest RD, Jackson CA. Microalbuminuria as predictor of vascular disease in non- diabetic subjects. Islington Diabetes Survey. Lancet 1988; 2(8610):530-533.

32   Bonner G. Risk evaluation and therapeutical implications of pulse pressure in primary arterial hypertension. Dtsch Med Wochenschr 2002; 127(45):2396-2399.

33   Pedrinelli R, Dell'Omo G, Di B, V, Pontremoli R, Mariani M. Microalbuminuria, an integrated marker of cardiovascular risk in essential hypertension. J Hum Hypertens 2002; 16(2):79-89.

34   Baldoncini R, Desideri G, Bellini C, Valenti M, Mattia G, Santucci A, Ferri C. High plasma renin activity is combined with elevated urinary Kidney International 1999; 56 (4) 1523-1755

35   Hishiki S, Tochikubo O, Miyajima E, Ishii M. Circadian variation of urinary microalbumin excretion and ambulatory blood pressure in patients with essential hypertension. J Hypertens 1998; 16(12 Pt 2):2101-2108.

36   Bianchi S, Bigazzi R, Baldari G, Sgherri G, Campese VM. Diurnal variations of blood pressure and microalbuminuria in essential hypertension. Am J Hypertens 1994; 7(1):23-29.

37   Nishimura M, Uzu T, Fujii T, Kimura G. Disturbed circadian rhythm of urinary albumin excretion in non-dipper type of essential hypertension. Am J Nephrol 2002; 22(5-6):455-462.

38   Agewall S, Fagerberg B, Attvall S, Ljungman S, Urbanavicius V, Tengborn L et al. Microalbuminuria, insulin sensitivity and haemostatic factors in non- diabetic treated hypertensive men. Risk Factor Intervention Study Group. J Intern Med 1995; 237(2):195-203.

39   Ruilope LM, Campo C, Rodriguez-Artalejo F, Lahera V, Garcia-Robles R, Rodicio JL. Blood pressure and renal function: therapeutic implications [editorial]. [Review] [54 refs]. J Hypertens 1996; 14(11):1259-1263.

40   Tomura S, Kawada K, Saito K, Lin YL, Endou K, Hirano C et al. Prevalence of microalbuminuria and relationship to the risk of cardiovascular disease in the Japanese population. Am J Nephrol 1999; 19(1):13-20.

41   Nilsson T, Svensson A, Lapidus L, Lindstedt G, Nystrom E, Eggertsen R. The relations of microalbuminuria to ambulatory blood pressure and myocardial wall thickness in a population. J Intern Med 1998; 244(1):55-59.

42   Leoncini G, Sacchi G, Viazzi F, Ravera M, Parodi D, Ratto E et al. Microalbuminuria identifies overall cardiovascular risk in essential hypertension: an artificial neural network-based approach. J Hypertens 2002; 20(7):1315-1321.

43   Bulatov VA, Stenehjem A, Os I. Left ventricular mass assessed by electrocardiography and albumin excretion rate as a continuum in untreated essential hypertension. J Hypertens 2001; 19(8):1473-1478.

44   Agewall S, Persson B, Samuelsson O, Ljungman S, Herlitz H, Fagerberg B. Microalbuminuria in treated hypertensive men at high risk of coronary disease. The Risk Factor Intervention Study Group. J Hypertens 1993; 11(4):461-469.

45   Agrawal B, Berger A, Wolf K, Luft FC. Microalbuminuria screening by reagent strip predicts cardiovascular risk in hypertension. J Hypertens 1996; 14(2):223-228.

46   Mykkanen L, Zaccaro DJ, O'Leary DH, Howard G, Robbins DC, Haffner SM. Microalbuminuria and carotid artery intima-media thickness in nondiabetic and NIDDM subjects. The Insulin Resistance Atherosclerosis Study (IRAS). Stroke 1997; 28(9):1710-1716.

47   Jensen JS, Feldt-Rasmussen B, Borch-Johnsen K, Jensen G. Urinary albumin excretion in a population based sample of 1011 middle aged non-diabetic subjects. The Copenhagen City Heart Study Group. Scand J Clin Lab Invest 1993; 53(8):867-872.

48   Bigazzi R, Bianchi S, Baldari D, Campese VM. Microalbuminuria predicts cardiovascular events and renal insufficiency in patients with essential hypertension. J Hypertens 1998; 16(9):1325-1333.

49   Gerstein HC, Mann JF, Yi Q, Zinman B, Dinneen SF, Hoogwerf B et al. Albuminuria and risk of cardiovascular events, death, and heart failure in diabetic and nondiabetic individuals. JAMA 2001; 286(4):421-426.

50   Ravera M, Ratto E, Vettoretti S, Viazzi F, Leoncini G, Parodi D et al. Microalbuminuria and subclinical cerebrovascular damage in essential hypertension. J Nephrol 2002; 15(5):519-524.

51   Bigazzi R, Bianchi S, Nenci R, Baldari D, Baldari G, Campese VM. Increased thickness of the carotid artery in patients with essential hypertension and microalbuminuria. Journal of Human Hypertension 1995; 9(10):827-833.

52   Erley CM, Risler T. Microalbuminuria in primary hypertension: is it a marker of glomerular damage? [editorial]. Nephrology, Dialysis, Transplantation 1994; 9(12):1713-1715.

53   Damsgaard EM, Froland A, Jorgensen OD, Mogensen CE. Microalbuminuria as predictor of increased mortality in elderly people. BMJ 1990; 300(6720):297-300.

54   Kuusisto J, Mykkanen L, Pyorala K, Laakso M. Hyperinsulinemic microalbuminuria. A new risk indicator for coronary heart disease. Circulation 1995; 91(3):831-837.

55   Morgan T, Anderson A. A comparison of candesartan, felodipine, and their combination in the treatment of elderly patients with systolic hypertension. Am J Hypertens 2002; 15(6):544-549.

56   Earle K, Walker J, Hill C, Viberti G. Familial clustering of cardiovascular disease in patients with insulin- dependent diabetes and nephropathy. N Engl J Med 1992; 326(10):673-677.

57   Earle K, Viberti GC. Familial, hemodynamic and metabolic factors in the predisposition to diabetic kidney disease. Kidney Int 1994; 45(2):434-437.

58   Barnes DJ, Pinto J, Viberti GC. The patient with diabetes mellitus. In: Cameron S, Davison AM, Grunfeld J-P, Kerr D, Ritz E, Winearls C , editors. Oxford Textbook of Clinical Nephrology. Oxford: Oxford Medical Publications , 1998: 723-777.

59   Predictors of the development of microalbuminuria in patients with Type 1 diabetes mellitus: a seven-year prospective study. The Microalbuminuria Collaborative Study Group. Diabet Med 1999; 16(11):918-925.

60   Gerstein HC, Mann JF, Pogue J, Dinneen SF, Halle JP, Hoogwerf B et al. Prevalence and determinants of microalbuminuria in high-risk diabetic and nondiabetic patients in the Heart Outcomes Prevention Evaluation Study. The HOPE Study Investigators. Diabetes Care 2000; 23 Suppl 2:B35-B39.

61   Jensen T, Stender S, Deckert T. Abnormalities in plasmas concentrations of lipoproteins and fibrinogen in type 1 (insulin-dependent) diabetic patients with increased urinary albumin excretion. Diabetologia 1988; 31(3):142-145.

62   Jones SL, Close CF, Mattock MB, Jarrett RJ, Keen H, Viberti GC. Plasma lipid and coagulation factor concentrations in insulin dependent diabetics with microalbuminuria. BMJ 1989; 298(6672):487-490.

63   Lahdenpera S, Groop PH, Tilly-Kiesi M, Kuusi T, Elliott TG, Viberti GC et al. LDL subclasses in IDDM patients: relation to diabetic nephropathy. Diabetologia 1994; 37(7):681-688.

64   Pontremoli R, Sofia A, Ravera M, Nicolella C, Viazzi F, Tirotta A et al. Prevalence and clinical correlates of microalbuminuria in essential hypertension: the MAGIC Study. Microalbuminuria: A Genoa Investigation on Complications. Hypertension 1997; 30(5):1135-1143.

65   Cirillo M, Senigalliesi L, Laurenzi M, Alfieri R, Stamler J, Stamler R et al. Microalbuminuria in nondiabetic adults: relation of blood pressure, body mass index, plasma cholesterol levels, and smoking: The Gubbio Population Study. Arch Intern Med 1998; 158(17):1933-1939.

66   Yip J, Mattock MB, Morocutti A, Sethi M , Trevisan R, Viberti G. Insulin resistance in insulin-dependent diabetic patients with microalbuminuria. Lancet 1993; 342(8876):883-887.

67   Groop L, Ekstrand A, Forsblom C, Widen E, Groop PH, Teppo AM et al. Insulin resistance, hypertension and microalbuminuria in patients with type 2 (non-insulin-dependent) diabetes mellitus. Diabetologia 1993; 36(7):642-647.

68   Bianchi S, Bigazzi R, Quinones Galvan A, Muscelli E, Baldari G, Pecori et al. Insulin resistance in microalbuminuric hypertension. Sites and mechanisms. Hypertension 1995; 26(5):789-795.

69   Trevisan R, Bruttomesso D, Vedovato M, Brocco S, Pianta A, Mazzon C et al. Enhanced responsiveness of blood pressure to sodium intake and to angiotensin II is associated with insulin resistance in IDDM patients with microalbuminuria. Diabetes 1998; 47(8):1347-1353.

70   Giner V, Coca A, de la SA. Increased insulin resistance in salt sensitive essential hypertension. J Hum Hypertens 2001; 15(7):481-485.

71   Pedrinelli R, Giampietro O, Carmassi F, Melillo E, Dell'Omo G, Catapano G et al. Microalbuminuria and endothelial dysfunction in essential hypertension. Lancet 1994; 344(8914):14-18.

72   Gruden G, Cavallo-Perin P, Bazzan M, Stella S, Vuolo A, Pagano G. PAI-1 and factor VII activity are higher in IDDM patients with microalbuminuria. Diabetes 1994; 43(3):426-429.

73   Stehouwer CD, Fischer HR, van Kuijk AW, Polak BC, Donker AJ. Endothelial dysfunction precedes development of microalbuminuria in IDDM. Diabetes 1995; 44(5):561-564.

74   Feldt-Rasmussen B. Increased transcapillary escape rate of albumin in type 1 (insulin-dependent) diabetic patients with microalbuminuria. Diabetologia 1986; 29(5):282-286.

75   Nannipieri M, Rizzo L, Rapuano A, Pilo A, Penno G, Navalesi R. Increased transcapillary escape rate of albumin in microalbuminuric type II diabetic patients. Diabetes Care 1995; 18(1):1-9.

76   Crook MA, Tutt P, Pickup JC. Elevated serum sialic acid concentration in NIDDM and its relationship to blood pressure and retinopathy. Diabetes Care 1993; 16(1):57-60.

77   Islam N, Kazmi F, Chusney GD, Mattock MB, Zaini A, Pickup JC. Ethnic differences in correlates of microalbuminuria in NIDDM. The role of the acute-phase response. Diabetes Care 1998; 21(3):385-388.

78   The Diabetes Control and Complications Trial Research Group. The effect of intensive treatment of diabetes on the development and progression of long term complications in insulin dependent diabetes mellitus. N Engl J Med 1993; 329:977-986.

79   UK Prospective Diabetes Study (UKPDS) Group. Intensive blood-glucose control with sulphonylureas or insulin compared with conventional treatment and risk of complications in patients with type 2 diabetes (UKPDS 33). UK Prospective Diabetes Study (UKPDS) Group. Lancet 1998; 352(9131):837-853.

80   Gaede P, Vedel P, Larsen N, Jensen GV, Parving HH, Pedersen O. Multifactorial intervention and cardiovascular disease in patients with type 2 diabetes. N Engl J Med 2003; 348(5):383-393.

81   MRC/BHF Heart Protection Study of cholesterol lowering with simvastatin in 20,536 high-risk individuals: a randomised placebo-controlled trial. Lancet 2002; 360(9326):7-22.

82   Velussi M. Long-term (18-month) efficacy of atorvastatin therapy in type 2 diabetics at cardiovascular risk. Nutr Metab Cardiovasc Dis 2002; 12(1):29-35.

83   UK Prospective Diabetes Study Group. Tight blood pressure control and risk of macrovascular and microvascular complications in type 2 diabetes: UKPDS 38. UK Prospective Diabetes Study Group. BMJ 1998; 317(7160):703-713.

84   Schrier RW, Estacio RO, Esler A, Mehler P. Effects of aggressive blood pressure control in normotensive type 2 diabetic patients on albuminuria, retinopathy and strokes. Kidney Int 2002; 61(3):1086-1097.

85   Heart Outcomes Prevention Evaluation Study Investigators. Effects of ramipril on cardiovascular and microvascular outcomes in people with diabetes mellitus: results of the HOPE study and MICRO-HOPE substudy. Lancet 2000; 355(9200):253-259.

86   Estacio RO, Jeffers BW, Hiatt WR, Biggerstaff SL, Gifford N, Schrier RW . The effect of nisoldipine as compared with enalapril on cardiovascular outcomes in patients with non-insulin-dependent diabetes and hypertension. N Engl J Med 1998; 338(10):645-652.

87   Bianchi S, Bigazzi R, Baldari G, Campese VM. Microalbuminuria in patients with essential hypertension. Effects of an angiotensin converting enzyme inhibitor and of a calcium channel blocker. Am J Hypertens 1991; 4(4 Pt 1):291-296.

88   Ruilope LM, Alcazar JM, Hernandez E, Praga M, Lahera V, Rodicio JL. Long-term influences of antihypertensive therapy on microalbuminuria in essential hypertension. Kidney International - Supplement 1994; 45:S171-3.

5

THE HEART IN DIABETES: RESULTS OF TRIALS

Giulio Zuanetti*°and Elena Sarugeri#°

°Adis International Ltd, Milano, Italy,
*Istituto di Ricerche Farmacologiche Mario Negri, Milano, Italy,
Istituto Scientifico Ospedale San Raffaele, Milano, Italy

INTRODUCTION

It has been known for many years that diabetes has profound consequences on the cardiovascular system, leading to increased cardiovascular morbidity and mortality in diabetic patients [1]. In the last years, the completion of several large trials (acronyms listed and explained in table 1) allowed to gather critical information on the efficacy and safety of different drugs in patients with a variety of cardiovascular diseases.

In most of these trials, the diabetic patients, generally identified on the basis of clinical history with no distinction between type 1 and type 2 diabetes, represented an important proportion of the randomised population, ranging between 10 and 25%.

In this brief review, we will focus on how these trials helped in widening our knowledge of the pathophysiology, prognosis and pharmacological treatment of diabetic patients with established cardiovascular disease.

Two specific settings will therefore be discussed: (a) acute coronary syndromes (ACS), including non ST-elevation myocardial infarction (non-STEMI) and ST-elevation myocardial infarction (STEMI), and (b) congestive heart failure (CHF).

ACUTE CORONARY SYNDROMES

Pathophysiology and prognosis
The introduction of aggressive pharmacological and non-pharmacological approaches for the treatment of ACS has led to a marked improvement in the patients prognosis.

This notwithstanding, the difference in survival between diabetic and non-diabetic patients, documented by several studies performed in the eighties [2,3], remains mostly unaffected. For example, data from GISSI-2 [4], the GUSTO-series [5] and ESPRIT [6] trials show a 30 to 100% higher in-hospital mortality in diabetic patients of both genders compared to non-diabetics.

The results from controlled clinical trials appear to mirror the real world situation, as documented by several observational studies. The recently reported data from MITRA plus [7], a registry of 50,000 patients hospitalised for ACS, have shown that among 28,000 consecutive patients admitted with STEMI, one quarter were diabetics. In these patients hospital mortality was increased by 30% and heart failure on discharge by 42%, with a poorer long term survival.

Efficacy of treatment

Intensive glucose control
Data from the pivotal DIGAMI trial [8] demonstrated that an intensive treatment with insulin-glucose infusion, targeted to achieve a tight control of blood glucose in patients with acute myocardial infarction, is associated with a lower long term morbidity and mortality.

However, control of glucose metabolism does not appear as the sole strategy to follow to prevent the progression of cardiovascular disease and its consequences in diabetic patients: in large prevention studies such as UGPD, DCCT and UKPDS, although tight glucose control was associated with a reduction of microvascular complications in both type 1 (DCCT) and type 2 (UKPDS) diabetes, the reduction of macrovascular complications did not always reach statistical significance, or was limited to specific patients or treatment groups (overweight patients treated with metformin in UKPDS), indicating that targeting abnormalities other than glucose metabolism is a key step in attempting to ameliorate prognosis of diabetics with cardiovascular diseases [9].

Table 1. Significance of acronyms of trials quoted

AIRE	The Acute Infarction Ramipril Efficacy
ASSENT	Assessment of the Safety and Efficacy of a New Thrombolytic
AWESOME	Angina with Extremely Serious Operative Mortality Evaluation
BARI	Bypass Angioplasty Revascularization Investigation
CAPRICORN	Carvedilol Post-Infarct Survival Control in Left Ventricular Dysfunction
CAPRIE	Clopidogrel versus Aspirin in Patients at Risk of Ischemic Events
CARE	Cholesterol and Recurrent Events
CCS	Chinese Cardiac Study Collaborative Groups
CIBIS	Cardiac Insufficiency Bisoprolol Study
CONSENSUS	Cooperative New Scandinavian Enalapril Survival Study
COPERNICUS	Carvedilol Prospective Randomised Cumulative Survival
CURE	Clopidogrel in Unstable Angina to Prevent Recurrent Events
DCCT	Diabetes Control and Complication Trial
DIGAMI	Diabetes Mellitus Insulin-Glucose Infusion in Acute Myocardial Infarction
EPIC	Evaluation of c7E3 for the Prevention of Ischemic Complications
EPILOG	Evaluation of PTCA to Improve Long-Term Outcome by c7E3 GP IIb/IIIa Receptor Blockade
EPISTENT	Evaluation of Platelet IIb/IIIa Inihibitor for Stenting Trial
ESPRIT	Enhanced Suppression of the Platelet IIb/IIIa Receptor with Integrilin Therapy
4S	Scandinavian Simvastatin Survival Study
GISSI	Gruppo Italiano per lo Studio della Sopravvivenza nell'Infarto Miocardico
GUSTO	Global Utilization of Streptokinase and Tissue Plasminogen Activator for Occluded Coronary Arteries
HPS	Heart Protection Study
LIPID	Long-term Intervention with Pravastatin in Ischemic Disease
MERIT-HF	Metoprolol CR/XL Randomised Intervention Trial in Congestive Heart Failure
MITRA plus	Maximal Individual Optimized Therapy for Acute Myocardial Infarction
OPTIMAAL	Optimal Trial in Myocardial Infarction with the Angiotensin II Antagonist Losartan
PARAGON	Platelet IIb/IIIa Antagonism for the Reduction of Acute Coronary Syndrome Events in a Global Organization Network
PPP	Prospective Pravastatin Pooling Project
PRISM	Platelet Receptor Inhibition in Ischemic Syndrome Management
PRISM-PLUS	Platelet Receptor Inhibition in Ischemic Syndrome Management in Patients Limited by Unstable Signs and Symptoms
PURSUIT	Platelet IIb/IIIa in Unstable Angina: Receptor Suppression Using Integrilin Therapy
SAVE	Survival and Ventricular Enlargement
SOLVD	Studies of Left Ventricular Dysfunction
TARGET	Do Tirofiban and ReoPro Give Similar Efficacy Outcomes Trial
TRACE	Trandolapril Cardiac Evaluation
UGDP	University Group Diabetes Program
UKPDS	United Kingdom Perspective Diabetes Study
Val-HeFT	Valsartan Heart Failure Trial

Fibrinolytic agents

Fibrinolytic treatment is similarly effective in diabetic and non-diabetic patients. The overview of fibrinolytic trials in acute MI [10] found that fibrinolytic treatment was associated with a 35 days mortality of 13.6% vs. 17.3% in diabetics (-21.7%, or 37 lives saved per 1000 treated patients) and 8.7% vs. 10.2% in non-diabetics (-14.3% or 15 lives saved per 1000 treated patients). The incidence of stroke in diabetics (1.9% in fibrinolytic treated patients vs. 1.3% in control subjects) was higher than in non-diabetics (1.0% vs. 0.6% respectively); however, this increased risk was by far outweighed by the beneficial effect on mortality. On the basis of the available data, in February 2003 the European Committee of Proprietary Medicinal Products (CPMP) issued a position statement highlighting that the increased chance of survival and reduced cardiac morbidity in diabetic patients treated with fibrinolytics outweighs the risk of intraocular haemorrhage. The relative efficacy of newer fibrinolytic treatment regimens has been determined in several trials, such as GUSTO-IV, ASSENT-2 and others, all showing that there was no specific clinical advantage of newer fibrinolytics such as reteplase or tecneteplase over standard thrombolytic treatment.

Aspirin, glycoprotein IIb/IIIa antagonists and clopidogrel

The role of aspirin as first-line therapy in the treatment of ACS patients with diabetes has been firmly established. The antiplatelet trialists' collaboration overview on patients with unstable angina, acute MI, prior MI, stroke or transient ischemic attack indicated a similar benefit (38 vs. 36 vascular events saved /1000 treated patients) in diabetics vs. non-diabetics [11]. However, the optimal dosage in the diabetic population remains unclear, since these patients tend to have a higher platelet aggregability. In the last years research has focussed on selective antiplatelet agents, such as the glycoprotein (GP) IIb/IIIa antagonists, particularly in patients with non-STEMI. A meta-analysis [12], including data on a total of 6458 diabetic patients (22% of the enrolled population) from the 6 large-scale platelet GP IIb/IIIa inhibitor non-STEMI ACS trials (i.e. PRISM, PRISM-PLUS, PARAGON A, PARAGON B, PURSUIT and GUSTO-IV) demonstrated that these agents may significantly reduce mortality at 30 days among diabetic patients. Platelet GP IIb/IIIa inhibition was associated with a significant mortality reduction at 30 days in diabetic (from 6.2 to 4.6%, p = 0.007), but not in non-diabetic patients (3.0 vs. 3.0%). The most marked benefit from active therapy was documented in 1279 diabetic patients undergoing percutaneous interventions (PCI) during hospitalisation (20% of the diabetic population), with a significant mortality reduction at 30 days in patients treated with these agents (from 4.0 to 1.2%). These observations confirm and expand the results of previous studies, showing a mortality reduction with abciximab, eptifibatide and tirofiban in diabetic patients undergoing coronary stenting. A pooled analysis of EPIC, EPILOG and EPISTENT showed a mortality reduction from 4.5% to 2.5% (p = 0.031) at 1 year in diabetic patients undergoing PCI [13]. Results from the ESPRIT trial [6] suggest that selective GP IIb/IIIa inhibition with eptifibatide is equally effective in ACS patients with or without diabetes undergoing coronary stenting in reducing the composite endpoint of death, MI, urgent target vessel revascularisation or thrombotic bailout at 48 hours.

Data from comparative trials indicate that there are no major differences among GP IIb/IIIa antagonists: results from the TARGET trial [14] suggest that tirofiban and abciximab are equally effective and well-tolerated in patients with coronary disorders and diabetes undergoing PCI, with comparable 1-year mortality rates.

Other antiplatelet agents, like the thienopyridine derivatives ticlopidine and clopidogrel, have been shown to reduce the recurrence of ischemic events in ACS patients: the CAPRIE study [15] demonstrated that clopidogrel reduced the combined risk of ischemic stroke, myocardial infarction, and vascular death to a greater extent than aspirin in patients with recent ischaemic stroke, recent myocardial infarction or peripheral arterial disorders (RR = 19%, p < 0.01). A subgroup analysis of the CAPRIE results, limited to patients with diabetes (n = 3866), confirmed the superiority of clopidogrel in reducing ischemic events in this high-risk population (RR = 13%, p < 0.05) [16].

In patients undergoing percutaneous coronary angioplasty (PTCA) with stenting (see also paragraph below), short-term aspirin treatment plus clopidogrel resulted in a substantial lower rate of myocardial infarction than did either aspirin alone or warfarin [17]. The role of long term combined therapy with aspirin and an antiplatelet agent like clopidogrel in ACS patients with non-STEMI has been investigated by the CURE trial [18]: the first primary outcome, death from cardiovascular causes, non-fatal myocardial infarction or stroke, was significantly reduced in the clopidogrel group as compared with the placebo group (RR = 0.80, p < 0.001). The benefits of adding clopidogrel to the standard treatment regimen for ACS patients were in addition to those of aspirin and were consistent in a number of patient subgroups, including that of patients with diabetes.

Percutaneous Coronary Angioplasty and Coronary Artery Bypass Grafting
A history of diabetes is associated with a higher incidence of complications during PTCA and to increased morbidity and mortality during follow-up. Interestingly, in the BARI trial [19] in patients with multivessel disease, diabetic patients treated with PTCA had a higher incidence of 5-year mortality as compared with patients undergoing coronary artery bypass grafting (CABG) (34.5 vs. 19.4%, RR = 1.87, p < 0.01), whereas no difference was observed in non-diabetic patients using the two different approaches. Based on these results, current guidelines favour CABG over percutaneous interventions (PCI) for the treatment of diabetics with multivessel coronary artery disease. However, the recent findings of the AWESOME randomised trial and registry [20] challenge this approach, showing that diabetic patients with medically refractory unstable angina and risk factors for adverse outcomes with bypass have a similar short- and long-term survival whether they undergo PCI or CABG (97 vs. 92% at 30 days; 81 vs. 72% at 36 months). The difference between the results of the BARI and AWESOME trials likely resides in the fact that the BARI study compared CABG with baloon angioplasty rather than contemporary PCI (including stenting and GP IIb/IIIa receptor blockers), and excluded patients who were at higher risk of adverse outcomes with bypass surgery. In light of the AWESOME results, PCI appears as a relatively safe alternative to CABG for diabetic patients with medically refractory unstable angina who are at high risk for CABG.

Beta-blockers
Beta-blockers are able to reduce post-MI mortality in diabetic patients, with an absolute and relative beneficial effect in most cases larger than that observed in non-diabetics. Current evidence is based on subgroup analysis of several trials performed during the eighties and on non-randomized studies [21], in which the population of patients with diabetes was scarcely represented. However, the pooled data indicate a 37% mortality reduction during the acute phase (13% in non-diabetics) and a 48% mortality reduction post-discharge (33% in non-diabetics). Since all these studies were performed before the advent of fibrinolytic therapy, the question remains whether this marked beneficial effect is still present in more "updated" populations. In a recent observational study conducted on 613 MI survivors with diabetes [22], use of beta-blockers (recorded in 53% of patients with diabetes) was associated with a 27% risk reduction in the incidence of a new coronary event, adjusted for age, sex, history of hypertension, body mass index (BMI) and blood lipids (p = 0.0001).

The use of beta-blockers in diabetic patients post-MI also decreases the risk for the development of heart failure, as documented by a large observational study of more than 13,600 patients with a mean age of 76 years and a high co-morbidity index (including diabetes), documenting a 43% reduction of 1-year hospital admissions for heart failure in patients given beta-blockers compared with those not receiving these agents [23]. The results of the CAPRICORN trial [24] recently provided further evidence of the benefits of beta-blockers in patients post-MI with high risk of heart failure and left ventricular systolic dysfunction. Treatment with carvedilol 6.25-25 mg/day, started 3-21 days after the onset of MI, significantly decreased all-cause mortality (RR = 0.77, p = 0.03) as well as cardiovascular mortality and recurrence of non-fatal MI. Although 22% of patients in this study had diabetes, no subgroup analysis on diabetic patients has been published so far.

Agents acting on renin-angiotensin system
The studies in which ACE-inhibitors have been started within 24 to 36 hrs after the onset of acute MI symptoms showed an overall reduction of about 5 deaths for 1000 treated patients. In the GISSI-3 study [25], treatment with lisinopril was associated with a decreased 6-week mortality both in type 1 (11.8% vs. 21.1%, p < 0.05) and in type 2 diabetes (8.0% vs. 10.6%, p < 0.05), corresponding to a 44.1 and 24.5% reduction, respectively. The meta-analysis by the "ACE-inhibitor in MI Collaborative Group" [26], including data from GISSI-3, CCS-1 and CONSENSUS-2, confirmed that the subgroup of patients with diabetes experienced a 30 days lower mortality (10.3 vs. 12.0%, or 17.3 lives saved per 1000 patients) when treated early with an ACE-inhibitor.

The one and only head to head trial of ACE-inihbibitors vs. angiotensin II receptor antagonists (AIIRA) currently available in the post-MI setting is OPTIMAAL [27], a multicentre study comparing the treatment effects of losartan 50 mg once daily and of captopril 50 mg three times daily on mortality and morbidity in patients with evidence of heart failure or left ventricular dysfunction after acute myocardial infarction. A non significant trend toward lower total mortality (the primary endpoint) was seen in favour of captopril; however, in the subgroup of diabetic patients risk ratio was very close to one, suggesting a substantial equivalence of the two therapeutic options in this subgroup of patients.

Statins
Three studies, the 4S [28], CARE [29] and LIPID [30] trials, evaluated the effect of statins in reducing morbidity and mortality in patients with an history of

ischemic heart disease (mainly previous MI). The main difference among these trials lies in the cut-off of cholesterol level for enrolment, that was much tighter for 4S than for CARE or LIPID. In all trials diabetics had a worse outcome compared to non-diabetics; also, in all trials, the reduction in mortality was proportionally at least similar to that observed in non-diabetics. A subsequent pooled analysis of data from CARE and LIPID, prospectively combined in the PPP Project [31], showed a significant reduction of coronary events in patients treated with pravastatin irrespective of diabetes status, with relative risk reductions ranging from 17 to 25%.

Finally, in the HPS trial [32], comparing simvastatin 40 mg daily to placebo in high risk patients irrespective of their cholesterol levels, the rate of first occurence of any major vascular event (non-fatal myocardial infarction or coronary death, non-fatal or fatal stroke, coronary or non-coronary revascularisation) was significantly reduced by simvastatin. The beneficial effect was maintained also in the different subgroups of high risk patients and particularly in diabetics with prior MI or other CHD (33.4% vs. 37.8%).

CONGESTIVE HEART FAILURE

Pathophysiology and Prognosis
The interest toward this clinical condition has grown recently mainly due to the increasing prevalence of this disease as a consequence of chronic ischemic heart disease, to the better understanding of pathophysiological mechanisms responsible for its evolution and to the availability of drugs that appear to markedly improve prognosis.

Again, data obtained in diabetic patients with CHF have been gathered mainly through the post-hoc analysis of clinical trials in patients with overt or silent CHF. There is strong evidence indicating that ischemic heart disease in diabetics, particularly in the post-MI setting, is associated with an increased incidence of CHF, which is not explained by a greater propensity for left ventricular remodelling, as shown by the echocardiographic substudy of the SAVE trial [33]: among post-MI patients, left ventricular enlargement between baseline and 2 years was lower in diabetic than non-diabetic patients (p < 0.05), although CHF developed in 30% of diabetic and in 17% of non-diabetic patients during follow-up (p<0.001). Moreover, in patients who developed CHF, left ventricular diastolic and systolic dilatation were greater in non-diabetic than in diabetic patients. These data suggest that the diabetic heart may be less capable of adapting to the loss of stroke volume by dilating than non-diabetic heart and thus may be less able to restore stroke volume after MI, leading to increased filling pressures with the same degree of contractile loss.

Analysis of crude mortality and morbidity rates in diabetics vs. non-diabetics with CHF indicates that diabetics have a worse outcome. For example, a meta-analysis of the major trials in this setting [34], including about 13,000 patients from SAVE, AIRE, TRACE, and a subpopulation of SOLVD trials, showed mortality of 36.4% in diabetics and 24.7% in non-diabetics. The relative role of concomitant risk factors in this setting remains undefined.

Efficacy of treatment

Together with diuretics, two classes of drugs are critical in the management of patients with heart failure: agents acting on renin-angiotensin system (ACE-inhibitors and AIIRA), which are now indicated in all classes of CHF patients, and beta-blockers, whose efficacy in reducing morbidity and mortality has rapidly emerged from the latest trials.

Agents acting on renin-angiotensin system

The landmark studies in the evaluation of the efficacy of ACE-inhibitors were performed in the eighties and early nineties, when the CONSENSUS, SOLVD treatment and SOLVD prevention trials were completed. A sub-analysis of the SOLVD trial showed that ACE-inhibitors are as effective in diabetics as in non-diabetics in reducing mortality and hospitalisation rates [35]. More recently, the attention of researchers shifted toward patients with overt CHF and/or left ventricular dysfunction resulting from acute MI. All the "long-term" studies enrolling patients with left ventricular dysfunction some time after MI have shown a significant benefit of ACE-inhibitor therapy, with a risk reduction in mortality of 19 to 27% over a 2.5-4 years follow-up. The meta-analysis of the major trials in this setting mentioned earlier [34] indicates that the beneficial effect of ACE-inhibitors documented in the overall population is present also when limiting the analysis to patients with a history of diabetes. More in detail, the benefit per 1000 patients was 36 in the 10,501 non-diabetics and 48 in the 2282 diabetics.

The recently published VaAlL-HeEFT trial [36] evaluated the long-term effects of the addition of the AIIRA valsartan to standard therapy for heart failure in a total of 5010 patients with CHF (NYHA class II-IV), randomly assigned to receive 160 mg of valsartan or placebo twice daily. The primary outcomes were overall mortality and the combined endpoint of mortality and morbidity. Overall mortality was similar in the two groups, whereas the incidence of the combined endpoint was 13.2% lower in the valsartan than in the placebo group (RR= 0.87, p = 0.009), predominantly because of a lower number of patients hospitalised for heart failure (13.8 vs. 18.2%, p < 0.0001). The beneficial effect of valsartan on the combined mortality-morbidity endpoint was generally consistent among predefined subgroups of patients, although the effect in diabetics seemed less pronounced than in non-diabetics.

Beta-blockers

For many years beta-blockers have been contraindicated in CHF patients, and even more so in diabetic patients, where the accentuation of altered lipid levels induced by these drugs and the fear of masking hypoglycaemic episodes have been considered strong contraindications to their use; however, the pioneering work performed in the seventies and the eighties particularly by Scandinavian groups led the way to their targeted use in patients with asymptomatic or overt CHF. A variety of large randomized trials on beta-blockers have included diabetic patients groups. In the MERIT-HF study [37], the proportional effect of the beta-blocker metoprolol was similar in diabetics as in non-diabetics. Consistent results were obtained with bisoprolol in CIBIS II [38] and carvedilol in COPERNICUS [39]. In this latter trial, enrolling patients with severe CHF, the risk reduction of total mortality was identical (35%) in both non-diabetic and diabetic patients. Therefore, it seems that the effect of beta-blockers is prominent irrespective of the diabetic status.

Table 2. Pharmacological agents in diabetic patients with ACS, post-MI, and overt CHF

	Prevention of ACS in high-risk patients	Treatment of ACS in-hospital	Treatment of MI post-discharge	Treatment of overt CHF
Fibrinolytics	NA	++	NA	NA
Aspirin	++	+	++	NA
GP IIb/IIIa antagonists	NA	+++	NA	NA
Clopidogrel	NA	++	NA	NA
ACE-inhibitors	+++	+++	++*	++
AIIRA	NA	NA	++*	++
Beta-blockers	++	+++	++	++
Statins	+++	NA	+++	NA

*   efficacy evaluated only in patients with left ventricular dysfunction
+++ efficacy higher than that in non-diabetics
++   efficacy similar to that in non-diabetics
+   efficacy lower than that in non-diabetics
NA   not applicable

IMPLICATIONS FOR CLINICAL PRACTICE

The continuous progresses in the management of patients with established cardiovascular diseases have radically changed their prognosis. This is particularly true for diabetic patients, whose rate of morbidity and mortality has been shown to be beneficially affected by a variety of interventions (table 2). Recent data from registries such as MITRA also confirm that, when used in standard clinical practice, intervention such as percutaneous coronary interventions, beta-blockers, statins and ACE-inhibitors are all able to decrease mortality in diabetics [7]. However, the application of these findings in clinical practice remains a major challenge, since interventions consistently documented to be effective in specific patients populations are often underused.

Finally, the burden of morbidity and mortality of diabetic patients with cardiovascular disease remains high, and deserves testing novel therapeutic approaches targeting the several pathophysiological alterations present in diabetic patients with cardiovascular diseases.

REFERENCES

1   Haffner SM, Lehto S, Ronnemaa T, Pyorala K, Laakso M. Mortality from coronary heart disease in subjects with type 2 diabetes and in nondiabetic subjects with and without prior myocardial infarction. N Engl J Med 1998; 339(4):229-234.
2   Smith JW, Marcus FI, Serokman R. Prognosis of patients with diabetes mellitus after acute myocardial infarction. Am J Cardiol 1984; 54(7):718-721.
3   Stone PH, Muller JE, Hartwell T, York BJ, Rutherford JD, Parker CB et al. The effect of diabetes mellitus on prognosis and serial left ventricular function after acute myocardial infarction: contribution of both coronary disease and diastolic left ventricular dysfunction to the adverse prognosis. The MILIS Study Group. J Am Coll Cardiol 1989; 14(1):49-57.
4   Zuanetti G, Latini R, Maggioni AP, Santoro L, Franzosi MG. Influence of diabetes on mortality in acute myocardial infarction: data from the GISSI-2 study. J Am Coll Cardiol 1993; 22(7):1788-1794.
5   Lee KL, Woodlief LH, Topol EJ, Weaver WD, Betriu A, Col J et al. Predictors of 30-day mortality in the era of reperfusion for acute myocardial infarction. Results from an international trial of 41,021 patients. GUSTO-I Investigators. Circulation 1995; 91(6):1659-1668.
6   Labinaz M, Madan M, O'Shea JO, Kilaru R, Chin W, Pieper K et al. Comparison of one-year outcomes following coronary artery stenting in diabetic versus nondiabetic patients (from the Enhanced Suppression of the Platelet IIb/IIIa Receptor With Integrilin Therapy [ESPRIT] Trial). Am J Cardiol 2002; 90(6):585-590.
7   Senges J. Diabetes mellitus and coronary syndromes in clinical practice. Presentation at European Society of Cardiology Annual Meeting, Berlin, Germany, 31 August-4 September, 2002. (quoted in www.incirculation.net/congress_report).

8   Malmberg K. Prospective randomised study of intensive insulin treatment on long term survival after acute myocardial infarction in patients with diabetes mellitus. DIGAMI (Diabetes Mellitus, Insulin Glucose Infusion in Acute Myocardial Infarction) Study Group. BMJ 1997; 314(7093):1512-1515.

9   Libby P, Plutzky J. Diabetic macrovascular disease: the glucose paradox? Circulation 2002; 106(22):2760-2763.

10   Indications for fibrinolytic therapy in suspected acute myocardial infarction: collaborative overview of early mortality and major morbidity results from all randomised trials of more than 1000 patients. Fibrinolytic Therapy Trialists' (FTT) Collaborative Group. Lancet 1994; 343(8893):311-322.

11   Collaborative overview of randomised trials of antiplatelet therapy—I: Prevention of death, myocardial infarction, and stroke by prolonged antiplatelet therapy in various categories of patients. Antiplatelet Trialists' Collaboration. BMJ 1994; 308(6921):81-106.

12   Roffi M, Chew DP, Mukherjee D, Bhatt DL, White JA, Heeschen C et al. Platelet glycoprotein IIb/IIIa inhibitors reduce mortality in diabetic patients with non-ST-segment-elevation acute coronary syndromes. Circulation 2001; 104(23):2767-2771.

13   Bhatt DL, Marso SP, Lincoff AM, Wolski KE, Ellis SG, Topol EJ. Abciximab reduces mortality in diabetics following percutaneous coronary intervention. J Am Coll Cardiol 2000; 35(4):922-928.

14   Roffi M, Moliterno DJ, Meier B, Powers ER, Grines CL, DiBattiste PM et al. Impact of different platelet glycoprotein IIb/IIIa receptor inhibitors among diabetic patients undergoing percutaneous coronary intervention: : Do Tirofiban and ReoPro Give Similar Efficacy Outcomes Trial (TARGET) 1-year follow-up. Circulation 2002; 105(23):2730-2736.

15   A randomised, blinded, trial of clopidogrel versus aspirin in patients at risk of ischaemic events (CAPRIE). CAPRIE Steering Committee. Lancet 1996; 348(9038):1329-1339.

16   Bhatt DL, Marso SP, Hirsch AT, Ringleb PA, Hacke W, Topol EJ. Amplified benefit of clopidogrel versus aspirin in patients with diabetes mellitus. Am J Cardiol 2002; 90(6):625-628.

17   Mehta SR, Yusuf S. The Clopidogrel in Unstable angina to prevent Recurrent Events (CURE) trial programme; rationale, design and baseline characteristics including a meta-analysis of the effects of thienopyridines in vascular disease. Eur Heart J 2000; 21(24):2033-2041.

18   Yusuf S, Zhao F, Mehta SR, Chrolavicius S, Tognoni G, Fox KK. Effects of clopidogrel in addition to aspirin in patients with acute coronary syndromes without ST-segment elevation. N Engl J Med 2001; 345(7):494-502.

19   Comparison of coronary bypass surgery with angioplasty in patients with multivessel disease. The Bypass Angioplasty Revascularization Investigation (BARI) Investigators. N Engl J Med 1996; 335(4):217-225.

20   Sedlis SP, Morrison DA, Lorin JD, Esposito R, Sethi G, Sacks J et al. Percutaneous coronary intervention versus coronary bypass graft surgery for diabetic patients with unstable angina and risk factors for adverse outcomes with bypass: outcome of diabetic patients in the AWESOME randomized trial and registry. J Am Coll Cardiol 2002; 40(9):1555-1566.

21   Kendall MJ, Lynch KP, Hjalmarson A, Kjekshus J. Beta-blockers and sudden cardiac death. Ann Intern Med 1995; 123(5):358-367.

22   Aronow WS, Ahn C. Effect of beta blockers on incidence of new coronary events in older persons with prior myocardial infarction and diabetes mellitus. Am J Cardiol 2001; 87(6):780-1, A8.

23   Rochon PA, Tu JV, Anderson GM, Gurwitz JH, Clark JP, Lau P et al. Rate of heart failure and 1-year survival for older people receiving low-dose beta-blocker therapy after myocardial infarction. Lancet 2000; 356(9230):639-644.

24   Dargie HJ. Effect of carvedilol on outcome after myocardial infarction in patients with left-ventricular dysfunction: the CAPRICORN randomised trial. Lancet 2001; 357(9266):1385-1390.

25   GISSI-3: effects of lisinopril and transdermal glyceryl trinitrate singly and together on 6-week mortality and ventricular function after acute myocardial infarction. Gruppo Italiano per lo Studio della Sopravvivenza nell'infarto Miocardico. Lancet 1994; 343(8906):1115-1122.

26   Zuanetti G. Cardiovascular Disease and Diabetes. Belfiore F, Mogensen CE Eds. New Concept in Diabetes and its treatment. Basel Karger, 2000:186-198.

27   Dickstein K, Kjekshus J. Effects of losartan and captopril on mortality and morbidity in high-risk patients after acute myocardial infarction: the OPTIMAAL randomised trial. Optimal Trial in Myocardial Infarction with Angiotensin II Antagonist Losartan. Lancet 2002; 360(9335):752-760.

28   Pyorala K, Pedersen TR, Kjekshus J, Faergeman O, Olsson AG, Thorgeirsson G. Cholesterol lowering with simvastatin improves prognosis of diabetic patients with coronary heart disease. A subgroup analysis of the Scandinavian Simvastatin Survival Study (4S). Diabetes Care 1997; 20(4):614-620.

29   Sacks FM, Pfeffer MA, Moye LA, Rouleau JL, Rutherford JD, Cole TG et al. The effect of pravastatin on coronary events after myocardial infarction in patients with average cholesterol levels. Cholesterol and Recurrent Events Trial investigators. N Engl J Med 1996; 335(14):1001-1009.

30   Prevention of cardiovascular events and death with pravastatin in patients with coronary heart disease and a broad range of initial cholesterol levels. The Long-Term Intervention with Pravastatin in Ischaemic Disease (LIPID) Study Group. N Engl J Med 1998; 339(19):1349-1357.

31   Sacks FM, Tonkin AM, Shepherd J, Braunwald E, Cobbe S, Hawkins CM et al. Effect of pravastatin on coronary disease events in subgroups defined by coronary risk factors: the Prospective Pravastatin Pooling Project. Circulation 2000; 102(16):1893-1900.

32   MRC/BHF Heart Protection Study of cholesterol lowering with simvastatin in 20,536 high-risk individuals: a randomised placebo-controlled trial. Lancet 2002; 360(9326):7-22.

33   Solomon SD, St John SM, Lamas GA, Plappert T, Rouleau JL, Skali H et al. Ventricular remodeling does not accompany the development of heart failure in diabetic patients after myocardial infarction. Circulation 2002; 106(10):1251-1255.

34   Flather MD, Yusuf S, Kober L, Pfeffer M, Hall A, Murray G et al. Long-term ACE-inhibitor therapy in patients with heart failure or left-ventricular dysfunction: a systematic overview of data from individual patients. ACE-Inhibitor Myocardial Infarction Collaborative Group. Lancet 2000; 355(9215):1575-1581.

35   Shindler DM, Kostis JB, Yusuf S, Quinones MA, Pitt B, Stewart D et al. Diabetes mellitus, a predictor of morbidity and mortality in the Studies of Left Ventricular Dysfunction (SOLVD) Trials and Registry. Am J Cardiol 1996; 77(11):1017-1020.

36   Cohn JN, Tognoni G. A randomized trial of the angiotensin-receptor blocker valsartan in chronic heart failure. N Engl J Med 2001; 345(23):1667-1675.

37   Effect of metoprolol CR/XL in chronic heart failure: Metoprolol CR/XL Randomised Intervention Trial in Congestive Heart Failure (MERIT-HF). Lancet 1999; 353(9169):2001-2007.

38   Erdmann E, Lechat P, Verkenne P, Wiemann H. Results from post-hoc analyses of the CIBIS II trial: effect of bisoprolol in high-risk patient groups with chronic heart failure. Eur J Heart Fail 2001; 3(4):469-479.

39   Mohacsi P, Fowler MB, Krum H, Tendera M, Coats A, Rouleau JL et al. Should physicians avoid the use of beta-blockers in patients with heart failure who have diabetes? Results of the COPERNICUS study. Circulation 2001; 104[17 (Suppl. II)]: 754 (Abstract 3551).

6

MICROALBUMINURIA AND GFR IN TYPE 1 AND TYPE 2 DIABETES

George Jerums, Sianna Panagiotopoulos and Richard MacIsaac
Endocrinology Unit & Department of Medicine, University of Melbourne, Austin Hospital, Studley Rd, Heidelberg, Victoria 3084, Australia,

INTRODUCTION

Microalbuminuria is an early component in a continuum of progressive increases in albumin excretion rate (AER) associated with diabetic nephropathy. The development of microalbuminuria has been equated with incipient nephropathy but microalbuminuria is also a risk factor for macrovascular disease, especially in patients with type 2 diabetes. Recent data suggest that a substantial minority of non-diabetic and diabetic people with impaired glomerular filtration rate (GFR) may not pass through the phase of microalbuminuria. This has led to the concept that both albuminuric and non-albuminuric pathways contribute to renal impairment in diabetic mephropathy.

This chapter will review the evidence linking changes in AER and GFR, both temporally as well as causatively in people with microalbuminuria. The data presented are based on a review of publications over the last 10 years, identified by the Ovid search engine, using the key words 'microalbuminuria' and 'GFR'.

Additional publications were found by searching for GFR data in the placebo or untreated arm of clinical trials lasting more than two years in people with microalbuminuria, and comparing these with data obtained from similar trials in normo- and macroalbuminuric patients. The following aspects are covered: traditional concepts of diabetic nephropathy, methodology, changing treatment targets of microalbuminuria, the influence of hyperfiltration on AER, the influence of albuminuria on GFR, AER-GFR relationships in microalbuminuric patients with type 1 compared with type 2 diabetes, albuminuric and non-albuminuric pathways to impaired GFR, and new understanding of albumin handling by the kidney.

EVOLUTION OF DIABETIC NEPHROPATHY

Diabetic renal disease is characterised by changes in both AER and GFR in predisposed patients. The usual sequence starts with an increase in GFR (hyperfiltration), followed by an increase in AER leading to microalbuminuria. Hyperfiltration may persist through the phase of microalbuminuria or it may normalise prior to the onset of overt nephropathy (macroalbuminuria), which is accompanied by further increases in AER and a declining GFR. In parallel with these changes, there is a rise in blood pressure which may begin before the development of microalbuminuria in type 2 diabetes but usually occurs during the early microalbuminuric phase in type 1 diabetes.

The above process evolves over 10-15 years and is generally similar in type 1 and type 2 diabetes, with some differences (Figure 1).

The major clinically identifiable initiators are hyperglycaemia and blood pressure control. Increases in AER into the microalbuminuric range may occur transiently with exercise, urinary tract infection, uncontrolled hyperglycaemia and cardiac failure, and on a long-term basis with hypertension, non-diabetic renal disease, and in association with large vessel disease. However, progression to overt diabetic nephropathy does not occur without long-term hyperglycaemia. Following the onset of overt nephropathy there is usually a close coupling of increases in AER with decreases in GFR. The subsequent rate of decline of GFR is influenced by several progression promoters including the level of blood pressure, hyperglycaemia and proteinuria, as well as retinopathy and smoking. Recent evidence suggests that a decline in GFR may occur, less commonly, in subjects with minimal or no increases in AER. This raises the question of whether the sequence of microalbuminuria leading to macroalbuminuria is itself a cause of renal injury resulting in a GFR decline, or whether changes in AER and GFR are both secondary to underlying renal structural changes.

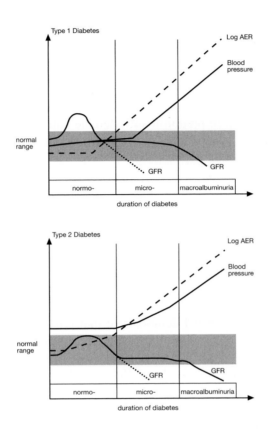

Figure 1. Blood pressure and GFR during normo-, micro- and macroalbuminuria in type 1 and type 2 diabetes.

HISTORICAL PERSPECTIVE

1982-84: Three studies in patients with type 1 diabetes demonstrate that microalbuminuria predicts the subsequent development of macroalbuminuria (overt diabetic nephropathy). This leads to the concept of microalbuminuria as a surrogate for diabetic nephropathy. Macroalbuminuria also becomes a surrogate for assessment of the onset of a decline in glomerular filtration rate. Despite early evidence that microalbuminuria predicts cardiovascular death to a greater extent than renal disease in type 2 diabetes [1] and in non-diabetic subjects [2], microalbuminuria becomes synonymous with early nephropathy in type 1 and type 2 diabetes.

1992: First publication by Lane, Steffes and Mauer [3] demonstrating the existence of a subgroup of predominantly female patients with type 1 diabetes and decreased creatinine clearance, normoalbuminuria and renal ultrastructural changes typical of diabetic nephropathy.

1994: First demonstration that a decrease in creatinine clearance associated with normoalbuminuria occurs in type 2 as well as type 1 diabetes and may occur in approximately 25% of diabetic patients with impaired creatinine clearance [4].

1994: Parving [5] demonstrates that non-diabetic (intrinsic) renal disease occurs more commonly in patients without diabetic retinopathy.

1996: Fioretto and Mauer [6] demonstrate that renal ultrastructure in type 2 diabetic patients with microalbuminuria and preserved renal function consists of not only typical (mainly glomerular) but also atypical (mainly extra-glomerular) pathology.

1996: Olsen and Mogensen [7] demonstrate that non-diabetic renal disease is uncommon if biopsies are performed randomly and from a diabetes clinic population as opposed to biopsies performed because of atypical clinical presentation in renal clinics.

2002: The Third National Health and Nutrition Examination Survey (NHANES III) reports a prevalence of renal insufficiency (GFR < 60 ml/min/1.73m^2) of 4.3% in the general population. In subjects aged 60-73 years 61% of people with renal insufficiency had normoalbuminuria [8].

2003: Prevention of Renal and Vascular End-stage Disease (PREVEND) Study shows prevalence of microalbuminuria is about 2 fold higher in men (16.4%) than women (9.4%) in a community-based sample of subjects aged 30-70 years [9].

2003: Studies in normoalbuminuric patients with type 1 diabetes and GFR < 90 ml/min/1.73 m^2 demonstrate typical ultrastructural changes of diabetic nephropathy [10].

METHODOLOGY

There are several methods of assessing or calculating GFR. The most accurate (isotopic) methods are also the most difficult to perform and the methods which are the easiest to perform are subject to lack of sensitivity (serum creatinine) or errors of urine collection (creatinine clearance). Although creatinine clearance may show good agreement with isotopic measurements of GFR using ^{51}Cr-EDTA or ^{99m}Tc-DTPA in people with mid-range renal function [11], creatinine clearance tends to underestimate hyperfiltration and to overestimate reduced GFR because of renal tubular secretion of creatinine [12]. For clinical purposes, the plasma disappearance of isotopic EDTA or DTPA is the best estimate of the true GFR when compared to the gold standard of inulin clearance using a constant infusion technique. The accuracy of single-shot plasma disappearance techniques is improved by use of the Brochner-Mortensen correction for the plasma decay rate of the isotope [13]. If this correction is not used, false high GFR data are obtained especially at higher absolute levels of GFR.

In expert hands, the mean day to day intra-individual coefficient of variation for isotopic measurements of GFR using a plasma decay technique ranges from 4%[14] to 7% [15]. By contrast, rates of decline of GFR measured over a median period of 2.4 years (range 1.9 to 5.5 years) may vary more than 3 fold, ranging from 5 to 17 ml/min/year in type 1 diabetic patients with overt diabetic nephropathy prior to antihypertensive treatment [14]. The highly variable rate of decline of GFR in individuals, coupled with short-term changes in GFR associated with initiation or cessation of antihypertensive therapy, suggests that GFR gradients calculated in 1-2 year studies may not accurately reflect the true rate of decline in renal function [16]. This is particularly important in microalbuminuric patients whose rates of decline of GFR may be less than 5 ml/min/1.73 m^2/year.

A further problem in interpreting changes in GFR is the acute effect of dietary protein intake and the reversible effects of antihypertensive therapy and glycaemic control which are observed over several weeks. A high protein meal may increase GFR by over 30% [17], and initiation of antihypertensive therapy usually lowers GFR by 5-10% [18]. Also, intensive glycaemic control may reverse hyperfiltration over 3-6 months [19]. Cessation of captopril based antihypertensive therapy has been shown to reverse the initial reduction in GFR after 8 years in patients with type 1 diabetes and microalbuminuria [20].

A similar 'treatment pause' has been shown to increase AER by over 20% one month after cessation of 1 year of antihypertensive therapy in hypertensive and normotensive microalbuminuric patients with type 1 or type 2 diabetes [21], and also after cessation of 3 years of therapy in normotensive microalbuminuric patients with type 1 diabetes [22].

The long-term response of GFR to antihypertensive therapy provides further difficulties in evaluating changes in GFR in microalbuminuric patients. Most studies have not detected significant changes over 2 years [23, 24], and some studies, using creatinine clearance as a surrogate for GFR, have failed to show significant changes over 5 years [11, 25].

The estimation of GFR from the Modification of Diet in Renal Disease (MDRD) formula [26] is simple but may be subject to two types of error. First, the MDRD data were obtained from a population with advanced renal disease, most of whom did not have diabetes. Extrapolation to diabetic patients with possible hyperfiltration may therefore be less accurate than direct measurement of GFR. Second, small errors in the measurement of serum creatinine can lead to large errors in the estimated GFR. For instance, serum creatinine levels in the NHANES III study had to be calibrated to MDRD levels by adding 20.3 μmol/L [8]. Without the calibration correction, approximately 3 fold higher prevalence data were obtained for impaired GFR in the United States (Table 1) [27].

There is a large intra-individual variation for AER as measured by using immunological techniques and recent studies have suggested that the renal handling of albumin is more complex than previously thought. Most albumin appears to be degraded to fragments (<10,000 Da) by lysosomal proteases prior to excretion and the fragments are not detected by conventional immunological techniques [28, 29]. Albumin also appears to be present in urine in an immuno-reactive and immuno-unreactive forms [30].

The concepts of microalbuminuria may change with time as these new techniques are used to explore the evolution of diabetic nephropathy.

Table 1.
Prevalence of impaired kidney function (according to GFR category) in NHANES III study

Study	Subgroup	n	GFR 30-59			GFR 15-30			GFR estimation
Garg 2002 [76]	Total	14,622	5.7			0.6			Serum Cr [96]
			AER			AER			
			N 77	μ 20	M 3	N 37	μ 37	M 26	
	Non-diabetic hypertensive	4,686	10.7			1.4			
	Non-diabetic normotensive	1,192	3.2			0.1			
	Non-diabetic		AER			AER			
			N 73	μ 23	M 4	N 43	μ 40	M 17	
	Diabetic	1,192	13.1			3.2			
			AER			AER			
			N 49	μ 43	M 8	N 20	μ 36	M 44	
Clase 2002 [27]	Non-diabetic	13,251	12.7			0.3			MDRD [26]
Coresh 2003 [8]	Total	15,600	4.3			0.2			MDRD simplified [97]
			AER			AER			
			N 61	μ 32	M 7	N 49	μ 43	M 8	
	Non-diabetic	14,341	3.7			0.2			
	Diabetic	1,201	14.2			0.9			

GFR category is expressed as ml/min/1.73m^2; GFR prevalence is shown as %;
N = normoalbuminuria; μ = microalbuminuria; M = macroalbuminuria; n = number of subjects

CHANGING TREATMENT TARGETS AND MICROALBUMINURIA

Since the initial concept of microalbuminuria in the early 1980's, there have been significant changes in approaches to the control of hyperglycaemia and hypertension. The DCCT (1997) [31] and UKPDS (1998) [32] studies were responsible for lowering HbA_{1c} targets to <7.0% and the captopril study (1993) [33] and IRMA-2 [24], IDNT [34] and RENAAL (2001) [35] studies were responsible for the widespread use of antihypertensive therapy based on inhibition of the renin angiotensin system with blood pressure targets to below 130/85 in patients with early and late diabetic nephropathy [36]. Although these targets are achieved in less than half of eligible patients in community based surveys, the earlier use of insulin in type 2 diabetes and the use of multiple antihypertensive agents are now part of 'standard' therapy, whereas they would have been considered inappropriate 20 years ago, when HbA_{1c} had just been introduced and blood pressure levels of less than 160/95 were considered normotensive. Since glycaemic control is critical in the initiation of nephropathy, and both glycaemic and blood pressure control determine the rate of progression of nephropathy, it follows that consideration of a calendar effect is important in evaluating AER and GFR studies during the last 20 years.

INFLUENCE OF GFR ON ALBUMINURIA

Hyperfiltration, defined as a GFR above the range observed in age matched non-diabetic subjects (>135 ml/min/1.73 m^2 in young subjects) occurs in approximately 20% of normo- and microalbuminuria patients with type 1 diabetes [37, 38] and 0-20% of patients with type 2 diabetes [39, 40] depending on the reference range used. Hyperfiltration occurs less commonly in some ethnic groups compared with others [40]. The increase in GFR usually starts at the stage of normoalbuminuria but may continue for several years into microalbuminuria [38] (Figure 1). Serial studies of GFR at the stage of hyperfiltration in type 1 diabetes have shown a decline towards the mid-normal range in both normoalbuminuric [41] and microalbuminuric [42] patients. In an 8 year study by Rudberg, 2 out of 5 patients progressing to macroalbuminuria did attain subnormal GFR levels. However, in 20 of 64 patients who progressed from normo- to micro- or macroalbuminuria GFR declined from ~148 to ~130 ml/min/1.73m^2 [42]. An observational study in 33 normotensive, normoalbuminuric patients with type 1 diabetes and with initial GFR of 137 ± 28 ml/min/1.73 m^2 reported a mean rate of decline of GFR of 2.4 ± 3.5 ml/min/1.73 m^2/year (p <0.05) over 8.4 years [43]. The changes of GFR in the last 2 studies probably represent resolution of hyperfiltration rather than the onset of impairment of renal function.

Timing of the onset of a decline in GFR is uncertain, in part because of the difficulty in separating the largely functional, reversible and potentially beneficial process represented by the resolution of hyperfiltration from the largely structural, irreversible and harmful process leading to a decline in GFR from normal to subnormal levels. In the absence of long-term studies unifying or separating rates of change of renal function at high and low levels of GFR, attempts have been made to link GFR to AER status. In a cross-sectional study of 84 patients with type 1 diabetes without antihypertensive treatment, GFR levels varied from normal to high and then to subnormal as AER increased from normo- to micro to macroalbuminuria [44]. The highest GFR level of 130 ml/min/1.73 m^2 corresponded to an AER of 34 mg/24 h. Interestingly, similar results were reported in the cross-sectional, population-based PREVEND Study from the city of Groningen [45]. In a sample of 7646 mainly non-diabetic subjects, creatinine clearance increased and then decreased in a parabolic fashion as AER increased from normo- to micro- to macroalbuminuria, with the highest levels corresponding to an AER in the range of 15-30 mg/24 h. The similarity between results in diabetic and non-diabetic subjects supports the possibility of a pathogenetic link between glomerular hyperfiltration and subsequent renal injury.

A study of changes in GFR and renal structure during the evolution of microalbuminuria in type 1 diabetes showed that patients with previous glomerular hyperfiltration had the steepest rate of decline in GFR of 11 ml/min/year over about 5 years compared with a rise of 0.8 ml/min/year in previously normo-filtering patients [46]. The rate of decline of GFR was positively correlated with glomerular basement membrane thickness and interstitial volume fraction and mean HbA_{1c} level. It was concluded that a decreasing GFR in the early stage of microalbuminuria may be due to more advanced glomerulopathy than in patients with stable GFR. This suggested that hyperfiltration is an independent risk factor for the development of overt nephropathy in patients with type 1 diabetes. By contrast, a case controlled prospective study of GFR in type 1 diabetic patients with normoalbuminuria did not support the concept that hyperfiltration predisposes to the development of microalbuminuria [41]. A similar number of hyperfiltering patients (4/25) progressed to microalbuminuria over 10 years compared with normofiltering patients (3/25). Baseline AER and blood pressure were the main predictors of final AER, with glomerular hyperfiltration playing a lesser role. However, neither of these studies was of sufficient duration to show whether patients with hyperfiltration develop an earlier onset of decline in GFR to subnormal levels. It is, therefore, not possible to link hyperfiltration to nephron dropout or to increases in fractional mesangial volume on present evidence.

INFLUENCE OF ALBUMINURIA ON GFR

The development of microalbuminuria usually precedes decreases in GFR in both type 1 and type 2 diabetes [47]. It has also been proposed that albuminuria itself contributes to the subsequent impairment of renal function [48]. Studies in isolated renal tubules have shown that exposure to albumin or other proteins promote renal injury [48]. A renal biopsy study in patients with type 2 diabetes and overt nephropathy has shown that the best predictor of later progression to impairment of renal function is the level of proteinuria rather than the type of renal lesion [49]. Patients with proteinuria >2 g/24 h had a 92% risk of progression to renal failure, whereas patients with <2 g proteinuria/24 h but matched for glycaemic and blood pressure control maintained stable serum creatinine levels. Data in Japanese patients with type 2 diabetes also support the possibility that protein traffic is a determinant of progression of renal disease [50]. Further support for this concept was provided by a study of the effects of ACE inhibition in patients with type 1 diabetes and overt diabetic nephropathy [51]. In the latter study a decrease in AER within 6 months of commencement of ACE inhibitor therapy predicted the degree of attenuation of the subsequent rate of decline of GFR over the ensuing 5 years.

Some, but not all, studies in patients with microalbuminuria have linked increases in AER to a decline in GFR. In middle-aged Israeli patients with type 2 diabetes and microalbuminuria, there was a progressive increase in serum creatinine levels over 5 years, implying a decrease in GFR of approximately 15% [52]. By contrast, no decline in GFR was observed in microalbuminuric Pima Indians over 3 years [53], and studies in type 1 diabetes have generally not shown a decline in GFR in microalbuminuric patients [54]. The relationship between microalbuminuria and GFR in type 2 diabetes is further complicated by the heterogeneity of renal structural lesions in these patients [6, 55, 56]. About one third of patients with type 2 diabetes and microalbuminuria show normal or near normal renal ultrastructure on biopsy [57] and microalbuminuria may also reflect large vessel disease rather that being a specific marker of renal damage [2]. This raises the possibility that these patients will manifest 'plateau' microalbuminuria without progressing to a decline in GFR. At present, renal biopsy is the only way to differentiate so-called 'benign' and 'malignant' microalbuminuria [58].

THE ROLE OF PROGRESSION PROMOTERS IN MICROALBUMINURIA

Changes in AER and/or GFR in patients with microalbuminuria may represent responses to one or more mediators of renal injury. Such 'progression promoters' could include glycaemic and blood pressure control as well as functional and structural changes within the kidney. For instance, there is strong evidence to indicate that glycaemic control determines the onset of microalbuminuria in both type 1 and type 2 diabetes [31, 32]. There is equally strong evidence to support a role for raised blood pressure as an initiator and progression promoter in diabetic nephropathy (Figure 2).

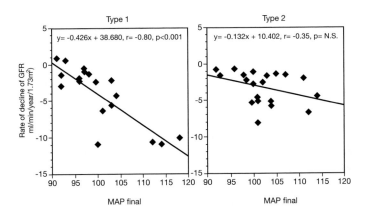

Figure 2. Relationship of rate of decline of GFR to MAP in type 1 and type 2 diabetes. Studies included for type 1 panel 2(A): [20, 22, 23, 33, 41, 43, 46, 71, 77, 78, 96-101], Studies included for type 2 panel 2(B): [5, 11, 24, 25, 34, 35, 68, 82-85, 87, 102-106]

However, the temporal relationship of hypertension to the onset of microalbuminuria differs in young patients with type 1 diabetes and older patients with type 2 diabetes. In type 1 diabetes microalbuminuria generally develops before increases in office blood pressure are detected [59], even though increases in nocturnal blood pressure occur much earlier [60]. In type 2 diabetes increases in blood pressure usually precede the development of microalbuminuria [61-63].

In both type 1 and type 2 diabetes the levels of systolic, diastolic and mean blood pressure have been associated with increases in AER and decreases in GFR in patients with microalbuminuria [64]. The relationship between the rate of decline of GFR and mean arterial pressure (MAP) is particularly strong in patients with type 1 diabetes and macroalbuminuria (Figures 1 and 2), but there is emerging evidence to support a similar relationship at the stage of microalbuminuria in type 1 and type 2 diabetes. However, increases in blood pressure may reflect diverse mechanisms, including an association with the metabolic syndrome in type 2 diabetes as well as a rise in blood pressure as a consequence of renal disease in both type 1 and type 2 diabetes. In addition to these systemic considerations, it is likely that intra-renal mechanisms involving cytokines and changes in glomerular and tubular ultrastructure mediate changes in AER and GFR in microalbuminuric patients [65].

RENAL ULTRASTRUCTURAL CHANGES AND GFR DECLINE

In overt nephropathy several studies have shown a close relationship between renal ultrastructural changes and a decline in GFR. In type 1 diabetes an increase in fractional mesangial volume and in glomerular basement membrane thickening has been associated with a decrease in creatinine clearance [66]. Increases in tubulo-interstitial fibrosis have also been linked to decreases in creatinine clearance in type 1 diabetes [67], but the possible pathogenetic role of extra-glomerular changes has not been investigated to the same degree as glomerular changes.

In type 2 diabetes a combination of glomerular structural changes, termed the glomerulopathy index, and the percentage of occluded glomeruli have been shown to correlate with the rate of GFR decline at the stage of overt nephropathy [68]. Another study in a subgroup of 47 patients with overt nephropathy from the IDNT Study showed that nodular intercapillary glomerulosclerosis, present in 17 patients, was associated with higher serum creatinine levels than the diffuse lesion alone, present in 15 patients [69]. Furthermore, diabetic retinopathy was more closely associated with the nodular form of diabetic glomerulosclerosis. In the IDNT study as a whole, the presence of retinopathy at baseline predicted a faster rate of doubling of serum creatinine levels [70].

Whether the above structure-function relationships exist before the onset of overt nephropathy is not clear. There is increasing evidence to support the concept that glomerular structural changes can exist in association with microalbuminuria in both type 1 [71] and type 2 diabetes [65], and that a significant decline in GFR may occur in type 1 and type 2 diabetes before the development of macroalbuminuria [10]. Furthermore, in normoalbuminuric patients with type 1 diabetes and subnormal GFR (< 90 ml/min/1.73 m^2) there is structural evidence of typical diabetic nephropathy [10]. In type 2 diabetes similar structure-function correlations have not yet been performed. Such studies are necessary to define the relative importance of renal haemodynamic as opposed to renal ultrastructural changes in determining the rate of decline of GFR in microalbuminuric patients [6].

The renal expression of cytokines is closely linked to structure-function relationships in microalbuminuric patients. Increased renal expression of TGF-ß has been linked to nephropathy in type 2 diabetes [72] and increased urinary expression of TGF-ß has been linked to nephropathy in type 1 diabetes [73]. Human studies linking AER and rates of decline in GFR at the stage of microalbuminuria will be necessary to delineate the role of new interventions which modulate the expression or action of specific cytokines in the kidney.

PREVALENCE OF IMPAIRED GFR DURING MICROALBUMINURIA IN TYPE 1 AND TYPE 2 DIABETES

Assessments of GFR in patients with microalbuminuria can be performed either cross-sectionally or longitudinally. The former yields data on prevalence and is heavily influenced by age, whereas the latter yields data on rate of GFR decline which is strongly influenced by blood pressure especially in type 2 diabetes. It follows that cross-sectional studies would be expected to show a higher prevalence of impaired GFR in elderly subjects with type 2 diabetes than in younger patients with type 1 diabetes. Also, longitudinal studies in elderly subjects with type 2 diabetes would be expected to show the age-related rate of decline of GFR of 1ml/min/year which has been documented in cross-sectional population studies [74, 75], in addition to any decline in GFR associated with diabetic nephropathy.

The first population-based study on the prevalence of impaired renal function in the United States was performed in NHANES III [8] (Table 1). Impairment of GFR in the range 15-60 ml/min/1.73m^2 was observed in 3.9% of non-diabetic and 15.1% of diabetic participants. The prevalence of impaired GFR < 60 ml/min/1.73m^2 in diabetic participants was too low to calculate in the 20-40 year age group, but increased from approximately 3% in the 40-59 year age group to approximately 35% in the > 70 year age group [8]. NHANES III also showed that impaired GFR is observed with a greater prevalence in older, hypertensive subjects without diabetes [76].

LONGITUDINAL STUDIES OF GFR IN MICROALBUMINURIC PATIENTS WITH TYPE 1 DIABETES (FIGURE 3)

In type 1 diabetes a few small studies have assessed rates of decline of GFR in microalbuminuric patients. In 1991 Mathiesen showed that GFR remained static over 4 years in 23 normotensive patients who were not treated with antihypertensive agents [77]. An extension of this study showed that mean GFR declined from 129 to 119 ml/min/1.73m^2 over 8 years but this failed to reach statistical significance for the group as a whole [20]. However, 8 patients progressing to macroalbuminuria did show a significant decline in GFR over the study period. The concept of AER progression being a determinant of a decline in GFR in microalbuminuric patients with type 1 diabetes is largely based on a 5 year study of 40 normotensive patients who did not receive antihypertensive therapy [78]. In 14/40 patients who progressed to macroalbuminuria the mean GFR decreased by 2.2 $\pm$ 3.8 ml/min/1.73m^2 (p = 0.05) compared with a rise of 0.5 $\pm$ 2.1 ml/min/1.73m^2 (p = NS) in the 26 non-progressors. There was a significant difference in the rate of change of GFR between the two groups (p < 0.05). Progressors showed a higher mean arterial pressure of 103 versus 93 mmHg in non-progressors, and the mean rate of decline of GFR was related to baseline systolic blood pressure. In addition, the rate of increase of AER was related to overall glycaemic control, supporting a role for glycaemic control as an initiator of the nephropathic process.

Other studies of placebo treated normotensive patients with type 1 diabetes and microalbuminuria who did not receive anti-hypertensive therapy have usually not shown significant rates of decline of GFR over intervals of 2 to 3 years. In 1994 a study of 46 placebo treated normotensive, microalbuminuric patients over 2 years reported a non-significant trend for GFR to decline by 3 ml/min/1.73m^2/year [23]. Twelve of the 46 patients developed macroalbuminuria but the rate of GFR change was not reported. In 1998 an Italian study of 34 placebo treated normotensive patients with type 1 diabetes and microalbuminuria showed no significant changes in GFR over 3 years [79]. In 2001, the Melbourne Diabetic Nephropathy Study Group reported the results of a study in normotensive patients with type 2 diabetes and microalbuminuria [22]. Seven placebo treated patients with an initial GFR of 90 ± 7 ml/min/1.73 m^2 showed a non-significant trend towards a decline in GFR of 1.3 ± 1.1 ml/min/1.73 m^2/year over a mean duration of follow-up of 65 ± 8 months.

Recent studies in hypertensive patients with microalbuminuria have not included an untreated or placebo treated control arm for ethical reasons. The rate of change of GFR may therefore reflect the level of blood pressure achieved as well as the type of antihypertensive therapy.

In 1994 a 2 year study in hypertensive patients with type 1 diabetes and microalbuminuria [80] showed a significant decline in GFR from baseline to 2 years during treatment with captopril (4.9 ± 2.1 ml/min/1.73m^2/year) or atenolol (3.7 ± 1.6 ml/min/1.73m^2/year). However, if the rate of decline of GFR was calculated from 6 months onwards it was no longer significant. A study in type 1 diabetic patients with hypertension and overt nephropathy had previously demonstrated a blunting of the rate of decline of GFR with increasing duration of antihypertensive therapy [18]. Further studies are required to determine if greater reductions in MAP are associated with reversal of the decline in GFR in hypertensive microalbuminuric patients with type 1 diabetes.

In summary, although cross-sectional studies have shown that GFR changes from hyperfiltration toward normofiltration when AER exceeds 50 µg/min [15], this has been difficult to demonstrate in longitudinal studies. However, the recent studies by Mauer's group indicate that even normoalbuminuria does not always ensure against reduction of GFR in type 1 diabetes which is associated with renal ultrastructural changes typical of diabetic nephropathy [65].

LONGITUDINAL STUDIES OF GFR IN MICROALBUMINURIC PATIENTS WITH TYPE 2 DIABETES (FIGURE 3)

There are at least 3 reasons why the rate of decline of GFR may differ in microalbuminuric patients with type 2 diabetes compared with type 1 diabetes. Firstly, there is an age related GFR decline of approximately 1 ml/min/1.73m^2/year after the age of 40 years [74, 75]. Secondly, there is a higher prevalence of hypertension in type 2 diabetes, which may accelerate renal injury [81]. Thirdly, a proportion of microalbuminuric patients with minimal or no detectable renal structural lesions may never progress to macroalbuminuria and may be expected to have stable GFR. Despite the above considerations, the rate of decline of GFR at the stage of overt nephropathy has been shown to be similar in type 2 and type 1 diabetes [81]. The available GFR data in microalbuminuric patients will be considered in the normotensive and then in the hypertensive setting.

The first study to suggest that a decline in GFR may occur in normotensive type 2 diabetic patients with microalbuminuria was reported by Ravid in 1993 [52]. The placebo group in this study included 45 middle-aged Israeli patients with mean baseline serum creatinine levels of 102 µmole/L. During 5 years of follow-up there was a 13% decrease in renal function as estimated by the inverse of the serum creatinine level, which represents a GFR decline of approximately 2.5 ml/min/year. However, other studies examining rates of decline in GFR in placebo treated normotensive patients have not detected any change. For instance, renal function as assessed by creatinine clearance was preserved over 4 years in 12 normotensive, microalbuminuric Japanese patients [82] and GFR remained stable over 5 years in 51 normotensive, microalbuminuric Indian patients [83].

Preservation of creatinine clearance was also observed during 5.3 years of antihypertensive therapy in the normotensive Appropriate Blood Pressure Control in Diabetes (ABCD) Study [11]. This study included 109 patients with microalbuminuria who were treated moderately or intensively with nisoldipine or enalapril based therapy. The mean arterial pressure achieved was 128/75 (MAP 93) mmHg in the intensive group and 137/81 (MAP 99) mmHg in the moderate group. Creatinine clearance fell by 5-10 ml/min in both study groups within 12 months of commencing antihypertensive therapy but there was no subsequent decline throughout the study. By contrast, creatinine clearance declined progressively by 4-6 ml/min/1.73m^2/year in patients with baseline macroalbuminuria in the same study [11].

Similar results were obtained in the hypertensive ABCD study using a moderate or intensive anti hypertensive regimen [25]. The mean blood pressure achieved was 132/78 (MAP 99) mmHg in the intensive group and 138/86 (MAP 103) mmHg in the moderate group in 150 hypertensive patients with baseline microalbuminuria. Creatinine clearance fell by about 5ml/min during the first year after initiation of antihypertensive therapy and thereafter stabilised in both treatment groups. As in the normotensive ABCD Study, there was a progressive decline in creatinine clearance of 5-6 ml/min/1.73m^2/year in hypertensive patients with macroalbuminuria at baseline. A study in a younger group of 50 microalbuminuric normotensive Pima Indians also demonstrated stable renal function during 4 years of follow-up [53]. By contrast, GFR decreased by 35% in 34 macroalbuminuric patients who were studied concurrently (p < 0.001).

In contrast to the above studies, several studies in hypertensive patients have reported a decline in GFR during microalbuminuria. In 1994, Lebovitz reported that GFR declined by 5 ml/min/year in 21 hypertensive microalbuminuric patients with a MAP of 101 mm Hg during a 3 year follow-up [84]. In 1997, Nielsen reported that GFR declined by approximately 1 ml/min/1.73m^2/year over 5.5 years in a group of normo- and microalbuminuric Danish patients with type 2 diabetes, some of whom were hypertensive [85]. However, this rate of GFR decline varied widely and did not exceed the age-related fall that is observed in non-diabetic subjects.

In 1996 Velussi reported a 3 year study of GFR in 18 hypertensive Italian patients with microalbuminuria [86]. Participants were treated with amlodipine or cilazapril to a target < 140 systolic and < 85 diastolic blood pressure (mmHg). The rate of GFR decline was significant in both groups, 2.33 ml/min/1.73m^2/year with amlodopine and 2.15 ml/min/1.73m^2/year with cilazapril, and was inversely related to MAP but not to HbA$_{1c}$.

In 2001 the IRMA-2 Study, which included 201 hypertensive patients with type 2 diabetes and microalbuminuria treated with conventional antihypertensive agents but not renin angiotensin system inhibitors, showed a biphasic decline in creatinine clearance from 109 to 105 ml/min/1.73m^2 over 2 years [24]. The decline in the initial 3 months was 0.9 ml/min/1.73m^2/month, compared with 0.1 ml/min/1.73m^2/month from 3 to 24 months.

There have been two other long-term studies of GFR decline in hypertensive Italian patients with microalbuminuria by Nosadini's group. In each study a renal biopsy was performed at baseline and all participants received antihypertensive therapy to achieve blood pressure levels less than 140/90 mmHg. In the first study there was a variable but significant decline of GFR of 1.3 ± 9.4 ml/min/1.73m^2/year (mean ± SD) [87]. The rate of GFR decline was strongly influenced by renal ultrastructural changes including fractional mesangial volume at baseline and by glycaemic control during follow-up, but not by MAP. The latter finding may have reflected good blood pressure control in all participants.

In 2001 the same group reported a 7 year follow-up of GFR decline in a group of micro- and macroalbuminuric type 2 diabetic patients [88]. In the first 4 years, 38 participants with normal renal ultrastructure at baseline showed no decline in GFR, whereas 50 participants with increased glomerular basement membrane thickness and fractional mesangial volume showed a significant change in GFR (increase of 1.21 vs decrease of 5.86 ml/min/1.73m^2/year, respectively). The two groups had near identical mean baseline AER of about 110 μg/min, but the range of baseline albuminuria extended to over 1000 μg/min. It is therefore difficult to assess the contribution of persistently microalbuminuric patients to the overall results. During a further 3 years of follow-up, half of the 50 participants with abnormal glomerular ultrastructure were treated with intensive glycaemic control (mean HbA$_{1c}$ 7.0%), while the remaining half were treated less intensively (mean HbA$_{1c}$ 8.0%) [88]. The rate of GFR decline in the intensive glycaemic control group was 1.8 versus 4.2 ml/min/1.73m^2/year in the less intensive group (p = 0.06). The rate of GFR decline during the last 3 years in the intensive glycaemic control group was significantly lower than in the first 4 years of the study.

The Melbourne Diabetic Nephropathy Study Group has studied 27 placebo treated normotensive, microalbuminuric patients with type 2 diabetes over 6 years. At baseline, mean age was 53 years and initial GFR was 98 ± 6 ml/min/1.73 m^2. The mean rate of decline of GFR was 4.2 ml/min/1.73 m^2 (p < 0.01) during a follow-up of 69 months. Thirteen of these patients developed hypertension during the study and were treated with either perindopril or nifedipine.

In summary, several studies ranging from 2 to 8 years in duration, have shown that GFR is stable in most normotensive patients with type 1 or type 2 diabetes as long as they remain normotensive and microalbuminuric. Significant but variable rates of GFR decline occur in hypertensive patients, those with intra-renal ultrastructural abnormalities and in patients progressing to macroalbuminuria. However, at least two methodological problems remain.

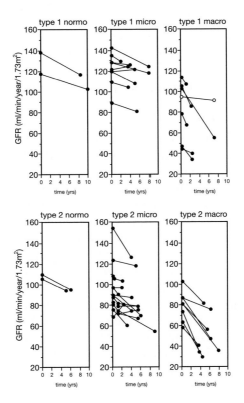

Figure 3. Longitudinal studies of changes in GFR according to AER status in type 1 and type 2 diabetes. Studies included for type 1 subjects with normoalbuminuria panel 3(A): [41, 43], Studies included for type 1 subjects with microalbuminuria panel 3(B): [20, 22, 23, 46, 71, 77-79], Studies included for type 1 subjects with macroalbuminuria panel 3(C): [33, 96-100], Studies included for type 2 subjects with normoalbuminuria panel 3(D): [103, 104], Studies included for type 2 subjects with microalbuminuria panel 3(E): [11, 14, 22, 24, 25, 53, 82-84, 107-109], Studies included for type 2 subjects with macroalbuminuria panel 3(F): [5, 34, 35, 68, 85, 105, 106].

First, it is difficult to differentiate the potentially reversible effect on GFR of initiation of antihypertensive therapy from the onset of nephron dropout or other renal ultastructural changes which imply permanent decline in renal function. Second, studies averaging 5 years in duration are still too short to reliably document a slow decline in GFR which may be in the range of 2-4 ml/min/1.73m^2/year and only marginally greater than the expected decline in GFR from aging alone.

EMERGING CONCEPTS REGARDING ALBUMIN HANDLING BY THE KIDNEY

A new understanding of the role of proximal tubular cells in the degradation of filtered proteins including albumin has been reached in the last 5 years. Studies by Comper's group and ourselves have shown that albumin is normally degraded in the kidney and that albumin-derived fragments are not detectable by standard immunological methods [89]. The normal renal handling of albumin involves its degradation through lysosomal uptake from the tubular fluid and subsequent exocytosis of the peptide products back into the urine [28, 90]. Our recent studies of ^{3}H-albumin handling in patients with type 1 diabetes have shown that albuminuria is also directly linked to changes in lysosomal mediated degradation of proteins [29]. These albumin-derived degradation products are found exclusively in the urine and not in blood. The above studies have shown that filtered albumin is fragmented to small peptides of <10-15 kD in size within minutes and that these albumin-derived fragments constitute >90-95% of urinary albumin compared with <5-10% of albumin that is in an intact form [91]. In general, the proportion of intact albumin increases as renal disease progresses from normo- to micro- to macroalbuminuria and may reflect renal tubular dysfunction.

In experimental and human diabetes, an increase in total albuminuria may reflect both an increase in the intact to fragment ratio of urinary albumin as well as alterations in the activity of a trans-tubular transport pathway [92]. By contrast, in experimental hypertension, increases in total albuminuria appear to be explained purely on the basis of a change in the intact:fragment ratio of urinary albumin [89]. The complexity of albumin-derived components in urine has recently been highlighted as intact albumin appears to be excreted in two forms, i.e. immuno-reactive and immuno-unreactive. Preliminary results have demonstrated a high prevalence of immuno-unreactive intact albumin, as measured by HPLC, in the early stages of diabetic renal disease. The exact nature and significance of immuno-unreactive intact urinary albumin is not known but elevated levels may possibly prove to be a useful early marker of renal disease that precedes an increase in immuno-reactive urinary albumin.

DISPARITY BETWEEN DECLINING GFR AND INCREASING AER

Most patients with diabetic renal disease display a decline in GFR that is preceded or accompanied by an increase in AER. However there is a growing body of evidence to suggest that some patients possibly follow an alternate, non-albuminuric pathway to renal impairment. The combination of impaired renal function in association with normoalbuminuria was first highlighted by Lane et al. [3] who identified eight women with type 1 diabetes who had low creatinine clearance but a normal AER. A recent study from this group has examined the clinical characteristics and renal ultrastructure in 105 normoalbuminuric type 1 diabetic patients [10]. A total of 23 (22 %) normoalbuminuric patients had a GFR < 90 ml/min/1.73 m^2 and a median AER of 7.7 (range 2.0-17.6) µg/min. These patients showed increased mesangial and mesangial matrix fractional volumes and glomerular basement membrane width when compared with age- and gender-matched controls. The glomerular lesions seen in normoalbuminuric patients with type 1 diabetes and a GFR < 90 ml/min/1.73 m^2 were also more advanced than those in normoalbuminuric patients with a GFR ≥ 90 ml/min/1.73 m^2. These investigators concluded that, in type 1 diabetes, low GFR could precede increases in AER, particularly in women with longstanding diabetes associated with retinopathy and hypertension.

Studies from our group have also shown that creatinine clearance can decline in patients with type 1 or type 2 diabetes, especially females without microalbuminuria [4]. More recently, we have explored the relationship between AER and isotopically measured GFR in a larger group of patients with type 2 diabetes [93]. Thirty-four percent of participants (109/301) had a GFR < 60 ml/min/1.73 m^2 (Figure 4). In patients with GFR ≥ 60 ml/min/1.73 m^2 the prevalence of normo-, micro- and macroalbuminuria was 115 (60 %), 64 (33 %) and 13 (7 %) respectively (Figure 4: zones 1, 2 and 3, respectively). For the 109 patients with a GFR < 60 ml/min/1.73 m^2 the prevalence of normo-, micro- and macroalbuminuria was 43 (39 %), 38 (35 %) and 28 (26 %) respectively (Figure 4: zones 4, 5 and 6 respectively). When the 301 patients were stratified according to their AER status regardless of their GFR, 158 (52%) had normo-, 102 (34 %) had micro- and 41 (14 %) had macroalbuminuria. For these normoalbuminuric patients, 115/158 (73%) had a corresponding GFR ≥ 60 ml/min/1.73m² and 43/158 (27%) had a GFR < 60 ml/min/1.73m².

The prevalence of a GFR < 60 ml/min/1.73m² and normoalbuminuria was also calculated after excluding patients whose normoalbuminuric status was possibly altered by the use of a renin angiotensin system inhibitor. After this adjustment the prevalence of a GFR < 60 ml/min/1.73 m² and normoalbuminuria was 20/86 (23%). Furthermore, after the additional exclusion of patients without retinopathy, the prevalence of a GFR < 60 ml/min/1.73 m² and normoalbuminuria was not altered, i.e. 8/35 (23%). Temporal changes in GFR were also calculated in a subset of 37/109 (34%) unselected patients with impaired renal function. The mean interval between GFR measurements (years) of 4.9 ± 0.5, 5.6 ± 0.6 and 6.6 ± 0.6 years and the rate of decline in GFR (ml/min/1.73m²/year) of 5.5 ± 1.0, 2.8 ± 1.0 and 3.0 ± 07 ml/min/1.73m²/year were not significantly different for normo- (n = 15), micro- (n = 12), and macro- (n = 10) albuminuric patients respectively.

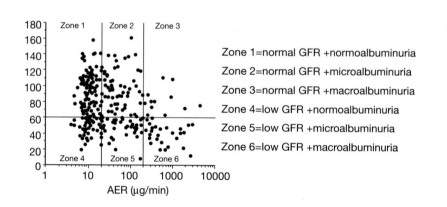

Figure 4. GFR and AER in 301 patients with type 2 diabetes subdivided according to level of albuminuria and GFR ≥ or < 60 ml/min/1.73m².

Similar cross-sectional data were obtained using the MDRD-6 formula [26] in a survey of 820 diabetic patients from our clinic. This showed that 102 normoalbuminuric patients, representing 12% of all survey participants, had a GFR < 60 ml/min/1.73m^2 [94].

Results from NHANES III suggest that the finding of non-albuminuric renal insufficiency in diabetes is not uncommon [76] (Table 1). The study included 14,622 non-institutionalised adult participants in the USA, of whom 8.3% demonstrated micro- and 1.0% macroalbuminuria. When albuminuria and renal insufficiency were considered together, 37% of participants with a low glomerular filtration rate (estimated GFR <30 ml/min/1.73 m^2) demonstrated no micro- or macroalbuminuria (i.e. non-albuminuric renal insufficiency). This was most evident in the age-group of 60-79 years: 34% of diabetic and 63% of non-diabetic hypertensive patients with a GFR < 30 ml/min/1.73m^2 demonstrated normoalbuminuria [76]. The prevalence of non-albuminuric renal insufficiency, when defined as a GFR < 60 ml/min/1.73m^2, for subjects with diabetes in this age group was 47%. Although this may be an overestimate because of a lack of calibration of serum creatinine levels to MDRD standards [8], this study nevertheless indicates that screening tests for albuminuria and renal insufficiency identify different segments of the population. The AUSDIAB study has recently inferred a similar discordance between albuminuria and GFR in the Australian population [95].

In conclusion whilst an increase in urinary albumin excretion remains the best non-invasive indicator of a patient's risk for progressive renal disease, its absence may not predict which patients are safe from a progressive decline in GFR. Females appear to be at a particularly increased risk for this non-albuminuric pathway to impaired renal function. It has been advocated that regular measurements of GFR should be performed in long-standing normoalbuminuric patients with type 1 diabetes, especially in females who also have with retinopathy or hypertension [10]. Our studies also suggest that the above should also apply to normoalbuminuric female patients with longstanding type 2 diabetes.

REFERENCES

1.   Mogensen CE, Christensen CK. Predicting diabetic nephropathy in insulin-dependent patients. N Engl J Med 1984; 311: 89-93.
2.   Yudkin JS, Forrest RD, Jackson CA. Microalbuminuria as predictor of vascular disease in non-diabetic subjects. Islington Diabetes Survey. Lancet 1988; 2: 530-533.

3. Lane PH, Steffes MW, Mauer SM. Glomerular structure in IDDM women with low glomerular filtration rate and normal urinary albumin excretion. Diabetes 1992; 41: 581-586.

4. Tsalamandris C, Allen TJ, Gilbert RE, et al. Progressive decline in renal function in diabetic patients with and without albuminuria. Diabetes 1994; 43: 649-655.

5. Christensen PK, Gall MA, Parving HH. Course of glomerular filtration rate in albuminuric type 2 diabetic patients with or without diabetic glomerulopathy. Diabetes Care 2000; 23 (Suppl 2): B14-20.

6. Fioretto P, Mauer M, Brocco E, et al. Patterns of renal injury in NIDDM patients with microalbuminuria. Diabetologia 1996; 39: 1569-1576.

7. Olsen S, Mogensen CE. How often is NIDDM complicated with non-diabetic renal disease? An analysis of renal biopsies and the literature. Diabetologia 1996; 39: 1638-1645.

8. Coresh J, Astor BC, Greene T, Eknoyan G, Levey AS. Prevalence of chronic kidney disease and decreased kidney function in the adult US population: Third National Health and Nutrition Examination Survey. Am J Kidney Dis 2003; 41: 1-12.

9. Verhave JC, Hillege HL, Burgerhof JG, et al. Cardiovascular risk factors are differently associated with urinary albumin excretion in men and women. J Am Soc Nephrol 2003; 14: 1330-1335.

10. Caramori ML, Fioretto P, Mauer M. Low glomerular filtration rate in normoalbuminuric type 1 diabetic patients: an indicator of more advanced glomerular lesions. Diabetes 2003; 52: 1036-1040.

11. Schrier RW, Estacio RO, Esler A, Mehler P. Effects of aggressive blood pressure control in normotensive type 2 diabetic patients on albuminuria, retinopathy and strokes. Kidney Int 2002; 61: 1086-1097.

12. Shemesh O, Golbetz H, Kriss JP, Myers BD. Limitations of creatinine as a filtration marker in glomerulopathic patients. Kidney Int 1985; 28: 830-838.

13. Brochner-Mortensen J, Rodbro P. Selection of routine method for determination of glomerular filtration rate in adult patients. Scand J Clin Lab Invest 1976; 36: 35-43.

14. Parving HH, Smidt UM, Hommel E, et al. Effective antihypertensive treatment postpones renal insufficiency in diabetic nephropathy. Am J Kidney Dis 1993; 22: 188-195.

15. Mogensen CE, Hansen KW, Nielsen S, et al. Monitoring diabetic nephropathy: glomerular filtration rate and abnormal albuminuria in diabetic renal disease—reproducibility, progression, and efficacy of antihypertensive intervention. Am J Kidney Dis 1993; 22: 174-187.

16. Levey AS. Assessing the effectiveness of therapy to prevent the progression of renal disease. Am J Kidney Dis 1993; 22: 207-214.

17. Mau Pedersen M, Mogensen CE, Jorgensen FS, et al. Renal effects from limitation of high dietary protein in normoalbuminuric diabetic patients. Kidney Int Suppl 1989; 27: S115-121.

18. Parving HH, Andersen AR, Smidt UM, Svendsen PA. Early aggressive antihypertensive treatment reduces rate of decline in kidney function in diabetic nephropathy. Lancet 1983; 1: 1175-1179.

19. Wiseman MJ, Saunders AJ, Keen H, Viberti G. Effect of blood glucose control on increased glomerular filtration rate and kidney size in insulin-dependent diabetes. N Engl J Med 1985; 312: 617-621.

20. Mathiesen ER, Hommel E, Hansen HP, Smidt UM, Parving HH. Randomised controlled trial of long term efficacy of captopril on preservation of kidney function in normotensive patients with insulin dependent diabetes and microalbuminuria. BMJ 1999; 319: 24-25.

21. Comparison between perindopril and nifedipine in hypertensive and normotensive diabetic patients with microalbuminuria. Melbourne Diabetic Nephropathy Study Group. BMJ 1991; 302: 210-216.

22. Jerums G, Allen TJ, Campbell DJ, et al. Long-term comparison between perindopril and nifedipine in normotensive patients with type 1 diabetes and microalbuminuria. Am J Kidney Dis 2001; 37: 890-899.

23. Viberti G, Mogensen CE, Groop LC, Pauls JF. Effect of captopril on progression to clinical proteinuria in patients with insulin-dependent diabetes mellitus and microalbuminuria. European Microalbuminuria Captopril Study Group. JAMA 1994; 271: 275-279.

24. Parving HH, Lehnert H, Brochner-Mortensen J, et al. The effect of irbesartan on the development of diabetic nephropathy in patients with type 2 diabetes. N Engl J Med 2001; 345: 870-878.

25. Estacio RO, Jeffers BW, Gifford N, Schrier RW. Effect of blood pressure control on diabetic microvascular complications in patients with hypertension and type 2 diabetes. Diabetes Care 2000; 23 (Suppl 2): B54-64.

26. Levey AS, Bosch JP, Lewis JB, et al. A more accurate method to estimate glomerular filtration rate from serum creatinine: a new prediction equation. Modification of Diet in Renal Disease Study Group. Ann Intern Med 1999; 130: 461-470.

27. Clase CM, Garg AX, Kiberd BA. Prevalence of low glomerular filtration rate in nondiabetic Americans: Third National Health and Nutrition Examination Survey (NHANES III). J Am Soc Nephrol 2002; 13: 1338-1349.

28. Osicka TM, Panagiotopoulos S, Jerums G, Comper WD. Fractional clearance of albumin is influenced by its degradation during renal passage. Clin Sci (Lond) 1997; 93: 557-564.

29. Osicka TM, Houlihan CA, Chan JG, Jerums G, Comper WD. Albuminuria in patients with type 1 diabetes is directly linked to changes in the lysosome-mediated degradation of albumin during renal passage. Diabetes 2000; 49: 1579-1584.

30. Comper WD, Osicka TM, Jerums G. High prevalence of immuno-unreactive intact albumin in urine of diabetic patients. Am J Kidney Dis 2003; 41: 336-342.

31. DCCT. The effect of intensive treatment of diabetes on the development and progression of long-term complications in insulin-dependent diabetes mellitus. The Diabetes Control and Complications Trial Research Group. N Engl J Med 1993; 329: 977-986.

32. UK Prospective Diabetes Study (UKPDS) Group. Intensive blood-glucose control with sulphonylureas or insulin compared with conventional treatment and risk of complications in patients with type 2 diabetes (UKPDS 33). Lancet 1998; 352: 837-853.

33. Lewis EJ, Hunsicker LG, Bain RP, Rohde RD. The effect of angiotensin-converting-enzyme inhibition on diabetic nephropathy. The Collaborative Study Group. N Engl J Med 1993; 329: 1456-1462.

34. Lewis EJ, Hunsicker LG, Clarke WR, et al. Renoprotective effect of the angiotensin-receptor antagonist irbesartan in patients with nephropathy due to type 2 diabetes. N Engl J Med 2001; 345: 851-860.

35. Brenner BM, Cooper ME, de Zeeuw D, et al. Effects of losartan on renal and cardiovascular outcomes in patients with type 2 diabetes and nephropathy. N Engl J Med 2001; 345: 861-869.

36. Bakris GL. A practical approach to achieving recommended blood pressure goals in diabetic patients. Arch Intern Med 2001; 161: 2661-2667.

37. Christiansen JS, Gammelgaard J, Tronier B, Svendsen PA, Parving HH. Kidney function and size in diabetics before and during initial insulin treatment. Kidney Int 1982; 21: 683-688.

38. Hansen KW, Mau Pedersen M, Christensen CK, et al. Normoalbuminuria ensures no reduction of renal function in type 1 (insulin-dependent) diabetic patients. J Intern Med 1992; 232: 161-167.

39. Vora JP, Dolben J, Dean JD, et al. Renal hemodynamics in newly presenting non-insulin dependent diabetes mellitus. Kidney Int 1992; 41: 829-835.

40. Schmitz A. Renal function changes in middle-aged and elderly Caucasian type 2 (non-insulin-dependent) diabetic patients—a review. Diabetologia 1993; 36: 985-992.

41. Yip JW, Jones SL, Wiseman MJ, Hill C, Viberti G. Glomerular hyperfiltration in the prediction of nephropathy in IDDM: a 10-year follow-up study. Diabetes 1996; 45: 1729-1733.

42. Rudberg S, Persson B, Dahlquist G. Increased glomerular filtration rate as a predictor of diabetic nephropathy—an 8-year prospective study. Kidney Int 1992; 41: 822-828.

43. Caramori ML, Gross JL, Pecis M, de Azevedo MJ. Glomerular filtration rate, urinary albumin excretion rate, and blood pressure changes in normoalbuminuric normotensive type 1 diabetic patients: an 8-year follow-up study. Diabetes Care 1999; 22: 1512-1516.

44. Marre M, Hadjadj S, Bouhanick B. The concept of incipient diabetic nephropathy and effect of early antihypertensive intervention, In: Mogensen C, ed. The Kidney and Hypertension in Diabetes Mellitus. (Fifth Ed). 2000 Kluwer Academic Publishers, Boston/Dordrecht/London, pp 423-433

45. de Jong PE, Hillege HL, Pinto-Sietsma SJ, De Zeeuw D. Screening for microalbuminuria in the general population: a tool to detect subjects at risk for progressive renal failure in an early phase? Nephrol Dial Transplant 2003; 18: 10-13.

46. Rudberg S, Osterby R. Decreasing glomerular filtration rate—an indicator of more advanced diabetic glomerulopathy in the early course of microalbuminuria in IDDM adolescents? Nephrol Dial Transplant 1997; 12: 1149-1154.

47. Mogensen CE, Keane WF, Bennett PH, et al. Prevention of diabetic renal disease with special reference to microalbuminuria. Lancet 1995; 346: 1080-1084.

48. Remuzzi G, Bertani T. Pathophysiology of progressive nephropathies. N Engl J Med 1998; 339: 1448-1456.

49. Ruggenenti P, Gambara V, Perna A, Bertani T, Remuzzi G. The nephropathy of non-insulin-dependent diabetes: predictors of outcome relative to diverse patterns of renal injury. J Am Soc Nephrol 1998; 9: 2336-2343.

50. Yokoyama H, Tomonaga O, Hirayama M, et al. Predictors of the progression of diabetic nephropathy and the beneficial effect of angiotensin-converting enzyme inhibitors in NIDDM patients. Diabetologia 1997; 40: 405-411.

51. Rossing P, Hommel E, Smidt UM, Parving HH. Reduction in albuminuria predicts a beneficial effect on diminishing the progression of human diabetic nephropathy during antihypertensive treatment. Diabetologia 1994; 37: 511-516.

52. Ravid M, Savin H, Jutrin I, et al. Long-term stabilizing effect of angiotensin-converting enzyme inhibition on plasma creatinine and on proteinuria in normotensive type II diabetic patients. Ann Intern Med 1993; 118: 577-581.

53. Nelson RG, Bennett PH, Beck GJ, et al. Development and progression of renal disease in Pima Indians with non-insulin-dependent diabetes mellitus. Diabetic Renal Disease Study Group. N Engl J Med 1996; 335: 1636-1642.

54. Mogensen CE, Christensen CK, Vittinghus E. The stages in diabetic renal disease. With emphasis on the stage of incipient diabetic nephropathy. Diabetes 1983; 32 (Suppl 2): 64-78.

55. Gambara V, Mecca G, Remuzzi G, Bertani T. Heterogeneous nature of renal lesions in type II diabetes. J Am Soc Nephrol 1993; 3: 1458-1466.

56. Fioretto P, Steffes MW, Mauer M. Glomerular structure in nonproteinuric IDDM patients with various levels of albuminuria. Diabetes 1994; 43: 1358-1364.

57. Fioretto P, Stehouwer CD, Mauer M, et al. Heterogeneous nature of microalbuminuria in NIDDM: studies of endothelial function and renal structure. Diabetologia 1998; 41: 233-236.

58. Stehouwer CD, Yudkin JS, Fioretto P, Nosadini R. How heterogeneous is microalbuminuria in diabetes mellitus? The case for 'benign' and 'malignant' microalbuminuria. Nephrol Dial Transplant 1998; 13: 2751-2754.

59. Mathiesen ER, Ronn B, Jensen T, Storm B, Deckert T. Relationship between blood pressure and urinary albumin excretion in development of microalbuminuria. Diabetes 1990; 39: 245-249.

60. Poulsen PL, Hansen KW, Mogensen CE. Ambulatory blood pressure in the transition from normo- to microalbuminuria. A longitudinal study in IDDM patients. Diabetes 1994; 43: 1248-1253.

61. Haneda M, Kikkawa R, Togawa M, et al. High blood pressure is a risk factor for the development of microalbuminuria in Japanese subjects with non-insulin-dependent diabetes mellitus. J Diabetes Complications 1992; 6: 181-185.

62. Schmitz A. Microalbuminuria, blood pressure, metabolic control, and renal involvement: longitudinal studies in white non-insulin-dependent diabetic patients. Am J Hypertens 1997; 10: 189S-197S.

63. Forsblom CM, Groop PH, Ekstrand A, et al. Predictors of progression from normoalbuminuria to microalbuminuria in NIDDM. Diabetes Care 1998; 21: 1932-1938.

64. Mogensen CE. Microalbuminuria as a predictor of clinical diabetic nephropathy. Kidney Int 1987; 31: 673-689.

65. Caramori ML, Fioretto P, Mauer M. The need for early predictors of diabetic nephropathy risk: is albumin excretion rate sufficient? Diabetes 2000; 49: 1399-1408.

66. Mauer SM, Steffes MW, Ellis EN, et al. Structural-functional relationships in diabetic nephropathy. J Clin Invest 1984; 74: 1143-1155.

67. Bader R, Bader H, Grund KE, et al. Structure and function of the kidney in diabetic glomerulosclerosis. Correlations between morphological and functional parameters. Pathol Res Pract 1980; 167: 204-216.

68. Gall MA, Nielsen FS, Smidt UM, Parving HH. The course of kidney function in type 2 (non-insulin-dependent) diabetic patients with diabetic nephropathy. Diabetologia 1993; 36: 1071-1078.

69. Schwartz MM, Lewis EJ, Leonard-Martin T, Lewis JB, Batlle D. Renal pathology patterns in type II diabetes mellitus: relationship with retinopathy. The Collaborative Study Group. Nephrol Dial Transplant 1998; 13: 2547-2552.

70. Rodby R, Gilbert R, for the Collaborative Study Group. The presence of retinopathy is associated with poor renal and cardiovascular outcomes in type II diabetic nephropathy. J Am Soc Nephrol 2002; 13: 644A (abstract).

71. Bangstad HJ, Osterby R, Rudberg S, et al. Kidney function and glomerulopathy over 8 years in young patients with Type I (insulin-dependent) diabetes mellitus and microalbuminuria. Diabetologia 2002; 45: 253-261.

72. Sharma K, Ziyadeh FN, Alzahabi B, et al. Increased renal production of transforming growth factor-beta1 in patients with type II diabetes. Diabetes 1997; 46: 854-859.

73. Gilbert RE, Akdeniz A, Allen TJ, Jerums G. Urinary transforming growth factor-beta in patients with diabetic nephropathy: implications for the pathogenesis of tubulointerstitial pathology. Nephrol Dial Transplant 2001; 16: 2442-2443.

74. Davis D, Shock N. Age changes in glomerular filtration rate, effective plasma renal flow, and tubular excretory capacity in adult males. J Clin Invest 1950; 29: 496-507.

75. Kesteloot H, Joossens JV. On the determinants of the creatinine clearance: a population study. J Hum Hypertens 1996; 10: 245-249.

76. Garg AX, Kiberd BA, Clark WF, Haynes RB, Clase CM. Albuminuria and renal insufficiency prevalence guides population screening: results from the NHANES III. Kidney Int 2002; 61: 2165-2175.

77. Mathiesen ER, Hommel E, Giese J, Parving HH. Efficacy of captopril in postponing nephropathy in normotensive insulin dependent diabetic patients with microalbuminuria. BMJ 1991; 303: 81-87.

78. Mathiesen ER, Feldt-Rasmussen B, Hommel E, Deckert T, Parving HH. Stable glomerular filtration rate in normotensive IDDM patients with stable microalbuminuria. A 5-year prospective study. Diabetes Care 1997; 20: 286-289.

79. Crepaldi G, Carta Q, Deferrari G, et al. Effects of lisinopril and nifedipine on the progression to overt albuminuria in IDDM patients with incipient nephropathy and normal blood pressure. The Italian Microalbuminuria Study Group in IDDM. Diabetes Care 1998; 21: 104-110.

80. Elving LD, Wetzels JF, van Lier HJ, de Nobel E, Berden JH. Captopril and atenolol are equally effective in retarding progression of diabetic nephropathy. Results of a 2-year prospective, randomized study. Diabetologia 1994; 37: 604-609.

81. Ritz E, Stefanski A. Diabetic nephropathy in type II diabetes. Am J Kidney Dis 1996; 27: 167-194.

82. Sano T, Kawamura T, Matsumae H, et al. Effects of long-term enalapril treatment on persistent micro- albuminuria in well-controlled hypertensive and normotensive NIDDM patients. Diabetes Care 1994; 17: 420-424.

83. Ahmad J, Siddiqui MA, Ahmad H. Effective postponement of diabetic nephropathy with enalapril in normotensive type 2 diabetic patients with microalbuminuria. Diabetes Care 1997; 20: 1576-1581.

84. Lebovitz HE, Wiegmann TB, Cnaan A, et al. Renal protective effects of enalapril in hypertensive NIDDM: role of baseline albuminuria. Kidney Int Suppl 1994; 45: S150-155.

85. Nielsen S, Schmitz A, Rehling M, Mogensen CE. The clinical course of renal function in NIDDM patients with normo- and microalbuminuria. J Intern Med 1997; 241: 133-141.

86. Velussi M, Brocco E, Frigato F, et al. Effects of cilazapril and amlodipine on kidney function in hypertensive NIDDM patients. Diabetes 1996; 45: 216-222.

87. Nosadini R, Velussi M, Brocco E, et al. Course of renal function in type 2 diabetic patients with abnormalities of albumin excretion rate. Diabetes 2000; 49: 476-484.

88. Brocco E, Velussi M, Cernigoi AM, et al. Evidence of a threshold value of glycated hemoglobin to improve the course of renal function in type 2 diabetes with typical diabetic glomerulopathy. J Nephrol 2001; 14: 461-471.

89. Russo LM, Bakris GL, Comper WD. Renal handling of albumin: a critical review of basic concepts and perspective. Am J Kidney Dis 2002; 39: 899-919.

90. Burne MJ, Osicka TM, Comper WD. Fractional clearance of high molecular weight proteins in conscious rats using a continuous infusion method. Kidney Int 1999; 55: 261-270.

91. Eppel GA, Pratt LM, Greive KA, Comper WD. Exogenous albumin peptides influence the processing of albumin during renal passage. Nephron 2002; 92: 156-164.

92. Eppel GA, Osicka TM, Pratt LM, et al. The return of glomerular-filtered albumin to the rat renal vein. Kidney Int 1999; 55: 1861-1870.

93.   MacIsaac R, McNeil K, Soo G, et al. The finding of normoalbuminuria does not ensure normal renal function in patients with type 2 diabetes. Diabetes 2002; 51 Suppl 2: A186 (abstract).

94.   Thomas MC, MacIsaac RJ, Tsalamandris C, Power D, Jerums G. Unrecognized anemia in patients with diabetes: a cross-sectional survey. Diabetes Care 2003; 26: 1164-1169.

95.   Atkins R, Briganti E, Shaw J, Zimmet P, Chadban S. Population prevalence of proteinuria and albuminuria - The AUSDIAB Kidney Study. J Am Soc Nephrol 2002; 13: 645A (abstract).

96.   Parving HH, Hommel E, Damkjaer Nielsen M, Giese J. Effect of captopril on blood pressure and kidney function in normotensive insulin dependent diabetics with nephropathy. BMJ 1989; 299: 533-536.

97.   Parving HH, Andersen AR, Smidt UM, et al. Effect of antihypertensive treatment on kidney function in diabetic nephropathy. Br Med J (Clin Res Ed) 1987; 294: 1443-1447.

98.   Parving HH, Smidt UM, Friisberg B, Bonnevie-Nielsen V, Andersen AR. A prospective study of glomerular filtration rate and arterial blood pressure in insulin-dependent diabetics with diabetic nephropathy. Diabetologia 1981; 20: 457-461.

99.   Hovind P, Rossing P, Tarnow L, Smidt UM, Parving HH. Progression of diabetic nephropathy. Kidney Int 2001; 59: 702-709.

100.   Bjorck S, Mulec H, Johnsen SA, Norden G, Aurell M. Renal protective effect of enalapril in diabetic nephropathy. BMJ 1992; 304: 339-343.

101.   Mogensen CE. Progression of nephropathy in long-term diabetics with proteinuria and effect of initial anti-hypertensive treatment. Scand J Clin Lab Invest 1976; 36: 383-388.

102.   Rachmani R, Levi Z, Lidar M, et al. Considerations about the threshold value of microalbuminuria in patients with diabetes mellitus: lessons from an 8-year follow-up study of 599 patients. Diabetes Res Clin Pract 2000; 49: 187-194.

103.   Silveiro SP, Friedman R, de Azevedo MJ, Canani LH, Gross JL. Five-year prospective study of glomerular filtration rate and albumin excretion rate in normofiltering and hyperfiltering normoalbuminuric NIDDM patients. Diabetes Care 1996; 19: 171-174.

104.   Ravid M, Brosh D, Levi Z, et al. Use of enalapril to attenuate decline in renal function in normotensive, normoalbuminuric patients with type 2 diabetes mellitus. A randomized, controlled trial. Ann Intern Med 1998; 128: 982-988.

105.   Trevisan R, Vedovato M, Mazzon C, et al. Concomitance of diabetic retinopathy and proteinuria accelerates the rate of decline of kidney function in type 2 diabetic patients. Diabetes Care 2002; 25: 2026-2031.

106.   Christensen PK, Rossing P, Nielsen FS, Parving HH. Natural course of kidney function in Type 2 diabetic patients with diabetic nephropathy. Diabet Med 1999; 16: 388-394.

107.   Lemley KV, Abdullah I, Myers BD, et al. Evolution of incipient nephropathy in type 2 diabetes mellitus. Kidney Int 2000; 58: 1228-1237.

108.   Berrut G, Bouhanick B, Fabbri P, et al. Microalbuminuria as a predictor of a drop in glomerular filtration rate in subjects with non-insulin-dependent diabetes mellitus and hypertension. Clin Nephrol 1997; 48: 92-97.

109.   Mosconi L, Ruggenenti P, Perna A, Mecca G, Remuzzi G. Nitrendipine and enalapril improve albuminuria and glomerular filtration rate in non-insulin dependent diabetes. Kidney Int Suppl. Vol. 55; 1996:S91-93

7

SERUM CREATININE AND OTHER MEASURES OF GFR IN DIABETES

Peter Rossing

Steno Diabetes Center, Niels Steensens Vej 2, 2820 Gentofte, Denmark

The measurement of renal function or the glomerular filtration rate (GFR) in diabetes can be used

1) to estimate the renal clearance of drugs to guide dosing or to identify patients at increased risk for radiocontrast-induced acute renal failure,
2) for confirming the need for treatment of end stage renal disease, or
3) to measure progression of chronic renal disease i.e. diabetic nephropathy.

The evaluation of progression in renal disease is important in the clinical setting for the monitoring of development of renal insufficiency and evaluation of the effectiveness of treatment in the individual. In research it is important to evaluate the impact of putative promoters of progression in renal disease in observational studies or to assess and compare the rate of progression in experimental groups in clinical trials. In order to obtain a valid assessment of the rate of decline in GFR it is necessary with regular measurements of GFR over a period of at least (2)-3 years applying a method with high precision and accuracy [1]. This is due to the usually rather slow rate of decline in GFR in diabetic nephropathy. The ideal method for assessing GFR does not exist and the available methods differ regarding precision and accuracy, cost, inconvenience and safety. In general the more precise methods are being more expensive and inconvenient. Thus one has to select a method according to the clinical situation.

SERUM CREATININE AS A MEASURE OF GFR

The level of serum creatinine is the most widely used measure of renal function in clinical practice. Serum creatinine can be assessed at a low cost and with little inconvenience for the patient. The reciprocal relationship between serum creatinine and the creatinine clearance allows a simple estimation of renal function (Figure 1). When progression in renal disease is evaluated the slope of either 1/serum creatinine or log (serum creatinine) is used. This is particularly useful when serum creatinine exceeds 200 µmol/l [2].

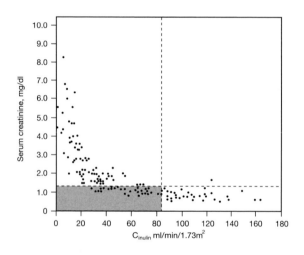

Figure 1 Simultaneous mesurement of serum creatinine and inulin clearance in 171 patients with glomerular disease. Vertical dashed line correspond to the lower limit of inulin clearance (82 ml/min/1.73 m²), the horizontal line corresponds to the upper limit for serum creatinine (1.4 mg/dl). The shaded area includes values for patients in whom inulin clearance is educed but serum creatinine is normal. (From Shemesh et al [4]).

There are however several problems related to the use of serum creatinine as a marker of renal function as reviewed by Levey [3]. Firstly there are technical difficulties with interfering substances (glucose, ketones) that can be solved by the use of a reaction kinetic principle, high performance liquid chromatography (HPLC) or gas chromatography with mass spectrometry (GC-MS) [4]. Secondly the level of serum creatinine is not only dependent on the GFR: the generation of creatinine is influenced by changes in muscle mass and dietary intake of protein. In particular the ingestion of cooked meat may lead to a fast increase in serum creatinine [5]. There may also be racial differences in serum creatinine for a given GFR level [6]. Furthermore creatinine does not behave like an ideal filtration marker, there is tubular secretion leading to an overestimation of GFR by a factor of at least 1.2, and the proportion of tubular secretion to glomerular filtration changes with variation in the level of GFR [7], and it is affected by several drugs (e.g. cimetidine, salicylates and trimethoprim). Furthermore the production of creatinine may be affected by lipid lowering drugs [8]. In addition there is extra-renal elimination of creatinine particularly in patients with low GFR. These conditions make it difficult to use serum creatinine to correctly estimate the level of renal function.

Problems related to differences in creatinine production affecting serum creatinine as well as the influence of extra-renal creatinine elimination, can be avoided by measuring creatinine clearance which in addition to the blood sample requires a 24 hour urine collection. However this adds the problem with accuracy of timed urine collections. The problems with tubular secretion can be avoided if the tubular secretion is blocked, for instance with the use of cimetidine [4, 9], but this further adds to the complexity of the measurement.

Because of the difficulties with urine collections, it has been attempted to solve the problems due to sex and age related changes in muscle mass with formulas like that of Cockroft and Gault [10] using serum creatinine to estimate creatinine clearance (Cl_{crea}) taking sex, age and body weight into account: Cl_{crea}=(140-Age)*K*body weight*(1/p-creatinine), (K=1.23 for men, 1.05 for women, p-creatinine in μmol/l, weight in kg and age in years). Cross-sectional data suggest that the formula gives an accurate estimate of glomerular filtration rate in diabetic nephropathy in some [11] but not all studies [12,13]. In a study evaluating the formula in type 2 diabetic patients with normal renal function the formula significantly underestimated GFR [14]. It has been suggested that very accurate results are obtained from the formula, if the methods for the measurement of creatinine are improved by the use of HPLC or enzymatic assays in combination with blockade of tubular creatinine secretion by administration of cimetidine over 24 hours [15]. Only few studies have evaluated if the formulas for estimation of GFR can be used to predict the decline in renal function. In a cohort of type 1 diabetic patients with nephropathy and long follow up, the mean decline of the cohort could be predicted using the Cockroft–Gault formula, but it was not accurate in the individual patient [13] and similarly poor results were found in a study of normoalbuminuric type 2 diabetic patients, in particular when the decline in GFR was small [15].

Recently Levey et al. suggested a more accurate prediction equation to estimate GFR, rather than Cl_{Crea}, based on data from 1628 patients in the MDRD study, using age, sex, race, serum creatinine, urea nitrogen and albumin concentration [16]. The MDRD study only included very few diabetic patients, and in a recent study of type 1 diabetic patients with normal or increased GFR it was found that this new equation offered no advantage to creatinine clearance or the Cockroft–Gault formula [17].

In patients with very advanced nephropathy approaching dialysis it may be necessary to use other formulas, due to the changes in creatinine metabolism [18]. In patients with declining renal function there is an increase in fractional tubular secretion and extrarenal elimination [7]. Usually there is a lowering in muscle mass and often a restriction in protein intake. All of which will tend to preserve the level of serum creatinine despite declining GFR. Accordingly Shemes et al. [7] found that patients with a GFR as low as ~30 ml/min/$1.73m^2$ may have normal serum creatinine, and in their follow up study [7] reductions in GFR of 50% were not associated with increases in serum creatinine of the expected magnitude, and even a lack of increase in some patients, thus when evaluating progression in renal disease, an increase in serum creatinine is not a very sensitive measurement of a decrease in renal function. This is in particular the case in patients with normal renal function due to the reciprocal relationship between serum creatinine and GFR, large variations in GFR are only associated with small changes in serum creatinine. On the other hand an elevation in serum creatinine is very specific for a decline in GFR. Thus an elevated serum creatinine or a doubling of the baseline serum creatinine have been used as endpoints in clinical trials [19], and it has been suggested that a threshold analysis instead of a slope analysis is more informative from a public health perspective since the adverse consequences of renal failure appear mostly in those whose renal function falls below a certain threshold [6]. This is only valid if changes in serum creatinine are not due to changes in therapy, muscle mass or diet. Illustrating this problem the Modification of Diet in Renal Disease study [20] concluded, that while a significant beneficial effect of low protein diet could not be demonstrated when using a true marker of GFR (^{125}I-iothalamate), such an effect would erroneously have been found if creatinine data had been used [21].

Other endogenous markers of GFR have been evaluated including ß$_2$-microglobulin which seems to be a more reliable method for evaluation of GFR than serum creatinine in cross sectional as well as longitudinal studies [22, 23] but determination of ß$_2$-microglobulin is expensive and not a routine method at most laboratories. In addition very high levels are found in serum in patients with certain malignant disorders or immunological diseases.

Recently there has been increasing interest for the use of serum cystatin C as a marker of GFR. Cystatin C is a low molecular weight nonglycosylated plasma protein that is freely filtered through the glomerulus and almost completely reabsorbed and catabolised by renal tubular cells. The production is constant and not altered by inflammatory conditions, not related to lean body mass and concentration is stable in stored plasma. It has been found to be a better marker for GFR than creatinine clearance or serum creatinine in type 1 [24] and type 2 diabetic patients [25]. In particular it was found that cystatin C was elevated in patients having impaired renal function but normal serum creatinine. Longitudinal studies are necessary to determine if changes in cystatin C is useful as a marker of progression in kidney disease.

GLOMERULAR FILTRATION RATE

An ideal marker for determination of glomerular filtration rate should fulfil the following requirements: it should be freely filtered at the glomerulus, no tubular secretion or re-absorption, it should not be metabolised, and it should be physiologically inert without affecting renal function, distribute instantaneously and freely in the extracellular volume, and should be easily measured [26]. Such a marker does not exist. However the renal clearance of inulin during constant infusion has been considered the gold standard for determination of GFR. The clearance is corrected for body surface area and normalised to 1.73 m^2 to take into account the relationship between kidney and body size and permit comparisons between patients. The renal clearance (Cl) during constant infusion is calculated from the plasma inulin level (P), urinary inulin concentration (U) and urine flow rate (V) as Cl=UV/P. The clearance is measured in three to five 30-minute periods during an oral water load. If during a constant infusion both distribution volume and plasma inulin concentration are constant the rate of infusion equals the rate of excretion. Then inulin clearance can be calculated from inulin infusion rate and plasma inulin concentration. However it is difficult to obtain constant inulin concentrations thus this technique is rarely used. The cumbersome procedures, difficulties with measuring inulin and its limited availability and cost has encouraged the search for alternative filtration markers.

The radioisotope-labelled markers ^{125}I-Iothalamate, ^{99m}Tc-DTPA and ^{51}Cr-EDTA have been found to give accurate and precise estimates of GFR [27] when used with constant infusion renal clearance techniques. To avoid problems with incomplete urine collections, a frequent phenomenon in diabetic patients due to cystopathy [28], plasma clearance techniques can be applied. The radioactive markers have particularly been used with such techniques. With these methods the GFR is determined without urine sampling as total plasma clearance from the declining plasma concentration followed as a function of time after injection of a bolus of the marker [29]. The clearance is calculated as the ratio of the injected amount of marker (Q) and the area under the plasma curve (A) (Cl=Q/A). Determination of the entire area under the plasma curve requires the drawing of many blood samples (10 to 20) during a time period of several hours depending on the level of renal function (three to five hours in normal to moderately decreased renal function, but up to 24 hours is recommended if GFR is below 15 ml/min). The final elimination follows a mono-exponential curve that is extrapolated to infinity. Simplified methods have been developed using the final slope only, determined by two to seven blood samples, the calculated area can be mathematically corrected to the total area under the curve preserving very high precision and accuracy which is necessary in longitudinal studies [30-33]. The simplified single injection technique has frequently been used in clinical studies or as a routine method for determination of GFR [29, 34].

The correction used in the simplified methods has the greatest influence at high clearance values being particularly important in microalbuminuric diabetic patients who are often hyperfiltering, where the initial part of the disappearance curve contributes to a larger extent to the total area under the curve. In accordance with this is has been found that the simpler methods lacked accuracy in diabetic patients with elevated GFR [35,36]. In these patients at least seven blood sampling times were recommended.

[51]Cr-EDTA (ethylenediaminetetraacetic acid) has been extensively used for plasma clearance studies and has been found to have a renal clearance ~10% lower than clearance of inulin [37], the difference has not been explained but could be due to plasma protein binding, tubular reabsorption or dissociation of the radio nuclide from EDTA. The plasma clearance is slightly higher than the renal clearance due to extrarenal elimination (~4 ml/min) [31]. The half-life of the isotope is 27 days. ^{125}I-Iothalamate can be administered as subcutaneous or intravenous injection. Due to a half-life of radioactive ^{125}I of 60 days, samples can be stored before radioisotope counting, which makes it useful for multicenter studies with a central laboratory as demonstrated in the MDRD study [20]. ^{99m}Tc-DTPA (diethylenetriaminepenta-acetic acid) is also used for renal scans, and it is inexpensive compared to the rather expensive ^{125}I-Iothalamate. Protein binding is potentially of concern and radiochemical instability varies among DTPA kits making quality control critical [38]. The radiolabelling of DTPA has to be carried out immediately before use due to instability. The half life of ^{99m}Tc is only 6 hours thus samples must be counted soon after the procedure.

Plasma clearance can be measured without drawing plasma samples at all, with the use of a gamma camera measuring renal elimination of a radioactive marker such as ^{99m}Tc-DTPA [39]. This technique is not as accurate as when plasma samples are collected, but it is possible to determine the contribution from each kidney, which is particularly useful when reno-vascular disease or unilateral nephrectomy is considered.

The use of radioactive markers exposes the patients to radiation, but the radiation dose is very small and for one measurement of GFR with ^{51}Cr-EDTA it is comparable to the daily background radiation dose (Effective dose equivalent <0.01 mSv.). But even if the radiation doses are small, the use of radioactive isotopes is usually avoided in children and pregnant women. As a non-radioactive alternative the radiocontrast agents such as iohexol have been suggested [40] . Iohexol has been compared with ^{51}Cr-EDTA in diabetic patients and excelent agreement was found over a wide range of GFR values [35]. It has also been possible to measure small concentrations of inulin with HPLC methods making plasma clearance of inulin after a single injection a possibility [41].

SUMMARY

The selection of method for assessment of GFR depends on the situation. In many clinical situations the use of serum creatinine or estimated creatinine clearance based on formulas or nomograms is sufficient if the limitations are recalled. In clinical studies a more accurate and precise method is warranted. In case of severe oedema, ascites or if the renal haemodynamics are changing within hours, renal clearance methods have to be used. Apart from these special situations the simplified single injection plasma clearance methods yield sufficiently accurate and precise assessments of GFR with a minimum of inconvenience, and is particularly useful in long-term follow-up studies evaluating the decline in renal function.

REFERENCES

1   Levey AS, Gassman J, Hall PM, Walker WG. Assessing the progression of renal disease in clinical studies: effects of duration of follow-up and regression to the mean. J Am Soc Nephrol 1991; 1:1087-1094.
2   Mitch WE, Walser M, Buffington GA, Lemann J. A simple method of estimating progression of chronic renal failure. Lancet 1976; ii:1326-1328.
3   Levey AS, Perrone RD, Madias NE. Serum creatinine and renal function. Ann Rev Med 1988; 39:465-490.
4   Kemperman FAW, Silberbusch J, Slaats EH, van Zanten AP, Weber JA, Krediet RT et al. Glomerular filtration rate estimation from plasma creatinine after inhibition of tubular secretion: relevance of the creatinine assay. Nephrol Dial Transplant 1999; 14:1247-1251.
5   Jacobsen FK, Christensen CK, Mogensen CE, Andreasen F, Hejlskov NSC. Pronounced increase in serum dreatinine concentration after eating cooked meat. Br Med J 1979;(I):1049-1050.
6   Hsu CY, Chertow GM, Curhan GC. Methodological issues in studying the epidemiology of mild to moderate chronic renal insufficiency. Kidney Int 2002; 61(5):1567-1576.
7   Shemesh O, Golbetz HV, Kriss JP, Myers BD. Limitations of creatinine as a filtration marker in glomerulopathic patients. Kidney Int 1985; 28:830-838.
8   Perlemoine C, Rigalleau V, Baillet L, Barthe N, Delmas-Beauvieux MC, Lasseur C et al. Cockcroft's formula underestimates glomerular filtration rate in diabetic subjects treated by lipid-lowering drugs. Diabetes Care 2002; 25(11):2106-2107.
9   van Acker BAC, Koome GCM, Koopman MG, de Waart DR, Arisz L. Creatinine clearance during cimetidine administration for measurement of glomerular filtration rate. Lancet 1992; 340:1326-1329.
10   Cockcroft DW, Gault MH. Prediction of creatinine clearance from serum creatinine. Nephron 1976; 16:31-41.
11   Sampson MJ, Drury PL. Accurate estimation of glomerular filtration rate in diabetic nephropathy from age, body weight, and serum creatinine. Diabetes Care 1992; 15:609-612.

12   Waz WR, Qattrin T, Feld LG. Serum creatinine, height, and weight do not predict glomerular filtration rate in children with IDDM. Diabetes Care 1993; 16:1067-1070.

13   Rossing P, Astrup A-S, Smidt UM, Parving H-H. Monitoring kidney function in diabetic nephropathy. Diabetologia 1994; 37:708-712.

14   Nielsen S, Rehling M, Schmitz A, Mogensen CE. Validity of rapid estimation of glomerular filtration rate in type 2 diabetic patients with normal renal function. Nephrol Dial Transplant 1999; 14:615-619.

15   Kemperman FAW, Krediet RT, Arisz L. Validity of rapid estimation of glomerular filtration rate in type 2 diabetic patients with normal renal function (Letter). Nephrol Dial Transplant 1999; 14:2964.

16   Levey AS, Bosch JP, Breyer JA, Greene T, Rogers N, Roth D et al. A more accurate method to estimate glomerular filtration rate from serum creatinine: a new prediction equation. Ann Intern Med 1999; 130:461-470.

17   Vervoort G, Willems HL, Wetzels JF. Assessment of glomerular filtration rate in healthy subjects and normoalbuminuric diabetic patients: validity of a new (MDRD) prediction equation. Nephrol Dial Transplant 2002; 17(11):1909-1913.

18   Walser M, Drew HH, Guldan JL. Prediction of glomerular filtration rate from serum creatinine concentration in advanced chronic renal failure. Kidney Int 1993; 44:1145-1148.

19   Lewis E, Hunsicker L, Bain R, Rhode R. The effect of angiotensin-converting-enzyme inhibition on diabetic nephropathy. N Engl J Med 1993; 329:1456-1462.

20   Klahr S, Levey AS, Beck GJ, Caggiula AW, Hunsicker L, Kusek JW et al. The effects of dietary protein restriction and blood-pressure control on the progression of chronic renal disease. N Engl J Med 1994; 330:877-884.

21   Levey AS, Bosch JP, Coggins CH, Greene T, Mitch WE, Schluchter MD et al. Effects of diet and antihypertensive therapy on creatinine clearance and serum creatinine concentration in the modification of diet in renal disease study. J Am Soc Nephrol 1996; 7:556-565.

22   Parving H-H, Andersen AR, Smidt UM. Monitoring progression of diabetic nephropathy. Upsala J Med Sci 1985; 90:15-23.

23   Viberti GC, Bilous RW, Mackintosh D, Keen H. Monitoring glomerular function in diabetic nephropathy. Am J Med 1983; 74:256-264.

24   Tan GD, Lewis AV, James TJ, Altmann P, Taylor RP, Levy JC. Clinical usefulness of cystatin C for the estimation of glomerular filtration rate in type 1 diabetes: reproducibility and accuracy compared with standard measures and iohexol clearance. Diabetes Care 2002; 25(11):2004-2009.

25   Mussap M, Dalla VM, Fioretto P, Saller A, Varagnolo M, Nosadini R et al. Cystatin C is a more sensitive marker than creatinine for the estimation of GFR in type 2 diabetic patients. Kidney Int 2002; 61(4):1453-1461.

26   Kasiske BL, Keane WF. Laboratory assessment of renal disease: clearance, urinalysis and renal biopsy. In: Brenner BM, editor. The Kidney. Philadelphia: Saunders, 1997: 1137-1174.

27   Levey AS. Assessing the effectiveness of therapy to prevent the progression of renal disease. Am J Kidney Dis 1993; 22:207-214.

28   Frimondt-Møller C. Diabetic cystopathy. Dan Med Bull 1978; 25:49-60.

29   Bröchner-Mortensen J. Current status on assessment and measurement of glomerular filtration rate. Clin Physiol 1985; 5:1-17.

30   Bröchner-Mortensen J. Routine methods and their reliability for assessment of glomerular filtration rate in adults with special reference to total [^{51}Cr]EDTA plasma clearance. Dan Med Bull 1978; 25:181-202.

31   Bröchner-Mortensen J, Rödbro P. Selection of routine method for determination of glomerular filtration rate in adult patients. Scand J Clin Lab Invest 1976; 36:35-45.

32   Bröchner-Mortensen J. A simple method for the determination of glomerular filtration rate. Scand J Clin Lab Invest 1972; 30:271-274.

33   Sambataro M, Tomaseth K, Pacini G, Robaudo C, Carraro A, Bruseghin M et al. Plasma clearance rate of 51 Cr-EDTA provides a precise and convenient technique for measurement of glomerular filtration rate in diabetic humans. J Am Soc Nephrol 1996; 7:118-127.

34   Parving H-H, Smidt UM, Hommel E, Mathiesen ER, Rossing P, Nielsen FS et al. Effective Antihypertensive Treatment Postpones Renal Insufficiency in Diabetic Nephropathy. Am J Kidney Dis 1993; 22:188-195.

35   Pucci L, Bandinelli S, Pilo M, Nannipieri M, Navalesi R, Penno G. Iohexol as a marker of glomerular filtration rate in patients with diabetes: comparison of multiple and simplified sampling protocols. Diabet Med 2001; 18(2):116-120.

36   Hansen HP, Rossing P, Mathiesen ER, Hommel E, Smidt UM, Parving HH. Assessment of glomerular filtration rate in diabetic nephropathy using the plasma clearance of 51Cr-EDTA. Scand J Clin Lab Invest 1998; 58(5):405-413.

37   Chantler C, Garnett ES, Parsons V, Veall N. Glomerular filtration rate measurement in man by the single injection method using ^{51}Cr-EDTA. Clin Sci 1969; 37:169-180.

38   Carlsen JE, Lehd Møller M, Lund JO, Trap-Jensen J. Comparison of four commercial Tc-99 (sn) DTPA preparations used for the measurement of glomerular filtration rate: concise communication. Journal of Nuclear Medicine 1980;126-129.

39   Rodby RA, Ali A, Rohde RD, Lewis E. Renal scanning ^{99m}Tc diethylene-triamine pentaacetic acid glomerular filtration rate (GFR) determination compared with iothalamate clearance GFR in diabetics. Am J Kidney Dis 1992; 20:569-573.

40   Stake G, Moon E, Rootwell IT, Monclair T. The clearance of iohexol as a measure of glomerular filtration rate in children with chronic renal failure. Scand J Clin Lab Invest 1991; 51:729-734.

41   Jung K, Henke W, Schulze BD, Sydow K, Precht K, Klotzek S. Practical approach for determining glomerular filtration rate by single injection inulin clearance. Clin Chem 1992; 38(3):403-407.

8

FAMILIAL FACTORS IN DIABETIC NEPHROPATHY

Giuseppina Imperatore[1], David J Pettitt[2], Robert L Hanson[3], William C. Knowler and Robert G. Nelson[3]

[1]Division of Diabetes Translation, Centers for Disease Control and Prevention, Atlanta, Georgia, US; [2]Sansum Medical Research Institute, Santa Barbara, California, USA; [3]Phoenix Epidemiology and Clinical Research Branch, NIDDK, Phoenix, USA

Reports of nephropathy developing in some patients with apparently well controlled diabetes and not developing in some patients even after years of severe hyperglycemia lead to the conclusion, expressed by several researchers [1-5], that some, but not all, individuals are predisposed to the development of diabetic renal disease. This chapter reviews some of the data, which indicate that there are familial differences in the predisposition to diabetic renal disease. If this familial predisposition is genetic, there must be an interaction between the genes and the environment, and it is often difficult to differentiate between genetic inheritance and the effect of a common environment shared by family members.

RACIAL DIFFERENCES IN PREVALENCE OF RENAL DISEASE

Some familial clustering of diabetic nephropathy may be accounted for by racial background, as diabetic nephropathy occurs at different rates in different racial groups. Several inter-racial comparisons have been made [6-10]. Rostand et al. [6] and Cowie et al. [9] both reported higher rates of end-stage renal disease in African American than Whites, and Pugh et al. [7] reported higher rates in

Mexican Americans than in Non-Hispanic Whites. Diabetes duration, which is a strong risk factor for end-stage renal disease, may account for some of the racial differences in these studies. However, with diabetes duration accounted for, Haffner et al. [8] found higher rates of proteinuria among Mexican Americans, and there are several reports of very high rates of renal disease among the Pima Indians [11-14], a population that has high rates of type 2 diabetes [15,16]. The incidence of end-stage renal disease in Pima Indians was similar to that in subjects with type1 diabetes in Boston, Massachusetts [11], but almost four times as high as in Caucasians with type 2 diabetes in Rochester, Minnesota [14].

The reasons for inter-population differences in rates of renal disease are unclear. Rostand [10] has argued that barriers to medical care for African Americans and Mexican Americans may impede early detection, and therefore, control of microalbuminuria and hypertension with a consequent adverse effect on the prevalence of renal disease. However, the cost, one of the major barriers to medical care, is not a factor for the Pima Indians, who have access to free medical care by providers who are well aware of the high risk of diabetic renal disease in this population. Thus, cost of medical care cannot be the only reason for racial differences. However, other aspects of access to medical care, such as transportation or cultural barriers, could be important.

Genes predisposing to renal disease might well exist at different frequencies in different races resulting in differences in susceptibility. Thus, if renal disease is genetic, its prevalence might be expected to differ by race. However, finding different rates in different races is consistent not only with genetic inheritance but also with differing environmental exposures or with differences in competing causes of death.

SIBLINGS OF AFFECTED INDIVIDUALS

Diabetic siblings of individuals with diabetic nephropathy are at higher risk for nephropathy than are diabetic siblings of diabetic individuals without nephropathy. This familial aggregation has been found in diverse populations with both type 1 and type 2 diabetes. Seaquist et al. [17] reported familial clustering of nephropathy among diabetic siblings of diabetic probands recruited from either the University of Minnesota kidney transplant registry or from a family diabetes study. Nephropathy was found among 83% of the diabetic siblings of diabetic probands with nephropathy but among only 17% of siblings of probands without nephropathy (figure 1). Furthermore, 41% of the siblings of probands with nephropathy had end-stage renal disease. Clustering of diabetic nephropathy among siblings was confirmed by Borch-Johnsen et al. [18], and higher albumin excretion was found in the nondiabetic siblings of probands with type 2 diabetes than of those without [19]. Quinn et al. [20] examined 110 probands for nephropathy status and found that the cumulative incidence of nephropathy for siblings of probands with diabetic nephropathy was 71.5% and only 25.4% for siblings of probands without nephropathy. The magnitude of the risk difference between the two groups of siblings suggests that genetic factors are very important. Similar results were observed in Brazilian and Indian subjects with type 2 diabetes [21,22]. Furthermore, Fioretto et al. [23] observed strong concordance in severity and patterns of glomerual lesions among sibling pairs with type 1 diabetes, despite lack of concordance in glycemia. These data, which are consistent with the hypothesis that genetic heredity is a major determinant of diabetic nephropathy, are also consistent with the hypothesis that an environmental factor or factors shared by siblings is responsible for the development of nephropathy in some families.

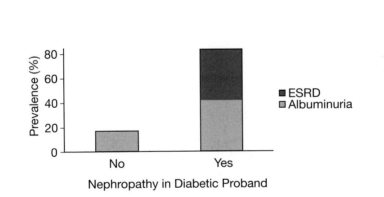

Figure 1. Prevalence of albuminuria and end-stage renal disease (ESRD) in diabetic siblings of diabetic probands with or without nephropathy. Adapted from Seaquist et al. [17].

OFFSPRING OF AFFECTED INDIVIDUALS

Proteinuria was studied in Pima Indian families with diabetes in two generations [24]. Proteinuria occurred among 14% of the diabetic offspring of diabetic parents if neither parent had proteinuria, 23% if one parent had proteinuria, and 46% if both parents had diabetes with proteinuria (figure 2). Moreover, a Finnish study showed that non-diabetic offspring of albuminuric type 2 diabetic parents had higher albumin excretion rates and a higher frequency of microalbuminuria than offspring of normoalbuminuric parents [25]. These data demonstrate that proteinuria aggregates in families and suggest that the susceptibility to renal disease is inherited independently of the diabetes. As with the sibling concordance described above, the inheritance could be a consequence of a shared environment, but since the environments of parents and of their children are very likely to differ more than those of siblings, a genetic inheritance is a strong possibility.

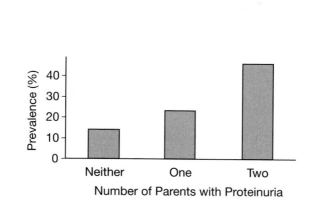

Figure 2. Prevalence of proteinuria by number of parents with proteinuria adjusted for age, sex, blood pressure, diabetes duration and glucose concentration. Adapted from Pettitt et al. [24].

A useful approach for discriminating between environmental and genetic factors is performing segregation analysis. This statistical method is used to determine the mode of inheritance of a disease from family data. Recently, Imperatore et al. [26] conducted a segregation analysis to determine the extent to which the major effect of a single gene might be responsible for the familial aggregation of nephropathy, defined as the presence of protein-to-creatinine ratio ≥ 500 mg/g, among Pima Indians with type 2 diabetes. The analysis included 715 nuclear families, containing 2,107 individuals. The results of this analysis were consistent with a major genetic effect on the prevalence of diabetic nephropathy, after accounting for duration of diabetes (figure 3). The model suggests that individuals homozygous (AA) or heterozygous (AB) for the putative high risk allele have a high risk of diabetic nephropathy, particularly after many years of diabetes, while those homozygous for the low risk allele (BB) have very little nephropathy, regardless of duration of diabetes. Similarly, segregation analysis in European Americans with type 2 diabetes provided some evidence for a genetic effect [27]. While it can be difficult with segregation analysis to distinguish the effect of a single major locus from that of a small number of loci, these analyses suggest that some of the genetic determinants of diabetic nephropathy may have effects of sufficient magnitude to be detected by conventional genetic techniques. Accordingly, a genome scan approach may be suitable for unfolding the genetics of this complication. However, to obtain significant results it requires collection of a large number of families with well-characterized phenotype. To address this need, the U.S. National Institute of Diabetes and Digestive and Kidney Diseases (NIDDK) is sponsoring a collaborative project to identify susceptibility genes for diabetic nephropathy: the Family Investigation of Nephropathy and Diabetes (FIND). This study includes families of African American, American Indian, Hispanic, and non-Hispanic White origin that are informative for nephropathy. In addition, the National Center for Research Resources and the Juvenile Diabetes Research Foundation are sponsoring the genetics of kidneys in diabetes (GoKinD) study. The GoKinD study is recruiting approximately 2,100 patients (1,100 patients with nephropathy and 1,000 without nephropathy) with type 1 diabetes and their parents. Hopefully all these efforts will result in the identification of loci conferring susceptibility to diabetic nephropathy and, ultimately, to a better understanding of the pathogenesis of this complication.

Other data from the Pima Indians indicate that diabetic nephropathy in parents is a risk factor for diabetes in the offspring [28]. The prevalence of diabetes at 25 to 34 years of age was 46% among the offspring of two diabetic parents if one had proteinuria and only 18% if neither had proteinuria. Corresponding rates among subjects with one diabetic and one nondiabetic parent were 29% if the diabetic parent had proteinuria and 11% if not. Thus, multiple loci or homozygosity at a single locus may determine susceptibility to both diabetes and renal disease. In other words, parents with diabetes and renal disease may have a higher genetic load, which increases the risk of diabetes in the offspring as well as increasing the risk of nephropathy once the diabetes develops.

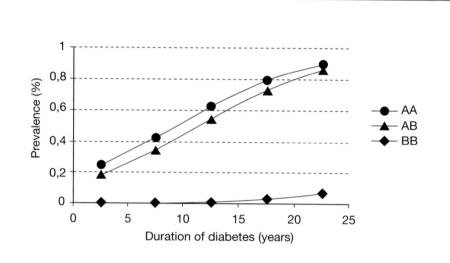

Figure 3. Prevalence of diabetic nephropathy, predicted by a segregation model, according to duration of diabetes and genotype at the putative disease locus. AA, homozygous for the disease allele A; AB, heterozygote; BB, subjects without the A allele. Adapted from Imperatore et al. [26]

FAMILIAL HYPERTENSION AND RENAL DISEASE

The frequent association of renal disease with hypertension has led to the examination of blood pressure in non-diabetic family members of persons with diabetes and in individuals thought to be at high risk of developing diabetes in the future. Viberti et al. found that both systolic and diastolic blood pressures were significantly higher in the parents of diabetic subjects with proteinuria than in the parents of diabetic subjects without proteinuria [29]. The difference between the mean blood pressures averaged 15 mmHg. Similarly, Krolewski et al. [30] reported that the risk of nephropathy among subjects with type 1 diabetes was three times as high in those having a parent with a history of hypertension as in those whose parents had no such history, and Takeda et al. [31] found evidence suggesting that paternal hypertension might be related to the development of nephropathy in patients with type 2 diabetes. Beatty et al. [32] found more insulin resistance as well as higher blood pressures in the offspring of hypertensive than of normotensive parents. These offspring, therefore, are presumably at increased risk of developing diabetes. Since they already have significantly higher blood pressures, they may be at particular risk of renal disease if they do develop diabetes.

Among diabetic Pima Indians whose parents did not have proteinuria, those with hypertensive parents had a higher prevalence of proteinuria than those with normotensive parents [33]. This finding was observed even among those with nondiabetic parents (figure 4). Moreover, higher mean blood pressure measured at least one year prior to the onset of diabetes predicted an abnormal urinary excretion of albumin determined after the diagnosis of diabetes [34]. Thus, the hypertension so often associated with diabetic nephropathy cross-sectionally does not appear to be entirely a result of the renal disease. This hypertension, which appears to be familial in several studies, may precede and contribute to the renal disease seen after several years of diabetes in some subjects.

MODIFICATION OF DISEASE

Environmental factors, most of which probably remain unknown, that influence the development or progression of renal disease in subjects with diabetes are likely to be shared with other family members resulting in concordance of renal disease. Therapeutic manipulations of several factors alter the course of diabetic renal disease in individuals, but it will take family studies to see if the response to therapies is also genetic or influenced by other environmental factors.

Various treatments, which will be discussed in detail in subsequent chapters, may alter the familial aggregation of renal disease. Reichard et al. [35] showed that intensive insulin therapy in type 1 diabetes can reduce the development of microvascular complications including diabetic kidney disease. Similar results were reported by the Diabetes Control and Complications Trial [36]. The results of the United Kingdom Prospective Diabetes Study, also, showed that intensive blood glucose control decreases the risk of microvascular complications, in patients with type 2 diabetes [37].

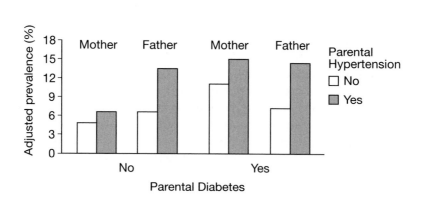

Figure 4. Prevalence of proteinuria according to parental hypertension and diabetes, adjusted for age, sex, diabetes duration and post-load plasma glucose Adapted from Nelson et al. [33].

Dietary protein may induce glomerular hyperfiltration [38], and beneficial effects of dietary protein restriction have been described [39-43]. As the renal effects differ with different types of protein [44], familial aggregation of renal disease may be due to a common diet rather than to genetics. Likewise, the beneficial effects of protein restriction may differ in different families depending, not only on genetic differences, but also on the type and the amount of protein consumed before the intervention.

Treatment of hypertension in subjects with diabetic nephropathy retards the progression of the renal disease [45], especially when drugs that block the renin-angiotensin system are used [46]. In several randomized trials, angiotensin converting enzyme inhibitors and angiotensin receptor blockers were shown to slow the progression of renal disease and reduce mortality in subjects with proteinuria, regardless of hypertension [47-54]. It is of interest to note that there is evidence suggesting that ACE insertion/deletion polymorphism may be involved in the responsiveness to the ACE inhibitors [55,56].

In summary, much of the intriguing information regarding the familial occurrence of diabetic renal disease suggests a genetic component for this disorder but is also consistent with environmental effects. The epidemiology of renal disease is complicated by the fact that several forms of therapy currently employed to treat hyperglycemia, proteinuria and hypertension can alter the progression of renal disease and may, in some cases, even prevent its development. Selective prevention of renal disease will likely alter the familial aggregation of the disease. If there are important genes providing susceptibility to renal disease or influencing the response to treatment, even if the contribution is small, their identification could increase the clinician's knowledge about the risk for a given patient and help identify those for whom intensive therapy may be most beneficial.

REFERENCES

1   Deckert T, Poulsen JE: Diabetic nephropathy: fault or destiny? Diabetologia 21:178-183, 1981.
2   Moloney A, Tunbridge WMG, Ireland JT, Watkins PJ: Mortality from diabetic nephropathy in the United Kingdom. Diabetologia 25:26-30, 1983.
3   Krolewski AS, Warram JH, Christlieb AR, Busick EJ, Kahn CR: The changing natural history of nephropathy in type I diabetes. Am J Med 78:785-794, 1985.
4   Seaquist ER, Goetz FC, Povey S: Diabetic nephropathy: an hypothesis regarding genetic susceptibility for the disorder. Minnesota Med 69:457-459, 1986.
5   What causes diabetic renal failure? [Editorial] Lancet 1:1433-1434, 1988.
6   Rostand SG, Kirk KA, Rutsky EA, Pate BA: Racial differences in the incidence of treatment for end-stage renal disease. N Engl J Med 306:1276-1279, 1982.
7   Pugh JA, Stern MP, Haffner SM, Eifler CW, Zapata M: Excess incidence of treatment of end-stage renal disease in Mexican Americans. Am J Epidemiol 127:135-144, 1988.
8   Haffner SM, Mitchell BD, Pugh JA, Stern MP, Kozlowski MK, Hazuda HP, Patterson JK, Klein R: Proteinuria in Mexican Americans and non-Hispanic Whites with NIDDM. Diabetes Care 12:530-536, 1989.

9   Cowie CC, Port FK, Wolfe RA, Savage PJ, Moll PP, Hawthorne VM: Disparities in incidence of diabetic end-stage renal disease according to race and type of diabetes. N Engl J Med 321:1074-1079, 1989.

10   Rostand SG: Diabetic renal disease in blacks? inevitable or preventable? [Editorial] N Engl J Med 321:1121-1122, 1989.

11   Nelson RG, Newman JM, Knowler WC, Sievers ML, Kunzelman CL, Pettitt DJ, Moffett CD, Teutch SM, Bennett PH: Incidence of end-stage renal disease in type 2 (non-insulin-dependent) diabetes mellitus in Pima Indians. Diabetologia 31:730-736, 1988.

12   Kunzelman CL, Knowler WC, Pettitt DJ, Bennett PH: Incidence of proteinuria in type 2 diabetes mellitus in the Pima Indians. Kidney Int 35:681-687, 1989.

13   Nelson RG, Knowler WC, Pettitt DJ, Saad MF, Bennett PH: Diabetic kidney disease in Pima Indians. Diabetes Care [Suppl 1] 16:335-341, 1993.

14   Nelson RG, Knowler WC, McCance DR, Sievers ML, Pettitt DJ, Charles MA, Hanson RL, Liu QZ, Bennett PH: Determinants of end-stage renal disease in Pima Indians with Type 2 (non-insulin-dependent) diabetes mellitus and proteinuria. Diabetologia 36:1087-1093, 1993.

15   Bennett PH, Burch TA, Miller M. Diabetes mellitus in American (Pima) Indians. Lancet 2:125-128, 1971.

16   Knowler WC, Pettitt DJ, Saad MF, Bennett PH: Diabetes mellitus in the Pima Indians: incidence, risk factors and pathogenesis. Diabetes Metab Rev 6:1-27, 1990.

17   Seaquist ER, Goetz FC, Rich S, Barbosa J: Familial clustering of diabetic kidney disease: evidence for genetic susceptibility to diabetic nephropathy. N Engl J Med 320:1161-1165, 1989.

18   Borch-Johnsen K, Nørgaard, Hommel E, Mathiesen ER, Jensen JS, Deckert T, Parving H-H: Is diabetic nephropathy an inherited complication? Kidney Int 41:719-722, 1992.

19   Faronato PP, Maioli M, Tonolo G, Brocco E, Noventa E, Piarulli F, Abaterusso C, Modena F, de Bigontina G, Velussi M, Inchiostro S, Santeusanio F, Bueti KA, Nosadini R. Clustering of albumin excretion rate abnormalities in Caucasian patients with NIDDM. Diabetologia 40:816-823, 1997.

20   Quinn M, Angelico MC, Warram JH, Krolewski AS: Familial factors determine the development of diabetic nephropathy in patients with IDDM. Diabetologia 39:940-945, 1996.

21   Canani LH, Gerchman F, Gross JL: Familial clustering of diabetic nephropathy in Brazilian type 2 diabetic patients. Diabetes 48:909-913, 1999.

22   Vijay V, Snehalatha C, Shina K, et al.: Familial aggregation of diabetic kidney disease in Type 2 diabetes in south India. Diabetes Res Clin Pract 1999, 43:167-171

23   Fioretto P, Steffes MW, Barbosa J, Rich SS, Miller ME, Mauer M: Is diabetic nephropathy inherited? Studies of glomerular structure in type 1 diabetic sibling pairs. Diabetes 48:865-869, 1999.

24   Pettitt DJ, Saad MF, Bennett PH, Nelson RG, Knowler WC: Familial predisposition to renal disease in two generations of Pima Indians with type 2 (non-insulin-dependent) diabetes mellitus. Diabetologia 33:438-443, 1990.

25   Forsblom CM, Kanninen T, Lehtovirta M, et al.: Heritability of albumin excretion rate in families of patients with Type II diabetes. Diabetologia 1999, 42:1359-1366

26   Imperatore G, Knowler WC, Pettitt DJ, Kobes S, Bennett PH, Hanson RL: Segregation analysis of diabetic nephroapthy in Pima Indians. Diabetes 49:1049-1056, 2000.

27   Fogarty DG, Rich SS, Wantman M, Warram JH, Krolewski AS: Segregation analysis of albumin excretion in families with type 2 diabetes. Diabetes 49:1057-1063, 2000.

28   McCance DR, Hanson RL, Pettitt DJ, Jacobsson LTH, Bennett PH, Bishop DT, Knowler WC. Diabetic nephropathy: a risk factor for diabetes mellitus in offspring. Diabetologia 38:221-226, 1995.

29   Viberti GC, Keen H, Wiseman MJ: Raised arterial pressure in parents of proteinuric insulin dependent diabetics. Br Med J 295:515-517, 1987.

30   Krolewski AS, Canessa M, Warram JH, Laffel LMB, Christlieb AR, Knowler WC, Rand LI: Predisposition to hypertension and susceptibility to renal disease in insulin-dependent diabetes mellitus. N Engl J Med 318:140-145, 1988.

31   Takeda H, Ohta K, Hagiwara M, Hori K, Watanabe K, Suzuki D, Tanaka K, Machimura H, Ya-Game M, Kaneshige H, Sakai H. Genetic predisposing factors in non-insulin-dependent diabetes with persistent albuminuria. Tokai J Exp Clin Med 17:199-203, 1992.

32   Beatty OL, Harper R, Sheridan B, Atkinson AB, Bell PM: Insulin resistance in offspring of hypertensive parents. Br Med J 307:92-96, 1993.

33   Nelson RG, Pettitt DJ, de Courten MP, Hanson RL, Knowler WC, Bennett PH: Parental hypertension and proteinuria in Pima Indians with NIDDM. Diabetologia 39:433-438, 1996.

34   Nelson RG, Pettitt DJ, Baird HR, Charles MA, Liu QZ, Bennett PH, Knowler WC: Pre-diabetic blood pressure predicts urinary albumin excretion after the onset of type 2 (non-insulin-dependent) diabetes mellitus in Pima Indians. Diabetologia 36:998-1001, 1993.

35   Reichard P, Nilsson B-Y, Rosenqvist U: The effect of long-term intensified insulin treatment on the development of microvascular complications of diabetes mellitus. N Engl J Med 329:304-309, 1993.

36   The Diabetes Control and Complications Trial Research Group: The effect of intensive treatment of diabetes on the development and progression of long-term complications in insulin-dependent diabetes mellitus. N Engl J Med 329:977-986, 1993.

37   UK Prospective Diabetes Study (UKPDS) Group: Intensive blood-glucose control with sulphonylureas or insulin compared with conventional treatment and risk of complications in patients with type 2 diabetes (UKPDS 33). Lancet 352:837-853, 1998.

38   Krishna GP, Newell G, Miller E, Heeger P, Smith R, Polansky M, Kapoor S, Hoeldtke R: Protein-induced glomerular hyperfiltration: role of hormonal factors. Kidney Int 33:578-583, 1988.

39   Wiseman MJ, Dodds R, Bending JJ, Viberti GC: Dietary protein and the diabetic kidney. Diabetic Med 4:144-146, 1987.

40   Walker JD, Dodds RA, Murrells TJ, Bending JJ, Mattock MB, Keen H, Viberti GC: Restriction of dietary protein and progression of renal failure in diabetic nephropathy. Lancet 2:1411-1415, 1989.

41   Mitch WE: Dietary protein restriction in chronic renal failure: nutritional efficacy, compliance, and progression of renal insufficiency. J Am Soc Nephrol 2:823-831, 1991.

42   Zeller K, Whittaker E, Sullivan L, Raskin P, Jacobson HR: Effect of restricting dietary protein on the progression of renal failure in patients with insulin-dependent diabetes mellitus. N Engl J Med 324:78-84, 1991.

43   Hansen HP, Tauber-Lassen E, Jensen BR, Parving HH. Effect of dietary protein restriction on prognosis in patients with diabetic nephropathy. Kidney Int 62:220-228,2002.

44   Nakamura H, Ito S, Ebe N, Shibata A: Renal effects of different types of protein in healthy volunteer subjects and diabetic patients. Diabetes Care 16:1071-1075, 1993.

45   Mogensen CE: Long-term antihypertensive treatment inhibiting progression of diabetic nephropathy. Br Med J 285:685-688, 1982.

46 Parving H-H, Hommel E, Smidt UM: Protection of kidney function and decrease in albuminuria by captopril in insulin dependent diabetics with nephropathy. Br Med J 297:1086-1091, 1988.

47 Marre M, Chatellier G, Leblanc H, Guyene TT, Menard J, Passa P: Prevention of diabetic nephropathy with enalapril in normotensive diabetics with microalbuminuria. Br Med J 297:1092-1095, 1988.

48 Mathiesen ER, Hommel E, Giese J, Parving H-H: Efficacy of captopril in postponing nephropathy in normotensive insulin dependent diabetic patients with microalbuminuria. Br Med J 303:81-87, 1991.

49 Ravid M, Savin H, Jutrin I, Bental T, Katz B, Lishner M: Long-term stabilizing effect of angiotensin-converting enzyme inhibition on plasma creatinine and on proteinuria in normotensive type II diabetic patients. Ann Int Med 118, 577-581, 1993.

50 Lewis EJ, Hunsicker LG, Bain RP, Rohde RD: The effect of angiotensin-converting-enzyme inhibition on diabetic nephropathy. N Engl J Med 329:1456-1462, 1993.

51 The Microalbuminuria Captopril Study: Captopril reduces the risk of nephropathy in IDDM patients with microalbuminuria. Diabetologia 39:587-593, 1996.

52 Lewis EJ, Hunsicker LG, Clarke WR, Berl T, Pohl MA, Lewis JB, Ritz E, Atkins RC, Rohde R, Raz I, for the Collaborative Study Group: Renoprotective effect of the angiotensin-receptor antagonist irbesartan in patients with nephropathy due to type 2 diabetes. N Engl J Med 345:851-860, 2001.

53 Brenner BM, Cooper ME, de Zeeuw Dick, Keane WF, Mitch WE, Parving H-H, Remuzzi G, Snapinn SM, Zhang Z, Shahinfar S, for the RENAAL Study Investigators: Effects of losartan on renal and cardiovascular outcomes in patients with type 2 diabetes and nephropathy. N Engl J Med 345:861-869, 2001.

54 Parving H-H, Lehnert H, Bröchner-Mortensen, Gomis R, Andersen Steen, Arner P, for the Irbesartan in Patients with Type 2 Diabetes and Microalbuminuria Study Group: The effect of irbesartan on the development of diabetic nephropathy in patients with type 2 diabetes. N Engl J Med 345:870-878, 2001.

55 van Essen GG, Rensma PL, de Zeeuw D, Sluiter WJ, Scheffer H, Apperloo AJ, de Jong PE: Association between angiotensin-converting-enzyme gene polymorphism and failure of renoprotective therapy. Lancet 347:94-95, 1996.

56 Penno G, Chaturvedi N, Talmud PJ, Cotroneo P, Manto A, Nannipieri M, Luong LA, Fuller JH: Effect of angiotensin-converting enzyme (ACE) gene polymorphism on progression of renal disease and the influence of ACE inhibition in IDDM patients: findings from the EUCLID Randomized Controlled Trial. EURODIAB Controlled Trial of Lisinopril in IDDM. Diabetes 47:1507-1511, 1998.

9

GENETICS AND DIABETIC NEPHROPATHY

Lise Tarnow
Steno Diabetes Center, 2820 Gentofte, Denmark

GENETIC SUSCEPTIBILITY

As reviewed in the previous chapter, the first suggestion of variable susceptibility to diabetic nephropathy emerged from epidemiological studies of the incidence rates suggesting the existence of a subset of type 1 diabetic patients, who are susceptible to develop diabetic nephropathy during the first and second decades of diabetes. In addition, a marked racial variation in the prevalence rates of diabetic nephropathy has been described. Furthermore, the unanimously reported familial clustering of diabetic nephropathy and the observations of elevated blood pressure and increased cardiovascular morbidity and early mortality among parents of type 1 diabetic patients with diabetic nephropathy support the hypothesis, that hereditary factors are involved in the liability to develop diabetic nephropathy.

GENETIC APPROACHES TO DIABETIC NEPHROPATHY

Diabetic nephropathy is likely to be a complex genetic trait, i.e. a phenotype that does not exhibit classic Mendelian recessive or dominant inheritance attributable to a single locus. Thus a combination of susceptibility alleles at several genes provides a risk of developing the disease. The relative high cumulative incidence (25-35%) of the disease can be accounted for if predisposing alleles with modest effects are common at several independent loci, since then their combination in a given person is expected to occur frequently. There are two basic strategies for characterising genes that influence complex genetic traits: association analyses and random marker approaches.

Association analysis

In candidate gene analysis one tests the association between a particular genetic variant and a trait, e.g. diabetic nephropathy, with the hope of identifying a variant that is more frequent among individuals with than those without the trait due to a causal relationship between the variant and the trait.

The choice of candidate genes and variants should make biological sense and be physiological meaningful. A problem with this approach is that there are numerous candidate genes for a given trait, and within each of these genes a large number of variants (e.g. deletions, micro-satellites, single nucleotide polymorphisms (SNPs)). In addition, since there is likely to be a great deal of heterogeneity, both with respect to the genes that predispose one to diabetic nephropathy and the environments that one may be exposed to, finding appropriate homogeneous case and control groups might be problematic.

To prevent spurious association due to population admixture, the use of parental non-transmitted alleles as an ethnical well-matched "internal" control group has been suggested[1;2]. However, in an ethnical homogenous population this design offers little advantage over traditional case-control studies and furthermore, this approach: transmission-disequilibrium test (TDT) is cumbersome because it involves genotyping of at least three individuals (proband and both parents) for the identification of a case and a control group, since only heterozygous parents are informative. Finally, a survival bias is introduced in the classical study of trios since parents of probands with diabetic nephropathy are at increased risk of early mortality[3] and only trios with two living parents can be included. The TDT is basically a test for association, however, if an associated allele is a susceptibility factor or is in linkage disequilibrium with a nearby disease gene, the TDT can be used to establish linkage[2].

Random marker approach

Random marker approaches involve gathering a large number of related individuals thought to be segregating for genes that influence a trait (e.g. diabetic nephropathy) and then trace the putative parent-to-offspring co-transmission of variants at landmark spots along the genome (marker loci) with possible trait-influencing variants. There are two general approaches to linkage analysis: 1] parametric pedigree analysis investigating co-segregation in large pedigrees. These can be very powerful provided that one specifies the correct model of inheritance. However, in the study of diabetic nephropathy, the fact that presence of diabetes is mandatory for the expression of the disease causing gene(s) makes collection of multiplex families difficult. A task further complicated by the increased mortality not merely among probands with type 1 diabetes and nephropathy[4] but also among their parents [3]. However, the main methods applied to genome searches are 2] allele-sharing methods, by which one tries to prove that the inheritance pattern is not consistent with random Mendelian segregation. Since no model is assumed these methods are more robust and affected relatives should show excess allele sharing even in the presence of incomplete penetrans, phenocopy, genetic heterogeneity and high-frequency disease alleles[5]. One major problem with pedigree and allele-sharing analyses is the focus on a single locus. In addition, linkage strategies are not powerful for detecting genes with small to moderate effects[6]. Sampling of sib-pairs concordant for high values (e.g. urinary albumin excretion rate) is most powerful for the detection of low frequency alleles which increase the trait, whereas sampling from the bottom tail of the distribution is the more powerful approach for detecting low-frequency protective alleles. However, sampling siblings discordant for a given trait is the uniformly best approach when allele frequencies are equal, studying co-dominant inheritance[7], and for the study of quantitative trait loci, i.e. urinary albumin excretion rate.

Association and linkage studies are two complementary analyses, each providing its own brand of information. Whereas association is simply a statistical statement about the co-occurrence of alleles and phenotypes, linkage is a specific genetic relationship between loci (not alleles or phenotypes). One may be able to detect linkage without association, e.g. where there are many independent trait causing genes, so that association with any particular allele is weak. Or association can be found without linkage, e.g. when an allele explains only a minor proportion of the variance for a given trait and thus by itself is a poor predictor of disease within a pedigree.

Statistical significance is another problem in genetic analysis since modern techniques allow for the testing of many chromosomal regions across the genome and testing of multiple models of inheritance. The choice of large sample sizes – more than 1000 cases and controls [8] – and stringent criteria for significance levels with lod scores >3.3 and p-values $<10^{-4}$ to 10^{-8} have been suggested to overcome this problem[5;8]. Furthermore, in studies where many and highly polymorphic markers are tested the obtained p-values should be adjusted for the number of comparisons. Finally, all positive genetic associations should be replicated in other data sets and by family-based association studies [8].

STUDIES ON THE GENETICS OF DIABETIC NEPHROPATHY

The search for genetic markers that would allow early diagnosis and identification of patients at risk has accelerated during the last decade. The vast majority of studies performed so far have been cross sectional association studies investigating candidate genes, and results from case-control studies have been reported from all over the world. Future studies of longitudinal design will enable investigators to take time course and environmental factors into account.

Candidate genes have been chosen based on the conception of a multifactorial aetiology of the structural and functional changes of diabetic glomerulopathy with contributions from metabolic abnormalities, haemodynamic alterations, cytokines, growth factors, and a genetic susceptibility[9]. This includes

1) diabetes susceptibility genes,
2) genes involved in regulation of blood pressure,
3) genes regulating cardiovascular risk factors,
4) glomerular structure, inflammation and growth factor genes, and
5) genes involved in glucose metabolism (Table 1).

Table 1. Putative candidate genes for diabetic nephropathy.

Gene	Association
1) Diabetes susceptibility genes	
- HLA	-
- Insulin	(+)
- Complement C4	(-)

Table 1. (cont.)

Gene	Association
2) Genes involved in regulation of blood pressure	
- ACE	+
- Angiotensinogen	-
- AGT$_1$R	-
- Renin	(+)
- Nitric oxide synthases	(+/-)
- Atrio natriuretic peptide	(+)
- G-protein ß3 subunit	(-)
- Bradykinin receptors	(-)

3) Genes regulating cardiovascular risk factors

- Apolipoprotein E	(+/-)
- Apolipoprotein(a)	(+)
- Paraoxonase	(+/-)
- Von Willebrand factor	NA
- PAI-1	(-)
- MTHFR	(+)
- Lipoprotein lipase	(+)

4) Glomerular structure, inflammation and growth factor genes

- Heparansulphat core protein (Perlecan)	(+)
- Collagen type IV α1-chain	(-)
- Matrix metallo protease 9	(+)
- Chemokine receptor	(+)
- Interleukin-1 gene cluster	(+/-)
- Interleukin-6	(+)
- TGF-ß	(+/-)
- Decorin	(-)
- VEGF	(+)
- N-acetyltransferase	(-)

5) Genes involved in glucose metabolism

- Aldose reductase	(+/-)
- AGE receptors	(+)
- ß3 adrenergic receptor	(-)
- GLUT1	(+/-)
- PC-1	(+/-)
- PPAR-γ	(+)

+: possible; -: unlikely; () data are sparse; NA: data not available

Genes involved in regulation of blood pressure

Among the candidate genes suggested for nephropathy, genes of the renin-angiotensin system and especially the gene coding for ACE, have attracted most interest. In addition to the circulating renin-angiotensin system, recent studies have demonstrated local gene expression of both renin, angiotensinogen, and ACE genes in the kidneys, adrenals, heart and blood vessels. Although vascular ACE activity is regulated at a considerably slower rate than that of renin, the enzyme is nevertheless a determinant of local angiotensin II production[13]. Thus, locally generated components of the renin-angiotensin system may play important roles in the function of these target organs, and may even reach the circulating blood and thus contribute to the levels found in plasma.

Angiotensin converting enzyme gene

Plasma concentration of ACE is remarkably stable within individual subjects, however large inter-individual differences exist. Rigat et al[14] detected an insertion (I) / deletion (D) polymorphism within the human ACE gene (ACE/ID), that accounts for half of the phenotypic variation of serum ACE. Based on the presence or absence of a 287 base pair sequence in intron 16 (a non-coding DNA-sequence), three genotypes are found (DD and II homozygotes and ID heterozygotes).

Subsequently, the polymorphic locus was sequenced and a 14 base pair repeat sequence flanking the insertion and potentially capable of producing a 'loop-out' of the intervening 287 base pair fragment was found[15]. Furthermore, the insertion contains a sequence with remarkable homology with a negative regulatory element in the mouse REN-1 gene suggesting this sequence as a potential silencer motif in the regulation of renin-angiotensin system activity.

An alternative explanation would be that the ACE/ID polymorphism is not the locus directly involved in regulating the variability of circulating ACE concentration, but merely a marker for a nearby unknown functional variant located within or near the ACE gene.

The quantitative expression of the ACE/ID polymorphism differ between subjects, since circulating ACE levels in non-diabetic healthy subjects homozygous for the D-allele was about twice that of II subjects with ID genotype subjects having intermediate values[14]. In diabetic populations a similar co-dominant relationship was found [16;17]. In addition to the findings that circulating levels of ACE are associated with the ACE/ID polymorphism, studies of ACE gene expression in human kidneys revealed highest tissue ACE and mRNA levels in glomeruli and tubuli of subjects with DD genotype as compared with other genotypes[18].

For the study of physiological consequences of the ACE/ID polymorphism the response to exogenous angiotensin I infusion was studied in normotensive men homozygotes for either allele[19]. Interestingly, recent studies[20] of endothelial-dependent vasodilatation with acetylcholine demonstrated a blunted response by strain gauge plethysmography in normo- and hypertensive subjects with the DD genotype, suggesting an angiotensin-II induced increased breakdown and/or reduced bradykinin mediated nitric oxide (NO) release in these subjects.

Within the diabetic kidney, elevated renal artery resistance[21] and lower GFR values[22] were demonstrated in uncomplicated type 1 diabetic patients with DD genotype. Recently, Marre et al[23] studied the effect of acute hyperglycaemia in normotensive normoalbuminuric type 1 diabetic patients, and found that those with DD or ID genotypes displayed alterations in glomerular haemodynamics consistent with preglomerular vasodilatation and resulting rise in glomerular capillary pressure during elevated blood glucose, while this was not observed in patients with II genotype

Originally, Cambien et al found the DD genotype to be a new potent risk factor for myocardial infarction in Caucasian middle-aged men, particularly in subjects considered to be at low cardiovascular risk[24]. This association with coronary heart disease has been confirmed by some and challenged by others. Two meta-analyses [25;26] both concluded that the D-allele of the ACE/ID polymorphism is a marker of atherosclerotic cardiovascular complications.

Published results describing an association between the ACE/ID genotype and blood pressure are as numerous as those that have not found such an association. However, more recent studies of human monogenic hypertension, studies in essential hypertension and in normotensive subjects, and from the rat model of hypertension all point to the ACE locus on human chromosome 17, or its homologous rat locus, as reviewed by Soubrier[27].

In diabetes, the initial report from Marre et al in 1994 proposed a protective effect of the II genotype against development of elevated urinary albumin excretion rate in type 1 diabetic patients[16]. A substantial number of association studies have been conducted to investigate the possible relationship between elevated urinary albumin excretion rate and the ACE/ID polymorphism in patients with diabetes. The results of the different studies have been conflicting for a number of reasons: *a)* the phenotypic characterisation of cases and controls is heterogenous, *b)* a variety of selection criteria have been applied, and *c)* the number of subjects studied is limited. Regarding *a)* Substantial ethnic differences in ACE/ID genotype frequency exists[28]. Criteria for the diagnosis of diabetic nephropathy differ substantially between studies. The majority of studies include patients with both micro- and macroalbuminuria among cases, despite the knowledge that not all type 1 diabetic patients with microalbuminuria will progress to overt nephropathy and some might even regress to normoalbuminuria[29;30]. Major differences with respect to type and interval of urine collections and determination of urinary albumin concentration/excretion rate may further contribute to the observed heterogeneity between studies. In addition, by selection of controls with microalbuminuria or relatively short duration of diabetes some studies actually can not exclude that a number of their controls will eventually develop diabetic nephropathy. *b)* Application of additional inclusion/exclusion criteria e.g proliferative retinopathy[31], normotensive cases[32], and patients treated with ACE inhibitors[33] increases the risk of population stratification and reduces generalisability. *c)* Furthermore, the number of patients studied in many of the trials is far too small to detect minor differences in risk of nephropathy in association studies. As pointed out recently, about 1200 cases and a similar number of controls is necessary to obtain sufficient power to detect a difference of the magnitude reported in a meta-analysis[34]. Finally, since the ACE/ID polymorphism is probably merely a marker for a nearby functional polymorphism[14] the degree of linkage disequilibrium between the two may vary from population to population resulting in an observed association in some, but not in other populations.

During 1997–98 four meta-analyses of various cardiovascular-renal disorders in diabetes and the ACE/ID polymorphism were published[26;34-36]. Given the limitations of available data and the inevitable heterogeneity of a meta-analysis they all proposed the D-allele to be associated with increased risk of diabetic nephropathy, though the effect might be overestimated due to preferential publication of positive results. In our review[35] of studies of Caucasian type 1 diabetic patients (n=2688) comparison of data is complicated by differences between study populations. However, a trend towards a protective effect of the II genotype on the development of increased urinary albumin excretion rate was observed with a pooled odds ratio of 0.72, (0.51-1.01), p=0.06. In type 2 diabetic patients this association was confined to Japanese populations[35]. Thus, the D-allele of the ACE/ID polymorphism is suggested to be a new risk factor for the development of diabetic nephropathy in Caucasian type 1 diabetic patients, although the effect is modest – supporting the concept of a complex genetic trait.

Logically, we can conclude from case-control studies only, that patients with diabetic nephropathy are at slightly increased risk of carrying the D-allele. For the definite answer to the question of the risk of development of diabetic nephropathy in patients with a given ACE/ID genotype we are awaiting prospective observational studies of large, unselected cohorts of uncomplicated type 1 diabetic patients followed for a long time (>15 years). At present, only few short-term studies applying a prospective longitudinal design have been reported. In the EUCLID trial progression from normo- to microalbuminuria did not differ between genotypes, however a beneficial effect of the ACE inhibitor, lisinopril on urinary albumin excretion rate was found only in the II group[37]. In accordance, a smaller proportion of patients with II genotype progressed from one stage of albuminuria to a higher in an observational study of 310 type 1 diabetic patients followed for a median of 6 years (range:2-9) [38].

Of interest, once overt diabetic nephropathy is present, several studies on the progression of kidney disease have demonstrated the ACE/ID polymorphism to play a role as progression promoter. Originally, we reported patients homozygous for the D-allele to have an accelerated loss of glomerular filtration rate during 7 years of ACE-inhibition in 35 type 1 patients with diabetic nephropathy[39]. Furthermore, in a prospective follow-up study of 56 type 2 diabetic patients the DD genotype was associated with increased loss of calculated creatinine clearance and increased 3 year mortality[40]. Other studies[31;41] did not find a similar effect on established diabetic nephropathy and thus the topic remains open for debate.

With respect to another microvascular complication of type 1 diabetes, e.g. diabetic retinopathy, no association between the ACE/ID polymorphism was found in our study[17], nor in other studies[34]. One major confounder to studies addressing this topic has been the co-existing presence of diabetic nephropathy, especially among patients with proliferative retinopathy.

Angiotensinogen gene

Linkage to hypertension was demonstrated[48] and an association between blood pressure and a molecular variant of the gene encoding the presence of a threonine instead of a methionine at residue 235 of mature angiotensinogen (T235 versus M235) was reported in several populations[48]. Furthermore, this molecular variant (M235T-polymorphism) was closely associated with a functional effect, plasma angiotensinogen concentrations being highest in T235 homozygotes[48]. Recently, a biological mechanism was suggested by the observation, that a variant in the proximal promoter of the angiotensinogen gene, known to be in very tight linkage disequilibrium with the M235T polymorphism, influenced the basal transcription rate of the gene[49].

In the study of the angiotensinogen gene and diabetic nephropathy results from case-control studies have been conflicting[50], though the majority of studies have found no association between the M235T polymorphism and diabetic nephropathy in type 1 or type 2 diabetic populations. Reasons for discrepancies between reports are numerous, e.g. degree of linkage disequilibrium, population admixture, phenotypic characterisation of cases and controls, selection criteria, and the small number of subjects studied.

In an attempt to reduce population stratification a family-based study was performed to investigate the M235T polymorphism for a possible role in the pathogenesis of diabetic nephropathy[51]. The heterozygous parents of 148 type 1 diabetic probands with and 62 probands without urinary albumin/creatinine rate >65 µg/mg were included in a TDT analysis. In aggregate, the transmission of the T-allele occurred at a similar frequency to probands with and to those without elevated urinary albumin excretion rate.

Angiotensin II Type 1 receptor gene

Most of the known actions of angiotensin II in adult humans are mediated by the angiotensin II type 1 receptor (AGT_1R), a G-protein coupled receptor expressed on cell surfaces of vascular smooth muscle, myocardium, adrenal cortex, and the kidney. A polymorphism has been described in the AGT_1R gene, corresponding to a transversion of adenine to cytosine (AC) at position 1166 in the 3' untranslated region of the gene[52]. The functional significance of this non-coding polymorphism had not been investigated until recently, when Miller et al[53] demonstrated an association between renal haemodynamic function and the AGT_1R^{1166} polymorphism in healthy subjects, constitutive and during treatment with a AGT_1R blocker or during angiotensin II infusion. Their renal findings are consistent with the hypothesis that the C-allele is related to augmented angiotensin II activity. Whether the AGT_1R^{1166} polymorphism is in linkage equilibrium with a functional variant within or in proxy of the AGT_1R gene, or influences directly the regulation of AGT_1R gene expression or receptor number remains to be elucidated.

Association between the AGT_1R^{1166} polymorphism and essential hypertension, aortic stiffness and cardiac hypertrophy have been reported [52]. Furthermore, a synergistic interaction between the AGT_1R^{1166} polymorphism and the ACE/ID polymorphism on the risk of myocardial infarction was suggested[54].

In diabetes, we found no differences in AGT_1R^{1166} genotype or allele distribution between type 1 diabetic patients with or without diabetic nephropathy[55]. This finding was subsequently confirmed in several other large case-control studies[31;56]. One study[57] found no significant association between the AGT_1R^{1166} polymorphism and elevated urinary albumin excretion rate per se either, but suggested a synergistic effect of this polymorphism and poor metabolic control on risk of nephropathy in type 1 diabetic patients. A finding, which could not be supported in a subsequent study from Northern Ireland[58] nor in a Danish study of interaction between the AGT_1R^{1166}, ACE/ID and M235T polymorphisms and long-term glycaemic control[59].

The first report applying a genome screening approach on sibling pairs concordant for type 1 diabetes, but discordant for nephropathy came from the Joslin clinic[60]. In this study of 66 sibpairs informative DNA markers were investigated in the regions containing genes encoding proteins of the renin-angiotensin system. No distortion in allele sharing for markers flanking the ACE or angiotensinogen genes was seen, and the proportions sharing 0, 1, and 2 alleles were close to the expected 0.25, 0.50, and 0.25 under the hypothesis of no linkage. On the contrary, the region containing the AGT_1R locus showed linkage with diabetic nephropathy with a surprisingly high peak maximum lod score of 3.1. To investigate whether the AGT_1R gene could account for the observed linkage, six new and previously known polymorphisms of the AGT_1R gene were examined in a TDT analysis of heterozygous parents of 147 type 1 diabetic patients with and 64 without elevated urinary albumin excretion rate. Neither the AGT_1R^{1166} polymorphism nor any of the other polymorphisms were associated with diabetic nephropathy in this study population[60]. In type 2 diabetic Pima Indians a tentative linkage with nephropathy (lod score 1.48) was found close to the AGT_1R gene on chromosome 3 as well[61]. Though for stringent threshold of a type 1 error (lod score=3.3), a study of 98 sib pairs concordant for nephropathy renders the power to detect loci of moderate effects on the susceptibility to microvascular complications relatively low.

Thus, the AGT_1R^{1166} polymorphism does not seem to be associated with diabetic nephropathy in type 1 diabetes. Preliminary studies suggesting linkage of persistently elevated urinary albumin excretion rate with the region containing the AGT_1R locus remains to be confirmed and further explored.

Renin gene
Although the renin gene is a very plausible candidate gene for diabetic nephropathy, like in essential hypertension no confirmed evidence for positive associations between renin gene polymorphisms and diabetic nephropathy in type 1 diabetic populations is available[62;63].

Genes regulating cardiovascular risk factors
Since endothelial dysfunction and dyslipidaemia are commonly observed in type 1 diabetic patients with elevated urinary albumin excretion rate[64;65], genes involved in regulation of the fibrinolytic cascade and lipid metabolism are plausible candidate genes for diabetic nephropathy and have been studied. However, the majority of observed associations between genetic variants and presence of diabetic microangiopathy have not been confirmed in studies of other populations – as indicated in table 1.

Glomerular structure, inflammation and growth factor genes

The 'Steno hypothesis' suggests that loss of the proteoglycan, heparan sulphate, from the basement membrane may be of major importance in the pathogenesis of diabetic nephropathy, and might be due to genetic polymorphisms in genes responsible for synthesis and degradation of glomerular structure proteins[66]. In one study[67] the first part of the Perlecan gene, encoding the heparan sulphate core protein, was screened for restriction fragment length polymorphisms. A *bam*HI polymorphism located within a domain responsible for binding of the heparan sulphate side chains was found to be significantly associated with diabetic nephropathy in two independent case-control studies[67]. Findings remain to be confirmed or refuted in other study populations.

Polymorphisms of the IL-1 gene cluster have also been examined, as this locus is involved in mesangial cell proliferation and extracellular matrix production. An association with the natural endogenous inhibitor of IL-1 was proposed[68], but could not be confirmed neither in our case-control study[69], nor in a study from Northern Ireland[70]. However, in their material an association between diabetic nephropathy and the B*2 allele of the IL-1ß gene was found, which we did not find in the Danish study[69].

In addition, recent studies have investigated the association between genes encoding IL-6, matrix metallo protease 9 and several growth factors thought to be involved in the pathogenesis of diabetic glomerulosclerosis e.g. TGF-ß and VEGF[71;72] so far without conclusive answers.

Genes involved in glucose metabolism

The enzyme aldose reductase has been implicated in several microvascular complications of diabetes, and a dinucleotide repeat polymorphism in the 5'end of the aldose reductase gene has been suggested to be strongly associated with nephropathy in type 1 diabetes[73]. A finding based on the observation of a decreased frequency of the Z+2 allele in patients with nephropathy. Subsequent case-control studies in type 1 and type 2 diabetic patients with and without elevated urinary albumin excretion rate and/or retinopathy have however reported conflicting results regarding the role of this promoter repeat polymorphism in the development of diabetic microvascular complications[74].

Interestingly, in 98 Pima Indian siblings concordant for type 2 diabetes and nephropathy the strongest evidence for linkage (lod score 2.73) was found in a genetic element on chromosome 7, encompassing the aldose reductase gene[61]. Linkage data from this region was not reported in the paper reporting on type 1 diabetic sib-pairs discordant for nephropathy[60]. Advanced glycation end-products (AGEs) may play an important role in the mechanisms by which chronic hyperglycaemia exerts its adverse effects in the kidneys. The four receptors for AGE have been scanned and 19 polymorphisms identified. The minor allele of a promoter polymorphism were reported to confer a weak protective effect and to be associated with longer duration of nephropathy free type 1 diabetes[75].

Genetic variation leading to deficiency in insulin secretion, action, or glucose uptake and utilization may be involved in the development of renal complications in type 1 and type 2 diabetes. The identified contributions from studied polymorphisms are disappointingly modest[76-79].

FUTURE PERSPECTIVES FOR THE STUDY OF GENETICS OF DIABETIC NEPHROPATHY

Numerous association studies have been carried out in a large number of small patient populations with predictable conflicting results. The D-allele of the ACE/ID polymorphism is suggested to be a new risk factor, although the effect is modest and prospective data are sparse. The M235T polymorphism in the angiotensinogen gene and the AGT_1R^{1166} polymorphism are unlikely to contribute, whereas the promoter variant in the aldose reductase gene might turn out to contribute to the genetic susceptibility of diabetic nephropathy.

In the mean time, the human genome project has identified and sequenced 50 to 100 000 human genes, including numerous new candidate genes for diabetic nephropathy. Large collaborative and prospective studies are required to determine which associations may be of relevance. Though cumbersome, family-based studies for linkage analyses are complementary and require multi-national collaborations for the collection of large enough numbers of families to allow confident results.

Considering diabetic nephropathy as a complex genetic trait, future studies on the interactions between different gene polymorphisms and environmental factors, and studies of gene expression and pharmaco-genetic functions will offer valuable information for the study of renal involvement in patients with type 1 diabetes. The ability to identify patients at inherited risk for or resistance to development of diabetic nephropathy would help considerably to augment current screening methods and influence initiation and intensity of new and already well-established treatment modalities.

REFERENCES

1   Thomsen G. HLA disease associations: models for insulin dependent diabetes mellitus and the study of complex human genetic disorders. Annual Reviews of Genetics 1988; 22:31-50.

2   Spielman RS, McGinnis RE, Ewens WJ. Transmission test for linkage disequilibrium: the insulin gene region and insulin-dependent diabetes mellitus (IDDM). American Journal of Human Genetics 1993; 52:506-516.

3   Earle K, Walker J, Hill C, Viberti GC. Familial clustering of cardiovascular disease in patients with insulin-dependent diabetes and nephropathy. N Engl J Med 1992; 326:673-677.

4   Borch-Johnsen K, Andersen PK, Deckert T. The effect of proteinuria on relative mortality in Type 1 (insulin-dependent) diabetes mellitus. Diabetologia 1985; 28:590-596.

5   Lander ES, Schork NJ. Genetic dissection of complex traits. Science 1994; 265:2037-2048.

6   Risch N, Merikangas K. The future of genetic studies of complex human diseases. Science 1996; 273:1516-1517.

7   Risch N, Zhang H. Extreme discordant sibpairs for mapping quantitative trait loci in humans. Science 1995; 268:1584-1589.

8   Todd JA. Interpretation of results from genetic studies of multifactorial diseases. Lancet 1999; 354(suppl I):15-16.

9   Parving H-H, Østerby R, Ritz E. Diabetic nephropathy. In: Brenner BM, editor. The Kidney. Philadelphia: WB Saunders, 2000: 1731-1773.

10   Barbosa J, Saner B. Do genetic factors play a role in the pathogenesis of diabetic microangiopathy? Diabetologia 1984; 27:487-492.

11   Chowdhury TA, Dyer PH, Mijovic CH, Dunger DB, Barnett AH, Bain SC. Human leukocyte antigen and insulin gene regions and nephropathy in type 1 diabetes. Diabetologia 1999; 42:1017-1020.

12   Raffel LJ, Vadheim CM, Roth M-P, Klein R, Moss SE, Rotter JI. The 5'insulin gene polymorphism and the genetics of vascular complications in type 1 (insulin-dependent) diabetes mellitus. Diabetologia 1991; 34:680-683.

13   Müller DN, Bohlender J, Hilgers KF, Dragun D, Costerousse O, Ménard J et al. Vascular angiotensin-converting enzyme expression regulates local angiotensin II. Hypertension 1997; 29:98-104.

14   Rigat B, Hubert C, Alhenc-Gelas F, Cambien F, Corvol P, Soubrier F. An insertion/deletion polymorphism in angiotensin I converting enzyme gene accounting for half the variance of serum enzyme levels. J Clin Invest 1990; 86:1343-1346.

15   Hunley TE, Julian BA, Philips JA, Summar ML, Yoshida H, Horn RG et al. Angiotensin converting enzyme gene polymorphism: potential silencer motif and impact on progression in IgA nephropathy. Kidney Int 1996; 49:571-577.

16   Marre M, Bernadet P, Gallois Y, Savagner F, Guyenne T-T, Hallab M et al. Relationships between angiotensin I converting enzyme gene polymorphism, plasma levels, and diabetic retinal and renal complications. Diab 1994; 43:384-388.

17   Tarnow L, Cambien F, Rossing P, Nielsen FS, Hansen BV, Lecerf L et al. Lack of relationship between an insertion/deletion polymorphism in the angiotensin-I-converting enzyme gene and diabetic nephropathy and proliferative retinopathy in IDDM patients. Diab 1995; 44:489-494.

18   Mizuiri S, Hemmi H, Kumanomidou H, Iwamoto M, Miyagi M, Sakai K et al. Angiotensin-converting enzyme (ACE) I/D genotype and renal ACE gene expression. Kidney Int 2001; 60:1124-1130.

19   Ueda S, Elliott HL, Morton JJ, Connell JMC. Enhanced pressor response to angiotensin I in normotensive men with the deletion genotype (DD) for angiotensin-converting enzyme. Hypertension 1995; 25:1266-1269.

20   Perticone F, Ceravolo R, Maio R, Ventura G, Zingone A, Perrotti N et al. Angiotensin-converting enzyme gene polymorphism is associated with endothelium-dependent vasodilatation in never treated hypertensive patients. Hypertension 1998; 31:900-905.

21   Fukumoto S, Ishimura E, Hosoi M, Kawagishi T, Kawamura T, Isshiki G et al. Angiotensin converting enzyme gene polymorphism and renal artery resistance in patients with insulin dependent diabetes mellitus. Life Sciences 1996; 59(8):629-637.

22   Miller JA, Scholey JW, Thai K, Pei YPC. Angiotensin converting enzyme gene polymorphism and renal hemodynamic function in early diabetes. Kidney Int 1997; 51:119-124.

23   Marre M, Bouhanick B, Berrut G, Gallois Y, Le Jeune J-J, Chatellier G et al. Renal changes on hyperglycemia and angiotensin-converting enzyme in type 1 diabetes. Hypertension 1999; 33:775-780.

24   Cambien F, Poirier O, Lecerf L, Evans A, Cambou JP, Arveiler D et al. Deletion polymorphism in the gene for angiotensin-converting enzyme is a potent risk factor for myocardial infarction. Nature 1992; 359-60:641-644.

25   Samani NJ, Thompson JR, O'Toole L, Channer K, Woods KL. A meta-analysis of the association of the deletion allele of the angiotensin-converting enzyme gene with myocardial infarction. Circulation 1996; 94:708-712.

26   Staessen JA, Wang JG, Ginocchio G, Petrov V, Saavedra AP, Soubrier F et al. The deletion/insertion polymorphism of the angiotensin converting enzyme gene and cardiovascular-renal risk. J Hypertens 1997; 15:1579-1592.

27   Soubrier F. Blood pressure gene at the angiotensin I-converting enzyme locus - chronicle of a gene foretold. Circulation 1998; 97:1763-1765.

28   Johanning GL, Johnston KE, Tamura T, Goldenberg RL. Ethnic differences in angiotensin converting enzyme gene polymorphism. J Hypertens 1995; 13(6):710-711.

29   Almdal T, Nørgaard K, Feldt-Rasmussen B, Deckert T. The predictive value of microalbuminuria in IDDM. Diabetes Care 1994; 17:120-125.

30   Forsblom CM, Groop P-H, Ekstrand A, Groop L. Predictive value of microalbuminuria in patients with insulin-dependent diabetes of long duration. Br Med J 1992; 305:1051-1053.

31   Marre M, Jeunemaitre X, Gallois Y, Rodier M, Chatellier G, Sert C et al. Contribution of genetic polymorphism in the renin-angiotensin system to the development of renal complications in insulin-dependent diabetes. J Clin Invest 1997; 99(7):1585-1595.

32   Chowdhury TA, Dronsfield MJ, Kumar S, Gough SLC, Gibson SP, Khatoon A et al. Examination of two genetic polymorphisms within the renin-angiotensin system: no evidence for an association with nephropathy in IDDM. Diabetologia 1996; 39:1108-1114.

33   Doi Y, Yoshizumi H, Yoshinari M, Iino K, Yamamoto M, Ichikawa K et al. Association between a polymorphism in the angiotensin-converting enzyme gene and microvascular complications in Japanese patients with NIDDM. Diabetologia 1996; 39:97-102.

34   Fujisawa T, Ikegami H, Kawaguchi Y, Hamada Y, Ueda H, Shintani M et al. Meta-analysis of association of insertion/deletion polymorphism of angiotensin I-converting enzyme gene with diabetic nephropathy and retinopathy. Diabetologia 1998; 41(1):47-53.

35   Tarnow L, Gluud C, Parving H-H. Diabetic nephropathy and the insertion/deletion polymorphism of the angiotensin-converting enzyme gene. Nephrol Dial Transplant 1998; 13:1125-1130.

36   Kunz R, Bork JP, Fritsche L, Ringel J, Sharma AM. Association between the angiotensin-converting enzyme-insertion/deletion polymorphism and diabetic nephropathy: a methodological appraisal and systematic review. J Am Soc Nephrol 1998; 9:1653-1663.

37   Penno G, Chaturvedi N, Talmud PJ, Cotroneo P, Manto A, Nannipieri M et al. Effect of angiotensin-converting enzyme (ACE) gene polymorphism on progression of renal disease and the influence of ACE inhibition in IDDM patients - findings from the EUCLID randomized controlled trial. Diab 1998; 47:1507-1511.

38   Hadjadj S, Belloum R, Gallois Y, Bouhanick B, Berrut G, Weekers L et al. Contribution of angiotensin I converting enzyme I/D polymorphism to the development and progression of nephropathy in type 1 diabetes. Diabetologia 42[suppl 1], A269. 1999. Ref Type: Abstract

39   Parving H-H, Jacobsen P, Tarnow L, Rossing P, Lecerf L, Poirier O et al. Deleterious effect of a deletion polymorphism in angiotensin-converting enzyme (ACE) gene on progression of diabetic nephropathy during ACE inhibition. Br Med J 1996; 313:591-594.

40   Fava S, Azzopardi J, Ellard S, Hattersley AT. ACE gene polymorphism as a prognostic indicator in patients with type 2 diabetes and established renal disease. Diabetes Care 2001; 24(12):2115-2120.

41   Björck S, Blohmé G, Sylvén C, Mulec H. Deletion insertion polymorphism of the angiotensin converting enzyme gene and progression of diabetic nephropathy. Nephrol Dial Transplant 1997; 12(suppl 2):67-70.

42   Tarnow L, Cambien F, Rossing P, Nielsen FS, Hansen BV, Lecerf L et al. Insertion/deletion polymorphism in the angiotensin-I-converting enzyme gene is associated with coronary heart disease in IDDM patients with diabetic nephropathy. Diabetologia 1995; 38:798-803.

43   Rasmussen LM, Ledet T. Aortic atherosclerosis in diabetes mellitus is associated with an insertion/deletion polymorphism in the angiotensin I-converting enzyme gene. Diabetologia 1996; 39:696-700.

44   Tarnow L, Rossing P, Nielsen FS, Fagerudd JA, Poirier O, Parving H-H. Cardiovascular morbidity and early mortality cluster in parents of type 1 diabetic patients with diabetic nephropathy. Diabetes Care 2000; 23:30-33.

45   Ruiz J, Blanché H, Cohen N, Velho G, Cambien F, Cohen D et al. Insertion/deletion polymorphism of the angiotensin-converting enzyme gene is strongly associated with

coronary heart disease in non-insulin-dependent diabetes mellitus. Proc Natl Acad Sci USA 1994; 91:3662-3665.

46   Keavney BD, Dudley CRK, Stratton IM, Holman RR, Matthews DR, Ratcliffe PJ et al. UK prospective diabetes study (UKPDS) 14: association of angiotensin-converting enzyme insertion/deletion polymorphism with myocardial infarction in NIDDM. Diabetologia 1995; 38:948-952.

47   Fujisawa T, Ikegami H, Shen G-Q, Yamato E, Takekawa K, Nakagawa Y et al. Angiotensin I-converting enzyme gene polymorphism is associated with myocardial infarction, but not with retinopathy or nephropathy, in NIDDM. Diabetes Care 1995; 18:983-985.

48   Jeunemaitre X, Soubrier F, Kotelevtsev YV, Lifton RP, Williams CS, Charru A et al. Molecular basis of human hypertension: Role of angiotensinogen. Cell 1992; 71:169-180.

49   Inoue I, Nakajima T, Williams CS, Quackenbush J, Puryear R, Powers M et al. A nucleotide substitution in the promoter of human angiotensinogen is associated with essential hypertension and affects basal transcription in vitro. J Clin Invest 1997; 99:1786-1797.

50   Staessen JA, Kuzentsova T, Wang JG, Emelianov D, Vlietinck R, Fagard R. M235T angiotensinogen gene polymorphism and cardiovascular renal risk. J Hypertens 1999; 17:9-17.

51   Rogus JJ, Moczulski D, Freire MBS, Yang Y, Warram JH, Krolewski AS. Diabetic nephropathy is associated with AGT polymorphism 235 - results of a family-based study. Hypertension 1998; 31:627-631.

52   Bonnardeaux A, Davies E, Jeunemaitre X, Fery AC, Clauser E, Tiret L et al. Angiotensin II Type 1 Receptor Gene Polymorphism in Human Essential Hypertension. Hypertension 1994; 24:63-69.

53   Miller JA, Thai K, Scholey JW. Angiotensin II type 1 receptor gene polymorphism predicts response to losartan and angiotensin II. Kidney Int 1999; 56:2173-2180.

54   Tiret L, Bonnardeaux A, Poirier O, Ricard S, Marques-Vidal P, Evans A et al. Synergistic effects of angiotensin-converting enzyme and angiotensin-II type 1 receptor gene polymorphisms on risk of myocardial infarction. Lancet 1994; 344:910-913.

55   Tarnow L, Cambien F, Rossing P, Nielsen FS, Hansen BV, Ricard S et al. Angiotensin II type 1 receptor gene polymorphism and diabetic microangiopathy. Nephrol Dial Transplant 1996; 11:1019-1023.

56   Chowdhury TA, Dyer PH, Kumar S, Gough SCL, Gibson SP, Rowe BR et al. Lack of association of angiotensin II type 1 receptor gene polymorphism with diabetic nephropathy in insulin-dependent diabetes mellitus. Diabetic Med 1997; 14:837-840.

57   Doria A, Onuma T, Warram JH, Krolewski AS. Synergistic effet of angiotensin II type 1 receptor genotype and poor glycaemic control on risk of nephropathy in IDDM. Diabetologia 1997; 40:1293-1299.

58   Savage DA, Feeney SA, Fogarty DG, Maxwell AP. Risk of developing diabetic nephropathy is not associated with synergism between the angiotensin II (type 1) receptor C1166 allele and poor glycaemic control. Nephrol Dial Transplant 1999; 14:891-894.

59   Tarnow L, Kjeld T, Knudsen E, Major-Pedersen A, Parving H-H. Lack of synergism between long-term poor glycaemic control and three gene polymorphisms of the renin angiotensin system on risk of developing diabetic nephropathy in Type 1 diabetic patients. Diabetologia 2000; 43:794-799.

60   Moczulski DK, Rogus JJ, Antonellis A, Warram JH, Krolewski AS. Major susceptibility locus for nephropathy in type 1 diabetes on chromosome 3q - results of novel discordant sib-pair analysis. Diab 1998; 47:1164-1169.

61   Imperatore G, Hanson RL, Pettitt DJ, Kobes S, Bennett PH, Knowler WC et al. Sib-pair linkage analysis for susceptibility genes for microvascular complications among Pima Indians with type 2 diabetes. Diab 1998; 47:821-830.

62   Angelico MC, Laffel L, Krolewski AS. Application of denaturing gradient gel electrophoresis to detect DNA polymorphisms in the renin gene in IDDM patients with and without diabetic nephropathy. In: Belfiore F, Bergman RN, Molinatti GM, editors. Current topics in diabetes research. Basel: Karger, 1993: 227-230.

63   Deinum J, Tarnow L, van Gool JM, de Bruin RA, Derkx FHM, Schalekamp MADH et al. Plasma renin and prorenin and renin gene variation in patients with insulin-dependent diabetes mellitus and nephropathy. Nephrol Dial Transplant 1999; 14:1904-1911.

64   Feldt-Rasmussen B. Microalbuminuria and clinical nephropathy in type 1 (insulin-dependent) diabetes mellitus: pathophysiological mechanisms and intervention studies. Dan Med Bull 1989; 36:405-415.

65   Jensen T, Stender S, Deckert T. Abnormalities in plasma concentrations of lipoproteins and fibrinogen in type 1 (insulin-dependent) diabetic patients with increased urinary albumin excretion. Diabetologia 1988; 31:142-145.

66   Deckert T, Feldt-Rasmussen B, Borch-Johnsen K, Jensen T, Kofoed-Enevoldsen A. Albuminuria reflects widespread vascular damage. The Steno hypothesis. Diabetologia 1989; 32:219-226.

67   Hansen PM, Chowdhury TA, Deckert T, Hellgren A, Bain SC, Pociot F. Genetic variation of the heparan sulfate proteoglycan gene (Perlecan gene) - association with urinary albumin excretion in IDDM patients. Diab 1997; 46:1658-1659.

68   Blakemore AIF, Cox A, Gonzalez A-M, Maskill JK, Hughes ME, Wilson RM et al. Interleukin-1 receptor antagonist allele (IL1RN*2) associated with nephropathy in diabetes mellitus. Hum Genet 1996; 97:369-374.

69   Tarnow L, Pociot F, Hansen PM, Rossing P, Nielsen FS, Hansen BV et al. Polymorphisms in the interleukin-1 gene cluster do not contribute to the genetic susceptibility of diabetic nephropathy in Caucasian patients with IDDM. Diab 1997; 46:1075-1076.

70   Loughrey BV, Maxwell AP, Fogarty DG, Middleton D, Harron JC, Patterson CC et al. An interleukin 1B allele, which correlates with a high secretor phenotype, is associated with diabetic nephropathy. Cytokine 1998; 10(12):984-988.

71   Pociot F, Hansen PM, Karlsen AE, Langdahl BL, Johannesen J, Nerup J. TGF-beta1 gene mutations in insulin-dependent diabetes mellitus and diabetic nephropathy. J Am Soc Nephrol 1998; 9:2302-2307.

72   Ng DPK, Warram JH, Krolewski AS. TGF-beta 1 as a genetic susceptibility locus for advanced diabetic nephropathy in type 1 diabetes mellitus: An investigation of multiple known DNA sequence variants. Am J Kidney Diseases 2003; 41(1):22-28.

73   Heesom AE, Hibberd ML, Millward A, Demaine AG. Polymorphism in the 5'-end of the aldose reductase gene is strongly associated with the development of diabetic nephropahty in type 1 diabetes. Diab 1997; 46:287-291.

74   Neamat-Allah M, Feeney S, Savage DA, Maxwell AP, Hanson RL, Knowler WC et al. Analysis of the association between diabetic nephropathy and polymorphisms in the aldose reductase gene in type 1 and type 2 diabetes mellitus. Diabet Med 2001; 18:906-914.

75   Poirier O, Nicaud V, Vionnet N, Raoux S, Tarnow L, Vlassara H et al. Polymorphism screening of four genes encoding advanced glycation end-product putative receptors - association study with nephropathy in type 1 diabetic patients. Diab 2001; 50:1214-1218.

76   Tarnow L, Grarup N, Hansen T, Parving H-H, Pedersen O. Diabetic microvascular complications are not associated with two polymorphisms in the GLUT-1 and PC-1 genes regulating glucose metabolism in Caucasian type 1 diabetic patients. Nephrol Dial Transplant 2001; 16:1653-1656.

77   Ng DPK, Canani LH, Araki S, Smiles A, Moczulski D, Warram JH et al. Minor effect of GLUT1 polymorphisms on susceptibility to diabetic nephropathy in type 1 diabetes. Diab 2002; 51:2264-2269.

78   Canani LH, Ng DPK, Smiles A, Rogus JJ, Warram JH, Krolewski AS. Polymorphism in ecto-nucleotide pyrophosphodiesterase 1 gene (ENPP1/PC-1) and early development of advanced diabetic nephropathy in type 1 diabetes. Diab 2002; 51:1188-1193.

79   Herrmann S-M, Ringel J, Wang J-G, Staessen JA, Brand E. Peroxisome Proliferator-activated receptor-gamma2 polymorphism Pro12Ala is associated with nephropathy in type 2 diabetes. Diab 2002; 51:2653-2657.

10

LOW BIRTH WEIGHT AND DIABETIC NEPHROPATHY

Susan E Jones and Jens R Nyengaard
University Hospital of Hartlepool, UK, and Aarhus University, Denmark

INTRODUCTION

Traditional risk factors for the development and progression of diabetic nephropathy include male sex, ethnicity, family history of hypertension or nephropathy, smoking and poor glycaemic control [1]. The genetics of diabetic nephropathy are incompletely understood the condition can develop in individuals in whom no 'traditional' risk factors are present.

Barker et al proposed that an individual could be 'programmed' in-utero to develop chronic diseases in adulthood such as hypertension [2], diabetes [3], and ischaemic heart disease [4]. Brenner proposed that essential hypertension was the result of reduction in glomerular number, which resulted in reduced total glomerular filtration surface area [5]. A unification of the Barker and Brenner hypotheses would be that individuals of low birth weight (LBW) would, due to adverse intra-uterine environment, have reduced glomerular number and if they developed diabetes in adulthood they would be more likely to develop diabetic nephropathy.

Both prospective animal and retrospective human studies have attempted address the role of intra-uterine environment in the development of diabetic nephropathy and this review will outline these.

EMBRYOLOGY AND INFLUENCES ON NEPHROGENESIS

The embryological development of the kidney is tightly regulated and involves a variety of cytokines and growth factors [6]. In vitro studies have shown that manipulation of matrix during glomerular morphogenesis may generate less developed nephrons [7]. In vivo studies have shown that a variety of intra-uterine insults such as gentamicin [8, 9] number and protein restriction [10, 11] can reduce glomerular number in rats.

THE BARKER HYPOTHESIS

Malnutrition in early pregnancy may result in symmetrically small babies with LBW. Mid-pregnancy malnutrition, the time of maximal placental growth, may result in a small baby and placental hypertophy. Final trimester malnutrition, the time of maximal fetal weight gain, may produce thin babies. Thus, there are a variety of markers of intra-uterine malnutrition: low birth weight, low birth weight relative to placental weight or low ponderal index (birth weight / length^3) [12].

A retrospective study among 5,664 men born in Hertfordshire, UK between 1911 and 1930 demonstrated an association between those of lowest birth weight, or lowest weight at age 1 year and deaths from ischaemic hear disease. This suggested a link between intra-uterine environment and cardiovascular disease [4] and this study also demonstrated that low ponderal index (abnormal thinness) was associated with cardiovascular disease in adulthood.

A further series of retrospective studies using a cohort on 449 men and women born between 1935 and 1942 in Preston, Lancashire, UK who still lived in the area were studied because there were extremely detailed maternity records for these people. Systolic and diastolic blood pressure, were strongly associated with placental weight at birth in both men and women [2]. An association between the development of both impaired glucose tolerance and Type 2 diabetes mellitus and LBW was also demonstrated [3].

Changes in hormone levels occur during fetal life [13]. Extensive research has focused upon changes in maternal glucocorticoids [14, 15] to explain the association between LBW and hypertension. It is hypothesised that dysfunction of the placental glucocorticoid barrier results in increased fetal exposure to maternal glucocorticoids which, in turn, effects the development of fetal vessels and thus increases the risk of adulthood hypertension [14].

STUDIES INVESTIGATING THE BARKER HYPOTHESIS

Large epidemiological studies of offspring of mothers exposed to malnutrition whilst pregnant include the Dutch Hunger Winter Study [16] and the Leningrad Siege Study [17].

The Dutch Hunger Winter Study (a cohort born between 1944 and 1946 in Amsterdam) demonstrated that first trimester exposure to intra-uterine malnutrition was associated with increased waist-hip ratio in adulthood but there was no effect on birth weight. In contrast, third trimester malnutrition reduced both birth weight and adulthood adiposity. A follow-up study of offspring of mothers from the original cohort demonstrated that infants born to these women did not show the expected increase in birth weight with increasing birth order [18]. This effect was observed in those offspring of mothers who were exposed to intra-uterine malnutrition during the first trimester and suggests that there are long-term biological effects that are independent of maternal birth weight which influence subsequent generations.

The Leningrad Siege Study compared two groups of offspring from Leningrad; those born during the siege (1941 – 1944) as an intra-uterine malnutrition group, those born before the siege as an infant malnutrition group; and a group from outside the city as an unexposed group. In contrast to Barker's studies there was no difference between the intra-uterine and infant groups with respect to the following: glucose intolerance, insulin concentration, blood pressure and lipid levels. Despite the problems of the lack of accurate birth weight data and low case ascertainment (only 44% of eligible subjects were screened) this study subjects that intra-uterine malnutrition does not have a major role in the pathogenesis of adulthood glucose intolerance and hypertension [17].

Extreme malnutrition may have little relevance to the general population and a number of studies have retrospectively examined the effects of birth weight on the development of chronic disease in adulthood using normal subjects. Results from large studies are shown in Table 1.

Table 1: Summary of large studies investigating the Barker Hypothesis

Study	Subjects and design	Ascertainment	Source data	Outcome measures	Conclusion
Health Professionals Follow-up Study USA [19]	22,846 males Postal questionnaire.	60%	Self reported BW.	Self reported BP Self reported DM Self reported weight.	LBW associated with hypertension Diabetes Obesity.
Nurses' Health Study [20, 21]	70,297 Postal questionnaire.	60%	Self reported BW.	As above.	As above.
Uppsala Sweden [22]	13,282 singleton births surviving beyond 1 yr. Born 1915 – 1929.	97%	Detailed maternity Records Linkage and census data.	CV mortality	LBW males have: Reduced fetal growth associated with: Increased CV mortality.
Helsinki Finland [23]	3,302 males Born 1924 – 1933.	92%	Detailed maternity records.	CV Mortality	LBW not associated with increased CV mortality Low ponderal index and low maternal BMI associated with increased CV mortality.
Stockholm Sweden [24]	2,237 males Born 1938 – 1957.	79%	Self reported BW.	DM IGT	Association with LBW strongest in those with a family history of diabetes.
Israel [25]	19,734 males, 12, 846 females. Born 1964 – 1971.	95.2%	Maternity records.	Blood pressure	Current BMI predicted BP.
Israel [26]	6,684 males, 4,199 females. Born 1974 – 1976.	97.1%	As above Maternal BMI.	Blood pressure	Low maternal BMI correlated with BP.

THE BRENNER HYPOTHESIS

Glomerular number shows wide biological variation in both humans (400,000 – 1,200,000) [27, 28] and rats (20,000 – 35,000) [11, 29]. Brenner et al, proposed that individuals with a mean glomerular number at the lower end of or below the physiological range are at increased risk of developing hypertension [5], due to a reduction in total filtration surface area. During the growth phase of a human being, hypertension may result in glomerular capillary hypertension and later on in glomerular sclerosis, which will further reduce the total glomerular filtration surface area, thus perpetuating a vicious cycle [30].

A variety of post-mortem studies in neonates have shown that intra-uterine growth retardation is associated with a reduction in glomerular number [31 – 33]. These studies may not be relevant to the general population because retrospective post mortem studies in adults with a higher birth weights do not show a relationship between birth weight and glomerular number [34]. The lack of relationship between birth weight and glomerular number is also demonstrated in animal studies [35, 36] and even in the IUGR studies there is no linear relationship between birth weight and glomerular number [33].

The mechanism by which glomerular number is reduced is uncertain but exogenous factors acting on the fetus may be important. Vitamin A and its derivatives play a role in nephrogenesis [37] and vitamin A deficiency is associated with renal abnormalities [38] and reduced glomerular number [39]. Low circulating levels of Vitamin A occur in women who smoke, abuse alcohol or adopt extreme weight reducing diets [40, 41]. Whether this reduction in Vitamin A levels is sufficient to reduce glomerular number is uncertain. Maternal smoking reduces birth weight [42] and in Manalich's study [33] maternal smoking status was a stronger determinant of glomerular number than birth weight itself.

Surgical reduction in glomerular number by unilateral nephrectomy in childhood [43], and unilateral renal agenesis [44] are associated with increased risk of hypertension but the prevalence of hypertension in adults undergoing nephrectomy are small [43]. These findings suggest that the early reduction in glomerular number in the pathogenesis of hypertension but the majority of people with hypertension have not undergone nephrectomy and do not have renal agenesis.

THE RELATIONSHIP BETWEEN LOW BIRTH WEIGHT, SYSTOLIC BLOOD PRESSURE AND GLOMERULAR NUMBER

Hypertension is an independent risk factor for the development of chronic diseases in adulthood such as ischaemic heart disease [45, 46] and its presence prior to the development of diabetes increases the risk of developing diabetic nephropathy [47 – 49]. All of the large epidemiological studies investigating the link between hypertension and LBW have been unable to determine whether this association was due to a reduction in glomerular number. It is likely that other factors such as family history, adulthood obesity and smoking are much more important in the pathogenesis of hypertension.

Very few published animal studies have measured systolic blood pressure and estimated glomerular number in LBW rats. In studies using intra-uterine low protein diet, rats exposed to low protein diet have reduced glomerular number, raised systolic blood pressure and lower birth weights compared to controls [36, 50]. This suggests that the relationship between LBW and systolic blood pressure may only hold true in a LBW individual was exposed to an abnormal intra-uterine environment, which in turn impaired renal development and reduced glomerular number. Even if this is true, interaction with other risk factors may be required to develop hypertension.

A small post-mortem study estimated glomerular number and volume in hypertensive Caucasian men (age range 35 – 59) and compared results to age height and weight matched normotensive controls [51]. This study demonstrated a reduction in glomerular number (median 702,379 Vs 1,429,200) and an increase in glomerular volume (median 6.50 x10-3 mm^3 Vs 2.79 x 10-3 mm^3) and there did not appear to be an increase in glomerular sclerosis in the hypertensive group. This study did not control for smoking status or family history of hypertension and the methodology used could have led to underestimation of glomerular volume. Birth weight data were not available for the subjects in this study and as such it is difficult to determine whether the reduction in glomerular number was due to adverse intra-uterine environment or as a consequence of hypertension itself.

Studies in populations with high rates of renal disease may provide more insight into the link between glomerular number and hypertension and one such population is the Aboriginals of Australia. An ultrasound study of 174 Aboriginal children and adolescents aged 5 – 18 years showed that the average renal size, corrected for current body size, was reduced in LBW children [52].

Obviously, this study could not estimate glomerular number. The authors suggested that the reduction in renal size with reduced birth weight may be a mechanism to explain the increased incidence of renal disease in this community, but the lack of estimation of renal size in age matched Caucasian controls weakens this augment. Autopsy studies have shown that Aboriginals have increase glomerular volume compared to Caucasians [53] but this population have high rates of post-streptococcal glomerulonephritis and this could have influenced the results. A study using a single albumin: creatinine ratio and self reported birth weights suggested that, amongst the Aboriginal population, increasing body mass index, blood pressure and LBW act together to increase urine albumin excretion with age [54]. This study was limited by incomplete ascertainment of birth weight amongst the older subjects in the study.

LOW BIRTH WEIGHT, GLOMERULAR NUMBER AND DIABETIC NEPHROPATHY

The variation in expression of renal disease among, for example, diabetic patients could be explained by the large variation in glomerular number and size within these patients [55, 56, 57]. The unification of the Barker and Brenner hypotheses is that intrauterine compromise, by whatever mechanism, generates LBW babies, which have smaller kidney with fewer glomeruli and / or smaller glomeruli.

These glomerular changes result in decreased total glomerular filtration surface area, giving rise to reduced total filtration surface area resulting in glomerular hypertension due to reduced renal functional reserve. The diabetic patients with the least and / or smallest glomeruli will then be more prone to develop irreversible renal failure when exposed to a renal insult in later life. Such a unification of the Barker and Brenner hypothesis within respect to diabetic nephropathy is disputed.

Rats exposed to low protein diet (LPD) in utero have reduced birth weight, smaller kidneys and hypertension compared to those exposed to normal protein diet (NPD) in utero [36, 50]. One study has examined the acute renal response to streptozotocin diabetes in LPD rats [36]. LPD rats demonstrate a greater proportional increase in glomerular volume and renal size in response to diabetes compared to NPD rats and they fail to normalise glomerular volume with insulin. Human studies suggest that persistent renal enlargement following normalisation of blood glucose in newly diagnosed Type 1 diabetes predisposes to the development of diabetic nephropathy [58] but long term data of renal changes diabetes in LPD rats is awaited. Despite the lack of long-term data the LPD rat study supports the unification of the Barker and Brenner and hypotheses.

Only one human study demonstrates a direct relationship between birth weight and proteinuria in diabetic subjects [59] and short stature, a putative marker of LBW, has been linked to the development of diabetic nephropathy [60].

Other retrospective studies in diabetic subjects challenge the unification of the Barker and Brenner and hypotheses: 1) there was no difference in birth weight between 25 Type 1 diabetic patients and 22 patients without diabetic nephropathy [61]. 2) There was no correlation between LBW, few and / or small glomeruli or low kidney weight and there was no difference in the four parameters in 19 control subjects and 22 Type 2 diabetic patients [34], see also figures 1 and 2 and table 2. 3) A large epidemiological study of 620 Caucasian non-diabetic subjects showed no correlation between birth weight, blood pressure and urinary albumin excretion [62] 4) Subjects in the Leningrad Siege study showed no relationship between intra-uterine malnutrition and urine albumin excretion [63] 5) Birth weight was not associated with progression of established diabetic nephropathy in 161 type 1 diabetic patients [64].

Table 2. The sex, age, kidney weight, glomerular number and size, and birth weight on 19 normal persons and 26 Type 2 diabetic patients (from ref 34). Data are expressed as mean + SD and (range) unless otherwise stated

	Controls	Type 2 Diabetes
Sex (m = males f = females)	8m / 11f	14m / 12f
Age (years)	59 ± 16 (34 – 87)	63 ± 11 (35 – 85)
Kidney Weight (grams)	137 ± 36 (91 – 206)	150 ± 38 (82 – 228)
Glomerular number per kidney (10^3)	670 ± 176 (393 – 1056)	673 ± 200 (379 – 1124)
Mean glomerular volume ($10^6 \ \mu m^3$)	6.25 ± 1.48 (3.95 – 8.97)	5.71 ± 1.74 (2.81 – 9.18)
Birth weight (grams)	$3\ 577 \pm 400$ (2 900 – 4 250)	$3\ 489 \pm 429$ (2 750 – 4 500)

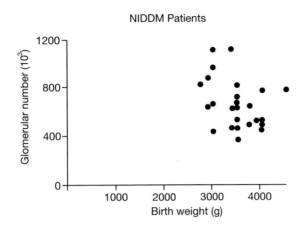

Fig 1. There is no significant correlation (r = -0.33, p = 0.10) between birth weight and total glomerular number per kidney in 26 Type 2 diabetic subjects (from ref. 34 with permission)

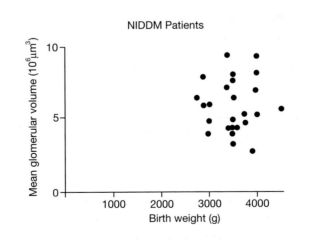

Fig 2. There is no significant correlation (r = 0.06, p = 0.78) between birth weight and mean glomerular volume in 26 Type 2 diabetic subjects (from ref. 34 with permission)

CONCLUSION

The unification of the Brenner and Barker hypotheses is based on observations that LBW results in high blood pressure and impaired glucose tolerance in adult life; that LBW results in low nephron number; and that low nephron number results in high blood pressure. It is likely that infants of very LBW at term (<2,500g) and those with intra-uterine growth retardation may have fewer and/or smaller glomeruli. In the developed world the incidence of LBW is approximately 7% of all live birth births [65] but the prevalence of diabetes is 2 – 3% per population [66] and approximately one third of diabetic subjects will develop diabetic nephropathy [1]. These figures suggest that intra-uterine environment on its own is not a major risk factor for the development of diabetic nephropathy. Thus, it remains difficult to support the unification of the Barker and Brenner hypotheses with respect to diabetic nephropathy in the developed world. However, It may turn out to be different in third world countries.

REFERENCES

1.   Viberti G-C, Walker J, Pinto J. Diabetic Nephropathy. In: Alberti K, Defronzo R, Keen H and Zimmet P, eds. The International Textbook of Diabetes. 1992; Vol 2: 1267 – 1328. John Wiley & Sons, Chichester.
2.   Barker D, Bull A, Osmond C, Simmonds S. Fetal and placental size and risk of hypertension in adult life. Br Med J 1990; 302: 259 – 262
3.   Barker D, Hales C, Fall C, Osmond C, Phipps K, Clark P. Type 2 (non-insulin dependent) diabetes mellitus, hypertension and hyperlipidaemia (syndrome X): relation to reduced fetal growth. Diabetologia 1993; 36: 62 – 67
4.   Barker D, Osmond C, Winter P, Margetts B, Simmonds S. Weight in infancy and death from ischaemic heart disease. Lancet 1989: 577 – 580
5.   Brenner B, Garcia D, Anderson S. Glomeruli and blood pressure: less of one and more of the other? Am J Hypertension 1988; 1: 335 – 347
6.   Bard J, Wolf A. Nephrogenesis and the development of renal disease. Nephrol Dial Transplant 1992; 7: 563 – 572
7.   Bard J. traction and the formation of mesenchymal condensations in vitro. BioEssays 1990; 12: 389 – 393
8.   Gilbert T, Lelièvre-Pérgorier M, Merlet-Bénichou C. Immediate and long-term renal effects of fetal exposure to gentamicin. Pediatric Nephrol 1990; 8: 175 – 180
9.   Gilbert T, Lelièvre-Pérgorier M, Merlet-Bénichou C. Long-term effects of mild oligonephronia induced in utero by gentamicin in the rat. Pediatric Res 1991; 30: 450 – 456
10. Zeman F. Effects of maternal protein restriction on the kidneys of newborn young of rats. J Nutrition 1968; 94: 111 – 116

11. Merlet-Bénichou C, Gilbert T, Muffat-Joly M, Lelièvre-Pérgorier M, Leroy B. Intra-uterine growth retardation leads to permanent nephron deficit in the rat. Pediatric Nephrol 1994; 8: 175 – 180

12. Barker D. Mothers, babies and disease in later life. Churchill Publishing. London 1994

13. Edwards C, Benediktsson R, Lindsay R, Seckle J. Dysfunction of the placental glucocorticoid barrier: link between fetal environment and adult hypertension? Lancet 1993; 341: 355 – 357

14. Garrett P, Bass P, Sanderman D. Barker and babies – early environment and renal disease in adulthood. J Pathol 1994; 173: 299 – 300

15. Benedicktsson R, Lindsay R, Noble J, Seckle J, Edwards C. Glucocorticoid exposure in utero: new model for adult hypertension. Lancet 1993; 341: 339 – 341

16. Jackson A, Langley-Evans S, McCarthy H. Nutritional influences in early life upon obesity and other body proportions. Ciba Foundation Symposium 1996; 201: 118 – 129

17. Stanner S, Bulmer K, Andres C, Lantseva O, Borodina V, Poteen V, Yudkin J. Does malnutrition in utero determine diabetes mellitus and coronary heart disease in adulthood? Results from the Leningrad siege, a cross sectional study. Br Med J 1997; 315: 1342 – 1348

18. Lumey L, Stein A. Offspring birth weights after maternal intrauterine undernutrition: a comparison within sibships. Am J Epidemiol 1997; 146: 801 – 809

19. Curhan G, Willett W, Rimm E, Spiegelman D, Ascherio A, Stampfer M. Birth weight and adult hypertension, diabetes mellitus and obesity in US men. Circulation 1996; 94: 1310 – 1315

20. Curhan G, Chetow G, Willett W, Spiegleman D, Colditz G, Manson J, Lithell U-B, McKeigue P. Birth weight and adult hypertension and obesity in US women. Circulation 1996; 94: 1310 – 1315

21. Rich-Edwards J, Stampfer M, Manson J Rosner B, Hankinson S, Colditz G, Willett W, Hennekens CH. Birth weight and risk of cardiovascular disease in a cohort of women followed up since 1976. Br Med J 315; 396 – 400

22. Leon D, Lithell H, Vagero D, Koupilova I, Mohsen R, Berglund L, Lithell U-B, McKeigue P. Reduced fetal growth rate and increased risk of death from ischaemic heart disease: cohort study of 15 000 Swedish men and women born 1915 – 29. Br Med J 1998; 317: 241 – 245

23. Forsén T, Eriksson J, Toumielehto J, Teramo K, Osmond C, Barker D. Mother's weight in pregnancy and coronary heart disease in a cohort of Finnish men: follow up study. Br Med J 1997; 315: 837 – 840

24. Carlsson S, Persson P-G, Alvarsson M, Efendic S, Norman A, Svanström L, Östenson C-G, Grill V. Low birth weight and family history of diabetes and glucose intolerance in Swedish middle aged mean. Diabetes Care 1999; 22: 1043 – 1047

25. Seidman D, Laor A, Galc R, Stevenson D, Mashiach S, Danon Y,. Birth weight, current body weight and blood pressure in late adolescence. Br Med J 1991; 302: 1235 – 1237

26. Laor A, Stevenson D, Sherner J, Gale R, Seidman D. Size at birth, maternal nutritional status in pregnancy and blood pressure at age 17: a population based analysis. Br Med J 1997; 48: 153 – 168

27. Moor R. The total number of glomeruli in the normal human kidney. Anat Rec 1931; 48:153 – 168

28. Tischer C, Madsen K. Anatomy of the kidney. In: Brenner B, Rector F, eds. The Kidney 3rd edition. 1986: 3 – 60. WB Saunders, Philadelphia:

29. Larsson L, Aperia A, Wilton P. Effect of normal development on compensatory renal growth. Kidney Int. 1980; 18: 29 – 35

30. Brenner B, Chertow G. Congenital oligonephropathy and the etiology of adult hypertension and progressive renal injury. Am J Kidney Dis 1994; 23: 171 – 175

31. Hinchcliffe S, Lynch M, Sargent P, Howard C, van Velzen D. The effect of intra-uterine growth retardation on the development of nephrons. Br J Obstet Gynaecol 1992; 99: 296 – 301

32. Leroy B, Josset P, Morgan G, Costill J, Merlet-Benichou C. Intrauterine growth retardation (IUGR) and nephron deficit: Preliminary study in man. Pediatric Nephrol 1992; 6: 21C

33. Manalich R, Reeves L, Herrara M, Melendi C, Fundora I. Relationship between weight at birth and the number and size of renal glomeruli in humans: a histomorphometric study. Kidney Int 2000; 58: 770 – 773

34. Nyengaard J, Bendtsen T, Mogensen C. Low birth weight – is it associated with few and small glomeruli in normal subjects and NIDDM patients? Diabetologia 1996; 39:1634 – 1637

35. Jones S, Nyengaard R, Flyvbjerg A, Bilous R, Marshall S. Birth weight has no influence on glomerular number and volume. Pediatric Nephrol 2001; 16: 340 – 345

36. Jones S, Bilous R, Flyvbjerg A, Marshall S. Intra-uterine environment influences glomerular number and the acute renal adaptation to experimental diabetes. Diabetologia 2001; 44: 721 – 728

37. Vilar J, Gilbert T, Moreau E, Merlet- Bénichou C. Metanephros organogenesis is highly stimulated by vitamin A derivatives in organ culture. Kidney Int 1996; 49: 1478 – 1487

38. Wilson J, Warkney J. Malformations in the genito-urinary tract induced by maternal Vitamin A deficiency in the rat. Am J Anat 1948; 83: 357 – 407

39. Lelièvere-Pégorier M, Villar J, Ferrier M, Moreau E, Freund N, Gilbert T, Merlet-Bénichou C. Mild Vitamin A deficiency leads to inborn nephron deficit in the rat. Kidney Int 1998; 54: 1455 – 1462

40. Gerster H. Vitamin A: Functions, dietary requirements and safety in humans. Int J Vitam Nutr Res 1997; 67: 71 – 90

41. Bonjour J. Vitamins and alcoholism IX. Vitamin A. Int J Vitam Nutr Res 1981; 51: 166 – 177

42. Baeulac-Baillargeon L, Desrosiers C. Caffeine – cigarette interaction on fetal growth. Am J Obstet Gynae 1987; 157: 1236 – 1240

43. Hakim R, Goldszer R, Brenner B. Hypertension and proteinuria; Long-term sequelae of unilateral nephrectomy. Kidney Int 1984; 25: 930 – 936

44. Argueso L, Richley M, Boyle E, Milliner D, Bergstrahl E, Kramer S. Prognosis of patients with unilateral agenesis. Pediatric Nephrol 1992; 6: 412 – 416

45. Shaper A, Pocock S, Walker M et al British Regional Heart Study: cardiovascular risk factors in middle aged men in 24 towns. Br Med J 1981; 283: 179 – 186

46. Stamler S, Bulmer K, Andres C et al. Diabetes, other risk factors and 12 – yr cardiovascular mortality for men screened in the Multiple Risk Factor Intervention Trial. Diabetes Care 1993; 16: 434 – 444

47. Viberti G, Keen H, Wiseman M. Raised arterial blood pressure in the parents of proteinuric insulin dependent diabetics. Br Med J 1985 295 515 - 517

48. Krolewski A, Canessa M, Warram J et al. Predisposition to hypertension and susceptibility to renal disease in insulin-dependent diabetes mellitus. New Engl J Med 1988; 318: 140 – 145

49. Nelson R, Bennett P, Beck G et al. Development and progression of renal disease in Pima Indians with non-insulin dependent diabetes mellitus. New Engl J Med 1996; 335: 1636 – 1642

50. Langley- Evans S, Welham S, Jackson A. Fetal exposure to low protein diet impairs nephrogenesis and promotes hypertension in the rat. Life Sci 1999; 64: 965 – 974

51. Keller G, Zimmer G, Mall G, Ritz E, Amann K. Nephron number in patients with primary hypertension. New Engl J Med 2003; 348: 101 – 108

52. Spencer J, Wang Z, Hoy W. Low birth weight and reduced renal volume in Aboriginal children. Am J Kidney Dis 2002; 37: 915 - 920

53. Young R, Hoy W, Kincaid-Smith P, Seymour A, Bertram J. Glomerular size and glomerulosclerosis in Australian Aborigines. AM J Kidney Dis 2000; 36: 481 – 489

54. Hoy W, Mathews J Pugsley D, Hayhurst B, Rees M, Kile E, Walker K, Wang Z. The multi-dimensional nature of renal disease: Rates and associations of albuminuria in an Australian Aboriginal community. Kidney Int 1998; 54: 1296 – 1304

55. Bendtsen T, Nyengaard J. The number of glomeruli in Type 1 (insulin dependent) and Type 2 (non-insulin dependent) diabetic patients. Diabetologia 1992; 35: 844 – 850

56. Nyengaard J, Bendsten T. Glomerular number and size in relation to age, kidney weight and body surface area in normal man. Anat Rec 1992; 35: 844 – 850

57. Wendy EH, Douglas-Denton RN, Hughson MD, Cass A, Johnson K, Bertram JF. A stereological study of glomerular number and volume: Preliminary findings in a multiracial study of kidneys at autopsy. Kidney Int 2003; 63: S31-S37

58. Baumgartl H, Banholzer P, Sigl G et al. On the prognosis of IDDM patients with large kidneys. The role of large kidneys for the development of diabetic nephropathy. Nephrol Dial Transplant 1998; 13: 630 – 634

59. Sanderman D, Reza M, Philips D, Barker D, Osmond C, Leatherdale B. Why do some diabetics develop nephropathy? A possible role of birth weight. Diabetic Med 1992; 9(Suppl 1); 36A

60. Rossing P, Tarnow L, Neilsen F, Boelskiftes S, Brenner B, Parving H-H. Short stature and diabetic nephropathy. Br Med J 1995; 310: 296 – 297

61. Eshøj O, Vaag A, Feldt-Ramussen B, Borch-Johnsen K, Beck-Neilsen H. No evidence of low birth weight as a risk factor for diabetic nephropathy in type 1 diabetic patients. Diabetologia 1995; 38 (Suppl 1): A 222

62. Vestbo E, Damsgaard E, Frøland A, Mogensen CE. Birth weight and cardiovascular factors in an epidemiological study. Diabetologia 1996; 39: 1598 – 1602

63. Yudkin J, Philips D, Stanner S. Proteinuria and progressive renal disease: birth weight and microalbuminuria. Nephol Dial Trans 1997; 12 (Supp 2): 10 – 13

64. Jacobsen P, Rossing P, Tarnow L, Hovind P, Parving H-H Birth weight – a risk factor for progression in diabetic nephropathy? J Int Med 2003; 253: 343-350

65. Macfarlane A, Mugford M. Birth Counts. Statistics of pregnancy and childbirth. 2000 Vol 1 & 2 HMSO Books: London

66. Amos A, McCarty D, Zimmet P The rising global burden of diabetes and its complications: Estimates and projections to the year 2010. Diabetic Med 1997; 14: S1 - 85

11

EFFECTS OF INSULIN ON THE CARDIOVASCULAR SYSTEM AND THE KIDNEY

Andrea Natali, Monica Nannipieri, and Ele Ferrannini
Department of Internal Medicine and Metabolism Unit, C N R Institute of Clinical Physiology at the University of Pisa School of Medicine, Pisa, Italy.

THE CARDIOVASCULAR SYSTEM

While *in vitro* studies have long considered the vascular effects of insulin (with a focus on the vascular complications of diabetes), at the physiological level the concept that exogenous insulin administration may be associated with haemodynamic changes [1] have mostly been circumscribed to the counter-regulatory (mainly adrenergic) hormonal response to insulin-induced hypoglycaemia. It has not been until the introduction of the glucose clamp technique, by which hyperinsulinaemia can be uncoupled from hypoglycaemia, that the existence of vascular actions of the hormone has been recognised. Interest has initially focused on insulin-induced vasodilatation [2]; more recently, a wider range of effects of insulin on microcirculation, vascular reactivity and central haemodynamics has been characterised, and their possible physiological significance is beginning to be appreciated.

Peripheral vascular resistance
The effect of pharmachologic concentrations of insulin has been assessed in various vascular preparations (aortic rings, mesenteric arteries, cremastere arteries) and all studies agree on a direct vasodilatatory effect of insulin [3-6]. Also in humans several studies [7,8] have established that insulin infusion with maintenance of glycaemia is followed by an increase in limb blood flow in healthy, young volunteers. Typically in these studies, sustained

hyperinsulinaemia (in the range of 300-700 pmol/l for 3-4 h) was followed by an increase in leg or forearm blood flow, as measured by thermodilution or pletysmography, amounting to 30-100% above baseline values. This effect was found to be blunted in patients with insulin resistance of glucose uptake (i.e, in obese [7], hypertensive [9] or diabetic subjects [10,11]). The relevance of this effect in explaining the reduced peripheral tissues insulin sensitivity has been challenged by the observation that it occurs only for unphysiologic insulin exposures. By compiling a vast amount of data in the literature [12], the relationship between insulin exposure (concentration x time) and changes in blood flow can be schematised as depicted in Fig. 1: within the physiological range of insulin exposure (the darker shade), limb blood flow may rise up to 30% of its baseline value, with a rather wide scatter depending on the experimental circumstances.

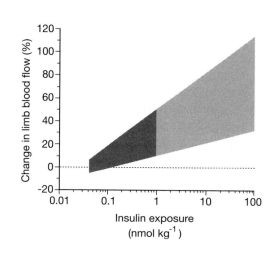

Fig. 1 Relationship between insulin exposure (expressed as total amount infused per kilogram body weight or per 10 kg of forearm muscle, for systemic intravenous and local intra-arterial administration, respectively) and percent change in limb blood flow (re-calculated from ref. [12]).

The few studies that have measured blood flow in response to a meal have consistently failed to observe significant peripheral vasodilatation [13-15]. On these grounds, it has been argued that insulin-induced vasodilatation is not an important determinant of insulin's metabolic effects. A possible objection is that if tissue perfusion increases in insulin sensitive but decreases in non-insulin sensitive tissues then total blood flow will not be substantially altered. Recent PET studies [16] have indeed shown that leg muscle blood flow is distributed in a heterogeneous pattern, and that glucose uptake tends to co-localise with higher perfusion rates in response to strong insulin stimulation. However, no difference between normal subjects and insulin resistant type 2 diabetic patients has been observed. These findings may simply reflect regional differences in muscle fibre composition, as oxidative type I fibres are both more sensitive to insulin and more richly capillarised [17]. By itself, co-localisation of flow and metabolism does not prove that insulin actually recruits previously unperfused or underperfused areas, thereby exposing more tissue to its metabolic action. Indeed, when a quantitative analysis of the co-localisation of insulin-stimulated blood flow and glucose uptake was performed the two were found to be spatially dissociated [18]. An increase in muscle tissue perfusion (nutritive blood flow) after insulin exposure has been observed in some studies, but not in all, probably depending on the intrinsic difficulty of blood flow measurement as well as methodological differences (glucose tracers [19], echographic indices of tissue perfusion [20], microdialysis [21], capillary microscopy [22], positron emission tomography [23]). The relevance of vasodilatation to the metabolic tissue response to insulin has been challenged also by a series of studies that have unsuccessfully tried to improve insulin action by acutely increasing tissue perfusion. Thus, in insulin resistant patients with essential hypertension the intra-arterial infusion of an endogenous vasodilator, adenosine [24], or of a direct nitric oxide (NO) donor, sodium nitroprusside [25], fails to overcome the metabolic insulin resistance. On the other hand, local infusion of high doses of vitamin C, by removing the inhibitory effect of oxidative stress on endothelial NO synthase, induces an increase in forearm blood flow during systemic insulin infusion also in insulin resistant subjects; this response, however, is not accompanied by an enhancement in glucose uptake [26]. Collectively, these observations indicate that exposure to acute insulinisation is followed by a modest increase in limb blood flow and this haemodynamic effect in humans is of limited consequence for insulin stimulation of glucose uptake at least within the physiological range of insulin concentrations.

The mechanisms by which insulin increases blood flow are not entirely clear. Neither adrenergic nor cholinergic blockade abolishes insulin-induced stimulation of calf blood flow [27], whilst both NG-monomethyl-L-arginine (L-NMMA), a competitive inhibitor of NO synthase [28,29], and ouabain [30], which blocks the insulin-stimulatable sodium potassium pump, have been shown to antagonise the vasodilatation induced by systemic hyperinsulinaemia. When infused locally insulin shows vascular effects that are blocked by propranolol, suggesting a ß-adrenergic component to the vasoactive action of insulin [31,32]. Therefore at least three pathways appear to be involved in the direct vascular action of insulin: hyperpolarization, NO/cGMP, and ß-adrenergic/cAMP. This heterogeneous effect of insulin has been confirmed *in vitro*: in smooth muscle cells, insulin induces an increase in both cAMP and cGMP that is receptor mediated and, for cGMP only, in part NO-dependent [33]. At pharmacologic concentrations, insulin stimulates NO synthesis in human endothelial cells; this effect is dependent on the number of insulin receptors, on their tyrosine kinase activity, and, downstream to the receptor, on both PI3 kinase and *Akt* signaling [34]. Insulin's effect on the endothelium is not limited to the stimulation of NO synthesis. In rat mesenteric arteries insulin vasodilatation is a transient phenomenon due to a parallel slow-onset stimulation of endothelin synthesis [5].

Therefore, the vascular net effect effect of insulin results from the combination of the two opposite vasoactive stimuli (Fig. 2). In elegant experiments *in vitro* and in man, it has been recently shown that concurrent endothelin production masks the vasodilatatory effect of low physiologic hyperinsulinaemia [35,36]; this could be the mechanism underlying the reduced vascular effect of insulin in insulin resistant rats [6], which have an increased responsiveness to endothelin [37].

Thus, the two effects appear to have not only different time-course but also different dose-response characteristics, and may be differentially active depending on the associated conditions. Finally, a further degree of complexity stems from the observation that the effect of insulin might be different, and based on different mechanisms, at different levels along the arterial tree, with the smaller arterioles being more sensitive to insulin's vascular effect and their vasodilatation depending almost entirely on hyperpolarization and prostanoids [4,6].

Vascular reactivity

A number of *in vitro* studies have consistently shown that insulin attenuates the effect of various vasoconstrictors (norepinephrine [38], arginine vasopressin [39], angiotensin II [40], and serotonin [40]), and that this effect is not present in insulin resistant animals [41,42]. The mechanisms through which this anti-vasoconstrictor action is exerted is largely dependent on the calcium antagonistic properties of the hormone [43,44] although a role for endothelium-derived NO cannot be ruled out [35]. Insulin has been found to blunt agonist-evoked intracellular calcium excursions by interfering with both the receptor-operated and the voltage-operated channels [40, 45]. Interestingly, both *ex vivo* [46] and *in vitro* insulin induces a small increase in unstimulated calcium concentration [44].

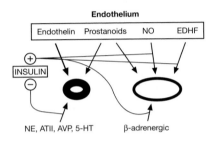

Fig. 2 Schematic summary of insulin effects on vascular reactivity. The principal vasoactive substances released by the vascular rendothelium exert vasoconstrictive (endothelin), vasodilating (NO and endothelium-derived hyperpolarizing factor [EDHF]) or mixed influences (prostanoids) on vascular tone. With the exception of potentiation of basal endothelin release, insulin generally interferes with this system both by potentiating vasodilating influences and by inhibiting vasoconstrictive actions. NE: norepinephrine, AVP: arginine vasopressine.

Although less consistently [47, 48], also in man insulin was found to counteract –α-adrenergic [32] and angiotensin II-mediated [49] vasocostriction when given intra-arterially. In the only study in which insulin and norepinephrine were given systemically, the former was able to blunt the rise in arterial blood pressure elicited by the latter, and this action of insulin was not present in the insulin resistant subjects [50]. All in all, the ability of insulin to blunt intracellular calcium transients makes the vasculature less sensitive to multiple vasoconstrictive agonists.

On the other hand, the vasodilatation induced by acetylcholine is enhanced by insulin while the effect of nitroprusside is not [51]. The mechanisms behind this potentiation are peculiar in that they appear to be influenced by the clinical condition. In fact, in normal subjects insulin potentiation of acetylcholine-induced vasodilatation is canceled by co-infusion of L-NAME, and thus involves facilitation of NO availability. In contrats, in patients with essential hypertension insulin potentiation of acetylcholine-induced vasodilatation is inhibited by ouabain. Both *in vitro* and *in vivo* insulin also facilitates the vasodilatation elicited by ß-adrenoceptor stimulation [32] and this effect is dependent on the presence of the endothelium [3].

In summary, insulin generally favours vasodilatation and blunts vasoconstriction (Fig. 2); however, the relevance of these actions to vascular homeostasis can be extremely variable since the three main effectors involved – NO, Na^+-K^+-ATPase and endothelin – show complex interactions [52] and are strongly modulated by genetic and environmental factors. Nevertheless, if insulin resistance extends to vascular tissues - as suggested by a study in genetically insulin resistant (fa/fa) rats in wich a selective impairment of the PI_3K/*Akt* pathway was observed in vascular endothelium [53] – then the vasculature of subjects with insulin resistance would be missing a protective factor. On the other hand, the possibility that vascular dysfunction causes insulin resistance, although theoretically plausible, has not found support in clinical studies in normal subjects and in patients with essential hypertension or obesity where vascular reactivity was found neither to segregate with insulin resistance of glucose metabolism nor with insulin resistance of vasodilatation [54-56].

Blood volume
Recent studies [57] have shown that administration of insulin in physiological doses under euglycaemic conditions leads to a 3% rise in haematocrit and a 7% reduction in blood volume, ie haemoconcentration. This effect, if small in size, is consistent, and closely related to the concomitant change in diastolic blood pressure levels (Fig. 3).

Loss of intravascular water to the extravascular space could be due to redistribution of blood flow to capillary beds with higher hydrostatic or lower oncotic pressure. Alternatively, insulin could vasoconstrict post-capillary venules, thereby leading to a generalised increase of the hydrostatic pressure in the capillary bed. The latter explanation is compatible with insulin-induced activation of the adrenergic nervous system (see below).

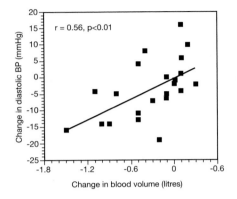

Fig. 3 Direct relationship between concomitant changes in blood volume and diastolic pressure induced by physiological hyperinsulinaemia (~600 pm~I1) under euglycaemic conditions. Note that the regression line predicts a 1 mmHg fall in blood pressure for each 0.1 litre decrease in blood volume.

Cardiac output and blood pressure

During systemic insulin administration at physiological doses, cardiac output increases by 10-15% as a result of a slight but consistent acceleration of heart rate (2 bpm on average) coupled with an increase in stroke volume [58]. These haemodynamic responses are mediated by adrenergic activation, as documented by a dose-dependent rise in circulating norepinephrine concentrations [59], an enhanced firing rate in the sympathetic fibres of the peroneal nerve, as measured by microneurography [8], and an upward shift in the sympathetic/vagal activity ratio, as measured by spectral analysis of heart rate variability [58]. The overall effect of simultaneous changes in cardiac output, blood volume, and peripheral vascular resistance in response to euglycaemic hyperinsulinaemia is maintenance of mean arterial blood pressure. This, however, is a compound of opposite changes in systolic and diastolic blood pressure. The former, in fact, tends to increase as cardiac dynamics are excited by enhanced adrenergic discharge, while the latter decreases due to the drop in peripheral vascular resistances (Table 1). It is interesting to note that the effects of insulin on the cardiovascular system are mediated by both peripheral reflexes and direct central neural influences.

Table 1. Haemodynamic effects of insulin under euglycaemic conditions

Effect	Change	Mechanism
Stroke volume	↑	Adrenergic stimulation
Heart rate	↑	Adrenergic stimulation
Blood volume	↑	Haemoconcentration
Peripheral vascular resistance	↓	Vasodilatation
Systolic blood pressure	↑	Adrenergic stimulation
Diastolic blood pressure	↓	Vasodilatation
Mean blood pressure	~	

Thus, direct relaxation of resistance arteries by insulin evokes tachycardia through the unloading of arterial baroreceptors, a reflex arch that involves central relays. In addition, insulin appears to directly desensitise the sinoatrial node to the baroreflex control of heart rate [58]. Mounting evidence [60], however, indicates that insulin, by trespassing (by transcytosis) the blood-brain barrier in the peri-ventricular area, binds to neurons in the arcuate and paraventricular nuclei, which then send inhibitory impulses to the vagus and excitatory impulses to the sympathetic nuclei. This reaction is completed by the release of corticotropin releasing hormone (CRH), which orchestrates a response including stimulation of cortisol and prolactin release and depression of growth hormone and thyroid-stimulating hormone [58,61]. Overall, even in the absence of hypoglycaemia the cardiovascular system responds to acute insulin administration with a moderate, specific stress reaction. Of note is that the pattern of haemodynamic responses to euglycaemic, physiologic hyperinsulinaemia is maintained in obesity, an insulin resistant state with a high-output, low-resistance haemodynamic pattern (Fig. 4) [58,62].

THE KIDNEY

Insulin and glomerular function
With regard to the effect of insulin on glomerular filtration rate (GFR), observations in the isolated kidney, in experimental animals, and in humans have yielded contradictory results, as decreased, increased or unchanged GFRs

have all been reported (reviewed in [63]). In healthy subjects under conditions of forced water diuresis - when changes in plasma volume are prevented - euglycaemic hyperinsulinaemia did not affect GFR [64]. Likewise, in a dose-response study in type I diabetic patients under fasting conditions, insulin was without significant effect on GFR [65]. Neither renal plasma flow (as measured with ^{131}I-hippuran) nor renal vascular resistances were affected by acute insulin administration. The role of plasma glucose concentration itself in the induction and/or maintenance of hyperfiltration has been controversial. During oral glucose loading, if large fluid volumes are co-administered, plasma volume and, in turn, GFR will increase.

On the other hand, a large glucose delivery to the proximal tubule could increase hydrostatic pressure in the tubular lumen, thereby leading to decreased GFR. Collectively, it appears that hyperglycaemia may be associated with small changes in GFR in either direction depending on factors such as duration of hyperglycaemia, hydration, and urine flow. An important question is whether insulin affects glomerular permeability to albumin and other proteins. We examined the acute effect of insulin on the systemic transcapillary escape rate (as measured by the ^{131}I-labelled albumin technique) and the excretion of albumin under time-controlled, steady-state conditions of glucose concentrations, urine output, blood pressure, and creatinine clearance [57]. While producing no significant change in albumin exit from the vascular compartment, physiological hyperinsulinaemia increased urinary albumin excretion by 50% in normoalbuminuric patients with type 2 diabetes but not in healthy subjects. In these patients, this effect was accompanied by an enhanced excretion of N-acetyl-β-D-glucosaminidase and retinol-binding protein - which are released and reabsorbed in the proximal tubule, respectively -, whereas the excretion of two proteins handled by the distal tubule (Tamm-Horsfall protein and epidermal growth factor) was unaffected (Fig. 4). These findings lend support to the notion that even modest increments in the glomerular permeability of albumin decrease the reabsorptive capacity of the proximal tubules, thereby leading to leakage of other tubular proteins. Moreover, this tubular albumin overload is intrinsically toxic to the interstitium, where it leads to the overexpression of inflammatory and vasoactive molecules [66,67]. Thus, perturbation of the glomerulo-tubular feed-back, rather than solely an increase in glomerular permeability, may be the trigger for nephropathy. In this context, the interaction between insulin and byperglycaemia on glomerulo-tubular function deserves further investigation as it may be an early sign of renal involvement in diabetes.

Insulin and tubular function

Specific binding of insulin is greatest in the thick ascending limb and distal convoluted tubules [68]. Insulin has been found to stimulate sodium transport in proximal tubules in the rabbit [69], and to increase chloride reabsorption by the loop segment in the rat [70]. Human studies, however, have indicated that the anti-natriuretic action of insulin takes place in the distal tubule [71,72]. Whether insulin affects sodium absorption by a direct effect on the renal tubules or through modulation of local or systemic factors that control sodium chloride reabsorption is still uncertain. Friedberg et al. [73], for example, reported that the anti-natriuretic effect of insulin could no longer be observed when insulin-induced hypokalaemia was prevented by simultaneous intravenous potassium administration. To test this hypothesis, we performed oral glucose tolerance tests with or without potassium replacement in a group of healthy subjects [74].

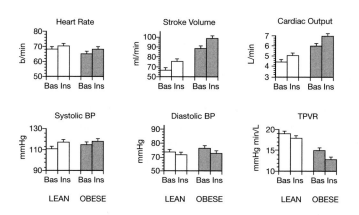

Fig. 4 Haemodynamic parameters in lean (empty bars) or obese (tinted bars) non-diabetic subjects in response to euglycaemic hyperinsulinaemia.

Moreover, to determine whether the anti-natriuretic effect of insulin is preserved in patients with impaired insulin action on glucose metabolism, a group of non-diabetic patients with essential hypertension was also studied. We found that healthy individuals and hypertensive patients exhibited similar insulin anti-natriuresis whether or not exogenous potassium was given to clamp serum potassium at basal levels. Also, insulin anti-natriuresis was independent of the presence of metabolic (=glucose metabolism) insulin resistance. The discordance with the results of Friedberg et al. [73] may depend on the differences between their experimental conditions (forced water diuresis, euglycaemic insulin clamp) and ours (maintenance of basal urine output, OGTT). In fact, *in vitro* studies have shown glucose increases anti-natriuresis due to enhanced glucose-sodium co-transport at the level of the convoluted proximal tubule [69]. *In vivo* studies using lithium clearance have demostrated that proximal sodium reabsorption is stimulated by hyperglycaemia in rats [75]; in patients with type 1 diabetes, sodium excretion is lower under hyperglycaemic than euglycaemic conditions [76]. At least in part, the effect of hyperglycaemia can be ascribed to the brush-border sodium co-transport, where glucose:sodium stoichiometry is 1:2 [77]. In a series of elegant studies, Nosadini et al. [78] found that patients with type 2 diabetes and metabolic insulin resistance retained more sodium than non-diabetic subjects at similar plasma glucose concentrations and filtered glucose. Moreover, at comparable degrees of hyperglycaemia the more insulin resistant patients exhibited more sodium retention, suggesting that metabolic insulin resistance may be coupled with an intrinsic renal abnormality.

In summary, both insulin alone and hyperglycaemia restrain renal sodium excretion; the most probable sites of action are the proximal tubule for hyperglycaemia, the distal portions of the nephron for insulin (though the latter is still somewhat uncertain). These two actions are combined in the physiological response to feeding [74]. Most importantly, in individuals with insulin resistance of glucose metabolism – i.e., diabetic [78], hypertensive [79], or obese [80] patients – insulin anti-natriuresis is preserved. Thus, the compensatory hyperinsulinaemia of insulin resistant subjects imposes a chronic anti-natriuretic pressure on the kidney. This may play a role in the development or maintenance of high blood pressure.

Insulin has a major role in potassium homeostasis. In dose-response studies in humans [81], euglycaemic hyperinsulinaemia stimulated potassium uptake by both liver and peripheral tissues. Insulin-induced hypokalemia is accompanied by a reduction in urinary potassium excretion. Insulin does not appear to have a direct effect on renal potassium handling, however. Thus, in our own studies [74] the anti-kaliuretic response to oral glucose was abolished when insulin-induced hypokalaemia was prevented by exogenous potassium supplementation. Importantly, when plasma potassium concentrations were clamped at their basal levels, glucose-induced insulin secretion was significantly heightened [74]. Thus, insulin modulates renal potassium excretion and its own release by the β-cell through the same signal, i.e., hypokalaemia. This dual feedback loop, or glucose-potassium cycle [82], explains the improvement in insulin secretion, and therefore in glucose tolerance, observed with the chronic use of ACE-inhibitors [83].

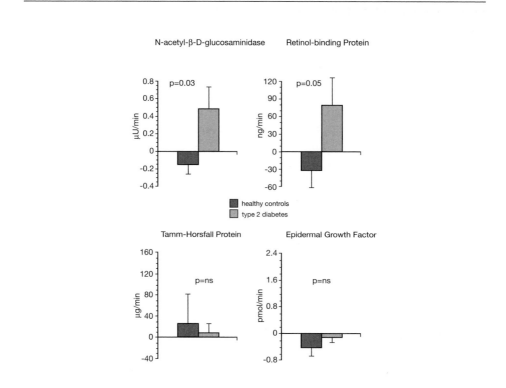

Fig. 5 Renal excretion of tubular proteins in response to isoglycaemic hyperinsulinaemia in subjects and patients with type 2 diabetes. Bars are mean (±1 SE) changes in excretion between normoinsulinaemia and hyperinsulinaemia under steady-state conditions [redrawn from reference 57].

The glucose-potassium cycle may also account for the opposing effects of potassium-losing diuretics and ACE-inhibitors on the risk of incident diabetes [84]. Sodium and uric acid excretion parallel one another under many physiological conditions [85, 86]. During euglycaemic hyperinsulinaemia, serum uric acid levels and creatinine clearance do not change, whereas the clearance rate and fractional excretion of uric acid decrease by 30%. The change in uric acid excretion is significantly related to the concomitant fall in urinary sodium excretion [87]. In patients with essential hypertension [79] and in obese subjects, we have found that the anti-uricosuric effect of insulin is maintained, and thus is independent of metabolic insulin resistance. The finding that uric acid and sodium urinary excretion are both restrained by physiological hyperinsulinaemia provides an explanation for the clustering of hyperuricaemia with insulin resistant states such as hypertension, obesity, and diabetes mellitus [88].

REFERENCES

1. Zierler KL. Theory of the use of arteriovenous concentration differences for measuring metabolism in steady and non-steady states. *J Clin Invest.* 1961;40:2111-2125.

2. Steinberg HO, Chaker H, Leaming R, Johnson A, Brechtel G, Baron A. Obesity insulin resistance is associated with endothelial dysfunction. Implication for the syndrome of insulin resistance. *J Clin Invest.* 1996;97:2061-2610.

3. Gros R, Borkowski KR, Feldman RD. Human insulin-mediated enhancement of vascular beta-adrenergic responsiveness. *Hypertension.* 1994;23:551-5.

4. McKay MK, Hester RL. Role of nitric oxide, adenosine, and ATP-sensitive potassium channels in insulin-induced vasodilation. *Hypertension.* 1996;28:202-8.

5. Misurski DA, Wu SQ, McNeill JR, Wilson TW, Gopalakrishnan V. Insulin-induced biphasic responses in rat mesenteric vascular bed: role of endothelin. *Hypertension.* 2001;37:1298-302.

6. Miller AW, Tulbert C, Puskar M, Busija DW. Enhanced endothelin activity prevents vasodilation to insulin in insulin resistance. *Hypertension.* 2002;40:78-82.

7. Laakso M, Edelman SV, Brechtel G, Baron AD. Decreased effect of insulin to stimulate skeletal muscle blood flow in obese man. *J Clin Invest.* 1990;85:1844-1852.

8. Anderson EA, Hoffman RP, Balon TW, Sinkey CA, Mark AL. Hyperinsulinemia produces both sympathetic neural activation and vasodilation in normal humans. *J Clin Invest.* 1991;87:2246-2252.

9. Baron AD, Brechtel-Hook G, Johnson A, Hardin D. Skeletal muscle blood flow. A possible link between insulin resistance and blood pressure. *Hypertension.* 1993;21:129-135.

10. Baron AD, Laakso M, Brechtel G, Edelman SV. Mechanism of insulin resistance in insulin-dependent diabetes mellitus: a major role for reduced skeletal muscle blood flow. *J Clin Endocrinol Metab.* 1991;73:637-643.

11. Laakso M, Edelman SV, Brechtel G, Baron AD. Impaired insulin-mediated skeletal muscle blood flow in patients with NIDDM. *Diabetes*. 1992;41:1076-1083.

12. Yki-Jarvinen H, Utriainen T. Insulin induced vasodilatation: physiology or pharmacology? *Diabetologia*. 1998;41:369-79.

13. Baron AD, Laakso M, Brechtel G, Hoit B, Watt C, Edelman SV. Reduced postprandial skeletal muscle blood flow contributes to glucose intolerance in human obesity. *J Clin Endocrinol Metab*. 1990;70:1525-33.

14. Dela F, Larsen J, Galbo H. Normal effect of insulin to stmulate blood flow in NIDDM. *Diabetes*. 1995;44:221-226.

15. Capaldo B, Gastaldelli A, Antoniello S, Auletta M, Pardo F, Ciociaro D, Guida R, Ferrannini E, Sacca L. Splanchnic and leg substrate exchange after ingestion of a natural mixed meal in humans. *Diabetes*. 1999;48:958-66.

16. Utriainen T, Nuutila P, Takala T, Vicini P, Ruotsalainen U, Ronnemaa T, Tolvanen T, Raitakari M, Haaparanta M, Kirvela O, Cobelli C, Yki-Jarvinen H. Intact insulin stimulation of skeletal muscle blood flow, its heterogeneity and redistribution, but not of glucose uptake in non-insulin-dependent diabetes mellitus. *J Clin Invest*. 1997;100:777-85.

17. Utriainen T, Holmang A, Bjorntorp P, Makimattila S, Sovijarvi A, Lindholm H, Yki-Jarvinen H. Physical fitness, muscle morphology, and insulin-stimulated limb blood flow in normal subjects. *Am J Physiol*. 1996;270:E905-11.

18. Raitakari M, Nuutila P, Ruotsalainen U, Laine H, Teras M, Iida H, Makimattila S, Utriainen T, Oikonen V, Sipila H, Haaparanta M, Solin O, Wegelius U, Knuuti J, Yki-Jarvinen H. Evidence for dissociation of insulin stimulation of blood flow and glucose uptake in human skeletal muscle: studies using [15O]H2O, [18F]fluoro-2-deoxy-D-glucose, and positron emission tomography. *Diabetes*. 1996;45:1471-7.

19. Bonadonna RC, Saccomani MP, Del Prato S, Bonora E, DeFronzo RA, Cobelli C. Role of tissue-specific blood flow and tissue recruitment in insulin-mediated glucose uptake of human skeletal muscle. *Circulation*. 1998;98:234-41.

20. Rattigan S, Clark MG, Barrett EJ. Hemodynamic actions of insulin in rat skeletal muscle: evidence for capillary recruitment. *Diabetes*. 1997;46:1381-8.

21. Holmang A, Muller M, Andersson OK, Lonnroth P. Minimal influence of blood flow on interstitial glucose and lactate-normal and insulin-resistant muscle. *Am J Physiol*. 1998;274:E446-52.

22. Serné EH, Stehouwer CDA, Maaten J, Wee PM, Rauwerda JA, Donker AJM, Gans R. Microvascular Function Relates to Insulin Sensitivity and Blood Pressure in Normal Subjects. *Circulation*. 1998:896-901.

23. Laine H, Knuuti MJ, Ruotsalainen U, Utriainen T, Oikonen V, Raitakari M, Luotolahti M, Kirvela O, Vicini P, Cobelli C, Nuutila P, Yki-Jarvinen H. Preserved relative dispersion but blunted stimulation of mean flow, absolute dispersion, and blood volume by insulin in skeletal muscle of patients with essential hypertension. *Circulation*. 1998;97:2146-53.

24. Natali A, Bonadonna R, Santoro D, Quiñones Galvan A, Baldi S, Frascerra S, Palombo C, Ghione S, Ferrannini E. Insulin resistance and vasodilation in essential hypertension: studies with adenosine. *J Clin Invest*. 1994;94:1570-1576.

25. Natali A, Quinones Galvan A, Pecori N, Sanna G, Toschi E, Ferrannini E. Vasodilatation with sodium nitroprusside does not improve insulin action in essential hypertension. *Hypertension*. 1998;31:632-636.

26. Natali A, Sironi A, Toschi E, Camastra S, Sanna G, Perissinotto A, Taddei S, Ferrannini E. Effect of vitamin C on forearm blood flow and glucose metabolism in essential hypertension. *Arterioscler Thromb Vasc Biol*. 2000;20:2401-6.

27. Randin D, Vollenweider P, Tappy L, Jequier E, Nicod P, Scherrer U. Effects of adrenergic and cholinergic blockade on insulin-induced stimulation of calf blood flow in humans. *Am J Physiol*. 1994;266:R809-16.

28. Steinberg H, Brechtel G, Johnson A, Fineberg N, Baron A. Insulin-mediated skeletal muscle vasodilatation is nitric oxide dependent. A novel action of insulin to increase nitric oxide release. *J Clin Invest*. 1994;94:1172-1179.

29. Scherrer U, Randin D, Vollenweider P, Vollenweider L, Nicod P. Nitric oxide release accounts for insulin's vascular effects in humans. *J Clin Invest*. 1994;94:2511-5.

30. Tack CJ, Lutterman JA, Vervoort G, Thien T, Smits P. Activation of the sodium-potassium pump contributes to insulin-induced vasodilation in humans. *Hypertension*. 1996;28:426-32.

31. Creager MA, Liang CS, Coffman JD. Beta adrenergic-mediated vasodilator response to insulin in the human forearm. *J Pharmacol Exp Ther*. 1985;235:709-14.

32. Lembo G, Iaccarino G, Vecchione C, Rendina V, Parrella L, Trimarco B. Insulin modulation of beta-adrenergic vasodilator pathway in human forearm. *Circulation*. 1996;93:1403-10.

33. Trovati M, Massucco P, Mattiello L, Cavalot F, Mularoni E, Hahn A, Anfossi G. Insulin increases cyclic nucleotide content in human vascular smooth muscle cells: a mechanism potentially involved in insulin-induced modulation of vascular tone. *Diabetologia*. 1995;38:936-41.

34. Zeng G, Nystrom FH, Ravichandran LV, Cong LN, Kirby M, Mostowski H, Quon MJ. Roles for insulin receptor, PI3-kinase, and Akt in insulin-signaling pathways related to production of nitric oxide in human vascular endothelial cells. *Circulation*. 2000;101:1539-45.

35. Verma S, Yao L, Stewart DJ, Dumont AS, Anderson TJ, McNeill JH. Endothelin antagonism uncovers insulin-mediated vasorelaxation in vitro and in vivo. *Hypertension*. 2001;37:328-33.

36. Cardillo C, Nambi SS, Kilcoyne CM, Choucair WK, Katz A, Quon MJ, Panza JA. Insulin stimulates both endothelin and nitric oxide activity in the human forearm. *Circulation*. 1999;100:820-5.

37. Juul K, Nielsen Lars B, Munkholm K, Stender S, Nordestgaard Borge G. Oxidation of plasma low density lipoprotein accelerates its accumulation and degradation in the arterial wall in vivo. *Circulation*. 1996;94:1698-04.

38. Yagi S, Takata S, Kiyokawa H, Yamamoto M, Noto Y, Ikeda T, Hattori N. Effects of insulin on vasoconstrictive responses to norepinephrine and angiotensin II in rabbit femoral artery and vein. *Diabetes*. 1988;37:1064-7.

39. Wu HY, Jeng YY, Yue CJ, Chyu KY, Hsueh WA, Chan TM. Endothelial-dependent vascular effects of insulin and insulin-like growth factor I in the perfused rat mesenteric artery and aortic ring. *Diabetes*. 1994;43:1027-32.

40. Kahn AM, Seidel CL, Allen JC, O'Neil RG, Shelat H, Song T. Insulin reduces contraction and intracellular calcium concentration in vascular smooth muscle. *Hypertension*. 1993;22:735-42.

41. Zemel MB, Reddy S, Sowers JR. Insulin attenuation of vasoconstrictor responses to phenylephrine in Zucker lean and obese rats. *Am J Hypertens*. 1991;4:537-9.

42. Lembo G, Iaccarino G, Vecchione C, Rendina V, Trimarco B. Insulin modulation of vascular reactivity is already impaired in prehypertensive spontaneously hypertensive rats. *Hypertension*. 1995;26:290-293.

43. Kahn A, Lichtemberg R, Allen J, Seidel C, Song T. Insulin-stimulated glucose transport inhibits Ca2+ influx and contraction in vascular smooth muscle. *Circulation.* 1995;92:1597-1603.

44. Touyz R, Tolloczko B, Shiffrin E. Insulin attenuates agonist-evoked calcium transients in vascular smooth muscle cells. *Hypertension.* 1994;23:25-28.

45. Standley PR, Zhang F, Ram JL, Zemel MB, Sowers JR. Insulin attenuates vasopressin-induced calcium transients and a voltage-dependent calcium response in rat vascular smooth muscle cells. *J Clin Invest.* 1991;88:1230-6.

46. Baldi S, Natali A, Buzzigoli G, Quinones Galvan A, Sironi A, Ferrannini E. In vivo effect of insulin on intracellular calcium concentrations: relation to insulin resistance. *Metabolism.* 1996;45:1-8.

47. Neahring JM, Stepniakowski K, Greene AS, Egan BM. Insulin does not reduce forearm alpha-vasoreactivity in obese hypertensive or lean normotensive men. *Hypertension.* 1993;22:584-90.

48. Tack CJ, Heeremans M, Thien T, Lutterman JA, Smits P. Regional hyperinsulinemia induces vasodilation but does not modulate adrenergic responsiveness in humans. *J Cardiovasc Pharmacol.* 1996;28:245-51.

49. Sakai K, Imaizumi T, Masaki H, Takeshita A. Intra-arterial infusion of insulin attenuates vosoreactivity in human forearm. *Hypertension.* 1993;22:67-73.

50. Baron AD, Brechtel G, Johnson A, Fineberg N, Henry DP, Steinberg HO. Interactions between insulin and norepinephrine on blood pressure and insulin sensitivity. *J Clin Invest.* 1994;93:2453-2462.

51. Taddei S, Virdis A, Mattei P, Natali A, Ferrannini E, Salvetti A. Effect of insulin on acetylcholine-induced vasodilation in normal subjects and in patients with essential hypertension. *Circulation.* 1995;92:2911-2918.

52. Gupta, McArthur C, Grady C, Ruderman N. Stimulation of vascular Na+/K+/ATPase activity by nitric oxide: a cGMP-independent effect. *Am J Physiol.* 1994;146:H146-H151.

53. Jiang Z, Lin Y, Clemont A, Feener E, Hein K, Igarashi M, Yamamuchi T, King G. Characterization of selective resistance to insulin signaling in the vasculature of obese Zuker (fa/fa) rats. *J Clin Invest.* 1999;104:447-457.

54. Utrianen T, Makimattila S, Virkamaki A, Bergholm R, Yki-Jarvinen H. Dissociation between insulin sensitivity of glucose uptake and endothelial function in normai subjects. *Diabetologia.* 1996;39:1477-82.

55. Natali A, Taddei S, Quinones-Galvan A, Camastra S, Baldi S, Frascerra S, Virdis S, Sudano I, Salvetti A, Ferrannini E. Insulin sensitivity, vascular reactivity, and clamp-induced vasodilatation in essential hypertension. *Circulation.* 1997;96:849-855.

56. Laine H, Yki-Jarvinen H, Kirvela O, Tolvanen T, Raitakary M, Solin O, Haaparanta M, Knuuti J, Nuutila P. Insulin resistance of glucose uptake in skeletal muscle cannot be ameliorated by enhancing endothelium-dependent blood flow in obesity. *J Clin Invest.* 1998;101:1156-1162.

57. Catalano C, Muscelli E, Quinones G, Baldi S, Masoni A, Gibb I, Torffvit O, Seghieri G, Ferrannini E. Effect of insulin on systemic and renal handling of albumin in nondiabetic and NIDDM subjects. *Diabetes.* 1997;46:868-875.

58. Muscelli E, Emdin M, Natali A, Pratali L, Camastra S, Gastaldelli A, Baldi S, Carpeggiani C, Ferrannini E. Autonomic and haemodynamic responses to insulin in lean and obese humans. *J Clin Endocrnol Metab.* 1998;83:2084-2090.

59. Rowe JW, Young JB, Minaker KL, Stevens AL, Pallotta J, Landsberg L. Effects of insulin and glucose infusions on sympathetic nervous system activity in normal man. *Diabetes.* 1981;30:219-225.

60. Davis S, Colburn C, Robbins R, Nadeau S, Neal D, Williams P, Cherrington A. Evidence that the brain of the conscious dog is insulin sensitive. *J Clin Invest*. 1995;95:593-602.

61. Schwartz M, Figlewitz D, Baskin D, Woods S, Porte DJ. Insulin in the brain: a hormonal regulator of energy balance. *Endocrin Rev*. 1992;13:387-414.

62. Ferrannini E. The haemodynamics of obesity: a theoretical analysis. *J Hypertens*. 1992;10:1417-23.

63. Quinones-Galvan A, Ferrannini E. Renal effects of insulin in man. *J Nephrol*. 1997;10:188-191.

64. DeFronzo RA, Cooke CR, Andres R, Faloona GR, Davis PJ. The effect of insulin on renal handling of sodium, potassium, and phosphate in man. *J Clin Invest*. 1975;55:845-855.

65. Christiansen JS, Frandsen M, Parving HH. The effect of intravenous insulin infusion on kidney function in insulin-dependent diabetes mellitus. *Diabetologia*. 1981;20:199-204.

66. Tucker BJ, Rasch R, Blantz RC. Glomerular filtration and tubular reabsorption of albumin in preproteinuric and proteinuric diabetic rats. *J Clin Invest*. 1993;92:686-94.

67. Benigni A, Remuzzi G. Glomerular protein trafficking and progression of renal disease to terminal uremia. *Semin Nephrol*. 1996;16:151-9.

68. Butlen D, Vadrot S, Roseau S, Morel F. Insulin receptors along the rat nephron: [125I] insulin binding in microdissected glomeruli and tubules. *Pflugers Arch*. 1988;412:604-12.

69. Baum M. Insulin stimulates volume absorption in the rabbit proximal convoluted tubule. *J Clin Invest*. 1987;79:1104-9.

70. Kirchner KA. Insulin increases loop segment chloride reabsorption in the euglycemic rat. *Am J Physiol*. 1988;255:F1206-13.

71. DeFronzo RA, Goldberg M, Agus ZS. The effects of glucose and insulin on renal electrolyte transport. *J Clin Invest*. 1976;58:83-90.

72. Skott P, Vaag A, Bruun NE, Hother-Nielsen O, Gall MA, Beck-Nielsen H, Parving HH. Effect of insulin on renal sodium handling in hyperinsulinaemic type 2 (non-insulin-dependent) diabetic patients with peripheral insulin resistance. *Diabetologia*. 1991;34:275-81.

73. Friedberg CE, Koomans HA, Bijlsma JA, Rabelink TJ, Dorhout Mees EJ. Sodium retention by insulin may depend on decreased plasma potassium. *Metabolism*. 1991;40:201-204.

74. Natali A, Quiñones Galvan A, Santoro D, Pecori N, Taddei S, Salvetti A, Ferrannini E. Relationship between insulin release, antinatriuresis and hypokalemia after glucose ingestion in normal and hypertensive man. *Clinical Science*. 1993;85:327-335.

75. Bank N, Aynedjian HS. Progressive increases in luminal glucose stimulate proximal sodium absorption in normal and diabetic rats. *J Clin Invest*. 1990;86:309-16.

76. Hannedouche TP, Delgado AG, Gnionsahe DA, Boitard C, Lacour B, Grunfeld JP. Renal hemodynamics and segmental tubular reabsorption in early type 1 diabetes. *Kidney Int*. 1990;37:1126-33.

77. Turner RJ, Moran A. Further studies of proximal tubular brush border membrane D-glucose transport heterogeneity. *J Membr Biol*. 1982;70:37-45.

78. Nosadini R, Sambataro M, Thomaseth K, Pacini G, Cipollina MR, Brocco E, Solini A, Carraro A, Velussi M, Frigato F, et al. Role of hyperglycemia and insulin resistance in determining sodium retention in non-insulin-dependent diabetes. *Kidney Int*. 1993;44:139-46.

79. Muscelli E, Natali A, Bianchi S, Bigazzi R, Quinones Galvan A, Sironi A, Frascerra S, Ciociaro D, Ferrannini E. Effect of insulin on renal sodium and uric acid handling in essential hypertension. *Am J Hypertens*. 1996;9:34-39.

80. Rocchini AP, Katch V, Kveselis D, Moorehead C, Martin M, Lampman R, Gregory M. Insulin and renal sodium retention in obese adolescents. *Hypertension.* 1989;14:367-374.

81. DeFronzo RA, Felig P, Ferrannini E, Wahren J. Effects of graded doses of insulin on splachnic and peripheral potassium metabolism in man. *Am J Physiol* 1980;238:E421-E427.

82. Ferrannini E, Galvan AQ, Santoro D, Natali A. Potassium as a link between insulin and the renin-angiotensin-aldosterone system. *J Hypertens Suppl.* 1992;10:S5-10.

83. Santoro D, Natali A, Palombo C, Brandi LS, Piatti M, Ghione S, Ferrannini E. Effects of chronic angiotensin converting enzyme inhibition on glucose tolerance and insulin sensitivity in essential hypertension. *Hypertension.* 1992;20:181-191.

84. Major outcomes in high-risk hypertensive patients randomized to angiotensin-converting enzyme inhibitor or calcium channel blocker vs diuretic: The Antihypertensive and Lipid-Lowering Treatment to Prevent Heart Attack Trial (ALLHAT). *Jama.* 2002;288:2981-97.

85. Cannon PJ, Svahn DS, Demartini FE. The influence of hypertonic saline infusions upon the fractional reabsorption of urate and other ions in normal and hypertensive man. *Circulation.* 1970;41:97-108.

86. Holmes EW, Kelley WN, Wyngaarden JB. Editorial: The kidney and uric acid excretion in man. *Kidney Int.* 1972;2:115-8.

87. Quinones Galvan A, Natali A, Baldi S, Frascerra S, Sanna G, Ciociaro D, Ferrannini E. Effect of insulin on uric acid excretion in humans. *Am J Physiol.* 1995;268:E1-5.

88. Modan M, Halkin H, Karasik A, Lusky A. Elevated serum uric acid—a facet of hyperinsulinaemia. *Diabetologia.* 1987;30:713-8.

12

VALUE OF SCREENING FOR MICROALBUMINURIA IN PATIENTS WITH DIABETES MELLITUS AS WELL AS IN THE GENERAL POPULATION

Bo Feldt-Rasmussen, Jan Skov Jensen and Knut Borch-Johnsen
Rigshospitalet University Hospital, Department of Nephrology, Copenhagen, Department of Cardiology, Gentofte Hospital, and Steno Diabetes Center, Gentofte, Denmark

The concept of microalbuminuria was first introduced among diabetologists [1,2]. It is diagnosed when the urinary albumin excretion rate (UAER) is slightly elevated compared with a normal reference range but lower than what is seen when the classical dipstix are positive for protein or albumin. Microalbuminuria is a marker of an increased risk of diabetic nephropathy and of cardiovascular disease in patients with Type 1 as well as Type 2 diabetes mellitus [1-18]. A high number of studies of the pathophysiology and of interventional measures in these patients have been published, and so has many sets of recommendations on the prevention of diabetic nephropathy, with special reference to microalbuminuria [19-34] (chapters 4, 6, 17, 26,31, 41, 46, 47 of this book). More recently microalbuminuria have shown to be a *risk factor* of cardiovascular disease also among otherwise apparently healthy persons (35-53). Furthermore, various intervention measures in patients with microalbuminuria and diabetes Type 1 and Type 2 have proven effective (54-57). Therefore, at least among diabetic patients, screening for microalbuminuria is of great value. This statement will be corroborated in the following sections of this chapter.

DEFINING MICROALBUMINURIA

Microalbuminuria has been defined using different units of measurement. According to the Gentofte-Montecatini convention [58] microalbuminuria is present when the UAER in a 24-hour urine or a short time collected urine during daytime is in the range of 30 to 300 mg/24h (20 to 200 mg/min) equivalent to 0.46 to 4.6 μmol/24h [58,59]. If a timed collection cannot be obtained, an index of albumin/creatinine (μg/mmol) can be calculated. Microalbuminuria is present at an index >3.5 (sensitivity > 95%, specificity >65%) [34]. The upper level is corresponding to a total urinary protein concentration of approximately 0.5 g/l which was previously considered to be the first marker of clinical diabetic nephropathy. The lower limit predicting nephropathy was defined on the basis of the results of four prospective studies in type 1 diabetic patients [1-4] (table 1). As shown in the table the studies have used different sampling periods, number of urine samples, reference range and they differed with respect to the length of the follow up periods. Nevertheless an international agreement was made on a lower predictive level of 30 mg/24h (20 μg/min) in order to make it possible to compare the outcome of studies from the various international study groups [58].

In the non-diabetic population clinical cardiovascular disease is often already present in subjects with an UAER in the range of 30 to 300 mg/24h [35-52] (table 2). Therefore the level of microalbuminuria must be lower if the measuring of UAER also should *predict* cardiovascular disease in the population. This will be discussed at the end of this chapter.

METHODOLOGICAL PROBLEMS

The concentration of albumin in the urine can be assayed using a number of immunoassays [20]. The major problem is the day to day variation of 23 to 52 %.

This variation is similar regardless of the urine collection procedure used: 24h, overnight collection, timed collection at daytime, during water diureses or by calculating an albumin/creatinine-ratio [4,20,22,59]. It is therefore recommended that presence of microalbuminuria is confirmed in at least two more urine collections [58].

Table 1. Four prospective studies demonstrating that an increased urinary albumin excretion rate (UAER) is a predictor of nephropathy in IDDM patients.

	Gentofte (1)[*]	London (2)	Aarhus (3)	Gentofte 2 (4)
Number of patients	23	63	44	71
Method for collecting urine	24 hours			24 hours
UAER				
Predictive Value for nephropathy (µg/min)	30	30	15	70
Observation (years)	6	14	10	6
Number of patients with UAER above the predictive value who progressed to nephropathy	5/8	7/8	12/14	7/7

*) The patients from this study were also included as a part of Gentofte 2.

The UAER is increased in the presence of urinary tract infections, menstrual bleedings, nephrological diseases other than diabetic nephropathy, severe hypertension and severe cardiac disease which all have to be excluded. It is also elevated during heavy physical exercise but not significantly affected in healthy subjects during normal daily life activities [20,22]. The UAER is elevated in diabetic patients in very poor glycaemic control with ketonuria and during episodes of ketoacidoses [20].

The collection period is also of importance. The level is similar in urines collected over 24-h and in timed daytime urine collections but reduced by 25% in urines collected overnight. Therefore the range of microalbuminuria in overnight urines should be an UAER of 23 to 230 mg/24h (15 to 150 µg/min) [20].

A close time-relationship between increase in UAER and increase in blood pressure has been demonstrated (60). The increase in UAER may precede the increase in blood pressure [61].

MICROALBUMINURIA AS A RISK FACTOR

Type 1 diabetes
The prevalence of microalbuminuria is 16 to 22% (27, 62) and the incidence over 7.3 years were recently demonstrated to be 12.6% [63]. Normally no other signs of micro- or macroangiopathy are present at the first diagnosis of

microalbuminuria. Later on with higher levels of microalbuminuria retinopathy will become much more frequent, and in fact microalbuminuria is a strong risk marker of severe retinopathy [20,22,23]. The blood-pressure is usually below 160/95 mmHg, but the mean blood-pressure is increasing by 3 mmHg per year [20,22,65]. The kidney function in terms of S-creatinine and glomerular filtration rate (GFR) are normal. The loss of kidney function is observed only in patients with the highest levels of UAER in the microalbuminuric range in whom a decline rate of GFR of 3 to 4 ml/(min*year) has been described [20,22,62]. The risk of clinical diabetic nephropathy is the highest among patients with an UAER in the range of 100 to 300 mg/24h (70 to 200 µg/min) [64,65]. The classical definition of clinical diabetic nephropathy at levels of UAER above 300 mg/24h therefore seems to be historical and dictated by the low sensitivity of the older methods for determining protein in urine.

Type 1 diabetic patients with classical proteinuria >0.5g/l are carrying almost the entire burden of the overmortality of diabetic patients [19]. This overmortality is only to a small extent caused by end stage renal failure. By far most of the patients are dying from cardiovascular diseases [19]. It is therefore widely accepted that microalbuminuria in the Type 1 diabetic patient is a valuable diagnostic parameter being highly predictive of excess mortality and cardiovascular morbidity [7-10]. The predictive value of microalbuminuria for cardiovascular diseases seems to be independent of conventional atherosclerotic risk factors, diabetic nephropathy, and diabetes duration and control [7].

It is important to identify all Type 1 diabetic patients with microalbuminuria because the progression of their disease can be delayed. Antihypertensive treatment reduces the fall rate of GFR by 50 % from 10 to less than 5 ml/(min*year) as observed in patients with clinical nephropathy [66-69]. The effect may be even more impressive when treatment is started at the first signs of an increasing blood-pressure but before development of overt hypertension [56, 70]. The effect of antihypertensive treatment is further emphasized by the important observation of an increased patient survival following the implementation in the late seventies of early antihypertensive treatment [71].

Optimizing the glycaemic control has also shown to be effective in arresting the progression of diabetic renal disease in its early stages i.e. delaying development and in some cases also the progression of microalbuminuria [57, 64, 72-75].

Non-insulin-dependent diabetes mellitus (Type 2 diabetes)
The prevalence of microalbuminuria is also high in Type 2 diabetic patients : 30 to 40 % [24,25,76]. Microalbuminuria is often present at diagnosis of the diabetic state. It is primarily associated to cardiovascular disease and Type 2 diabetic patients with microalbuminuria are at an increased risk of cardiovascular death compared with patients with a normal UAER [11-18,25].

End stage renal failure only occurs in 3 to 8 % of Type 2 diabetic patients despite the high prevalence of microalbuminuria. On the other hand microalbuminuria is a predictor of increasing levels of very low density lipoprotein cholesterol and a decrease of high density lipoprotein cholesterol [77]. Microalbuminuria therefore seems to be a *risk factor* of generalized disease to an even higher extent than in Type 1 diabetic patients and in fact microalbuminuria appears to be an independent risk factor as is the case in Type 1 diabetic patients [53, 78].

Also in Type 2 diabetic patients the causal link between microalbuminuria and generalized vascular disease is unknown. It is likely that a link should be found in alterations in the composition of the basal membranes of the capillaries and of the extracellular matrices as also hypothesized in Type 1 diabetic patients. In any case presence of the well-known risk factors is not sufficient to explain the entire overmortality of patients with Type 2 diabetes: hypertension, dyslipidaemia, atherogenic changes in the haemostatic system (increased von Willebrand factor and plasma fibrinogen) [24,25]. In a 10-year follow-up of 328 Type 2 diabetic patients it has recently been shown that increased UAER, endothelial dysfunction, and chronic inflammation are interrelated processes that develop in parallel, progress with time and are strongly and independently associated with risk of death [78].

Treating normotensive Type 2 diabetic patients with microalbuminuria with ACE inhibitors delays the progression to diabetic nephropathy [79, 80]. In 2001 it was convincingly demonstrated that treatment with Angiotensin 2 receptor antagonists also delays the progression from microalbuminuria to clinical nephropathy [54]. Furthermore in early 2003 the Steno 2 study clearly demonstrated the effect of multifactorial intervention and cardiovascular diseases in patients with Type 2 diabetes and microalbuminuria [55].

Non-diabetics

Microalbuminuria is also present in the non-diabetic population. This has been described in a number of studies [35-52]. Whenever mentioned, the reference range of the UAER seems to be rather low in relation to the classical definition of microalbuminuria. In table 3 is shown the reference range of UAER in 10 different studies. Except for one study with a higher level, the median or mean value of UAER is given from 2.6 to 8 µg/min and the upper 95% percentile in more than 50% of the studies as 15 µg/min or below [36, 37, 41, 43, 44, 46, 48, 81-84]. Microalbuminuria in its classical definition therefore seems to represent a relatively high UAER among non-diabetics. In an English 4-year follow-up study microalbuminuria, however, increased the mortality rate 24 times [36]. In a Danish study UAER was measured in 216 non-diabetic subjects, 60 to 74 years of age [37]. The median UAER was 7.52 µg/min (25 and 75 percentiles were 4.77 and 14.85 µg/min). The subjects were reexamined 7 years later. Among the 107 subjects with an initial UAER above the median value 23 had died in contrast to 8 out of 107 below the median UAER (p<0.008). In both studies the predictive effect of microalbuminuria was independent of the conventional atherosclerotic risk factors [36,37], which are usually increased among non-diabetic subjects with microalbuminuria (table 2).

Two larger scaled population based studies have also confirmed that a UAER above a certain level is predictive of developing ischaemic heart disease and increased mortality [47]. In a Finnish study of Kuusisto et al, 1.069 elderly inhabitants were followed for 3-4 years. Those who at baseline had an A/C ratio above the upper quintile (>3.2 mg albumin/mmol creatinine) had a higher morbidity and mortality from ischaemic heart disease (odds ratio 2.2) [49]. In our own study of 2.181 participants of the 1st Monica Population Study, Glostrup, Copenhagen County, an A/C ratio above the upper decile (>0.65 mg albumin/mmol creatinine) was significantly associated with an increased relative risk of 2.3 for development of ischaemic heart disease [47]. Also in the two latter studies, the predictive effect of microalbuminuria was independent of the conventional atherosclerotic risk factors.

Finally, a sub-analysis of the Heart Outcomes Prevention Evaluation Study (HOPE) indicated that any degree of albuminuria is a risk factor for cardiovascular events in individuals with or without diabetes; the risk increased at levels of UAER well below the microalbuminuric cut off [53].

It is likely that the link between microalbuminuria and cardiovascular disease may be explained by other pathophysiologic mechanisms, e.g. an universally increased transvascular albumin leakage [85,86] as well as other signs of endothelial dysfunction [87,88].

Prospective population studies including our own are in progress aiming to further clarify the role of UAER as a predictor of premature death of cardiovascular disease in apparently healthy subjects.

Table 2. Associations between microalbuminuria and atherosclerotic risk factors

Author	Haffner	Winocour	Woo	Metcalf	Gould	Dimmitt	Beatty	Mykkänen	Jensen
Publication year	1990	1992	1992	1992 & 1993	1993	1993	1993	1994	1997
Microalbuminuria	U_{alb}>30 mg/l	U_{alb}>20 mg/l	U_{alb}/U_{Creat}>90%-ile	U_{alb} continuous variable	UAER 20-200 µg/min	U_{alb}> medial	UAER 20-200 µg/min	U_{alb}/U_{create}>2	UAER >90%-ile
Sample size	316	447	1.333	5.349	959	474	264	1.068	2.613
Male sex					↑	↑			↑
Age					↑	↓		↑	
Blood pressure	↑	↑	↑	↑	↑			↑	↑
S-insulin	↑		↑					↑	
P-lipids	↑			↑		↑	↑	↑	
Body mass index				↑					↑
Smoking				↑					↑
Height				↓					
B-glucose					↑		↑		

↑, microalbuminuria is assoiated with increased levels of the risk factor; ↓, microalbuminuria is assoiated with increased levels of the risk factor.

U_{alb}, urinary albumin concentretion; U_{creat}, urinary creatinine concentretion; UAER, urinary albumin excretion rate.

Table 3. Reference values of urinary excretion in non-diabetic individuals.

Study (Author, country, publication year)	Urine collection	Sample size (Numbers)	Age (Years)	Sex (M/F)	Urinary albumin excretion
Marre et al, France (1987)	Timed overnight	60	40±13	28/32	4.2±4.1 µ/min[a]
Marre et al, France (1987)	Timed daytime	60	40±13	28/32	6.6 ±7.7 µ/min[a]
Marre et al, France (1987)	Timed 24-hours	60	40±13	28/32	8.0±8.1 µ/[a]min
Watts et al, UK (1988)	Morning spot	127	33±12	59/68	3.9(0.9-16.2)[a] mg/l [f]
Watts et al, UK (1988)	Timed overnight	127	33±12	59/68	3.2(1.2-8.6) µg/[a]min [f]
Watts et al, UK (1988)	Timed daytime	127	33±12	59/68	4.5(1.0-9.1) µg/[a]min [f]
Yudkin et al, UK (1988)	Timed daytime	184	60±12	68/116	2.8(0.09-154.6) [a] µg/min [c]
Gosling & Beevers, UK (1989)	Timed 24-hours	199	40±11	99/100	3.7(0.1-22.9) µg[a]/min [c]
Damsgaard et al, Denmark (1990)	Timed daytime	223	68(64-71)	89/134	7.5(4.8-14.9) µg/[b]min [b]
Metcalf et al, New Zealand (1992)	Morning spot	5.670	49(40-78)	4.106/1.564	5.2(5.1-5.4) mg/l[c] [g]
Dimmitt et al, Australia (1993)	Morning spot	474	34(17-64)	241/233	5.3 mg/ [ch]
Mykkänen et al, Finland (1994)	Morning spot	826	69.0± 0.1	312/514	23.7±2.5mg/l[d] [d]
Gould et al, UK (1994)	Timed overnight	812	40-75	359/453	2.6(0.1-148.8)[e] µg/min [c]
Gould et al, UK (1994)	Timed daytime	913	40-75	411/502	4.1(0.1-165.6) µg/min [c]
Jensen et al, Denmark (1997)	Timed overnight	2.613	30-70	1.340/1.273	2.8(1.2-7.0)µg/[e]min [I]

[a]Mean±SD [b]Median (1-3. Interquartile range) [c]median (range) [d]mean± SE [e]range [f]mean (95% C.I.) [g]geometric mean (95% C.I.) [h]median [i]median(10-90 interpercentile range)

CONCLUSIONS AND RECOMMENDATIONS

Measuring the UAER is a well documented and a well established part of monitoring *Type 1 diabetic patients*. The most simple urine sampling procedures can be used as long as the UAER is not significantly elevated i.e. as long as the albumin/ creatinine index is below 3.5 µg/mmol. It should be examined at least once a year. When microalbuminuria is suspected, a method of quantitating the UAER should be used at all subsequent visits in the outpatient clinic or until it is found normal at three consecutive visits. Presence of microalbuminuria warrants intensified follow up in order to diagnose and to intervene against retinopathy, nephropathy, hypertension and, if necessary to optimize the glycaemic control [89].

In *patients with Type 2 diabetes*, the UAER should be measured at diagnosis and once a year. Measuring the UAER is part of the general description of the cardiovascular risk profile of the individual patient. If the UAER is elevated treatment with ACE inhibitors or AII antagonists should be started; a multifactorial intervention strategy should be implemented [55].

Among non-diabetic subjects an increased UAER is a marker of cardiovascular disease as well as a risk factor of premature death. Examining the UAER is recommended as part of the routine medical check up of the adult and to replace the less sensitive examination for protein in the urine, which after all only serves to disclose diseases of the kidneys and the urinary tract. Examining of UAER should be restricted to those with presence of other modifyable risk factors such as dyslipidemia, arterial hypertension and other signs of the metabolic syndrome. As was the case in Type 2 diabetic patients presence of increased values will reinforce the need to intervene against any other risk factor present. Values of UAER above the microalbuminuric range should obviously lead to routine examinations to exclude nephro-urological diseases. The significance of an increased UAER on development of cardiovascular disease is to some extent clarified but so far no direct clinical consequences should be drawn of microalbuminuria per se.

Among non-diabetic subjects the present indications are that UAER is significantly elevated and predictive of disease at a much lower level than in diabetic patients i.e. at a level below the classical definition of microalbuminuria. Further research is needed for this clarification as well as for the investigation of interventional measures. Microalbuminuria is therefore still in focus in numerous epidemiological and pathophysiological studies.

REFERENCES

1. Parving H-H, Oxenbøll B, Svendsen PAa, Christiansen JS, Andersen AR. Early detection of patients at risk of developing diabetic nephropathy. Acta Endocrinol (Copenh) 1982; 100: 550-555.
2. Viberti GC, Hill RD, Jarret RJ, Argyropoulos A, Mahmud U, Keen H. Microalbuminuria as a predictor of clinical nephropathy in insulin-dependent diabetes mellitus. Lancet 1982; i: 1430-1432.
3. Mogensen CE, Christensen CK. Predicting diabetic nephropathy in insulin-dependent patients. N Engl J Med 1984; 311: 89-93.
4. Mathiesen ER, Oxenbøll B, Johansen K , Svendsen PA, Deckert T. Incipient nephropathy in Type 1 (insulin-dependent) diabetes. Diabetologia 1984; 26: 406-410.
5. Mogensen CE. Microalbuminuria predicts clinical proteinuria and early mortality in maturity onset diabetes. N Engl J Med 1984; 310: 356-360.
6. Jarrett RJ, Viberti GC, Argyropoulos A, Hill RD, Mahmud U, Murrels TJ. Microalbuminuria predicts mortality in non-insulin-dependent diabetes. Diabetic Med 1984; 1: 17-19.
7. Deckert T, Yokoyama H, Mathiesen ER, Rønn B, Jensen T, Feldt-Rasmussen B, Borch-Johnsen K, Jensen JS. Cohort study of predictive value of urinary albumin excretion for atherosclerotic vascular disease in patients with insulin dependent diabetes. BMJ 1996; 312: 871-874.
8. Messent JWC, Elliot TG, Hill RD, Jarrett RJ, Keen H, Viberti GC. Prognostic significance of microalbuminuria in insulin-dependent diabetes mellitus: A twenty-three year follow-up study. Kidney Int 1992; 41: 836-839.
9. Torffvit O, Agardh C-D. The predictive value of albuminuria for cardiovascular and renal disease. A 5-year follow-up study of 476 patients with type 1 diabetes mellitus. J Diabetic Compl 1993; 7: 49-56.
10. Jensen T, Borch-Johnsen K, Kofoed-Enevoldsen A, Deckert T. Coronary heart disease in young type 1 (insulin-depedent) diabetic patients with and without diabetic nephropathy: Incidence and risk factors. Diabetologia 1987; 30: 144-148.
11. Schmitz A, Vaeth M. Microalbuminuria: A major risk factor in non-insulin-dependent diabetes. A 10-year follow-up study of 503 patients. Diabetic Med 1988; 5: 1126-1134.
12. Mattock MB, Morrish NJ, Viberti GC, Keen H, Fitzgerald AP, Jackson G. Prospective study of microalbuminuria as predictor of mortality in NIDDM. Diabetes 1992; 41: 736-741.
13. Neil A, Hawkins M, Potok M, Thororgood M, Cohen D, Mann J. A prospective population-based study of microalbuminuria as a predictor of mortality in NIDDM. Diabetes Care 1993; 16: 996-1003.
14. Gall M-A, Borch-Johnsen K, Hougaard P, Nielsen FS, Parving H-H. Albuminuria and poor glycemic control predict mortality in NIDDM. Diabetes 1995; 44: 1303-1309.
15. Rossing P, Hougaard P, Borch-Johnsen K, Parving H-H. Predictors of mortality in insulin dependent diabetes: 10 year observational follow up study. BMJ 1996; 313: 779-784.
16. Damsgaard EM, Frøland A, Jørgensen OD, Mogensen CE. Eight to nine year mortality in known non-insulin dependent diabetics and controls. Kidney Internat 1992; 41: 731-735.
17. MacLeod JM, Lutale J, Marshall SM. Albumin excretion and vascular deaths in NIDDM. Diabetologia 1995; 38: 610-616.

18. Beilin J, Stanton KG, McCann VJ, Knuiman MW, Divitini ML. Microalbuminuria in type 2 diabetes: an independent predictor of cardiovascular mortality. Aust Nz J Med 1996; 26: 519-525.

19. Borch-Johnsen K. The prognosis of insulin-dependent diabetes - an epidemiological approach (Thesis). Dan Med Bull 1989; 36: 336-348.

20. Feldt-Rasmussen B. Microalbuminuria and clinical nephropathy in Type 1 (insulin-dependent) diabetes mellitus: Pathophysiological mechanisms and intervention studies (Thesis). Dan Med Bull 1989; 36: 405-415.

21. Jensen T. Albuminuria - a marker of renal and general vascular disease in IDDM (Thesis). Dan Med Bull 1991; 38: 134-144.

22. Christensen CK. The pre-proteinuric phase of diabetic nephropathy (Thesis). Dan Med Bull 1991; 38: 145-159.

23. Mathiesen ER. Prevention of diabetic nephropathy: Microalbuminuria and perspectives for intervention in insulin-dependent diabetes (Thesis). Dan Med Bull 1993; 40: 273-285.

24. Schmitz A. The kidney in non-insulin-dependent diabetes. Studies on glomerular structure and function and the relationship between microalbuminuria and mortality. Acta Diabetologica 1992; 29: 47-69.

25. Gall M. Albuminuria in non-insulin-dependent diabetes mellitus: prevalence, causes and consequences (Thesis). Dan Med Bull 1997: 44: 465-485.

26. Deckert T, Feldt-Rasmussen B, Borch-Johnsen K, Jensen T, Kofoed-Enevoldsen A. Albuminuria reflects widespread vascular damage. The Steno hypothesis. Diabetologia 1989; 32: 219-226.

27. Mogensen CE, Hansen KW, Sommer S et al. Microalbuminuria: studies in diabetes, essential hypertension and renal disease as compared with the background population. In *Advances in Nephrology*. Grunfeld JP, ed. Mosby Year Book, 1991; vol 20: 191-228.

28. Viberti GC, Mogensen CE, Passa P, Bilous R, Mangili R. St Vincent Declaration, 1994: Guidelines for the prevention of diabetic renal failure. In *The Kidney and Hypertension in Diabetes Mellitus*, 2nd ed. Mogensen CE, ed. Boston, Dordrecht, London: Kluwer Academic Publishers, 1994; pp 515-527.

29. Anon. Prevention of diabetes mellitus: report of a WHO study group. WHO Tech Rep Ser 844. Geneva: WHO, 1994: 55-59.

30. Jerums G, Cooper M, Gilbert R, O'Brien R, Taft J. Microalbuminuria in diabetes. Med J Aust 1994; 161: 265-268.

31. Consensus development conference on the diagnosis and management of nephropathy in patients with diabetes mellitus. Diabetes Care 1994; 17: 1357-1361.

32. Bennett PH, Haffner S, Kaiske BL, et al. Screening and management of microalbuminuria in patients with diabetes mellitus: recommendations to the scientific advisory board of the National Kidney Foundation from an ad hoc committee of the council on diabetes mellitus of the National Kidney Foundation. Am J Kidney Dis 1995; 25: 107-112.

33. Striker GE. Report on a workshop to develop management recommendations for the prevention of progression in chronic renal disease (Bethesda, April, 1994). Nephrol Dial Transplant 1995; 10: 290-292.

34. Mogensen CE, Keane WF, Bennett PH, Jerums G, Parving H-H, Passa P, Steffes MW, Striker GE, Viberti GC. Prevention of diabetic renal disease with special reference to microalbuminuria. Lancet 1995; 346: 1080-1084.

35. Jensen JS. Microalbuminuria and the risk of atherosclerosis. Dan Med Bull 2000;47:63-78.

36. Yudkin JS, Forrest RD, Jackson CA. Microalbuminuria as predictor of vascular disease in non-diabetic subjects: Islington diabetes survey. Lancet 1988; ii: 530-533.
37. Damsgaard EM, Frøland A, Jørgensen OD, Mogensen CE. Microalbuminuria as predictor of increased mortality in elderly people. BMJ 1990; 300: 297-300.
38. Haffner SM, Stern MP, Gruber KK, Hazuda HP, Mitchell BD, Patterson JK. Microalbuminuria. Potential marker for increased cardiovascular risk factors in non-diabetic subjects. Arteriosclerosis 1990; 10: 727-731.
39. Winocour PH, Harland JOE, Millar JP, Laker MF, Alberti KGMM. Microalbuminuria and associated cardiovascular risk factors in the community. Atherosclerosis 1992; 93: 71-81.
40. Woo J, Cockram CS, Swaminathan R, Lau E, Chan E, Cheung R. Microalbuminuria and other cardiovascular risk factors in non-diabetic subjects. Int J Cardiol 1992; 37: 345-350.
41. Metcalff P, Baker J, Scott A, Wild C, Scragg R, Dryson E. Albuminuria in people at least 40 years old: Effect of obesity, hypertension and hyperlipidemia. Clin Chem 1992; 38: 1802-1808.
42. Metcalff PA, Baker JR, Scragg RKR, Dryson E, Scott AJ, Wild CJ. Albuminuria in people at least 40 years old. Effect of alcohol consumption, regular exercise, and cigarette smoking. Clin Chem 1993; 39: 1793-1797.
43. Gould MM, Mohamed-Ali V, Goubet SA, Yudkin JS, Haines AP. Microalbuminuria: associations with height and sex in non-diabetic subjects. BMJ 1993; 306: 240-242.
44. Dimmitt SB, Lindquist TL, Mamotte CDS, Burke V, Beilin LJ. Urine albumin excretion in healthy subjects. J Human Hypertens 1993; 7: 239-243.
45. Beatty OL, Atkinson AB, Browne J, Clarke K, Sheridan B, Bell PM. Microalbuminuria does not predict cardiovascular disease in a normal general practice population. Ir J Med Sci 1993; 163: 140-142.
46. Mykkänen L, Haffner SM, Kuusisto J, Pyörälä K, Laakso M. Microalbuminuria precedes the development of NIDDM. Diabetes 1994; 43: 552-557.
47. Jensen JS, Borch-Johnsen K, Feldt-Rasmussen B, Jensen G, Feldt-Rasmussen B. Atherosclerotic risk factors are increased in clinically healthy subjects with microalbuminuria. Atherosclerosis 1995; 112: 245-252.
48. Gould MM, Mohamed-Ali V, Goubet SA, Yudkin JS, Haines AP. Associations of urinary albumin excretion rate with vascular disease in Europid nondiabetic subjects. J Diabetic Compl 1994; 8: 180-188.
49. Kuusisto J, Mykkänin L, Pyörälä K, Laakso M. Hyperinsulinemic microalbuminuria. A new risk indicator for coronary heart disease. Ciculation 1995: 91: 831-837.
50. Jensen JS, Borch-Johnsen K, Feldt-Rasmussen B, Appleyard M, Jensen G. Urinary albumin excretion and history of acute myocardial infarction in a cross-sectional population study of 2613 individuals. Journal of Cardiovascular Risk 1997; 4: 121-125.
51. Borch-Johsen K, Feldt-Rasmussen B, Strandgaard S, Schroll M, Jensen SR. Urinary albumin excretion. An independent predictor of ischemic heart disease. Aterioscler Thromb Vasc Biol 1999, 19:1992-1997.
52. Jensen JS, Feldt-Rasmussen B, Clausen P, Borch Johnsen K, Jensen G. Arterial hypertension, microalbuminuria, and the risk of ischaemic heart disease. Hypertension 2000;35:898-903.
53. Gerstein HC, Mann JFE, Yi Q, Zinman B, Dinneen SF, Hoogwerf B et al. Albuminuria and risk of cardiovascular events, death, and heart failure in diabetic and nondiabetic individuals. JAMA 2001;286:421-426.

54. Parving H-H, Lehnert H, Bröchner-Mortensen J, Gomis R, Andersen S, Arner P. The effect of Irbesartan in patients with Type 2 diabetes. N Engl J Med 2001;345:870-8.

55. Gaede P, Vedel P, Larsen N, Jensen GVH, Parving H-H, Pedersen O. Multifactorial intervention and cardiovascular disease in patients with type 2 diabetes. N Engl J Med 2003;348:383-93.

56. Mathiesen ER, Hommel E, Hansen HP, Smidt UM, Parving H-H. Randomised controlled trial of long term efficacy of captopril on preservation of kidney function in normotensive patients with insulin dependent diabetes and microalbuminuria. BMJ 1999; 319: 24-25.

57. Microalbuminuria Collaborative Study Group, United Kingdom. Intensive therapy and progression to clinical albuminuria in patients with insulin dependent diabetes mellitus and microalbuminuria. BMJ 1995; 311: 973-977.

58. Mogensen CE, Chachati A, Christensen CK, Close CF, Deckert T, Hommel E, Kastrup J, Lefebvre P, Mathiesen ER, Feldt-Rasmussen B, Schmitz A, Viberti GC. Microalbuminuria: an early marker of renal involvement in diabetes. Uremia Invest 1985-86; 9: 85-95.

59. Feldt-Rasmussen B, Dinesen B, Deckert M. Enzyme immuno assay. an improved determination of urinary albumin in diabetics with incipient nephropathy. Scand J Clin Lab Invest 1985; 45: 539-544.

60. Thomas W, Shen Y, Molicath ME, Steffes MW. Rise in albumiuria and blood pressure in patients who progressed to diabetic nephropathy in the Diabetes Control and Complications Trial. J Am Soc Nephrol 2001;12:333-340.

61. Mathiesen ER, Rønn B, Jensen T, Storm B, Deckert T. The relationship between blood pressure and urinary albumin excretion in the development of microalbuminuria. Diabetes 1990; 39: 245-249.

62. Parving H-H, Hommel E, Mathiesen ER, Skøtt P, Edsberg B, Bahnsen M et al. Prevalence of microalbuminuria, arterial hypertension, retinopathy and neuropathy in patients with insulin dependent diabetes. BMJ 1988; 296: 157-160.

63. Chaturvedi N, Bandinelli S, Mangili R, Penno G, Rottiers RE, Fuller JH on behalf of the EURODIAB Prospective Complications Study Group. Microalbuminuria in type 1 diabetes: Rates, risk factors and glycemic threshold. Kidney International 2001; 60:219-227.

64. Feldt-Rasmussen B, Mathiesen ER, Jensen T, Lauritzen T, Deckert T. Effect of improved metabolic control on loss of kidney function in insulin-dependent diabetic patients. Diabetologia 1991; 34: 164-170.

65. Mathiesen ER, Feldt-Rasmussen B, Hommel E, Deckert T, Parving H-H. Stable glomerular filtration rate in normotensive IDDM patients with stable microalbuminuria: A 5-year prospective study. Diabetes Care 1997; 20/3: 286-289.

66. Bjorck S, Mulec H, Johnsen SA et al. Renal protective effect of Enalapril in diabetic nephropathy. BMJ 1992; 304: 339-343.

67. Lewis EJ, Hunsicker LG, Bain RP, Rohde RD, for the Collaborative Study Group. The effect of angiotensin-converting-enzyme inhibition on diabetic nephropathy. N Engl J Med 1993; 329: 1456-1462.

68. Parving H-H, Andersen AR, Schmidt UM, Hommel E, Mathiesen ER, Svendsen PAa. Effect of antihypertensive treatment on kidney function in diabetic nephropathy. BMJ 1987; 294: 1443-1447.

69. Mathiesen ER, Hommel E, Giese J, Parving H-H. Efficacy of captopril in postponing nephropathy in normotensive insulin-dependent diabetic patients with microalbuminuria. BMJ 1991; 303: 81-87.

70. Viberti GC, Mogensen CE, Groop L, Pauls JF, for the European Microalbuminuria Captopril Study Group. Effect of captopril on progression to clinical proteinuria in patients with insulin-dependent diabetes mellitus and microalbuminuria. JAMA 1994; 271: 275-279.

71. Parving H-H, Hommel E. Prognosis in diabetic nephropathy. BMJ 1989; 299: 230-233.

72. Dahl-Jørgensen K, Hanssen KF, Kierulf P, Bjøro T, Sandvik L, Aagenaess Ø. Reduction of urinary albumin excretion after 4 years of continuous subcutaneous insulin infusion in insulin-dependent diabetes mellitus. Acta Endocrinol (Copenh) 1988; 117: 19-25.

73. Reichard P, Berglund B, Britz A, Cars I, Nilsson BY, Rosenqvist U. Intensified conventional insulin treatment retards the microvascular complications of insulin-dependent diabetes mellitus (IDDM). The Stockholm Diabetes Intervention Study after five years. J Intern Med 1991; 230: 101-108.

74. The Diabetes Control and Complications Trial Research Group. The effect of intensive treatment of diabetes on the development and progression of long-term complications in insulin-dependent diabetes mellitus. N Engl J Med 1993; 329: 977-986.

75. Diabetes Control and Complications (DCCT) Research Group. Effect of intensive therapy on the development and progression of diabetic nephropathy in the diabetes control and complications trial. Kidney Int 1995; 42: 1703-1720.

76. Gall M, Rossing P, Skøtt P, Damsbo P, Vaag A, Bech K et al. Prevalence of micro- and macro-albuminuria, arterial hypertension, retinopathy and large vessel disease in European Type 2 (non-insulin-dependent) diabetic patients. Diabetologia 1991; 34: 655-661.

77. Niskanen L, Uusitupa M, Sarlund H, Siitonen O, Voutilainen E, Penttila I et al. Microalbuminuria predicts the development of serum lipoprotein abnormalities favouring atherogenesis in newly diagnosed Type 2 (non-insulin-dependent) diabetic patients. Diabetologia 1990; 33: 237-243.

78. Stehouwer CDA, Gall M-A, Twisk JWR, Knudsen E, Emeis JJ, Parving H-H. Increased urinary albumin excretion, endothelial dysfunction, and chronic low-grade inflammation in type 2 diabetes. Diabetes 2002;51:1157-1165.

79. Ravid M, Savin H, Jutrin I, Bental T, Katz B, Lishner M. Long-term stabilizing effect of angiotensin-converting enzyme inhibition on plasma creatinine and on proteinuria in normotensive type II diabetic patients. Ann Intern Med 1993; 118: 577-581.

80. Gaede P, Vedel P, Parving H-H, Pedersen O. Intensified multifactorial intervention in patients with type 2 diabetes mellitus and microalbuminuria: The Steno type 2 randomised study. Lancet 1999; 353: 617-622.

81. Gosling P, Beevers DG. Urinary albumin excretion and blood pressure in the general population. Clin Sci 1989; 76: 39-42.

82. Marre M, Claudel J-P, Ciret P, Luis N, Suarez L, Passa P. Laser immunonephelometry for routine quantification of urinary albumin excretion. Clin Chem 1987; 33: 209-213.

83. Watts GF, Morris RW, Khan K, Polak A. Urinary albumin excretion in healthy adult subjects: reference values and some factors affectin their interpretation. Clin Chim Acta 1988; 172: 191-198.

84. Jensen JS, Feldt-Rasmussen B, Borch-Johnsen K, Jensen G and the Copenhagen City Heart Study Group. Urinary albumin excretion in a population based sample of 1011 middle aged non-diabetic subjects. Scand J Clin Lab Invest 1993; 53: 867-872

85. Jensen JS, Borch-Johnsen K, Jensen G, Feldt-Rasmussen B. Microalbuminuria reflects a generalized transvascular albumin leakiness in clinically healthy subjects. Clin Sci 1995; 88: 629-33.

86. Jensen JS, Borch-Johnsen K, Deckert T, Deckert M, Jensen G, Feldt-Rasmussen B. Reduced glomerular size- and charge-selectivity in clinically healthy individuals with microalbuminuria. Eur J Clin Invest 1995; 25: 608-614.

87. Clausen P, Feldt-Rasmussen B, Jensen G, Jensen JS. Endothelial haemostatic factors are associated with progression of urinary albumin excretion in clinically healthy subjects: a 4-year prospective study. Clinical Science 1999; 97: 37-43.

88. Stehouwer CDA, Lambert J, Donker AJM, van Hinsbergh VWM. Endothelial dysfunction and pathogenesis of diabetic angiopathy. Cardiovascular Research 1997; 34: 55-68.

89. Borch-Johnsen K, Wenzel H, Viberti GC, Mogensen CE. Is screening and intervention for Microalbuminuria worthwhile in patients with insulin dependent diabetes? BMJ 1993; 306: 1722-1725.

13

DYSFUNCTION OF THE VASCULAR ENDOTHELIUM AND THE DEVELOPMENT OF RENAL AND VASCULAR COMPLICATIONS IN DIABETES

Coen D.A. Stehouwer

Department of Internal Medicine and Institute for Cardiovascular Research, VU University Medical Centre, 1081 HV Amsterdam, the Netherlands

INTRODUCTION

The risk of microangiopathy in diabetic patients is highest in those with the most severe hyperglycaemia. Hyperglycaemia, however, is a necessary but not a sufficient cause of clinically important microangiopathy. Hypertension is an additional major cause, and smoking, hypercholesterolaemia, diabetic dyslipidaemia (i.e., low high density lipoprotein (HDL) cholesterol and high triglycerides), obesity and hyperhomocysteinaemia may also contribute. Risk of macroangiopathy, as in non-diabetic individuals, is related to general risk factors for atherothrombosis, such as age, smoking, hypertension, hypercholesterolaemia, dyslipidaemia, obesity and hyperhomocysteinaemia. Risk factors for micro- and macroangiopathy thus show much overlap except that risk of macroangiopathy does not appear to be strongly related to hyperglycaemia, although this is controversial [1-8]. Hypertension, dyslipidaemia and obesity are seen more often in patients with type 2 than in those with type 1 diabetes. In addition, the latter three risk factors occur together more commonly than expected by chance and are thus said to *cluster* in the metabolic syndrome, which further consists of insulin resistance, hyperinsulinaemia, and impaired fibrinolysis. In both types of diabetes, risk of macroangiopathy is strongly determined by the presence of nephropathy, even in its early stages (microalbuminuria), which identifies a group of patients at very high risk of developing severe complications, i.e., proliferative retinopathy, renal insufficiency, severe neuropathy, and cardiovascular disease. On the other hand, a substantial fraction of diabetic patients, perhaps 50%, will never develop this cluster of severe complications, i.e. they appear "protected".

Dysfunction of the vascular endothelium is thought to play a key role in the pathogenesis of micro- and macroangiopathy in diabetes. This chapter will review how endothelial dysfunction relates to the pattern of disease occurrence described above and what current biochemical mechanisms have been proposed as an explanation for the development of endothelial dysfunction in diabetes.

WHAT IS ENDOTHELIAL DYSFUNCTION AND HOW CAN IT BE MEASURED IN HUMANS?

The endothelium is an important locus of control of vascular and thus organ functions [9-21]. To carry out its functions, the endothelium produces components of the extracellular matrix and a variety of regulatory mediators, such as nitric oxide, prostanoids, endothelin, angiotensin-II, tissue-type plasminogen activator (t-PA) and plasminogen activator inhibitor-1 (PAI-1), von Willebrand factor (vWF), adhesion molecules and cytokines.

Normal functions of the endothelium include the following:

- it actively decreases vascular tone;
- it limits leukocyte adhesion and thus inflammatory activity in the vessel wall;
- it maintains vascular permeability to nutrients, hormones, other macromolecules, and leukocytes within narrow bounds;
- it inhibits platelet adhesion and aggregation by producing prostacyclin, nitric oxide and ectonucleotidases;
- it limits activation of the coagulation cascade by the thrombomodulin-protein C, heparan sulphate-antithrombin and tissue factor-tissue factor pathway inhibitor interactions; and
- it regulates fibrinolysis by producing t-PA and its inhibitor, PAI-1.

Nitric oxide is a particularly important endothelium-derived mediator, because of its vasodilator, anti-platelet, anti-proliferative, permeability-decreasing and anti-inflammatory properties. Nitric oxide inhibits leukocyte adhesion and rolling as well as cytokine-induced expression of vascular cell adhesion molecule-1

(VCAM-1) and monocyte chemotactic protein-1, effects that are at least in part attributable to inhibition of the transcription factor NF-κB through increased expression of its inhibitor, IκB.

Dysfunction of the endothelium can be considered present when its properties have changed in a way that is inappropriate with regard to the preservation of organ function. For example, basement membrane synthesis may be altered, resulting in changes in cell-matrix interactions which can contribute to arterial stiffening and increased microvascular permeability; vascular tone and permeability may increase, which contributes to increased blood pressure and atherogenesis; and the endothelium may lose its antithrombotic and profibrinolytic properties and may instead acquire prothrombotic and antifibrinolytic properties. Such alterations *(endothelial dysfunctions)* do not necessarily occur simultaneously. Furthermore, they may differ according to the nature of the injury and may depend on the intrinsic properties of the endothelium (e.g., arterial versus microvascular endothelium). Endothelial *activation* designates one specific set of dysfunctions characterised by (usually inflammatory-cytokine-induced) increased interactions with blood leukocytes, in which adhesion molecules (such as E-selectin and VCAM-1) and chemoattractants (such as monocyte chemotactic protein-1 and interleukin-8) are essential.

Endothelial dysfunctions are thought to play important roles not only in the initiation of atherosclerosis, but also in its progression and clinical sequelae, and can be conceptualised as transducers of atherogenic risk factors. In this view, risk factors such as oxidatively modified low density lipoprotein (LDL) cholesterol, smoking and diabetes initiate atherosclerosis through endothelial activation, whereas the protective effect of HDL is mediated by its ability to decrease LDL oxidation. The predilection to atherosclerosis of arterial branching points, bifurcations and convexities is explained by the fact that blood flow there is non-laminar or even turbulent and shear stress low or oscillatory, and that these conditions increase endothelial activation, effects that are enhanced by high blood pressure. Experimental models of hypercholesterolaemia, hypertension and diabetes also have in common that endothelial nitric oxide availability is decreased, whether through decreased production or through increased degradation. For example, high LDL cholesterol increases the production of reactive oxygen species and thus nitric oxide scavenging, but also increases the interaction between nitric oxide synthase and caveolin-1, which decreases nitric oxide production. Another important example is angiotensin-II, which increases activity of vascular NAD(P)H oxidases, superoxide production and nitric oxide scavenging, and thus decreases nitric oxide availability. These processes will increase endothelial activation.

Endothelial function cannot be measured directly in humans. Estimates of different types of endothelial dysfunction may be obtained indirectly by measuring endothelium-dependent vasodilation, plasma levels of endothelium-derived mediators (e.g., regulatory proteins) and, possibly, the transcapillary escape rate of albumin and microalbuminuria. Some other vascular properties, such as arterial stiffness, are probably in part endothelium-dependent [16,21]. It should be emphasised that several assumptions are implicit in the use of such estimates of endothelial function in humans. Firstly, tests intended to estimate nitric-oxide-mediated endothelium-dependent vasodilation in part measure effects of other endothelial vasodilators such as prostacyclin and endothelium-derived hyperpolarising factor, and in part may be confounded by impaired vascular smooth muscle function. Secondly, the concept that high plasma levels of endothelium-derived mediators reflect endothelial dysfunction in clinically relevant arteries (such as the coronary and carotid) requires (a) that other cell types are not an important source; (b) that synthesis is more important than clearance, unless the latter is endothelium-dependent; and (c) that endothelial function in the microvasculature parallels that in large arteries, because microvascular endothelium, with its very large surface area and synthetic capacity, is the most important determinant of plasma levels of endothelium-derived mediators. Information on the validity of these assumptions is as yet scarce. In some cases, the assumptions are clearly invalid, e.g. for PAI-1, which is produced by many cell types. Thirdly, it is likely that the transcapillary escape rate of albumin is determined not only by the endothelium, but also by the biochemical and biophysical properties of the extracellular matrix and by haemodynamic forces. Finally, it is unlikely that the presence of microalbuminuria always and exclusively reflects a generalised increase of endothelial permeability; it may be wholly or partly a local renal haemodynamic phenomenon in at least some cases. Thus, the estimates which exist for assessing endothelial function in vivo in humans are reasonable but not perfect.

ENDOTHELIAL DYSFUNCTION IN DIABETES: CURRENT ISSUES

Endothelial function in diabetes has been studied to answer several distinct questions, namely [22-27]:

- Is the occurrence of microalbuminuria accompanied by severe endothelial dysfunction, and, if so, can this explain why microalbuminuria is accompanied by an increased risk of other microangiopathic complications and of atherothrombotic disease?
- Is hyperglycaemia a sufficient cause of at least some types of endothelial dysfunction and is diabetes therefore usually a state of endothelial dysfunction?
- What is the significance of the finding that insulin resistance (regardless of the presence of diabetes) is associated with endothelial dysfunction?
- What are the mechanisms that cause diabetes-associated endothelial dysfunction?

The importance of these questions lies in the expected consequences of persistent endothelial dysfunction, which include

- increased blood pressure through increased peripheral arteriolar resistance, impaired renal function and increased large arterial stiffness;
- increased susceptibility to microangiopathy through both haemodynamic (increased microvascular pressure and permeability) and other mechanisms, such as inflammation; and
- increased susceptibility to atherothrombosis through increases in blood pressure, vascular permeability, leukocyte adhesion and inflammation, and procoagulant and antifibrinolytic changes.

GENERALISED ENDOTHELIAL DYSFUNCTION, CHRONIC, LOW-GRADE INFLAMMATION, MICROALBUMINURIA AND ATHEROTHROMBOSIS

In both type 1 and type 2 diabetes, patients with advanced nephropathy (macroalbuminuria) have a greatly increased risk of severe retinopathy, neuropathy and atherothrombotic disease. This pattern can be observed even in early nephropathy, i.e. microalbuminuria, which has raised the question of what common mechanisms may be at work [1,2,22]. Because (micro-)albuminuria is often associated with classic risk factors for microangiopathy and atherothrombosis, notably poor glycaemic control, hypertension, obesity, dyslipidaemia and smoking, an obvious possibility is that such risk factors cause both (micro-)albuminuria and atherothrombosis and thus explain their association. Many studies have investigated this and have concluded that common risk factors explain at most a small part of the association between (micro-) albuminuria and atherothrombosis [28]. Other mechanisms must therefore be at work, which may include severe, generalised endothelial dysfunction and chronic, low-grade inflammation.

Indeed, endothelial dysfunction in type 1 and 2 diabetes complicated by micro- or macroalbuminuria is generalised, in that it affects many aspects of endothelial function and occurs both in the kidney and elsewhere [22]. Such data, together with more limited data showing that microalbuminuria is also associated with endothelial dysfunction in the absence of diabetes, have led to the concept that microalbuminuria itself is a marker of generalised renal and extrarenal endothelial dysfunction. Endothelial dysfunction is a central feature of the pathogenesis of atherothrombosis and could thus explain the latter's association with (micro)albuminuria. It is less clear how endothelial dysfunction might cause (micro)albuminuria. Theoretically, endothelial dysfunction could contribute to the pathogenesis of albuminuria both directly, by causing increased glomerular pressure and the synthesis of a leaky glomerular basement membrane, and indirectly, by influencing glomerular mesangial and epithelial cell function in a paracrine fashion (e.g. through inflammatory mechanisms). Importantly, the molecular pathways by which endothelial dysfunction causes (micro) albuminuria have yet to be worked out.

Chronic, low-grade inflammation (as assessed from markers such as plasma C-reactive protein (CRP) concentration) is another candidate to explain the association between (micro-)albuminuria and extrarenal complications [29-31]. Indeed, regardless of the presence of diabetes, chronic, low-grade inflammation is associated with the occurrence and progression of (micro)albuminuria [30], and with risk of atherothrombotic disease [9]. In addition, chronic, low-grade inflammation can be both cause and consequence of endothelial dysfunction, and the two appear tightly linked [29-31]. Nevertheless, recent data indicate that the association between (micro)albuminuria and atherothrombotic disease cannot be explained entirely by markers of endothelial dysfunction and chronic inflammation [30,31]. One (likely) possibility is that such markers do not fully capture the processes they are meant to reflect; but an alternative or additional explanation is that there are other pathways that link (micro)albuminuria to extrarenal complications, such as autonomic neuropathy [32,33] or prothrombotic mechanisms (Figure 1).

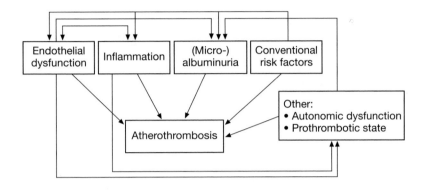

Figure 1. Postulated pathways linking conventional risk factors, endothelial dysfunction, inflammatory activity, (micro-)albuminuria and atherothrombosis in diabetes

Diabetes is associated with activation of the coagulation cascade (1). Hyperglycaemia, non-enzymatic glycation and oxidative stress increase tissue factor activity and factor VII activity, decrease antithrombin activity and impair heparan sulphate synthesis. Initially, anticoagulant defenses such as the response to activated protein C and the secretion of tissue factor pathway inhibitor may be enhanced. In patients with micro- and macroalbuminuria, i.e. in those with severe endothelial dysfunction, activation of the coagulation cascade increases further and endothelial anticoagulant defenses may be overwhelmed. In addition, patients with the metabolic syndrome have high PAI-1 levels and thus impaired fibrinolysis. Importantly, increased coagulation and impaired fibrinolysis may increase thrombus formation and persistence after plaque rupture, and in part explain the poor prognosis of diabetic patients after myocardial infarction.

AT WHAT STAGE OF DIABETES DOES ENDOTHELIAL DYSFUNCTION BECOME MANIFEST?

Type 1 diabetes

Patients who have had type 1 diabetes for more than 5 to 10 years and who have normal urinary albumin excretion, as compared to non-diabetic individuals, are characterised by subtle increases in blood pressure and large artery stiffness and by autonomic dysfunction, and some or perhaps most have impaired endothelial function and increased low-grade inflammation. All these abnormalities are worse in the microalbuminuric stage [22,29,34,35]. It is not clear how they interact nor whether impaired endothelial function is a common antecendent or a consequence, but these data illustrate that cardiovascular function, including endothelial function, does become impaired before the onset of microalbuminuria, at least when the latter is defined as ≥30 mg per 24h. The possibility remains, however, that patients with 'normal' urinary albumin excretion who show such cardiovascular abnormalities are those in whom urinary albumin excretion is in fact increased albeit within the normal range as conventionally defined, i.e. the (arbitrary) cutoff of 30 mg per 24h may be too high. This has a parallel in type 2 diabetes and in non-diabetic individuals, in whom *any* increase in microalbuminuria appears associated with increased risk of atherothrombosis [28].

Endothelial dysfunction thus occurs before microalbuminuria sets in. However, is endothelial dysfunction a feature of type 1 diabetes per se and is moderate hyperglycaemia sufficient to impair endothelial function? It has been argued that nitric-oxide-mediated, endothelium-dependent vasodilation is impaired in short-term uncomplicated diabetes and that hyperglycaemia, in the absence of other factors, acutely impairs endothelium-dependent vasodilation in non-diabetic individuals [22,36,37]. Several findings are however in conflict with these concepts [38-42]. Firstly, studies that carefully stratified patients according to the presence or absence of a normal urinary albumin excretion rate have concluded that, in reasonably well-controlled type 1 diabetes, endothelium-dependent and -independent vasodilation of resistance and conduit arteries are neither impaired nor enhanced [38,39]. Secondly, early uncomplicated type 1 diabetes is accompanied by dilation, not constriction, of small and large blood vessels, and an increase in microvascular blood flow [1,39]. Microvascular dilation may cause capillary hypertension, and, according to the so-called haemodynamic hypothesis of the pathogenesis of microangiopathy, capillary hypertension will, in time, damage the microvascular endothelium and thus set the stage for more advanced stages of microangiopathy, such as microalbuminuria. It is at this stage that a general impairment of endothelial function can usually be clearly observed, although endothelial function may sometimes be normal even among microalbuminuric individuals [43]. Notably, the mediators responsible for the vasodilation typical of early type 1 diabetes remain to be identified, and it is not known whether the endothelium is involved. Taken together, these data suggest that the diabetic state predisposes to the development of endothelial dysfunction, but in and of itself is not a sufficient cause. Other factors, genetic or environmental, are likely to play a role in determining who among type 1 diabetic patients goes on to develop aggressive angiopathy and who does not [44].

Type 2 diabetes

Endothelial dysfunction is common in early and otherwise uncomplicated type 2 diabetes, perhaps especially among women [45], and is associated with an increased risk of cardiovascular mortality and with an increased risk of development and progression of microalbuminuria [20,22,30,31]. It is not clear to what extent this endothelial dysfunction is caused by hyperglycaemia. Endothelial dysfunction in type 2 diabetes appears to be independent of that induced by hypertension and obesity [45,46], but the role, versus hyperglycaemia, of other diabetes-associated variables, such as high triglyceride levels, low HDL cholesterol levels, abnormal LDL composition, hyperinsulinaemia, insulin resistance, and chronic low-grade inflammation remains to be established [31,47]. An important contender is increased inflammatory activity. Endothelial dysfunction, inflammation and urinary albumin excretion in type 2 diabetes are progressive and closely interrelated [31]. Nevertheless, as in type 1 diabetes, microalbuminuria in type 2 diabetes can occur in the absence of severe endothelial dysfunction [43,48], and then has a relatively good prognosis [49].

ENDOTHELIAL DYSFUNCTION, INSULIN RESISTANCE AND THE METABOLIC SYNDROME

Insulin resistance usually precedes the development of type 2 diabetes and is often accompanied by a cluster of other risk factors (see above). The mechanisms underlying this clustering are still unclear, but all elements of the cluster share two important pathophysiological features, namely insulin resistance and endothelial dysfunction. A widely accepted theory states that insulin resistance is the primary abnormality that gives rise to type 2 diabetes, hypertension and dyslipidaemia, and that endothelial dysfunction merely represents the impact of hyperglycaemia and other features of the metabolic syndrome. An alternative concept is that endothelial dysfunction is at the heart of the metabolic syndrome. According to this concept, the endothelial dysfunction in large arteries that is an early and prominent event in atherothrombotic disease is parallelled by endothelial dysfunction in resistance vessels and metabolically important capillary beds that contributes to the development of the metabolic syndrome [50].

How can endothelial dysfunction impair insulin-induced glucose disposal? Firstly, insulin is a vasoactive hormone. Insulin increases muscle blood flow in a time- and concentration-dependent fashion through a mechanism that involves binding to the insulin receptor on the endothelial cell membrane and that can be abolished by inhibiting nitric oxide synthase. Nevertheless, insulin-induced increases in glucose uptake and total blood flow have different concentration-effect curves as well as time kinetics. Therefore, it is unlikely that a simple insulin-induced increase in total blood flow per se can increase glucose disposal. Secondly, however, in a process termed capillary recruitment, insulin can redirect blood flow in skeletal muscle from non-nutritive capillaries (those that are not coupled to muscle cells) to nutritive capillaries (those that are) and thus increase glucose disposal even without increasing total blood flow [51,52]. In this way, physical integrity and normal function of the arteriolar and capillary endothelium are prerequisites for normal metabolic insulin action. Indeed, insulin's vasodilator actions have been shown to be impaired in classic insulin-resistant states, notably type 2 diabetes, obesity and hypertension, and to be decreased by mediators closely associated with insulin resistance, namely tumour necrosis factor-α (TNF-α) and free fatty acids [53-55]. Taken together, these data suggest that endothelial dysfunction and impaired capillary recruitment can cause insulin resistance with respect to glucose disposal both when the microvascular endothelium is otherwise healthy but cannot react properly to insulin ('endothelial insulin resistance') and when the microvascular endothelium is injured through other mechanisms, such as age-related capillary drop-out ('rarefaction', i.e. reduced capillary density per volume of tissue).

Decreased capillary density and impaired capillary recruitment may in part explain why insulin resistance is associated with hypertension [56-58], as capillaries can contribute to control of peripheral vascular resistance by virtue of their narrow caliber and relative non-distensibility; by rarefaction (modelling indicates that for ~40% rarefaction, there is a ~20% increase in peripheral vascular resistance); and through active deformations, i.e. contractility [59]. In turn, the association of decreased capillary density and impaired recruitment with low birth weight [60,61] and increasing age may help explain the propensity of such individuals both to insulin resistance and hypertension.

Decreased capillary density and impaired capillary recruitment may also play a role in the development of atherogenic changes in lipoprotein concentrations, through impaired action of endothelium-bound lipoprotein lipase [50].

The molecular pathways through which insulin increases nitric oxide synthesis, endothelium-dependent vasodilation and capillary recruitment have not yet been fully elucidated, nor how TNF-α, free fatty acids and perhaps hyperinsulinaemia itself [62,63] impair these actions of insulin. Firstly, insulin can act on insulin receptors on endothelial cells to produce nitric oxide but also endothelin-1, a potent vasoconstrictor. Endothelial insulin resistance can thus be conceptualised as a shift in the balance between vasodilators and vasoconstrictors produced by insulin, with vasodilation as the normal response and impaired vasodilation or even net vasoconstriction as abnormal responses. Secondly, although insulin's endothelial actions have been shown to occur in cell culture and in isolated vessels, this does not exclude that, in vivo, insulin may act at insulin receptors on vascular smooth cells to cause vasodilation and (or) on skeletal muscle to activate glucose metabolism to produce a metabolite (e.g., adenosine) that then acts on local endothelial and (or) smooth muscle cells. Thirdly, regardless of the presence of diabetes, chronic, low-grade inflammation is closely associated with, and may link, endothelial dysfunction and metabolic insulin resistance [64-67]. These postulated pathways are summarised in Figure 2.

MOLECULAR CELL BIOLOGY OF ENDOTHELIAL DYSFUNCTION IN DIABETES

General remarks
Endothelial dysfunction in diabetes originates from three main sources [1,3,68-76]. Firstly, hyperglycaemia and its immediate biochemical sequelae *directly* alter endothelial function. Glucose transport into endothelial and vascular smooth muscle cells is insulin-independent and is autoregulated in smooth muscle cells, but not in endothelial cells, in which an increase in blood glucose

concentration will thus increase the intracellular accumulation of glucose and its metabolites.

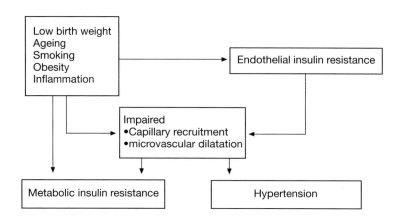

Figure 2. Postulated pathways linking cardiovascular risk factors, insulin resistance and microvascular function

Thus, endothelial cells exposed to high glucose in vitro increase the production of extracellular matrix components, such as collagen and fibronectin, and of procoagulant proteins, such as vWF and tissue factor, and show decreased proliferation, migration and fibrinolytic potential, and increased apoptosis. Secondly, high glucose influences endothelial cell functioning *indirectly* by the synthesis of growth factors (e.g., transforming growth factor-β (TGF-β) and vascular endothelial growth factor (VEGF), cytokines (e.g., TNF-α) and vasoactive agents in other cells. Thirdly, the components of the metabolic syndrome can affect endothelial function.

Hyperglycaemia and its immediate biochemical sequelae
An increase in intracellular glucose will lead to an increase in the flux of glucose to sorbitol via the polyol pathway, an increase in glucosamine-6-phosphate via the hexosamine pathway, and the activation of protein kinase C

(PKC) via de novo synthesis of diacylglycerol (DAG). In addition, glucose and glucose-derived dicarbonyl compounds react non-enzymatically with the basic amino acids, lysine and arginine, in proteins to form advanced glycation endproducts (AGEs) both extra- and intracellularly. Figure 3 shows how, intracellularly, these four biochemical mechanisms may all be the consequence of hyperglycaemia-induced overproduction of reactive oxygen species in mitochondria [68,74].

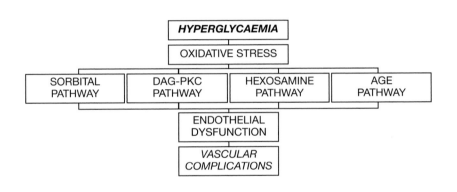

Figure 3. Four biochemical pathways through which hyperglycaemia can cause endothelial dysfunction and vascular complications

The sorbitol pathway. In most cells, excess glucose can be metabolised to sorbitol and fructose by aldose reductase and sorbitol dehydrogenase, which is accompanied by increased oxidation of NADPH to NADP+ and increased reduction of NAD+ to NADH. This pathway is thought to impair endothelial function because the increase in the cytosolic NADH/NAD+ ratio results in a redox imbalance that resembles that which occurs in tissue hypoxia and therefore is termed *hyperglycaemic pseudohypoxia*. It increases the formation of methylglyoxal and AGEs and enhances oxidative stress [1]. The full impact of the sorbitol pathway in vascular dysfunction is, however, not completely understood and the role of inhibition of aldose reductase in the prevention and treatment of diabetic complications remains unclear [1].

The DAG-PKC pathway. The cellular pathogenic consequences of hyperglycaemia-induced synthesis of DAG and activation of PKC are multiple and include dysregulation of vascular permeability directly or indirectly (the latter through the induction of VEGF in smooth muscle cells); dysregulation of blood flow by decreasing endothelial nitric oxide synthase activity and (or) increasing endothelin-1 synthesis; basement membrane thickening through TGF-β-mediated increased synthesis of type IV collagen and fibronectin; impaired fibrinolysis through increased expression of PAI-1; and increased oxidative stress by the regulation of several NADPH oxidases.

In vascular cells, the PKCβII isoform appears preferentially activated. In diabetic animals, an oral PKCβ inhibitor prevented diabetes-induced abnormalities in mRNA expression of TGF-β1, type IV collagen and fibronectin, ameliorated increases in glomerular filtration rate and accelerated glomerular mesangial expansion, and partly corrected urinary albumin excretion. Studies to evaluate the importance of the DAG-PKC pathway in humans are underway [1].

The hexosamine pathway. The vascular effects of the hexosamine pathway, in which fructose-6-phosphate is converted to glucosamine-6-phosphate by the enzyme glutamine:fructose-6-phosphate amidotransferase, are just beginning to be understood but may be profound. In aortic endothelial cells, hyperglycaemia was shown to increase levels of hexosamine-6-phosphate and subsequently N-acetylglucosamine (GlcNAc). This, by the addition of GlcNAc to serine and threonine residues, increased O-linked glycosylation of the transcription factor SP-1, which decreased SP-1 phosphorylation and increased SP-1 activity, which in turn can increase transcription of PAI-1 and TGF-β1 [74]. Other proteins, such as PKC and endothelial cell nitric oxide synthase can be modified in a similar way. For example, such a modification of the Akt site of endothelial cell nitric oxide synthase has been shown to decrease enzyme activity [75].

Non-enzymatic glycation. Non-enzymatic glycation of proteins is the condensation reaction of the carbonyl group of sugar aldehydes with the Nterminus of free amino acids of proteins and initially leads to a Schiff base, which then undergoes rearrangement to early glycation Amadori-adducts such as fructosamine. Amadori-adducts are relatively stable and only a small fraction undergoes rearrangements to irreversible AGEs. AGEs are a mixture of different moieties. When oxidation is involved in their formation, so-called glycoxidation products such as pentosidine and N^{ε}-(carboxymethyl)lysine result. Initially, AGEs were thought to form only on long-lived extracellular molecules, because of the slow rate of reaction of glucose with proteins. However, intracellular and short-lived molecules have now also been shown to be targets for AGE formation through reactions with other sugars such as glucose-6-phosphate and glyceraldehyde-3-phosphate, which form AGEs at a much faster rate than glucose. In addition, the highly reactive dicarbonyl compounds methylglyoxal, glyoxal and 3-deoxyglucosone, which are formed from the degradation of glycolytic intermediates, are believed to contribute importantly to the formation of AGEs in vivo. This so-called carbonyl stress has been implicated in the accelerated vascular damage in both diabetes and uraemia. In endothelial cells, methylglyoxal is probably the main AGE-forming compound and can be degraded to D-lactate by the glyoxylase system [69,70].

The introduction of AGEs in the extracellular matrix can interfere with endothelial function in several ways. AGE-modified type I and IV collagen inhibit normal matrix formation and cross-linking, and decrease arterial elasticity; AGE-modified matrix stimulates interactions with mononuclear cells and macromolecules such as LDL; and AGEs may act as oxidants. In addition, AGE-modified plasma proteins can bind to the receptor for AGE (RAGE) [76], which has been shown to mediate signal transduction via a receptor-mediated induction of reactive oxygen species and activation of the transcription factors NF-κB and p21[ras]. In animal models, blockade of RAGE inhibited the development of macrovascular disease and diabetic nephropathy [76].

Many aspects of diabetic complications are thus potentially related to the effect of Amadori-adducts [77] and AGEs. Clinical trials with aminoguanidine, an AGE formation inhibitor that had shown promise in animal experiments, have unfortunately been halted because of unforeseen side effects, but trials with other AGE formation inhibitors and with AGE cross-link breakers are underway or are being planned.

Oxidative stress as a final common pathway of hyperglycaemia-induced vascular dysfunction. Hyperglycaemic pseudohypoxia, glucose autooxidation and AGE formation increase oxidative stress. In addition, hyperglycaemia impairs endothelial free radical scavenging by reducing the activity of the pentose phosphate pathway and thus decreasing the availability of NADPH to the glutathione redox cycle [70].

Reactive oxygen species can affect many signalling pathways, such as G-proteins, protein kinases, ion channels and transcription factors, and may modify endothelial function by a variety of mechanisms. These include direct effects on the endothelium such as peroxidation of membrane lipids, activation of NF-κB, and interference with the availability of nitric oxide; and indirect effects such as increasing the oxidation of LDL and the activation of platelets and monocytes. On the other hand, endothelial cells can respond to high glucose levels by increasing the expression of antioxidant enzymes such as superoxide dismutase, catalase and glutathione peroxidase.

It is not known whether oxidative stress causes endothelial dysfunction in human diabetes. It has been difficult to assess the presence of increased oxidative stress in vivo, mainly because of questionable specificity and reproducibility of the methods used. In short-term experiments, high doses of vitamin C can improve some aspects of endothelial dysfunction in diabetes [1].

On the other hand, randomised clinical trials of anti-oxidants have failed to show a decrease in macrovascular disease. The reasons for this discrepancy are unclear.

Growth factors and cytokines: TGF-β, VEGF and TNF-α

TGF-β. TGF-β plays a major role in diabetic nephropathy [78]. It mediates glomerular capillary basement thickening and mesangial matrix expansion. Its role in the thickening of capillary basement membranes elsewhere (e.g., in the retina) is less well established. TGF-β1 is increased through hyperglycaemia-induced PKC activation; through Amadori-albumin and AGEs; through stretch and angiotensin-II; and through cytokine activation of endothelial cells. TGF-β1 stimulates the production of matrix components such as type I and IV collagen, fibronectin, laminin, and proteoglycans in cultured glomerular mesangial cells and epithelial cells; is involved in the regulation of glomerular endothelial, epithelial and mesangial proliferation; and also has potent anti-inflammatory effects on vascular cells, down-regulating cytokine-induced expression of E-selectin, VCAM-1 and monocyte chemotactic protein-1 [78].

VEGF. VEGF is a potent and apparently endothelium-specific mitogenic cytokine, whose expression can be induced by hypoxia through hypoxia-inducible factor-1, but also by insulin-like growth factor-1 and TGF-β1. VEGF can induce the proliferation and migration of vascular endothelial cells leading to angiogenesis, neovascularisation and increased vascular permeability. Several studies have shown increased vitreous VEGF levels in patients with proliferative diabetic retinopathy, and antagonists of VEGF and its receptors have been shown to reduce retinopathy in animal models. The role of increased or decreased VEGF in other diabetic complications is the subject of much ongoing research [79].

TNF-α and inflammation. TNF-α is an inflammatory cytokine produced by neutrophils, macrophages and, importantly, adipocytes. TNF-α can induce other powerful cytokines such as interleukin-6, which in turn regulates the expression of CRP. These mediators alone or in combination can impair endothelial function and contribute to atherothrombosis. In addition, TNF-α can induce insulin resistance, which may at least in part explain why insulin resistance, endothelial dysfunction and atherothrombosis are so closely related (see above). Finally, recent studies have shown that TNF-α and inflammation in general can contribute to the pathogenesis of diabetic nephropathy.

Vascular cells are both a target for cytokines and a source. The spectrum of endothelial cell responses elicited by cytokines is varied. Briefly, inflammatory cytokines increase vascular permeability; alter vasoregulatory responses; increase leukocyte adhesion to endothelium; and facilitate thrombus formation by inducing procoagulant activity, by inhibiting anticoagulant pathways and by impairing fibrinolysis via stimulation of PAI-1. Activation of the transcription factor NF-κB is crucial in cytokine regulation of gene expression in endothelial cells [12]. NF-κB is activated not only by TNF-α and interleukin-1, but also by hyperglycaemia, AGEs, angiotensin II, oxidised lipids and insulin. Taken together, these data suggest that NF-κB pathway is an important contributor to the pathogenesis of vascular disease in diabetes mellitus.

The metabolic syndrome: insulin resistance, insulin, hypertension, dyslipidaemia, and obesity

Insulin resistance. How metabolic and endothelial insulin resistance occur and why they are closely related is not fully understood (see above). Endothelial insulin resistance, whether primary or secondary (Figure 2), can be regarded as a form of endothelial dysfunction and conceivably contributes to both atherothrombosis and microangiopathy. Both TNF-α and free fatty acids can cause metabolic and endothelial insulin resistance. TNF-α may induce endothelial insulin resistance through its ability to impair intracellular signalling by inhibition of insulin-stimulated autophosphorylation and phosphorylation of insulin receptor substrate-1. How non-esterified fatty acids impair insulin's endothelial actions is not clear.

Insulin. Both type 2 and type 1 diabetes are usually accompanied by chronic hyperinsulinaemia. Whether insulin has atherogenic effects is controversial, mainly because it is not clear whether effects such as increased vascular permeability to macromolecules and increased vascular smooth muscle cell proliferation occur at physiological concentrations. In addition, insulin can increase nitric oxide synthesis and may have anti-inflammatory and anti-atherogenic effects [80]. Taken together, these data raise the possibility that insulin may have adverse effects when insulin signalling in vascular cells is abnormal.

Hypertension. Hypertension is a major determinant of microangiopathy and atherothrombosis in diabetes. Hypertension causes endothelial activation and impaired nitric oxide availability (see above); whether the latter then contributes to increased blood pressure is not clear. Experimental data indicate that decreased nitric oxide availability in the kidney may contribute to vasoconstriction and decreased glomerular filtration; impaired tubuloglomerular feedback; decreased medullary blood flow and impaired pressure natriuresis; and progressive proteinuria. Salt sensitivity of blood pressure may denote an inability to increase nitric oxide availability in response to increased blood pressure [81].

Dyslipidaemia. The effects of LDL cholesterol (see above) may be enhanced in type 2 diabetes, which is associated with increased small dense LDL particles. In addition, type 2 diabetes, especially when glycaemic control is poor, is characterised by increased postprandial triglyceride-rich lipoproteins (chylomicrons and VLDL particles), which can enhance oxidative stress and impair endothelial function both directly and indirectly (by increasing the production of small dense LDL particles and by reducing HDL [82,83]). These changes contribute to atherothrombosis and may also play a role in nephropathy, as such dyslipidaemia can damage glomerular podocytes and mesangial cells [84]. Dyslipidaemia has been associated with increases in urinary albumin excretion in both type 1 and type 2 diabetes [85,86].

Obesity. Obesity, especially visceral obesity, is associated with increased risk of atherothrombosis and microangiopathy. These effects may be mediated through the associations of obesity with hypertension, dyslipidaemia and insulin resistance, and also through mediators directly secreted by adipocytes, such as TNF-α, leptin and PAI-1. For example, obesity-associated proteinuria may be related to hyperfiltration, increased renal venous pressure, glomerular hypertrophy and increased matrix production through increased synthesis of vasoactive and fibrogenic mediators, such as angiotensin-II, insulin, leptin and TGF-β1 [87].

Asymmetric dimethylarginine (ADMA). There is some evidence that levels of ADMA, an endogenous inhibitor of nitric oxide, are associated with the metabolic syndrome [88], which may in part be caused by hyperglycaemia-induced impairment of ADMA breakdown [89]. This is an area of active investigation.

CONCLUSIONS

The endothelium is an important locus of control of vascular functions, and reasonable but not perfect methods exist for assessing endothelial function in vivo in humans. Endothelial dysfunction in diabetes complicated by micro- or macroalbuminuria is generalised, in that it affects many aspects of endothelial function. The close linkage between microalbuminuria and endothelial dysfunction in diabetes is an attractive explanation for the fact that microalbuminuria is a risk marker for atherothrombosis. In type 1 diabetes, endothelial dysfunction precedes and may cause diabetic microangiopathy, but it is not clear whether endothelial dysfunction is a feature of the diabetic state per se. In type 2 diabetes, endothelial function is impaired from the onset of the disease and is strongly related to adverse outcomes. It is not clear whether impaired endothelial function is cause by hyperglycaemia or by other factors. Regardless of the presence of diabetes, impaired endothelial function is closely associated with and may contribute to insulin resistance. Endothelial dysfunction in diabetes originates from three main sources. Firstly, hyperglycaemia and its immediate biochemical sequelae *directly* alter endothelial function. Secondly, hyperglycaemia influences endothelial cell functioning *indirectly* by the synthesis of growth factors, cytokines and vasoactive agents in other cells. Thirdly, the components of the metabolic syndrome can impair endothelial function.

REFERENCES

(References are preferentially to reviews and articles published after 1996.)

1. Tooke JE (ed). Diabetic angiopathy. London: Arnold, 1999.
2. Mogensen CE (ed). The kidney and hypertension in diabetes mellitus (5th edition). Boston: Kluwer, 2000.
3. Stehouwer CDA, Yudkin JS (eds). Diabetic angiopathy. Semin Vasc Med 2002;2:1-228.
4. Jager A, Kostense PJ, Nijpels G, Dekker JM, Heine RJ, Bouter LM, Donker AJM, Stehouwer CDA. Serum homocysteine levels are associated with the development of (micro)albuminuria. The Hoorn Study. Arterioscler Thromb Vasc Biol 2001;21:74-81.
5. Stehouwer CDA, Gall MA, Hougaard P, Jakobs C, Parving HH. Plasma homocysteine concentration predicts mortality in non-insulin-dependent diabetic patients with and without albuminuria. Kidney Int 1999;55:308-14.
6. Hoogeveen EK, Kostense PJ, Jakobs C, Dekker JM, Nijpels G, Heine RJ, Bouter LM, Stehouwer CDA. Hyperhomocysteinemia increases risk of death, especially in type 2 diabetes: 5-year follow-up of the Hoorn Study. Circulation 2000;101:1506-11.
7. Epidemiology of diabetes intervention and complications (EDIC) research group. Effect of intensive diabetes treatment on carotid artery wall thickness in the epidemiology of diabetes interventions and complications. Diabetes 1999;48:383-90.
8. Laakso M. Hyperglycemia and cardiovascular disease in type 2 diabetes. Diabetes 1999;48:937-42.
9. Ross R. Atherosclerosis - an inflammatory disease. N Engl J Med 1999;340:115-26.
10. Cines DB, Pollak E, Buck CA, Loscalzo J, Zimmerman GA, McEver RP, Pober JS, Wick TM, Konkle BA, Schwartz BS, Barnathan ES, McCrae KR, Hug BA. Schmidt AM, Stern DM. Endothelial cells in the physiology and in the pathophysiology of vascular disorders. Blood 1998;91:3527-61.
11. De Caterina R. Endothelial dysfunctions: common denominators in vascular disease. Curr Opin Lipidol 2000;11:9-23.
12. de Martin R, Hoeth M, Hofer-Warbinek R, Schmid JA. The transcription factor NF-κB and the regulation of vascular cell function. Arterioscler Thromb Vasc Biol 2000;20:e83-8.
13. John S, Schmieder RE. Impaired endothelial function in arterial hypertension and hypercholesterolemia: potential mechanisms and differences. J Hypertens 2000;18:363-74.
14. Berry C, Brosnan MJ, Fennell J, Hamilton CA, Dominiczak AF. Oxidative stress and vascular damage in hypertension. Curr Opin Nephrol Hypertens 2001;10:247-55.
15. Sowers JR. Hypertension, angiotensin II, and oxidative stress. N Engl J Med 2002;346:1999-2001.
16. McVeigh GE, Hamilton PK, Morgan DR. Evaluation of mechanical arterial properties: clinical, experimental and therapeutic aspects. Clin Sci 2002;102:51-67.
17. Stehouwer CDA. Is measurement of endothelial dysfunction clinically useful? Eur J Clin Invest 1999;29:459-61.
18. Cannon RO. Cardiovascular benefit of cholesterol-lowering therapy: does improved endothelial vasodilator function matter? Circulation 2000;102:820-2.
19. Jager A, van Hinsbergh VWM, Kostense PJ, Emeis JJ, Yudkin JS, Nijpels G, Dekker JM, Heine RJ, Bouter LM, Stehouwer CDA. Von Willebrand factor, C-reactive protein and 5-year mortality in diabetic and nondiabetic subjects: the Hoorn Study. Arterioscler Tromb Vasc Biol 1999;19:3071-8.

20. Jager A, van Hinsbergh VWM, Kostense PJ, Emeis JJ, Nijpels G, Dekker JM, Heine RJ, Bouter LM, Stehouwer CDA. Increased levels of soluble vascular cell adhesion molecule 1 are associated with risk of cardiovascular mortality in type 2 diabetes. Diabetes 2000;49:485-91.

21. JKinlay S, Creager MA, Fukumoto M, Hikita H, Fang JC, Selwyn AP, Ganz P. Endothelium-derived nitric oxide regulates arterial elasticity in human arteries in vivo. Hypertension 2001;38:1049-53.

22. JStehouwer CDA, Lambert J, Donker AJM, van Hinsbergh VWM. Endothelial dysfunction and the pathogenesis of diabetic angiopathy. Cardiovasc Res 1997;34:55-68.

23. JFlyvbjerg A. Putative pathophysiological role of growth factors and cytokines in experimental diabetic kidney disease. Diabetologia 2000;43:1205-23.

24. JCooper ME. Interaction of metabolic and haemodynamic factors in mediating experimental diabetic nephropathy. Diabetologia 2001;44:1957-72.

25. JLorenzi M, Cerhardinger C. Early cellular and molecular changes induced by diabetes in the retina. Diabetologia 2001;44:791-804.

26. JCameron NE, Eaton SEM, Cotter MA, Tesfaye S. Vascular factors and metabolic interactions in the pathogenesis of diabetic neuropathy. Diabetologia 2001;44:1973-88.

27. JBeckman JA, Creager MA, Libby P. Diabetes and atherosclerosis. Epidemiology, pathophysiology, and management. JAMA 2002;287:2570-81.

28. JGerstein HC, Mann JFE, Yi Q, Zinman B, Dinneen SF, Hoogwerf B, Hallé JP, Young J, Rashkwo A, Joyce C, Nawaz S, Yusuf S, for the HOPE Study Investigators. Albuminuria and risk of cardiovascular events, death, and heart failure in diabetic and nondiabetic individuals. JAMA 2001;286:421-6.

29. JSchalkwijk CG, Poland DCW, van Dijk W, Kok A, Emeis JJ, Dräger AM, Doni A, van Hinsbergh VWM, Stehouwer CDA. Plasma concentration of C-reactive protein is increased in Type I diabetic patients without clinical macroangiopathy and correlates with markers of endothelial dysfunction: evidence for chronic inflammation. Diabetologia 1999;42:351-7.

30. JJager A, van Hinsbergh VWM, Kostense PJ, Emeis JJ, Nijpels G, Dekker JM, Heine RJ, Bouter LM, Stehouwer CDA. C-reactive protein and soluble vascular cell adhesion molecule-1 are associated with elevated urinary albumin excretion but do not explain its link with cardiovascular risk. Arterioscler Thromb Vasc Biol 2002;22:593-8.

31. JStehouwer CDA, Gall MA, Twisk JWR, Knudsen E, Emeis JJ, Parving HH. Increased urinary albumin excretion, endothelial dysfunction, and chronic low-grade inflammation in type 2 diabetes. Progressive, interrelated, and independently associated with risk of death. Diabetes 2002;51:1157-65.

32. Smulders YM, Jager A, Gerritsen J, Dekker JM, Nijpels G, Heine RJ, Bouter LM, Stehouwer CDA. Cardiovascular autonomic function is associated with (micro-) albuminuria in elderly Caucasian subjects with impaired glucose tolerance or type 2 diabetes: the Hoorn Study. Diabetes Care 2000;23:1369-74.

33. Gerritsen J, Dekker JM, TenVoorde BJ, Kostense PJ, Heine RJ, Bouter LM, Heethaar RM, Stehouwer CDA. Impaired autonomic function is associated with increased mortality, especially in subjects with diabetes, hypertension, or a history of cardiovascular disease. Diabetes Care 2001;24:1793-8

34. van Ittersum FJ, Spek JJ, Praet IJA, Lambert J, IJzerman RG, Fischer HRA, Nikkels RE, Van Bortel LMAB, Donker AJM, Stehouwer CDA. Ambulatory blood pressures and autonomic nervous function in normoalbuminuric type I diabetic patients. Nephrol Dial Transplant 1998;13:326-32.

35. Vervoort G, Lutterman JA, Smits P, Berden JHM, Wetzels JF. Transcapillary escape rate of albumin is increased and related to haemodynamic changes in normo-albuminuric type 1 diabetic patients. J Hypertens 1999;17:1911-6.

36. Dogra G, Rich L, Stanton K, Watts GF. Endothelium-dependent and -independent vasodilation studied at normoglycaemia in type I diabetes mellitus with and without microalbuminuria. Diabetologia 2001;44:593-601.

37. Giugliano D, Marfella R, Coppola L, Verazzo G, Acampora R, Giunta R, Nappo F, Lucarelli C, D'Onofrio F. Vascular effects of acute hyperglycemia in humans are reversed by L-arginine: evidence for reduced availability of nitric oxide during hyperglycemia. Circulation 1997;95:1783-90.

38. Chan NN, Vallance P, Colhoun HM. Nitric oxide and vascular responses in type 1 diabetes. Diabetologia 2000;43:137-47.

39. Vervoort G, Wetzels JF, Lutterman JA, van Doorn LG, Berden JHM, Smits P. Elevated skeletal muscle blood flow in uncomplicated type 1 diabetes mellitus. Role of nitric oxide and sympathetic tone. Hypertension 1999;34:1080-5.

40. O'Byrne S, Forte P, Roberts LJ, Morrow JD, Johnston A, Änggard E, Leslie RDG, Benjamin N. Nitric oxide synthesis and isoprostane production in subjects with type 1 diabetes and normal urinary albumin excretion. Diabetes 2000;49:857-62.

41. Chiarelli F, Cipollone F, Romano F, Tumini S, Costantini F, di Ricco L, Pomilio M, Pierdomenico SD, Marini M, Cuccurullo F, Mezzetti A. Increased circulating nitric oxide in young patients with type 1 diabetes and persistent microalbuminuria. Diabetes 2000;49:1258-63.

42. Pieper GM. Enhanced, unaltered and impaired nitric oxide-mediated endothelium-dependent relaxation in experimental diabetes mellitus: importance of disease duration. Diabetologia 1999;42:204-13.

43. Stehouwer CDA, Yudkin JS, Fioretto P, Nosadini R. How heterogeneous is microalbuminuria? The case for 'benign' and 'malignant' microalbuminuria. Nephrol Dial Transplant 1998;13:2751-4

44. Miller JA, Thai K, Scholey JW. Angiotensin II type 1 receptor gene polymorphism and the response to hyperglycemia in early type 1 diabetes. Diabetes 2000;49:1585-9.

45. Steinberg HO, Paradisi G, Cronin J, Crowde K, Hempfling A, Hook G, Baron AD. Type II diabetes abrogates sex differences in endothelial function in premenopausal women. Circulation 2000;101:2040-6.

46. Hogikyan RV, Galecki AT, Pitt B, Halter JB, Greene DA, Supiano MA. Specific impairment of endothelium-dependent vasodilation in subjects with type 2 diabetes independent of obesity. J Clin Endocrinol Metab 1998;83:1946-52.

47. Bagg W, Ferri C, Desideri G, Gamble G, Ockelford P, Braatvedt G. The influences of obesity and glycemic control on endothelial activation in patients with type 2 diabetes. J Clin Endocrinol Metab 2001;86:5491-7.

48. Fioretto P, Stehouwer CDA, Mauer M, Chiesura-Corona M, Brocco E, Carraro A, Bortoloso E, van Hinsbergh VWM, Crepaldi G, Nosadini R. Heterogeneous nature of microalbuminuria in non-insulin-dependent diabetes: studies of endothelial function and renal structure. Diabetologia 1998;41:233-6.

49. Jager A, Hinsbergh VWM van, Kostense PJ, Nijpels G, Emeis JJ, Dekker JM, Heine RJ, Bouter LM, Stehouwer CDA. Prognostic implications of retinopathy and a high plasma von Willebrand factor concentration in type 2 diabetic subjects with microalbuminuria. Nephrol Dial Transplant 2001;16:529-536.

50. Pinkney JH, Stehouwer CDA, Coppack SW, Yudkin JS. Endothelial dysfunction: cause of the insulin resistance syndrome. Diabetes 1997;46(suppl 2):S9-13.

51. Coggins M, Lindner J, Rattigan S, Jahn L, Fasy E, Kaul S, Barrett E. Physiologic hyperinsulinemia enhances human skeletal muscle perfusion by capillary recruitment. Diabetes 2001;50:2682-90.

52. Serné EH, IJzerman RG, Gans ROB, Nijveldt R, de Vries G, Evertz R, Donker AJM, Stehouwer CDA. Direct evidence for insulin-induced capillary recruitment in skin of healthy subjects during physiological hyperinsulinemia. Diabetes 2002;51:1515-22.

53. Youd JM, Rattigan S, Clark MG. Acute impairment of insulin-mediated capillary recruitment and glucose uptake in rat skeletal muscle in vivo by TNF-a. Diabetes 2000;49:1904-9.

54. Steinberg HO, Baron AD. Vascular function, insulin resistance and fatty acids. Diabetologia 2002;45:623-34.

55. Clerk LH, Rattigan S, Clark MG. Lipid infusion impairs physiologic insulin-mediated capillary recruitment and muscle glucose uptake in vivo. Diabetes 2002;51:1138-45.

56. Serné EH, Stehouwer CDA, ter Maaten JC, ter Wee PM, Rauwerda JA, Donker AJM, Gans ROB. Microvascular function relates to insulin sensitivity and blood pressure in normal subjects. Circulation 1999;99:896-902.

57. Serné EH, Gans ROB, Maaten JC ter, Wee PM ter, Donker AJM, Stehouwer CDA. Capillary recruitment is impaired in essential hypertension and relates to insulin's metabolic and vascular actions. Cardiovasc Res 2001;49:161-8.

58. Serné EH, Gans ROB, Maaten JC ter, Tangelder GJ, Donker AJM, Stehouwer CDA. Impaired skin capillary recruitment in essential hypertension is caused by both functional and structural capillary rarefaction. Hypertension 2001;38:238-42.

59. Levy BI, Ambrosio G, Pries AR, Struijker Boudier HAJ. Microcirculation in hypertension. A new target for treatment? Circulation 2001;104:735-40.

60. Serné EH, Stehouwer CDA, ter Maaten JC, ter Wee PM, Donker AJM, Gans ROB. Birth weight relates to blood pressure and microvascular function in normal subjects. J Hypertens 2000;18:1421-7.

61. IJzerman RG, Voordouw JJ, Weissenbruch MM, Delemarre-van der Waal HA, Stehouwer CDA. The association between birth weight and capillary recruitment is independent of blood pressure and insulin sensitivity: a study in prepubertal children. J Hypertens 2002;20:1957-63.

62. Eringa EC, Stehouwer CDA, Merlijn T, Westerhof N, Sipkema P. Physiological concentrations of insulin induce endothelin-mediated vasoconstriction during inhibition of NOS or PI3-Kinase in skeletal muscle arterioles. Cardiovasc Res 2002;56:464-71.

63. Arcaro G, Cretti A, Balzano S, Lechi A, Muggeo M, Bonora E, Bonadonna RC. Insulin causes endothelial dysfunction in humans. Sites and mechanisms. Circulation 2002;105:576-82.

64. Fernández-Real JM, Ricart W. Insulin resistance and inflammation in an evolutionary perspective: the contribution of cytokine genotype/phenotype to thriftiness. Diabetologia 1999;42:1367-74.

65. Yudkin JS, Stehouwer CDA, Emeis JJ, Coppack SW. C-reactive protein in healthy subjects: associations with obesity, insulin resistance and endothelial dysfunction. A potential role for cytokines originating from adipose tissue? Arterioscler Thromb Vasc Biol 1999;19:972-8.

219

66. Perticone F, Ceravolo R, Candigliota M, Ventura G, Iacopino S, Sinopoli F, Mattioli PL. Obesity and body fat distribution induce endothelial dysfunction by oxidative stress. Diabetes 2001;50:159-65.

67. Festa A, D'Agostino R, Tracy RP, Haffner SM. Elevated levels of acute-phase proteins and plasminogen activator inhibitor-1 predict the development of type 2 diabetes. The Insulin Resistance Atherosclerosis Study. Diabetes 2002;51:1131-7.

68. Brownlee M. Biochemistry and molecular cell biology of diabetic complications. Nature 2001;414:813-20.

69. Singh R, Barden A, Mori T, Beilin L. Advanced glycation end-products: a review. Diabetologia 2001;44:129-46.

70. Baynes JW, Thorpe SR. Role of oxidative stress in diabetic complications. Diabetes 1999;48:1-9.

71. Spitaler MM, Graier WF. Vascular targets of redox signalling in diabetes mellitus. Diabetologia 2002;45:476-94.

72. Saltiel AR, Kahn CR. Insulin signalling and the regulation of glucose and lipid metabolism. Nature 2001;414:799-806.

73. Ginsberg HN. Insulin resistance and cardiovascular disease. J Clin Invest 2000;106:453-8.

74. Du XL, Edelstein D, Dimmeler S, Ju Q, Sui C, Brownlee M. Hyperglycemia inhibits endothelial nitric oxide synthase activity by posttranslational modification at the Akt site. J Clin Invest 2001;108:1341-8.

75. Du XL, Edelstein D, Rossetti L, Fantus IG, Goldberg H, Ziyadeh F, Wu J, Brownlee M. Hyperglycemia-induced mitochondrial superoxide overproduction activates the hexosamine pathway and induces plasminogen activator inhibitor-1 expression by increasing Sp1 glycosylation. Proc Natl Acad Sci USA 2000;97:12222-6.

76. Stern DM, Yan SD, Yan SF, Schmidt AM. Receptor for advanced glycation endproducts (RAGE) and the complications of diabetes. Ageing Res Rev 2002;1:1-15.

77. Schalkwijk CG, Ligtvoet N, Twaalfhoven H, Jager A, Blaauwgeers HGT, Schlingemann RO, Tarnow L, Parving HH, Stehouwer CDA, van Hinsbergh VWM. Amadori-albumin in type 1 diabetic patients: correlation with markers of endothelial function, association with diabetic nephropathy and localization in retinal capillaries. Diabetes 1999;48:2446-53.

78. Chen S, Hong SW, Iglesias-de la Cruz MC, Isono M, Casaretto A, Ziyadeh FN. The key role of the transforming growth factor-beta system in the pathogenesis of diabetic nephropathy. Renal Fail 2002;23:471-81.

79. Duh E, Aiello LP. Vascular endothelial growth factor and diabetes. Diabetes 1999;48:1899-906.

80. Dandona P, Aljada A, Mohanty P. The anti-inflammatory and potential anti-atherogenic effect of insulin: a new paradigm. Diabetologia 2002;45:924-30.

81. Leclercq B, Jaimes EA, Raij L. Nitric oxide synthase and hypertension. Curr Opin Nephrol Hypertens 2002;11:185-9.

82. Hayden JM, Reaven PD. Cardiovascular risk factors in diabetes mellitus type 2: a potential role for novel cardiovascular risk factors. Curr Opin Lipidol 2000;11:519-28.

83. Nappo F, Esposito K, Cioffi M, Giugliano G, Molinari AM, Paolisso G, Marfella R, Giugliano D. Postprandial endothelial activation in healthy subjects and in type 2 diabetic patients: role of fat and carbohydrate meals. JACC 2002;39:1145-50.

84. Sahadevan M, Kasiske BL. Hyperlipidemia in kidney disease: causes and consequences. Curr Opin Nephrol Hypertens 2002;11:323-9.

85. Chaturvedi N, Bandinelli S, Mangili R, Penno G, Rottiers RE, Fuller JH, on behalf of the EURODIAB Prospective Complications Study Group. Microalbuminuria in type 1 diabetes: rates, risk factors and glycemic threshold. Kidney Int 2001;60:219-27.

86. Smulders YM, Rakic M, Stehouwer CDA, Weijers RNM, Slaats EH, Silberbusch J. Determinants of progression of microalbuminuria in patients with non-insulin-dependent diabetes mellitus. Diabetes Care 1997;20:999-1005.

87. Adelman RD. Obesity and renal disease. Curr Opin Nephrol Hypertens 2002;11:331-5.

88. Chan NN, Chan JCN. Asymmetric dimethylarginine (ADMA): a potential link between endothelial dysfunction and cardiovascular diseases in insulin resistance syndrome? Diabetologia 2002;45:1609-16.

89. Lin KY, Asagami T, Tsao PS, Adimoolam S, Kimoto M, Tsuji H, Reaven GM, Cooke JP. Impaired nitric oxide synthase pathway in diabetes mellitus. Role of asymmetric dimethylarginine and dimethylarginine dimethylaminohydrolase. Circulation 2002;106:987-92.

14

PATHOGENESIS AND MANAGEMENT OF BACTERIAL URINARY TRACT INFECTIONS IN ADULT PATIENTS WITH DIABETES MELLITUS

Andy I.M. Hoepelman

Department of Medicine, Division Acute Medicine & Infectious Diseases, University Medical Center Utrecht, Utrecht, The Netherlands

INTRODUCTION

Urinary tract infections (UTIs) are among the most common bacterial infections [1]. Up to 50 percent of women report having had at least one UTI in their lifetimes.[2] Uncomplicated UTIs occur most often in young healthy adult women and are easy to treat. However, in other patient groups, UTIs can have a complicated course, are more difficult to treat, and often recur. Complicated UTIs occur most commonly in patients with abnormalities of the genitourinary tract. However, also other subtle conditions such as age over 65 years, treatment with immunosuppressive drugs, the presence of Human Immunodeficiency Virus (HIV)-infection and last but not least diabetes mellitus (DM) predispose to an enhanced susceptibility for the development of a UTI with a complicated course.[3,4]

DM is the most common endocrine disease. Besides organ complications as retinopathy, nephropathy and neuropathy, diabetic patients also suffer more frequently from (complicated) infections compared to nondiabetic patients. In a large study of bacteremic patients, it was demonstrated that two thirds of the patients had DM; the urinary tract was the most prevalent infection site.[5]

In this chapter we focus on UTIs, although we are aware that infections elsewhere are also very important, particularly in men with DM. Furthermore it is important to realize that most of the research described here, has been performed in female patients, who have a higher prevalence of UTIs than men. First, this article describes shortly the specific aspects on the epidemiology, pathogenesis, clinical presentation and consequences of asymptomatic and symptomatic UTIs in adult patients with DM, followed by a more extensive description of the management of bacteriuria in these patients. Because of the specialized character, the treatment of the complications of UTIs will not be described.

EPIDEMIOLOGY

The majority of the infections in diabetic patients are localized in the urinary tract.[5] An autopsy study in 1940 showed that approximately 20 percent of the patients with DM had a serious infection of the urinary tract. The authors stated that this prevalence was 5 times higher than found in studies with non-diabetic patients.[6] Although different studies show a wide range, nearly all investigators report that the prevalence of asymptomatic bacteriuria (ASB) in women with DM is 3-4 times higher than in women without DM [7,8]. In men results are more consistent, a frequency between 1-2% has been found, with no difference between diabetic and non-diabetic men [9]. The frequency of symptomatic infections in women with DM is also increased [10]. Both men and women with diabetes have an increased risk of acute pyelonephritis requiring hospital admission. In a recent study diabetes was estimated to increase the probability 20 to 30-fold under the age of 44, and 3 to 5-fold over the age of 44 [11]. Furthermore, complications of an upper UTI are more likely to occur in diabetic patients. For example, emphysematous pyelonephritis is seen almost exclusively in diabetic patients, and, although uncommon, half of the patients with papillary necrosis have diabetes.[12]

PATHOGENESIS

Pathogenesis in general
UTIs almost exclusively result from the ascending route. Bacteria colonizing the perineum and vagina can enter the bladder and further ascend to the kidneys. The most important defense mechanisms of the host, are the urine

flow from the kidneys to the bladder and the intermittent voiding, resulting in complete emptying of the bladder. Patients with urinary obstruction, stasis and reflux have more difficulty in clearing bacteria and these conditions also seem to predispose to the development of a UTI, although exact data are lacking [13].

The essential step in the pathogenesis of UTIs, is the adherence of uropathogens to the bladder mucosa. Adhesins (fimbriae) are therefore important virulence factors. Although virulence factors have been characterized best in *E. coli* (the most common uropathogen), many of the same principles may be applicable to other gram-negative uropathogens, for example *Klebsiella* [14]. Type 1 fimbriae mediate the adherence of *E. coli* to glycoprotein receptors (uroplakins) on the uroepithelial cells, whereas P fimbriae bind to glycolipid receptors in the kidney [15].

Pathogenesis in patients with DM

The increased frequency of UTIs in diabetic patients is likely due to several factors (table 1). Suggested host-related mechanisms are a) the presence of glycosuria; b) defects in neutrophil function and c) increased adherence to uroepithelial cells. Our in vitro studies indeed showed that glycosuria enhances the growth of different *E. coli*-strains, [16] however this was not confirmed by in vivo studies, which failed to show a higher prevalence of bacteriuria among diabetic patients with compared to patients without glycosuria [8,17].

The data on impaired neutrophil function are contradictory [18,19]. Moreover, the incidence of UTIs is not increased in other groups of patients with neutrophil defects or neutropenia [20]. Local cytokine secretion might be of importance. Cytokines are small proteins, which play an important role in the regulation of host defenses against systemic and local bacterial infections [21]. Therefore, we investigated urinary cytokine excretion in diabetic patients and found lower urinary IL-8 and IL-6 concentrations (p=0.1 and p<0.001 respectively) in diabetic women than in nondiabetic controls. A lower urinary leukocyte cell count correlated with lower urinary IL-8 and IL-6 concentrations (p<0.05)[22]. This might contribute to the increased incidence of UTIs in this patient group.

Most interestingly, we have found that the adherence of type 1-fimbriated *E. coli* to uroepithelial cells of women with DM is increased, compared to the adherence to uroepithelial cell of women without DM [23]. So, it seems that this increased adherence plays an important role in the pathogenesis of UTIs in women with DM.

Table 1. Host factors associated with an increased risk for symptomatic or asymptomatic urinary tract infections (UTIs) in women with diabetes mellitus (DM)

General
sexual intercourse[17]
history of (recurrent) UTIs[8]
obstruction, urine stasis, reflux, instrumentation of urinary tract[13] [a]
Associated with (complications of) DM
peripheral neuropathy[8]
macroalbuminuria[8]
longer duration of DM[8]
glycosuria (in vitro)[16]
decreased urinary cytokine secretion[22]
increased adherence of *E. coli* to uroepithelial cells[23]
Genetic factors[a]
secretor status[68]
blood group[68]
history of UTIs of the mother[69]

[a] Not studied specifically in diabetic patients

As part of the immune response, infection and adherence of the bacteria to uroepithelial cells stimulates cytokine and chemokine secretion, as well as exfoliation of the superficial cells. It has long been thought that uropathogenic *E. coli* are non-invasive pathogens. However, a recent study in mice has shown that type-1 fimbriated *E. coli* can not only lead to exfoliation, but can also invade the uroepithelial cells, replicate and form quiescent intracellular reservoirs which can serve as a possible source for recurrent UTIs [24]. Because we found lower urinary cytokine concentrations in women with DM [22], we hypothesized that in these patients bacteria might invade uroepithelial cells more easily, and, by an impaired inflammatory response, evade the innate host defenses [15]. This would explain why relapses of UTIs occur often in these patients [25]. Future studies will have to provide the evidence for this phenomenon.

Associated risk factors
Factors that have been proposed constituting an enhanced risk for UTIs in diabetics include: age, metabolic control, duration of DM, diabetic cystopathy,

more frequent hospitalization and instrumentation of the urinary tract, recurrent vaginitis and vascular complications [10,26]. However, different studies show conflicting results. Moreover, most of them do not differentiate between patients with DM type 1 and type 2. We have determined the risk factors for the prevalence of ASB and the incidence of symptomatic UTIs in a large cohort of 636 diabetic women. We found that women with DM type 1 with a longer duration of diabetes, or the presence of peripheral neuropathy and macroalbuminuria had an increased risk on ASB. In women with DM type 2, a higher age, macroalbuminuria, and a recent symptomatic UTI predisposed for ASB. There was no association between the diabetes regulation and the presence of ASB [8]. Equally to healthy women, the most important risk factor for the development of a symptomatic UTI for women with DM type 1 was recent sexual intercourse. For women with DM type 2, the most important risk factor of a symptomatic UTI was the presence of ASB [27,17]. Thirty-four percent of the women with DM type 2 with ASB developed a symptomatic UTI compared to 19% of the women without ASB [28].

It has been suggested that diabetic cystopathy and peripheral neuropathy are associated with the pathogenesis of UTIs in diabetic patients [10]. However, we and others could not find a correlation between the presence of peripheral neuropathy and a bladder residue after micturition nor with the presence of ASB [8,29,30].

BACTERIOLOGY

The bacteria isolated from diabetic patients with a UTI are similar as found in nondiabetic patients with a <u>complicated</u> UTI [31]. As in uncomplicated UTIs, *E. coli* causes the majority of infections. However, other strains are relatively more frequently cultured in these patients. For example, one study reported *E. coli* to be the causative uropathogen in 47% of the UTIs in diabetic patients and in 68% of the UTIs in nondiabetic patients [32]. Non-*E. coli* uropathogens, found in patients with DM, include *Klebsiella* species, *Enterobacter* species, *Proteus* species, Group B Streptococci and *Enterococcus faecalis* [7,12,26]. Some authors found that diabetic patients are more likely to be infected with a resistant uropathogen [32,33]. However, we could not confirm this finding in our cohort of diabetic women with ASB. A total of 135 *E. coli* were isolated from women with diabetes mellitus (mean age 57 ± 14 years) were compared to 5907 routine isolates of *E. coli* obtained from female patients visiting an outpatient department (mean age 52 ± 17). The resistance rates of *E. coli* isolated from diabetic patients and the routine isolates of *E. coli* to trimethoprim-sulfamethoxazole were 19% and 23%, respectively, to amoxicillin 16% and 32%, to nitrofurantoin 1% and 3%, to ciprofloxacin 0% and 4%, to ofloxacin 0% and 5%, and to norfloxacin 1% and 4%. (Meiland et al , unpublished information).

CONSEQUENCES OF ASYMPTOMATIC BACTERIA

Recently, a large study among 796 sexually active, non-pregnant women without DM (age 18-40 years old), identified ASB as a strong predictor of a subsequent symptomatic UTI [34] In (other) studies of non-diabetic patients, it was suggested that ASB can lead to recurrent UTIs, progressive renal impairment, hypertension, and an increased mortality [35], although most authors agree that ASB per se in a healthy individual causes no harm [36,37]. However, despite the high prevalence of ASB among women with DM, little is known about the consequences in this specific population [12,7]. In the study mentioned earlier, we have shown that women with DM type 2 with ASB at baseline had an increased risk of developing a UTI during the 18-month follow-up, compared to women with DM type 2 without ASB at baseline (17% without ASB versus 27% with ASB, p=0.02). In contrast, we did not find a difference in the incidence of asymptomatic UTI between DM type 1 women with and without ASB. However, a more interesting finding was that women with DM type 1 and ASB had tendency to a faster decline in renal function than those without ASB (relative increase in creatinin 4.6% versus 1.5%, p=0.2) [28]. If longer follow-up studies, as ongoing in our center, show that ASB contributes to the development of diabetic nephropathy, this would have important consequences. Diabetes now accounts for 35% of all new cases of end-stage renal disease in the United States, and persons with DM make up the fastest growing group of renal dialysis and transplant recipients [38,39].

CLINICAL PRESENTATION

UTIs in diabetic patients can be either asymptomatic or symptomatic. ASB is defined as the presence of at least 10^5 colony-forming units of the same urinary tract pathogen per milliliter in two consecutive clean voided midstream urine cultures. Several studies have shown that the presence of ASB is a predictor of symptomatic infections, in patients with as well as in patients without DM [17,34]. The presentation of a lower (symptomatic) UTI can be accompanied by classical symptoms as dysuria, frequency, urgency, hematuria, and/or abdominal discomfort. However, the same symptoms may be produced by inflammation in the urethra or by infective agents as *Chlamydia trachomatis*, herpes simplex or by a vaginitis (e.g. *Candida albicans)* which also occur frequently in women with DM. Therefore a urine specimen should be checked for leukocyturia (the presence, in uncentrifuged urine, of ≥5 leukocytes/high power field or 10 leucocytes/mm^3) and bacteriuria. Upper tract involvement is common in patients with DM [9,40].

Acute pyelonephritis is a clinical syndrome characterized by fever and chills, flank pain, costovertebral angle tenderness, and other general symptoms, such as nausea and vomiting. There may or may not be symptoms of lower UTI, such as dysuria. Some patients, however, only present with symptoms of a lower UTI but nevertheless have upper tract involvement (subclinical pyelonephritis) [10]. Bilateral involvement is more common in diabetic patients [41]. Infection leads to bacteremia relatively often in these patients. There are exceptional cases of renal abscesses, papillary necrosis and emphysematous pyelonephritis [12,42]. Renal abscess formation should be suspected in patients who do not respond to antimicrobial therapy after 72 hours. Therefore, if symptoms do not resolve within this time period, ultrasonography or CT-scanning of the kidneys should be performed [10]. Papillary necrosis is also a complication of UTI in diabetic patient, which is important to recognize. Symptoms consist of flank pain, chills, fever and renal insufficiency develops in 15% of the cases. Therefore the diagnosis should be suspected in patients responding poorly to antimicrobial therapy. Emphysematous pyelonephritis is a necrotizing infection characterized by gas production within the renal parenchyma. The disease is seen almost exclusively in diabetic patients. Gram-negatives are the most common isolates but multiple organisms occur. Clinical features include fever, flank pain and a palpable mass in 45% of the patients. Bacteremia is a frequent complication of emphysematous pyelonephritis. Diagnosis is made radiographically, starting with a plain abdominal film of the kidney, ureter and bladder, which detects renal emphysema in 85%. Ultrasound can be useful, especially in diagnosing obstructive complications. However, CT-scanning (without contrast) is the study of choice because of its high sensitivity and because it precisely defines the localization and extension of the gas formation, which is important in determining the optimal therapeutic strategy [10].

TREATMENT

Despite the high prevalence of the disease, clinical trials specifically dealing with the treatment of UTIs in diabetic patients are rare. No randomized trials are available comparing the optimal duration and the choice of the treatment. Therefore most recommendations for treatment of UTIs in diabetic patients are based on expert opinions more than on scientific evidence.

Discussion exists whether all UTIs in patients with DM should be considered and subsequently treated as complicated infections. Do the vast majority of UTIs in diabetic patients need to be labeled 'complicated' with the resulting more aggressive management? Why not be more conservative, get the data from prospective studies and not create 'disease' when there is none in many patients? Some authors indeed state that the term 'complicated' should be reserved for (diabetic) patients with therapy failure (persistent or recurrent infection) or with the presence of other conditions which in itself would lead to categorization as 'complicated UTI' (eg. abnormalities of urinary tract, impaired renal function) [43,44].However, others [33,45] mean that all UTIs in patients with DM should be treated as complicated infections, in order to avoid the development of possible dangerous complications.

Antimicrobial treatment
Few clinical trials have dealt with the outcome of treatment of ASB in patients with DM [40,9]. From these studies, the authors conclude that 1) two weeks of treatment is as effective as 6 weeks treatment; 2) the recurrence rate is high, even after prolonged antibiotic treatment; and 3) recurrences (4-8 weeks post-therapy) are mostly re-infections and not relapses with the same microorganism (which occur earlier). In addition, physicians should be aware of the high prevalence of underlying structural genitourinary abnormalities among bacteriuric women with DM [40].

The need for screening of ASB in diabetic (female) patients, with the intention to treat, depends on the question whether or not ASB per se can lead to serious complications as renal function deterioration [46]. Since such evidence is not yet available, we and several authors [36], but not all [10,37], believe that a restrictive policy towards the treatment of ASB is justified. A recently published randomized controlled trial sheds some new light on this. In this study of Harding et al [73], 108 diabetic women with ASB (diagnosed by 2 urine cultures showing $\geq 10^5$ CFU) were randomized to receive a 3- or 14-day course of either trimethoprim-sulfamethoxazole or placebo. Ciprofloxacin was provided to patients in the antibiotic-treatment group who were infected with a resistant organism. Because the first 6 patients assigned to a 3-day antibiotic regimen had early relapses, this study arm was discontinued. All patients were subsequently screened every 3 months for bacteriuria, and women in the antibiotic therapy group were given further suppressive antimicrobial therapy if they were bacteriuric. Four weeks after the end of the initial course of therapy, 78 percent of placebo recipients had bacteriuria, as compared with 20 percent of women who received antimicrobial agents (P<0.001). During a mean follow-up of 27 months, 20 of 50 women in the placebo group (40 percent) and 23 of 55 women in the antimicrobial-therapy group (42 percent) had at least one episode of symptomatic urinary tract infection. The time to a first symptomatic episode was similar in the placebo group and the antimicrobial-therapy group, as were the rates of any symptomatic urinary tract infection and hospitalization for urinary tract infection. The authors concluded that treatment of asymptomatic bacteriuria in women with diabetes does not appear to reduce complications and diabetes itself should not be an indication for screening for or treatment of asymptomatic bacteriuria [73].

However, in our previous paper [28] we described that women with diabetes type 1 and ASB had a tendency to a decline in renal function during the short follow-up. Since diabetes type 1 and type 2 are considered different disease's, separate analyses of these patient groups are warranted. In the study of Harding et al. [73] all patients were analyzed together and only 17 (20%) had type 1. We think therefore, that the conclusion of this very interesting study, should be that it is difficult to keep these patients non-bacteriuric. Furthermore, we think that it is premature to conclude that screening and treatment of ASB in diabetic women is not needed because we must await the results of our 5 year follow-up study with nearly 200 women with diabetes type 1, which has renal function development as primary outcome parameter. [75].

For <u>uncomplicated</u> acute bacterial cystitis (i.e. in otherwise healthy young women) the Infectious Diseases Society of America (IDSA) recommends a 3 days course with trimethoprim-sulfamethoxazole (TMP-SM2) as standard therapy. Alternatively, one can prescribe trimethoprim alone or a fluoroquinolon, for example ofloxacin. Other fluoroquinolones have similar effectiveness, but regarding the higher costs and the increasing problem of resistant microorganisms, these should only be used as an alternative in communities with high rates of resistance to TMP-SMX [48]. However, the guidelines do not include recommendations for complicated infections.

Few therapeutic trials have specifically been performed among diabetic patients. Because of the frequent (asymptomatic) upper tract involvement and the possible serious complications, many experts recommend a 7- to 14-day oral antimicrobial regimen for bacterial cystitis in diabetic patients, instead of the recommended 3-day course for uncomplicated cystitis [10,27,49]. In a recent double-blind study, the efficacy in the treatment of complicated urinary lower UTIs of a 5-day ofloxacin treatment was compared to a 10-day regimen. Four hundred and sixteen women were studied of whom an unknown percentage had DM. The authors concluded that both regimens were equally effective [50].

Although some authors state that in diabetic patients the choice of agent does not differ from the treatment in otherwise healthy patients [31,44], most authors prefer antimicrobial agents which achieve high levels not only in the urine but also in the urinary tract tissues: e.g. fluoroquinolones, TMP-SMX and amoxicillin-clavulanic acid [27,51].This may especially hold true given the recent data indicating invasion of *E. coli* into the bladder cells [24]. A recent randomized, double-blind study including 85 (20%) women with DM, has shown that a 7-day regimen with ciprofloxacin or with ofloxacin resulted in a cure rate of 90 and 87 %, respectively, 5-9 days after treatment of a complicated lower UTI [52]. In the group of women with DM the success rates were comparable (87 and 85)[50,52]. Given these data, the mouse data of the group of Hultgren, showing a potential intraepithelial reservoir, our own data showing a very high relapse rate in ASB and the data of the group of Nicolle, showing a 10% failure rate in the 6 women treated for ASB, in our opinion indicates that treatment guidelines for uncomplicated UTI in diabetic women should differ from those in the IDSA guidelines (Table 3). We would recommend a 7-day regimen with an agent that penetrates epithelial cells.

Both TMP-SMZ and the fluoroquinolones have proven to be effective, both are more effective than beta-lactam agents are [48]. In areas with a resistance rate over 20% for TMP-SMZ the primary choice would be a fluoroquinolon because low resistance rates are found at least all over Europe [74]. To prevent resistance development against the agents mentioned above studies with both nitrofurantoin and fosfomycin are warranted. Noteworthy is the possible hypoglycemic effect of TMP-SM2, which has been observed using (higher doses of) this agent [51,49].

In all cases of suspected pyelonephritis in diabetic patients a culture of urine before starting therapy is indicated, as well as blood cultures if the patient is severely ill [10]. The treatment of uncomplicated pyelonephritis does not differ for patients with or without DM. For treatment of mild acute pyelonephritis the IDSA recommends an oral fluoroquinolon, possibly after an initial single parenteral dose of an antimicrobial. Diabetic patients are usually treated within the hospital, with a parenteral fluoroquinolon or a cefalosporine as initial therapy. In communities with a resistance rate of <15% of *E. coli* to TMP-SMX, TMP-SMX is considered a suitable alternative. After 48-72 hours, if symptoms have resolved, oral therapy may be started. These recommendations rely on clinical practice, since all randomized studies comparing oral with intravenous therapy have excluded patients with underlying systemic illnesses as DM. The current standard duration of therapy for uncomplicated pyelonephritis in both diabetic as in nondiabetic patients is 14 days [53,51,27,48]. In a recent randomized trial a 7-day oral ciprofloxacin regimen was more effective than a 14-day TMP-SMX regimen for the treatment of uncomplicated pyelonephritis, as indicated by greater bacteriologic and clinical cure rates [54]. This was probably due to a high resistance rate (18%) to TMP-SMX in this study. However, this study tells us that in uncomplicated pyelonephritis a treatment duration of 7-days is enough. Although highly interesting, comparable studies will have to be performed specifically enrolling patients with DM, before such a regimen can be advised in these patients.

In patients with DM, a follow-up urine culture (2-4 weeks post-therapy) is considered useful to detect early relapses and because of the higher treatment failure[33]. Considering the text mentioned above, it is clear that clinical trials specifically dealing with the treatment of UTIs in diabetic patients, comparing the optimal duration and the choice of the therapy, are needed.

The traditional treatment of emphysematous pyelonephritis is nephrectomy of the affected kidney. Surgery has been reported to lower the mortality from 80% in patients treated with antimicrobial treatment alone, to 20% [10]. Although an increasing number of cases are reported of successful conservative management, antibiotic therapy combined with percutaneous drainage,[55] no consensus exists whether this strategy should replace (or proceed) the standard nephrectomy.

Non-antimicrobial treatments and preventive strategies

The worldwide increasing problem of resistant uropathogens [56] calls for additional non-antimicrobial strategies, both for the treatment as for the prevention of UTIs (table 2). General advises include sufficient fluid intake, complete emptying of the bladder during voiding, less use of spermicides, and restrictive catheter use.

Table 2. Non-antimicrobial treatments and strategies that possibly reduce the incidence of urinary tract infections[a]

General preventive strategies [70]
sufficient fluid intake complete emptying of bladder during voiding less use of spermicides restrictive catheter use [71]
cranberry juice (oral) [59]
lactobacilli (oral or vaginal) [59,72]
Estrogen suppletion in postmenopausal women (oral or vaginal)) [61,60,62]
Vaccines (both currently on halt)
Urovac [66] FimH-adhesin-based [64,65]

[a] the strategies mentioned have been studied in nondiabetic patients

Cystitis in diabetic women. Treatment guidelines
3-day therapy is probably not effective [12, 25, 73]
Treat with agents that penetrate the urothelium [24]
Trimethoprim-(sulfamethoxazole) is the agent of choice in areas with low resistance rates (<20%) [54,74]
Fluoroquinolones are effective [52]
Beta-lactam antibiotics are less effective [48]
Short course therapy with nitrofurantoin and fosfomycin should be evaluated

An interesting possible preventive or treatment option is ingestion of cranberry juice. At first, the beneficial effect of cranberry juice was thought to be the result of acidification of the urine. More recently, in vitro studies have identified the inhibition of bacterial adherence to the uroepithelial cells as the most plausible mechanism of action [57]. Another possible preventive strategy is the oral or vaginal administration of lactobacilli. Lactobacilli are part of the commensal vaginal flora and are thought to protect against UTIs by competitive exclusion of uropathogens [58]. In a recent randomized trial, regular drinking of cranberry juice but not of *lactobacillus* GG drink reduced the recurrence of UTIs in women with *E. coli* infection [59]. In addition, several investigators have studied the influence of estrogen administration. Estrogen deficiency in postmenopausal women has been implicated in the pathogenesis of recurrent UTI, apparently due to an increase in vaginal pH and the subsequent reduction in number of lactobacilli [60]. Several randomized trials of estrogen administration have been performed, mostly including small numbers of patients, and with conflicting results. In a recent review, the authors conclude that estrogen administration is of benefit in decreasing the recurrence rate of UTIs in postmenopausal women, especially if administered vaginally [61]. A randomized, blinded study among 2763 postmenopausal women who participated in a study on coronary heart disease, reported no reduction of the frequency of UTIs in patients with oral hormone therapy (estrogen plus medroxyprogesterone acetate) compared to women who received a placebo [62]. All strategies mentioned have been studied in nondiabetic patients, but we think that the results will be comparable in patients with DM. A randomized study comparing estrogens and cranberry juice in elderly non-diabetic women is currently underway. However, one should realize that cranberry juice is difficult to take (large volume), contains a lot of calories and is expensive.

Since the adherence of *E. coli* to the uroepithelial cell is an essential step in the pathogenesis of UTIs, prevention of this would theoretically lead to a decreased incidence of UTIs. Therefore the attention has shifted towards the development of a vaccine, based on the FimH adhesin of type 1 fimbriae of *E. coli*. In vitro and animal studies have shown that this vaccine can prevent adherence of *E. coli* to uroepithelial cells and decrease incidence of UTIs in vaccinated monkeys [63,64]. We have demonstrated that addition of vaccine-induced antiserum to uroepithelial cells isolated from diabetic women, also decreases the adherence of type-1 fimbriated *E. coli* to diabetic uroepithelial cells [65]. At this moment, clinical studies have been discontinued, because although safe, the vaccine proved only 30% effective in young sexually active women. In addition, another vaccine under study in women with recurrent UTIs. This vaccine is based on immunization by vaginal suppositories containing heat-killed uropathogenic bacteria from 10 different isolates [66]. Also this vaccine is no longer available.

In the last years, more research has been done in the area of prevention of post-operative infections in diabetic patients. Although non-randomized, these studies confirm the hypothesis that hyperglycemia is associated with an increased risk of post-operative infection. The authors recommend optimal peri-operative glycemic control (glucose levels <200 mg/dl) [67,44].

FUTURE ISSUES

Longer follow-up studies among diabetic patients (as ongoing in our center) analyzing the effects of ASB on renal function should answer the question whether women (especially type-1) with DM should be kept non-bacteriuric. Furthermore, randomized therapeutic trials specifically enrolling patients with DM will have to define the best therapeutic management, focussing on type of antimicrobial agent and optimal treatment duration. New developments on non-antimicrobial approaches must show their value in preventing UTIs in diabetic patients.

SUMMARY

Urinary tract infections (UTIs) are more common and tend to have a more complicated course in patients with diabetes mellitus (DM). The mechanisms, which potentially contribute to the increased prevalence of both asymptomatic and symptomatic bacteriuria in these patients are defects in the local urinary cytokine secretions and an increased adherence of the microorganisms to the uroepithelial cells. The need for treatment of asymptomatic bacteriuria (ASB) remains controversial. No evidence is available on the optimal treatment of acute cystitis and pyelonephritis in patients with DM. Because of the frequent (asymptomatic) upper tract involvement and the possible serious complications, many experts recommend a 7- to 14-day oral antimicrobial regimen for bacterial cystitis in these patients, with an antimicrobial agent that achieves high levels both in the urine and in urinary tract tissues. Current data suggest that shorter regimens will lead to failure also in uncomplicated UTI in women.

The recommended treatment of acute pyelonephritis does not differ from that in nondiabetic patients. Clinical trials specifically dealing with the treatment of UTIs in diabetic patients, comparing the optimal duration and choice of antimicrobial agent, are needed. Besides that, new approaches to preventive strategies must prove their value in this specific patient group.

REFERENCES

1. Hooton TM, Stamm WE. Diagnosis and treatment of uncomplicated urinary tract infection. Infect Dis Clin North Am 1997 Sep; 11 (3): 551-81
2. Barnett BJ, Stephens DS. Urinary tract infection: an overview. Am J Med Sci 1997 Oct; 314 (4): 245-9
3. Johnson JR, Roberts PL, Stamm WE. P fimbriae and other virulence factors in *Escherichia coli* urosepsis: Association with patients' characteristics. J Infect Dis 1987 Jul; 156 (1): 225-9
4. Hoepelman AIM, Van Buren M, Van den Broek PJ, et al. Bacteriuria in men infected with HIV-1 is related to their immune status (CD4+ cell count). AIDS 1992; 6 (2): 179-84
5. Carton JA, Maradona JA, Nuno FJ, et al. Diabetes mellitus and bacteraemia: A comparative study between diabetic and non-diabetic patients. Eur J Med 1992 Jul; 1 (5): 281-7
6. Baldwin AD, Root HF. Infections of the upper urinary tract in the diabetic patient. N Engl J Med 1940 Aug 15; 223 (7) 244-250
7. Zhanel GG, Harding GK, Nicolle LE. Asymptomatic bacteriuria in patients with diabetes mellitus. Rev Infect Dis 1991; 13 (1): 150-4
8. Geerlings SE, Stolk RP, Camps MJL, et al. Asymptomatic bacteriuria may be considered a complication in women with diabetes. Diabetes Care 2000 May; 23 (6): 744-9
9. Forland M, Thomas V, Shelokov A. Urinary tract infections in patients with diabetes mellitus. Studies on antibody coating of bacteria. JAMA 1977 Oct 31; 238 (18): 1924-6
10. Patterson JE, Andriole VT. Bacterial urinary tract infections in diabetes. Infect Dis Clin North Am 1997 Sep; 11 (3): 735-750
11. Nicolle LE, Friesen D, Harding GK, et al. Hospitalization for acute pyelonephritis in Manitoba, Canada, during the period from 1989 to 1992; impact of diabetes, pregnancy, and aboriginal origin. Clin Infect Dis 1996 Jun; 22 (6): 1051-6
12. Wheat LJ. Infection and diabetes mellitus. Diabetes Care 1980 Jan; 3 (1): 187-97
13. Sobel JD, Kaye D, Urinary tract infections. In: Principles and practice of infectious diseases. Mandell GL, Bennett JE, Dolin R, eds. New York (NY) 1995: 662-90
14. Podschun R, Sievers D, Fischer A, et al. Serotypes, hemagglutinins, siderophore synthesis, and serum resistance of *Klebsiella* isolates causing human urinary tract infections. J Infect Dis 1993 Dec; 168 (6): 1415-21
15. Mulvey MA, Schilling JD, Martinez JJ, et al. Bad bugs and beleaguered bladders: Interplay between uropathogenic *Escherichia coli* and innate host defenses. Proc Natl Acad Sci U S A 2000 Aug 1; 97 (16): 8829-35
16. Geerlings SE, Brouwer EC, Gaastra W, et al. Effect of glucose and pH on uropathogenic and non-uropathogenic *Escherichia coli*: studies with urine from diabetic and non-diabetic individuals. J Med Microbiol 1999; 48 (6): 535-9

17. Geerlings SE, Stolk RP, Camps MJL, et al. Risk factors for symptomatic urinary tract infection in women with diabetes mellitus. Diabetes Care 2000 Dec; 23 (12): 1737-41
18. Delamaire M, Maugendre D, Moreno M, et al. Impaired leucocyte functions in diabetic patients. Diabet Med 1997; 14 (1): 29-34
19. Balasoiu D, Van Kessel KC, Van Kats-Renaud HJ, et al. Granulocyte function in women with diabetes and asymptomatic bacteriuria. Diabetes Care 1997 Mar; 20 (3): 392-5
20. Wang QN, Qiu ZD. Infection in acute leukemia: an analysis of 433 episodes. Rev Infect Dis 1989 Nov; 11 (Suppl 7): S1613-S1620
21. Luster AD. Chemokines - Chemotactic cytokines that mediate inflammation. N Engl J Med 1998; 338 (7): 436-445
22. Geerlings SE, Brouwer EC, Van Kessel KCPM, et al. Cytokine secretion is impaired in women with diabetes mellitus. Eur J Clin Invest 2000 Nov; 30 (11): 995-1001
23. Geerlings SE, Meiland R, Van Lith EC, et al. Adherence of type 1-fimbriated *Escherichia coli* to uroepithelial cells: more in diabetic women than in controls. Diabetes Care, 2002,:25; 1405-09
24. Mulvey MA, Schilling JD, Hultgren SJ. Establishment of a persistent *Escherichia coli* reservoir during the acute phase of a bladder infection. Infect Immun 2001 Jul; 69 (7): 4572-9
25. Geerlings SE, Brouwer EC, Gaastra W, et al. Is a second urine necessary for the diagnosis of asymptomatic bacteriuria? Clin Infect Dis 2000; 31 (3): E3-4
26. Zhanel GG, Nicolle LE, Harding GKM, et al. Prevalence of asymptomatic bacteriuria and associated host factors in women with diabetes mellitus. Clin Infect Dis 1995 Aug; 21 (2): 316-22
27. Stamm WE, Hooton TM. Management of urinary tract infections in adults. N Engl J Med 1993 Oct 28; 329 (18): 1328-34
28. Geerlings SE, Stolk RP, Camps MJL, et al. Consequences of asymptomatic bacteriuria in women with diabetes mellitus. Arch Intern Med 2001 Jun 11; 161 (11): 1421-7
29. Frimodt-MØller C. Diabetic cstopathy: epidemiology and related disorders. Ann Intern Med 1980; 92 (2 Part 2): 318-21
30. Vejlsgaard R. Studies on urinary infection in diabetics. II Significant bacteriuria in relation to long-term diabetic manifestations. Acta Med Scand 1966; 179: 183-8
31. Nicolle LE. A practical guide to antimicrobial management of complicated urinary tract infection. Drugs & Aging 2001; 18 (4): 243-54
32. Lye WC, Chan RKT, Lee EJC, et al. Urinary tract infections in patients with diabetes mellitus. J Infect 1992; 24: 169-74
33. Johnson JR, Stamm WE. Urinary Tract Infections in Women: Diagnosis and Treatment. Ann Intern Med 1989 Dec 1; 111 (11): 906-17
34. Hooton TM, Scholes D, Stapleton AE, et al. A prospective study of asymptomatic bacteriuria in sexually active young women. N Engl J Med 2000 Oct 5; 343 (14): 992-7
35. Ronald AR, Patullo LS. The natural history of urinary infections in adults. Infect Dis Clin North Am 1991 Mar; 75 (2): 299-312
36. Stein G, Funfstuck R. Asymptomatic bacteriuria-what to do. Nephrol Dial Transplant 1999; 14 (7): 1618-21
37. Zhanel GG, Harding GKM, Guay DRP. Asymptomatic bacteriuria. Which patients should be treated? Arch Intern Med 1990 Jul; 150 (7): 1389-96
38. Nelson RG, Knowler WC, Pettitt DJ, et al. Kidney diseases in diabetes. In: Diabetes in America. National Diabetes Data Group, eds. Bethesda (MD) 1995: 349-401

39. Ritz E, Orth SR. Nephropathy in patients with type 2 diabetes mellitus. N Engl J Med 1999 Oct 7; 341 (15): 1127-33

40. Forland M, Thomas VL. The treatment of urinary tract infections in women with diabetes mellitus. Diabetes Care 1985 Sep; 8 (5): 499-506

41. Calvet HM, Yoshikawa TT. Infections in diabetes. Infect Dis Clin North Am 2001 Jun; 15 (2): 407-21

42. Saiki J, Vaziri ND, Barton C. Perinephric and intranephric abscesses: a review of the literature. West J Med 1982 Feb; 136 (2): 95-102

43. Ronald AR, Harding GKM. Complicated urinary tract infections. Infect Dis Clin North Am 1997; 11 (3): 583-93

44. Ronald A, Ludwig E. Urinary tract infections in adults with diabetes. Int J Antimicrob Agents 2001 Apr; 17 (4): 287-92

45. Melekos MD, Naber KG. Complicated urinary tract infections. Int J Antimicrob Agents 2000 Aug; 15 (4): 247-56

46. Nicolle LE. Asymptomatic bacteriuria in diabetic women. Diabetes Care 2000 Jul; 23 (6): 722-3

47. Deresinski S. Infections in the diabetic patient: Strategies for the clinician. Infectious Disease Reports 1995 Jan; 1 (1): 1-12

48. Warren JW, Abrutyn E, Hebel JR, et al. Guidelines for antimicrobial treatment of uncomplicated acute bacterial cystitis and acute pyelonephritis in women. Clin Infect Dis 1999 Oct; 29 (4): 745-58

49. Poretsky L, Moses AC. Hypoglycemia associated with trimethoprim/sulfamethoxazole therapy. Diabetes Care 1984 Sep; 7 (5): 508-9

50. Veyssier P, Botto H, Jean C, et al. 5 Day- versus 10 Day- Ofloxacin (OFL) treatment in complicated lower urinary tract infections (LUTI) in women (W) [abstract L1057]. 41th Interscience Congres on Antimicrobial Agents and Chemotherapy, 2001 Dec 16-19; American Society for Microbiology; Chicago: 464

51. Schaeffer AJ. Bacterial urinary tract infections in diabetes. J Urol 1998 Jul; 160 (1): 293

52. Raz R, Naber KG, Raizenberg C, et al. Ciprofloxacin 250 mg twice daily versus ofloxacin 200 mg twice daily in the treatment of complicated urinary tract infections in women. Eur J Clin Microbiol Infect Dis 2000 May; 19 (5): 327-31

53. Rubin RH, Shapiro ED, Andriole VT, et al. Evaluation of new anti-infective drugs for the treatment of urinary tract infection. Clin Infect Dis 1992; 15 (Suppl 1): S216-27

54. Talan DA, Stamm WE, Hooton TM, et al. Comparison of ciprofloxacin (7 days) and trimethoprim-sulfamethoxazole (14 days) for acute uncomplicated pyelonephritis in women: a randomized trial. JAMA 2000 Mar 22; 283 (12): 1583-90

55. Chen MT, Huang CN, Chou YH, et al. Percutaneous drainage in the treatment of emphysematous pyelonephritis: 10-year experience. J Urol 1997 May; 157 (5): 1569-73

56. Gupta K, Scholes D, Stamm WE. Increasing prevalence of antimicrobial resistance among uropathogens causing acute uncomplicated cystitis in women. JAMA 1999 Feb 24; 281 (8): 736-8

57. Lowe FC, Fagelman E. Cranberry juice and urinary tract infections: What is the evidence? Urology 2001 Mar; 57 (3): 407-13

58. Boris S, Suarez JE, Vazquez F, et al. Adherence of human vaginal lactobacilli to vaginal epithelial cells and interaction with uropathogens. Infect Immun 1998 May; 66 (5): 1985-9

59. Kontiokari T, Sundqvist K, Nuutinen M, et al. Randomised trial of cranberry-lingonberry juice and *Lactobacillus* GG drink for the prevention of urinary tract infections in women. BMJ 2001 Jun 30; 322 (7302): 1571-3

60. Raz R, Stamm WE. A controlled trial of intravaginal estriol in postmenopausal women with recurrent urinary tract infection. N Engl J Med 1993; 329 (11): 753-6

61. Hextall A. Oestrogens and lower urinary tract function. Maturitas 2000 Aug 31; 36 (2): 83-92

62. Brown JS, Vittinghoff E, Kanaya AM, et al. Urinary tract infections in postmenopausal women: effect of hormone therapy and risk factors. Obstet Gynecol 2001 Dec; 98 (6): 1045-52

63. Langermann S, Palaszynski S, Barnhart M, et al. Prevention of mucosal *Escherichia coli* infection by FimH-adhesin-based systemic vaccination. Science 1997 Apr 25; 276 (5312): 607-11

64. Langermann S, Mollby R, Burlein JE, et al. Vaccination with FimH adhesin protects cynomolgus monkeys from colonization and infection by uropathogenic *Escherichia coli*. J Infect Dis 2000 Feb; 181 (2): 774-8

65. Meiland R, Geerlings SE, Brouwer EC, et al. Adherence of *Escherichia coli* to uroepithelial cells of women with diabetes mellitus (DM) can be inhibited by vaccine-induced anti-FimCH antiserum [abstract L1349]. 41th Interscience Congres on Antimicrobial Agents and Chemotherapy; 2001 Dec 16-19; American Society for Microbiology; Chicago: 468

66. Uehling DT, Hopkins WJ, Beierle LM, et al. Vaginal mucosal immunization for recurrent urinary tract infection: extended phase II clinical trial. J Infect Dis 2001 Mar 1; 183 (Suppl 1): S81-3

67. Golden SH, Peart-Vigilance C, Kao WH, et al. Perioperative glycemic control and the risk of infectious complications in a cohort of adults with diabetes. Diabetes Care 1999 Sep; 22 (9): 1408-14

68. Kinane DF, Blackwell CC, Brettle RP, et al. ABO blood group, secretor state, and susceptibility to recurrent urinary tract infection in women. Br Med J 1982; 285: 7-9

69. Scholes D, Hooton TM, Roberts PL, et al. Risk factors for recurrent urinary tract infection in young women. Journal of Infectious Diseases 2000 Oct; 182 (4): 1177-82

70. Stapleton A, Stamm WE. Prevention of urinary tract infection. Infect Dis Clin North Am 1997 Sep; 11 (3): 719-33

71. Nicolle LE. Prevention and treatment of urinary catheter-related infections in older patients. Drugs & Aging 1994; 4 (5): 379-91

72. Reid G, Bruce AW, Taylor M. Influence of three-day antimicrobial therapy and *lactobacillus* vaginal suppositories on recurrence of urinary tract infections. Clin Ther 1992 Jan; 14 (1): 11-6

73. harding GK, Zhanel GG, Nicolle LE, Cheang M; Manitoba Diabetes Urinary Tract Infection Study Group. Antimicrobial treatment in diabetic women with asymptomatic bacteriuria. N Engl J Med 2002 Nov 14;347(20):1617-8

74. Kahlmeter G. An international survey of the antimicrobial susceptibility of pathogens from uncomplicated urinary tract infections: the ECO.SENS Project. J Antimicrob Chemother. 2003 Jan;51(1):69-76.

75. Geerlings SE, R Meiland, IM Hoepelman, Antimicrobial treatment in diabetic women with asymptomatic bacteriuria New Engl J Med, 2003; 348(10): 957–8.

15

PATHOLOGY OF THE KIDNEY IN DIABETES MELLITUS

Steen Olsen

Professor Emeritus, Department of Pathology, Herlev Hospital, DK-2730 Herlev, Denmark.

The history of our knowledge of the light microscopy of diabetic glomerulopathy began with the famous paper by Kimmelstiel and Wilson in 1936 [1]. With some justification, it can be said that it has been completed by the careful analysis of large series by Thomsen 1965 [2] and Ditscherlein 1969 [3], the first mentioned taking advantage of the introduction of percutaneous renal biopsies.

Histologic lesions of the renal glomerulus in diabetics were not totally unknown when Kimmelstiel and Wilson reported their findings, but the exact relationship of these alterations to the diabetic state was unclear. Kimmelstiel and Wilson were the first investigators to draw attention to the characteristic »intercapillary«, nodular thickening of mesangial regions and its association with a clinical syndrome consisting of severe proteinuria, edema, hypertension, and eventually a decrease in renal function.

The histology of diabetic glomerulopathy described here rests upon the cornerstones mentioned above and other important classical contributions [4-9] as well as more recent data. Arteriolar changes are included due to the close anatomic and functional connection of arterioles with the glomerulus. Some differential diagnostic problems are discussed, and a brief review of tubulointerstitial lesions is also provided since it is still not known whether they are secondary to vascular changes or have other pathogenesis.

DIABETIC GLOMERULOPATHY

The diffuse lesion

This consists of a uniform widening of the mesangial regions (figure 1). It is particularly well exhibited in sections stained by periodic acid-Schiff (PAS) or by silver methenamine that display structures often described as finger-like radiations from the glomerular hilum.

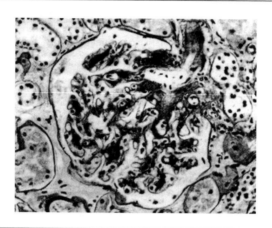

Fig. 1. Diabetic glomerulopathy, diffuse type. There is a slight increase of PAS-positive material in all mesangial regions, radiating from the vascular pole (*upper right*). PAS-haematoxylin.

The nodular lesion

As the volume of the mesangial matrix increases, some mesangial regions become more prominent than others and may take on a globular shape (figure 2). The mesangial nodule is thus created by a gradual increase of the diffuse lesion and the distinction between them is arbitrary. Several nodules may be present in each glomerulus, but usually only a few of the mesangial regions are affected in this way

The nodules are distributed in a horseshoe-shaped area corresponding to the peripheral mesangium [12]. The other mesangial regions present the diffuse lesion. Small nodules contain evenly distributed mesangial cells, but in medium-sized or large nodules, the central areas are almost always acellular.

The periphery of the nodule contains one or a few layers of mesangial cells. Around the nodule, a ring of capillaries is present and they may be dilated. It has been suggested that the formation of the nodule is preceded by focal mesangiolysis [13,14].

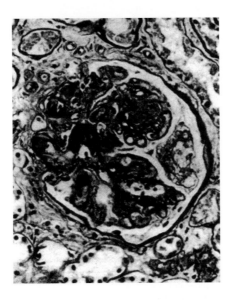

Fig. 2. Diabetic glomerulopathy. The diffuse component is more marked than in figure 1 and a nodule has been formed from a particulary voluminous region. PAS-haematoxylin.

The fibrinous cap

Insudative or exudative lesions consists of deposits of plasma proteins and lipids within renal arterioles (arteriolar hyalinosis), glomerular capillaries (fibrinoid or fibrin cap) and Bowman's capsule (capsular drop). The fibrin cap [8,9,15-17] is situated in the peripheral capillary wall and has a crescentic shape (figure -3).

If the basement membrane is stained by silver methenamine, the cap appears to be situated between this and the endothelium. Its structure is homogeneous although small vacuoles may be seen in which lipids can be demonstrated in frozen sections stained by oil-red.

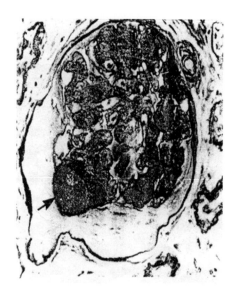

Fig. 3. Fibrinoid cap in diabetic glomerulopathy. Totally obsolescent glomerulus with several fibrinoid caps, one of them indicated by an arrow. The crescent-shaped pale area to the left is subcapsular, fibrotic tissue. The PAS-positive glomerular basement membranes form a solid, retracted tuft. PAS-haematoxylin.

The capsular drop

This lesion [1,3] is situated on the inner side of the capsule of Bowman. It sometimes looks like a drop (figure 4), but it may also be more extended, as a slender, fusiform deposit. Its outer border is formed by the capsule of Bowman; its inner projects toward the urinary space.

Arteriolar hyalinosis

In the early stage of arteriolar hyalinosis (or hyaline arteriolosclerosis), small drops of strongly eosinophilic material accumulate in the wall of the juxtaglomerular arterioles. They may be situated in the intima or in the media. They gradually increase in size and eventually involve the whole arteriolar wall, which then appears as a strongly thickened, homogeneous structure. Arteriolar hyalinosis in diabetes involves the afferent arteriole as well as the efferent arteriole (figure 5).

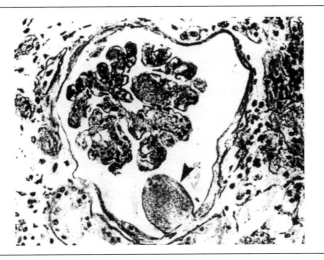

Fig. 4. Capsular drop in diabetic glomerulopathy. A large, drop-shaped deposit *(arrow)*. PAS-haematoxylin.

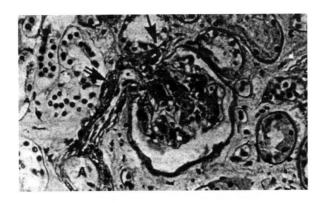

Fig. 5. Arteriolosclerosis in diabetes. There is moderate hyaline arteriolosclerosis in both the afferent *(double arrow)* and the efferent *(arrow)* arterioles. A, interlubular artery. PAS-haematoxylin.

Staining characteristics and histochemistry
Histochemical studies have been published by several authors [10,17,18]. The most important results are presented in table 1. The fibrinoid cap, capsular drop, and arteriolar hyalinosis are identical in staining characteristics, which is why some authors have included them in one group.

Immunoflourescence microscopy (IF) shows often IgG in a fine linear pattern along the glomerular capillary walls [19-21]. This reaction is considered to be unspecific since albumin can also be detected in the same location and IgG cannot be eluded. The nodules are negative. Exudative lesions are positive for C3, β-lipoprotein and (weakly) for IgG [21]. Insulin or anti-insulin is not detectable by IF in the glomeruli [20,21].

Table 1 Staining characteristics of diabetic glomerular lesions

Stain	Diffuse	Nodular	Exudative[a]
Haematoxylineosin	+red	+red	++red
V. Gieson-Hansen	+red	+red	++yellow
Masson-trichrome	++blue	++blue	+++red
Phosphotungstic acid-haematoxylin	0	0	+++deep blue
PAS after diastase	++	++	+++
Silver-methenamine	++black	+/- black fibrils in pale matrix	0
Alcian-blue	+	0	0
Congo red, other amyloid stains	0	0	0
Neutral fat	0	(+) occasionally	+ fat vacuoles

[a]Exudative lesions are fibrinoid caps, capsular drops, and arteriolar hyalinosis

Ultrastructure
A wealth of important morphometric data have been published on glomerular ultrastructural lesions in DM and their relation to duration of disease, presence of micro- or macroalbuminuria and other clinical parameters. A review of these are presented in other chapters in this book. The following is a brief discussion of the main glomerular lesions seen on electron microscopy [22 – 24].

Glomerular ultrastructure is normal at the onset of IDDM. After about two years, widening of the glomerular basement membrane and expansion of mesangial matrix (increased volume fraction of matrix per mesangium) can be demonstrated by morphometry. The fraction of the glomerular tuft occupied by mesangium, which is normal at the beginning of the disease, begins to increase and this becomes marked after 5 - 10 years in patients with microalbuminuria. Most of this expansion is due to matrix accumulation, but there is some participation of cell volume. A decrease of capillary filtration surface can be demonstrated later on. Nodules are composed of mesangial matrix containing very few clefts with cytoplasm of mesangial cells. Foot process width is increased in microalbuminuric compared with normoalbuminuric diabetics and the width of filtration slits is increased in normo- as well as microalbuminuric diabetics compared with control subjects.

Development of the lesions by time
The most powerful determinant for the appearance and development of glomerular and vascular lesions in diabetes is duration of the diabetic state [2]. Diffuse glomerulopathy can be demonstrated by ultrastructural morphometry after a few years of diabetes [26], but is usually not distinct light-microscopically until 5-10 years after the onset of the disease. Nodular glomerulosclerosis demands at least 15 years of diabetes to develop. The nodules tend to disappear with marked glomerular obsolescence. Whereas the precise onset of the diabetic disease is known in insulin dependent diabetes (IDDM) this is not the case with non-insulin dependent diabetes (NIDDM) in which the disease may have been present several years before diagnosis. This is why glomerular nodules may occasionally be seen in patients with a *known* duration of diabetes of less than 15 years, and they may even occur at the time diagnosis is made. The diffuse lesion and arteriolosclerosis occur in 20% of patients before 5 years have elapsed from the apparent onset [2]. These lesions are non-specific, and thus their presence in a patient suffering from diabetes may be unrelated to the diabetic state.

The fibrinoid cap occurs most frequently in the later stages of glomerulopathy, but, in contradistinction to all other glomerular lesions in this disease, the capsular drop is found almost as often in earlier as in later stages [2].

A peculiar and as yet unexplained fact is that about 60% of patients with long-standing diabetes do *not* develop clinical nephropathy or diabetic glomerular changes.

247

The development of glomerulopathy is associated with increasing albuminuria. At the onset of microalbuminuria there is on electron microscopy significant increase in peripheral basement membrane thickness and mesangial volume in relation to glomerular volume. In the stage of macroalbuminuria there is usually distinct light-microscopic glomerular changes. While this is the normal sequence, macroalbuminuria may occur in spite of normal glomerular structure. The situation is not rare, we found it in 13 % of our NIDDM patients with macroalbuminuria [25]. So far no explanation has been given for the increased glomerular capillary permeability in these patients, but endothelial dysfunction or biochemical glomerular basement membrane changes caused by sustained hyperglycemia are obvious candidates

Glomerular structure in the terminal phase

The appearance of glomeruli in advanced diabetic glomerulopathy presents a broad spectrum ranging from totally occluded to almost normal glomeruli. Glomeruli, which are still open, may be hypertrophic and often present global mesangial hypercellularity. Totally occluded glomeruli are not evenly distributed, but tend to be concentrated in radiating stripes parallel to the medullary rays [28]. There is no difference in the severity of glomerular involvement between deep and superficial cortical zones. The total number of glomeruli decreases with progression of the diabetic nephropathy, at least in IDDM [29].

It is important to realize that this terminal pattern is not exclusively due to glomerular alterations specific for diabetes. Ischemic scarring and focal glomerular sclerosis occur and may indicate that causes other than progression of diabetic glomerular lesion may be partially responsible for the development of renal failure, such as vascular constriction with glomerular ischemia and lesions due to hyperfunction of remaining glomeruli.

Specificity of the lesions

The diffuse lesion is completely non-specific and may be present in older people without diabetes. The combination of arteriolosclerosis and the diffuse lesion often occurs in hypertension, but involvement of both the afferent arteriole and the efferent arteriole is regarded as a strong indication of diabetes [6, 30, 31] although even this combination is not entirely specific [15].

All insudative lesions are much more numerous and/or larger in diabetics than in controls but they are not specific. Even capsular drops and hyalinosis of efferent arterioles which have traditionally been regarded as specific lesions may be seen in small numbers in some non-diabetic controls [15].

The nodular lesion is often regarded as pathognomonic for diabetes. It is true that numerous reports of nodular lesions in non-diabetic patients have been published [for a list, see ref. 3]. Most of these reports can be criticized, however, either because of doubt as to absence of diabetes or to lack of application of precise criteria for the morphologic diagnosis. There are, however, well documented cases on record with typical nodular glomerulopathy without diabetes [32, 33].

Although the *typical* nodular lesion is very strongly associated with diabetes, there exist nevertheless other conditions in which glomerular nodules may occur. Since these may present diagnostic difficulties, they will be briefly mentioned here. For a detailed report and illustrations, the reader is referred to an earlier publication [34].

In renal *amyloidosis*, abnormal homogeneous substance is deposited in the peripheral as well as mesangial parts of the glomerular capillary walls. In rare cases, the deposits may take on the shape of typical diabetic nodules with an acellular center. They can be correctly classified by the use of amyloid stains and by demonstration of typical fibrils on electron microscopy.

Some types of advanced *glomerulonephritis* (mesangial proliferative, membrano-proliferative) have a histology that resembles nodular glomerulosclerosis. In glomerulonephritis, however, there is a distinct hypercellularity and the central, acellular area that is so characteristic for diabetes is not present. Nodules in glomerulonephritis involve all mesangial areas and are of almost equal size. Immunodeposits are usually present, but are faint or absent in diabetes.

Glomerular nodules may also be present in various *dysproteinemias* (e.g. multiple myeloma and heavy-chain disease [35-40].

The clinical picture may often solve the diagnostic problem, but the occurrence of glomerular nodules in these diseases should be a reminder to the pathologist not to postulate the presence of diabetes on the prima facie detection of nodular structures in the glomeruli.

249

GLOMERULONEPHRITIS AND OTHER COMPLICATING DISEASES

Glomerulonephritis has been thought to occur more frequently in patients with diabetic renal disease than could be explained by mere coincidence [39, 40]. Autopsy studies have, however, shown that complicating glomerular disease is rare and probably not exceeding prevalence in the general population [41]. In biopsy studies of patients with IDDM glomerulonephritis seems to be comparatively rare [42, 43], probably around 2-3% in unselected cases with proteinuria and duration of diabetes of more than 10 years. It has recently been reported that it may be more common in NIDDM [for literature see ref 44], but data from different series are conflicting. The rates of glomulonephritis in these studies vary between 0 and 69% and those of other complicating renal diseases between 0 and 20%. Geographical differences and variable criteria for histopathological diagnosis may be partly responsible, but the main cause of the diverging results is probably selection of patients for renal biopsy. Most of the investigations are based upon biopsies from patients referred to a nephrologic clinic and in some reports it was explicitly stated that the biopsies were made due to presence of symptoms and signs considered to be caused by other diseases than diabetes. It is clear that this will favor inclusion of patients with complicating renal disease. Pinel et al [45] on the other hand, in their investigation of patients with NIDDM, have excluded all patients with clinical renal disease other than the presence of micro- or macroalbuminuria and found no complicating renal disease. Investigating a consecutive series of renal biopsies from 53 patients with NIDDM and microalbuminuria. Brocco et al did not find any with complicating glomerulonephritis [46]. Only one study, that of Parving et al., was population-based and cross sectional [47]. In this series of patients with macroalbuminuria, 23% had non diabetic glomerular disease. Half of these had, however, no glomerular lesions by light microscopy (LM) or IF and were thought to have a complicating minor change nephropathy. While most types of glomerulitis can be confidently diagnosed by proliferative or membranous glomerular changes and deposits of immunoglobulin, this is not the case with minor change disease. Albuminuria in a diabetic patient with normal glomeruli by LM and IF may be due to the still unknown factor responsible for minor change disease, to focal and segmental glomerular sclerosis missed due to sampling problems, to early diffuse diabetic glomerulopathy, not detectable by LM, or to other, hypothetical causes (vascular permeability factors? Biochemical alterations of the glomerular basement membrane?) [48]. We have at the moment no explanation of albuminuria in diabetic patients with normal glomerular structure. This group of patients should be investigated further.

Other complicating diseases. Atheroma emboli may be found in the intrarenal vessels as a complication to diabetic macroangiopathy (atherosclerosis in the aorta and renal arteries). Papillary necrosis is also a well known complication. Other renal diseases occurring in the same age as NIDDM such as amyloidosis and myeloma are probably unrelated to the diabetic state.

TUBULOINTERSTITIAL LESIONS

It is well established that long term diabetic nephropathy is associated with marked *interstitial fibrosis, tubular atrophy* and *mononuclear cell infiltration.* Formerly these changes were interpreted as evidence of complicating chronic pyelonephritis [3]. Since they were shown to be correlated to the renal microvascular alterations characteristic for long term diabetes, it was later on suggested that they were due to chronic ischemia [47, 48]. Lane et al [49] found in IDDM that mesangial volume fraction, severity of arteriolar hyalinosis, percentage of globally sclerosed glomeruli, and interstitial volume fraction for total renal cortex were significantly correlated and all four structural parameters correlated with glomerular filtration rate and urinary albumin excretion. Stepwise multiple regression analysis suggested, however, that they are partially independent. Gambara et al [50] described a special subgroup of patients with diabetic renal disease in which the severe interstitial changes were not clearly correlated with glomerular or vascular lesions. Similar observations were reported by another group of investigators who analysed patients with microalbuminuria [46] and described three patterns of renal morphology. One had normal structure, another had typical diabetic glomerular changes and a third group had absent or mild glomerular changes together with disproportionately severe tubulointerstitial changes and/or arteriolar hyalinosis. Conceivably such changes may not be due to ischemia but to the diabetic metabolic abnormality, like diabetic glomerulopathy although with other pathogenesis.

REFERENCES

1.   Kimmelstiel P, Wilson C. Intercapillary lesions in the glomeruli of the kidney. Am J Pathol 1936; 12: 83-105.

251

2. Thomsen AC. *The Kidney in Diabetes Mellitus* (thesis). Copenhagen: Munksgaard, 1965.
3. Ditscherlein G. *Nierenveränderungen bei Diabetikern*. Jená: G. Fischer, 1969.
4. Allen AC. So-called intercapillary glomerulosclerosis: a lesion associated with diabetes mellitus. Arch Pathol Lab Med 1941; 32: 33-51.
5. Bell ET. Renal lesions in diabetes mellitus. Am J Pathol 1942; 18: 744-745.
6. Bell ET. Renal vascular disease in diabetes mellitus. Diabetes 1953; 2: 376-389.
7. Bell ET. *Diabetes Mellitus: A Clinical and Pathological Study of 2529 Cases*. Springfield IL: Thomas, 1960.
8. Fahr T. Über Glomerulosklerose. Virschows Arch (Pathol Anat) 1942; 309: 16-33.
9. Spühler O, Zollinger HU. Die diab. Glomerulosklerose. Dtsch Arch Klin Med 1943; 190: 321-379.
10. Muirhead EE, Montgomery POB, Booth E. The glomerular lesions of diabetes mellitus: cellular hyaline and acellular hyaline lesions of »intercapillary glomerulosclerosis« as depicted by histochemical studies. Arch Intern Med 1956; 98: 146-161.
11. Randerath E. Zur Frage der intercapillären (diabetischen) Glomerulosklerose. Virchows Arch (Pathol Anat) 1953; 323: 483-523.
12. Sandison A, Newbold KM, Howie AJ. Evidence for unique distribution of Kimmelstiel-Wilson nodules in glomeruli. Diabetes 1992; 41: 952-955.
13. Stout LC, Kumar S, Whorton EB. Focal mesangiolysis and the pathogenesis of the Kimmelstiel-Wilson nodule. Hum Pathol 1993; 24: 77-89.
14. Yafumi S, Hiroshi K, Shin-Ichi T, Mitsuhiro Y, Hitoshi Y, Yoshitaka K, Nobu H. Mesangiolysis in diabetic glomeruli: Its role in the formation of nodular lesions. Kidney Int 1988; 34: 389-396.
15. Stout LC, Kumar S, Whorton EB. Insudative lesions - their pathogenesis and association with glomerular obsolescence in diabetes: A dynamic hypothesis based on single views of advancing human diabetic nephropathy. Hum Pathol 1994; 25: 1213-1227.
16. Barrie HJ, Aszkanazy CL, Smith GW. More glomerular changes in diabetics. Can Med Assoc J 1952; 66: 428-431.
17. Koss LG. Hyaline material with staining reaction of fibrinoid in renal lesions in diabetes mellitus. Arch Pathol Lab Med 1952; 54: 528-547.
18. Rinehart JF, Farquhar MG, Jung HC, Abul-Haj SK. The normal glomerulus and its basic reactions in disease. Am J Pathol 1953; 29: 21-31.
19. Gallo GR. Elution studies in kidneys with linear deposition of immunoglobulin in glomeruli. Am J Pathol 1970; 61: 377-394.
20. Westberg NG, Michael AF. Immunohistopathology of diabetic glomerulosclerosis. Diabetes 1972; 21: 163-174.
21. Frøkjær Thomsen O. Studies of diabetic glomerulosclerosis using an immunofluorescent technique. Acta Pathol Microbiol Scand (A) 1972; 80: 193-200.
22. Østerby R. Early phases in the development of diabetic glomerulopathy. A quantative electron microscopic study. Acta Med Scandinav, 1975 (S:574) thesis.
23. Østerby R. Glomerular structural changes in type 1 (insulin-dependent) diabetes mellitus – causes, consequences, and prevention. Diabetologia, 1992; 35: 803-12.
24. Björn S, Bangstad HJ, Hanssen K, et al. Glomerular epithelial foot processes and filtration slits in IDDM patients. Diabetologia, 1995; 38: 1197-1204.
25. Christensen P, Larsen S, Horn T, Olsen S, Parving HH. Causes of albuminuria in patients with type 2 diabetes without diabetic retinopathy. Kidney International, 2000; 58: 1719-31.

26. Østerby R, Gundersen HJG, Nyberg G, Aurell M. Advanced diabetic glomerulopathy. Quantitative structural characterization of nonoccluded glomeruli. Diabetes 1987; 36: 612-619.

27. Hørlyck A, Gundersen HJG, Østerby R. The cortical distribution pattern of diabetic glomerulopathy. Diabetologia 1986; 29: 146-150.

28. Bendtsen TF, Nyengaard JR. The number of glomeruli in Type 1 (insulin-dependent) and Type 2 (non-insulin dependent) diabetic patients. Diabetologia 1992; 35: 844-850.

29. Allen AC. *The Kidney: Medical and Surgical Diseases*, 2nd ed. London: Churchill, 1962; pp 38.

30. Heptinstall RH. *Pathology of the Kidney*, 3rd ed. Boston: Little, Brown and Company, 1983; Ch. 26

31. Olsen S. The renal structure damage in patients with type 2 diabetes. In: Mogensen CE (ed.). *Diabetic Nephropathy in Type 2 Diabetes*. London: Science Press Ltd, 2002, p.31–40.

32. Da-Silva EC, Saldanha LB, Pestalozzi MS, Del-Bueno IJ, Barros RT, Marcondes M, Nussenzveig I. Nodular diabetic glomerulosclerosis without diabetes mellitus. Nephron 1992; 62: 289-291.

33. Kanwar YS, Garces J, Molitch ME. Occurrence of intercapillary nodular glomerulosclerosis in the absence of glucose intolerance. Am J Kidney Dis 1990; 15: 281-283.

34. Olsen TS. Mesangial thickening and nodular glomerular sclerosis in diabetes mellitus and other diseases. Acta Pathol Microbiol Scand (A) 1972; 80: 203-216.

35. Sølling K, Askjær S-A. Multiple myeloma with urinary excretion of heavy chain components of IgG and nodular glomerulosclerosis. Acta Med Scand 1973; 194: 23-30.

36. Gallo GR, Feiner HD, Katz LA, Feldman GM, Correa EB, Chuba JV Buxbaum JN. Nodular glomerulopathy associated with nonamyloidotic kappa light chain deposits and excess immunoglobulin light chain synthesis. Am J Pathol 1980; 99: 621-644.

37. Sølling K, Sølling J, Jacobsen NO, Frøkjær Thomsen O. Nonsecretory myeloma associated with nodular glomerulosclerosis. Acta Med Scand 1980; 207: 137-143.

38. Schubert GE, Adam A. Glomerular nodules and long-spacing collagen in kidneys of patients with multiple myeloma. J Clin Pathol 1974; 27: 800-805.

39. Wehner H, Bohle A. The structure of the glomerular capillary basement membrane in diabetes mellitus with and without nephrotic syndrome. Virchows Arch (Pathol Anat) 1974; 364: 303-309.

40. Yum M, Maxwell DR, Hamburger R, Kleit SA. Primary glomerulonephritis complicating diabetic nephropathy. Hum Pathol 1984; 15: 921-927.

41. Waldherr R, Ilkenhans C, Ritz E. How frequent is glomerulonephritis in diabetes mellitus type II ? Clin Nephrol 1992; 37: 271-273.

42. Mauer SM, Steffes MW, Ellis EN, Sutherland DER, Brown DM, Goetz FC. Structural-functional relationships in diabetic nephropathy. J Clin Invest 1984; 74: 1143-1155.

43. Richards N, Greaves I, Lee S, Howie A, Adu D, Michael J. Increased prevalence of renal biopsy findings other than diabetic glomerulopathy in type II diabetes mellitus. Nephrol Dial Transplant 1992; 7: 397-399.

44. Olsen S, Mogensen CE. How often is type II diabetes mellitus complicated with non-diabetic renal disease? A material of renal biopsies and an analysis of the literature. Diabetologia 1996; 39: 1638-1645.

45. Pinel NBF, Bilous R, Corticelli P, Halimi S, Cordonnier D. Renal Biopsies in 30 Micro- and Macroalbuminuric Non-Insulin Dependent (NIDDM) Patients: Heterogeneity of Renal Lesions. Heidelberg: European Diabetic Nephropathy Study Group, 1995.

46. Brocco E, Fioretto P, Mauer M, Saller A, Carraro A, Frigato C, Chiesura-Corona M, Bianchi L, Baggio B, Maioll M, Abaterusso C, Velussi M, Sambatoro M, Virgili F, Ossi E, Nosadini R. Renal structure and function in non-insulin dependent diabetic patients with microalbuminuria. Kidney Int. 1997; 52: Suppl. 63: S40-S44

47. Parving H-H, Gall M-A, Skøtt P,Jørgensen HE, Løkkegaard H, Jørgensen F, Nielsen B, Larsen S. Prevalence and causes of albuminuria in non-insulin-dependent diabetic patients. Kidney Int, 1992; 41: 758-762

48. Olsen S. Identification of non-diabetic glomerular disease in renal biopsies from diabetics – a dilemma. Neprol Dial Transplant 1999; 13: 1846-49.

49. Lane PH, Steffes M, Fioretto P, Mayer SM. Renal interstitial expansion in insulin-dependent diabetes mellitus. Kidney Int 1993; 43: 661-667.

50. Gambara V, Remuzzi G, Bertani T. Heterogenous nature of renal lesions in type II diabetes. J Am Soc Nephrol 1993; 3: 1458-1466.

16

RENAL STRUCTURAL CHANGES IN PATIENTS WITH TYPE 1 DIABETES AND MICROALBUMINURIA

Hans-Jacob Bangstad and Susanne Rudberg

Department of Paediatrics, Aker and Ullevål Diabetes Research Centre, Ullevål University Hospital, Oslo, Norway, and The Department of Woman and Child Health, Karolinska Institute, Stockholm, Sweden

Associations between early stages of diabetic nephropathy and structural changes is far from clarified since some reports present rather marked changes in patients in the preclinical stage whereas others found very moderate changes in the early stage of nephropathy. Hence the issue is still a challenge to further studies. This chapter concentrates on the renal morphological changes in patients with Type 1 diabetes and early nephropathy and the possibilities of influencing the progression by blood glucose control and antihypertensive treatment.

STRUCTURES IN QUESTION

Structural changes in glomeruli, termed <u>diabetic glomerulopathy</u> is the aspect that ha attracted most attention. The increased thickness of the glomerular basement membrane (BMT) and the mesangial expansion with accumulation of matrix is the fundamental change [1]. The relative increase of mesangium and of mesangial matrix is expressed as volume fractions, e.g. mesangium per glomerulus, matrix per mesangium or per glomerulus. The volume fractions are relative measures, estimating the composition of glomeruli and mesangial regions. These parameters are the quantitative expressions of the characteristic appearance of diabetic glomerulopathy. An overall estimate of the glomerulopathy may be expressed by a structural index (e.g. BMT/10+Vv (matrix/glom)%). Of decisive importance for obtaining reliable data describing the earliest stages is a sufficient and unbiased sampling. In order to reduce the imprecision in the estimates of the mesangial volume fraction a method with complete cross-sections at 3 levels per glomerulus has been applied [2].

Another glomerular structural change of completely different nature is the glomerular hypertrophy present in the earliest phase of diabetes [3]. In advanced stages it is further expressed as a compensatory enlargement, accompanying the developing glomerulopathy [4].

Further, extra-glomerular changes may play an important role. Rather characteristic is the arteriolar hyalinosis affecting afferent and efferent arterioles. This arteriolopathy can be expressed as the volume fraction of extra-cellular material (matrix) per media. Also, expansion of the cortical interstitium is part of the whole picture. Further, measurable enlargement has been described in the juxta-glomerular apparatus and the vascular pole region.

The frequency of glomerular occlusions, capsular drops and fibrinoid lesions will not be dealt with in detail, but still after 20 years duration of diabetes only 3.8 % of the glomeruli seem to be occluded and no association between number of occluded glomeruli and glomerulopathy was found [5].

PATIENTS WITH MICROALBUMINURIA VS. HEALTHY CONTROLS

We studied two series of kidney biopsies from 38 normotensive young patients with Type 1 diabetes as baseline data for prospective studies [6,7]. Most of the diabetic patients had AER in the low range with a median of 31 μg/min (range 15-194). Their mean age was 19 years (14-29) and diabetes duration 11 years (6-18). The microalbuminuric (MA) patients showed a clear increment in BMT with a mean of 586 nm (95% confidence interval 553-619 nm) versus 350 nm (315-384) in the control group. All of the MA patients had BMT above the normal range. The average BM thickening during the years with diabetes was approximately 20 nm per year. This approximation was based on the assumption that the patients had a BM thickness at onset of diabetes corresponding to the mean BMT of the control group, i.e. 350 nm. A significant parallel matrix expansion in the microalbuminuric patients vs. the normal controls was observed. Matrix/glomerular volume fraction was 0.12 (0.11-0.13) vs. 0.09 (0.08-0.10) in the two groups respectively [8]. The findings are confirmed in a large study recently presented [9].

It is hardly surprising that it is possible with sensitive methods to show morphological changes in Type 1 patients with clinical indications of renal impairment (microalbuminuria) when compared to healthy controls, but the extent of the changes should be emphasized.

MICROALBUMINURIA VS. NORMOALBUMINURIA

In the 60s several reports indicated that morphological changes were present at the onset of Type 1 diabetes. Later studies clearly showed that the glomeruli are normal at that time [10] and the impact of that observation was supported by studies of identical twins discordant for Type 1 diabetes [11]. In a clinical setting the transition from normo- to microalbuminuria is of utmost importance. Walker et al. compared two groups of Type 1 diabetes patients [12]. One with normoalbuminuria (n=9, AER <20 µg/min) and one with microalbuminuria (n=6). Even though the number of patients was low, a significant increment in BM thickness, mesangial/glomerular volume fraction and also the matrix parameters was found in patients with MA compared to those with NA. The patients in the normoalbuminuric (NA) group were slightly younger and had a shorter duration of diabetes than the MA-group, although the differences were not statistically significant. The group of patients with microalbuminuria was rather heterogeneous with a wide range in diabetes duration. These results differ from those presented by Fioretto et al. [13], who found no difference between patients with normo- and low-grade microalbuminuria (<32 µg/min). In the study by Caramori et al [9] comprising patients with longstanding diabetes, 88 with NA and 17 with MA, a considerable overlap in the two groups was observed concerning both BMT and mesangial/glomerular volume fraction, but still the difference between the groups was significant. A large proportion of the NA-patients had BMT and mesangial/glomerular volume fraction in the normal range, 240-424 nm and 0.14 – 0.26 respectively. In a fairly large study of normoalbuminuric adolescents [14] also abnormal levels of BMT and mesangial volume fraction were found in some cases, but concurrent controls were not studied, and advanced glomerulopathy was not observed.

An American study reported findings in children and adolescents with diabetes duration five to twelve years [15]. They found a high frequency of BM-thickening and increased mesangial/glomerular volume fraction in more than fifty percent of the group, most of which (48/59) had normal AER. It is obvious that measurable changes can be found in the normoalbuminurics, - the conflicting findings may depend on the selection of patients or the quantitative methodology.

EXTRA-GLOMERULAR CHANGES

In advanced stages of nephropathy several structural compartments in the kidney display distinct abnormalities. The hyalinosis of efferent and afferent arterioles was described a long time ago. Increase in the interstitial tissue has in fact been incriminated as a very important determinant of the late fall in renal function [16]. Some information on these structures during earlier phases of nephropathy has been obtained in recent years.

Semi-quantitative studies of the hyalinosis of arterioles have dealt with a very broad clinical range. The results showed that the score of arteriolar lesions correlated with the severity of glomerulopathy and interstitial expansion and also with renal function [17]. Clearly in this composite picture with affection of all compartments it is not possible to determine which is the most important in terms of the further progression of nephropathy, in particular since abnormalities in one compartment may be very closely and causally related to that in others.

In quantitative ultrastructural studies the composition of arteriolar walls was estimated in NA and MA IDDM patients and in controls [18]. All of the patients had clinical blood pressure within the normal range. Increased matrix per media was found in afferent and efferent arterioles in the MA patients, showing that matrix abnormalities have developed in this location at the earliest stage of nephropathy. The matrix/media volume fraction of the afferent arterioles correlated with glomerular parameters, both BMT and matrix/glomerular volume fraction. Quantitative data are now available in one follow-up study, before and after antihypertensive treatment [19]. At baseline highly significant alterations were present in afferent and efferent arterioles. In the follow-up period of 2,5 years a moderate progression was observed in matrix/media volume fraction in afferent arterioles, but no significant worsening in the efferent arterioles. After 8 years a large increase in the matrix/media volume fraction both in the afferent and the efferent arterioles ($p<0.001$) and a decline in the endothelial cell thickness was found. The arteriolar parameters correlated with AER and inversely with GFR [20].

Another structural change has recently been demonstrated in young Type 1 patients with MA. The volume of the juxta-glomerular apparatus is increased compared with that in non-diabetic controls. Furthermore, also the size expressed relative to glomerular volume, is increased. The interrelationship with functional variables, whether causative or consequent, is not known at the present time [21]. However, after a follow-up of 8 years the JGA-size remained stable, but decreased relative to the glomerular size [22]. The connection between the changes in the afferent and the efferent arterioles, the JGA and possibly the RAS-system, may explain the haemodynamic changes found in early nephropathy [14].

Interstitial expansion is a companion of advanced glomerulopathy and vasculopathy. The interstitium expressed as fraction of cortical space has been shown to correlate with AER and creatinine clearance, as well as with glomerular and arteriolar changes, considering a wide range of functional impairment [17]. We estimated the interstitial volume fraction in the MA patients with low grade albuminuria, and found that it was increased compared to controls already in this early phase [6]. A positive correlation with the degree of glomerulopathy was found, indicating parallel or maybe even interactive processes.

GLOMERULOPATHY AND BLOOD GLUCOSE CONTROL

The impact of long-term hyperglycaemia on the development of structural changes has been demonstrated in several animal studies [23-26]. One study in man showed that in renal allografts no significant increase in BM thickness and mesangial volume fraction was found 2-10 years after pancreas transplantation in 11 patients [27]. Specific mesangial matrix parameters were not investigated. In a prospective long term (12 years) study of renal allografts, the increment of the mesangial volume fraction, but not the BM thickening, was prevented when blood glucose control was improved [28]. Similar results have been demonstrated in patients receiving simultaneous pancreas- and kidney transplantation [29]. Those patients with a well-functioning pancreas transplant seemed to be spared the development of diabetic glomerulopathy. Very intriguing data has been published in pancreas transplanted patients with native kidneys who were followed with kidney biopsies at transplantation and after five and ten years [30]. Whereas the glomerulopathy seemed to progress from 0-5 years, less severe affection was observed after ten years, indicating that long-term metabolic normalisation may entail reversion of established lesions. However, the patients studied after 10 years were the survivors, some patients had dropped out due to renal failure.

In our own series we studied the relationship between structural changes and preceding blood glucose control. The estimated yearly increment of BMT and matrix volume fraction from the start of diabetes correlated with mean HbA_{1c} from the year preceding the study, which probably reflects the long term blood glucose control [6]. Another study in adolescents confirmed this by finding that 5-year mean HbA1c in addition to diabetes duration and GFR, was a variable with an independent influence on the glomerulopathy index [7].

The prospective study dealing with metabolic control was concluded after 2 and a half years period [31]. The patients were randomised to either intensive insulin treatment by continuous subcutaneous insulin infusion (CSII) or conventional treatment (CT, - mostly multiple injections). It should be noticed that the mean HbA_{1c}-values in the two groups were rather high, and that the difference between the groups was modest, although significant, 8.7% and 9.9% respectively (normal range 4.3-6.1%). The AER was for most of the patients in the low microalbuminuric range throughout the study. In fact, 38 % of the patients had AER <15 µg/min at the end of the study and thus by definition had no longer microalbuminuria. The main finding of the study was that in the CSII-group none of the matrix-parameters increased, whereas they all increased (not significantly for matrix/glomerular volume fraction) in the CT-group. The BM thickness increased in both groups, - but the increment during the study period was significantly larger in the CT-group [140 nm (50-230) vs. 56 nm (27-86)]. The association between blood glucose control and structure was confirmed when all the patients were considered together. A strong correlation was found between mean HbA_{1c} during the study and increase in BM thickness and matrix/glomerular volume fraction (figure 1). We thus showed that the progression of morphological changes in the glomerulus could be identified within a short period of only 2-3 years. Furthermore, we observed that reduced mean blood glucose levels clearly retarded the progression of morphological changes in the glomeruli. However, the glycated haemoglobin level achieved in the CSII-treated group (8.7%) was not sufficient to stop the progression of morphological changes.

In the long term follow-up of the prospective study, the patients did not adhere to the randomisation after 2,5 years, but in the total group we found that the severity of the glomerulopathy presented at baseline predicted the AER six years later [32]. In the multiple regressions analysis mean 8-years HbA1c and baseline matrix/glomerular volume fraction and BMT accounted for 70 % of the AER-level after 8 years. At that time the diabetes duration was 20 years. Only 3 of the 18 patients had a significant increase in AER (> 25 % per year) and five turned normoalbuminuric during these 8 years [33]

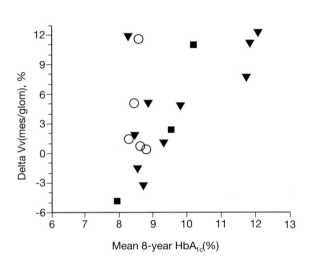

Figure 1. Absolute change in Vv(mes/glom) vs. mean 8 year HbA1c, r=0.57, p=0.01. Three subjects with AER-increment > 25% per year (■), 10 subjects with no significant increment of AER during the study (▼), and five subjects with normoalbuminuria at the end of the study (○) [33].

GLOMERULOPATHY AND ANTIHYPERTENSIVE TREATMENT

Glomerulopathy is observed as early as 2 years after onset of diabetes [34] and is associated with the level of nocturnal diastolic blood pressure after 10 years in children and adolelescents in whom persistent microalbuminuria has not developed [35]. Antihypertensive treatment has been shown to have a beneficial effect on the course of nephropathy. Further, several recent data present evidence that administration of this treatment regimen in the stage of microalbuminuria to normotensive patients has protective effect [36].

To investigate the influence of angiotensin converting enzyme inhibitors

(ACEI) or beta-blockers on renal structural changes in Type I diabetes, we studied 13 young normotensive patients with microalbuminuria [37]. Patients were randomised to either an ACE-inhibitor (enalapril 20 mg daily, n=7) or a beta-blocker (metoprolol 100 mg daily, n=6), and renal biopsies were taken before and after 36-48 months´ treatment. As a reference group we used 9 patients on conventional insulin treatment and without antihypertensive treatment (AHT) that had renal biopsies previously taken with 26-34 months´ intervals [31]. These patients had similar age, duration of diabetes and degree of microalbuminuria as those on AHT. We found that BMT, diabetic glomerulopathy index (DGP, figure 2) [i.e. BMT/10+Vv(mat/glom)%] and interstitial fractional volume increased during follow-up in the reference group only. Microalbuminuria was normalised in both the ACEI-treated and the beta-blocker-treated groups, but not in the reference group. Mean HbA_{1c} during the study period did not differ significantly between groups, whereas mean diastolic blood pressure was significantly lower in the antihypertensive groups than in the reference group. It was also found that mean diastolic blood pressure correlated significantly to the changes in BMT, DGP index and the interstitial expansion.

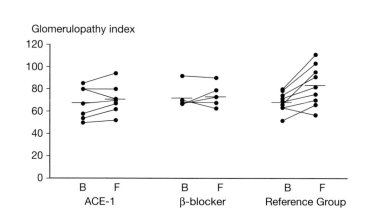

Fig 2. Glomerulopathy index (BMT/10 + Vv(matrix/glom) %) in baseline (B) and follow-up biopsies (F) in three groups treated with ACEI, beta-blocker or conventional insulin treatment. The increase in the reference group is statistically significant (p=0.007) and this group is significantly different from the two other groups (p=0.02 and 0.03 respectively) [37].

Thus our data suggest that progression of *early* renal structural changes may be prevented or delayed during a 3 year period, by the use of either ACEI *or* beta-blocker. It is likely that this effect is due to maintenance of a normal or low blood pressure.

These results are in contrast to the data from the ESPRIT study where neither ACEI (enalapril 10 mg once daily) nor Ca-antagonist (nifedipine 10 mg twice daily) did affect the glomerulopathy changes [38]. It should be kept in mind though, that patients in the ESPRIT study had a longer diabetes duration and were older, but more important, they were in a more advanced stage of diabetic nephropathy and the dosage of enalapril was lower than in those included in our study.

We also studied the association between I/D polymorphism of the ACE-gene and progression of diabetic glomerulopathy in the same groups of patients referred to above, i.e those treated with either ACE-I or betablocker, and those without AHT. To extend the number of subjects another group of 9 patients on insulin pump treatment but without AHT, who likewise had renal biopsies previously performed, were included [31]. We found that eight patients had II-, 19 had ID-, and 3 had DD-genotypes, but only those with ID-or DD-genotypes showed any progression in BMT or DGP-index. Among patients with ID-or DD-genotypes progression of BM thickening and DGP-index was more marked in those without AHT than in those with any AHT. However, presence of the D-allele and not having AHT were both variables with an independent influence on the progression of BM thickening. These data indicate that microalbuminuric type 1 diabetic patients who are carriers of the D-allele do benefit from the use ACEI as well as beta-blockers [39].

GLOMERULAR STRUCTURAL CHANGES VERSUS ALBUMIN EXCRETION

AER is an important parameter of kidney function in the early stages of nephropathy. In groups of diabetic patients representing a wide range of renal functional impairment significant correlations between glomerulopathy parameters and AER are found [1], and especially the correlation between mesangial expansion and AER has been underlined. This seems to reflect the fact that in the very advanced stages with marked proteinuria mesangial expansion is the dominant feature of the glomerulopathy. Within the range of microalbuminuria the correlation is less tight; however, positive associations have been described [6].

In a study dealing with young normoalbuminuric patients it was found that a subset exhibiting MA at the time of kidney biopsy, had more advanced changes than those patients in the lower normoalbuminuric range [35]. One of our series has been followed for six years after the baseline biopsy. It was revealed that primarily BMT, but also systolic blood pressure and mean 6-year HbA_{1c} contributed to the variation in AER [32]. In conflict with these observations are the reports mentioned above of rather advanced glomerulopathy in cases with low grade microalbuminuria [13,40,41], and even in normoalbuminuria [13,14]. It seems that these somewhat atypical cases with concurrently rather low GFR and AER are predominantly female Type 1 diabetes patients with long duration. In one of the series [41] a high frequency of totally occluded glomeruli was found, and enlargement of the vascular pole area in the open glomeruli was marked [42]. This change may represent a compensation to falling GFR and might influence the level of AER. Diabetic patients with a slow development of nephropathy may exhibit a deviating structural pattern where changes of arterioles and arteries (diabetic macroangiopathy) play an important role.

It is still unclear whether the elevation of blood pressure observed in diabetic nephropathy precedes, develops in parallel with or follows the initial increment of AER [36]. In our prospective study none of the patients had arterial hypertension (>150/90 mmHg), but 24 hours ambulatory blood pressure was not measured [31]. No associations between blood pressure (BP) and glomerular parameters were found, neither at baseline nor at follow-up, but all patients had BP within a fairly narrow range. Thus we cannot speculate upon the role of BP on the initiation of structural lesions. However, recent findings of a Swedish group indicate such an impact [35].

MECHANISMS OF ALBUMINURIA

Even if correlation between albumin excretion and structural lesions have been observed we still lack the deeper insight into the mechanisms behind the increment in albumin leakage. The increase in BM thickness in itself is unlikely to be responsible for the increased albumin excretion rate, but qualitative changes, e.g. reduced negative charge and/or presence of large pores, which develop concomitantly with the increase in thickness, may be decisive.

The urinary excretion of negatively charged proteins, e.g. albumin, is restricted by the negatively charged basement membrane. In the aforementioned prospective study [6] the charge selectivity index (clearances of IgG/IgG_4) was not associated with BM thickness at the beginning of the study. However, a striking correlation was found between the increase of BM thickness and the loss of charge selectivity during the study [43]. This may imply that the increase in BM thickness takes place concomitant with qualitative changes (e.g. loss of negative charge).

It is not known which substances that are responsible for the early thickening of BM and matrix expansion in diabetes. In the BM collagen IV predominates quantitatively, while laminin and heparan-sulphate proteoglycan probably play an important role as well. The mesangial matrix contains in addition collagen V, fibronectin, and chondroitin/dermatan sulfate proteoglycans [44]. Short-term experimental studies show that hyperglycaemia induces increased production of most of the aforementioned proteins [45-47], increased levels of the proteins' respective mRNA [48,49], increased matrix synthesis [50], and reduced amount of heparan-sulphate proteoglycan [51,52]. Furthermore, hyperglycaemia leads to accumulation of advanced glycated end products of proteins (AGE). These glycated proteins do contribute to the formation of pathological tissue deposits [53]. In our study [31] the level of serum-AGEs at the start of the study was related to the changes in structural parameters during the study period [54]. In experimental diabetes accumulation of AGE was inhibited by aminoguanidin and ACEI [55].

An interesting observation in advanced glomerulopathy [56] and in the early stage in microalbuminuric patients [57] is capillary loops with extremely thin and fluffy BM, contrasting markedly the other capillaries in the biopsies. They may be an expression of a compensatory glomerular growth, setting in at this early stage, and could represent the large pores.

The BM-thickening develops in parallel with matrix expansion. Matrix changes, quantitative and qualitative, may interfere with the function of the mesangial cells [58]. Mesangial cell function plays a role in many aspects of glomerular physiology [59] and one immediate consequence of the matrix expansion is that the distance between mesangial cells increases. This may impair the cell-to-cell interaction.

A rather new area of interest in diabetic nephropathy is the podocytes and the slit diaphragms. A longitudinal study provided evidence for an association between loss of podocytes and AER [60]. In young patients with normo- and microalbuminuria Berg et al found a positive correlation between AER and foot process (nm) width and a negative correlation with the slit pore (μm^{-2}), [14]. In experimental diabetic nephropathy amelioration of the podocyte foot process broadening was obtained by RAS-blockade [61] and in biopsies from patients with type-2 diabetes, the expression of messenger-RNA of one of the slit pore membrane proteins, nephrin, was modulated by ACEI [62]. Hyperglycaemia and TGF-β1 in concert seem to induce the production of collagen IV and VEGF in the podocytes [63].

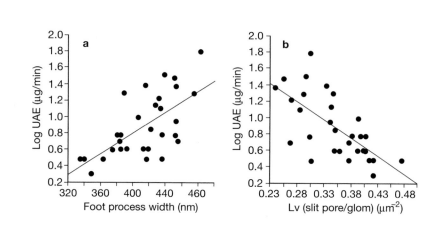

Fig. 3 Urinary albumin excretion (UAE) expressed in log values, in relation to **a**. foot process width (r=0.645, n=30, p<0.001) and **b**. length density of filtration slits Lv (slit pore/glom) (r=0.683, n=30, p<0.001)

Altogether, the present data indicate that the increased loss of albumin across the glomerular filtration barrier is a sign associated with early structural lesions of diabetic glomerulopathy and that the further development can be arrested or at least slowed by intensive insulin and/or antihypertensive treatment.

REFERENCES

1. Mauer SM, Steffes MW, Ellis EN, Sutherland DE, Brown DM, Goetz FC. Structural-functional relationships in diabetic nephropathy. J Clin Invest 1984; 74:1143-1155.

2. Østerby R. Research methodologies related to renal complications: structural changes. In Research Methodologies in Human Diabetes, Part 2, Mogensen CE, Standl E, eds. Berlin, New York: Walter de Gruyter, 1995; pp 289-09

3. Østerby R, Gundersen HJ. Glomerular size and structure in diabetes mellitus. 1. Early abnormalities. 1975; 11:229-229.

4. Gundersen HJ, Østerby R. Glomerular size and structure in diabetes mellitus. 2. Late abnormalities. Diabetologia 1977;13:43-48.

5. Østerby R, Hartman A, Nyengaard JR, Bangstad, H-J Development of renal structural lesions in Type 1 diabetic patients with microalbuminuria. Observations by light microscopy in 8-years' follow-up biopsies. Virchows Arch; 2002: 449: 94-101.

6. Bangstad H-J, Østerby R, Dahl-Jørgensen K, et al. Early glomerulopathy is present in young Type 1 (insulin-dependent) diabetic patients with microalbuminuria. Diabetologia 1993; 36: 523-529.

7. Rudberg S, Østerby R, Dahlquist G, Nyberg G, Persson B. Predictors of renal morphological changes in the early stage of microalbuminuria in adolescents with IDDM. Diabetes Care 1997;20:265-271.

8. Østerby R, Bangstad H-J, Rudberg S. Structural changes in microalbuminuria. Effect of intervention. Nephrology Dialysis Transplantation [Abstract] 1998; 13: 1067-68.

9. Caramori ML, Kim Y, Huang C, Fish AJ, Rich SS, Miller ME, Russell G, Mauer M. Cellular basis of diabetic nephropathy: 1. Study design and renal structural-functional relationships in patients with long-standing type 1 diabetes. Diabetes. 2002 Feb;51(2):506-13

10. Østerby R. Early phases in the development of diabetic nephropathy. Acta Med Scand 1975; Suppl.574 : 1-80.

11. Steffes MW, Sutherland DER, Goetz FC, Rich SS, Mauer SM. Studies of kidney and muscle biopsies in identical twins discordant for type 1 diabetes mellitus. N Engl J Med 1985; 312: 1281-1287.

12. Walker JD, Close CF, Jones SL, et al. Glomerular structure in type I (insulin-dependent) diabetic patients with normo- and microalbuminuria. Kidney Int 1992; 41: 741-748.

13. Fioretto P, Steffes MW, Mauer SM. Glomerular structure in nonproteinuric IDDM patients with various levels of albuminuria. Diabetes 1994; 43: 1358-1364.

14. Berg UB, Torbjørnsdotter TB, Jaremko G, Thalme B. Kidney morphological changes in relation to long-term renal function and metabolic control in adolescents with IDDM. Diabetologia 1998; 41. 1047-1056.

15. Ellis EN, Warady BA, Wood EG, Hassanein R, Richardson WP, Lane PH et al. Renal structural-functional relationship in early diabetes mellitus. Pediatr Nephrol 1997;11:584-591.

16. Ziyadeh FN, Goldfarb S. The diabetic renal tubulointerstitium. In Dodd S, ed: Current topics in pathology. Springer-Verlag, Berlin; 1995: 175-201.

17. Lane PH, Steffes MW, Fioretto P, Mauer SM. Renal interstitial expansion in insulin-dependent diabetes mellitus. Kidney Int 1993; 43: 661-667.

18. Østerby R, Bangstad H-J, Nyberg G, Walker JD, Viberti GC. A quantitative ultrastructural study of juxtaglomerular arterioles in IDDM patients with micro- and normoalbuminuria. Diabetologia 1995; 38: 1320-1327.

19. Gulmann C, Rudberg S, Østerby R. Renal arterioles in patients with type I diabetes and microalbuminuria before and after treatment with antihypertensive drugs. Virchows Arch 1999; 434: 523-528.

20. Østerby R, Hartmann A, Bangstad, H-J. Structural changes in renal arterioles in Type 1 diabetic patients. Quantitative electron microscopy findings in 8 years follow-up biopsies. Diabetologia 2002; 45:542-549.

21. Gulmann C, Rudberg S, Nyberg G, Østerby R. Enlargement of the juxtaglomerular apparatus in insulin-dependent diabetes mellitus patients with microalbuminuria. Virchows Arch 1998; 433: 63-67.

22. Gulman C, Østerby R, Bangstad H-J. Long-term studies of the juxtaglomerular apparatus in young microalbuminuric Type 1 diabetic patients. APMIS 2001:109;767-73

23. Rasch R. Prevention of diabetic glomerulopathy in streptozotocin diabetic rats by insulin treatment. Glomerular basement membrane thickness. Diabetologia 1979; 16: 319-324.

24. Rasch R. Prevention of diabetic glomerulopathy in streptozotocin diabetic rats by insulin treatment. The mesangial region. Diabetologia 1979; 17: 243-248.

25. Kern TS, Engerman RL. Kidney morphology in experimental hyperglycemia. Diabetes 1987; 36: 244-249.

26. Petersen J, Ross J, Rabkin R. Effect of insulin therapy on established diabetic nephropathy in rats. Diabetes 1988; 37: 1346-1350.

27. Bilous RW, Mauer SM, Sutherland DER, Najarian JS, Goetz FC, Steffes MW. The effect of pancreas transplantation on the glomerular structure of renal allografts in patients with insulin-dependent diabetes. N Engl J Med 1989; 321: 80-85.

28. Barbosa J, Steffes MW, Connett J, Mauer M. Hyperglycemia is causally related to diabetic renal lesions. Diabetes 1992; 41: 9A.

29. Wilczek H, Jaremko G, Tyden G, Groth CG. Evolution of diabetic nephropathy in kidney grafts. Transplantation 1995; 59: 51-57.

30. Fioretto P, Steffes MW, Sutherland DER, Goetz FC, Mauer M. Reversal of lesions of diabetic nephropathy after pancreas transplantation. N Eng J Med 1998; 339: 69-75.

31. Bangstad H-J, Østerby R, Dahl-Jørgensen K, Berg KJ, Hartmann A, Hanssen KF. Improvement of blood glucose control retards the progression of morphological changes in early diabetic nephropathy. Diabetologia 1994; 37: 483-490

32. Bangstad H-J, Østerby R, Hartmann A, Berg TJ, Hanssen KF. Severity of glomerulopathy predicts long-term urinary albumin excretion rate in patients with Type 1 diabetes and microalbuminuria. Diabetes Care 1999; 22: 314-319.

33. Bangstad H-J, Østerby R, Rudberg S, Hartmann A, Hanssen KF. Kidney function and glomerulopathy over 8 years in young patients with type 1 (insulin-dependent9 diabetes and microalbuminuria. Diabetologia 2002.;45:253-261

34. Drummond K, Mauer M. The early natural history of nephropathy in type 1 diabetes: II. Early renal structural changes in type 1 diabetes. Diabetes 2002; 51: 1580-1587.

35. Torbjornsdotter TB, Jaremko GA, Berg UBAmbulatory blood pressure and heart rate in relation to kidney structure and metabolic control in adolescents with Type 1 diabetes. Diabetologia. 2001; 44: 865-873

36. Mogensen CE. Microalbuminuria, blood pressure and diabetic renal disease. Origin and development of ideas. Diabetologia 1999; 42: 263-285.

37. Rudberg S, Østerby R, Bangstad HJ, Dahlquist G, Persson B. Effect of angiotensin converting enzyme inhibitor or beta-blocker on glomerular structural changes in young microalbuminuric patients with Type I (insulin-dependent) diabetes mellitus. Diabetologia 1999; 42: 589-595.

38. No author listed Effect of 3 years of antihypertensive therapy on renal structure in type 1 diabetic patients with albuminuria: the European Study for the Prevention of Renal Disease in Type 1 Diabetes (ESPRIT). Diabetes 2001; 50: 843-850.

39. Rudberg S, Rasmussen LM, Bangstad H-J, Østerby R. Influence of insertion/deletion polymorphism in the angiotensin converting enzyme gene on the progression of diabetic glomerulopathy in IDDM patients with microalbuminuria. Diabetes Care 2000; 23: 544-548

40. Lane PH, Steffes MW, Mauer SM. Glomerular structure in IDDM women with low glomerular filtration rate and normal urinary albumin excretion. Diabetes 1992; 41: 581-586.

41. Østerby R, Schmitz A, Nyberg G, Asplund J. Renal structural changes in insulin dependent diabetic patients with albuminuria. Comparison of cases with onset of albuminuria after short and long duration. APMIS 1998; 106: 361-370.

42. Østerby R, Asplund J, Bangstad H-J et al. Glomerular volume and the glomerular vascular pole area in patients with insulin-dependent diabetes mellitus. Virchow Arch 1997; 431:351-357.

43. Bangstad H-J, Kofoed-Enevoldsen A, Dahl-Jørgensen K, Hanssen KF. Glomerular charge selectivity and the influence of improved blood glucose control in Type 1 diabetic patients with microalbuminuria. Diabetologia 1992; 35: 1165-1170.

44. Silbiger S, Crowley S, Shan Z, Brownlee M, Satriano J, Schlondorff D. Nonenzymatic glycation of mesangial matrix and prolonged exposure of mesangial matrix to elevated glucose reduces collagen synthesis and proteoglycan charge. Kidney Int 1993; 43: 853-864.

45. Brownlee M, Spiro RG. Glomerular basement membrane metabolism in the diabetic rat: in vivo studies. Diabetes 1979; 28: 121-125.

46. Cagliero E, Roth T, Roy S, Lorenzi M. Characteristics and mechanisms of high-glucose-induced overexpression of basement membrane components in cultured human endothelial cells. Diabetes 1991; 40: 102-110.

47. Roy S, Sala R, Cagliero E, Lorenzi M. Overexpression of fibronectin induced by diabetes or high glucose: phenomenon with a memory. Proc Natl Acad Sci USA 1990; 87: 404-408.

48. Ledbetter S, Copeland EJ, Noonan D, Vogeli G, Hassel JR. Altered steady-state mRNA levels of basement membrane proteins in diabetic mouse kidneys and thromboxane synthase inhibition. Diabetes 1990; 39: 196-203.

49. Poulsom R, Kurkinen M, Prockop DJ, Boot-Handford RP. Increased steady-state levels of laminin B1 mRNA in kidneys of long term streptozotocin-diabetic rats. J Biol Chem 1988; 263: 10072-10076.

50. Ayo SH, Radnik RA, Garoni JA, Glass II WF, Kreisberg JI. High glucose causes an increase in extracellular matrix proteins in cultured mesangial cells. Am J Pathol 1990; 136: 1339-1348.

51. Shimomura H, Spiro RG. Studies on the macromolecular components of human glomerular basement membrane and alterations in diabetes: decreased levels of heparan sulfate proteoglycan and laminin. Diabetes 1987; 36: 374-381.

52. Olgemöller B, Schwabbe S, Gerbitz KD, Schleicher ED. Elevated glucose decreases the content of a basement associated heparan sulphate proteoglycan in proliferating cultured porcine mesangial cells. Diabetologia 1992; 35: 183-186.

53. Brownlee M, Vlassara H, Cerami A. Nonenzymatic glycosylation and the pathogenesis of diabetic complications. Ann Intern Med 1984; 101: 527-537.

54. Berg TJ, Torjesen PA, Bangstad H-J, Bucala R, Østerby R, Hanssen KF. Advanced glycosylation end products predict changes in the kidney morphology in patients with insulin dependent diabetes mellitus. Metabolism 1997; 46: 661-665.
55. Forbes JM, Cooper ME, Thallas V, Burns WC, Thomas MC, Brammar GC, Lee F, Grant SL, Burrell LA, Jerums G, Osicka TM Reduction of the accumulation of advanced glycation end products by ACE inhibition in experimental diabetic nephropathy. Diabetes 2002: 51: 3274-3282.
56. Østerby R, Nyberg G. New vessel formation in the renal corpuscles in advanced diabetic glomerulopathy. J Diabetic Compl 1987; 1: 122-127.
57. Østerby R, Asplund Jonasson, Bangstad H-J, Nyberg G, Rudberg S, Viberti GC, Walker JD. Neovascularisation at the vascular pole region in diabetic glomerulopathy. Nephrology Dial Transplant 1999; 14: 348-352
58. Kashgarian M, Sterzel RB. The pathobiology of the mesangium. Kidney Int 1992; 41: 524-529.
59. Hawkins NJ, Wakefield D, Charlesworth JA. The role of mesangial cells in glomerular pathology. Pathology 1990; 22: 24-32.
60. White KE, Bilous RW, Marshall SM, El Nahas M, Remuzzi G, Piras G, De Cosmo S, Viberti G.Podocyte number in normotensive type 1 diabetic patients with albuminuria. Diabetes 2002; 51: 3083-3089.
61. Bonnet F, Cooper ME, Kawachi H, Allen TJ, Boner G, Cao Z. Irbesartan normalises the deficiency in glomerular nephrin expression in a model of diabetes and hypertension. Diabetologia 2001; 44:874-877
62. Milsrud SA, Allen TJ, Bertram JF, Hulthen UL, Kelly DJ, Cooper ME, Wilkinsom-Berka JL, Gilbert RE. Podocyte foot process broadening in experimental diabetic nephropathy: amelioration with renin-angiotensin blockade. Diabetologia 2001; 44: 878-882.
63. Langham RG, Kelly DJ, Cox AJ, Thomson NM, Holthofer H, Zaoui P, Pinel N, Cordonier DJ, Gilbert RE. Proteinuria and the expression of the podocyte slit diaphragm protein, nephrin, in diabetic nephropathy: effects of angiotensin converting enzyme inhibition. Diabetologia 2002; 45: 1572-1576.
64. Iglesias-de la Cruz MC, Ziyadeh FN, Isono M, Kouahou M, Han DC, Kalluri R, Mundel P, Chen S. Effects of high glucose and TGF-beta1 on the expression of collagen IV and vascular endothelial growth factor in mouse podocytes. Kidney Int 2002; 62: 901-913.

17

RENAL STRUCTURE IN TYPE 2 DIABETES

Paola Fioretto, Michele Dalla Vestra and Michael Mauer
Department of Medical and Surgical Sciences, University of Padova, Italy;Department of Pediatrics, University of Minnesota, Minneapolis, MN, USA.

INTRODUCTION

Although 80 % or more of diabetic patients receiving renal replacement therapy have type 2 diabetes [1-5], the renal pathology and natural history of diabetic nephropathy (DN) in type 2 diabetes has been studied much less intensely than in type 1 diabetes and thus many important questions remain unclear. The clinical manifestations of DN, proteinuria, declining glomerular filtration rate (GFR) and increasing blood pressure, are similar in type 1 and type 2 diabetes [6-7], as they are in many other renal diseases; nevertheless whether these clinical features are the consequences of similar underlying renal lesions is not entirely known. In type 1 diabetes it is generally accepted that the most important structural changes, leading to progressive renal function loss occur in the glomeruli [8-13]; concomitantly and roughly in proportion to the degree of glomerulopathy, the glomerular arterioles, tubules and interstitium also undergo structural changes, including hyalinosis of the arteriolar wall, thickening and reduplication of tubular basement membranes, tubular atrophy and interstitial expansion and fibrosis [8-14].

These extraglomerular lesions become progressive and severe only when glomerulopathy is far advanced. Quantitative morphometric studies have demonstrated that the lesion most closely related to the decline in renal function in type 1 diabetes is mesangial expansion, caused predominantly by mesangial matrix accumulation [12, 15]. We have also observed, in sequential renal biopsies of type 1 diabetic patients performed 5 years apart, that the only structural change associated with increasing albuminuria was mesangial

Mogensen CE (ed.) THE KIDNEY AND HYPERTENSION IN DIABETES MELLITUS. Copyright©
2004 by Martin Dunitz, a member of the Taylor & Francis Group, plc. All rights reserved.

expansion [13]; glomerular basement membrane (GBM) width, interstitial expansion and the number of globally sclerosed glomeruli did not change over 5 years in this group of patients in transition from normo to microalbuminuria or from microalbuminuria to overt nephropathy. Thus, in type 1 diabetes severe arteriolar, tubular and interstitial lesions are rare unless advanced diabetic glomerulopathy is present.

When overt nephropathy develops in patients with type 1 diabetes for at least 10 years, advanced diabetic glomerulopathy is almost always present, while non-diabetic renal diseases are very uncommon in such patients [Fioretto and Mauer, unpublished data]. In proteinuric type 2 diabetic patients, in contrast, the prevalence of non-diabetic renal lesions has been reported to be high (approximately 20-30%). Parving et al reported that 23% of type 2 diabetic patients with proteinuria had non-diabetic glomerulopathies, which these authors classified as minimal lesion nephropathy, mesangio-proliferative glomerulonephritis (GN) and sequelae of GN [16]. Heterogeneity in renal lesions has also been reported by Gambara et al, who found that only 37 % of proteinuric type 2 diabetic patients had typical changes of DN [17]. In a more recent study from the same authors, 46% of the patients had typical diabetic nephropathy, whereas 18% had superimposed non-diabetic renal diseases [18]. Khan et al observed the presence of non-diabetic renal disease in 42% of 153 type 2 patients with overt nephropathy [19]; the occurrence of non diabetic renal disease was much lower (12%) in the series of 33 proteinuric patients studied by Olsen and Mogensen [20]. However in all these studies, with the exception of the study of Parving, patients were referred to the nephrologist and kidney biopsies were performed for clinical indications; thus many of these renal biopsies were presumably performed because the patient's clinical course was considered to be atypical for diabetic nephropathy. These studies, therefore, may not describe the usual type 2 patients with diabetic nephropathy, but rather those with an unusual clinical course. The different results may reflect also differences in the indications for kidney biopsy. A large autopsy study on type 2 diabetic patients did not confirm a high incidence of non-diabetic renal diseases [21]. Moreover, hospitals using more as compared to less restricted clinical indicators for renal biopsies in type 2 diabetic patients have a higher fraction of cases with typical diabetic nephropathology [22]. Thus, the available data suggests that the heretofore-contradictory results regarding renal structure in type 2 diabetic patients are, in substantial part, the consequence of selection bias. Consequently, the natural history of nephropathy in type 2 diabetes is best-investigated using research patients rather than those acquired through clinical biopsy indications.

ELECTRON MICROSCOPY STUDIES

Quantitative morphometric studies in type 2 diabetes are scarce; in Japanese type 2 diabetic patients with a wide range of renal function, morphometric measures of diabetic glomerulopathy showed correlations to renal functional parameters similar to those observed in type 1 diabetes [23]. However, more recent studies suggest a significant incidence of normal glomerular structure among microalbuminuric and proteinuric Japanese type 2 diabetic patients [24]. Diabetic glomerulopathy was estimated by Østerby et al. in Caucasian type 2 proteinuric diabetic patients [25]. All the morphometric glomerular parameters were, on average, abnormal. However some patients had glomerular structural measures within the normal range. In type 1 diabetic patients with overt nephropathy, on the other hand, glomerular structure was always severely altered [12, 25, 26, and Fioretto and Mauer, unpublished data]. We have studied a large group of Caucasian type 2 diabetic patients recruited for research studies, and found that, although diabetic glomerular structural parameters were, on average, more altered in patients with microalbuminuria and macroalbuminuria than in those with normoalbuminuria, several patients had normal glomerular structure despite increased albumin excretion rates [27]. Also, compared to patients with type 1 diabetes and similar renal function, diabetic glomerulopathy was less advanced in patients with type 2 diabetes. Albumin excretion rate was directly related to both GBM width ($r=0.47$, $p<0.001$) and Vv(mes/glom) ($r=0.44$, $p<0.001$); GFR was inversely related to Vv(mes/glom) ($r=0.47$, $p<0.001$) but not to GBM width. Although these structural/functional relationships were statistically significant in type 2 diabetes, they were imprecise and less strong than in type 1 diabetes [12, 26].

Thus, these findings suggest that mesangial expansion is a crucial structural change, leading to loss of renal function in type 2, as in type 1, diabetes. However glomerular lesions are less advanced in type 2 than type 1 diabetic patients and a substantial number of type 2 diabetic patients have normal glomerular structure despite abnormal albumin excretion rate. These data are in agreement with those in Pima Indians where, in a much smaller group, there was no significant difference in glomerular ultrastructure between patients with long-term type 2 diabetes with normoalbuminuria and those with microalbuminuria [28]. Diabetic glomerulopathy parameters were more severely altered only in patients with proteinuria. These results were true for mesangial fractional volume, GBM width and also for foot process width and the number of podocytes per glomerulus [28].

IS PODOCYTE INJURY RELEVANT?

In type 2 diabetic Pima Indian patients podocyte loss and increased foot process width have been hypothesized to play a role in the progression to overt nephropathy. Nevertheless, as in patients with type 1 diabetes [29], the changes in podocytes had been thought to occur late in the course of diabetic renal disease, and to be more involved in mechanisms of progression rather than in those of genesis and early development [28].

However, in a recent longitudinal study, Meyer et al found that the number of podocytes per glomerulus was the strongest predictor of the changes in albuminuria and that fewer cells predicted more rapid progression during the follow up of microalbuminuric type 2 diabetic Pima Indian patients [30].

We studied podocyte structure in 67 Caucasian type 2 diabetic patients [31]. The numerical density of podocytes per glomerulus (Nv(epi/glom)) was significantly decreased in all diabetic patients compared to controls, and was lower in microalbuminuric and proteinuric than in normoalbuminuric patients. The absolute number of podocytes per glomerulus (Epi N/glom) was lower in MA and P patients compared to controls; however there were no significant differences among the diabetic groups. In addition microalbuminuric and proteinuric patients had decreased length density of filtration slits over the peripheral GBM (FSLv/glom), and increased foot process width (FPW) compared to normoalbuminuric. AER was inversely related to Nv[epi/glom] and FSLv/glom and directly to FPW ($p<0.0005$ for all), while there was no correlation with Epi N/glom. GFR was related only to FSLv/glom ($p<0.05$). Since 16 pts with abnormal AER had normal Vv(mes/glom) (≤ 0.25) we compared their podocyte structure to that of 16 NA with normal Vv(mes/glom). Patients with abnormal AER had lower Nv(epi/glom) and FSLv/glom ($p<0.05$ and $p<0.02$, respectively) and higher FPW ($p<0.01$) than NA. These results suggest that changes in podocyte structure and density occur the early stages of diabetic nephropathy and might contribute to increasing albuminuria in these in Caucasian type 2 diabetic patients. Moreover, podocyte structural changes could in part explain abnormal albuminuria in patients without diabetic glomerulopathy. These findings also suggest that in Caucasian type 2 diabetic patients the density of podocytes may be more functionally relevant than the absolute number.

LIGHT MICROSCOPY STUDIES: HETEROGENEITY IN RENAL STRUCTURE IN MICROALBUMINURIC PATIENTS

Microalbuminuria (MA) antedates clinical proteinuria in both type 1 [32-34] and type 2 diabetes [35, 36]. The predictive value of MA was thought to be quite different in type 1 and type 2 diabetes in that only approximately 20% of type 2 patients with MA progressed to overt nephropathy over a decade of follow-up in contrast to over 80% of type 1 diabetic patients [36]. However, in more recent studies, approximately 30% of type 2 diabetic patients with MA progressed to overt nephropathy over a decade and a similar progression rate was observed in patients with type 1 diabetes [37]. The different predictive value of MA to overt nephropathy in the studies performed 2 decades ago and in the more recent ones may reflect a change in the natural history of renal disease in diabetes. The low predictive value of MA for overt nephropathy in type 2 diabetes may in part be accounted for by the high mortality from cardiovascular disease, which can interrupt the progression to clinical nephropathy. However, other explanations are tenable, including the possibility that MA in type 2 diabetes, at least in a subset of patients, may not be associated with the same underlying abnormalities, which are so common in patients with type 1 diabetes and MA.

Nonetheless, to date there is no full explanation to the clinical observation that only a subgroup of type 2 and type 1 diabetic patients with MA progresses to overt nephropathy, while in one-half or more renal function remains stable. It can be hypothesized that MA in type 2 patients may be either consequent to diabetic glomerulopathy, as in type 1 diabetes, and progress to overt nephropathy, or be due to other renal lesions or reflect altered vascular permeability due to regional or generalized endothelial dysfunction [7, 38]. The structural basis for MA in type 1 diabetes has been studied by us and others and it is now established that, when albuminuria exceeds 20 µg/min, diabetic glomerulopathy, with thickening of the GBM and mesangial expansion, is usually well established [39]. In type 2 diabetes, we have described the light microscopy results in the largest cohort of microalbuminuric patients studied so far [40, 41]. Kidney biopsies were performed in 53 patients (all Caucasians). Age was 58±8 years (Mean±1SD), known diabetes duration was 11±7 years and HbA1c was 8.3±1.8%. GFR, determined by the plasma clearance of [51] Cr-EDTA, was 99±28 ml/min/1.73 m^2 and AER was 61 [20-199] µg/min (median, range). Patients were defined hypertensive when blood pressure values exceed 140/85 mm Hg, or when on antihypertensive therapy regardless of BP levels. Using these criteria all but 9 patients were receiving antihypertensive therapy, and the majority of them were on ACE-inhibitors. Overall, according to the criteria described above, 78% of these patients were hypertensive. For comparison, kidney biopsies were obtained from 36 (17 M/19F) kidney donors at the time of renal transplantation, at the University of Minnesota; these controls were matched for age with the diabetic patients (age: 55.7±7 years).

Light microscopy. The initial reading of the biopsy material made apparent the inadequacy of existing descriptive systems, which had largely been based on observations of research biopsies in type 1 diabetes. In this series, however, many type 2 patients with MA either did not have glomerulopathy, or had only mild mesangial expansion by light microscopy; in fact the majority of the MA type 2 diabetic patients had normal or near normal glomerular structure, with or without tubulo-interstitial and arteriolar changes.

Thus we proposed a new classification system, which included 3 major groups:

Category I: Normal or near normal renal structure. These patients (15 M/7F, 41%) had biopsies which were normal or showed mild mesangial expansion, tubulo-interstitial changes or arteriolar hyalinosis (Figure 1A).

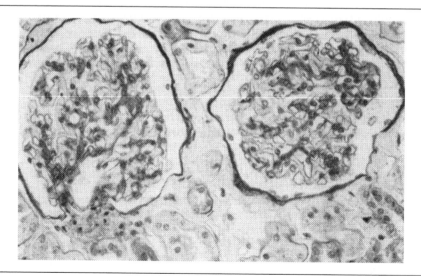

Figure 1A. Glomeruli from a patient in category C I. Glomerular structure is near normal with mild mesangial expansion (PAS).

Category II: Typical diabetic nephropathology. These patients (9M/5F, 26%) had established diabetic lesions with approximately balanced severity of glomerular, tubulo-interstitial and arteriolar changes. This picture is typical of that seen in type 1 diabetic patients with obvious light microscopic DN changes (Figure 1B).

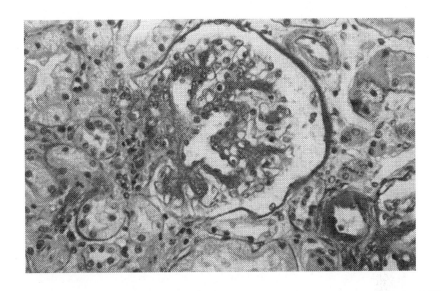

Figure 1B. Glomerulus from a patient in category C II, with well established diabetic glomerulopathy. Diffuse mesangial expansion, moderate arteriolar hyalinosis, and mild interstitial fibrosis are present (PAS).

Category III: Atypical patterns of renal injury. These patients (11M/6F, 33%) had relatively mild diabetic glomerular changes with disproportionately severe renal structural changes including:

(a) Tubular atrophy, tubular basement membrane thickening and reduplication and interstitial fibrosis (tubulo-interstitial lesions) (Figure 1C).
(b) Advanced glomerular arteriolar hyalinosis commonly associated with atherosclerosis of larger vessels (Figure 1D).
(c) Global glomerular sclerosis.

In Category III group these patterns were present in all possible combinations (Figures 1C and 1D); however important tubulo-interstitial changes were observed in all but 1 patient who had very severe arteriolar hyalinosis lesions. These tubulo-interstitial lesions were often associated with arteriolar changes and in some patients with global glomerulosclerosis.

In the age matched control group, 3/36 subjects had important tubulo-interstitial changes. Several normal controls had mild arteriolar hyalinosis lesions; 6 controls had more advanced arteriolar lesions, sometimes comparable to those observed in patients in categories II and III.

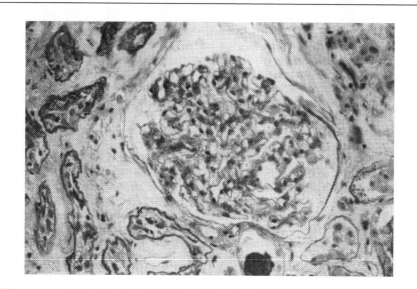

Figure 1C. Glomerulus from a patient in category C III (a) with near normal glomerular structure and TBM thickening, tubular atrophy and severe interstitial fibrosis (PAS).

We found no cases of definable non-diabetic renal disease in this series of 53 patients.

Age was similar in the three groups; known duration of type 2 diabetes was longer in CII and CIII patients than CI (14 ± 6 and 13 ± 8 yrs vs 7 ± 3, $p<0.05$ for both). HbA1c levels were significantly different among groups with CII patients having the highest HbA1c values. BMI was only mildly increased in CII patients (26±4) and was significantly greater in CI (30±4) and CIII (29±3) than in CII patients (p<0.05 for both). AER levels were similar in the three groups; GFR was lower in CII (86±37 ml/min/1.73 m^2) than in CI (109±19) and CIII patients (96±20, p<0.05 for both). Systolic and diastolic blood pressure values were similar in the three groups as was the prevalence of hypertension (84%, 73% and 79%, respectively).

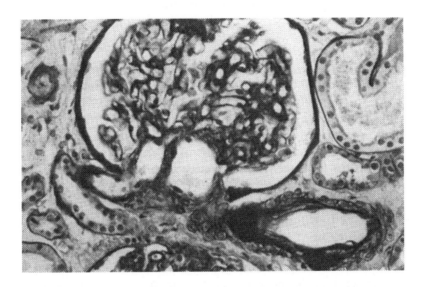

Figure 1D. Glomerulus from a patient in category C III (b) with mild mesangial expansion and severe arteriolar hyalinosis, affecting both afferent and efferent glomerular arterioles (PAS).

Diabetic retinopathy was present in all CII patients (background in 6 and proliferative in 8). None of the patients in CI and CIII had proliferative retinopathy, while background diabetic retinopathy was observed in 9 of 22 CI and 6 of 17 CIII patients. Thus, all CII patients had diabetic retinopathy and all patients with proliferative retinopathy had "typical" diabetic nephropathy lesions.

Given the clinical features of the three groups we hypothesize that the "atypical" patterns of renal injury observed in many type 2 diabetic patients are probably related to hyperglycemia. Thus, hyperglycemia may cause different patterns of renal injury in older type 2 compared to younger type 1 diabetic patients. The tubulo-interstitial and vascular changes could also be related to aging, atherosclerosis and systemic hypertension. However, hypertension was present in almost all patients in all 3 structural categories, and cannot, *per se*, account for the different lesions observed in category III. Further, mean age was similar in category II and III patients (60 years), despite the different patterns of renal injury in the two groups, and our observations in a large number of age-matched normal controls argue that normal aging is not sufficient to explain most of the renal structural changes observed in C III patients. One possibility is that the heterogeneity in renal structure might reflect the heterogeneous nature of type 2 diabetes. Thus, patients with "typical" DN lesions had longer known diabetes duration, worse metabolic control and all had diabetic retinopathy. Interestingly, their BMI only slightly exceeded normal values, as opposed to the clearly increased BMI values in CI and CIII patients. This suggests that the different underlying pathophysiologic mechanisms responsible for type 2 diabetes in these groups of patients may also underlie different renal pathophysiologic mechanisms or responses. Another possibility is that some of the heterogeneity in renal structure seen in these studies may represent interactions of diabetes and aging, particularly among CIII patients.

A remarkably high number of MA type 2 patients (41%) had normal or near normal renal structure (C I). They tended to be younger and to have shorter diabetes duration than patients with renal lesions (categories II and III). Changes in podocyte structure may in part explain the abnormal AER in these patients; however, it is also possible that MA in this subset is a manifestation of generalized endothelial dysfunction rather than of established renal structural damage. The predictive elucidation of the significance of MA on the subsequent development of renal, retinal and macrovascular complications in these patients would be of great clinical and theoretical interest.

ENDOTHELIAL FUNCTION IN RELATION TO RENAL STRUCTURE

Since MA is not associated with renal structural changes in a substantial subset of type 2 diabetic patients, we considered the possibility that MA in these patients could be consequent to endothelial dysfunction. To test this hypothesis we measured von Willebrand factor (vWF) plasma levels, an endothelial-derived protein indicative of endothelial function, in a group of MA patients who also had a research kidney biopsy performed [42]. Thirty-two patients were studied and, contrary to our hypothesis, vWF plasma levels were significantly increased only in patients with renal structural abnormalities (both CII [typical] and CIII [atypical] patterns) and was normal in patients with normal renal structure (CI) [42]. The results of this study do not provide an explanation for MA in patients without renal injury, and the nature of MA in these patients remains unknown. vWF plasma levels, however, represent only one measure of endothelial function, and further studies are necessary. Nevertheless, from these studies on vWF and renal structure we suggest that there are two types of MA in type 2 diabetes: one associated with increased vWF plasma levels, established renal structural lesions and, frequently, diabetic retinopathy, and the other characterized by normal vWF plasma levels, normal renal structure and absent or mild diabetic retinopathy [42, 43]. Whether these two types of MA have different prognostic implications for end stage renal disease and cardiovascular events deserves longitudinal studies.

LONGITUDINAL STUDIES

Our long-term follow-up studies with repeated measures of renal filtration function suggest that the heterogeneity in renal structure has an important prognostic value. The results in 108 type 2 diabetic patients with microalbuminuria or proteinuria, with repeated measures of GFR over a follow-up of 4 years suggest that the severity of glomerulopathy has a strong impact on the course of kidney function. Patients with more advanced diabetic glomerulopathy had a faster decline of GFR over time compared to patients with absent or with mild glomerulopathy [44]. This study also found that baseline AER and GFR at and mean blood pressure levels during follow-up did not significantly influence the change in GFR. In contrast, patients with faster GFR decline had the worst metabolic control [44]. These findings were similar also when the light microscopy categories were used, in that patients with typical diabetic glomerulopathy (Category II) had the fastest GFR decline.

ACE GENE POLYMORPHISM

As suggested for type 1 diabetes, genetic factors may be important in conferring diabetic nephropathy risk/protection also in type 2 diabetic patients. We studied the relationships between the I/D polymorphism of the ACE gene and diabetic glomerulopathy in 77 type 2 diabetic patients with microalbuminuria or proteinuria [45]. Despite similar renal function among patients with II, ID or DD genotypes, glomerulopathy was more severe in DD patients. Moreover, when subdivided in tertiles of increasing values of GBM width and mesangial matrix fractional volume, the DD carriers had an odds ratio (OR) of 6.11 (CI: 1.84-20.3) and 10.67 (CI: 2.51-45.36) of being in the tertile III than in I for GBM width and mesangial matrix fractional volume [45]. Given that patients with more advanced glomerulopathy have faster progression of their renal disease. These results are in keeping with the observation that the I/D polymorphism of the ACE gene is associated with the rate of progression of diabetic nephropathy. Another study in type 1 diabetes also showed that D allele carriers had more severe diabetic glomerulopathy and more rapid progression of glomerular structural lesions [46]. Thus, among patients with type 2 diabetes and abnormal albumin excretion rate, the presence of the DD genotype is associated with a high risk for the presence of advanced diabetic glomerulopathy lesions. Genotyping patients for the ACE gene might be helpful in clinical practice in identifying those type 2 diabetic patients at greater risk of serious renal lesions, so they could be targeted for intensive metabolic and blood pressure control.

These findings might also partially explain the contradictory results of case-control studies on the association between the ACE gene I/D polymorphism [and other genes] and nephropathy risk in type 2 diabetes. In fact, although all our patients had abnormal albumin excretion rates, only a subset had advanced diabetic glomerulopathy, and those patients more frequently carried the DD genotype; had we not performed the kidney biopsies, these associations would not have easily emerged. Thus, when planning to study the association of candidate gene polymorphisms with nephropathy risk/progression in type 2 diabetes, it is necessary to define the patients' phenotype as precisely as possible. The phenotype of increased albumin excretion rate in type 2 diabetes is probably too 'distant' from the ACE or other genotype to be used in genetic association studies.

CONCLUSIONS

These studies, far from clarifying the mechanisms responsible for increased albuminuria in type 2 diabetic patients, clearly demonstrate the complexity and the problematic nature of diabetic nephropathy in these patients. These results will hopefully stimulate further investigations and new directions of research.

For example, to better understand the pathophysiologic mechanisms responsible for MA and P in type 2 diabetes we are currently studying the relationships between renal lesions and macrovascular disease [47]. Studies on the interaction of aging and type 2 diabetes on renal structure and function would also be of interest particularly in the subset of MA patients with disproportionally severe tubulo-interstitial lesions. Also a better understanding of tubular function needs to be developed in these patients [39]. Finally, longitudinal detailed renal structural and functional studies of type 2 diabetic patients are crucial to the understanding of the clinical implications of these complex processes.

REFERENCES

1. US Renal Dara System annual report. Bethesda, MD: National Institute of Health and National Institute of Diabetes and Digestive and Kidney Diseases, 2000.
2. Cordonnier DJ, Zmirou D, Benhamou PY, Halimi S, Ledoux F, Guiserix J. Epidemiology, development and treatment of end-stage renal failure in type 2 diabetes. The case of mainland France and of overseas French territories. Diabetologia 1993; 36: 1109-1112.
3. Ritz E, Nowack R, Fliser D, et al. Type II diabetes mellitus: is the renal risk adequately appreciated? Nephrol Dial Transplant 1991; 6: 679-682.
4. Catalano C, Postorino M, Kelly PJ. Diabetes mellitus and renal replacement therapy in Italy: prevalence, main characteristic and complications. Nephrol Dial Transplant 1990; 5: 788-796.
5. Mauer M, Fioretto P, Woredekal Y, Friedman E. Diabetic Nephropathy. In: Schrier RW, Gottschalk CW [eds]. Diseases of the kidney, 7th edn. Little Brown& Co. 2001, Vol 3, 2083-2127.
6. Mogensen CE, Shmitz A, Christiensen CK. Comparative renal pathophysyology relevant to IDDM and NIDDM patients. Diabetes Metab Rev 1988; 4: 453.
7. Shmitz A. Nephropathy in non-insulin dependent diabetes mellitus and perspectives for intervention. Diab Nutr Metab 1995; 7: 135-148.
8. Mauer SM, Steffes MW, Brown DM. The kidney in diabetes. Am J Med 1981; 70: 603-612.
9. Fioretto P, Mogensen CE, Mauer SM. Diabetic nephropathy. In: Pediatric nephroplogy, ed by Holliday MA, Barratt TM, Avner ED, New York, Williams and Wilkins, 1994; 576-585.
10. Lane PH, Steffes MW, Fioretto P, Mauer SM. Renal interstitial expansion in insulin-dependent diabetes mellitus. Kidney Int 1993; 43: 661-67.
11. Gellman DD, Pirani CL, Soothill JF, Muehrcke RC, Maduros W, Kark RM. Structure and funtion in diabetic nephropathy: the importance of diffuse glomerulosclerosis. Diabetes 1959; 8: 251-256.
12. Mauer SM, Steffes MW, Ellis EN, Sutherland DER, Brown DM, Goetz FC. Structural functional relationships in diabetic nephropathy. J Clin Invest 1984; 74: 1143-1155.

13. Fioretto P, Steffes MW, Sutherland DER, Mauer M. Sequential renal biopsies in IDDM patients: structural factors associated with clinical progression. Kidney Int 1995; 48:1929-1935.
14. Brito P, Fioretto P, Drummund K, Kim Y, Steffes MW, Basgen JM, Sisson-Ross S, Mauer M. Proximal tubular basement membrane width in insulin-dependent diabetes mellitus. Kidney Int 1998; 53: 754-761.
15. Steffes MW, Bilous RW, Sutherland DER, Mauer SM. Cell and matrix components in the glomerular mesangium in type I diabetes. Diabetes 1992; 41: 679-84.
16. Parving H-H, Gall M-A, Skøtt P, Jørgensen HE, Løkkegaard H, Jørgensen F, Nielsen B, Larsen S. Prevalence and causes of albuminuria in non-insulin-dependent diabetic patients. Kidney Int 1992; 41: 758-762.
17. Gambara V, Mecca G, Remuzzi G, Bertani T. Heterogeneous nature of renal lesions in type II diabetes. JASN 1993; 3: 1458-1466.
18. Ruggenenti P, Gambara V, Perna A, Bertani T, Remuzzi G. The nephropathy of NIDDM: predictors of outcome relative to diverse patterns of renal injury. J Am Soc Nephrol 1998; 9: 2336-2343.
19. Kahn S, Seghal V, Appel GB, D'Agati V. Correlates of diabetic and non-diabetic renal disease in NIDDM. JASN 1995; 6: 451 [Abs].
20. Olsen S, Mogensen CE. Non-diabetic renal disease in NIDDM proteinuric patients may be rare in biopsies from clinical practice. Diabetologia 1996; 39: 1638-1645.
21. Waldherr R, Ilkenhans C, Ritz E. How frequent is glomerulonephritis in diabetes mellitus type II? Clinical Nephrology 1992; 37: 271-273.
22. Mazzucco G, Bertani T, Fortunato M, Bernardi M, Leutner M, Boldorini R, Monga G. Different patterns of renal damage in type 2 diabetes mellitus: a multicentric study on 393 biopsies. Am J Kidney Dis 2002; 39: 713-720.
23. Hayashi H, Karasawa R, Inn H et al. An electron microscopic study of glomeruli in Japanese patients with non-insulin dependent diabetes. Kidney Int 1992; 41: 749-757.
24. Moiya T, Moriya R, Yajima Y, Steffes MW, Mauer M. Urinary albumin excretion is a weaker predictor of diabetic nephropathy lesions in Japanese NIDDM patients than in Caucasian IDDM patients. JASN, 1997, 8: 116A [abs].
25. Østerby R, Gall MA, Schmitz A, Nielsen FS, Nyberg G, Parving HH. Glomerular structure and function in proteinuric type 2 [non insulin dependent] diabetic patients. Diabetologia 1993; 36: 1064-1070.
26. Caramori ML, Kim Y, Huang C, Fish AJ, Rich SS, Miller ME, Russell G, Mauer M. Cellular basis of diabetic nephropathy: 1. Study design and renal structural-functional relationships in patients with long-standing type 1 diabetes. Diabetes 2002; 51: 506-513.
27. Fioretto P, Mauer M, Bortoloso E, Barzon I, Saller A, Dalla Vestra M, Abaterusso C, Baggio B, Nosadini R. Glomerular ultrastructure in type 2 diabetes. JASN 1998, 9: 114 A [abs].
28. Patgalunan ME, Miller PL, Jumping-Eagle S, Nelson RG, Myers BD, Rennke HC, Coplon NS, Meyer TW. Podocyte loss and progressive glomerular injury in type 2 diabetes. J Clin Invest 1997; 99: 342-348.
29. Ellis EN, Steffes MW, Chavers BM, Mauer SM. Observations of glomerular epithelial cell structure in patients with type 1 diabetes mellitus. Kidney Int 1987; 32: 736-741.
30. Meyer TW, Bennett PH, Nelson RG. Podocyte number predicts long-term urinary albumin excretion in Pima Indians with Type II diabetes and microalbuminuria. Diabetologia 1999; 42: 1341-1344.

31. Dalla Vestra M, Masiero A, Roiter AM, Saller A, Crepaldi G, Fioretto P. Is Podocyte Injury Relevant In Diabetic Nephropathy? Studies in Type 2 Diabetic Patients. Diabetes 2003 in press.

32. Viberti GC, Hill RD, Jarrett RJ, Argyropoulos A, Mahmud U, Keen H. Microalbuminuria as a predictor of clinical nephropathy in insulin-dependent diabetes mellitus. Lancet 1982 i: 1430-32.

33. Parving H-H, Oxenbøll B, Svensen PAA, Christiansen JS, Andersen AR. Early detection of patients at risk of developing diabetic nephropathy: a longitudinal study of urinary albumin excretion. Acta Endocrinol Copenh 1982; 7, 100: 550-52.

34. Mogensen CE, Christensen CK. Predicting diabetic nephropathy in insulin-dependent diabetic patients. N Engl J Med 1986; 331: 89-93.

35. Mogensen CE. Microalbuminuria predicts clinical proteinuria and early mortality in maturity-onset diabetes. N Engl J Med 1984; 310: 356-360.

36. Mogensen CE. Microalbuminuria as a predictor of clinical diabetic nephropathy. Kidney Int 1987; 31: 673-689.

37. Camamori ML, Fioretto P, Mauer M. The need for early predictors of diabetic nephropathy risk: is albumin excretion rate sufficient? Diabetes 2000; 49: 1399-1408.

38. Stehouwer CDA, Nauta JJP, Zeldenrust GC, Hackeng WHL, Donker AJM, den Ottolander GJH [1992]. Urinary albumin excretion, cardiovascular disease, and endothelial dysfunction in non-insulin dependent diabetes mellitus. Lancet 1992; 340: 319-323.

39. Fioretto P, Steffes MW, Mauer M. Glomerular structure in non proteinuric IDDM patients with various levels of albuminuria. Diabetes 1994; 43: 1358-1364.

40. Fioretto P, Mauer M, Brocco E, Velussi M, Frigato F, Muollo B, Sambataro M, Abaterusso C, Baggio B, Crepaldi G, Nosadini R. Patterns of renal injury in type 2 [non insulin dependent] diabetic patients with microalbuminuria. Diabetologia 1996; 39: 1569-1576.

41. Brocco E, Fioretto P, Mauer M, Saller A, Carraro A, Frigato F, Chiesura-Corona M, et al. Renal structure and function in non-insulin dependent diabetic patients with microalbuminuria. Kidney Int 1997; 63: S155-158.

42. Fioretto P, Stehouwer CDA, Mauer M, Chiesura-Corona M, Brocco E, Carraro A, Bortoloso E, van Hinsberg V, Crepaldi G, Nosadini R. Heterogeneous nature of microalbuminuria in NIDDM: studies of endothelial function and renal structure. Diabetologia 1998; 41: 233-236.

43. Stehower CDA, Yudkin JS, Fioretto P, Nosadini R. How heterogeneous is microalbuminuria in diabetes mellitus? The case for 'benign' and 'malignant' microalbuminuria. Nephrol Dial Transplant 1998; 13: 2751-2754.

44. Nosadini R, Velussi M, Brocco E, Bruseghin M, Abaterusso C, Saller A, Dalla Vestra M, Carraro A, Bortoloso E, Sambataro M, Barzon I, Frigato F, Muollo B, Chiesura-Corona M, Pacini G, Baggio B, Piarulli F, Sfriso A, Fioretto P: Course of renal function in type 2 diabetic patients with abnormalities of albumin excretion rate. Diabetes 2000; 49: 476-484.

45. Solini A, Dalla Vestra M, Saller A, Nosadini R, Crepaldi G, Fioretto P. The Angiotensin-Converting Enzyme DD Genotype is Associated with Glomerulopathy lesions in Type 2 Diabetes. Diabetes, 2002; 51: 251-255.

46. Rudberg S, Rasmussen L, Bangstad H-J, Østerby R. Influence of insertion/deletion polymorphism in the ACE-I gene on the progression of diabetic glomerulopathy in type 1 diabetic patients with microalbuminuria. Diabetes Care 2000; 23: 544-548.

47.   Saller A, Dalla Vestra M, Bombonato G, Sacerdoti D, Chiesura-Corona M, Marangon A, Fioretto P, Crepaldi G, Nosadini R. The role of macrovascular disease in the pathogenesis of renal damage in type 2 diabetic patients. Diabetologia 1999; 42, S1: A268 [abs].

18

NEPHROPATHY IN TYPE 2 DIABETIC PATIENTS, PREDICTORS OF OUTCOME

[1, 2] Gozewijn D. Laverman, [2,3] Piero Ruggenenti and [2,3] Giuseppe Remuzzi

[1] Department of Internal Medicine, Division of nephrology, University Hospital Groningen, Groningen, The Netherlands; [2] Mario Negri Institute for Pharmacological Research, Bergamo, Italy; [3] Unit of Nephrology and Dialysis, Azienda Ospedaliera Ospedali Riuniti di Bergamo, Bergamo, Italy

THE RELEVANCE OF THE PROBLEM

Nephropathy is a major cause of illness and death of patients with type 2 diabetes mellitus (DM), the excess being confined to proteinuric patients due to complications of end-stage renal disease (ESRD) and particularly due to cardiovascular events [1]. Diabetic nephropathy is the single most common cause of ESRD in the United States and more than one third of all patients enrolled in the Medicare ESRD program are actually diabetics [2]. It derives that costs of renal replacement therapy for diabetics alone is a major public health issue, approaching almost epidemic proportions for type 2 DM in Western countries [3;4].

The continuous increase in the number of diabetics needing renal replacement therapy (twice the annual rate of ESRD from other conditions [2;3] depends on one hand from a growing number of patients suffering diabetes (in particular type 2), as well as from the constant improvement in health care facilities that allows more and more patients to live long enough to progress to ESRD. Once on renal replacement therapy, however, mortality among diabetic patients is 1.5 to 2.5 times higher than in non-diabetics [4] so that less than 20% of diabetics survive for 5 years on dialysis [3;4]. This disturbing epidemiology underscores the urgent need to identify potentially treatable risk factors in order to delay or even completely halt the progression of diabetic nephropathy towards ESRD and need of replacement therapy.

Traditionally, the natural history of nephropathy in type 2 DM has been more difficult to characterize than in type 1 DM. This is particularly true for Caucasians in whom the onset of type 2 DM is difficult to detect and occurs at an advanced age. The confounding factors include an effect of aging per se to lower the glomerular filtration rate (GFR) [5] and a high frequency of co-existent renal disease unrelated to DM beyond the age of 50 years [6-8]. Furthermore, premature cardiovascular death, occurring in the majority of these patients before they reach ESRD [9] limits the full expression of the natural history of the renal disease.

Yet, the outcome in terms of ESRD, cardiovascular events and death is becoming predictable from the constellation of risk factors. The pivotal role of albuminuria has been further elaborated. In addition, the classical cardiovascular risk factors hypertension, dyslipidemia, obesity and smoking all seem to be involved in progression of renal disease.

ALBUMINURIA

Microalbuminuria
In addition to the increased risk of progression to nephropathy, microalbuminuria also predicts cardiovascular disease. Actually, the "Steno hypothesis" has postulated that microalbuminuria points to a widespread disturbance of the endothelial cell function in diabetic and perhaps in non-diabetic patients [10]. Thus, endothelial cell barrier dysfunction in the macrocirculation may allow the transudation of plasma proteins (including lipoproteins) into the vessel wall to promote the atherogenetic process and predispose to cardiovascular events.

The presence of microalbuminuria as a predictor of progression to macroalbuminuria has been recognized since several years and applies to both type 1 and type 2 DM [11]. In 1984 Mogensen found that over 9 years the risk of progression to macroalbuminuria was only 22% in type 2 DM [9] as compared with 80% in type 1 DM patients with microalbuminuria. However, later studies in non-European series found that the predictive value of microalbuminuria is comparable in type 1 and type 2 DM. Indeed, Nelson and coworkers found that over four year the cumulative incidence of macroalbuminuria was 37% in microalbuminuric Pima Indians [12]. This is in agreement with the five-year incidence of 42% reported by Ravid et al [13] in young Jewish patients with type 2 DM and microalbuminuria at baseline. Probably, the younger age of patients in both these series as compared to that in the Mogensen study (approximately 20 years difference) allowed a larger proportion of diabetics to live enough to progress to overt nephropathy [14].

Whether the onset of microalbuminuria predicts a progressive fall in GFR is less clear. Although the Nelson's study found that in microalbuminuric Pima Indians the GFR was stable over time [12], a progressive decline in renal function, reflected by an increase in serum creatinine concentration, was reported in the Ravid's series [13].

Apart from predicting overt nephropathy, microalbuminuria also predicts cardiovascular mortality in type 2 DM [9;15]. The competing risk of cardiac death and progression to renal failure may explain, at least in part, the Mogensen's findings of a lower predictive value of microalbuminuria for the development of overt nephropathy in type 2 DM as compared with type 1 DM [9]. Indeed, in one series, over 10 years only 3% of microalbuminuric type 2 diabetic patients died from uremia, while 58% died from cardiac causes [16]. Higher urinary albumin excretion rates were found in type 2 diabetic patients with coronary heart disease both at the time the diagnosis of diabetes was made and later on. Meanwhile, in the general population too, the association between microalbuminuria and cardiovascular risk [17] and mortality [18] has been recognized.

Macroalbuminuria
In established nephropathy due to type 1 DM [19] and in non-diabetic nephropathies [20], the severity of macroalbuminuria (or proteinuria) is the strongest known predictor of progressive renal function loss. Moreover, in non-diabetic renal disease, during treatment with renin-angiotensin system (RAS) blockade (i.e. ACE inhibition or angiotensin receptor blockade, ARB), the improved renal outcome is strongly related to the effect on proteinuria [20]. Similarly, ACE inhibitors slow progression of type 1 diabetic nephropathy [19] together with usually considerable reduction of proteinuria in these patients [21]. These findings are all consistent with the view that proteins, once leaked through the glomerular barrier, are tubulotoxic and that proteinuria thus is a true mediator of disease progression [22].

In contrast, the role of proteinuria in type 2 DM has been less well-studied –until recently. Notably, type 2 diabetic patients usually are resistant to antihypertensive therapy, often requiring several drugs to control blood pressure. This therapy-resistance also applies to the antihypertensive and antiproteinuric effect of ACE inhibitors and ARBs: these effects are considerably smaller in type 2 DM than usually observed in non-diabetics or type 1 DM and this has previously prevented the possibility to study the role of proteinuria and proteinuria reduction in nephropathy due to type 2 DM.

However, two recent large double-blind, randomized trials, the Irbesartan in Diabetic Nephropathy Trial (IDNT)[23] and the Reduction of Endpoints in TYPE 2 with the Angiotensin II Antagonist Losartan (RENAAL) trial [24] have demonstrated that ARB, compared with non-RAS blocking agents, reduced the number of renal endpoints (e.g. doubling of serum creatinine and progression to ESRD) in type 2 diabetic patients with nephropathy. These studies provided an excellent opportunity to study risk factors in a time-dependent fashion, because both were prospective studies including over 1500 patients.

The issue whether proteinuria is an independent risk marker for renal –and also cardiovascular- endpoints, has specifically been addressed in the RENAAL-dataset (RENAAL study group, unpublished data). First, the predictive value of a series of putative risk factors, including blood pressure, cholesterol, HbA1C, hemoglobin, serum creatinine and proteinuria was evaluated at baseline. This analysis demonstrated that proteinuria not only is an independent risk factor, but, moreover, proteinuria is the strongest of all putative risk factors tested - both for renal as well as cardiovascular endpoints.

Together with previous findings in Caucasian [25] and Asian [26] proteinuric type 2 diabetic patients, this proves that baseline proteinuria has important predictive value, not only in non-diabetic and type 1 diabetic nephropathy, but also in type 2 DM. Moreover, in type 2 diabetic nephropathy, baseline proteinuria is to be considered also a cardiovascular risk factor.

Second, to study which changes induced by therapy predicted the renal and cardiovascular outcome, several parameters (including blood pressure, proteinuria, body weight and GFR), measured six months after randomisation, were tested in a multivariate model. This showed that suppression of proteinuria by losartan was the strongest predictor of long-term protection from renal and cardiovascular events. If proteinuria reduction was considered as the percentage change from baseline, again more benefit was achieved with a higher antiproteinuric response. Patients with more than 30% reduction of proteinuria, i.e. the average reduction observed in studies with type 1 DM and non-diabetic renal patients, had a considerably lower risk to reach renal or cardiovascular endpoints than patients with less effective proteinuria reduction –even after correction for other cardiovascular risk factors.

On the same line, a similar analysis, performed in the IDNT data-set [27], found that baseline proteinuria predicts cardiovascular and renal endpoints. Again, also the residual proteinuria and percentage change of proteinuria (measured twelve months after randomisation), were strong predictors of outcome and it was estimated that approximately 35-40% of the renoprotective effect of ARB is accounted for by the antiproteinuric effect.

TRADITIONAL CARDIOVASCULAR RISK FACTORS

Hypertension, dyslipidemia, obesity and smoking, that is, the classic cardiovascular risk factors, each contribute to the risk profile in the patient with type 2 DM.

Blood pressure
Hypertension develops in about half of the patients with type 2 DM. This is important, not only because increased systemic blood pressure is a cardiovascular risk factor, but also because of the association between hypertension and accerated renal function loss. Moreover, effective blood pressure control is associated with a slower disease progression, possibly because of a concomitant amelioration of intracapillary hypertension and protein ultrafiltration in the kidneys. Thus, patients in the IDNT who had lower systolic blood pressure levels during treatment also had a markedly lower risk to reach a renal endpoint [28]. Although the study was not designed to compare the renal effects of different levels of achieved blood pressure control, the findings do favour an important effect of lowering systolic blood pressure in macroalbuminuric type 2 diabetic patients, at least to 130 mm Hg –and possibly lower.

Dyslipidemia
Dyslipidemia is a clear cardiovascular risk factor and lipid-lowering therapy reduces the risk of cardiovascular events in diabetic patients with coronary heart disease [29]. Moreover, there is also evidence, both in type 1 [30] and type 2 DM [31], that lipid abnormalities are associated with progressive renal function

loss. Actually, hypercholesterolemia might merely be an epiphenomenon of overt proteinuria, which, in turn, would be the major independent promoter of progression because of the chronic nephrotoxic effect of enhanced protein traffic [22]. Nevertheless, lipid particles may have a specific nephrotoxic effect by their proinflammatory actions elicited once having been deposited in kidney tissue [32] and this may contribute to chronic tubulointerstitial damage and scarring. The lipid lowering class of HmGCoA inhibitors ("statins") is of particular importance, first because of the striking protective effects on cardiovascular morbidity and mortality in a wide array of high risk patients, including type 1 and type 2 DM, achieved irrespective of the baseline plasma LDL [33]. On the same line, statins do have a specific renoprotective effect in experimental disease of diabetic [34] and non-diabetic [35] origin. Together with these experimental findings, independent proteinuria-lowering effects in hypertensive patients [36;37], underline the need for randomized clinical trials to test whether therapy aimed at reducing cholesterol has renoprotective potential also in human renal diseases.

Obesity and insulin resistance
Obesity plays a role in the pathophysiology of insulin resistance leading to type 2 DM and is in addition an independent risk factor for cardiovascular disease. Moreover, obesity appears to have impact on the kidneys since, regardless of diabetes, it is associated with microalbuminuria [38] and occasionally severely obese subjects display overt proteinuria [39]. This so-called obesity-associated glomerulopathy, histologically characterized by focal segmental glomerulosclerosis, is considered as an independent disease entity [40].

What could be the mechanism behind proteinuria in obese non-diabetic subjects? It is known that, consistent with a condition of increased renal RAS activity, obese persons display glomerular hyperfiltration [41]. It might be argued that this results from increased local renal ACE activity in the kidney, as found in obese mice [42]. Interestingly, however, fat cells have the machinery to synthesize several RAS components, such as angiotensinogen, ACE and the AT1R [43] and this may influence systemic and renal RAS activity. Thus, in subjects who carry excessive amounts of fat cells, this may result in an unfavourable environment for initiation or progression of renal damage.

Alternatively, in obese subjects, decreased insulin sensitivity is a common finding and this is a fortiori true in the severe obese. Thus, an alternative view is that insulin resistance -that is, the disorder ultimately leading to diabetes- might be the determinant of obesity-related glomerulopathy. In this respect, it is noteworthy that Praga et al. found in a series of obese patients with glomerulopathy that type 2 DM developed in five out of fifteen individuals after up to ten years follow-up [44]. Also, isolated case-reports have described insulin-resistant patients with biopsy-findings typical for diabetic glomerulosclerosis without frank diabetes [45;46]. These findings suggest that the conditions to develop diabetic nephropathy are already apparent in the stage of insulin-resistance, and insulin resistance or the metabolic environment associated with insulin-resistance may initiate or sustain progressive renal damage.

Smoking

It is increasingly recognized that smoking is not only a cardiovascular risk factor, but also a risk factor for development and progression of diabetic nephropathy [47-49]. Of note, even in the general population, smoking is associated with microalbuminuria and renal function abnormalities [50]. Smoking-induced increase of systemic blood pressure and/or glomerular hyperfiltration (as documented in type 1 DM [51]) could be a mechanism behind this. In line with this, a cross-sectional study at renal biopsy findings in type 2 diabetic patients showed that glomerular alterations –and not interstitial fibrosis- were associated with smoking [52]. Thus, smoking cessation is not only important to prevent malignancies and cardiovascular disease, but, in addition, it should also be part of any renoprotective regimen.

GLYCEMIC CONTROL

Poor glycemic control predicts subsequent chronic complications of type 1 and type 2 DM, including the development of nephropathy. Although the role of chronic hyperglycemia in the progression of type 2 diabetic nephropathy has long remained obscure [53], recent evidence has shown that better glycemic control is associated with a lower incidence of progression of albuminuria [31;54;55] and of reaching the endpoint doubling of serum creatinine [54]. The "AGE hypothesis" [56] postulates that a major mechanism behind diabetic complications is the impaired function and/or tissue deposition of irreversibly modified proteins, also called advanced glycation end-products (AGES), the formation of which appears to be favoured by persistent hyperglycemia. This obviously urges for strict glycemic control to prevent this process. Also, animal experimental evidence has now shown that therapy aimed to degradate AGES has the potential to inhibit progression of diabetic nephropathy [57].

HISTOLOGICAL ALTERATIONS

At variance with type 1 DM -where overt proteinuria is almost invariably the clinical counterpart of typical diabetic glomerulopathy- in type 2 DM the appearance of macroalbuminuria may reflect different patterns of renal injury, including typical diabetic-like lesions (in one- to two-thirds of cases), nephroangiosclerosis, or forms of glomerular disease of non-diabetic type [7;8]. It might therefore be suggested that, at the stage of clinically overt nephropathy, renal structural changes may already be very advanced and diffuse in type 2 diabetic patients and the glomerular lesions may evolve to an extent that prevents pharmacological treatments from achieving the desired effect on membrane sieving functional properties [58]. This would, in turn explain the relatively poor response to RAS blockade in overt nephropathy due to type 2 DM [23;24] compared with type 1 DM [19] and non-diabetic nephropathy [59].

Considering the predictive value of renal lesions for renal outcome, it has been shown that in proteinuric type 2 DM patients, the rate of renal disease progression was rather independent of the type of underlying glomerular lesions [25]. Instead, the course of disease was consistently predicted by the amount of proteinuria in these patients and a cut-off value of baseline proteinuria was identified that segregated progressors from non-progressors: Patients with proteinuria below 2 g/24h had stable serum creatinine and a 100% kidney survival at 5 years, whereas those with proteinuria above >2 g/24h had a 92 % risk to progress to ESRD over the same period. Quantification of a global score of tissue injury was of further help to predict disease outcome, only in progressors. Of interest, in the same study, proteinuria was, in addition to serum creatinine, the only independent clinical predictor of disease progression –which is in line with the recent findings from RENAAL and IDNT, as discussed above.

Based on these data, in type 2 DM nephropathy, quantification of urinary protein excretion is enough to identify patients at risk of progression. Among progressors, a renal biopsy in addition to precise quantification of proteinuria, can help predicting the risk of terminal renal failure and the median time to dialysis. In particular, patients at low risk and patients inexorably destined to ESRD can be reliably identified.

HOW COULD THE RISK FACTORS OF TYPE 2 DM BE MODIFIED: FUTURE PERSPECTIVES

If one thing has become clear from recent trials such as RENAAL and IDNT, it is the finding that mortality, cardiovascular events and risk of ESRD remain alarmingly high in type 2 diabetic patients with nephropathy –even in patients treated with RAS blockade and several other antihypertensive agents [23;24]. Thus, much more efforts are required to reduce these risks to acceptable proportions.

Early treatment in type 2 diabetic patients without complications
The high risks in the patients with type 2 diabetic nephropathy is in sharp contrast with the outspoken benefits of RAS blockade in the normoalbuminuric and microalbuminuric stage [60-64]. Therefore, early detection of increased urinary albumin excretion rate, followed by early treatment of microalbuminuria is imperative. Today, microalbuminuria can be measured with tests that are reproducible, acceptable, and harmless to the patient. In addition, the cost-benefit ratio in screening and early treatment seems to be advantageous. Thus, the World Health Organization and the International Diabetes Federation have recommended (St. Vincent Declaration) that all diabetics aged 12 to 70 years should be screened for microalbuminuria at least once a year. Regular monitoring of patients who result positive ensures that renal and extra-renal complications are identified early and preventive intervention therapy instituted, including good metabolic control, raised blood pressure correction, and Renin Angiotensin System inhibition [65].

With the clues of harmful effects of decreased insulin-sensitivity and/or its metabolic consequences in mind, it is promising that type 2 DM itself is in principle preventable by restoring decreased insulin-sensitivity with life style intervention or pharmacotherapy [66]. It will also be important to evaluate whether restoring insulin sensitivity has renoprotective potential in people who have type 2 DM. Interestingly, in type 1 DM, early glomerular and tubulointerstitial lesions seem to be reversible by rescueing the kidney from the diabetic environment by means of a pancreas transplantation [67]. Because in type 2 DM, the core defect is insulin resistance, the insulin-sensitizing thiazolidinediones [68] provide a new class of drugs that could demonstrate the proof of principle. Preliminary evidence from diabetic rats has now shown that, indeed, these drugs may have renoprotective effects [69].

Type 2 diabetic patients with established nephropathy: aggressive treatment
In the past, once hypertension and increased serum cholesterol had been identified as risk factors, the effect of treatment specifically aimed to lower these risk factors was tested in randomized trials –and several antihypertensive and cholesterol lowering drugs proved to be effective in reducing end-organ damage. Evidence from the large trials in type 2 diabetic nephropathy is now available showing the importance of proteinuria as a modifiable risk factor. In particular, this is underscored by the finding that the degree of proteinuria reduction predicts the efficacy of end-organ protection.

Thus, to follow the generally appropriate approach once a risk factor has been identified, the next step must be to test the effect of treatment, specifically aimed to reach predefined proteinuria targets in the setting of randomized trials. For clinical practice, the optimal renoprotective treatment will require a multi-drug approach [70].

Recent studies suggest that the view on "normal" ranges for blood pressure, albuminuria, and cholesterol needs to be reconsidered. Data from the Framingham Heart study in persons without apparent cardiovascular disease show that even within the normal range for blood pressure, those persons with a "high-normal" blood pressure (average: 132/81 mm Hg) have an increased cardiovascular risk [71]. In the same line, the Groningen population-based "PREVEND" study has shown that not only micro-albuminuria, but even "high-normal" albuminuria (i.e., 15-30 mg/24h) is clearly associated with increased cardiovascular risk [17] and renal function abnormalities [72]. Considering cholesterolemia, treatment with statins effectively reduced cardiovascular events in high-risk patients, including diabetics, and this was found irrespective whether cholesterol was elevated or not [33].

Thus, the use of cut-off values does not identify "safe" blood pressure or cholesterol levels, but rather results in high risk-patients being withheld from effective therapy.

In contrast with the other parameters, proteinuria is zero in the normal situation. Even in the microalbuminuric range, proteinuria is associated with increased cardiovascular and renal risk. In patients with nephropathy, it is therefore approriate to aim for complete annihilation of albuminuria. The finding that this is an achievable goal even in patients with long-lasting nephrotic-range proteinuria should encourage nephrologists and diabetologists to pursue this target in every patient with diabetes and renal disease.

REFERENCES

1. Striker GE, Agodoa LL, Held P, Doi T, Conti F, Striker LJ: Kidney disease of diabetes mellitus (diabetic nephropathy): perspectives in the United States. J Diabet.Complications 5:51-52, 1991

2. The United States Renal Data System. USRDS 1994 Annual Data Report, The National Institutes of Health, National Institute of Diabetes and Digestive and Kidney Diseases. 1994. Bethesda, MD.

3. The United States Renal Data System. USRDS 1997 Annual Data Report. National Institute of Diabetes and Digestive and Kidney Diseases. 1997. Bethesda, MD.

4. Pastan S, Bailey J: Dialysis therapy. N.Engl.J Med. 338:1428-1437, 1998

5. Palmer BF, Levi M: Effect of aging on renal function and disease, in Brenner's & Rector's *The Kidney*, 5th ed., edited by Brenner BM, Philadelphia, W.B. Saunders Company, 1996, pp 2274-2296

6. Ruggenenti P, Remuzzi G: The diagnosis of renal involvement in non-insulin-dependent diabetes mellitus. Curr.Opin.Nephrol.Hypertens. 6:141-145, 1997

7. Gambara V, Mecca G, Remuzzi G, Bertani T: Heterogeneous nature of renal lesions in type II diabetes. J Am.Soc.Nephrol. 3:1458-1466, 1993

8. Parving HH, Gall MA, Skott P, Jorgensen HE, Lokkegaard H, Jorgensen F, Nielsen B, Larsen S: Prevalence and causes of albuminuria in non-insulin-dependent diabetic patients. Kidney Int. 41:758-762, 1992

9. Mogensen CE: Microalbuminuria predicts clinical proteinuria and early mortality in maturity-onset diabetes. N.Engl.J.Med. 310:356-360, 1984

10. Deckert T: Nephropathy and coronary death—the fatal twins in diabetes mellitus. Nephrol.Dial.Transplant. 9:1069-1071, 1994

11. Mogensen CE, Keane WF, Bennett PH, Jerums G, Parving HH, Passa P, Steffes MW, Striker GE, Viberti GC: Prevention of diabetic renal disease with special reference to microalbuminuria. Lancet 346:1080-1084, 1995

12. Nelson RG, Bennett PH, Beck GJ, Tan M, Knowler WC, Mitch WE, Hirschman GH, Myers BD: Development and progression of renal disease in Pima Indians with non-insulin-dependent diabetes mellitus. Diabetic Renal Disease Study Group.

13. Ravid M, Savin H, Jutrin I, Bental T, Katz B, Lishner M: Long-term stabilizing effect of angiotensin-converting enzyme inhibition on plasma creatinine and on proteinuria in normotensive type II diabetic patients. Ann.Intern.Med. 118:577-581, 1993

14. Parving HH: Initiation and progression of diabetic nephropathy. N.Engl.J Med. 335:1682-1683, 1996

15. Nelson RG, Pettitt DJ, Carraher MJ, Baird HR, Knowler WC: Effect of proteinuria on mortality in NIDDM. Diabetes 37:1499-1504, 1988

16. Schmitz A, Vaeth M: Microalbuminuria: a major risk factor in non-insulin-dependent diabetes. A 10-year follow-up study of 503 patients. Diabet.Med. 5:126-134, 1988

17. Janssen WM, Hillege H, Pinto-Sietsma SJ, Bak AA, De Zeeuw D, De Jong PE: Low levels of urinary albumin excretion are associated with cardiovascular risk factors in the general population. Clin.Chem.Lab Med. 38:1107-1110, 2000

18. Hillege HL, Fidler V, Diercks GF, van Gilst WH, De Zeeuw D, van Veldhuisen DJ, Gans RO, Janssen WM, Grobbee DE, De Jong PE: Urinary albumin excretion predicts cardiovascular and noncardiovascular mortality in general population. Circulation 106:1777-1782, 2002

19. Lewis EJ, Hunsicker LG, Bain RP, Rohde RD: The effect of angiotensin-converting-enzyme inhibition on diabetic nephropathy. The Collaborative Study Group. N.Engl.J.Med. 329:1456-1462, 1993

20. Ruggenenti P, Perna A, Mosconi L, Pisoni R, Remuzzi G: Urinary protein excretion rate is the best independent predictor of ESRF in non-diabetic proteinuric chronic nephropathies. "Gruppo Italiano di Studi Epidemiologici in Nefrologia" (GISEN). Kidney Int. 53:1209-1216, 1998

21. Weidmann P, Boehlen LM, de Courten M: Effects of different antihypertensive drugs on human diabetic proteinuria. Nephrol.Dial.Transplant. 8:582-584, 1993

22. Remuzzi G, Bertani T: Pathophysiology of progressive nephropathies. N.Engl.J Med. 339:1448-1456, 1998

23. Lewis EJ, Hunsicker LG, Clarke WR, Berl T, Pohl MA, Lewis JB, Ritz E, Atkins RC, Rohde R, Raz I: Renoprotective effect of the angiotensin-receptor antagonist irbesartan in patients with nephropathy due to type 2 diabetes. N.Engl.J.Med. 345:851-860, 2001

24. Brenner BM, Cooper ME, De Zeeuw D, Keane WF, Mitch WE, Parving HH, Remuzzi G, Snapinn SM, Zhang Z, Shahinfar S: Effects of losartan on renal and cardiovascular outcomes in patients with type 2 diabetes and nephropathy. N.Engl.J.Med. 345:861-869, 2001

25. Ruggenenti P, Gambara V, Perna A, Bertani T, Remuzzi G: The nephropathy of non-insulin-dependent diabetes: predictors of outcome relative to diverse patterns of renal injury. J Am.Soc.Nephrol. 9:2336-2343, 1998

26. Yokoyama H, Tomonaga O, Hirayama M, Ishii A, Takeda M, Babazono T, Ujihara U, Takahashi C, Omori Y: Predictors of the progression of diabetic nephropathy and the beneficial effect of angiotensin-converting enzyme inhibitors in NIDDM patients. Diabetologia 40:405-411, 1997

27. Atkins RC, Briganti EM, Wiegmann TB: Effect of baseline proteinuria and change in proteinuria with treatment on the risk of renal endpoints in the irbesartan diabetic nephropathy trial (IDNT). (abstract) J Am.Soc.Nephrol. 13:7A, 2002

28. Pohl MA, Blumenthal S, Hunsicker LG: Impact of achieved systolic blood pressure on renal function in type 2 diabetic nephropathy. (abstract) J Am.Soc.Nephrol. 13:644A, 2002

29. Pyorala K, Pedersen TR, Kjekshus J, Faergeman O, Olsson AG, Thorgeirsson G: Cholesterol lowering with simvastatin improves prognosis of diabetic patients with coronary heart disease. A subgroup analysis of the Scandinavian Simvastatin Survival Study (4S). Diabetes Care 20:614-620, 1997

30. Breyer JA, Bain RP, Evans JK, Nahman NS, Jr., Lewis EJ, Cooper M, McGill J, Berl T: Predictors of the progression of renal insufficiency in patients with insulin-dependent diabetes and overt diabetic nephropathy. The Collaborative Study Group. Kidney Int. 50:1651-1658, 1996

31. Ravid M, Brosh D, Ravid-Safran D, Levy Z, Rachmani R: Main risk factors for nephropathy in type 2 diabetes mellitus are plasma cholesterol levels, mean blood pressure, and hyperglycemia. Arch.Intern.Med. 158:998-1004, 1998

32. Keane WF: The role of lipids in renal disease: future challenges. Kidney Int. 57 Suppl 75:27-31, 2000

33. Heart Protection Study Collaborative Group: MRC/BHF Heart Protection Study of cholesterol lowering with simvastatin in 20,536 high-risk individuals: a randomised placebo-controlled trial. Lancet 360:7-22, 2002

34. Kim SI, Han DC, Lee HB: Lovastatin inhibits transforming growth factor-beta1 expression in diabetic rat glomeruli and cultured rat mesangial cells. J.Am.Soc.Nephrol. 11:80-87, 2000

35. Lee SK, Jin SY, Han DC, Hwang SD, Lee HB: Effects of delayed treatment with enalapril and/or lovastatin on the progression of glomerulosclerosis in 5/6 nephrectomized rats. Nephrol.Dial.Transplant. 8:1338-1343, 1993

36. Lee TM, Su SF, Tsai CH: Effect of pravastatin on proteinuria in patients with well-controlled hypertension. Hypertension 40:67-73, 2002

37. Nakamura T, Ushiyama C, Hirokawa K, Osada S, Shimada N, Koide H: Effect of cerivastatin on urinary albumin excretion and plasma endothelin-1 concentrations in type 2 diabetes patients with microalbuminuria and dyslipidemia. Am.J Nephrol. 21:449-454, 2001

38. Tozawa M, Iseki K, Iseki C, Oshiro S, Ikemiya Y, Takishita S: Influence of smoking and obesity on the development of proteinuria. Kidney Int. 62:956-962, 2002

39. Weisinger JR, Kempson RL, Eldridge FL, Swenson RS: The nephrotic syndrome: a complication of massive obesity. Ann.Intern.Med. 81:440-447, 1974

40. Kambham N, Markowitz GS, Valeri AM, Lin J, D'Agati VD: Obesity-related glomerulopathy: an emerging epidemic. Kidney Int. 59:1498-1509, 2001

41. Chagnac A, Weinstein T, Korzets A, Ramadan E, Hirsch J, Gafter U: Glomerular hemodynamics in severe obesity. Am.J.Physiol Renal Physiol 278:F817-F822, 2000

42. Barton M, Carmona R, Morawietz H, D'Uscio LV, Goettsch W, Hillen H, Haudenschild CC, Krieger JE, Munter K, Lattmann T, Luscher TF, Shaw S: Obesity is associated with tissue-specific activation of renal angiotensin-converting enzyme in vivo: evidence for a regulatory role of endothelin. Hypertension 35:329-336, 2000

43. Giacchetti G, Faloia E, Mariniello B, Sardu C, Gatti C, Camilloni MA, Guerrieri M, Mantero F: Overexpression of the renin-angiotensin system in human visceral adipose tissue in normal and overweight subjects. Am.J.Hypertens. 15:381-388, 2002

44. Praga M, Hernandez E, Morales E, Campos AP, Valero MA, Martinez MA, Leon M: Clinical features and long-term outcome of obesity-associated focal segmental glomerulosclerosis. Nephrol.Dial.Transplant. 16:1790-1798, 2001

45. Altiparmak MR, Pamuk ON, Pamuk GE, Apaydin S, Ozbay G: Diffuse diabetic glomerulosclerosis in a patient with impaired glucose tolerance: report on a patient who later develops diabetes mellitus. Neth.J Med. 60:260-262, 2002

46. Yoshida A, Morozumi K, Oikawa T, Suganuma T, Aoki J, Sugito K, Koyama K, Fujinami T, Shigematsu H: Nodular glomerulosclerosis in a patient showing impaired glucose tolerance. Nippon Jinzo Gakkai Shi 32:877-884, 1990

47. Orth SR, Ritz E, Schrier RW: The renal risks of smoking. Kidney Int. 51:1669-1677, 1997

48. Sawicki PT, Didjurgeit U, Muhlhauser I, Bender R, Heinemann L, Berger M: Smoking is associated with progression of diabetic nephropathy. Diabetes Care 17:126-131, 1994

49. Ritz E, Ogata H, Orth SR: Smoking: a factor promoting onset and progression of diabetic nephropathy. Diabetes Metab 26 Suppl 4:54-63, 2000

50. Pinto-Sietsma SJ, Mulder J, Janssen WM, Hillege HL, De Zeeuw D, De Jong PE: Smoking Is Related to Albuminuria and Abnormal Renal Function in Nondiabetic Persons. Ann.Intern.Med. 133:585-591, 2000

51. Hansen HP, Rossing K, Jacobsen P, Jensen BR, Parving HH: The acute effect of smoking on systemic haemodynamics, kidney and endothelial functions in insulin-dependent diabetic patients with microalbuminuria. Scand.J Clin.Lab Invest 56:393-399, 1996

52. Baggio B, Budakovic A, Dalla Vestra M, Saller A, Bruseghin M, Fioretto P: Effects of Cigarette Smoking on Glomerular Structure and Function in Typer 2 Diabetic Patients. (abstract) J Am.Soc.Nephrol. 13:2730-2736, 2002

53. Parving HH: Renoprotection in diabetes: genetic and non-genetic risk factors and treatment. Diabetologia 41:745-759, 1998

54.   Intensive blood-glucose control with sulphonylureas or insulin compared with conventional treatment and risk of complications in patients with type 2 diabetes (UKPDS 33). UK Prospective Diabetes Study (UKPDS) Group. Lancet 352:837-853, 1998

55. Tanaka Y, Atsumi Y, Matsuoka K, Onuma T, Tohjima T, Kawamori R: Role of glycemic control and blood pressure in the development and progression of nephropathy in elderly Japanese NIDDM patients. Diabetes Care 21:116-120, 1998

56. Thorpe SR, Baynes JW: Role of the Maillard reaction in diabetes mellitus and diseases of aging. Drugs Aging 9:69-77, 1996

57. Degenhardt TP, Alderson NL, Arrington DD, Beattie RJ, Basgen JM, Steffes MW, Thorpe SR, Baynes JW: Pyridoxamine inhibits early renal disease and dyslipidemia in the streptozotocin-diabetic rat. Kidney Int. 61:939-950, 2002

58. Ruggenenti P, Mosconi L, Sangalli F, Casiraghi F, Gambara V, Remuzzi G, Remuzzi A: Glomerular size-selective dysfunction in NIDDM is not ameliorated by ACE inhibition or by calcium channel blockade. Kidney Int. 55:984-994, 1999

59. Ruggenenti P, Perna A, Gherardi G, Garini G, Zoccali C, Salvadori M, Scolari F, Schena FP, Remuzzi G: Renoprotective properties of ACE-inhibition in non-diabetic nephropathies with non-nephrotic proteinuria. Lancet 354:359-364, 1999

60. Ruggenenti P, Remuzzi G: Anti-hypertensive agents and incipient diabetic nephropathy, in The Diabetes Annual/9, edited by Marshall SM, Home PD, Rizza RA, Amsterdam, Elsevier Science B.V., 1995, pp 295-317

61. Ruggenenti P, Remuzzi G: The renoprotective action of angiotensin-converting enzyme inhibitors in diabetes. Exp.Nephrol. 4 Suppl 1:53-60, 1996

62. Lebovitz HE, Wiegmann TB, Cnaan A, Shahinfar S, Sica DA, Broadstone V, Schwartz SL, Mengel MC, Segal R, Versaggi JA: Renal protective effects of enalapril in hypertensive NIDDM: role of baseline albuminuria. Kidney Int.Suppl 45:S150-S155, 1994

63. Trevisan R, Tiengo A: Effect of low-dose ramipril on microalbuminuria in normotensive or mild hypertensive non-insulin-dependent diabetic patients. North-East Italy Microalbuminuria Study Group. Am.J Hypertens. 8:876-883, 1995

64. Sano T, Kawamura T, Matsumae H, Sasaki H, Nakayama M, Hara T, Matsuo S, Hotta N, Sakamoto N: Effects of long-term enalapril treatment on persistent micro- albuminuria in well-controlled hypertensive and normotensive NIDDM patients. Diabetes Care 17:420-424, 1994

65. Nielsen FS, Rossing P, Gall MA, Skott P, Smidt UM, Parving HH: Long-term effect of lisinopril and atenolol on kidney function in hypertensive NIDDM subjects with diabetic nephropathy. Diabetes 46:1182-1188, 1997

66. Knowler WC, Barrett-Connor E, Fowler SE, Hamman RF, Lachin JM, Walker EA, Nathan DM: Reduction in the incidence of type 2 diabetes with lifestyle intervention or metformin. N.Engl.J Med. 346:393-403, 2002

67. Fioretto P, Steffes MW, Sutherland DE, Goetz FC, Mauer M: Reversal of lesions of diabetic nephropathy after pancreas transplantation. N.Engl.J.Med. 339:69-75, 1998

68. Schoonjans K, Auwerx J: Thiazolidinediones: an update. Lancet 355:1008-1010, 2000

69. McCarthy KJ, Routh RE, Shaw W, Walsh K, Welbourne TC, Johnson JH: Troglitazone halts diabetic glomerulosclerosis by blockade of mesangial expansion. Kidney Int. 58:2341-2350, 2000

70. Ruggenenti P, Schieppati A, Remuzzi G: Progression, remission, regression of chronic renal diseases. Lancet 357:1601-1608, 2001

71. Vasan RS, Larson MG, Leip EP, Evans JC, O'Donnell CJ, Kannel WB, Levy D: Impact of high-normal blood pressure on the risk of cardiovascular disease. N.Engl.J.Med. 345:1291-1297, 2001

72. Pinto-Sietsma SJ, Janssen WM, Hillege HL, Navis G, Zeeuw DD, Jong PE: Urinary albumin excretion is associated with renal functional abnormalities in a nondiabetic population. J.Am.Soc.Nephrol. 11:1882-1888, 2000

19

ADVANCED GLYCATION END-PRODUCTS AND DIABETIC RENAL DISEASE

Merlin C Thomas[1], Mark E Cooper[1], George Jerums[2],
[1]Danielle Alberti Memorial Centre for Diabetes Complications, Baker Heart Research Institute, Melbourne 8008, Victoria, AUSTRALIA;
[2]University of Melbourne, Director of Endocrinology, Endocrine unit, Austin and Repatriation Medical Centre (Austin Campus), West Heidelberg, Victoria, AUSTRALIA

Prolonged hyperglycemia and oxidative stress in diabetes result in the production and accumulation of advanced glycation end products (AGEs) [1]. AGEs are formed via the *Maillard* or 'browning' reaction between reducing sugars and amine residues on proteins, lipids or nucleic acids. Under normal circumstances, this reaction is slow, meaning that AGE-modification predominantly occurs in long-lived molecules such as collagen and lens proteins [1]. The degree of AGE-modification therefore represents one mechanism to judge the '*age*' of a molecule allowing the recognition of senescent targets for excretion or catabolism [2]. In addition, as molecular turnover is reduced with increasing chronological age [3], the amount and variety of AGE-modified tissue increases, contributing to many of the changes recognised as signs of *ageing* (such as cataracts and stiffness). In diabetes, prolonged hyperglycemia and oxidative stress hasten the formation of AGEs [4], meaning not only that long-lived proteins become more heavily modified but also that shorter-lived molecules such as apolipoproteins become targets for *de novo* advanced glycation [1,2]. In addition, the intracellular formation of AGEs from reactive carbonyl intermediates may occur at a much faster rate than glucose-derived AGE formation that occurs outside the cell. These intracellular AGEs potentially represent an important source of glycation products, as AGE levels may be increased after only days of hyperglycemia, well before similar changes can be demonstrated in vitro.

Mogensen CE (ed.) THE KIDNEY AND HYPERTENSION IN DIABETES MELLITUS. Copyright©
2004 by Martin Dunitz, a member of the Taylor & Francis Group, plc. All rights reserved.

AGEs have been shown to have a wide range of chemical, cellular and tissue effects implicated in the development and progression of diabetic nephropathy (*Table 1*).

Table 1. Effects of AGEs that potentially contribute to diabetic nephropathy

Extracellular matrix:
Intermolecular and intramolecular cross-linking [22,33-36]
Disruption of cell-matrix and matrix-matrix interactions [38-40]
Increased ECM synthesis [43-48]
Tubuloepithelial-mesenchymal transdifferentiation [22]
Reduced metalloprotease activity [52,53]

Induction of oxidative stress:
Increased generation of reactive oxygen species [58]
Activation of NADPH oxidase [59]
Mitochondrial dysfunction [1,60]
Depletion of endogenous anti-oxidants [57]

Induction of cytokines and growth factors including:
TGFβ1, CTGF, VEGF, IGF-1, PDGF
TNFα, IL-1B, IL-6 [1,2,19,22]

Activation of cellular pathways:
PKC-MAPK pathway [64]
Tyrosine kinase pathway [1]
NFκB [19-22]

Other effects :
Altered expression of nephrin [70-73]
Disruption of vaso-relaxation [2]

The accumulation of AGEs in diabetes is closely linked to the presence and duration of hyperglycemia. For example, the DCCT demonstrated a close association between hyperglycemia and AGEs levels, with significant reductions in skin AGE concentrations after intensive glycaemic intervention [5]. However, AGEs may be considered downstream mediators of renal injury in diabetes. This is illustrated by studies showing that inhibition of advanced glycation is able to attenuate renal injury, without influencing glycaemic control [6]. In addition, administration of exogenous AGEs in non-diabetic animals is able to generate lesions similar to those seen in diabetic nephropathy

[7]. In the DCCT study, AGE levels were a better predictor for the development of complications of diabetes than glycated haemoglobin, with over a third of the variance in complications in that study attributable to differences in AGE indices. Notably, the influence of AGEs was even greater in the intensive control cohort, suggesting that while glycaemic control is important, it is not sufficient to prevent complications [5]. Taken together, these studies suggest that AGEs represent a potent common mechanism by which hyperglycemia and oxidative stress may induce renal injury in patients with diabetes.

AGEs are a chemically heterogeneous group of compounds, many of which are poorly defined or remain to be identified [8]. While AGE-modification usually commences at one amino-group, some of the best-characterised AGEs, such a pentosidine and pyrroline, form intermolecular cross-links between modified proteins. These cross-links can result in significant changes in protein structure and function, such as increased stiffness and resistance to proteolytic digestion. In addition, many of these compounds have intrinsic fluorescence, meaning that tissue fluorescence may be used as a marker for the presence of AGE modifications. For example, tissue fluorescence has been shown to increase with *ageing* [9]. With the development of diabetes, there is a marked increase in tissue fluorescence in the kidney [6], the retina [10] and other sites of diabetic microvascular disease [11]. Renal and hepatic impairment are also associated with increased tissue fluorescence, reflecting the role of these organs in the catabolism and excretion of AGEs [12].

Other AGEs, such as carboxymethyllysine (CML), are neither cross-links nor fluorescent. However, CML constitutes the main epitope for recognition by most commercially available antibodies used for the detection and quantification of AGEs. In clinical studies, Makita *et al* have reported increased serum CML-AGE levels in diabetic patients [13]. Notably, the greatest increase in CML-AGE staining in diabetes appears to occur in the diabetic glomerulus [14], particularly in the expanded mesangial matrix and nodular lesions of diabetic nephropathy [15].

The molecular identity of the AGEs that most contribute to the development of diabetic complications including nephropathy has not been clearly determined. In recent studies, Miura *et al* found that fluorescent AGEs better correlated with complications in patients with type I diabetes than levels of pentosidine or non-fluorescent AGEs like CML [16]. However, in a study of patients with type II diabetes, Beisswenger *et al* reported that non-fluorescent CML-AGE levels were better associated with the presence of complications including retinopathy and nephropathy [17]. It is possible that both these measured AGEs may be a marker for the presence of (unmeasured) reactive AGE intermediates [1]. In addition, if the majority of AGE-mediated injury occurs via activation of multi-ligand AGE receptors (see below), it is possible that the accumulation of AGEs via a variety of pathways and in a variety of molecular forms may be similarly pathogenic.

AGE-RECEPTORS

Many of the effects of AGEs appear to be mediated by interaction with specific AGE receptors and binding proteins. These receptors are present on various renal cell types [2], including mesangial cells [18] and podocytes [11, 19]. Over the last decade, a number of AGE binding sites have been identified. The first binding site to be cloned, the receptor for AGE (RAGE), was initially identified in endothelial cells [20]. Our group has detected RAGE in other sites including the kidney, retina, nerve and blood vessels [10]. Activation of the RAGE receptor is also linked to increased production of fibrogenic growth factors and cytokines (see below). Further studies have suggested that RAGE has a central role in the many of these changes [19,21]. For example, AGE- and CML- modified proteins promote the activation and expression of IL-6 and TGFb1 in tubular cells. This effect may be inhibited using the soluble form of the RAGE or a RAGE-specific antibody [21,22].

In addition to RAGE, many other AGE receptors have also been identified. These include AGE-R1 (p60), AGE-R2 (protein kinase-C substrate), AGE-R3 (galectin-3) [23], lysozyme [24] as well as the macrophage scavenger receptors [25] and lectin-like oxidized low density lipoprotein receptor-1 (LOX-1) [26] and CD-36 [27].

Most of these AGE-binding proteins are constitutively expressed in a limited number of cell types and only at low levels in the absence of injury and inflammation. Expression is enhanced in response to metabolic states such as diabetes and uraemia possibly due to high levels of AGEs in these conditions. In particular, activated cells at sites of diabetes-associated renal and vascular injury often show high level expression of these binding proteins that co-localise with AGE deposition [11]. The role of these receptors remains an area of active investigation. One view is that AGE-receptors identify senescent tissue elements for excretion or catabolism. The specific up-regulation of AGE-receptors at sites of injury also suggests a role in mediating inflammation, cell differentiation and tissue repair.

The importance of AGE-receptor mediated pathways in the pathogenesis of diabetic nephropathy is illustrated by studies in which specific AGE-receptors have been genetically modified. For example, galectin-3-deficient mice develop accelerated glomerulopathy, as evidenced by the increase in proteinuria, matrix gene expression, and mesangial expansion [28]. Similarly, attenuation of AGE R1-dependent uptake and degradation is associated with accelerated glomerular pathology in the spontaneously diabetic non-obese diabetic (NOD) strain of mice [29]. Low AGE R1 expression has also been associated with patients with severe nephropathy [30].

It is likely that AGE-receptors interact, in so far as they share the same substrate. In addition, expression levels may also be closely linked. For example, the galectin-3 knockout model is associated with *reduced* expression of scavenger receptor A and AGE-R1 yet increased expression of RAGE and AGE-R2 [28]. These results suggest that the AGE-R1 and R3 receptor pathways may protect against AGE-mediated tissue injury, while RAGE-mediated signalling augments it. This conclusion is further supported by studies performed in mice over-expressing the RAGE gene. These mice have been shown to have accelerated renal damage following the induction of diabetes [31]. Similarly RAGE knockout mice appear to be protected against the development of mesangial expansion in diabetes [19]. These experimental studies have also been supported by recent clinical studies demonstrating that functional polymorphisms in the promoter of the RAGE gene (-374 T/A) are associated with proteinuria and cardiovascular disease in patients with type 1 diabetes, particularly those with poor metabolic control [32].

ACEs AND EXTRACELLUAR MATRIX PROTEINS

Diabetic nephropathy is characterised by the accumulation of extracellular matrix (ECM) protein in the glomerular mesangium and tubulo-interstitium. Because of their slow turnover, ECM proteins are especially susceptible to AGE-modification, resulting in alterations of both structure and function. For example, the formation of inter-and intramolecular cross-links following the glycation of collagen leads to structural alterations including changes in packing and surface charge [1,33]. Matrix cross-links may act as a 'sticky web' resulting in non-specific trapping of macromolecules and contributing to mesangial expansion. The increased number of acid-stable cross-links by diabetic collagen is reflected in a marked increase in acid-insoluble collagen in diabetic tissues [34]. Cleavage of AGE-induced cross-links by agents such as N-phenacylthiazolium bromide (PTB) and ALT-711 restores collagen solubility [22,35,36] and is associated with a reduction in matrix accumulation within the diabetic tissues including the kidney and the heart [22,36].

Cell-matrix interactions may also be disrupted by matrix glycation contributing to changes in cellular adhesion [37], altered cell growth and loss of the epithelial cell phenotype [22]. In addition, heterotypic interactions between matrix proteins are disturbed by AGE-modifications [38]. The affinity of laminin and fibronectin for type IV collagen and heparan sulphate proteoglycan is decreased following AGE-modification [39,40]. Glycation also inhibits the homotypic interactions required for polymeric self-assembly of type IV collagen [40] and laminin [41]. These changes may be particularly apparent in the glomerular basement membrane, where the induction of chemical cross-links between amines leads to an increase in protein permeability [42]. Cross-link breakers, on the other hand, are able to prevent the development of albuminuria in experimental diabetes [22].

ECM composition may also be substantially altered by AGEs. The expression of extracellular proteins such as fibronectin, type I and type IV collagen is increased by AGEs in a dose and time dependent manner, in the presence [43] or absence of hyperglycemia [44-46]. For example, the glomerular expression of type IV collagen and laminin is increased following the direct injection of AGEs into mice [45]. This has been considered to be a direct effect via AGE-specific receptors involving activation of the JAK/STAT signal transcription pathway [46], leading to the induction of profibrotic cytokines and growth factors including TGFb1, VEGF and CTGF [1,2,19,22]. CTGF (also known as IGF-binding protein-related protein-2) is a potent profibrotic agent and is increased in diabetic nephropathy [47]. Inhibitors of advanced glycation such as aminoguanidine can prevent increased expression of CTGF in diabetes, associated with a reduction in tissue AGE levels and the prevention of mesangial expansion [18]. In addition, we have recently demonstrated that soluble AGEs including carboxymethyllysine (CML) containing proteins are able to induce the expression of CTGF and fibronectin production in cultured human mesangial cells [18]. Similar changes have also been reported in human dermal fibroblasts, where the AGE-induced up-regulation of CTGF is mediated through the receptor for advanced glycation (RAGE) [48].

Excessive ECM production is also compounded by the increased numbers of interstitial fibroblasts, myofibroblasts and infiltrating macrophages in diabetic nephropathy. While some of these cells migrate to the interstitium due to chemokines released in response to injury, the transdifferentiation of tubular epithelial cells into a mesenchymal phenotype (tubuloepithelial-mesenchymal transdifferentiation, TEMT) has also been implicated in the accelerated fibrogenesis seen in diabetic nephropathy [49]. TEMT is regulated by several growth factors and cytokines including TGFβ1, FGF, interleukin-1 and EGF [49]. In addition, we have reported that AGEs may also induce TEMT, potentially contributing to their profibrotic action [22]. The mechanism of this action is the subject of ongoing research but it appears to be receptor mediated, as blockade of the RAGE receptor prevents TEMT, implying a crucial role for the AGE/RAGE interaction in cell differentiation. This process appears to be dependent on the activation of TGFβ1, since a neutralising antibody to TGFβ1 can block AGE-induced TEMT [22]. This downstream signalling pathway may be further regulated by intracellular mediators of the Smad family, in particular Smad 2 or Smad 3 which are phosphorylated by the type I TGFβ receptor [50]. Recent reports also suggest that basement membrane composition and integrity is also important for the maintenance of epithelial phenotype. Zisberg *et al* describe how type 1 collagen (known to be upregulated by AGEs and diabetes) promotes TEMT [51].

In addition, inhibition of assembly of type IV collagen NC1 hexamers (as occurs with collagen glycation [41]) facilitates TEMT in vitro, possibly through the up-regulation of TGFβ1 in tubular epithelial cells that follows the disruption of basement membrane architecture [51].

At the same time that matrix synthesis is augmented by AGEs, the expression and activity of degradative matrix metalloproteinases are also reduced. Not only are AGE-modified proteins more resistant to enzymatic digestion, but experimental diabetes is associated with a reduction in the matrix-degradative capacity of the kidney [52]. This effect is replicated *in vitro*, with a 45% reduction in the matrix-degrading activity of matrix metalloproteinases secreted by mesangial cells following growth on glycated matrix [53]. In both instances, glycation results not only in a decrease in the expression and activity of matrix metalloproteinases secreted by mesangial cells but also the increased expression and activity of tissue metalloproteinase inhibitors.

AGEs AND OXIDATIVE STRESS

Increased production of reactive oxygen species (ROS) is recognised as a key component in the development of diabetic nephropathy leading to the production of cytokines, adhesion molecules and chemokines [1,54]. It is now apparent that there is a synergistic relationship between advanced glycation and oxidative stress. While AGEs can be slowly produced though non-oxidative pathways, this reaction is accelerated by oxidative stress through the formation of highly reactive *glycoxidation* and *lipoxidation* intermediates such as *methylglyoxal*. In experimental diabetes, oxidative stress is increased in proportion to AGE accumulation [55]. There is also evidence in human diabetic glomerular lesions of increased oxidative stress and AGE accumulation [14] both of which may be attenuated by good glycaemic control [56]. In addition, tissue accumulation of AGEs can be reduced in diabetic animals treated with anti-oxidants [57].

Elevated oxidative stress seen in diabetes is viewed to be the result of both an increase in ROS generation and a decrease in endogenous anti-oxidant activity including free radical scavengers and enzyme systems [54]. AGEs lead to enhanced formation of free radicals both directly through catalytic sites in their molecular structure [58] and via stimulation of membrane-bound NAD(P)H oxidase through the RAGE receptor [59]. In addition, AGE-dependent depletion of cellular anti-oxidant systems such as glutathione peroxidase are also inhibited by antibodies to AGER1, AGE-R2 as well as RAGE [57]. Mitochondrial dysfunction induced by AGEs and carbonyl intermediates may also contribute to the generation of superoxide [60]. Some studies have also suggested an important role for oxidative stress in RAGE-mediated signalling. This is illustrated by the finding that anti-oxidants are able to prevent the up-regulation of TGFβ1 following exposure to AGEs [61]. Similarly, depletion of the endogenous anti-oxidant activity increases their susceptibility to activation by AGEs [61].

AGEs AND CYTOKINES

AGEs result in the expression and activation of a number of pro-inflammatory cytokines, growth factors and adhesion molecules implicated in the pathogenesis of diabetic nephropathy (Table 1). These include VEGF, CTGF, TGFβ1, IGF-I, platelet-derived growth factor, TNF-α, IL-1β, and IL-6 [1,2,19,22]. The effect of AGEs may be both direct (through AGE receptors) and indirect, via generation of ROS and changes in the integrity of the extracellular matrix.

In particular, the induction of TGFβ1 appears to be the key intermediate step for many of the AGE-mediated effects on cell growth and matrix homeostasis. TGFβ1 expression is closely linked to AGE accumulation in the kidney [62]. Administration of exogenous AGEs in non-diabetic animals is able to increase the renal expression of TGFβ1 [22]. In addition, inhibitors of advanced glycation reduce the overproduction of TGFβ1 in diabetic animals, independent of glycaemic status [43,63]. We have recently shown that antibodies to TGFβ1 are able to block AGE-mediated transdifferentiation of renal tubular epithelial cells [22]. One explanation for this effect may be that the transcriptional up-regulation of TGFβ1 in diabetes appears to be mediated via PKC dependent pathways for which AGEs are a potent stimulus. Moreover, inhibitors of AGEs have been shown to attenuate renal PKC over-expression in diabetic rats [64]. Some studies have also suggested an important role for oxidative stress in AGE-induced TGFβ1 transcription. This is illustrated by the finding that anti-oxidants are able to prevent the up-regulation of TGFβ1 following exposure to AGEs [61].

INTERACTIONS BETWEEN AGEs and THE RENIN ANGIOTENSIN SYSTEM

Overactivity of the intra-renal renin-angiotensin system (RAS) has been strongly implicated in the pathogenesis of diabetic nephropathy, although the source of this activation is not yet established. AGEs significantly interact with the RAS as demonstrated by the reversal in AGE-induced collagen production by captopril *in vitro*, possibly by attenuating RAGE expression [46]. We have previously described the rapid development of glomerulosclerosis and tubulointerstitial fibrosis following the induction of diabetes in the Ren-2 rat, a strain with genetic overactivity of the RAS [65]. Interestingly, in this angiotensin-II dependent model, renal injury can be attenuated following treatment with an inhibitor of AGE formation, ALT-946 [66]. In addition, we have recently demonstrated that *in vivo* ACE inhibition significantly reduces the formation and accumulation of renal AGEs in experimental diabetes [67]. The major site of this action by ACE inhibitors is yet to be established. This may represent a direct effect, as simultaneous incubation of ACE inhibitors with glucose and protein prevents the *in vitro* formation of AGEs [68]. In addition, ACE inhibitors can attenuate the expression of NAPDPH oxidase [67, 69] and therein reduce AGEs formed via glycoxidation.

The overlapping activities of AGEs and the RAS in the development and progression of diabetic nephropathy is illustrated by the expression of nephrin, a slit-pore protein thought to play a role in proteinuria. The expression of nephrin is reduced in experimental diabetes and restored following treatment with an inhibitor of advanced glycation or blockade of the RAS [70]. Similarly, both glycated matrix and angiotensin II are able to reduce nephrin expression *in vitro* [71]. It seems likely that an interaction of metabolic and haemodynamic factors compound the deleterious effects of the diabetic milieu and reduce the threshold for injury via common mechanisms. However, it remains to be established whether a combination of haemodynamic and metabolic interventions are more effective than either individual therapy in preventing diabetes associated renal injury [72].

INTERVENTIONS TO REDUCE AGE ACCUMULATION

Interventions to reduce renal AGE accumulation appear to be renoprotective in the context of diabetes. A number of pharmacological inhibitors of AGE-dependent pathways have been developed (*Figure 1*). Aminoguanidine is a hydrazine derivative that acts to reduce AGE formation by binding to reactive dicarbonyl and aldehyde products of early glycation and glycoxidation such as 3-deoxyglucosone [6]. Aminoguanidine has been shown in experimental models of diabetes to not only reduce tissue AGE levels but also to retard the development of neuropathy, retinopathy and nephropathy [6,10,34]. Our studies in the streptozotocin diabetic rat have shown that aminoguanidine, administered from the induction of diabetes, attenuates diabetes-related increases in tissue AGEs and as well as retarding the development of albuminuria and mesangial expansion [6]. This effect is related to the duration of treatment with aminoguanidine, suggesting that the generation of AGEs in the kidney is time dependent and closely linked to the development of experimental diabetic nephropathy [73]. New, more selective, inhibitors of advanced glycation such as *ALT-946* [N-(2-Acetamidoethyl) hydrozinecarbox-imidamide hydrochloride] have been developed which, unlike aminoguanidine, do not appear to inhibit NO synthase [34,66,74]. This agent also significantly reduces renal AGE accumulation and albuminuria in models of experimental diabetes [66,75].

Pyridoxamine is a natural intermediate of vitamin B_6 metabolism, which has also been shown to reduce AGE levels and improve renal dysfunction associated with experimental diabetes [75]. Pyridoxamine reacts with carbonyl intermediates of the Maillard reaction, blocking the formation of advanced glycation and lipoxidation end products (AGEs and ALEs). In addition, pyridoxamine is able to scavenge reactive carbonyl products of glucose and lipid oxidation. By contrast to other AGE inhibitors, pyridoxamine has minimal toxicity and is now in Phase II clinical trials.

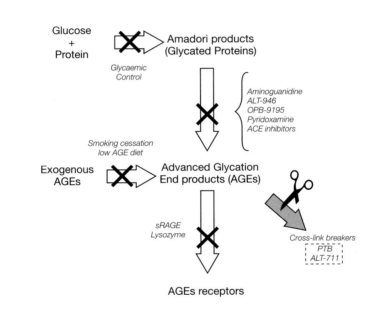

Figure 1. Treatment strategies to reduce AGE-mediated injury in diabetes

OPB-9195 [[(+/-)-2-isopropylidenehydrazono-4-oxo-thiazolidin-5-ylacetanilide] belongs to a group of thiazolidine derivatives, which are used predominantly as hypoglycaemic agents. Although OPB-9195 does not lower blood glucose levels, it significantly reduces serum concentrations and tissue deposition of AGEs, possibly though the trapping reactive carbonyl intermediates [63]. OPB-9195 has now been shown to prevent progression of mesangial expansion and glomerulosclerosis in experimental diabetes [63].

Another group of compounds that reduce AGE levels are the so called "cross-link breakers" These agents cleave pre-formed AGE cross-links thereby promoting the clearance of smaller AGE derived moieties by the kidney and liver [22,35,36]. The first cross-link breaker described was the thiazolium compound, phenacylthiazolium bromide (PTB) that has been shown to reduce the accumulation of vascular AGE in experimental diabetes [22]. More recently, another chemically related cross-link breaker, ALT-711 [4,5-Dimethyl-3-(2-oxo2-phenylethyl)-thiazolium chloride] has been reported to reverse diabetes-induced increases in large artery stiffness [35]. In addition, we have recently demonstrated that this agent is associated with reduced serum AGE levels and tissue AGE accumulation in animals with experimental diabetes [36]. If these AGE cross-link breakers can be shown to have similar effects in the kidney, this would provide a conceptual basis for the reversal of AGE-mediated tissue damage, which till now has been regarded as irreversible.

Another approach to reduce AGE levels has been to provide soluble AGE-receptors to compete with cellular receptors for AGE binding and thereby reduce endogenous activation. There have now been several studies that soluble RAGE is able to modify AGE-mediated activation of pathways implicated in the development of diabetic nephropathy [19,21,76]. Similarly, lysozyme has been shown to normalise serum AGE levels and improve albuminuria in murine models of diabetes [77].

There is accumulating evidence that, in addition to AGEs formed *in vivo*, exogenous AGEs acquired from the diet may contribute to the body AGE burden [78]. In particular, long-term storage or prolonged heating of foodstuffs in the presence of sugars (that results in appetising '*browning*') also generates a number of AGEs capable of activating AGE-receptors involved in the inflammatory response and fibrogenesis [78]. In addition, curing of tobacco produces a number of AGEs, which may be inhaled in cigarette smoke [79]. The importance of exogenous AGEs is especially apparent in the presence of impaired clearance of AGEs such as in patients with renal impairment. However, there is now evidence to suggest that exposure to high levels of exogenous AGEs may directly contribute to the development of albuminuria and atherosclerosis in otherwise normal animals [81]. Tissue and circulating AGEs are significantly higher in smokers and in patients on high AGE diets [82]. In addition, dietary interventions to reduce AGE intake reduce both serum AGE levels and result in reduced levels of inflammatory mediators in patients with diabetes [83]. Such diets may ultimately provide an important adjunct to interventions directed towards the inhibition of endogenous glycation.

CLINICAL STUDIES

Clinical studies in patients with diabetes clearly demonstrate a strong correlation between AGEs and the severity of microvascular complications. In particular, serum levels of AGEs are significantly increased with the progression to microalbuminuria and subsequently to overt nephropathy [2]. Similar results have been demonstrated correlating skin levels of AGEs with the severity of complications in patients with long-standing type I diabetes [3]. Some studies suggest that AGE levels may only loosely correlate with glycaemic control in the clinical setting [16]. This finding is consistent with the hypothesis that oxidative stress (in particular lipid oxidation) may be a more important mediator of advanced glycation than hyperglycemia *per se* in patients already receiving interventions directed towards improved glycaemic control [54].

While specific interventions to reduce AGE levels have proved highly successful in experimental diabetes, there have only been a few studies to translate these findings into clinical practice. Large clinical studies of pimagedine (aminoguanidine) in patients with type I diabetes (ACTION 1) and type II diabetes (ACTION 2) and overt nephropathy were terminated due to safety concerns and apparent lack of efficacy. Nonetheless, pimagedine was associated with a reduction in urine protein excretion in sub-population of patients with moderate renal impairment and a reduction in the progression of retinopathy [84]. Smaller studies with aminoguanidine have demonstrated significant improvements in red cell deformability and dyslipidaemia [84,85]. More promising have been studies with the cross-link breaker, ALT-711. In patients with isolated systolic hypertension (but not diabetes specifically) ALT-711 was associated with improvements in large artery stiffness [86]. Preliminary results from the DIAMOND (Distensibility Improvement and Remodelling in Diastolic Heart Failure) study also demonstrated reductions in left ventricular mass and improvement in left ventricular diastolic filling following treatment with ALT-711. This was manifested clinically by

315

improvements in their NYHA class and quality-of-life [87]. ALT-711 is currently in two additional human clinical trials, albeit not in patients with renal disease. Future studies of this agent in patients with diabetic nephropathy are keenly awaited.

REFERENCES

1. Brownlee M. Biochemistry and molecular cell biology of diabetic complications. Nature 2001; 414(6865):813-20
2. Vlassara H. The AGE-receptor in the pathogenesis of diabetic complications. Diabetes Metab Res Rev. 2001: 17(6):436-43
3. Szweda PA, Friguet B, Szweda LI. Proteolysis, free radicals, and aging. Free Radic Biol Med. 2002; 33: 29-36
4. Fu MX, Wells-Knecht KJ, Blackledge JA, Lyons TJ, Thorpe SR, Baynes JW. Glycation, glycoxidation, and cross-linking of collagen by glucose. Kinetics, mechanisms, and inhibition of late stages of the Maillard reaction. Diabetes 1994: 43: 676-683
5. Monnier VM, Bautista O, Kenny D, Sell DR, Fogarty J, Dahms W, Cleary PA, Lachin J, Genuth S.Skin collagen glycation, glycoxidation, and crosslinking are lower in subjects with long-term intensive versus conventional therapy of type 1 diabetes: relevance of glycated collagen products versus HbA1c as markers of diabetic complications. DCCT Skin Collagen Ancillary Study Group. Diabetes Control and Complications Trial. Diabetes 1999;48(4):870-80
6. Soulis-Liparota T, Cooper M, Papazoglou D, Clarke B, Jerums G. Retardation by aminoguanidine of development of albuminuria, mesangial expansion, and tissue fluorescence in streptozocin-induced diabetic rat. Diabetes 1991: 40: 1328-34
7. Vlassara H, Striker LJ, Teichberg S, Fuh H, Li YM, Steffes M. Advanced glycation end products induce glomerular sclerosis and albuminuria in normal rats. Proc Natl Acad Sci U S A 91: 11704-8, 1994
8. Raj DS, Choudhury D, Welbourne TC, Levi M. Advanced glycation end products: a Nephrologist's perspective. Am J Kidney Dis 2000;35(3):365-80
9. Dyer DG, Dunn JA, Thorpe SR, Bailie KE, Lyons TJ, McCance DR, Baynes JW. Accumulation of Maillard reaction products in skin collagen in diabetes and aging. J Clin Invest 1993; 91: 2463-9.
10. Hammes H, Martin S, Federlin K, Geisen K, Brownlee M. Aminoguanidine treatment inhibits the development of experimental diabetic retinopathy. Proc Natl Acad Sci USA; 88: 11555-11558,1991
11. Soulis T, Thallas V, Youssef S, Gilbert RE, McWilliam B, Murray-McIntosh RP, Cooper ME. Advanced glycation end products and the receptor for advanced glycated end products co-localise in organs susceptible to diabetic microvascular injury: immunohistochemical studies. Diabetologia 1997; 40: 619-628
12. Makita Z, Bucala R, Rayfield EJ, Friedman EA, Kaufman AM, Korbet SM, Barth RH, Winston JA, Fuh H, Manogue KR, et al. Reactive glycosylation endproducts in diabetic uraemia and treatment of renal failure. Lancet 1994; 343: 1519-22
13. Makita Z, Radoff S, Rayfield EJ, Yang Z, Skolnik E, Delaney V, Friedman EA, Cerami A, Vlassara H. Advanced glycosylation end products in patients with diabetic nephropathy. N Engl J Med 1991; 325: 836-842

14. Suzuki D, Miyata T, Saotome N, Horie K, Inagi R, Yasuda Y, Uchida K, Izuhara Y, Yagame M, Sakai H, Kurokawa K. Immunohistochemical evidence for an increased oxidative stress and carbonyl modification of proteins in diabetic glomerular lesions. *J Am Soc Nephrol* 1999;10:822-32

15. Soulis T, Cooper ME, Vranes D, Bucala R, Jerums G. The effects of aminoguanidine in preventing experimental diabetic nephropathy are related to duration of treatment. Kidney Int 1996; 50: 627-634

16. Miura J, Yamagishi S, Uchigata Y, Takeuchi M, Yamamoto H, Makita Z, Iwamoto Y. Serum levels of non-carboxymethyllysine advanced glycation endproducts are correlated to severity of microvascular complications in patients with Type 1 diabetes. J Diabetes Complications 2003:17(1):16-21

17. Beisswenger PJ, Makita Z, Curphey TJ, Moore LL, Jean S, Brinck Johnsen T, Bucala R, Vlassara H. Formation of immunochemical advanced glycosylation end products precedes and correlates with early manifestations of renal and retinal disease in diabetes. Diabetes 1995; 44: 824-9

18. Twigg SM, Cao Z, MCLennan SV, Burns WC, Brammar G, Forbes JM, Cooper ME. Renal connective tissue growth factor induction in experimental diabetes is prevented by aminoguanidine. Endocrinology 2002; 143(12):4907-15

19. Wendt TM, Tanji N, Guo J, Kislinger TR, Qu W, Lu Y, Bucciarelli LG, Rong LL, Moser B, Markowitz GS, Stein G, Bierhaus A, Liliensiek B, Arnold B, Nawroth PP, Stern DM, D'Agati VD, Schmidt AM.RAGE Drives the Development of Glomerulosclerosis and Implicates Podocyte Activation in the Pathogenesis of Diabetic Nephropathy.Am J Pathol. 2003; 162(4):1123-37

20. Schmidt A, Vianna M, Gerlach M, Brett J, Ryan J, Kao C, Esposito H, Hegarty W, Hurley W, Clauss M, Wang F, Pan Y, Tsang T, Stern D. Isolation and characterisation of two binding proteins for advanced glycation end products from bovine lung which are present on the endothelial cell surface. J Biol Chem 1992; 267: 14987-14997

21. Morcos M, Sayed AA, Bierhaus A, Yard B, Waldherr R, Merz W, Kloeting ISchleicher E, Mentz S, Abd el Baki RF, Tritschler H, Kasper M, Schwenger V, Hamann A, Dugi KA, Schmidt AM, Stern D, Ziegler R, Haering HU, Andrassy M, van der Woude F, Nawroth PP. Activation of tubular epithelial cells in diabetic nephropathy. Diabetes. 2002:51(12):3532-44

22. Oldfield MD, Bach LA, Forbes JM, Nikolic-Paterson D, McRobert A, Thallas V, Atkins RC, Osicka T, Jerums G, Cooper ME. Advanced glycation end products cause epithelial-myofibroblast transdifferentiation via the receptor for advanced glycation end products (RAGE). J Clin Invest 2001: 108: 1853-63

23. Li Y, Mitsuhashi T, Wojciechowicz D, Shimizu N, Li J, Stitt A, He C, Banerjee D, Vlassara H. Molecular identity and distribution of advanced glycation endproducts receptors: Relationship of p60 to OST-48 and p90 to 80K-H membrane proteins. Proc Natl Acad Sci USA 1996; 93: 11047-11052

24. Li YM, Tan AX, Vlassara H. Antibacterial activity of lysozyme and lactoferrin is inhibited by binding of advanced glycation-modified proteins to a conserved motif. Nature Medicine 1995; 1: 1057-1061

25. Miyazaki A, Nakayama H, Horiuchi S.Scavenger receptors that recognize advanced glycation end products. Trends Cardiovasc Med. 2002;12(6):258-62

26. Jono T, Miyazaki A, Nagai R, Sawamura T, Kitamura T, Horiuchi S. Lectin-like oxidized low density lipoprotein receptor-1 (LOX-1) serves as an endothelial receptor for advanced glycation end products (AGE).FEBS Lett. 2002; 511(1-3):170-4

27. Kuniyasu A, Ohgami N, Hayashi S, Miyazaki A, Horiuchi S, Nakayama H.CD36-mediated endocytic uptake of advanced glycation end products (AGE) in mouse 3T3-L1 and human subcutaneous adipocytes.FEBS Lett. 2003; 537(1-3):85-90

28. Pugliese G, Pricci F, Iacobini C, Leto G, Amadio L, Barsotti P, Frigeri L, Hsu DK, Vlassara H, Liu FT, Di Mario U. Accelerated diabetic glomerulopathy in galectin-3/AGE receptor 3 knockout mice. FASEB J. 2001: 15(13):2471-9

29. He CJ, Zheng F, Stitt A, Striker L, Hattori M, Vlassara H. Differential expression of renal AGE-receptor genes in NOD mice: possible role in non obese diabetic renal disease. Kidney Int. 58(5):1931-40, 2000

30. He CJ, Koschinsky T, Buenting C, Vlassara H.Presence of diabetic complications in type 1 diabetic patients correlates with low expressionof mononuclear cell AGE-receptor-1 and elevated serum AGE. Mol Med. 2001; 7(3):159-68

31. Yamamoto Y, Kato I, Doi T, Yonekura H, Ohashi S, Takeuchi M, Watanabe T, Yamagishi S, Sakurai S, Takasawa S, Okamoto H, Yamamoto H. Development and prevention of advanced diabetic nephropathy in RAGE-overexpressing mice. J Clin Invest. 2001;108(2):261-8

32. Pettersson-Fernholm K, Forsblom C, Hudson BI, Perola M, Grant PJ, Groop PH. The Functional -374 T/A RAGE Gene Polymorphism Is Associated With Proteinuria and Cardiovascular Disease in Type 1 Diabetic Patients. Diabetes. 2003; 52(3):891-894

33. Bai P, Phua K, Hardt T, Cernadas M, Brodsky B. Glycation alters collagen fibril organization. Connect Tissue Res 1992; 28(1-2): 1-12

34. Nyengaard JR, Chang K, Berhorst S, Reiser KM, Williamson JR, Tilton RG. Discordant effects of guanidines on renal structure and function and on regional vascular dysfunction and collagen changes in diabetic rats. Diabetes. 1997; 46(1): 94-106

35. Cooper ME, Thallas V, Forbes J, Scalbert E, Sastra S, Darby I, Soulis T: The cross-link breaker, N-phenacylthiazolium bromide prevents vascular advanced glycation end-product accumulation. Diabetologia 2000;43: 660-664

36. Candido R, Forbes JM, Thomas MC, Thallas V, Dean RG, Burns WC, Tikellis C,Ritchie RH, Twigg SM, Cooper ME, Burrell LM. A Breaker of Advanced Glycation End Products Attenuates Diabetes-Induced Myocardial Structural Changes. Circ Res. 2003, March

37. Krishnamurti U, Rondeau E, Sraer JD, Michael AF, Tsilibary EC. Alterations in human glomerular epithelial cells interacting with nonenzymatically glycosylated matrix. J Biol Chem 1997; 272(44): 27966-70

38. Tarsio JF, Wigness B, Rhode TD, Rupp WM, Buchwald H, Furcht LT. Nonenzymatic glycation of fibronectin and alterations in the molecular association of cell matrix and basement membrane components in diabetes mellitus. Diabetes 1985; 34(5):477-84

39. Charonis AS, Tsilbary EC. Structural and functional changes of laminin and type IV collagen after nonenzymatic glycation. Diabetes 1992; 41 Suppl 2:49-51

40. Raabe HM, Hopner JH, Notbohm H, Sinnecker GH, Kruse K, Muller PK. Biochemical and biophysical alterations of the 7S and NC1 domain of collagen IV from human diabetic kidneys. Diabetologia 1998; 41(9):1073-9

41. Charonis AS, Tsilbary EC. Structural and functional changes of laminin and type IV collagen after nonenzymatic glycation. Diabetes 1992; 41 Suppl 2:49-51

42. Walton HA, Byrne J, Robinson GB. Studies of the permeation properties of glomerular basement membrane: cross-linking renders glomerular basement membrane permeable to protein. Biochim Biophys Acta 1992; 1138(3):173-83

43. Kelly DJ, Gilbert RE, Cox AJ, Soulis T, Jerums G, Cooper ME. Aminoguanidine ameliorates over-expression of prosclerotic growth factors and collagen deposition in experimental diabetic nephropathy. J Am Soc Nephrol 2001;12(10):2098-107

318

44. Kim YS, Kim BC, Song CY, Hong HK, Moon KC, Lee HS. Advanced glycosylation end products stimulate collagen mRNA synthesis in mesangial cells mediated by protein kinase C and transforming growth factor-beta. J Lab Clin Med 2001;138(1):59-68

45. Yang CW, Vlassara H, Peten EP, He CJ, Striker GE, Striker LJ. Advanced glycation end products up-regulate gene expression found in diabetic glomerular disease. Proc Natl Acad Sci U S A 1994; 91(20): 9436-40

46. Huang JS, Guh JY, Chen HC, Hung WC, Lai YH, Chuang LY. Role of receptor for advanced glycation end-product (RAGE) and the JAK/STAT-signaling pathway in AGE-induced collagen production in NRK-49F cells. J Cell Biochem 2001; 81(1):102-13

47. Riser BL, Denichilo M, Cortes P, Baker C, Grondin JM, Yee J, Narins RG. Regulation of connective tissue growth factor activity in cultured rat mesangial cells and its expression in experimental diabetic glomerulosclerosis. J Am Soc Nephrol 2000; 11(1):25-38

48. Twigg SM, Chen MM, Joly AH, Chakrapani SD, Tsubaki J, Kim HS, Oh Y, Rosenfeld RG. Advanced glycosylation end products up-regulate connective tissue growth factor (insulin-like growth factor-binding protein-related protein 2) in human fibroblasts: a potential mechanism for expansion of extracellular matrix in diabetes mellitus. Endocrinology 2001; 142(5):1760-9

49. Lan HY. Tubular epithelial-myofibroblast transdifferentiation mechanisms in proximal tubule cells. Curr Opin Nephrol Hypertens 2003; 12(1):25-9

50. Li JH, Huang XR, Zhu HJ, Oldfield M, Cooper ME, Truong LC, Johnson RJ, Lan HY. AGEs activate Smad signalling via TGFB dependent and independent mechanisms: implications for diabetic nephropathy and vascular disease. FASEB J (in press) April 2003.

51. Zeisberg M, Bonner G, Maeshima Y, Colorado P, Muller GA, Strutz F, Kalluri R. Renal fibrosis: collagen composition and assembly regulates epithelial-mesenchymal transdif-ferentiation. Am J Pathol 2001; 159(4):1313-21

52. Zaoui P, Cantin JF, Alimardani-Bessette M, Monier F, Halimi S, Morel F, Cordonnier Role of metalloproteases and inhibitors in the occurrence and progression of diabetic renal lesions. Diabetes Metab 2000; 26 Suppl 4: 25-9

53. McLennan SV, Martell SK, Yue DK. Effects of mesangium glycation on matrix metalloproteinase activities: possible role in diabetic nephropathy. Diabetes 51(8):2612-8, 2002

54. Baynes JW, Thorpe SR. Role of oxidative stress in diabetic complications: a new perspective on an old paradigm. Diabetes 1999; 48(1):1-9

55. Sugimoto H, Shikata K, Wada J, Horiuchi S, Makino H.Advanced glycation end products-cytokine-nitric oxide sequence pathway in the development of diabetic nephropathy: aminoguanidine ameliorates the overexpression of tumour necrosis factor-alpha and inducible nitric oxide synthase in diabetic rat glomeruli. Diabetologia. 1999; 42(7):878-86

56. Odetti P, Traverso N, Cosso L, Noberasco G, Pronzato MA, Marinari UM. Good glycaemic control reduces oxidation and glycation end-products in collagen of diabetic rats. *Diabetologia*. 1996; 39:1440-7

57. Lander HM, Tauras JM, Ogiste JS, Hori O, Moss RA, Schmidt AM. Activation of the receptor for advanced glycation end products triggers a p21(ras)-dependent mitogen-activated protein kinase pathway regulated by oxidant stress. J Biol Chem. 1997; 11;272(28):17810-4

58. Yim MB, Yim HS, Lee C, Kang SO, Chock PB. Protein glycation: creation of catalytic sites for free radical generation. Ann N Y Acad Sci 2001; 928:48-53

59. Wautier JL, Wautier MP, Schmidt AM, Anderson GM, Hori O, Zoukourian C, Capron L, Chappey O, Yan SD, Brett J, Advanced glycation end products (AGEs) on the surface of diabetic erythrocytes bind to the vessel wall via a specific receptor inducing oxidant stress in the vasculature: a link between surface-associated AGEs and diabetic complications. Proc Natl Acad Sci U S A.1994 ;91(16):7742-6

60. Rosca MG, Monnier VM, Szweda LI, Weiss MF. Alterations in renal mitochondrial respiration in response to the reactive oxoaldehyde methylglyoxal. Am J Physiol Renal Physiol. 2002; 283(1):F52-9,

61. Lal MA, Brismar H, Eklof AC, Aperia A. Role of oxidative stress in advanced glycation end product-induced mesangial cell activation. Kidney Int 2002; 61(6): 2006-14

62. Yamagishi S, Inagaki Y, Okamoto T, Amano S, Koga K, Takeuchi M.Advanced glycation end products inhibit de novo protein synthesis and induce TGF-beta overexpression in proximal tubular cells. Kidney Int. 2003; 63(2):464-73

63. Tsuchida K, Makita Z, Yamagishi S, Atsumi T, Miyoshi H, Obara S, Ishida M, Ishikawa S, Yasumura K, Koike T. Suppression of transforming growth factor beta and vascular endothelial growth factor in diabetic nephropathy in rats by a novel advanced glycation end product inhibitor, OPB-9195. Diabetologia. 1999;42(5):579-88.

64. Osicka TM, Yu Y, Panagiotopoulos S, Clavant SP, Kiriazis Z, Pike RN, Pratt LM, Russo LM, Kemp BE, Comper WD, Jerums G. Prevention of albuminuria by aminoguanidine or ramipril in streptozotocin-induced diabetic rats is associated with the normalization of glomerular protein kinase C. Diabetes 2000;49(1):87-93

65. Mifsud SA, Skinner SL, Cooper ME, Kelly DJ, Wilkinson-Berka JL. Effects of low-dose and early versus late perindopril treatment on the progression of severe diabetic nephropathy in (mREN-2)27 rats. J Am Soc Nephrol. 2002; 13(3):684-92

66. Wilkinson-Berka JL, Kelly DJ, Koerner SM, Jaworski K, Davis B, Thallas V, Cooper ME. ALT-946 and aminoguanidine, inhibitors of advanced glycation, improve severe nephropathy in the diabetic transgenic (mREN-2)27 rat. Diabetes.2002; 51(11):3283-9

67. Forbes JM, Cooper ME, Thallas V, Burns WC, Thomas MC, Brammar GC, Lee F, Grant SL, Burrell LA, Jerums G, Osicka TM. Reduction of the accumulation of advanced glycation end products by ACE inhibition in experimental diabetic nephropathy. Diabetes 2002 ;51(11):3274-82

68. Miyata T, van Ypersele de Strihou C, Ueda Y, Ichimori K, Inagi R, Onogi H, Ishikawa N, Nangaku M, Kurokawa K. Angiotensin II receptor antagonists and angiotensin-converting enzyme inhibitors lower in vitro the formation of advanced glycation end products: biochemical mechanisms. J Am Soc Nephrol 2002;13(10):2478-87

69. Onozato ML, Tojo A, Goto A, Fujita T, Wilcox CS. Oxidative stress and nitric oxide synthase in rat diabetic nephropathy: effects of ACEI and ARB. Kidney Int 2002; 61(1):186-94

70. Cooper ME, Mundel P, Boner G. Role of nephrin in renal disease including diabetic nephropathy. Semin Nephrol. 2002;22(5):393-8

71. Doublier S, Salvidio G, Lupia E, Ruotsalainen V, Verzola D, Deferrari G, Camussi G. Nephrin Expression Is Reduced in Human Diabetic Nephropathy: Evidence for a Distinct Role for Glycated Albumin and Angiotensin II. Diabetes. 2003; 52(4):1023-1030

72. Cooper ME. Pathogenesis, prevention, and treatment of diabetic nephropathy. Lancet. 1998 ;352(9123):213-9.

73. Soulis T, Cooper ME, Vranes D, Bucala R, Jerums G.Effects of aminoguanidine in preventing experimental diabetic nephropathy are related to the duration of treatment. Kidney Int 1996;50(2):627-34,

74. Forbes JM, Soulis T, Thallas V, Panagiotopoulos S, Long DM, Vasan S,Wagle D, Jerums G, Cooper ME. Renoprotective effects of a novel inhibitor of advanced glycation.Diabetologia. 2001;44(1):108-14

75. Degenhardt TP, Alderson NL, Arrington DD, Beattie RJ, Basgen JM, Steffes MW, Thorpe SR, Baynes JW. Pyridoxamine inhibits early renal disease and dyslipidemia in the streptozotocin-diabetic rat. Kidney Int 2002;61(3):939-50

76. Bucciarelli LG, Wendt T, Qu W, Lu Y, Lalla E, Rong LL, Goova MT, Moser B,Kislinger T, Lee DC, Kashyap Y, Stern DM, Schmidt AM.RAGE blockade stabilizes established atherosclerosis in diabetic apolipoprotein E-null mice. Circulation. 2002;106(22):2827-3

77. Zheng F, Cai W, Mitsuhashi T, Vlassara H. Lysozyme enhances renal excretion of advanced glycation endproducts in vivo and suppresses adverse age-mediated cellular effects in vitro: a potential AGE sequestration therapy for diabetic nephropathy? Mol Med. 2001; 7(11):737-47

78. Koschinsky T, He CJ, Mitsuhashi T, Bucala R, Liu C, Buenting C, Heitmann K, Vlassara H. Orally absorbed reactive glycation products (glycotoxins): an environmental risk factor in diabetic nephropathy. Proc Natl Acad Sci U S A. 1997; 10;94(12):6474-9

79. Cerami C, Founds H, Nicholl I, Mitsuhashi T, Giordano D, Vanpatten S, Lee A, Al-Abed Y, Vlassara H, Bucala R, Cerami A. Tobacco smoke is a source of toxic reactive glycation products. Proc Natl Acad Sci U S A. 1997; 9;94(25):13915-20

80. Zheng F, He C, Cai W, Hattori M, Steffes M, Vlassara H. Prevention of diabetic nephropathy in mice by a diet low in glycoxidation products. Diabetes Metab Res Rev. 2002; 18(3):224-37

81. Vlassara H, Cai W, Crandall J, Goldberg T, Oberstein R, Dardaine V, Peppa M, Rayfield EJ. Inflammatory mediators are induced by dietary glycotoxins, a major risk factor for diabetic angiopathy. Proc Natl Acad Sci U S A. 2002 ; 99(24):15596-601

82. Nicholl ID, Stitt AW, Moore JE, Ritchie AJ, Archer DB, Bucala R. Increased levels of advanced glycation endproducts in the lenses and blood vessels of cigarette smokers. Mol Med. 1998; 4(9):594-601,

83. Uribarri J, Peppa M, Cai W, Goldberg T, Lu M, He C, Vlassara H. Restriction of dietary glycotoxins reduces excessive advanced glycation end products in renal failure patients. J Am Soc Nephrol. 2003; 14(3):728-31

84. Appel G, Bolton K, Freedman B, Wuerth JP, Cartwright K: Pimagedine lowers total urinary protein and slows progression of overt diabetic nephropathy in patients with type 1 diabetes mellitus. J Am SocNephrol 1999; 10:153A

85. Brown CD, Zhao ZH, Thomas LL, deGroof R, Friedman EA. Effects of erythropoietin and aminoguanidine on red blood cell deformability in diabetic azotemic and uremic patients. Am J Kidney Dis. 2001; 38(6):1414-20

86. Kass DA, Shapiro EP, Kawaguchi M, Capriotti AR, Scuteri A, deGroof RC, Lakatta EG. Improved arterial compliance by a novel advanced glycation end-product crosslink breaker. Circulation. 2001; 104(13):1464-70

87. Data Presented at Ninth Annual Scientific session of the Society of Geriatric Cardiology [http://www.pharmalive.com/news/show_article.asp?articleID=80504&catid=14]

PROTEIN KINASE C ACTIVATION AND ITS INHIBITION FOR THE TREATMENT OF DIABETIC RENAL PATHOLOGIES

Ronald Ma[1], Keiji Isshiki[2] and George L. King[3]

[1]*Department of Medicine and Therapeutics, Prince Of Wales Hospital, Hong Kong,*
[2]*Department of Medicine, Shiga University of Medical Science, Seta, Otsu Shiga 520-2192,*
Japan, [3]*Research Division, Joslin Diabetes Center, Department of Medicine, Harvard Medical*
School, Boston, MA 02215, USA

INTRODUCTION

The Diabetes Control and Complications Trial (DCCT) and the United Kingdom Prospective Diabetes Study (UKPDS) reported that the strict maintenance of euglycemia by intensive insulin treatment can delay the onset and slow the progression of diabetic nephropathy, respectively, in patients with type 1 and type 2 diabetes mellitus [1, 2]. These studies suggested that the adverse effects of hyperglycemia on metabolic pathways are the main causes of long-term complications in diabetes such as kidney disease. The importance of excessive glucose in the development of diabetic renal glomerular abnormalities is supported by the results of Heilig et al., who found that the overexpression of glucose transporter 1 (GLUT1) into glomerular mesangial cells enhanced the production of extracellular matrix components which may contribute to mesangial expansion [3]. Multiple biochemical mechanisms have been proposed to explain the adverse effects of hyperglycemia. Activation of diacylglycerol (DAG)-protein kinase C (PKC) pathway [4, 5], enhanced polyol pathway related with myo-inositol depletion [6], altered redox state [7], overproduction of advanced glycation end products [8], and enhanced growth factor and cytokine production [9, 10] have all been proposed as potential cellular mechanisms by which hyperglycemia induces the chronic diabetic complications.

In this article, evidence regarding the activation of DAG-PKC pathway will be briefly reviewed (Fig. 1) [11].

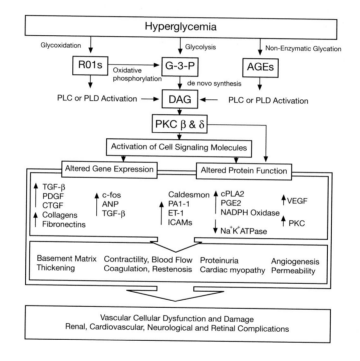

Figure 1. Diagram of the effects of DAG-PKC activation in diabetes vascular complications. ROI indicates reactive oxygen intermediate; G-3-P, glycerlaldehyde-3-phosphate; AGE, advanced glycation endproduct; DAG, diacylglycerol; PLC, phospholipase C; PLD, phospholipase D; PKC, protein kinase C; TGF-β, transforming growth factor-β; PDGF, platelet derived growth factor; CTGF, connective tissue growth factor; PLA$_2$, cytosolic phospholipase A$_2$; PGE$_2$, prostaglandin E$_2$; PAI-1, plasminogen activator inhibitor type-1; ET-1, endothelin-1; ICAM, intercellular adhesion molecule-1; ANP, atrial natriuretic peptide; VEGF, vascular endothelial growth factor.

The possibility that changes in PKC activities could be causing diabetic vascular complications has been discussed frequently due to the finding that PKC activation can increase vascular permeability, extracellular matrix synthesis, contractility, leukocyte attachment, cell growth, and angiogenesis [12-14]. All of these vascular functions have been reported to be abnormal in the diabetic state. When the DAG levels and PKC activities were first quantitated, we and Craven et al. showed that elevating glucose concentration from 5 to 20 mM increased both DAG and PKC levels in vascular cells or tissue including renal glomeruli, retina, and aorta [15-18]. Possible activation of DAG-PKC has also been reported in the liver and skeletal muscle of insulin resistant and diabetic animals, suggesting that the activation of DAG-PKC signal transduction pathway may also be induced in insulin resistance by other abnormal metabolites other than glucose such as the elevation of free fatty acids [19-23]. Activation of PKC, especially the β-isoform has been shown to be increased in monocytes from type 2 diabetic patients and in healthy people in which an acute rise of plasma glucose was induced [24]. Furthermore, the normalization of circulating plasma glucose by insulin infusion, in diabetic patients, resulted in a slight reduction of PKC activity. These data indicate that PKC activation in diabetes is largely accounted for by hyperglycemia and monocyte PKC activation may even be partly responsible for the accelerated atherosclerosis in type 2 diabetic patients [24].

It is not surprising that the activation of PKC could affect such a wide range of tissues and cellular activities since PKC is a family of serine and threonine kinases which act as intracellular signal transduction system for many cytokines and hormones [12, 13]. Different PKC isoforms are also one of the major downstream targets for lipid signaling molecules and can be classified according to their structure differences. Conventional PKC isoforms (α, β1, β2, γ) are sensitive to both Ca++ and DAG whereas new PKC isoforms (δ, ε, η/L, θ) are sensitive to DAG but insensitive to Ca++ due to the loss of Cl region. Atypical PKC isoforms (ς, ι/λ) may also be sensitive to other phospholipids such as the products of phosphatidylinositol-3-kinase [25, 26].

MECHANISMS OF PKC-ACTIVATION

The sources of cellular DAG are multiple with the majority derived from the hydrolysis of polyphosphoinositides or phosphatidylcholine by phospholipase C or D, respectively [12-14]. The mechanism by which PKC is activated by diabetes and by hyperglycemia appears to be related to increase in de novo synthesis of DAG through glycolytic pathway [15, 18]. It is also possible that the increases in free fatty acids in diabetic state may enhance the synthesis of DAG levels [25, 27-29].

We and others have found that the elevation of DAG level is directly responsible for the activation of PKC in glomeruli of diabetic rats and cultured mesangial cells exposed to high glucose concentrations [15, 17, 30]. The role of increasing DAG in causing PKC activation by hyperglycemia is support by the studies of using high doses of vitamin E or inhibitors of DAG kinase which decrease the metabolism of DAG to phosphatidic acid [31]. Vitamin E treatment at high doses, equivalent to 1500-1800 unit/day, in animal models of diabetes and in diabetic patients, improved renal hyperfiltration associated with normalization of DAG/PKC pathway through activation of DAG kinase [32, 33].

Multiple PKC isoforms are activated in each vascular tissue of diabetic animal models. Among them PKC-β isoforms appear to be most consistently increased. Using immunoblotting study we have reported that PKC-α and β1 isoforms exhibited a greater increase, in vivo, in membranous fractions isolated from diabetic rat glomeruli and, in vitro, in mesangial cells exposed to elevated glucose levels [30], whereas PKC-β2 was reported to be preferentially activated in aorta and heart of diabetic rats [16]. Interestingly, Kikkawa et al. have reported that PKC-ς as well as PKC-α was activated in rat glomerular mesangial cells exposed to high glucose concentrations [34], although the mechanism for PKC-ς activation, which is independent on DAG, is unclear. Whiteside et al reported the PKC-β-isoform was also increased in the membrane pool in the glomeruli of diabetic rats [35].

PATHOPHYSIOLOGY OF PKC ACTIVATION

Functionally, the activation of DAG-PKC pathway has been correlated with many vascular changes in enzymatic activities, gene expressions, contractility, extracellular matrix synthesis, and cell growth and differentiation. To determine those vascular or renal dysfunctions which are due to specifically the activation of PKC-β isoform, we have characterized a selective inhibitor to PKC-β isoform (LY333531) and studied its effect on glomerular cells or tissues from diabetic animals. The specificity of PKC-β inhibitor LY333531 was evaluated by in vitro study, which examined PKC isoform-induced phosphorylation of myelin basic protein. LY333531 inhibited PKC-β1 and β2 with a half-maximal inhibitory constant (IC50) of 4.5 and 5.9 nM, respectively, whereas the IC50 was 250 nM or greater for other PKC isoforms and over 1 μM for other non PKC kinases [17]. Furthermore, its specificity was confirmed in vivo study to examine the phosphorylation of PKC α and β1, which has been shown to correspond to PKC isoform specific activation, in isolated glomeruli from control and streptozotocin (STZ)-induced diabetic rats with or without LY333531 (10 mg/kg body wt/day) [30]. Diabetes enhanced phosphorylation of both PKC α and β1 by 60 and 75%, respectively. PKC-β specific inhibitor LY333531 prevented the increase in phosphorylation of PKC-β1 but not PKC-α in the glomeruli of diabetic rats, indicating the specific PKC-β isoform inhibition by LY333531 occurs in vivo [30].

INVOLVEMENT OF PKC IN RENAL HEMODYNAMICS

The effects of PKC-β isoform inhibitor, LY333531, on renal hemodynamics were examined first. These functional parameters included glomerular filtration rates (GFR) and urinary albumin excretion rates (UAE). Treatment with LY333531 orally at the onset of diabetes normalized GFR and glomerular PKC activity in a dose-dependent manner [17]. Intervention treatment with LY333531 also ameliorated the increase in urinary albumin excretion rate in diabetic rats 12 weeks after the onset of diabetes [17], suggesting that PKC-β activation may cause the early hemodynamic and histological abnormalities which have been implicated to be responsible for glomerular injury leading to the progression of diabetic nephropathy. Unlike PKC-β inhibitor, vitamin E treatment in diabetic rats reduced renal DAG levels, normalized PCK-β activation and glomerular filtration rates [32].

Treatment with high-dose of vitamin E in type 1 diabetic patients, with <10 years duration of disease and no microalbuminuria, significantly normalized renal hyperfiltration. Diabetic patients with the highest creatinine clearances and poorest glycemic control showed the most marked normalization in response to vitamin E treatment [33].

One possible mechanism to explain renal hyperfiltration in poorly controlled diabetes is the increase in vasodilatory prostanoids such as prostaglandin E_2 (PGE_2) which have been noted in the kidney of diabetic patients and animals with glomerular hyperfiltration [36, 37]. We have reported that the possible overproduction of glomerular PGE_2 in the glomeruli of diabetic rats could be due to an enhanced synthesis of arachidonic acid via the activation of cytosolic phospholipase A_2 ($cPLA_2$) by PKC since specific inhibitor of PKC-β isoform was able to decrease PGE_2 and arachidonic acid release by hyperglycemia [30]. Haneda et al. have found that the increase in mitogen-activated protein kinase (MAPK) activity, which was dependent on diabetes-induced activation of PKC pathway, was able to enhance $cPLA_2$ activity, resulting in increase in arachidonic acid release in glomerular mesangial cells exposed to elevated glucose levels [38]. Williams et al. have also reported similar findings showing that PKC activation by glucose increased PGE_2 production through $cPLA_2$ and it was normalized in the presence of general PKC inhibitors such as H-7 or staurosporine in glomerular mesangial cells [6].

These results strongly support that diabetes-induced hyperfiltration could be due to an overproduction of vasodilatory prostanoids through the activation of $cPLA_2$ which was due to the activation of PKC-MAPK pathway. In addition, Igarashi et al. identified p38 MAP kinase as a possible intermediate target, in vascular cells, which can be activated by high glucose levels and diabetes [39]. Its activation is mediated by either PKC-dependent or -independent pathways, with the latter induced significantly by levels of hyperglycemia not usually observed clinically. At moderate and commonly encountered levels of hyperglycemia, p38 MAP kinase was activated by PKC-β isoform-dependent processes [39].

Another important biochemical change induced by DAG-PKC activation is the inhibition of Na+-K+ ATPase, an integral component of the sodium pump, which is involved in the maintenance of cellular integrity and functions such as contractility, growth, and differentiation [40]. Its inhibition has been well established in the vascular and neural tissues of diabetic patients and diabetic experimental animals [6]. However, the mechanisms by which hyperglycemia can inhibit Na+-K+ ATPase is still unclear especially regarding the role of PKC. We have found that PKC activation induced by diabetes or hyperglycemia can lead to the inhibition of Na+-K+ ATPase. PKC-β inhibitor prevented the decrease of Na+-K+ATPase induced by hyperglycemia, suggesting the importance of PKC-β activation in the development of mesangial or glomerular dysfunctions which are due to the inhibition of Na+-K+ ATPase activity in diabetes [30].

INVOLVEMENT OF PKC IN GLOMERULAR STRUCTURAL CHANGES

One of the most important glomerular pathological changes in diabetic nephropathy is structural alterations including glomerular hypertrophy, basement membrane thickening, and mesangial expansion due to the accumulation of extracellular matrix components such as collagen and fibronectin [41]. A close relationship is also ovserved between mesangial expansion and the declining surface area available for glomerular filtration. Thus, the mechanisms responsible for mesangial expansion are closely related to the formation of nodular glomerulosclerosis, resulting in end stage diabetic nephropathy.

Although multiple mechanisms are probably involved in causing mesangial expansion, many studies have recently focused on the role of transforming growth factor β (TGF-β), a multifunctional cytokine, in the regulation of extracellular matrix production in diabetic nephropathy and other tissues where fibrosis is present [9, 10]. TGF-β can stimulate the production of extracellular matrix such as type IV collagen, fibronectin and laminin in cultured mesangial cells and epithelial cells [42-44]. Increase in gene and protein expressions of TGF-β were found in glomeruli from diabetic animal models as well as diabetic patients [45-49], suggesting that overexpression of TGF-β might be responsible for the development of mesangial expansion in diabetic nephropathy. This hypothesis was strengthen by the fact that inhibition of TGF-β activity with neutralizing antibody attenuates the increase in mRNA expressions of type IV collagen and fibronectin in renal cortex and glomeruli of diabetic animal models [50-53]. Since PKC is well-known stimulator for synthesis of type IV collagen and fibronectin [54], it has been postulated that PKC activation might be involved in the enhancement of TGF-β expression in diabetes. To substantiate this hypothesis, we have examined the effect of PKC-β inhibitor LY333531 on the gene expressions of TGF-β1, type IV collagen, and fibronectin in glomeruli of control and diabetic rats [30]. In the glomeruli of diabetic rats, the expression of TGF-β1 mRNA was significantly increased compared to control rats [30].

Treatment with LY333531 and other PKC inhibitors abrogated the enhanced glomerular expression of TGF-β mRNA in diabetic rats [30, 55, 56]. LY333531 also prevented mRNA overexpression of extracellular matrix components such as type IV collagen and fibronectin in the glomeruli of diabetic rats, again supporting the importance of PKC-β activation and TGF-β expression in causing extracellular matrix protein overproduction.

CTGF

TGF-β driven matrix synthesis has been recently showed to be mediated partly by connective tissue growth factor (CTGF), a pro-fibrotic factor, which Murphy et al showed to be expressed in renal cortex and glomeruli of rat kidneys with diabetic nephropathy and to be induced in primary human mesangial cells exposed to high glucose levels, through TGF-β1 and PKC dependent pathways [57]. Similar reports with regard to CTGF and TGF-β have been reported in other vascular tissues suggest that inhibition of the PKC-β isoform with LY333531 could prevent the increase in CTGF expression due to PKC-β activation and prevent the resultant extracellular matrix deposition [58, 59].

VEGF

An increase in vascular permeability is an important early manifestation of diabetic vascular dysfunction, especially in retinal vessels and kidneys. Marked increases in albumin permeation have been reported in the eye, sciatic nerve, aorta and kidney obtained from diabetic rats [60]. Vascular endothelial growth factor (VEGF) in a potent vascular permeability factor and can stimulate vascular endothelial cells to proliferate [61]. VEGF appears to be the primary mediator of the neovascularization observed in proliferative diabetic retinopathy [62], and could also be important in inducinge vascular permeability in diabetic nephropathy. VEGF could potentially contribute to renal pathology by induction of CTGF [63]. Chou et al [64] showed that in glomeruli from STZ-induced diabetic rats and insulin-resistant rats, there is a 2 fold increase in the expression of VEGF and its receptors. Increased expressions of VEGF and its receptor VEGF-R2 in distal tubules and collecting ducts have also been reported in experimental diabetes as demonstrated by using radiolabelled VEGF [65]. A recent study in rat mesangial cells found that high glucose can induce the expression of VEGF in cultured mesangial cells, and this was inhibited by a PKC inhibitor [66]. There is now accumulating evidence from studies on various microvascular tissues that VEGF action is mediated by PKC [67, 68]. Thus, it is possible that part of the protective effects of PKC beta inhibitor on diabetic nephropathy is due to the inhibition of VEGF action in the kidney. It is interesting to note that administration of neutralizing antibodies to VEGF for 6 weeks was associated with resolution of hyperfiltration and attenuation of albuminuria in a rat model of experimental diabetes [69] and a type 2 diabetes model using db/db mice [70].

OTHER AGENTS AND METABOLITES WHICH CAN ALTER

Thiazolidinediones

Thiazolidinedione (TZD) compounds are widely used as oral hypoglycemic agents. A recent study in diabetic rats and mesangial cells cultured under high glucose condition reported that treatment with troglitazone can ameliorate the increase in glomerular hyperfiltration, albumin excretion and extracellular matrix deposition associated with diabetes. This is attributed to the action of thiazolidinediones on activating a DAG kinase, which could metabolize DAG to phosphatidic acid and therefore avoid the accumulation of DAG and its subsequent activation of the DAG-PKC-ERK pathway. This finding suggests that TZDs potentially could be beneficial for diabetic nephropathy by preventing the activation of DAG-PKC-ERK pathway [71].

Vitamin E

Increase in oxidative stress is observed in renal glomeruli and many of the vascular and non-vascular tissues exposed to hyperglycemia. Evidence seems to suggest that oxidative stress may contribute to the properties of diabetic complications. Strong evidence also exists that oxidants could be mediating its their adverse effects activating DAG-PKC pathways. d-alpha-tocopherol (vitamin E) has been reported to reverse the changes in microvascular tissue in diabetes. In addition to its antioxidant properties, vitamin E has been reported to modulate the PKC signal transduction pathway [33]. Intraperitoneal administration of d-alpha-tocopherol to diabetic rats prevented the increased glomerular filtration and albumin excretion associated with diabetes [32]. This effect was also thought to be due to its antioxidant action and the modulation of DAG kinase activity, with vitamin E treatment leading to decreased DAG levels and reduced PKC activation [32, 72]. The effect of vitamin E was tested in a recent clinical trial in 36 patients with type 1 diabetes of less than 10 years duration with minimal diabetic retinopathy or microalbuminuria, where it was found that 4 month treatment with high-dose vitamin E (1800IU/day) lead to a significant reversal of the reduced retinal blood flow and a reduction in the hyperfiltration in diabetic subjects [33]. Gaede et al has reported that 800

IU/day of vitamin E decrease microalbuminuria in type 1 diabetes patients after only three months of treatment.

Advanced Glycation Endproducts (AGE) inhibitors, Soluble receptor of AGEs

Aminoguanidine, an inhibitor of AGE formation, can block the development of the microvascular complications of diabetes in animal models possibly by inhibiting PKC activation [8, 73, 74]. However, the effect of aminoguanidine cannot be interpreted as definitive in support of the AGE concept since it has parallel action as an inhibitor of inducible nitric oxidant [75, 76]. Clinical trials of aminoguanidine have been limited because of its toxicity. The receptors of AGEs (RAGE) interactions have been shown to include PKC activation in cultured cells [77]. The use of soluble RAGE to block binding to RAGE in animal models of diabetes has been reported to prevent several effects of hyperglycemia with some through inhibiting PKC activation [78].

Angiotensin converting enzyme inhibitors (ACEI)

ACEIs are anti-hypertensive drugs with a well known-effects in preventing the progression of chronic renal failure [79]. Numerous reports have documented the defensive effects of ACEIs in various abnormalities of diabetic nephropathy in both human and animals. In addition, some reports have shown that ACEI agents can decrease albuminuria through the inhibition of PKC activation in diabetic animal models [74, 80, 81]. However, it is possible that these effects of ACEI are related to angiotensin activities directly or to inhibitions of the PKC system [80, 82]. Recently, Kelly et al reported that PKCβ inhibitors can attenuate the progression of experimental nephropathy in transgenic rats, (mRen-2)27 rats, which are expressing the entire mouse renin gene (Ren-2) and develop many similar characteristics to human diabetic nephropathy when diabetes is induced with STZ [56]. Conversely, it is reported that activation of PKCβII can induce ACE expression in neonatal rat cardiomyocytes [83]. Thus, cross talk between the renin-angiotensin system and the PKC pathway appear to exist and may be significant in the development of diabetic nephropathy.

RESULTS FROM CLINICAL TRIALS

The safety and vascular effects of LY333531 were evaluated in a one month clinical study on 29 patients with type 1 or 2 diabetes of less than 10 years, with no or minimal retinopathy. This double-blind, placebo-controlled randomized trial showed significant improvement in retinal blood flow and mean circulation time with no change in glycemic indices [84]. Results of the clinical trial of

LY333531 in diabetic neuropathy have also been reported recently. A 1-year double-blind, randomized, placcbo-controled trial with LY333531 at 32mg or 64mg was carried out on 205 patients with type 1 or 2 diabetes and diabetic peripheral neuropathy. The results showed that LY333531 improved both symptoms of neuropathy and vibration detection threshold [85] as well as objective measures of nerve function by physician assessment. The Protein Kinase C Diabetic Retinopathy Study (PKC-DRS), a multi-national, multi-center, placebo-controlled, randomized, double-masked, 4-arm clinical trial designed to evaluate the effects of LY333531 on the progression of diabetic retinopathy is also nearing completion and its results should be available soon [84]. PKCβ isoform activation may induce endothelial dysfunction. Beckman et al have reported that PKCβ isoform inhibitor, LY333531, was able to normalize endothelial induced vasodilation in hyperglycemia-induced endothelial dysfunction [86].

SUMMARY

Great deal of evidence have accumulated to indicate that PKC, especially the β isoform, activation can cause many of the pathophysiological abnormalities associated with the development and progression of diabetic nephropathy and other vascular diseases in the diabetic states. The ability of PKC-β specific inhibitor LY333531 to prevent diabetes induced glomerular hyperfiltration, increase in albuminuria, inhibition of Na+-K+ ATPase and glomerular overexpression of TGF-β and extracellular matrix components suggested that PKC-β activation induced by diabetes and hyperglycemia lies in intracellular signaling pathway leading to these abnormalities. The availability of PKC-β inhibitor LY333531 provided an important tool to decipher insights into the molecular pathogenesis of diabetic nephropathy. Clinical studies using PKC-β inhibitor LY333531 which are ongoing will determine the therapeutic usefulness of PKC-β inhibition in diabetic complications. In addition, other isoforms of PKC such as α and δ isoform may also be important. Isoform selective inhibitors of these PKC's should be developed and tested for their in vivo activites.

Since vitamin E and thiazolidinedione treatments have been shown to be beneficial in normalizing renal hemodynamics without changing glycemic control in animal models of diabetes. It is possible that these agents may also decrease the risks of developing diabetic nephropathy by modulating the DAG-PKC pathway.

ACKNOWLEDGEMENTS

Dr. Ronald Ma is recipient of a Croucher Foundation Fellowship, a training fellowship form the Hong Kong Society of Endocrinology, Metabolism and Reproduction and a William Randolph Hearst Foundation Fellowship. Dr. Keiji Isshiki is recipient of a mentor fellowship from American Diabetes Association. Studies were supported by National Institutes of Health grants, NIH ROI-EY05110 and EY9178

REFERENCES

1   The Diabetes Control and Complications Trial Research Group: The effect of intensive treatment of diabetes on the development and progression of long-term complications in insulin-dependent diabetes mellitus. N Engl J Med 329: 977-86, 1993
2   UK Prospective Diabetes Study (UKPDS) Group: Intensive blood-glucose control with sulphonylureas or insulin compared with conventional treatment and risk of complications in patients with type 2 diabetes (UKPDS 33). UK Prospective Diabetes Study (UKPDS) Group. Lancet 352: 837-53, 1998
3   Heilig CW, Concepcion LA, Riser BL, Freytag SO, Zhu M and Cortes P: Overexpression of glucose transporters in rat mesangial cells cultured in a normal glucose milieu mimics the diabetic phenotype. J Clin Invest 96: 1802-14, 1995
4   King GL, Ishii H and Koya D: Diabetic vascular dysfunctions: a model of excessive activation of protein kinase C. Kidney Int Suppl 60: S77-85, 1997
5   Derubertis FR and Craven PA: Activation of protein kinase C in glomerular cells in diabetes. Mechanisms and potential links to the pathogenesis of diabetic glomerulopathy. Diabetes 43: 1-8, 1994
6   Greene DA, Lattimer SA and Sima AA: Sorbitol, phosphoinositides, and sodium-potassium-ATPase in the pathogenesis of diabetic complications. N Engl J Med 316: 599-606, 1987
7   Williamson JR, Chang K, Frangos M, Hasan KS, Ido Y, Kawamura T, Nyengaard JR, van den Enden M, Kilo C and Tilton RG: Hyperglycemic pseudohypoxia and diabetic complications. Diabetes 42: 801-13, 1993
8   Brownlee M, Cerami A and Vlassara H: Advanced glycosylation end products in tissue and the biochemical basis of diabetic complications. N Engl J Med 318: 1315-21, 1988
9   Sharma K and Ziyadeh FN: Hyperglycemia and diabetic kidney disease. The case for transforming growth factor-beta as a key mediator. Diabetes 44: 1139-46, 1995
10   Mogyorosi A and Ziyadeh FN: Update on pathogenesis, markers and management of diabetic nephropathy. Curr Opin Nephrol Hypertens 5: 243-53, 1996
11   Sheetz MJ and King GL: Molecular understanding of hyperglycemia's adverse effects for diabetic complications. Jama 288: 2579-88, 2002
12   Nishizuka Y: Intracellular signaling by hydrolysis of phospholipids and activation of protein kinase C. Science 258: 607-14, 1992

13   Nishizuka Y: Protein kinase C and lipid signaling for sustained cellular responses. Faseb J 9: 484-96, 1995

14   Liscovitch M and Cantley LC: Lipid second messengers. Cell 77: 329-34, 1994

15   Craven PA, Davidson CM and DeRubertis FR: Increase in diacylglycerol mass in isolated glomeruli by glucose from de novo synthesis of glycerolipids. Diabetes 39: 667-74, 1990

16   Inoguchi T, Battan R, Handler E, Sportsman JR, Heath W and King GL: Preferential elevation of protein kinase C isoform beta II and diacylglycerol levels in the aorta and heart of diabetic rats: differential reversibility to glycemic control by islet cell transplantation. Proc Natl Acad Sci U S A 89: 11059-63, 1992

17   Ishii H, Jirousek MR, Koya D, Takagi C, Xia P, Clermont A, Bursell SE, Kern TS, Ballas LM, Heath WF, Stramm LE, Feener EP and King GL: Amelioration of vascular dysfunctions in diabetic rats by an oral PKC beta inhibitor. Science 272: 728-31, 1996

18   Inoguchi T, Xia P, Kunisaki M, Higashi S, Feener EP and King GL: Insulin's effect on protein kinase C and diacylglycerol induced by diabetes and glucose in vascular tissues. Am J Physiol 267: E369-79, 1994

19   Heydrick SJ, Ruderman NB, Kurowski TG, Adams HB and Chen KS: Enhanced stimulation of diacylglycerol and lipid synthesis by insulin in denervated muscle. Altered protein kinase C activity and possible link to insulin resistance. Diabetes 40: 1707-11, 1991

20   Cortright RN, Azevedo JL, Jr., Zhou Q, Sinha M, Pories WJ, Itani SI and Dohm GL: Protein kinase C modulates insulin action in human skeletal muscle. Am J Physiol Endocrinol Metab 278: E553-62, 2000

21   Bell KS, Schmitz-Peiffer C, Lim-Fraser M, Biden TJ, Cooney GJ and Kraegen EW: Acute reversal of lipid-induced muscle insulin resistance is associated with rapid alteration in PKC-theta localization. Am J Physiol Endocrinol Metab 279: E1196-201, 2000

22   Ikeda Y, Olsen GS, Ziv E, Hansen LL, Busch AK, Hansen BF, Shafrir E and Mosthaf-Seedorf L: Cellular mechanism of nutritionally induced insulin resistance in Psammomys obesus: overexpression of protein kinase Cepsilon in skeletal muscle precedes the onset of hyperinsulinemia and hyperglycemia. Diabetes 50: 584-92, 2001

23   Dohm GL: Mechanisms of muscle insulin resistance in obese individuals. Int J Sport Nutr Exerc Metab 11 Suppl: S64-70, 2001

24   Ceolotto G, Gallo A, Miola M, Sartori M, Trevisan R, Del Prato S, Semplicini A and Avogaro A: Protein kinase C activity is acutely regulated by plasma glucose concentration in human monocytes in vivo. Diabetes 48: 1316-22, 1999

25   Newton AC: Regulation of the ABC kinases by phosphorylation: protein kinase C as a paradigm. Biochem J 370: 361-71, 2003

26   Parekh DB, Ziegler W and Parker PJ: Multiple pathways control protein kinase C phosphorylation. Embo J 19: 496-503, 2000

27   Evans L, Frenkel L, Brophy CM, Rosales O, Sudhaker CB, Li G, Du W and Sumpio BE: Activation of diacylglycerol in cultured endothelial cells exposed to cyclic strain. Am J Physiol 272: C650-6, 1997

28   Yu C, Chen Y, Cline GW, Zhang D, Zong H, Wang Y, Bergeron R, Kim JK, Cushman SW, Cooney GJ, Atcheson B, White MF, Kraegen EW and Shulman GI: Mechanism by which fatty acids inhibit insulin activation of insulin receptor substrate-1 (IRS-1)-associated phosphatidylinositol 3-kinase activity in muscle. J Biol Chem 277: 50230-6, 2002

29   Boden G and Shulman GI: Free fatty acids in obesity and type 2 diabetes: defining their role in the development of insulin resistance and beta-cell dysfunction. Eur J Clin Invest 32 Suppl 3: 14-23, 2002

30   Koya D, Jirousek MR, Lin YW, Ishii H, Kuboki K and King GL: Characterization of protein kinase C beta isoform activation on the gene expression of transforming growth factor-beta, extracellular matrix components, and prostanoids in the glomeruli of diabetic rats. J Clin Invest 100: 115-26, 1997

31   Bursell SE, Takagi C, Clermont AC, Takagi H, Mori F, Ishii H and King GL: Specific retinal diacylglycerol and protein kinase C beta isoform modulation mimics abnormal retinal hemodynamics in diabetic rats. Invest Ophthalmol Vis Sci 38: 2711-20, 1997

32   Koya D, Lee IK, Ishii H, Kanoh H and King GL: Prevention of glomerular dysfunction in diabetic rats by treatment with d-alpha-tocopherol. J Am Soc Nephrol 8: 426-35, 1997

33   Bursell SE, Clermont AC, Aiello LP, Aiello LM, Schlossman DK, Feener EP, Laffel L and King GL: High-dose vitamin E supplementation normalizes retinal blood flow and creatinine clearance in patients with type 1 diabetes. Diabetes Care 22: 1245-51, 1999

34   Kikkawa R, Haneda M, Uzu T, Koya D, Sugimoto T and Shigeta Y: Translocation of protein kinase C alpha and zeta in rat glomerular mesangial cells cultured under high glucose conditions. Diabetologia 37: 838-41, 1994

35   Whiteside CI and Dlugosz JA: Mesangial cell protein kinase C isozyme activation in the diabetic milieu. Am J Physiol Renal Physiol 282: F975-80, 2002

36   Perico N, Benigni A, Gabanelli M, Piccinelli A, Rog M, De Riva C and Remuzzi G: Atrial natriuretic peptide and prostacyclin synergistically mediate hyperfiltration and hyperperfusion of diabetic rats. Diabetes 41: 533-8, 1992

37   Craven PA, Caines MA and DeRubertis FR: Sequential alterations in glomerular prostaglandin and thromboxane synthesis in diabetic rats: relationship to the hyperfiltration of early diabetes. Metabolism 36: 95-103, 1987

38   Haneda M, Araki S, Togawa M, Sugimoto T, Isono M and Kikkawa R: Mitogen-activated protein kinase cascade is activated in glomeruli of diabetic rats and glomerular mesangial cells cultured under high glucose conditions. Diabetes 46: 847-53, 1997

39   Igarashi M, Wakasaki H, Takahara N, Ishii H, Jiang ZY, Yamauchi T, Kuboki K, Meier M, Rhodes CJ and King GL: Glucose or diabetes activates p38 mitogen-activated protein kinase via different pathways. J Clin Invest 103: 185-95, 1999

40   Vasilets LA and Schwarz W: Structure-function relationships of cation binding in the Na+/K(+)-ATPase. Biochim Biophys Acta 1154: 201-22, 1993

41   Ziyadeh FN: The extracellular matrix in diabetic nephropathy. Am J Kidney Dis 22: 736-44, 1993

42   Gilbert RE, Cox A, Wu LL, Allen TJ, Hulthen UL, Jerums G and Cooper ME: Expression of transforming growth factor-beta1 and type IV collagen in the renal tubulointerstitium in experimental diabetes: effects of ACE inhibition. Diabetes 47: 414-22, 1998

43   MacKay K, Striker LJ, Stauffer JW, Doi T, Agodoa LY and Striker GE: Transforming growth factor-beta. Murine glomerular receptors and responses of isolated glomerular cells. J Clin Invest 83: 1160-7, 1989

44   Nakamura T, Miller D, Ruoslahti E and Border WA: Production of extracellular matrix by glomerular epithelial cells is regulated by transforming growth factor-beta 1. Kidney Int 41: 1213-21, 1992

45   Hong SW, Isono M, Chen S, Iglesias-De La Cruz MC, Han DC and Ziyadeh FN: Increased glomerular and tubular expression of transforming growth factor-beta1, its type II receptor, and activation of the Smad signaling pathway in the db/db mouse. Am J Pathol 158: 1653-63, 2001

46   Isono M, Chen S, Hong SW, Iglesias-de la Cruz MC and Ziyadeh FN: Smad pathway is activated in the diabetic mouse kidney and Smad3 mediates TGF-beta-induced fibronectin in mesangial cells. Biochem Biophys Res Commun 296: 1356-65, 2002

47   Yamamoto T, Nakamura T, Noble NA, Ruoslahti E and Border WA: Expression of transforming growth factor beta is elevated in human and experimental diabetic nephropathy. Proc Natl Acad Sci U S A 90: 1814-8, 1993

48   Nakamura T, Fukui M, Ebihara I, Osada S, Nagaoka I, Tomino Y and Koide H: mRNA expression of growth factors in glomeruli from diabetic rats. Diabetes 42: 450-6, 1993

49   Sharma K and Ziyadeh FN: Renal hypertrophy is associated with upregulation of TGF-beta 1 gene expression in diabetic BB rat and NOD mouse. Am J Physiol 267: F1094-01, 1994

50   Chen S, Carmen Iglesias-de la Cruz M, Jim B, Hong SW, Isono M and Ziyadeh FN: Reversibility of established diabetic glomerulopathy by anti-TGF-beta antibodies in db/db mice. Biochem Biophys Res Commun 300: 16-22, 2003

51   Ziyadeh FN, Sharma K, Ericksen M and Wolf G: Stimulation of collagen gene expression and protein synthesis in murine mesangial cells by high glucose is mediated by autocrine activation of transforming growth factor-beta. J Clin Invest 93: 536-42, 1994

52   Sharma K, Jin Y, Guo J and Ziyadeh FN: Neutralization of TGF-beta by anti-TGF-beta antibody attenuates kidney hypertrophy and the enhanced extracellular matrix gene expression in STZ-induced diabetic mice. Diabetes 45: 522-30, 1996

53   Ziyadeh FN, Hoffman BB, Han DC, Iglesias-De La Cruz MC, Hong SW, Isono M, Chen S, McGowan TA and Sharma K: Long-term prevention of renal insufficiency, excess matrix gene expression, and glomerular mesangial matrix expansion by treatment with monoclonal antitransforming growth factor-beta antibody in db/db diabetic mice. Proc Natl Acad Sci U S A 97: 8015-20, 2000

54   Fumo P, Kuncio GS and Ziyadeh FN: PKC and high glucose stimulate collagen alpha 1 (IV) transcriptional activity in a reporter mesangial cell line. Am J Physiol 267: F632-8, 1994

55   Chen S, Cohen MP, Lautenslager GT, Shearman CW and Ziyadeh FN: Glycated albumin stimulates TGF-beta 1 production and protein kinase C activity in glomerular endothelial cells. Kidney Int 59: 673-81, 2001

56   Kelly DJ, Zhang Y, Hepper C, Gow RM, Jaworski K, Kemp BE, Wilkinson-Berka JL and Gilbert RE: Protein Kinase C beta Inhibition Attenuates the Progression of Experimental Diabetic Nephropathy in the Presence of Continued Hypertension. Diabetes 52: 512-518, 2003

57   Murphy M, Godson C, Cannon S, Kato S, Mackenzie HS, Martin F and Brady HR: Suppression subtractive hybridization identifies high glucose levels as a stimulus for expression of connective tissue growth factor and other genes in human mesangial cells. J Biol Chem 274: 5830-4, 1999

58   Way KJ, Isshiki K, Suzuma K, Yokota T, Zvagelsky D, Schoen FJ, Sandusky GE, Pechous PA, Vlahos CJ, Wakasaki H and King GL: Expression of connective tissue growth factor is increased in injured myocardium associated with protein kinase C beta2 activation and diabetes. Diabetes 51: 2709-18, 2002

59   Chen Y, Blom IE, Sa S, Goldschmeding R, Abraham DJ and Leask A: CTGF expression in mesangial cells: involvement of SMADs, MAP kinase, and PKC. Kidney Int 62: 1149-59, 2002

60   Williamson JR, Chang K, Tilton RG, Prater C, Jeffrey JR, Weigel C, Sherman WR, Eades DM and Kilo C: Increased vascular permeability in spontaneously diabetic BB/W rats and in rats with mild versus severe streptozocin-induced diabetes. Prevention by aldose reductase inhibitors and castration. Diabetes 36: 813-21, 1987

61   Neufeld G, Cohen T, Gengrinovitch S and Poltorak Z: Vascular endothelial growth factor (VEGF) and its receptors. Faseb J 13: 9-22, 1999

62 Aiello LP, Avery RL, Arrigg PG, Keyt BA, Jampel HD, Shah ST, Pasquale LR, Thieme H, Iwamoto MA, Park JE and et al.: Vascular endothelial growth factor in ocular fluid of patients with diabetic retinopathy and other retinal disorders. N Engl J Med 331: 1480-7, 1994

63 Suzuma K, Naruse K, Suzuma I, Takahara N, Ueki K, Aiello LP and King GL: Vascular endothelial growth factor induces expression of connective tissue growth factor via KDR, Flt1, and phosphatidylinositol 3-kinase-akt-dependent pathways in retinal vascular cells. J Biol Chem 275: 40725-31, 2000

64 Chou E, Suzuma I, Way KJ, Opland D, Clermont AC, Naruse K, Suzuma K, Bowling NL, Vlahos CJ, Aiello LP and King GL: Decreased cardiac expression of vascular endothelial growth factor and its receptors in insulin-resistant and diabetic States: a possible explanation for impaired collateral formation in cardiac tissue. Circulation 105: 373-9, 2002

65 Cooper ME, Vranes D, Youssef S, Stacker SA, Cox AJ, Rizkalla B, Casley DJ, Bach LA, Kelly DJ and Gilbert RE: Increased renal expression of vascular endothelial growth factor (VEGF) and its receptor VEGFR-2 in experimental diabetes. Diabetes 48: 2229-39, 1999

66 Cha DR, Kim NH, Yoon JW, Jo SK, Cho WY, Kim HK and Won NH: Role of vascular endothelial growth factor in diabetic nephropathy. Kidney Int Suppl 77: S104-12, 2000

67 Aiello LP, Bursell SE, Clermont A, Duh E, Ishii H, Takagi C, Mori F, Ciulla TA, Ways K, Jirousek M, Smith LE and King GL: Vascular endothelial growth factor-induced retinal permeability is mediated by protein kinase C in vivo and suppressed by an orally effective beta-isoform-selective inhibitor. Diabetes 46: 1473-80, 1997

68 Xia P, Aiello LP, Ishii H, Jiang ZY, Park DJ, Robinson GS, Takagi H, Newsome WP, Jirousek MR and King GL: Characterization of vascular endothelial growth factor's effect on the activation of protein kinase C, its isoforms, and endothelial cell growth. J Clin Invest 98: 2018-26, 1996

69 de Vriese AS, Tilton RG, Elger M, Stephan CC, Kriz W and Lameire NH: Antibodies against vascular endothelial growth factor improve early renal dysfunction in experimental diabetes. J Am Soc Nephrol 12: 993-1000, 2001

70 Flyvbjerg A, Dagnaes-Hansen F, De Vriese AS, Schrijvers BF, Tilton RG and Rasch R: Amelioration of long-term renal changes in obese type 2 diabetic mice by a neutralizing vascular endothelial growth factor antibody. Diabetes 51: 3090-4, 2002

71 Isshiki K, Haneda M, Koya D, Maeda S, Sugimoto T and Kikkawa R: Thiazolidinedione compounds ameliorate glomerular dysfunction independent of their insulin-sensitizing action in diabetic rats. Diabetes 49: 1022-32, 2000

72 Lee IK, Koya D, Ishi H, Kanoh H and King GL: d-Alpha-tocopherol prevents the hyperglycemia induced activation of diacylglycerol (DAG)-protein kinase C (PKC) pathway in vascular smooth muscle cell by an increase of DAG kinase activity. Diabetes Res Clin Pract 45: 183-90, 1999

73 Friedman EA: Advanced glycosylated end products and hyperglycemia in the pathogenesis of diabetic complications. Diabetes Care 22 Suppl 2: B65-71, 1999

74 Osicka TM, Yu Y, Panagiotopoulos S, Clavant SP, Kiriazis Z, Pike RN, Pratt LM, Russo LM, Kemp BE, Comper WD and Jerums G: Prevention of albuminuria by aminoguanidine or ramipril in streptozotocin-induced diabetic rats is associated with the normalization of glomerular protein kinase C. Diabetes 49: 87-93, 2000

75 Nilsson BO: Biological effects of aminoguanidine: an update. Inflamm Res 48: 509-15, 1999

76   Scivittaro V, Ganz MB and Weiss MF: AGEs induce oxidative stress and activate protein kinase C-beta(II) in neonatal mesangial cells. Am J Physiol Renal Physiol 278: F676-83, 2000

77   Schmidt AM and Stern DM: RAGE: a new target for the prevention and treatment of the vascular and inflammatory complications of diabetes. Trends Endocrinol Metab 11: 368-75, 2000

78   Wautier JL, Zoukourian C, Chappey O, Wautier MP, Guillausseau PJ, Cao R, Hori O, Stern D and Schmidt AM: Receptor-mediated endothelial cell dysfunction in diabetic vasculopathy. Soluble receptor for advanced glycation end products blocks hyperpermeability in diabetic rats. J Clin Invest 97: 238-43, 1996

79   Mackenzie HS and Brenner BM: Current strategies for retarding progression of renal disease. Am J Kidney Dis 31: 161-70, 1998

80   Ruiz-Munoz LM, Vidal-Vanaclocha F and Lampreabe I: Enalaprilat inhibits hydrogen peroxide production by murine mesangial cells exposed to high glucose concentrations. Nephrol Dial Transplant 12: 456-64, 1997

81   Pfaff IL and Vallon V: Protein Kinase C Beta Isoenzymes in Diabetic Kidneys and Their Relation to Nephroprotective Actions of the ACE Inhibitor Lisinopril. Kidney Blood Press Res 25: 329-40, 2002

82   Kim L, Lee T, Fu J and Ritchie ME: Characterization of MAP kinase and PKC isoform and effect of ACE inhibition in hypertrophy in vivo. Am J Physiol 277: H1808-16, 1999

83   Zhang Y, Bloem LJ, Yu L, Estridge TB, Iversen PW, McDonald CE, Schrementi JP, Wang X, Vlahos CJ and Wang J: Protein kinase C betaII activation induces angiotensin converting enzyme expression in neonatal rat cardiomyocytes. Cardiovasc Res 57: 139-46, 2003

84   Aiello LP: The Potential Role of PKC beta in Diabetic Retinopathy and Macular Edema. Surv Ophthalmol 47 Suppl 2: S263-9, 2002

85   Vinik AI: Neuropathy: new concepts in evaluation and treatment. South Med J 95: 21-3, 2002

86   Beckman JA, Goldfine AB, Gordon MB, Garrett LA and Creager MA: Inhibition of protein kinase Cbeta prevents impaired endothelium-dependent vasodilation caused by hyperglycemia in humans. Circ Res 90: 107-11, 2002

21

BIOCHEMICAL ASPECTS OF DIABETIC NEPHROPATHY

Cora Weigert and Erwin D. Schleicher

Department of Medicine, Division of Endocrinology, Metabolism and Pathobiochemistry, University of Tübingen, Germany

The dominant histological feature of diabetic nephropathy is the thickening of the glomerular basement membrane (GBM) and expansion of the mesangial matrix [1-3]. The changes correlate strongly with the clinical onset of proteinuria, hypertension and kidney failure. Although more than 60 years have elapsed since Kimmelstiel and Wilson [4] described in diabetic glomeruli the distinctive periodic acid-schiff (PAS)-reactive nodular deposits, progress in elucidating the pathobiochemistry has been slow. Recent investigations with electron microscopic, immunochemical and biochemical methods have led to an improved understanding of the structure-function relationship of the glomerular filtration unit in normal and pathological conditions [5].

MOLECULAR STRUCTURE AND FUNCTION OF GLOMERULAR EXTRACELLULAR MATRIX

The extracellular matrix of the glomerulus consists of the basement membrane interposed between endothelial and epithelial cells and the closely adjoining extracellular matrix surrounding the mesangial cells. The structural and functional properties of the matrix components are summarized in table 1. The basement membrane representing the size and charge selective area of the filtration unit is composed of a filamentous network of collagen type IV fibrils.

Immunohistochemical studies revealed that the collagen IV chains are inhomogenously distributed within the glomerulus. The α1,α2-chains are primarily detected in the mesangial matrix whereas the α3,α4-chains are exclusively found in the glomerular basement membrane [6]. The basement membranes also contain a proteoglycan which consists of three heparan sulfate side chains covalently attached to the protein core [10,11]. It has been convincingly shown that the negatively charged heparan sulfate chains form the anionic barrier of the glomerular filtration unit [5,12,13]. A detailed review of this heparan sulfate proteoglycan (HSPG) and its changes in diabetes is given in the following chapter. The traces of fibronectin found in normal glomerular matrices are probably derived from plasma since the tissue specific fibronectin A+ which contains the extra domain A is not detected in normal glomeruli [14]. The mesangial matrix, although developmentally and morphologically distinct from the glomerular basement membrane, contains essentially the same components but in different distributions.

Table 1. Structure and function of the major components of the glomerular basement membrane and mesangial matrix

Component	Structure	Function
Collagen type IV	Triplehelix with non-helical segments; 5 different chains with approximately 1700 amino acids are known [6,9] Chains are unequally distributed in the glomerular matrix [6]	Mechanical scaffold; Size selective filter; Binding to cell adhesion molecules
Collagen type VI	3 different chains [8]	Formation of microfibrils
Laminin	3 different poly-peptide chains MW 800 KD [9]	Cell adhesion Integrin binding
Heparan sulfate proteoglycan (HSPG) or agrin	Coreprotein MW 470 KD [7,10,18] 3 heparan sulfate side chains	Integrin binding Charge selective filter Antiproliferative Binding of humoral factors

Several functions of the matrix components can now be explained by features of these components on the molecular level. Specific cell-matrix adhesion molecules which are intercalated in the cellular plasma membrane recognize well-defined amino acid sequences found in collagen, laminin and fibronectin [9,15]. Furthermore, these adhesion molecules (integrins), which are in contact with the cytoskeleton influence cell migration and cell proliferation. Changes in matrix composition may therefore alter cellular adhesion, migration and proliferation and thus influencing repair processes [15]. The finding that HSPG by virtue of its side chains specifically binds polypeptide growth factors like basic fibroblast growth factor (bFGF) or transforming growth factor β (TGF-β) is important in this context. It has been suggested that the matrix-bound growth factors may act as a reservoir for vascular repair mechanisms [16]. The anti-proliferative role of heparan sulfate on mesangial cells underlines the possible importance of this proteoglycan in glomerular matrix [17].

STRUCTURAL AND FUNCTIONAL GLOMERULAR ALTERATIONS IN DIABETES

The first major change after the onset of diabetes is the increased volume of the whole kidney and the glomeruli [19]. These hypertrophical glomeruli have normal structural composition. After a few years the amount of glomerular matrix material is increased [1,3]. Biochemical determinations indicate an increased amount of collagen in the glomerular extracellular matrices [20]. More recently, an increase in collagen type VI in the glomerular matrix of diabetic patients has been documented [21]. On the basis of immunochemical measurement, it has become evident that the HSPG content of glomerular matrix is lower in diabetic patients [22] consistent with previous chemical analyses of the heparan sulfate chains [23,24]. These immunochemical measurements, although yielding reliable quantitative values, were performed with preparations of glomerular matrices which contain firstly, both the basement membrane and the mesangial matrix and secondly a mixture of glomeruli which may be affected to a variable degree. Therefore, immunohistochemical studies have been performed to distinguish the changes within the different compartments of the glomerulus and between the individual glomeruli.

These immunohistochemical studies, summarized in table 2, indicate that in diabetic kidneys with slight lesions only a minor increase in all basement membrane components was found except for HSPG. More pronounced diffuse glomerulosclerosis showed a further increase in basement membrane components, especially collagen IV α1,α2-chains in the expanded mesangial matrix. However, HSPG which was entirely absent from the enlarged matrix could only be observed in the periphery of the glomeruli. The staining of collagen IV α3,α4-chain showed a similar distribution as found for HSPG however, with intense staining of the thickened glomerular basement membrane [6]. To this stage of nephropathy the accumulation of excess matrix material can be attributed to quantitative changes of the components present in normal glomeruli. In contrast, pronounced nodular lesions exhibited a strong decrease of collagen IV α1,α2-chains, laminin, and HSPG, which were only detectable in the periphery of the noduli. Staining sequential sections with collagen VI antiserum or PAS revealed coincidence of both stainings indicating that the noduli consist mostly of collagen type VI [8]. Peripheral areas of these noduli were also positive for collagen III, which was not detected in earlier lesions. It appears that in diffuse glomerulosclerosis an increase in normal matrix components occurs while the nodular glomerulosclerosis is characterized by qualitative changes (table 2). Morphological and structural changes occurring in the interstitium, tubuli or glomerular arterioles are a concomitant of diabetic nephropathy [1].

Table 2. Changes of glomerular matrix composition in different stages of diabetic glomerulosclerosis (GS)*

| | Diffuse GS | | Nodular GS | |
	GBM	mesangium	GBM	mesangium
laminin	↑	↑	↑	↓
collagen IV				
α1,α2-chain	↑	↑	↑	↓
α3,α4-chain	↑	-	↑	↑
HSPG	↓→	↓	↓	-
fibronectin A+	-	n.d.	-	↑
collagen III	-	-[1]	-	↑[2]
collagen VI	↓	↑[3]	↓	↑↑

↑ = increased; ↓ = decreased; → = unchanged; - = not detectable; *see also [6-8]; n.d. = not determined; [1]traces in late diffuse GS; [2]only peripheral; [3]focally

In vivo and in vitro studies of collagen metabolism in glomeruli obtained from diabetic animals demonstrated that increased collagen deposition is caused by an increased synthesis and concomitant decreased degradation [20,25,26]. Fukui et al. [27] found an increased steady state mRNA levels of the collagen IV α1-chain, laminin B1 and B2 and fibronectin while the collagen I α1-chain was unchanged in the kidneys of diabetic rats after one month of diabetes. The message for HSPG was decreased after induction of diabetes and increased steadily afterwards. The changes in mRNA levels, which preceded the glomerular matrix expansion could be prevented by normalisation of blood glucose by insulin treatment. Recent *in situ* hybridization studies revealed that mRNA transcript levels of $\alpha_1(IV)$ collagen are increased more than twofold in glomerular and proximal tubular cells in long-term (12 months) diabetic rats [28]. In the glomerulum, mainly mesangial cells showed enhanced $\alpha_1(IV)$ collagen expression. The $\alpha_1(IV)$ collagen deposition in the mesangial matrix was similarly increased. Chronic treatment with a modified heparin preparation completely prevented the increased $\alpha_1(IV)$ collagen deposition and expression and the overt albuminuria in diabetic rats. Taken together, these results indicate that the increased synthesis of collagen IV, laminin and fibronectin is the biochemical correlate of the expansion of the mesangial matrix and the thickening of glomerular basement membrane observed histologically. The occurrence of decreased degradation of matrix components has also been documented [26].

Extensive studies have shown that the changes in glomerular ultrastructure are closely associated with renal function [2,3]. Comparing the immunohistochemical findings with clinical data Nerlich et al. [7] found that the increase in the glomerular matrix components was consistently associated with impaired renal filter function. Late stage nodular glomerulosclerosis associated with decrease of all basement membrane components, and increase in collagen III and VI coincided with severe renal insufficiency. In all cases, even in early diffuse glomerulosclerosis, HSPG was decreased.

ALTERED GENE EXPRESSION IN THE DIABETIC KIDNEY

The biochemical events leading to the quantitative and finally qualitative alterations of the glomerular matrix are currently under intensive investigation. The detrimental effects of the diabetic environment are translated into altered gene activation, thus preceeding or mediating the changes in glomerular matrix protein production. The first group of genes for which increases in gene expression were found in the diabetic kidney are several growth factors. Among them are components of the transforming growth factor-β1 (TGF-β1) system: TGF-β1 protein itself [14;29,30], the TGF-β1 activator thrombospondin-1 [31],

345

and the TGF-β1 receptor type 2 [32]; furthermore, the expression of the prosclerotic cytokine connective tissue growth factor (CTGF) [33], of platelet derived growth factor (PDGF) [34,35], and of vascular endothelial growth factor (VEGF) [36] was enhanced. Although the TGF-β1 cascade is considered to be the major key mediator implicated in the progression of renal disease [37], participation of the other cytokines could be demonstrated by several *in vivo* and *in vitro* studies: CTGF expression affects matrix synthesis and its turnover, thereby potentially acting as a downstream mediator of TGF-β1 [33]; *in vivo* transfection of PDGF induces glomerulosclerosis in the rat kidney [38]; administration of a neutralising antibody to VEGF ameliorate early and long-term renal changes in diabetic rodents [39,40]. Furthermore, activation of the IGF-pathway in the diabetic kidney has been reported [41,42]. The second group of genes for which gene activation was demonstrated include the matrix proteins themselves. In the following the pathobiochemical pathways responsible for this deranged transcriptional regulation in the diabetic kidney are discussed.

HYPERGLYCAEMIA AND THE PATHOGENESIS OF DIABETIC NEPHROPATHY

The main metabolic disorder occuring in diabetes is hyperglycaemia. Two landmark studies, the Diabetes Control and Complications Trial (DCCT) and the United Kingdom Prospective Diabetes Study (UKPDS) showed that intensive blood glucose control clearly reduces the development or progression of diabetic nephropathy [43,44]. Thus, the impact of extracellular high glucose concentrations on renal cell gene expression was investigated in detail:

Ayo and coworkers reported that prolonged exposure to high glucose concentrations leads to an increase in collagen IV, laminin and fibronectin synthesis on the protein and mRNA level in mesangial cells [45]. Furthermore, mesangial cells exposed to elevated glucose synthesize less HSPG [46]. Studies with epithelial, endothelial and mesangial cells revealed that all three cell types of the glomerulus produce more collagen type IV when exposed to elevated glucose levels [47]. Periodic changes in glucose concentration, simulating more closely disordered glucose homeostasis, lead to enhanced synthesis of collagen type III and IV compared to continuous low or high glucose environment. This data indicates the deleterious effects of fluctuating glucose levels on the development of diabetic glomerulosclerosis [48].

Similar effects of ambient high glucose conditions were shown on growth factor gene expression: Several groups reported the high glucose-induced upregulation of TGF-β1 gene expression in both, proximal tubular cells and glomerular mesangial cells [49,50]. Culture of mesangial cells in high glucose showed markedly increased CTGF mRNA levels [33]; PDGF and VEGF expression was also found to be elevated by ambient high glucose in mesangial cells [51,52]. Other components of the TGF-β1-system were also found to be induced by high glucose: increased expression of thrombospondin-1 contributes to the excessive TGF-β1 bioactivity by conversion of latent TGF-β1 protein to its biologically active form [31], and induction of TGF-β1 type 2 receptor amplifies the activation of the TGF-β1 cascade [32].

Recent data show that high glucose concentrations stimulate gene expression of matrix proteins, the extracellular matrix protease inhibitor plasminogen activator inhibitor-I (PAI-I) and TGF-β1 by increasing the activity of the corresponding promoters. These studies using promoter fragments fused to reporter genes such as luciferase indicate an activation of the murine and human TGF-β1 promoter [53,54] and of the TGF-β1 type II receptor promoter [32] by high glucose. PAI-I promoter activity is enhanced by high glucose [55]; the fibronectin promoter is stimulated additively by high glucose and TGF-β1 [56]. TGF-β1 itself is known to activate promoters of several genes, including the promoters for α2 collagen type I [57], type IV [58], laminin [59] and in an autocrine loop, transcription of its own gene [60]. Similarly TGF-β1 increases the activity of the HSPG promoter [61]. The most frequently found transcription factors which may mediate the high glucose- and TGF-β1-induced promoter activation are members of the AP-1 family and Sp1. Consensus sequences for AP-1 have been found in the promoters of the different collagen types, fibronectin and TGF-β1 and confirmed to be responsible for the high glucose- or TGF-β1-mediated transcriptional activation [54;56,57;59,60]. Sp1 binding sites have been shown to mediate the high glucose-induced PAI-I promoter upregulation [55].

How do these diverse transcription factor and gene activations all result from high glucose concentrations? A large amount of data have been accumulated, indicating the participation of four main biochemical pathways as mediators of the adverse effects of hyperglycaemia on gene regulation: the protein kinase C (PKC) pathway, the generation of advanced glycation end-products (AGEs), increased flux through the hexosamine biosynthetic pathway (HBP) and the aldose reductase pathway. The PKC and the AGE pathway are also illustrated in detail in other chapters of the book.

Activation of protein kinase C

The involvement of PKC in diabetic nephropathy is in accordance with several reports, which provide evidence for a role of glucose-induced activation of PKC in the elevated synthesis of matrix components [62,63]. Application of a PKC β isoform specific inhibitor ameliorated the changes in glomerular filtration rate, albumin excretion rate and retinal circulation in diabetic rats in a dose-responsive manner, in parallel with its inhibition of PKC activities [64]. Moreover, inhibition of PKC activities abrogated the high glucose-induced TGF-β1 promoter activation in mesangial cells [54]. The high glucose-induced activation of PKC isoforms can subsequently upregulate MAPK pathways, thus inducing the transcriptional activity of AP-1 proteins by enhanced gene expression or posttranslational modifications. The transcripts and protein levels of the AP-1 family members c-Jun and c-Fos are elevated in mesangial cells cultured in high glucose [65]. Posttranslational activation is shown by increased DNA binding activity of AP-1 proteins derived from mesangial cells exposed to elevated glucose concentrations, which is not due to differences in the protein level [66] and phosphorylation of the AP-1 related transcription factor CREB after treatment of mesangial cells with high glucose and TGF-β1 [67]. Hyperglycaemia has been reported to activate MAP kinases including ERK1/2 and p38 MAPK in glomeruli of diabetic rodents [68,69] and in mesangial cells [70,71] and the increase in MAPK activity has been shown to be PKC-dependent [54].

Increased formation of advanced glycation end-products

Recent approaches suggest that the development of diabetic late complications may be linked to the formation of advanced glycation end-products (AGE-products). These AGE-products, such as carboxymethyl-lysine, pentosidine and malondialdehyde-lysine, accumulate in expanded mesangial matrix and nodular lesions as shown in renal tissue from patients with diabetic nephropathy [72]. The cellular effects of AGE-products are mediated by specific binding to cell surface molecules of which the receptor for advanced glycation end-products (RAGE) is well characterized [73]. Expression of RAGE is increased in kidneys from patients with diabetic nephropathy [74]. Furthermore, AGE-products and their receptors co-localize in the renal glomerulus of rats with experimental diabetes [75]. Although upregulation of mesangial TGF-β1 synthesis with concomitant increase of extracellular matrix production by AGEs has been shown [76], and AGEs induced VEGF expression [77], the main action of the AGE-RAGE system not only in terms of diabetic nephropathy is to cause chronic cellular activation and oxidative stress. RAGE expression is enhanced by a positive feedback loop via activation of the transcription factor NF-κB [73], perpetuating the stimulatory event and leading to cellular perturbation [78]. In this stage the cells are highly susceptible to further stress stimuli resulting in chronic inflammation and accelerated sclerosis.

Increased flux through the hexosamine biosynthetic pathway

Hyperglycaemia increases the flux through the HBP; fructose-6-phosphate from glycolysis is thereby converted to glucosamine-6-phosphate, using glutamine as amino-group donor. The reaction is catalysed by glutamine:fructose-6-phosphate aminotransferase (GFAT), the rate-limiting enzyme of this pathway. The product glucosamine-6-phosphate is rapidly further converted to uridine-5'-diphosphate-N-acetylglucosamine (UDP-GlcNAc), the substrate for the nucleocytoplasmic enzyme O-GlcNAc transferase (OGT). The attachment of a single O-GlcNAc to serine or threonine residues of proteins is considered as a new regulatory modification important to signal transduction cascades [79]. The important function of the HBP in the initiation of the alteration of the glomerular matrix has been proven by inhibition of GFAT, which was shown to block hyperglycaemia-induced expression of TGF-β1 and PAI-I and subsequently the production of matrix proteins [80,81]. Moreover, overexpression of GFAT in mesangial cells enhances TGF-β1 gene activation and fibronectin accumulation [82]. Promoter-reporter gene-assays revealed that binding sites for the transcription factor Sp1 regulate the high glucose-induced promoter activation of PAI-I [55]. The mechanism by which increased flux through the HBP resulted in gene activation is not completely clarified, but the HBP-mediated, enhanced O-GlcNAc modification of Sp1 was suggested to activate its transcriptional activity [83] and DNA binding activity [84]. Thus, the promoter activity of Sp1-driven genes, e.g. PAI-I and TGF-β1, could be stimulated by the O-GlcNAc modification of this transcription factor.

Increased flux through the aldose reductase pathway

The aldose reductase pathway involves intracellular formation of sorbitol from glucose catalysed by aldose reductase. Chronic hyperglycaemia leads to sorbitol accumulation in a variety of tissues such as peripheral neurons, lens and renal tubuli [85]. The initial hypothesis that sorbitol accumulation causes tissue damage is unlikely to operate in the kidney [86]. The inositol depletion theory suggested by Greene and coworkers explains tissue damages as impairment of myo-inositol uptake leading to a decrease of phosphatidyl-inositides in the cell membrane [85]. Although the cellular inositol uptake is competitively inhibited by D-glucose [87] and non-competitively inhibited by hyperosmolar intracellular sorbitol [88], recent studies showed that cells may counterregulate inositol depletion [89,90]. Thus, it is not generally agreed that the increase in intracellular sorbitol is the cause of the impaired function of the affected tissues in diabetes. Furthermore, after treatment of diabetic rats for six months with the aldose reductase inhibitor tolrestat only a slight reduction in the urinary albumin excretion rate was observed indicating that other mechanism are operating in diabetic nephropathy [91].

The role of oxidative stress

Many studies have shown that diabetes and hyperglycaemia increase oxidative stress, but it was not known if it is an important early mediator of the high glucose effects on renal structures and functions. A recent study showed that high glucose increased the production of superoxide by the mitochondrial electron-transport chain in endothelial cells [81,92]. Inhibition of the generation of these reactive oxygen species (ROS) prevented the activation of PKC pathways, the increased flux through the HBP and the aldose reductase pathway, and the enhanced synthesis of AGEs. Whether this interference would also block high glucose-induced derranged production of glomerular matrix production is currently under investigation. It was demonstrated that mesangial cells grown in ambient high glucose produced ROS [93], thus leading to activation of PKC, AP-1 and NF-κB, and the up-regulation of TGF-β1 and of matrix protein expression. The existence of glucose-induced oxidative stress in mesangial cells was also shown by decreased glutathione (GSH) and elevated malondialdehyde (MDA) levels [94]. Addition of antioxidants caused the restorage of GSH and a clear reversal of fibronectin and collagen IV expression.

A scheme of the pathways mentioned above is depicted in figure 1.

Glucose transporter-1 as a permissive factor

Glucose transport is rate-limiting for glucose metabolism and the main glucose transporter (GLUT) on mesangial cells, GLUT1, is a high-affinity, low-capacity transporter [95]. Thus, mesangial glucose uptake appears to be essentially determined by the number of GLUT1 on the cell surface rather than by ambient glucose concentrations [96]. Accordingly, experimental work has recognized the upregulation of mesangial GLUT1 expression by ambient high glucose and IGF-1 [97]. The hyperglycaemia-induced TGF-β1 [98] and, similiarly, angiotensin II stimulate GLUT1 expression [99]. Furthermore, recent studies demonstrated a significant increase in GLUT1 protein in the renal cortex of diabetic animals [100] and in mesangial cells isolated from diabetic subjects [101].

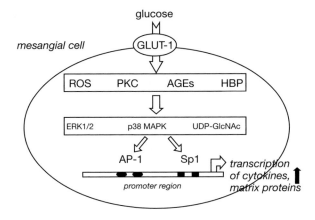

Fig. 1 Proposed molecular mechanism of the hyperglycaemia-induced matrix synthesis in mesangial cells. Elevated glucose concentrations entering the cell via the glucose transporter 1 (GLUT 1) activates the production of reactive oxygen species (ROS), protein kinase C (PKC), generation of advanced glycated end-products (AGEs) and the hexosamine biosynthetic pathway (HBP). Subsequently induced mitogen-activated protein kinases (MAPK)-dependent pathways or increases in UDP-GlcNAc are leading to enhanced expression and/or phosphorylation of proteins of the activating protein 1 complex (AP-1) or activation of Sp1. Since the promoters of extracellular matrix (ECM) proteins and of cytokines contain AP-1 and Sp1 binding sites the expression of these genes is induced.

The essential role of elevated GLUT1 levels in the development of the pathological changes in diabetic nephropathy was proven by a mesangial cell model stably transfected with human GLUT1 (GT1) [102]. These cells showed a five fold increased glucose uptake, a 2.1-fold increase in lactate production, and enhanced expression and net deposition of matrix proteins, e.g. fibronectin

351

when cultured in physiological levels of extracellular glucose. In a recent report we provide evidence for the activation of different intracellular signaling pathways in GT1 cells cultured in normal glucose concentrations and mesangial cells exposed to high glucose concentrations [103]. Our investigation of the molecular mechanism of the enhanced fibronectin production in these cells has revealed a protein kinase C-dependent, activated AP-1-mediated pathway, which acts independently of TGF-β1. In contrast to mesangial cells cultured in ambient high glucose, no production of reactive oxygen species, no activation of the p38 or ERK1/2 MAPK pathways nor any increase in TGF-β1 synthesis could be detected.

ANGIOTENSIN II AND DEVELOPMENT OF DIABETIC GLOMERULOPATHY

Angiotensin II is the dominant effector of the renin-angiotensin system (RAS). Angiotensin II regulates salt and water balance, blood pressure, and the vascular tone. Several recent studies have provided clear evidence that angiotensin-converting enzyme (ACE)-inhibitors slow the progression of diabetic nephropathy by mechanisms mainly independent from reduction of systemic blood pressure [104,105]. Thus, angiotensin II is a renal growth factor that exerts non-hemodynamic effects on the kidney and modulates cell growth and extracellular matrix synthesis and degradation [106]. The profibrogenetic actions of angiotensin II have been shown by several laboratories.

Angiotensin II stimulates TGF-β1 gene activation and synthesis and matrix component production through binding of the angiotensin type 1 (AT1)-receptor in mesangial cells. The increased extracellular matrix protein expression depends on bioactivity and *de-novo* synthesis of TGF-β, since administration of neutralizing antibodies to TGF-β or TGF-β antisense oligonucleotides blocked this cellular response to angiotensin II [106,107]. ACE-inhibitor-treated diabetic rats showed a normalisation of TGF-β1 type II receptor mRNA and protein [108]. Moreover, synthesis of the prosclerotic cytokine CTGF was increased by angiotensin II in cultured renal cells [109] and the transcriptional activation of the rate-limiting enzyme of the HBP, GFAT, was observed in angiotensin II-stimulated mesangial cells [110]. Matrix degradation was recognized to be affected by angiotensin II through induction of PAI-I [111].

In vitro and *in vivo* studies revealed striking similarities of the signal transduction pathways induced by high glucose exposure and angiotensin II treatment leading to the altered glomerular gene expression [106,107]. Results obtained with mesangial cells and renal tubular epithelial cells indicate an activation of PKC and p38 MAPK by angiotensin II through AT1-receptors [104], which was also found in glomeruli of hypertensive rodents [112]. Other reports have shown that angiotensin II induces the DNA-binding activity of AP-1 proteins [113,114], thereby mediating the TGF-β1 promoter activation by PKC- and p38 MAPK-dependent pathways [115]. Moreover, angiotensin II was recognized to generate oxidative stress via NADPH oxidase [116]. These data suggest that angiotensin II may regulate the fibrotic process via a AT1-receptor/AP-1 pathway.

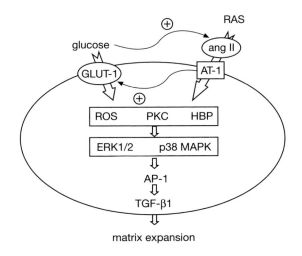

Fig. 2 Proposed molecular mechanism of the hyperglycaemia- and angiotensin II-induced TGF-β1 expression. After binding to the angiotensin receptor 1 (AT-1) angiotensin II (ang II) may stimulate the matrix synthesis by activation of the same signal transduction pathways as high glucose does. Elevated glucose may also increase ang II production, and ang II may activate glucose transport.

It remains open whether high glucose and angiotensin II potentiate the response of renal cells to the other signal. Results of *in vitro* studies in mesangial cells were ambiguous. The MAP kinases ERK1/2 and p38 are additively activated by both stimuli resulting in an enhanced effect on transcription factor AP-1 activity compared to high glucose or angiotensin II treatment alone [117]. Angiotensin II-induced growth and collagen IV synthesis also were increased under high glucose conditions [118]. However, no additive effect was found on TGF-β1 promoter activity [115]. Little is known about the interaction of hyperglycaemia and angiotensin II. The status of the renin-angiotensin system (RAS) in diabetes remains controversial and multiple investigations gave no clear hint that the intrarenal angiotensin II-system is activated in patients susceptible to diabetic nephropathy [104]. Moreover, some components of the RAS were reported to downregulated in diabetic renal disease [104]. A recent report linking hyperglycaemia to increased angiotensin II generation demonstrated that high glucose stimulates angiotensin II production in mesangial cells and that the high glucose-induced TGF-β1 synthesis, mesangial matrix accumulation, and decrease in collagenase activity is reversed by losartan, a AT1-receptor antagonist [119]. These data give rise to the hypothesis that antagonizing the effects of angiotensin II, e.g. in ACE-inhibitor therapy, interfere not only with the renin-angiotensin-system but may ameliorate hyperglycaemia-induced pathomechanisms which are mediated in part by angiotensin II and resulting in development of diabetic nephropathy. The proposed signal transduction pathways stimulated by hyperglycaemia and angiotensin II and possible interactions are summarized in figure 2.

ACKNOWLEDGEMENTS

The work from the author's laboratory was supported by the Deutsche Forschungsgemeinschaft (Schl 239-7). The critical comments of Drs. R. Lehmann, R. Lammers, and D. Burt are gratefully acknowledged.

REFERENCES

1.   Mauer SM, Ellis E, Bilous RW, Steffes MW. »The pathology of diabetic nephropathy.« In *Complications of Diabetes Mellitus*, Draznin B, Melmed S, LeRoith D, eds. New York: Alan R Liss Inc., 1989; pp 95-101.
2.   Mauer SM, Steffes MW, Ellis EN, Sutherland DER, Brown DM, Goetz FC. Structural-functional relationships in diabetic nephropathy. J Clin Invest 1984; 74: 1143-1155.

3. Østerby R, Gall MA, Schmitz A, Nielsen FS, Nyberg G, Parving H-H. Glomerular structure and function in proteinuric type 2 (non-insulin-dependent) diabetic patients. Diabetologia 1993; 36: 1064-1070.
4. Kimmelstiel P, Wilson C. Intercapillary lesions in the glomeruli of the kidney. Am J Pathol 1936; 12: 83-89.
5. Farquhar MG, Lemkin MC, Stow JL. »Role of proteoglycans in glomerular function and pathology.« In *Nephrology*, Robinson RR, ed. New York: Springer-Verlag,, 1985; pp 580-590.
6. Kim Y, Kleppel M, Butkowski R, Mauer M, Wieslander J, Michael A. Differential expression of basement membrane collagen chains in diabetic nephropathy. Am J Pathol 1991; 138: 413-420.
7. Nerlich A, Schleicher E. Immunohistochemical localization of extracellular matrix components in human diabetic glomerular lesions. Am J Pathol 1991; 139: 889-899.
8. Nerlich A, Schleicher ED, Wiest I, Specks U, Timpl R. Immunohistochemical localization of collagen VI in diabetic glomeruli. Kidney Int 1994, 45: 1648-1656.
9. Timpl R. Structure and biological activity of basement membrane proteins. Eur J Biochem 1989; 180: 487-503.
10. Kallunki P, Tryggvason K. human basement membrane heparan sulfate proteoglycan core protein: A 467-kD protein containing multiple domains resembling elements of the low density lipoprotein receptor, laminin, neural cell adhesion molecules, and epidermal growth factor. J Cell Biol 1992; 116: 559-571.
11. Schleicher ED, Wagner EM, Olgemöller B, Nerlich AG, Gerbitz KD. Characterization and localization of basement membrane-associated heparan sulphate proteoglycan in human tissues. Lab Invest 1989; 61: 323-332.
12. Stow JL, Sawada H, Farquhar MG. Basement membrane heparan sulfate proteoglycans are concentrated in the laminae rarae and in podocytes of the rat renal glomerulus. Proc Natl Acad Sci USA 1985; 82: 3296-3300.
13. van den Born J, van den Heuvel PWJ, Bakker MAH, Veerkamp JH, Assmann KJM, Berden JHM. A monoclonal antibody against GBM heparan sulfate induces an acute selective proteinuria in rats. Kidney Int 1992; 41: 115-123.
14. Yamamoto T, Nakamura T, Noble NA, Ruoslahti E, Border WA. Expression of transforming growth factor ß is elevated in human and experimental diabetic nephropathy. Proc Natl Acad Sci USA 1993; 90: 1814-1818.
15. Ruoslahti E. »Extracellular matrix in the regulation of cellular functions.« In *Cell to Cell Interaction*, Burger MM, Sordat B, Zinkernagel RM, eds. Basel: Karger, 1990; pp 88-98.
16. d'Amore PA. Modes of FGF release in vivo and in vitro Cancer and Metastasis Reviews 1990; 9: 227-238.
17. Wright TC, Casellot JJ, Diamond JR, Karnovsky MJ. »Regulation of cellular proliferation by heparin and heparan sulfate.« In *Heparin*, Lane DA, Lindahl U, eds. London: Edward Arnold, 1989; pp 295-316.
18. Raats CJI, van den Born J, Berden JHM. Glomerular heparan sulfate alterations: Mechanism and relevance for proteinuria. Kid. Int. 2000; 57: 385-400.
19. Dalla Vestra M, Saller A, Mauer M, Fioretto P. Role of mesangial expansion in the pathogenesis of diabetic nephropathy. J Nephrol 2001; 14: Suppl. 4: S51-57
20. Spiro RG. »Pathogenesis of diabetic glomerulopathy: a biochemical view.« In *The Kidney and Hypertension in Diabetes Mellitus*, Mogensen CE, ed. Boston: Martinus Nijhoff Publishing, 1988; pp 117-130.
21. Mohan PS, Carter WG, Spiro RG. Occurrence of type VI collagen in extracellular matrix of renal glomeruli and its increase in diabetes. Diabetes 1990; 39: 31-37.

22. Shimomura H, Spiro RG. Studies on macromolecular components of human glomerular basement membrane and alterations in diabetes: decreased levels of heparan sulfate proteoglycan. Diabetes 1987; 36: 374-381.

23. Parthasarathy N, Spiro RG. Effect of diabetes on the glycosaminoglycan component of the human glomerular basement membrane. Diabetes 1982; 31: 738-741.

24. Schleicher E, Wieland OH. Changes of human glomerular basement membrane in diabetes mellitus. Eur J Clin Chem Clin Biochem 1984; 22: 223-227.

25. Haneda M, Kikkawa R, Horide N, Togawa M, Koya D, Kajiwara N, Ooshima A, Shigeta Y. Glucose enhances type IV collagen production in cultured rat glomerular mesangial cells. Diabetologia 1991; 34: 198-200.

26. Schaefer RM, Paczek L, Huang S, Teschner M, Schaefer L, Heidland A. Role of glomerular proteinases in the evolution of glomerulosclerosis. Eur J Clin Chem Clin Biochem 1992; 30: 641-646.

27. Fukui M, Nakamura T, Ebihara I, Shirato I, Tomino Y, Koide H. ECM gene expression and its modulation by insulin in diabetic rats. Diabetes 1992; 41: 1520-1527.

28. Ceol M, Nerlich A, Baggio B, Anglani A, Sauer U, Schleicher E, Gambaro G. Increased glomerular α_1 (IV) collagen expression and deposition in long-term diabetic rats in prevented by chronic glycosminoglycan treatment. Lab Invest 1996; 74; 484-495.

29. Nakamura T, Fukui M, Ebihara I, Osada S, Nakaoka I, Tomino Y, Koide H. mRNA Expression of growth factors in glomeruli from diabetic rats. Diabetes 1993; 42: 450-456.

30. Park IS, Kiyomoto H, Abboud SL, Abboud HE. Expression of transforming growth factor-beta and type IV collagen in early streptozotocin-induced diabetes. Diabetes 1997; 46: 473-480.

31. Yevdokimova N, Wahab NA, Mason RM. Thrombospondin-1 is the key activator of TGF-beta1 in human mesangial cells exposed to high glucose. J Am Soc Nephrol. 2001; 12:703-712

32. Isono M, Mogyorosi A, Han DC, Hoffman BB, Ziyadeh FN. Stimulation of TGF-beta type II receptor by high glucose in mouse mesangial cells and in diabetic kidney. Am J Physiol Renal Physiol. 2000; 278:F830-838.

33. Wahab NA, Yevdokimova N, Weston BS, Roberts T, Li XJ, Brinkman H, Mason RM. Role of connective tissue growth factor in the pathogenesis of diabetic nephropathy. Biochem J. 2001; 359:77-87.

34. Kelly DJ, Gilbert RE, Cox AJ, Soulis T, Jerums G, Cooper ME. Aminoguanidine ameliorates overexpression of prosclerotic growth factors and collagen deposition in experimental diabetic nephropathy. J Am Soc Nephrol. 2001; 10:2098-2107

35. Nakamura T, Ebihara I, Fukui M, Tomino Y, Koide H. Effect of a specific endothelin receptor A antagonist on mRNA levels for extracellular matrix components and growth factors in diabetic glomeruli. Diabetes. 1995; 44:895-899.

36. Cooper ME, Vranes D, Youssef S, Stacker SA, Cox AJ, Rizkalla B, Casley DJ, Bach LA, Kelly DJ, Gilbert RE. Increased renal expression of vascular endothelial growth factor (VEGF) and its receptor VEGFR-2 in experimental diabetes. Diabetes. 1999; 48:2229-2239.

37. Sharma K, Ziyadeh FN. Perspectives in diabetes.Hyperglycemia and diabetic kidney disease. The case for transforming growth factor-β as a key mediator. Diabetes 1995; 44: 1139-1146.

38. Isaka Y, Fujiwara Y, Ueda N, Kaneda Y, Kamada T, Imai E. Glomerulosclerosis induced by in vivo transfection of transforming growth factor-beta or platelet-derived growth factor gene into the rat kidney. J Clin Invest. 1993; 92:2597-6012.

39. Flyvbjerg A, Dagnaes-Hansen F, De Vriese AS, Schrijvers BF, Tilton RG, Rasch R. Amelioration of long-term renal changes in obese type 2 diabetic mice by a neutralizing vascular endothelial growth factor antibody. Diabetes. 2002; 51:3090-3094.

40. de Vriese AS, Tilton RG, Elger M, Stephan CC, Kriz W, Lameire NH. Antibodies against vascular endothelial growth factor improve early renal dysfunction in experimental diabetes. J Am Soc Nephrol. 2001;12:993-1000.

41. Raz I, Rubinger D, Popovtzer M, Gronbaek H, Weiss O, Flyvbjerg A. Octreotide prevents the early increase in renal insulin-like growth factor binding protein 1 in streptozotocin diabetic rats. Diabetes. 1998; 47:924-930.

42. Bach LA, Cox AJ, Mendelsohn FA, Herington AC, Werther GA, Jerums G. Focal induction of IGF binding proteins in proximal tubules of diabetic rat kidney. Diabetes. 1992; 41:499-507.

43. The Diabetes Control and Complications Trial research group: The effects of intensive insulin treatment of diabetes on the development and progression of long-term complications in insulin-dependent diabetes mellitus. N. Engl. J. Med.1993; 329:977-986.

44. United Kingdom Prospective Diabetes Study Group. Intensive blood glucose control with sulphonylureas or insulin compared with conventional treatment and risk of complication in patients with type 2 diabetes (UKPDS 33). Lancet 1998; 352:837-853.

45. Ayo SH, Radnik RA, Glass IIWF, Garoni JA, Rampt ER, Appling DR, Kreisberg JI. Increased extracellular matrix synthesis and mRNA in mesangial cells grown in high-glucose medium. Am J Physiol 1990; 260: F185-F191.

46. Olgemöller B, Schwaabe S, Gerbitz KD, Schleicher ED. Elevated glucose decreases the content of a basement membrane associated proteoglycan in proliferating mesangial cells. Diabetologia 1992; 35: 183-186.

47. Danne T, Spiro MJ, Spiro RG. Effect of high glucose on type IV collagen production by cultured glomerular epithelial, endothelial, and mesangial cells. Diabetes 1993; 42: 170-177.

48. Takeuchi A, Throckmorton DC, Brogden AP, Yoshizawa N, Rasmussen H, Kashgarian M. Periodic high extracellular glucose enhances production of collagens III and IV by mesangial cells. Am Physiol Soc 1995; 268: F13-F19.

49. Ziyadeh FN, Sharma K, Ericksen M, Wolf G: Stimulation of collagen gene expression and protein synthesis in murine mesangial cells by high glucose is mediated by autocrine activation of transforming growth factor-beta. *J Clin Invest* 93:536-542, 1994

50. Kolm V, Sauer U, Olgemöller B, Schleicher ED. High glucose-induced TGF-beta 1 regulates mesangial production of heparan sulfate proteoglycan.Am J Physiol 1996; 270 : F812-21.

51. Di Paolo S, Gesualdo L, Ranieri E, Grandaliano G, Schena FP. High glucose concentration induces the overexpression of transforming growth factor-beta through the activation of a platelet-derived growth factor loop in human mesangial cells. Am J Pathol. 1996; 149:2095-2106.

52. Kim NH, Jung HH, Cha DR, Choi DS. Expression of vascular endothelial growth factor in response to high glucose in rat mesangial cells. J Endocrinol. 2000; 165:617-624.

53. Hofman BB, Sharma K, Zhu Y, Ziyadeh FN: Transcriptional activation of transforming growth factor-β1 in mesangial cell culture by high glucose concentration. Kidney Int 1998; 54:1107-1116.

54. Weigert C, Sauer U, Brodbeck K, Pfeiffer A, Haering HU, Schleicher ED: AP-1 proteins mediate hyperglycemia-induced activation of the human TGF-beta 1 promoter in mesangial cells. J. Am. Soc. Nephrol. 2000; 11:2007-2016.

55. Goldberg HJ, Scholey J, Fantus IG. Glucosamine activates the plasminogen activator inhibitor 1 gene promoter through Sp1 DNA binding sites in glomerular mesangial cells. Diabetes. 2000; 49:863-871.

56. Kreisberg JI, Garoni JA, Radnik R, Ayo SH: High glucose and TGF-β1 stimulate fibronectin gene expression through a cAMP response element. Kidney Int 1994, 46: 1019-1024.

57. Chung KY, Agarwal A, Uitto J, Mauviel A: An AP-1 binding sequence is essential for regulation of the human alpha2(I) collagen (COL1A2) promoter activity by transforming growth factor-beta. J Biol Chem 1996, 271: 3272-3278.

58. Kuncio GS, Alvarez R, Li S, Killen PD, Neilson EG: Transforming growth factor-beta modulation of the alpha 1(IV) collagen gene in murine proximal tubular cells. Am J Physiol 1996, 271: F120-125.

59. Virolle T, Monthouel MN, Djabari Z, Ortonne JP, Meneguzzi G, Aberdam D: Three activator protein-1-binding sites bound by the Fra2.JunD complex cooperate for the regulation of murine laminin alpha3A (lama3A) promoter activity by transforming growth factor-beta. J Biol Chem 1998, 273: 17318-17325.

60. Kim S-J, Angel P, Lafyatis R, Hattori K, Kim KY, Sporn MB, Karin M, Roberts AB: Autoinduction of transforming growth factor β1 is mediated by the AP-1 complex. Mol Cell Biol 1990,10: 1492-1497.

61. Iozzo RV, Pillarisetti J, Sharma B, Murdoch AD, Danielson KG, Uitto J, Mauviel A: Structural and functional characterization of the human perlecan gene promoter. Transcriptional activation by transforming growth factor-beta via a nuclear factor 1-binding element. J Biol Chem 1997, 272: 5219-28.

62. Ayo SH, Radnik R, Garoni JA, Troyer DA, Kreisberg JA. High glucose increases diacylglycerol mass and activates protein kinase C in mesangial cells. Am J Physiol 1991; 261: F571-F577.

63. Craven PA, DeRubertis FR. Protein kinase C is activated in glomeruli from streptozotocin diabetic rats. Possible mediation by glucose. J Clin Invest 1989; 83: 1667-1675.

64. Ishii H, Jirousek MR, Koya D, Takagi C, Xia P, Clermont A, Bursell SE, Kern TS, Ballas LM, Heath WF, Stramm LE, Feener EP, King GL. Amelioration of vascular dysfuntions in diabetic rats by an oral PKC beta inhibitor. Science 1996; 272: 728-731.

65. Kreisberg JI, Radnik RA, Ayo SH, Garoni J, Saikumar P: High glucose elevates c-fos and c-jun transcripts and proteins in mesangial cell cultures. Kidney Int 1994, 46: 105-112.

66. Wilmer WA, Cosio FG: DNA binding of activator protein-1 is increased in human mesangial cells cultured in high glucose concentrations. Kidney Int 1998, 53:1172-1181.

67. Kreisberg JI, Radnik RA, Kreisberg SH: Phosphorylation of cAMP responsive element binding protein after treatment of mesangial cells with high glucose plus TGFβ or PMA. Kidney Int 1996, 50: 805-810.

68. Haneda M, Araki S, Togawa M, Sugimoto T, Isono M, Kikkawa R: Mitogen-activated protein kinase cascade is activated in glomeruli of diabetic rats and glomerular mesangial cells cultured under high glucose conditions. Diabetes 1997; 46:847-853.

69. Igarashi M, Wakasaki H, Takahara N, Ishii H, Zhen YJ, Yamauchi T, Kuboki K, Meier M, Rhodes CJ, King GL: Glucose or diabetes activate p38 mitogen-activated protein kinase via different pathways. J Clin Invest 1999; 103: 185-195.

70. Kang MJ, Wu X, Ly H, Thai K, Scholey JW. Effect of glucose on stress-activated protein kinase activity in mesangial cells and diabetic glomeruli. Kidney Int. 1999; 55:2203-2214.

71. Isono M, Cruz MC, Chen S, Hong SW, Ziyadeh FN: Extracellular signal-regulated kinase mediates stimulation of TGF-beta 1 and matrix by high glucose in mesangial cells. J. Am. Soc. Nephrol. 2000; 11:2222-2230.

72. Suzuki D, Miyata T, Saotome N, Horie K, Inagi R, Yasuda Y, Uchida K, Izuhara Y, Yagame M, Sakai H, Kurokawa K: Immunohistochemical evidence for an increased oxidative stress and carbonyl modifications of proteins in diabetic glomerular lesions. J Am Soc Nephrol 1999, 10: 822-832

73. Schmidt AM, Yan SD, Wautier J-L, Stern D: Activation of receptor for advanced glycation end products. Circ Res 1999, 84: 489-497.

74. Bierhaus A, Ritz E, Nawroth PP: Expression of receptors for advanced glycation end-products in occlusive vascular and renal disease. Nephrol Dial Transplant 1996, 11 Suppl 5:87-90.

75. Soulis T, Thallas V, Youssef S, Gilbert RE, McWilliam BG, Murray-McIntosh RP, Cooper ME: Advanced glycation end products and their receptors co-localise in rat organs susceptible to diabetic microvascular injury. Diabetologia 1997, 40: 619-628

76. Pugliese G, Pricci F, Romeo G, Pugliese F, Mene P, Giannini S, Cresci B, Galli G, Rotella CM, Vlassara H, Di Mario U: Upregulation of mesangial growth factor and extracellular matrix synthesis by advanced glycation end products via a receptor-mediated mechanism. Diabetes 1997, 46: 1881-1887

77. Yamagishi S, Inagaki Y, Okamoto T, Amano S, Koga K, Takeuchi M, Makita Z. Advanced glycation end product-induced apoptosis and overexpression of vascular endothelial growth factor and monocyte chemoattractant protein-1 in human-cultured mesangial cells. J Biol Chem. 2002; 277:20309-20315.

78. Morcos M, Sayed AA, Bierhaus A, Yard B, Waldherr R, Merz W, Kloeting I, Schleicher E, Mentz S, Abd el Baki RF, Tritschler H, Kasper M, Schwenger V, Hamann A, Dugi KA, Schmidt AM, Stern D, Ziegler R, Haering HU, Andrassy M, van der Woude F, Nawroth PP. Activation of tubular epithelial cells in diabetic nephropathy. Diabetes. 2002; 51:3532-3544.

79. Wells L, Vosseller K, Hart GW. Glycosylation of nucleocytoplasmic proteins: signal transduction and O-GlcNAc. Science. 2001; 291:2376-2378.

80. Kolm-Litty V, Sauer U, Nerlich A, Lehmann R, Schleicher ED: High glucose-induced transforming growth factor β1 production is mediated by the hexosamine pathway in porcine glomerular mesangial cells. J Clin Invest 1998, 101:160-169.

81. Du XL, Edelstein D, Rossetti L, Fantus IG, Goldberg H, Ziyadeh F, Wu J, Brownlee M: Hyperglycemia-induced mitochondrial superoxide overproduction activates the hexosamine pathway and induces plasminogen activator inhibitor-1 expression by increasing Sp1 glycosylation. Proc. Natl. Acad. Sci. U S A 2000; 97:12222-12226.

82. Weigert C, Brodbeck K, Lehmann R, Haring HU, Schleicher ED. Overexpression of glutamine:fructose-6-phosphate-amidotransferase induces transforming growth factor-beta1 synthesis in NIH-3T3 fibroblasts. FEBS Lett. 2001; 488:95-99.

83. Kadonaga JT, Courey AJ, Ladika J, Tjian R. Distinct regions of Sp1 modulate DNA binding and transcriptional activation. Science. 1988; 242:1566-1570.

84. Weigert C, Klopfer K, Kausch C, Brodbeck K, Stumvoll M, Haring HU, Schleicher ED. Palmitate-induced activation of the hexosamine pathway in human myotubes: Increased expression of glutamine:fructose-6-phosphate aminotransferase. Diabetes 2003 (in press)

85. Greene D. The pathogenesis and its prevention of diabetic neuropathy and nephropathy. Metabolism 1988; 37: suppl. 1: 25-29.

86. Larkins RG, Dunlop ME. The link between hyperglycaemia and diabetic nephropathy. Diabetologia 1992; 35: 499-504.

87. Olgemöller B, Schwaabe S, Schleicher ED, Gerbitz KD. Competitive inhibition by glucose of myo-inositol incorporation into cultured porcine mesangial cells. Biophys Biochem Acta 1990; 1052: 47-52.

88. Li W, Chan LS, Khatami M, Rockey JH: Non-competitive inhibition of myo-inositol transport in cultured bovine retinal capillary pericytes by glucose and reversal by sorbinil. Biochim Biophys Acta 1986; 857: 198-208.

89. Guzman NJ, Crews FT. Regulation of inositol transport by glucose and protein kinase C in mesangial cells. Kidney Int 1992; 42: 33-40.

90. Olgemöller B, Schleicher E, Schwaabe S, Gerbitz KD. Upregulation of myo-inositol transport compensates for competitive inhibition by glucose. Diabetes 1993; 42:1119-1125.

91. Mc Caleb ML, Mc Kean ML, Hohman TC, Laver N, Robinson WG. Intervention with aldose reductase inhibitor, tolrestat, in renal and retinal lesions of streptozotocin diabetic rats. Diabetologia 1991; 34: 659-701.

92. Nishikara T, Edelstein D, Du XL, Yamagishi S, Matsumura T, Kaneda Y, Yorek MA, Beebe D, Oates PJ, Hammes HP, Giardino I, Brownlee M: Normalizing mitochondrial superoxide production blocks three pathways of hyperglycaemic damage. Nature 2000; 404:787-790.

93. Ha H, Lee HB. Reactive oxygen species as glucose signaling molecules in mesangial cells cultured under high glucose. Kidney Int Suppl. 2000; 77:S19-25.

94. Catherwood MA, Powell LA, Anderson P, McMaster D, Sharpe PC, Trimble ER. Glucose-induced oxidative stress in mesangial cells. Kidney Int. 2002; 61:599-608.

95. Mueckler M: Facilitative glucose transporters (Review). Eur J Biochem 1994; 219:713-725.

96. Mogyorosi A, Ziyadeh FN: GLUT1 and TGF-β: the link between hyperglycemia and diabetic nephropathy. Nephrol. Dial. Transplant. 1999; 14:2827-2829.

97. Heilig CW, Liu Y, England RL, Freytag SO, Gilbert JD, Heilig KO, Zhu M, Concepcion LA, Brosius III FC: D-Glucose stimulates mesangial cell GLUT1 expression and basal and IGF-1-sensitive glucose uptake in rat mesangial cells. Diabetes 1997; 46:1030-1039.

98. Inoki K, Haneda M, Maeda S, Koya D, Kikkawa R: TGF-β1 stimulates glucose uptake by enhancing GLUT1 expression in mesangial cells. Kidney Int. 1999; 55:1704-1712.

99. Quinn LA, McCumbee WD: Regulation of glucose transport by angiotensin II and glucose in cultured vascular smooth muscle cells. J. Cell. Physiol. 1998; 177:94-102.

100. D'Agord Schaan B, Lacchini S, Bertoluci MC, Irigoyen MC, Machado UF, Schmid H: Increased renal GLUT1 abundance and urinary TGF-beta 1 in streptozotocin-induced diabetic rats: implications for the development of nephropathy complicating diabetes. Horm Metab Res 2001; 33:664-669.

101. Liu ZH, Chen ZH, Li Y-J, Liu D, Li LS: Phenotypic alterations of live mesangial cells in patients with diabetic nephropathy obtained from renal biopsy specimen (Abstract). J. Am. Soc. Nephrol. 1999; 10:A0669.

102. Heilig CW, Conception LA, Riser BL, Freytag SO, Zhu M, Cordes P: Overexpression of glucose transporters in rat mesangial cells cultered in a normal glucose milieu mimics the diabetic phenotype. J. Clin. Invest. 1995; 96:1802-1814.

103. Weigert C, Brodbeck K, Brosius FC III, Huber M, Lehmann R, Friess U, Facchin S, Aulwurm S, Häring HU, Schleicher ED, Heilig CW: Evidence for a novel, TGF-β1-independent mechanism of fibronectin production in mesangial cells overexpressing glucose transporters. Diabetes 2003; 52:527-535.

104. Wolf G, Ziyadeh FN: The role of angiotensin II in diabetic nephropathy: emphasis on nonhemodynamic mechanisms. Am J Kid Disease 1997, 29: 153-163

105. Mogensen CE: Microalbuminuria, blood pressure and diabetic renal disease: origin and development of ideas. Diabetologia 1999, 42: 263-285.

106. Wolf G: Angiotensin II is involved in the progression of renal disease: importance of non-hemodynamic mechanisms. Nephrologie 1998, 19: 451-456

107. Kagami S, Border WA, Miller DE, Noble NA: Angiotensin II stimulates extracellular matrix protein synthesis through induction of transforming growth factor-beta expression in rat glomerular mesangial cells. J Clin Invest 1994, 93: 2431-2437

108. Hill C, Logan A, Smith C, Gronbaek H, Flyvbjerg A. Angiotensin converting enzyme inhibitor suppresses glomerular transforming growth factor beta receptor expression in experimental diabetes in rats. Diabetologia. 2001; 45:495-500.

109. Mezzano SA, Ruiz-Ortega M, Egido J. Angiotensin II and renal fibrosis. Hypertension. 2001; 38:635-638.

110. James LR, Fantus IG, Goldberg H, Ly H, Scholey JW. Overexpression of GFAT activates PAI-1 promoter in mesangial cells. Am J Physiol Renal Physiol. 2000; 279:F718-727.

111. Nakamura S, Nakamura I, Ma L, Vaughan DE, Fogo AB. Plasminogen activator inhibitor-1 expression is regulated by the angiotensin type 1 receptor in vivo. Kidney Int. 2000; 58:251-259.

112. Hamaguchi A, Shokei K, Izumi Y, Zhan Y, Yamanaka S, Iwao H: Contribution of extracellular signal-regulated kinase to angiotensin II-induced transforming growth factor-β1 expression in vascular smooth muscle cells. Hypertension 1999, 34: 126-131.

113. Ruiz-Ortega M, Lorenzo O, Ruperez M, Blanco J, Egido J. Systemic infusion of angiotensin II into normal rats activates nuclear factor-kappaB and AP-1 in the kidney: role of AT(1) and AT(2) receptors. Am J Pathol. 2001; 158:1743-1756.

114. Morishita R, Gibbons GH, Horiuchi M, Kaneda Y, Ogihara T, Dzau VJ. Role of AP-1 complex in angiotensin II-mediated transforming growth factor-β expression and growth of smooth muscle cells: using decoy approach against AP-1 binding site. Biochem Biophys Res Commun 1998; 243:361-367.

115. Weigert C, Brodbeck K, Klopfer K, Haring HU, Schleicher ED. Angiotensin II induces human TGF-beta 1 promoter activation: similarity to hyperglycaemia. Diabetologia. 2002; 45:890-898.

116. Griendling KK, Minieri CA, Ollerenshaw JD, Alexander RW. Angiotensin II stimulates NADH and NADPH oxidase activity in cultured vascular smooth muscle cells. Circ Res. 1994; 74:1141-1148.

117. Natarajan R, Scott S, Bai W, Yerneni KKV, Nadler J: Angiotensin II signaling in vascular smooth muscle cells under high glucose conditions. Hypertension 1999, 33: 378-384

118. Amiri F, Shaw S, Wang X, Tang J, Waller JL, Eaton DC, Marrero MB. Angiotensin II activation of the JAK/STAT pathway in mesangial cells is altered by high glucose. Kidney Int. 2002; 61:1605-1616.

119. Singh R, Alavi N, Singh AK, Leehey DJ: Role of angiotensin II in glucose-induced inhibition of mesangial matrix degradation. Diabetes 1999, 48: 2066-2073

22

PATHOGENESIS OF DIABETIC GLOMERULOPATHY: THE ROLE OF GLOMERULAR HEMODYNAMIC FACTORS

Sharon Anderson, [1] and Radko Komers, [1,2]
[1]Division of Nephrology and Hypertension, Oregon Health and Science University, Portland, OR, U.S.A. and
[2]Diabetes Center, Institute for Clinical Experimental Medicine, Prague, Czech Republic

INTRODUCTION

Glomerular hyperfiltration in Type 1 diabetes mellitus (DM) of short duration has been recognized for many years [1-3], with increments in renal plasma flow (RPF) and nephromegaly [3]. With the finding of early hyperfiltration, Stalder and Schmid proposed that these early functional changes may predispose the subsequent development of diabetic glomerulopathy [1]. Early support for the hypothesis that renal hyperperfusion and hyperfiltration contribute to diabetic glomerulopathy emanated from the finding of diabetic glomerulopathy only in the non-stenosed kidney in the setting of unilateral renal artery stenosis [4]. Similar studies have more recently been performed in the much larger patient population with Type 2 DM. Studies reveal a wide range of renal hemodynamics in this group, but provide clear evidence for elevations of glomerular filtration rate (GFR) and RPF in significant proportions of patients of Caucasian, Native- and African-American origin [5-12]. Furthermore, compelling evidence for the presence of renal hemodynamic abnormalities in Type 2 diabetes has been reported in Pima Indians [12]. In that study, transition from impaired glucose tolerance to Type 2 DM was accompanied by a 30% increase in GFR. An increase in GFR has been also reported in obesity [13], a condition which often accompanies Type 2 DM.

Alterations in renal hemodynamics in diabetes are also associated with loss of renal functional reserve, i.e., the ability to increase GFR in response to amino acid infusion or to ingestion of a meal rich in protein [14]. These maneuvers may identify altered renal hemodynamics in a subset of patients with GFR within the normal range.

It has been proposed that the glomerular hyperfunction of early Type 1 DM predicts the later development of overt nephropathy and diabetic glomerulopathy [15,16], though some have failed to document such a relationship [17-19]. The reasons for these disparate results are as yet unclear. Likewise, the role of the glomerular hyperfiltration observed in Type 2 diabetic patients in the subsequent development of nephropathy remains to be established in longitudinal studies. However, preliminary results indicate a reduction in GFR over the first 2 years after diagnosis, with the greatest changes in the younger patients with initial GFR values greater than 120 ml/min [20]. Despite the controversy in human diabetes concerning the significance of hyperfiltration in the subsequent development of overt nephropathy, extensive experimental data provides considerable insight into the importance of hemodynamic factors in the initiation and progression of diabetic glomerulopathy [21,22].

RENAL HEMODYNAMICS IN EXPERIMENTAL DIABETES MELLITUS

Several animal models of both Type 1 and Type 2 DM have been used to study the role of altered hemodynamics in the development of diabetic glomerulopathy [21-24]. As in diabetic patients, diabetic rats tend to exhibit reduced values for whole kidney GFR during periods of severe uncontrolled hyperglycemia; single nephron (SN) GFR and plasma flow rates are also normal or reduced in animals in such catabolic states [24]. In the more clinically applicable model of Type 1 diabetes with moderate hyperglycemia, whole kidney GFR and SNGFR increase by about 40% as compared to normal rats [24-26]. Reductions in intrarenal vascular resistances result in elevation of the glomerular capillary plasma flow rate, Q_A. Despite normal blood pressure levels, transmission of systemic pressures to the glomerular capillaries is facilitated by proportionally greater reductions in afferent compared to efferent arteriolar resistances. Consequently, the glomerular capillary hydraulic pressure (P_{GC}) rises. Thus, the observed single nephron hyperfiltration results from both glomerular capillary hyperperfusion and hypertension [24-26]. In longterm studies, diabetic rats develop morphologic changes reminiscent of those in the diabetic human, including glomerular basement membrane thickening, renal and glomerular hypertrophy, mesangial matrix thickening and hyaline deposition, and ultimately glomerular sclerosis [25-30].

Evidence that these glomerular hemodynamic maladaptations contribute to the development and progression of diabetic glomerulopathy has been shown by studies of maneuvers which aggravate or ameliorate glomerular hyperperfusion and hyperfiltration, without affecting metabolic control. Uninephrectomy, which increases SNGFR, Q_A and P_{GC} in normal rats, accelerates the development of albuminuria and glomerular sclerosis in diabetic rats [31]. Intensification of glomerular lesions is observed in the unclipped kidney of diabetic rats with two-kidney Goldblatt hypertension, while the clipped kidney is substantially protected from glomerular injury [32]. Diabetic renal injury is similarly amplified by augmentation of dietary protein content, which increases glomerular perfusion and filtration [25].

By contrast, dietary protein restriction, which reduces SNGFR, Q_A and P_{GC} in other models, has clarified the role of hemodynamic factors in diabetic glomerulopathy. In long-term diabetes, low protein diets limited SNGFR by reducing the elevated P_{GC} and Q_A, and virtually prevented albuminuria and glomerular injury. In contrast, diabetic rats fed a high protein diet exhibited glomerular capillary hyperfiltration, hyperperfusion and hypertension, and marked increases in albuminuria and glomerular morphologic injury [25]. As there were no differences in metabolic control between the various groups, this study provided clear evidence that amelioration of the maladaptive glomerular hemodynamic pattern could prevent diabetic renal disease could dramatically lower the risk of diabetic glomerulopathy.

MECHANISMS OF HYPERFILTRATION IN DIABETES

The pathogenesis of diabetic hyperfiltration is multifactorial. Numerous mechanisms and mediators for this effect have been proposed (Table 1), and are briefly reviewed here. For better clarity, these mechanisms are divided in five areas separately discussed below. However, the reader should be aware of overlap between these processes, and the fact that they act in concert to promote renal hemodynamic alterations in diabetes.

Table 1

POTENTIAL MEDIATORS OF DIABETIC HYPERFILTRATION
1. Factors affecting predominantly afferent arteriolar tone
        Hyperglycemia/insulinopenia
        Advanced glycosylation end products
        Atrial natriuretic peptide and extracellular fluid volume expansion
        Nitric oxide and blunted tubulo-glomerular feedback
        Vasodilator prostaglandins
        Increased plasma ketone bodies, organic acids
        Increased plasma glucagon levels
        Increased plasma levels of growth hormone and insulin-like growth factor-1
        Impaired afferent arteriolar voltage-gated calcium channels
        Altered responsiveness or receptor density to catecholamines/angiotensin II/TxA2

2. Factors affecting predominantly afferent arteriolar tone
        Increased activity of the RAS, endothelin, and vasoconstrictor prostanoids

3. Miscellaneous factors
        Protein kinase C
        Increased Na+ reabsorption upstream from macula densa
        Increased kallikrein-kinin activity
        Abnormalities in calcium metabolism
        Vascular endothelial growth factor
        Abnormal myo-inositol metabolism
        Tissue hypoxia/abnormalities in local vasoregulatory factors

---

Metabolic millieu

Considering the simple fact that without the hyperglycemia and other factors characteristic for the diabetic milieu there would be no hemodynamic changes or nephropathy, the diabetic metabolic milieu must contribute. Hyperglycemia and/or insulinopenia *per se* [20,33], together with augmented growth hormone and glucagon levels [34,35], have been invoked in this process. Reduction of plasma glucose with initial institution of therapy reduces GFR in both Type 1 and 2 DM [33,36]. In moderately hyperglycemic diabetic rats, normalization of blood glucose levels reverses hyperfiltration [37], and insulin infusion reduces P_{GC} [38]. By contrast, insulin infusion sufficient to produce hyperinsulinemia, with euglycemia, increases P_{GC} and hyperfiltration in normal rats [39]. Further, infusion of blood containing early glycosylation products reproduces glomerular hyperfiltration in normal rats [40]. However, it should be appreciated that the most pronounced changes in renal hemodynamics as compared to nondiabetic animals occur in moderately hyperglycemic rats treated with suboptimal doses of exogenous insulin. Hyperfiltration often does not develop in rats without exogenous insulin treatment, despite moderate hyperglycemia. This finding suggests that some insulin levels, in concert with hyperglycemia, are necessary for development of renal hemodynamic changes in diabetes. Whether these effects are linked to vasodilator actions of insulin remains to be established.

There is growing evidence suggesting separate physiological and pathophysiological effects of C-peptide [41], a part of the endogenous insulin molecule that is not contained in exogenous insulin preparations. In addition to alterations in plasma insulin levels and actions, it has been suggested that the lack of C-peptide in diabetic rats also contributes to hyperfiltration [42,43].

Vasoactive factors
Apart from the above-mentioned mechanisms which are closely related to the diabetic metabolic milieu, there is a substantial evidence suggesting that renal hemodynamic alterations are a consequence of imbalance between the vasoactive humoral systems controlling the glomerular circulation. It is assumed that the balance between factors influencing the afferent arteriolar tone is shifted towards vasodilators, whereas opposite could be expected on the efferent arteriole.

Atrial natriuretic peptide (ANP), which induces afferent dilation and efferent constriction, represents one such promising candidate for mediating diabetic hyperfiltration. Plasma ANP levels are elevated in diabetes [44], and blockade of the ANP action with an antibody [44] or a specific receptor antagonist [45] blunts hyperfiltration in diabetic rats. It is likely that altered levels of ANP in diabetes are a consequence of an increase in total exchangeable body sodium and the hypervolemic state [46,47], although resistance to ANP may be also involved [48]. In any case, these observations suggest that sodium homeostasis is an important factor in the pathogenesis of hyperfiltration.

Nitric oxide (NO) is a potent vasodilator acting on both afferent and efferent arterioles, presumably with predominant afferent actions *in vivo* [49]. In mammalian tissues, NO is synthesized by a family of isoenzymes known as nitric oxide synthases (NOS). Considering its renal actions, NO is a good candidate for mediating diabetic hyperfiltration. Paradoxically, diabetes is considered to be a state with reduced NO bioavailability [50,51]. However, as recently reviewed [52], the situation in the diabetic kidney, in particular at the early stages of diabetes, is more complex.

Most of the renal hemodynamic studies conducted in hyperfiltering rats demonstrated increased renal hemodynamic responses and near-normalization of renal hemodynamics in response to inhibition of NO synthesis with non-specific NOS inhibitors (i.e., affecting all NOS isoforms) [53-55]. More recent studies attempted to identify the contribution of individual NOS isoforms in the process. We have recently focused on renal hemodynamic roles of neuronal NOS (nNOS, NOS1). This isoform is particularly of interest in the diabetic kidney. Under physiological conditions, NOS1-derived NO counteracts afferent vasoconstrictor signals mediated by the tubuloglomerular feedback mechanism, thus contributing to the control of P_{GC} [56]. The renal vascular tree is more sensitive to the systemic NOS1 inhibition in diabetic rats, as compared to controls [57]. Furthermore, we observed complete amelioration of hyperfiltration in response to intrarenal selective NOS1 inhibition in conjunction with increased number of nNOS-positive cells in MD regions of diabetic kidneys [58]. These observations identified NOS1-derived NO as an important player in the pathogenesis of diabetic hyperfiltration, and are in accordance with previous reports showing blunting of the tubuloglomerular feedback in diabetic rats [59,60], as further discussed below. There is also evidence suggesting that activity of the endothelial NOS isoform (eNOS, NOS3) may be increased, and responsible for renal NO hyperproduction in diabetes [61,62].

In addition to possible direct effects of diabetes on NOS activities, the NO-mediated alterations in renal hemodynamics may be related to increased activity of factors, which act as NO-dependent vasodilators or activate NO-cGMP pathway as a part of their signal transduction. De Vriese, et al [63] reported that neutralization of vascular endothelial growth factor (VEGF) with an antibody ameliorated diabetic hyperfiltration. VEGF has been implicated with non-hemodynamic pathways in the pathogenesis of diabetic complications, and also possesses vasomotor effects mediated by NO. Some other factors implicated in the pathophysiology of diabetic glomerulosclerosis, such as TGF-beta and leptin, also signal in part via NO. However, whether these pathways may have impact on glomerular hemodynamics remains to be elucidated.

Enhanced production of reative oxygen species (ROS) appears to be an important mechanism in the pathophysiology of diabetic complications, including nephropathy. Their role has been validated in long-term studies [64,65]. ROS are involved in diabetes-induced alterations in lipids and proteins, cellular signaling [66], inactivation of NO [67], and hemodynamics, acting predominantly as vasoconstrictors [68].

Hemodynamically oriented studies have suggested that ROS, as renal vasoconstrictors, decrease bioavailability of NO or limit the buffering capacity of NO against vasoconstrictors [69-71]. Therefore, one would expect that the net effect of this imbalance would result in renal vasoconstriction. However, this is difficult to reconcile with the fact of diabetic hyperfiltration. Importantly, there is no evidence demonstrating the effect of ROS scavenging on basal arteriolar tone in diabetic rats [70]. Considering the NO-ROS interaction, one would expect enhanced afferent vasodilator responses to antioxidants in diabetes.

In contrast, *in vivo* studies demonstrated that antioxidant treatment may normalize hyperfiltration in diabetes [64]. Considering the decrease in filtration fraction (FF) in diabetic rats treated with antioxidants, which was observed, one would expect efferent arteriolar effects of antioxidant treatment. These data suggest that these renal microvascular effects are attributable not only to protection of NO from quenching, but also to other mechanisms. One of those mechanisms compatible with the long-term glomerular hemodynamic actions of antioxidants could be, for example, inhibition of angiotensin II (Ang II) signaling via ROS [66].

A role for cyclooxygenase (COX) metabolites of arachidonic acid in the pathogenesis of diabetic nephropathy has been suggested in a number of clinical and experimental studies. Schambelan, et al [72] demonstrated an increase in conversion of exogenous arachidonate to prostaglandin E2 (PGE2), prostaglandin F2alpha, prostaglandin D2, and thromboxane B2 (TxB2) in glomeruli from diabetic rats. In the early stages of nephropathy, vasodilatory prostaglandins, such as prostaglandin E2 and prostacyclin, have been implicated in mediating alterations in renal hemodynamics in humans with Type 1 DM [73-76], as well as in experimental models of diabetes [77-80]. As demonstrated by Jensen, et al [77], inhibition of PG synthesis results in significant reductions in SNGFR, Q_A and P_{GC}.

The above mentioned evidence about the role of PG in the renal hemodynamics in diabetes relied on measurements of renal function in response to non-specific inhibitors that inhibit both COX isoenzymes. More recent studies focused on contribution of individual isoforms in the development of renal hemodynamic changes in diabetes. These studies demonstrated increased expression of COX-2 isoform in the diabetic kidney, and a modest effect of the selective COX-2 inhibition on glomerular filtration rate in diabetic rats as compared to COX-1 expression and acute inhibition [81].

Diabetes-related abnormalities of other vasodilator mechanisms have also been suggested, with findings of activation of the kallikrein-kinin system [82-84]. However, studies with kinin receptor antagonists have thus far proven inconsistent [85-87]. Earlier studies suggested that diabetic hyperfiltration might be at least in part attributable to increases in growth hormone [35] and potentially insulin-like growth factor levels. Current evidence suggests that although active in the pathophysiology of glomerular hypertrophy, growth hormone contribution to renal injury in diabetes has a minor hemodynamic component [88].

With respect to the delicate balance between dilators and constrictors in the control of glomerular hemodynamics, reduced afferent or mesangial actions of vasoconstrictor systems may also contribute. These mechanisms include reduced glomerular receptor sites for the vasoconstrictors Ang II and thromboxane [89,90]; and altered vascular responsiveness to catecholamines and Ang II [91-93].

The role of vasoconstrictor systems is, however, more complex. In apparent contrast to the reduced preglomerular and glomerular actions of some of these systems, inhibition of vasoconstrictor systems such as the RAS [26], endothelin (ET) [94], or thromboxane A2 [95,96] has beneficial effects on the development of nephropathy including amelioration of diabetic hyperfiltration. The most plausible explanation for this phenomenon is that the reduction of hyperfiltration by inhibition of these substances is achieved, at least in part, by inhibition of their efferent arteriolar actions. This also suggests that, unlike the preglomerular vasculature, diabetes is associated with normal or increased efferent actions of vasoconstrictors. Supporting this view are our whole kidney data showing an increase in renal hemodynamic vasodilator response to Ang II [92] in conjunction with reduced FF in diabetic rats. In parallel, Hollenberg's group have repeatedly documented enhanced activity of the renal RAS in both types of diabetes by demonstrating enhanced hemodynamic responses in these patients as compared to non-diabetic subjects [97,98]. It should be noted that similar to the glomerular microcirculatory pattern in general, renal hemodynamic responses to various mediators in experimental diabetes are largely dependent upon the state of metabolic control and insulin treatment. These differences may explain some disparate findings of studies exploring the activities of vasoactive systems in diabetes.

Alterations in signal transduction
There is convincing evidence suggesting the role of activation of the protein kinase C (PKC) enzyme family in the pathogenesis of diabetic complications. Importantly, some of these iso-enzymes are not only activated by hyperglycemia via de-novo synthesis of diacylglycerol, but also operate in signaling cascades of some vasoactive peptides, such as Ang II. Amelioration of hyperfiltration, associated with an overall renoprotective effect in the diabetic kidney, was observed in studies with newly available inhibitors of PKC [99].

In addition to PKC, other signaling pathways that are involved in the control of vascular tone are also activated in renal cells in some models of diabetes. For example, the p38 module of mitogen-activated protein kinases and Akt/PKB fulfill those criteria [100-105]. The renal hemodynamic impact of increased activities of such pathways represents a promising direction for future research.

Renal sodium handling and tubuloglomerular feedback.
In the normal kidney, cells of the macula densa (MD) sense early distal intratubular concentrations of Na+ and Cl- and in response to increasing ion concentrations, they send vasoconstrictor signals to the afferent arterioles. This autoregulatory mechanism, known as tubuloglomerular feedback (TGF), prevents excessive NaCl losses from the organism. Earlier studies suggested blunting of the TGF in experimental diabetes, resulting in a reduction of afferent constrictor signals [59,60].

More recently Vallon, et al [106,107] demonstrated that reduced TGF activity may be simply a result of increased Na^+ tubular reabsorption via Na^+/glucose cotransport, leading to reduced electrolyte delivery to the distal nephron. The same group extended this concept by linking the increases in proximal tubular reabsorption in diabetes to tubular hypertrophy induced by enhanced activity of ornithine decarboxyase (ODC)[108]. The concept is further supported by clinical and experimental observations demonstrating paradoxical increase in

GFR in response to a low salt diet [109,110]. However, this complex of observations suggesting the role of distal sodium delivery into the MD region is in contradiction to findings by other groups. Long-term studies showed that amelioration of hyperfiltration with some degree of nephroprotection in diabetic rats can be achieved by sodium restriction [111,112]. It is possible that mechanisms described by Vallon and co-workers represent short-term adjustments of renal hemodynamics in diabetes, whereas long-term treatment with a low salt diet can ultimately reduce hyperfiltration and be beneficial via a wide spectrum of mechanisms.

Intrinsic defects in glomerular arterioles, electromechanical coupling
Using videomicroscpy in isolated blood-perfused juxtamedullary nephrons, Carmines and co-workers [113,114] described several diabetes-induced alterations in afferent arteriolar ion channels that can result in increased baseline diameter and impaired responses to vasoconstrictors. Diabetic rats have suppressed vasoconstrictor-induced increases in intracellular Ca^{2+} concentrations due to functional defects in afferent arteriolar L-type calcium channels [113]. Subsequent studies [114] implicated increased expression and function of the ATP-sensitive K(+) channels (K-ATPc) in the renal afferent arteriolar dilation which occurs in experimental diabetes.

ROLE OF GLOMERULAR CAPILLARY HYPERTENSION

Of the glomerular hemodynamic determinants of hyperfiltration, the available evidence suggests that glomerular capillary hypertension plays the key role in progression of renal injury. Long-term protection against albuminuria and glomerular sclerosis was obtained in normotensive diabetic rats by angiotensin converting enzyme inhibitor (ACEI) therapy in doses which modestly lowered systemic blood pressure, but selectively normalized P_{GC}, without affecting the supranormal SNGFR and Q_A [26]. Studies in a variety of experimental models, including diabetes, have consistently shown that interventions which control glomerular capillary hypertension are associated with marked slowing of the development of structural injury [115].

Until recently, little was known of the exact mechanism(s) by which glomerular capillary hypertension eventuates in structural injury. Recently, innovative new techniques using a variety of *in vitro* systems have been developed to address this question. These studies postulate that glomerular hemodynamic factors modify the growth and activity of glomerular component cells, inducing the elaboration or expression of cytokines and other mediators, which then stimulate mesangial matrix production and promote structural injury. For instance, increased shear stress on endothelial cells enhances activity of such mediators as endothelin [116], NO [117,118], transforming growth factor-ß [119], and several cellular adhesion molecules [120,121] and modulates release of platelet derived growth factor [122,123]. Altered hemodynamics also influence mesangial cells: it has been postulated that expansion of the glomerular capillaries, and stretching of the mesangium in response to hypertension, might translate high P_{GC} into increased mesangial matrix formation [124]. Evidence for this mechanism comes from observations in microperfused rat glomeruli, in which increased hydraulic pressure was associated with increased glomerular volume; and in cultured mesangial cells, where cyclic stretching resulted in enhanced synthesis of protein, total collagen, collagen IV, collagen I, laminin, fibronectin, and transforming growth factor-ß (TGF-ß)[125-128]. Of particular relevance to diabetes, the accumulation of extracellular matrix caused by any degree of mechanical strain is aggravated in a milieu of high glucose concentration [128].

Additionally, growing mesangial cells under pulsatile conditions has been reported to stimulate PKC, calcium influx, and proto-oncogene expression [129], and Ang II receptor and angiotensinogen mRNA levels [125], as well as altered extracellular matrix protein processing enzymes [130,131]. Mediators of oxidant stress are induced by shear stress in vascular smooth muscle cells [132], as well as mechanical stretch in proximal tubular cells [133]. More evidence comes from the recent finding that application of pressure (comparable to elevated glomerular pressures *in vivo*) enhances mesangial cell matrix synthesis in cultured cells [134]. Finally, application of stress reduces glomerular epithelial cell podocyte differentiation and [135] and induces F-actin reorganization [136], representing another pathway of cellular injury. Given these new techniques, the cellular and molecular mechanisms by which glomerular hyperfiltration and hypertension leads to structural injury are in process of being elucidated.

REFERENCES

1.   Stalder G, Schmid R. 1959. Severe functional disorders of glomerular capillaries and renal hemodynamics in treated diabetes mellitus during childhood. Ann Paediatr, 193:129-138.

2. Ditzel J, Junker K. 1972. Abnormal glomerular filtration rate, renal plasma flow and renal protein excretion in recent and short-term diabetes. Br Med J, 2:13-19.

3. Mogensen CE, Andersen MJF. 1973. Increased kidney size and glomerular filtration rate in early juvenile diabetes. Diabetes, 22:706-712.

4. Berkman J, Rifkin H. 1973. Unilateral nodular diabetic glomerulosclerosis (Kimmelstiel-Wilson). Metabolism, 22:715-722.

5. Vora J, Dolben J, Dean J, Williams JD, Owens DR, Peters JR. 1992. Renal hemodynamics in newly presenting non-insulin-dependent diabetics. Kidney Int, 41:829-835.

6. Myers BD, Nelson RG, Williams GW, et al. 1991. Glomerular function in Pima Indians with non-insulin-dependent diabetes mellitus of recent origin. J Clin Invest, 88:524-530.

7. Palmisano JJ, Lebovitz HE. 1989. Renal function in Black Americans with type II diabetes. J Diab Compl, 3:40-44.

8. Nelson RG, Bennett PH, Beck GJ, Tan M, Knowler WC, Mitch WE, Hirschman GH, Myers BD. 1996. Development and progression of renal disease in Pima Indians with non-insulin-dependent diabetes mellitus. New Engl J Med, 335:1636-1642.

9. Nowack R, Raum E, Blum W, Ritz E. 1992. Renal hemodynamics in recent-onset Type II diabetes. Am J Kidney Dis, 20:342-347

10. Ritz E, Stefanski A. 1996. Diabetic nephropathy in Type II diabetes. Am J Kidney Dis, 27:167-194.

11. Wirta O, Pasternack A, Laippala P, Turjanmaa V. 1996. Glomerular filtration rate and kidney size after six years disease duration in non-insulin-dependent diabetic subjects. Clin Nephrol, 45:10-71.

12. Nelson RG, Tan M, Beck GJ, Bennett PH, Knowler WC, Mitch WE, Blouch K, Myers BD. 1999. Changing glomerular filtration with progression from impaired glucose tolerance to Type II diabetes mellitus. Diabetologia, 42: 90-93.

13. Hall JE, Brands MW, Henegar JR, Sheck EW. 1998. Abnormal kidney function as a cause and a consequence of obesity hypertension. Clin Exp Pharmacol Physiol, 25: 58-64.

14. Sackmann H, Tran-Van T, Tack T, Hanaire-Broutin H, Tauber JP, Ader JL. 1998. Renal functional reserve in IDDM patients. Diabetologia, 41: 86-93.

15. Mogensen CE. 1986. Early glomerular hyperfiltration in insulin-dependent diabetics and late nephropathy. Scand J Clin Lab Invest, 46:201-206.

16. Rudberg S, Persson B, Dahlquist G. 1992. Increased glomerular filtration rate as a predictor of diabetic nephropathy - an 8 -year prospective study. Kidney Int, 41:822-828.

17. Lervang H-H, Jensen S, Borchner-Mortensen J, Ditzel J. 1988. Early glomerular hyperfiltration and the development of late nephropathy in type 1 (insulin-dependent) diabetes mellitus. Diabetologia, 31:723-729.

18. Yip JW, Jones SL, Wiseman M, Hill C, Viberti GC. 1996. Glomerular hyperfiltration in the prediction of nephropathy in IDDM. A 10-year followup study. Diabetes, 45:1729-1733.

19. Mogensen CE. 1994. Glomerular hyperfiltration in human diabetes. Diabetes Care, 17:770-775.

20. Vora JP, Leese GP, Peters JR, Owens DR. 1996. Longitudinal evaluation of renal function in non-insulin-dependent diabetic patients with early nephropathy: effects of angiotensin-converting enzyme inhibition. J Diab Complic 10:88-93

21. Anderson S. 1992. Antihypertensive therapy in experimental diabetes. J Am Soc Nephrol, 3 (Suppl 1):S86-S90.

22. O'Donnell MP, Kasiske BL, Keane WF. 1986. Glomerular hemodynamics and structural alterations in experimental diabetes. FASEB J, 2:2339-2347.

23. Park SK, Meyer TW. 1995. The effect of hyperglycemia on glomerular function in obese Zucker rats. J Lab Clin Med, 125:501-507.

24. Hostetter TH, Troy JL, Brenner BM. 1981. Glomerular hemodynamics in experimental diabetes mellitus. Kidney Int, 19:410-415.

25. Zatz R, Meyer TW, Rennke HG, Brenner BM. 1985. Predominance of hemodynamic rather than metabolic factors in the pathogenesis of diabetic glomerulopathy. Proc Natl Acad Sci (USA), 82:5963-5967.

26. Zatz R, Dunn BR, Meyer TW, Anderson S, Rennke HG, Brenner BM. 1986. Prevention of diabetic glomerulopathy by pharmacological amelioration of glomerular capillary hypertension. J Clin Invest, 77:1925-1930.

27. Seyer-Hansen K. 1983. Renal hypertrophy in experimental diabetes mellitus. Kidney Int, 23:643-646.

28. Seyer-Hansen K, Hansen J, Gundersen HJG. 1980. Renal hypertrophy in experimental diabetes. A morphometric study. Diabetologia, 18:501-505.

29. Steffes MW, Brown DM, Basgen JM, Mauer SM. 1980. Amelioration of mesangial volume and surface alterations following islet transplantation in diabetic rats. Diabetes, 29:509-515.

30. Mauer SM, Michael AF, Fish AJ, Brown DM. 1972. Spontaneous immunoglobulin and complement deposition in glomeruli of diabetic rats. Lab Invest, 27:488-494.

31. O'Donnell MP, Kasiske BL, Daniels FX, Keane WF. 1986. Effect of nephron loss on glomerular hemodynamics and morphology in diabetic rats. Diabetes, 35:1011-1015.

32. Mauer SM, Steffes MW, Azar S, Sandberg SK, Brown DM. 1978. The effect of Goldblatt hypertension on development of the glomerular lesions of diabetes mellitus in the rat. Diabetes, 27:738-744.

33. Christiansen JS, Gammelgaard J, Tronier B, Svendsen PA, Parving H-H. 1982. Kidney function and size in diabetics before and during initial insulin treatment. Kidney Int 21:683-8

34. Parving H-H, Christiansen JS, Noer I, Tronier B, Mogensen CE. 1980. The effect of glucagon infusion on kidney function in short-term insulin-dependent juvenile diabetics. Diabetologia, 19:350-354.

35. Christiansen JS, Gammelgaard J, Orskov H, Andersen AR, Telmer S, Parving H-H. 1980. Kidney function and size in normal subjects before and during growth hormone administration for one week. Eur J Clin Invest, 11:487-490.

36. Vora J, Dolben J, Williams JD, Peters JR, Owens DR. 1993. Impact of initial treatment on renal function in newly-diagnosed Type 2 (non-insulin-dependent) diabetes mellitus. Diabetologia, 36:734-740.

37. Stackhouse S, Miller PL, Park SK, Meyer TW. 1990. Reversal of glomerular hyperfiltration and renal hypertrophy by blood glucose normalization in diabetic rats. Diabetes, 39:989-95.

38. Scholey JW, Meyer TW. 1989. Control of glomerular hypertension by insulin administration in diabetic rats. J Clin Invest, 83:1384-1389.

39. Tucker BJ, Anderson CM, Thies RS, Collins RC, Blantz RC. 1992. Glomerular hemodynamic alterations during acute hyperinsulinemia in normal and diabetic rats. Kidney Int, 42:1160-1168

40. Sabbatini M, Sansone G, Uccello F, Giliberti A, Conte G, Andreucci VE. 1992. Early glycosylation products induce glomerular hyperfiltration in normal rats. Kidney Int 42:875-881.

41. Wahren J, Ekberg K, Johansson J, Henriksson M, Pramanik A, Johansson BL, Rigler R, Jornvall H. 2000. Role of C-peptide in human physiology. Am J Physiol, 278:E759-768

42. Huang DY, Richter K, Breidenbach A, Vallon V. 2002. Human C-peptide acutely lowers glomerular hyperfiltration and proteinuria in diabetic rats: a dose-response study. Naunyn-Schmied Arch Pharmacol, 365:67-73, 2002

43. Sjoquist M, Huang W, Johansson BL. 1998. Effects of C-peptide on renal function at the early stage of experimental diabetes. Kidney Int, 54: 758-764.

44. Ortola FV, Ballermann BJ, Anderson S, Mendez RE, Brenner BM. 1987. Elevated plasma atrial natriuretic peptide levels in diabetic rats. J Clin Invest, 80:670-674.

45. Zhang PL, Mackenzie HS, Troy JL, Brenner BM. 1994. Effects of an atrial natriuretic peptide receptor antagonist on glomerular hyperfiltration in diabetic rats. J Am Soc Nephrol, 4:1564-1570.

46. Feldt-Rasmussen B. 1987. Central role for sodium in the pathogenesis of blood pressure changes independent of angiotensin, aldosterone and catecholamines in Type 1 (insulin-dependent) diabetes mellitus. Diabetologia, 30: 610-617.

47. O'Hare JA, Ferris BJ, Brady D, Twomey B, O'Sullivan DJ. 1985. Exchangable sodium and renin in hypertensive diabetic patients with and without nephropathy. Hypertension, 7 [Suppl II]: II43-II48.

48. Fioretto P, Sambataro M, Cipollina MR, Giorato C, Carraro A, Opocher G, Sacerdoti D, Brocco E, Morocutti A, Mantero F. 1992. Role of atrial natriuretic peptide in the pathogenesis of sodium retention in IDDM with and without glomerular hyperfiltration. Diabetes, 41: 936-945.

49. Deng A, Baylis C. 1993. Locally produced EDRF controls preglomerular resistance and ultrafiltration coefficient. Am J Physiol, 264: F212-F215.

50. Pieper GM. 1998. Review of alterations in endothelial nitric oxide production in diabetes. Protective role of arginine on endothelial dysfunction. Hypertension, 31:1047-1060

51. Goligorsky MS, Chen J, Brodsky S. 2001. Workshop: endothelial cell dysfunction leading to diabetic nephropathy : focus on nitric oxide. Hypertension 37:744-748.

52. Komers R, Anderson S. 2003. The paradoxes of nitric oxide in the diabetic kidney. *Am J Physiol*, in press

53. Bank N, Aynedjian HS. 1993. Role of EDRF (nitric oxide) in diabetic renal hyperfiltration. Kidney Int, 43:1306-12.

54. Tolins JP, Shultz PJ, Raij L, Brown DM, Mauer SM. 1993. Abnormal renal hemodynamic response to reduced renal perfusion pressure in diabetic rats: role of NO. Am J Physiol, 265: F886-95.

55. Mattar AL, Fujihara CK, Ribeiro MO, de Nucci G, Zatz R. 1996. Renal effects of acute and chronic nitric oxide inhibition in experimental diabetes. Nephron, 74:136-43

56. Wilcox CS, Welch WJ, Murad F, Gross SS, Taylor G, Levi R, Schmidt HH. 1992. Nitric oxide synthase in macula densa regulates glomerular capillary pressure. Proc Natl Acad Sci, 89: 11993-11997.

57. Komers R, Oyama TT, Chapman JG, Allison KM, Anderson S. 2000. Effects of systemic inhibition of neuronal nitric oxide synthase on hemodynamics in diabetic rats. Hypertension, 35:655-661

58. Komers R, Lindsley JN, Oyama TT, Allison KM, Anderson S. 2000. Role of neuronal nitric oxide synthase (NOS1) in the pathogenesis of renal hemodynamic changes in diabetes. Am J Physiol, 279:F573-583

59. Blantz RC, Peterson OW, Gushwa L, Tucker BJ. 1982. Effect of modest hyperglycemia on tubuloglomerular feedback activity. Kidney Int, 22 (Suppl 12):S206-S212.

60. Vallon V, Blantz RC, Thomson S. 1995. Homeostatic efficiency of tubuloglomerular feedback is reduced in established diabetes mellitus in rats. Am J Physiol, 269:F876-F883.

61. Sugimoto H, Shikata K, Matsuda M, Kushiro M, Hayashi Y, Hiragushi K, Wada J, Makino H. 1998. Increased expression of endothelial cell nitric oxide synthase (ecNOS) in afferent and glomerular endothelial cells is involved in glomerular hyperfiltration of diabetic nephropathy. Diabetologia, 41: 1426-1434.

62. De Vriese AS, Stoenoiu MS, Elger M, Devuyst O, Vanholder R, Kriz W, Lameire NH. 2001. Diabetes-induced microvascular dysfunction in the hydronephrotic kidney: role of nitric oxide. Kidney Int, 60:202-210

63. De Vriese AS, Tilton RG, Elger M, Stephan CC, Kriz W, Lameire NH. 2001. Antibodies against vascular endothelial growth factor improve early renal dysfunction in experimental diabetes. J Am Soc Nephrol, 12:993-1000

64. Koya D, Lee IK, Ishii H, Kanoh H, King GL. 1997. Prevention of glomerular dysfunction in diabetic rats by treatment with d-alpha-tocopherol. J Am Soc Nephrol, 8:426-435

65. Melhem MF, Craven PA, Derubertis FR. 2001. Effects of dietary supplementation of alpha-lipoic acid on early glomerular injury in diabetes mellitus. J Am Soc Nephrol, 12:124-133

66. Griendling KK, Ushio-Fukai M. 2000. Reactive oxygen species as mediators of angiotensin II signaling. Regul Pept 91:21-27

67. Sugimoto H, Shikata K, Wada J, Horiuchi S, Makino H. 1999. Advanced glycation end products-cytokine-nitric oxide sequence pathway in the development of diabetic nephropathy: aminoguanidine ameliorates the overexpression of tumour necrosis factor-alpha and inducible nitric oxide synthase in diabetic rat glomeruli. Diabetologia, 42: 878-886.

68. Schnackenberg CG. 2002. Physiological and pathophysiological roles of oxygen radicals in the renal microvasculature. Am J Physiol, 282:R335-342

69. Ohishi K, Carmines PK. 1995. Superoxide dismutase restores the influence of nitric oxide on renal arterioles in diabetes mellitus. J Am Soc Nephrol, 5:1559-1566

70. Schnackenberg CG, Wilcox CS. 2001. The SOD mimetic tempol restores vasodilation in afferent arterioles of experimental diabetes. Kidney Int 59:1859-1864

71. Schoonmaker GC, Fallet RW, Carmines PK. 2000. Superoxide anion curbs nitric oxide modulation of afferent arteriolar ANG II responsiveness in diabetes mellitus. Am J Physiol 278:F302-F309.

72. Schambelan M, Blake S, Sraer J, Bens M, Nives MP, Wahbe F. 1985. Increased prostaglandin production by glomeruli isolated from rats with streptozotocin-induced diabetes mellitus. J Clin Invest 75:404-412

73. Esmatjes E, Fernandez MR, Halperin I, Camps J, Gaya J, Arroyo V, Rivera F, Figuerola D. 1985. Renal hemodynamic abnormalities in patients with short term insulin-dependent diabetes mellitus. J Clin Endocrinol Metab 60:1231-1236

74. Hommel E, Mathiesen E, Arnold-Larsen S, Edsberg B, Olsen UB, Parving H-H. 1987. Effects of indomethacin on kidney function in type 1 (insulin-dependent) diabetic patients with nephropathy. Diabetologia 30:78-81

75. Gambardella S, Andreani D, Cancelli A, Di Mario U, Cardamone I, Stirati G, Cinotti G, Pugliese F. 1988. Renal hemodynamics and urinary excretion of 6-keto-prostaglandin F1 alpha and thomboxane B2 in newly diagnosed type 1 diabetic patients. Diabetes 37:1044-1048

76. Viberti GC, Benigni A, Bognetti E, Remuzzi G, Wiseman MJ. 1989. Glomerular hyperfiltration and urinary prostaglandins in type 1 diabetes mellitus. Diab Med 6:219-223

77. Jensen PK, Steven K, Blaehr H, Christiansen JS, Parving H-H. 1986. Effects of indomethacin on glomerular hemodynamics in experimental diabetes. Kidney Int, 29:490-495.

78. Kasiske BL, O'Donnell MP, Keane WF. 1985. Glucose-induced increases in renal hemodynamic function. Possible modulation by renal prostaglandins. Diabetes 34:360-364

79. Craven PA, Caines MA, DeRubertis FR. 1987. Sequential alterations in glomerular prostaglandin and thromboxane synthesis in diabetic rats: relationship to the hyperfiltration of early diabetes. Metabolism 36:95-103

80. Perico N, Benigni A, Gabanelli M, Piccinelli A, Rog M, DeRiva C, Remuzzi G. 1992. Atrial natriuretic peptide and prostacyclin synergistically mediate hyperfiltration and hyperperfusion of diabetic rats. Diabetes 41: 533-538

81. Komers R, Lindsley JN, Oyama TT, Schutzer WE, Reed JF, Mader SL, Anderson S. 2001. Immunohistochemical and functional correlations of renal cyclooxygenase-2 in experimental diabetes. J Clin Invest 107:889-898

82. Mayfield RK, Margolius HS, Levine JH, Wohltmann HJ, Loadholt CB, Colwell JA. 1984. Urinary kallikrein excretion in insulin-dependent diabetes mellitus and its relationship to glycemic control. J Clin Endocrinol Metab 59:278-286.

83. Jaffa AA, Miller DH, Bailey GS, Chao J, Margolius HS, Mayfield RK. 1987. Abnormal regulation of renal kallikrein in experimental diabetes. Effects of insulin in prokallikrein synthesis and activation. J Clin Invest 80: 1651-1659.

84. Campbell DJ, Kelly DJ, Wilkinson-Berka JL, Cooper ME, Skinner SL. 1999. Increased bradykinin and "normal" angiotensin peptide levels in diabetic Sprague-Dawley and transgenic (mRen-2)27 rats. Kidney Int 56:211-21

85. Jaffa AA, Rust PF, Mayfield RK. 1995. Kinin, a mediator of diabetes-induced glomerular hyperfiltration. Diabetes, 44:156-160.

86. Vora JP, Oyama TT, Thompson MM, Anderson S. 1997. Interactions of the kallikrein-kinin and renin-angiotensin systems in experimental diabetes. Diabetes, 46:107-112.

87. Komers R, Cooper ME. 1995. Acute renal hemodynamic effects of ACE inhibition in diabetic hyperfiltration: role of kinins. Am J Physiol, 268:F588-F594.

88. Landau D, Israel E, Rivkis I, Kachko L, Schrijvers BF, Flyvbjerg A, Phillip M, Segev Y. 2003. The effect of growth hormone on the development of diabetic kidney disease in rats. Nephrol Dial Transplant 18:694-702.

89. Ballermann BJ, Skorecki KL, Brenner BM. 1984. Reduced glomerular angiotensin II receptor density in early untreated diabetes mellitus in the rat. Am J Physiol, 247:F110-F116.

90. Wilkes BM, Kaplan R, Mento PF, Aynedjian H Macica CM, Schlondorff D, Bank N. 1992. Reduced glomerular thromboxane receptor sites and vasoconstrictor responses in diabetic rats. Kidney Int, 41:992-999.

91. Christlieb AR. 1974. Renin, angiotensin and norepinephrine in alloxan diabetes. Diabetes, 23:962-970.

92. Kennefick TM, Oyama TT, Thompson MM, Vora JP, Anderson S. 1996. Enhanced renal sensitivity to angiotensin actions in diabetes mellitus in the rat. Am J Physiol, 271:F595-F602.

93. Ohishi K, Okwueze MI, Vari RC, Carmines PK. 1994. Juxtamedullary microvascular dysfunction during the hyperfiltration stage of diabetes mellitus. Am J Physiol, 267:F99-F105.

94. Benigni A, Colosio V, Brena C, Bruzzi I, Bertani T, Remuzzi G. 1998. Unselective inhibition of endothelin receptors reduces renal dysfunction in experimental diabetes. Diabetes 47: 450-456.

95. Kontessis PS, Jones SL, Barrow SE, Stratton PD, Alessandrini P, De Cosmo S, Ritter JM, Viberti JC. 1993. Effect of thromboxane sythase inhibitor on renal function in diabetic nephropathy. J Lab Clin Med 21: 415-423.

96. Uriu K, Kaizu K, Hashimoto O, Komine N, Etoh S. 1994. Acute and chronic effects of thromboxane A2 inhibition on the renal hemodynamics in streptozotocin-induced diabetic rats. Kidney Int 45:794-802

97. Price D, Porter L, Gordon M, Fisher N, De'Oliveira J, Laffel L, Passan D, Williams G, Hollenberg N. 1999. The paradox of the low-renin state in diabetic nephropathy. J Am Soc Nephrol 10:2382-2391

98. Lansang MC, Price DA, Laffel LM, Osei SY, Fisher ND, Erani D, Hollenberg NK. 2001. Renal vascular responses to captopril and to candesartan in patients with type 1 diabetes mellitus. *Kidney* International 59:1432-1438

99. Ishii H, Jirousek MR, Koya D, Takagi C, Xia P, Clermont A, Bursell SE, Kern TS, Ballas LM, Heath WF, Stramm LE, Feener EP, King GL. 1996. Amelioration of vascular dysfunctions in diabetic rats by an oral PKC beta inhibitor. Science 272:728-31

100. Meloche S, Landry J, Huot J, Houle F, Marceau F, Giasson E. 2000. p38 MAP kinase pathway regulates angiotensin II-induced contraction of rat vascular smooth muscle. Am J Physiol 279:H741-751, 2000

101. Igarashi M, Wakasaki H, Takahara N, Ishii H, Jiang ZY, Yamauchi T, Kuboki K, Meier M, Rhodes CJ, King GL. 1999. Glucose or diabetes activates p38 mitogen-activated protein kinase via different pathways. J Clin Invest 103:185-195

102. Kang SW, Adler SG, Lapage J, Natarajan R. 2001. p38 MAPK and MAPK kinase 3/6 mRNA and activities are increased in early diabetic glomeruli. Kidney Int 60:543-552

103. Fulton D, Gratton JP, McCabe TJ, Fontana J, Fujio Y, Walsh K, Franke TF, Papapetropoulos A, Sessa WC. 1999. Regulation of endothelium-derived nitric oxide production by the protein kinase Akt. Nature 399:597-601

104. Downward J. 1998. Mechanisms and consequences of activation of protein kinase B/Akt. Curr Opin Cell Biol 10:262-267

105. Feliers D, Duraisamy S, Faulkner JL, Duch J, Lee AV, Abboud HE, Choudhury GG, Kasinath BS. 2001. Activation of renal signaling pathways in db/db mice with type 2 diabetes. Kidney Int 60:495-504

106. Vallon V, Richter K, Blantz RC, Thomson S, Osswald H. 1999. Glomerular hyperfiltration in experimental diabetes mellitus: potential role of tubular reabsorption. J Am Soc Nephrol 10:2569-2576

107. Vallon V, Huang DY, Deng A, Richter K, Blantz RC, Thomson S. 2002. Salt-sensitivity of proximal reabsorption alters macula densa salt and explains the paradoxical effect of dietary salt on glomerular filtration rate in diabetes mellitus. J Am Soc Nephrol 13:1865-1871

108. Thomson SC, Deng A, Bao D, Satriano J, Blantz RC, Vallon V. 2001. Ornithine decarboxylase, kidney size, and the tubular hypothesis of glomerular hyperfiltration in experimental diabetes. J Clin Invest 107:217-224

109. Luik PT, Hoogenberg K, Van Der Kleij FG, Beusekamp BJ, Kerstens MN, De Jong PE, Dullaart RP, Navis GJ. 2002. Short-term moderate sodium restriction induces relative hyperfiltration in normotensive normoalbuminuric Type I diabetes mellitus. *Diabetologia* 45:535-541,

110. Vallon V, Wead LM, Blantz RC. 1995. Renal hemodynamics and plasma and kidney angiotensin II in established diabetes mellitus in rats: effect of sodium and salt restriction. J Am Soc Nephrol 5:1761-1767

111. Bank N, Lahorra MA, Aynedjian HS, Wilkes BM. 1988. Sodium restriction corrects hyperfiltration of diabetes. Am J Physiol 254: F668-F676.

112. Allen TJ, Waldron MJ, Casley D, Jerums G, Cooper ME. 1997. Salt restriction reduces hyperfiltration, renal enlargement, and albuminuria in experimental diabetes. Diabetes 46: 119-124.

113. Carmines PK, Ohishi K, Ikenaga H. 1996. Functional impairment of renal afferent arteriolar voltage-gated calcium channels in rats with diabetes mellitus. J Clin Invest, 98:2564-2571

114. Ikenaga H, Bast JP, Fallet RW, Carmines PK. 2000. Exaggerated impact of ATP-sensitive K(+) channels on afferent arteriolar diameter in diabetes mellitus. J Am Soc Nephrol 11:1199-1207

115. Anderson S. 1993. Pharmacologic interventions in experimental animals. In Prevention of Progressive Chronic Renal Failure. El Nahas AM, Mallick NP, Anderson S, eds. Oxford: Oxford Univ. Press

116. Kuchan MJ, Frangos JA. 1993. Shear stress regulates endothelin-1 release via protein kinase C and cGMP in cultured endothelial cells. Am J Physiol, 264:H150-H156.

117. Buga GM, Gold ME, Fukuto JM, Ignarro LJ. 1991. Shear stress-induced release of nitric oxide from endothelial cells grown on beads. Hypertension, 17:187-193.

118. Awolesi MA, Sessa WC, Sumpio BE. 1995. Cyclic strain upregulates nitric oxide synthesis in cultured bovine aortic endothelial cells. J Clin Invest, 96:1449-1454.

119. Ohno M, Cooke JC, Dzau VJ, Gibbons GH. 1995. Fluid shear stress induces endothelial transforming growth factor beta-1 transcription and production. Modulation by potassium-channel blockade. J Clin Invest, 95:1363-1369.

120. Nagel T, Resnick N, Atkinson WJ, Dewey CF, Jr, Gimbrone, MA, Jr. 1994. Shear stress selectively upregulates intercellular adhesion molecule-1 expression in cultured human vascular endothelial cells. J Clin Invest, 94:885-891.

121. Sugimoto H, Shikata K, Hirata K, Akiyama K, Matsuda M, Kushiro M, Hayashi Y, Miyatake N, Miyasaka M, Makino H. 1997. Increased expression of intercellular adhesion molecule-1 (ICAM-1) in dibetic rat glomeruli: glomerular hyperfiltration is a potential mechanism of ICAM-1 upregulation. Diabetes 46: 2075-2081

122. Ott MJ, Olson JL, Ballermann BJ. 1995. Chronic *in vitro* flow promotes ultrastructural differentiation of endothelial cells. Endothelium, 3:21-30.

123. Malek AM, Gibbons GH, Dzau VJ, Izumo S. 1993. Fluid shear stress differentially modulates expression of genes encoding basic fibroblast growth factor and platelet-derived growth factor B chain in vascular endothelium. J Clin Invest 92:2013-2021.

124. Riser BL, Cortes P, Zhao X, Bernstein J, Dumler F, Narins RG. 1992. Intraglomerular pressure and mesangial stretching stimulate extracellular matrix formation in the rat. J Clin Invest, 90:1932-1943.

125. Becker B, Yasuda T, Kondo S, Vaikunth S, Homma T, Harris RC. 1998. Mechanical stretch/relaxation stimulates a cellular renin-angiotensin system in cultured rat mesangial cells. Exp Nephrol 6:57-126. Harris RC, Haralson MA, Badr KF. 1992. Continuous stretch-relaxation in culture alters rat mesangial cell morphology, growth characteristics, and metabolic activity. Lab Invest, 66:548-554.

127. Riser BL, Cortes P, Heilig C, Grondin J, Ladson-Wofford S, Patterson D, Narins RG. Cyclic stretching force selectively up-regulates transforming growth factor-ß isoforms in cultured rat mesangial ells. Am J Pathol, 148:1915-1923.

128. Cortes P, Zhao X, Riser BL, Narins RG. 1997. Role of glomerular mechanical strain in the pathogenesis of diabetic nephropathy. Kidney Int, 51:57-68.

129. Homma T, Akai Y, Burns KD, Harris RC. 1992. Activation of S6 kinase by repeated cycles of stretching and relaxation in rat glomerular mesangial cells. J Biol Chem, 267:23129-23135.

130. Yasuda T, Kondo S, Homma T, Harris RC. 1996. Regulation of extracellular matrix by mechanical stress in rat glomerular mesangial cells. J Clin Invest 98:1991-2000

131. Harris RC, Akai Y, Yasuda T, Homma T. 1995. The role of physical forces in alterations of mesangial cell function. Kidney Int 45 (Suppl 45):S17, 1995

132. Wagner CT, Durante W, Christodoulide N, Hellums JD, Schafer AI. 1997. Hemodynamic forces induce the expression of heme oxygenase in cultured vascular smooth muscle cells. J Clin Invest, 100:589-596.

133. Ricardo SD, Ding G, Eufemio M, Diamond JR. 1997. Antioxidant expression in experimental hydronephrosis: role of mechanical stretch and growth factors. Am J Physiol, 272:F789-F798.

134. Mattana J, Singhal PC. 1995. Applied pressure modulates mesangial cell proliferation and matrix synthesis. Am J Hypertension, 8:1112-1120.

135. Petermann AT, Hiromura K, Blonski M, Pippin J, Monkawa T, Durvasalu R, Couser WG, Shankland SJ. 2002. Mechanical stress reduces podocyte proliferation in vitro. Kidney Int, 61:40-50

136. Endlich K, Kress KR, Reiser J, Uttenweiler D, Kriz W, Mundel P, Endlich K. 2001. Podocytes respond to mechanical stress in vitro. J Am Soc Nephrol, 12:413-422

23

THE EMERGING ROLE OF GROWTH HORMONE (GH) AND VASCULAR ENDOTHELIAL GROWTH FACTOR (VEGF) IN DIABETIC KIDNEY DISEASE

Allan Flyvbjerg, Dinah Khatir and Ruth Rasch
Medical Department M (Diabetes and Endocrinology), Medical Research Laboratories,
Institute of Experimental Clinical Research, Aarhus University Hospital, Aarhus, Denmark and
Department of Cell Biology, Institute of Anatomy, Aarhus University, Aarhus, Denmark

INTRODUCTION

The development of diabetic nephropathy in Type 1 and Type 2 diabetes mellitus is still a significant clinical problem associated with increased morbidity and mortality [1-4]. The well known early changes of the diabetic kidney disease are renal enlargement and hyperfiltration. Later on in the incipient stage an increase in urinary albumin excretion (UAE) is followed by increased basement membrane thickness (BMT), mesangial proliferation and glomerular sclerosis that may lead to overt diabetic nephropathy and progressive renal insufficiency [1-4]. Interestingly, the renal functional and structural changes in animal models of Type 1 and Type 2 diabetes have fundamental similarities to those occurring in diabetic patients and accordingly spontaneously developing or chemically-induced (i.e. streptozotocin (STZ)) diabetic rodents have been used to elucidate the pathogenesis of diabetic kidney disease. These diabetic animal models develop renal enlargement, glomerular hypertrophy and renal hyperfiltration within weeks after diabetes debut and increased UAE, increased glomerular BMT and mesangial expansion within months [5,6]. Due to their growth promoting and proliferative effects, several growth factors have attracted attention in various aspects of diabetes research including conceivable effects on functional and structural changes in the development of diabetic kidney disease [6]. The present review will present data on a definite role of the growth hormone (GH) and vascular endothelial growth factor (VEGF) in the pathogenesis of the renal changes in experimental diabetes.

GROWTH HORMONE (GH)

Viewed historically, GH is the growth factor with the longest association to diabetes. The anterior pituitary became interesting when Young in 1937 showed that anterior pituitary extracts precipitated diabetes in dogs [7] and attention was focused on GH 50 years ago, when Campbell et al. showed that daily injections of highly purified GH made dogs permanently diabetic [8]. The discovery that induced further interest in GH and diabetes was the observations by Yde [9] and Hansen et al. [10] that diabetic patients present with substantial GH hypersecretion. At the same time the 'GH-hypothesis' was launched by Lundbæk et al. suggesting GH to play an important role in the development of diabetic microangiopathy (i.e. retinopathy) [11]. The role of insulin-like growth factors (IGFs) and diabetes appears to be much shorter, although as early as 30 years ago studies on sulphation factor (SF) or non-suppressible insulin-like activity (NSILA) in diabetic patients were performed without awareness of their partial identity with IGFs [12]. Yde was the first to show that the SF was abnormal in diabetic serum, with a negative correlation with metabolic control [12]. Today it is generally believed that metabolic deterioration in diabetes first decreases hepatic IGF-I formation and serum IGF-I concentration, which then secondarily induces GH hypersecretion through an intact feedback mechanism [6,13-15]. Increased circulating GH concentrations are then believed to stimulate local IGF-I concentrations in non-hepatic tissues (e.g. in the kidney) as discussed below.

EVIDENCE FOR A ROLE OF GH IN DIABETIC KIDNEY DISEASE

As described above it is well-known that poorly controlled diabetes in man is characterized by GH hypersecretion [9-16], while the most widely used experimental animals model for Type 1 diabetes, the STZ-diabetic rats, is characterized by low circulating GH concentrations, with loss of the characteristic pulsatility early after induction of diabetes [17]. The reason for this discrepancy is still controversial as discussed in detail in [18]. Just recently we discovered that diabetic mice present with GH hypersecretion and low circulating IGF-I levels [19], indicating that this animal strain may be a better model for the circulating perturbations in the GH/IGF axis seen in human diabetes than the diabetic rat. It seems evident, however, that the difference between experimental diabetes in rats and human diabetes with respect to the GH/IGF axis is restricted to GH. Similar changes have been reported for other elements in the GH/IGF axis in poorly controlled diabetic rats and man, including changes in circulating concentrations of GHBP, IGF-I and IGFBPs [18-24]. In addition, specific changes occur locally in the diabetic kidney, involving a number of complex cellular mechanisms with changes in renal GHBP, IGF receptors and IGFBPs [25].

Decreased serum GHBP concentrations and low hepatic GHR number are well described features in experimental diabetes [16,17,23,24]. In contrast only few data have been published on the renal expression of GHR and GHBP in experimental diabetes. In a recent study including both short- and long-term diabetic rats, differential changes in kidney GHR and GHBP mRNA were observed [16]. In the cortex, no change was seen in the GHR mRNA throughout the observation period of six months, while a significant increase in the GHBP mRNA was observed 1 month after induction of diabetes and sustained for the rest of the study period [16]. No changes were seen in GHR or GHBP mRNA in the medullary regions [16]. These data indicate that although the GHR and GHBP mRNAs originate from the same gene, they are differentially regulated during the development of experimental diabetic kidney disease and furthermore imply a specific functional role for GHBP. Whether the increase in renal GHBP mRNA actually enhances renal GH availability to the GHR and thereby enhances a patho-physiological role of GH is still unknown.

It is well established today that the rapid increase in renal growth and function seen in various experimental models of Type 1 diabetes is preceded by a rise in renal tissue concentration of IGF-I [19-23, 25-30]. Further evidence that IGF-I, with the modulating effect of GH, may be involved in both the short- and long-term renal changes is given in a series of experiments in diabetic dwarf rats. The dwarf rat strain used in these experiments is characterized by having a inherited autosomally recessive gene [31]. Homozygous dwarf rats present with an isolated GH deficiency with about 5-10% of normal pituitary GH content, low circulating GH levels and reduced circulating and tissue concentrations of IGF-I, but otherwise normal pituitary function [31]. In short-term experiments, STZ-diabetic dwarf rats exhibit slower and lesser initial renal and glomerular hypertrophy as well as a smaller rise in kidney IGF-I than diabetic controls with intact pituitary, indicating that GH per se may be involved in the modulation of renal enlargement [26]. Furthermore, long-term diabetic dwarf rats, with a diabetes duration of six months, display a smaller degree of renal and glomerular hypertrophy and rise in UAE, when compared to the changes observed in pituitary intact diabetic rats [32].

TARGETING GH BY GH RECEPTOR ANTAGONISTS

Several experimental and clinical studies have previously examined the effect of partial blockade of GH by long-acting somatostatin analogues in diabetes (for review please see [6])). More recently a series of highly specific antagonists of the GH action has been developed for the potential therapeutic use in various patho-physiological conditions, including diabetes mellitus. Initially it was shown that alteration of single amino acids in the third α-helix of bovine (b)GH (residues 109-126) results in a GH antagonist (GHA)[33-34]. In vitro experiments showed that this new group of GHAs binds to the GH receptor with the same affinity as native GH, but in vivo a phenotypic dwarf animal characterized by low circulating IGF-I levels and a proportional body composition develops when the GHA is expressed in transgenic (TG) mice [33-34]. Studies in long-term diabetic GHA TG mice, that express the GHA (bGH-G119R or hGH-G120R), have shown that these animals are protected against development of diabetic renal changes [35,36]. When compared with TG diabetic mice expressing bGH, the diabetic mice expressing GHAs showed lesser glomerular damage, no increase in total urine protein, no glomerular hypertrophy and no increase in glomerular $\alpha 1$ type IV collagen mRNAs [35,36]. The inhibitory effects of GHAs in transgenic mice were seen without alteration in glycaemic control as similar concentrations in blood glucose, insulin and HbA1c were seen in the different diabetic animals expressing wild-type bGH, GHAs or bGH [35,36]. These results are further supported by data obtained in a recent study in diabetic GHR/GHBP knockout (KO) mice, where disruption of the GHR/GHBP gene was followed by protection against diabetes-induced renal changes, despite equivalent levels of hyperglycaemia [37]. Theoretically, however, GHA TG mice and GHR/GHBP KO mice may be less susceptible to diabetic renal changes because of effects of GHR blockade and low circulating IGF-I levels before the induction of diabetes. Furthermore, the renal effects might be mediated indirectly through the low serum IGF-I levels per se at the time of diabetes induction. In order to elucidate the potential usefulness of GHAs as a therapeutic agent in diabetic kidney disease in terms of tolerance and specificity, we recently performed a series of studies with exogenous administration of a long-acting GHA (G120K-PEG) to diabetic mice [19,38,39].

386

In the initial experiment non-diabetic and STZ-diabetic mice were treated with the GHA for one month after diabetes induction [19]. In GHA-treated diabetic mice, renal IGF-I accumulation, renal enlargement, and glomerular hypertrophy were abolished, and further the diabetes-associated increase in UAE was reduced [19] (Figure 1). These effects were achieved through a specific mechanism at the renal GHR level, as no effect of treatment was seen on changes in body weight, food consumption, metabolic control, serum GH or IGF-I [19]. These results have since been confirmed in non-obese diabetic (NOD) mice [37]. In a recently conducted experiment the effect of GH antagonism alone or in combination with angiotensin converting enzyme inhibition (ACEi) treatment was examined on manifest renal changes in NOD mice [39]. Preliminary results showed that GHA treatment was equally potent to ACEi treatment in reducing UAE [39]. No studies have so far appeared on the effects of GHAs in animal models of Type 2 diabetes or in Type 2 diabetic patients.

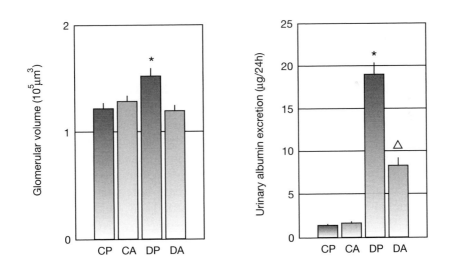

Figure 1. Inhibitory effect of a specific growth hormone receptor (GHR) antagonist of the diabetes induced glomerular hypertrophy and rise in urinary albumin excretion (UAE) in non-diabetic mice treated with placebo (CP) or GHR antagonist (CA) and diabetic mice treated with placebo (DP) or GHR antagonist (DA). Adapted from reference [19].

THE VEGF SYSTEM

The VEGF family consists of more than five different isoforms of highly conserved homodimeric glycoproteins, with heparin-binding properties [40-42]. VEGF was first recognized in 1983 and named vasopermeability factor due to its potent permeability-inducing properties. VEGF also exert potent mitogenic actions in endothelial cells [41] and has been shown to play an important role in pathological angiogenesis [43]. The most potent stimulus for VEGF is hypoxia and VEGF has been claimed to be a 'survival factor' during tissue ischemia [40]. Finally, VEGF is an important factor for normal nephrogenesis [40]. The two best-described VEGF receptors (VEGFR-1 and VEGFR-2), also known as the fms-like tyrosine kinase (Flt-1) and fetal liver kinase 1 (Flk-1), are high-affinity transmembrane tyrosine kinase receptors [40]. In the human kidney, VEGF has been demonstrated in the podocytes, distal tubular cells, and to a lesser extent in proximal tubular cells, while absent in mesangial and endothelial cells [43]. The VEGFRs are expressed predominantly in endothelium of preglomerular vessels, glomeruli and postglomerular vessels, but have also been identified in renal mesangial cells and tubules of normal kidney [43]. The specific mechanism by which VEGF may influence the glomerular fenestration is so far unknown.

EVIDENCE FOR A ROLE OF VEGF IN DIABETIC KIDNEY DISEASE

In vitro, mesangial cells, glomerular endothelial cells, vascular smooth muscle cells (VSMCs), proximal and distal tubular cells are capable of producing VEGF. Angiotensin II induces VEGF production in mesangial cells [43], and high glucose-induced VEGF production in VSMCs seems to be protein kinase C (PKC)-modulated and/or -dependent (44). VEGF upregulates the expression of endothelial nitric oxide (NO) synthase (NOS3) in endothelial cells and increases the production of NO, thus indicating that NO may act as a downstream mediator for VEGF [45]. In vivo, increased renal VEGF gene expression, glomerular immunoreactivity and VEGFR binding have been described both in animal models of Type 1 (i.e. STZ-diabetic animals), and Type 2 diabetes (i.e. Otsuka-Long-Evans-Tokushima-Fatty (OLETF) rats, and Zucker Diabetic Fatty (ZDF-rats))[46-48]. Data on serum VEGF levels obtained in Type 1 diabetic subjects have been controversial. One study reported comparable serum VEGF levels in diabetic and non-diabetic children and adolescents [49], whereas two other studies found increased serum [50] and plasma VEGF levels [51] in diabetic individuals. Serum VEGF levels were reported to be influenced by glycaemic control, and to be markedly increased in young patients with microvascular complications [50]. Further, a study in adult Type 1 diabetic men reported elevated plasma VEGF in the early course of diabetic nephropathy [52] while another study showed that plasma VEGF levels in adult Type 1 diabetic patients were neither correlated with the extent of diabetic microvascular complications nor with other key risk factors [53]. In Type 2 diabetic patients, plasma VEGF concentration tended to increase with increasing UAE [54]. Recently, urinary and plasma VEGF levels were studied in 73 Type 2 diabetic patients, and the relationship between these values and the severity of diabetic nephropathy [55]. Plasma VEGF concentration was significantly higher in Type 2 diabetic patients with overt proteinuria than in patients with normo- or microalbuminuria. The VEGF excretion increased according to the degree of proteinuria in diabetic subjects and further a weak but significant correlation was found between urinary VEGF excretion and the levels of serum creatinine, creatinine clearance, microalbuminuria, and proteinuria [55].

TREATMENTS TARGETING VEGF

Substantial research has been focused on the development of VEGF/VEGFR antagonists to block the VEGF mediated signaling pathway. These strategies include monoclonal antibodies directed against VEGF (VEGF-ab's), VEGFR inhibitors (VEGFR-TKi's), ACEi's, PKC-inhibitors (PKCi's), advanced glycation endproduct (AGE) inhibitors, VEGF aptamers and gene therapy by a soluble VEGFR.

In a series of recent studies the crucial role of VEGF in glomerular enlargement has been elucidated in non-diabetic models of glomerular hypertrophy. Administration of VEGF-ab to uninephrectomized mice blunted the compensatory renal enlargement and abolished the glomerular hypertrophy [56]. Likewise, administration of VEGF-ab in mice fed a high protein diet abolished the glomerular hypertrophy seen in placebo-treated animals on an identical diet, without affecting kidney enlargement or body weight [57]. Recently, two studies have been performed on the effect of VEGF-ab's in diabetic animal models. Administration of VEGF-ab to a model of Type 1 diabetes (i.e. STZ-diabetic rats) for 6 weeks abolished the diabetes-associated hyperfiltration and upregulation in NOS3 and partly the rise in glomerular enlargement, renal growth and the increase in UAE [58]. These effects were seen without any impact on metabolic control in diabetic animals and no renal effects of treatment were seen in non-diabetic controls [58]. Further, VEGF-ab administration in an obese mouse model of Type 2 diabetes (i.e. db/db mice) showed amelioration of diabetic renal changes by attenuation of the diabetes-associated increases in kidney weight, glomerular volume and UAE, while the increase in BMT and creatinine clearance was abolished [59] (Figure 2). Finally, VEGF-ab administration tended to reduce total mesangial volume expansion [59] (Figure 2). VEGFR-TKi's are rather newly developed substances designed primarily to block the angiogenic effect of VEGF in oncology, and accordingly no preclinical or clinical diabetes studies have yet been published. Studies on the renal effects of VEGFR-TKi's are currently being performed in animal models of Type 1 and Type 2 diabetes.

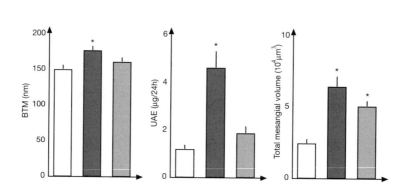

Figure 2. The effect of 2 months administration of a neutralizing VEGF-antibody (ab) on basement membrane thickness (BMT), urinary albumin excretion (UAE) and total mesangial volume in an animal model of type 2 diabetes (i.e. the db/db mice). Non-diabetic controls (open bars), placebo treated db/db mice (black bars) and VEGF-ab treated db/db mice (grey bars). *P < 0.05 vs. non-diabetic controls and VEGF-ab treated db/db mice; ΔP < 0.05 vs. non-diabetic controls and placebo treated db/db mice. Adapted from reference [59].

Administration of ACEi's in a model of Type 1 diabetes (i.e. STZ-rats) has been shown to reduce the diabetes associated elevation in retinal VEGF gene expression and vascular permeability to albumin [60]. Further, clinical studies in Type 1 and Type 2 diabetic patients with proliferative retinopathy have showed a strong negative correlation between vitreous VEGF levels and the daily enalapril dose used [61]. However, the EURODIAB controlled trial of lisinopril in insulin-dependent diabetes mellitus (EUCLID) demonstrated a weak association between treatment with lisinopril and circulating plasma VEGF levels, despite definite effects of these agents on retinopathy and nephropathy, suggesting that these effects may not predominantly be mediated through circulating VEGF [62].

Hyperglycaemia-induced activation of PKC and diacyl-glycerol has been suggested to be an important mechanism in endothelial dysfunction and microvascular changes in experimental animal studies. Long-term administration of a specific PKCβ inhibitor to both Type 1 and Type 2 diabetic animal models exerts beneficial renal effects. Interestingly, VEGF production in high glucose media is PKC dependent, therefore PKC inhibition might be a useful therapeutic strategy for the treatment of diabetic nephropathy [44]. Only a few number of studies have been published on the possible interrelationship between PKC and VEGF in vivo, and no studies with a renal focus have yet appeared. Of interest, however, it has been shown that a partially selective PKC inhibitor, that blocks phosphorylation by VEGF of several PKC isoforms, inhibits retinal neovascularization [63,64]. In addition, neutralizing PKC isoforms (i.e. ζ and δ) suppresses the aberrant VEGF overexpression in renal cell carcinoma cells and the resultant angiogenesis [65]. Administration of specific PKC isozyme inhibitors may be a novel approach in blocking the VEGF-mediated renal effects in diabetes.

In one study, using a Type 2 diabetic rat model [47], it is shown that long-term treatment with OPB-9195, a novel inhibitor of AGE formation, abolished the enhanced renal VEGF mRNA and protein overexpression along with renoprotection, by restoring diabetes-induced renal collagen IV accumulation to normal and reducing the rise in UAE [47].

Finally, VEGF aptamers [66] or treatment by gene therapy may be new promising tools to blunt patho-physiological effects of VEGF as indicated in a recent study, where retinal neovascularization in a non-diabetic rat model, was reduced by local application of soluble VEGFR producing vector [67].

SUMMARY AND CONCLUSIONS

Despite intensified metabolic control and antihypertensive treatment of diabetic patients, the development of diabetic nephropathy remains a serious problem. There is increasing evidence for a multifactorial pathogenesis of diabetic kidney disease, including various growth factors and cytokines as active players. This article has reviewed recent evidence for the significance of GH and VEGF in the development of experimental diabetic kidney disease. In addition, experimental data strongly suggest that GH and VEGF blockade may present new concepts in the treatment of diabetic renal complications. Future studies are warranted to fully characterize the clinical potential of GH and VEGF inhibitors as drugs for treatment of diabetic complications in general. Recent observations have suggested that there most likely in an important interaction or cross-talk among various growth factors that may promote the development of diabetic kidney disease. This would imply that strategies which involve multiple effects on the development of diabetic kidney disease may be more effective than drugs which influence one pathway. An increasing number of studies on the effects of combination of inhibitors with different points of action have the potential to provide new therapeutic strategies and experimental and clinical studies on combination therapies are expected to appear in the coming years.

REFERENCES

1. Deckert T, Poulsen JE, Larsfin M. Prognosis of diabetics with diabetes onset before age thirty one. Diabetologia 1978; 14: 363-370.
2. Mogensen E, Christensen CK. Predicting diabetic nephropathy in insulin dependent diabetes mellitus. N Engl J Med 1984; 311: 89-93.
3. Diabetes Control and Complications Trial Research Group. The effect of intensive treatment of diabetes on the development and progression of long-term complications in insulin-dependent diabetes mellitus. N Engl J Med 1993; 329: 977-986.
4. U.K. Prospective Diabetes Study (UKPDS) Group. Intensive blood-glucose control with sulphonylureas or insulin compared with conventional treatment and risk of complications in patients with type 2 diabetes (UKPDS 33). Lancet 1998; 352: 837-853.
5. McNeill JH (Ed). Experimental models of diabetes. CRC Press LLC, Boca Raton, Florida, USA, 1999; pp. 1-418.
6. Flyvbjerg A. Putative pathophysiological role of growth factors and cytokines in experimental diabetic kidney disease. Diabetologia 2000; 43:1205-1223
7. Young FG. Permanent diabetes produced by pituitary (anterior lobe) injections. Lancet 1937; ii: 372-374.
8. Campbell J, Davidson IWF, Lei HP. The production of permanent diabetes by highly purified growth hormone. Endocrinology 1950; 46: 588-590.

9. Yde H. Abnormal growth hormone response to ingestion of glucose in juvenile diabetics. Acta Med Scand 1969; 186: 499-504.

10. Hansen AaP, Johansen K. Diurnal pattern of blood glucose, serum FFA, insulin, glucagon and growth hormone in normals and juvenile diabetics. Diabetologia 1970; 6: 27-33.

11. Lundbæk K, Christensen HJ, Jensen VA, Johansen K, Olsen TS, Hansen AaP, Ørskov H, Østerby R. Diabetes, diabetic angiopathy and growth hormone (hypothesis). Lancet 1970; ii: 131-133.

12. Yde H. The growth hormone dependent sulphation factor in serum from patients with various types of diabetes. Acta Med Scand 1969; 186: 293-297.

13. Flyvbjerg A. Growth factors and diabetic complications. Diabetic Med 1990; 7: 387-399.

14. Janssen JAMJL, Lamberts SWJ. Circulating IGF-I and its protective role in the pathogenesis of diabetic angiopathy. Clin Endocrinol 2000; 52:1-9.

15. Møller N, Ørskov H. Growth hormone, IGF-I and diabetic angiopathy revisited. Clin Endocrinol 2000; 52: 11-12.

16. Landau D, Domene H, Flyvbjerg A, Grønbæk H, Roberts Jr CT, Argov S, LeRoith D. Differential expression of renal growth hormone receptor and its binding protein in experimental diabetes mellitus. GH and IGF Research 1998; 8: 39-45.

17. Tannenbaum GS. Growth hormone secretion dynamics in streptozotocin diabetes: Evidence of a role for endogenous somatostatin. Endocrinology 1981; 108: 76-82.

18. Marshall SM, Alberti KGMM. Alterations in the growth hormone/insulin-like growth factor axis in human and experimental diabetes: differences and similarities. In: Flyvbjerg A, Ørskov H, Alberti KGMM (eds) Growth hormone and insulin-like growth factor I in human and experimental diabetes. Chichester: John Wiley & Sons, 1993; pp. 23-46.

19. Flyvbjerg A, Bennett WF, Rasch R, Kopchick JJ, Scarlett JA. Inhibitory effect of a growth hormone receptor antagonist (G120K-PEG) on renal enlargement, glomerular hypertrophy and urinary albumin excretion in experimental diabetes in mice. Diabetes 1999; 48: 377-382.

20. Flyvbjerg A, Ørskov H, Alberti KGMM (Eds). Growth hormone and insulin-like growth factor I in human and experimental diabetes. John Wiley & Sons, Chichester, New York, Brisbane, Toronto, Singapore, 1993; pp. 1-322.

21. Flyvbjerg A. The role of insulin-like growth factor I in intial renal hypertrophy in experimental diabetes. In: Flyvbjerg A, Ørskov H, Alberti KGMM (eds) Growth hormone and insulin-like growth factor I in human and experimental diabetes. Chichester: John Wiley & Sons, 1993; pp. 271-306.

22. Flyvbjerg A, Alberti KGMM, Froesch ER, de Meyts P, von zür Mühlen A, Ørskov H (Eds). International symposium on glucose metabolism and growth factors. Metabolism 1995; 44: 1-123.

23. Massa G, Verhaeghe J, Vanderschueren-Lodeweyckx M, Bouillon R. Normalization of decreased plasma concentrations of growth hormone-binding protein by insulin treatment in spontaneously diabetic BB rats. Horm Metab Res 1993; 25: 325-326.

24. Maes M, Ketelslegers J-M, Underwood LE. Low plasma somatomedin-C in streptozotocin-induced diabetes mellitus. Correlation with changes in somatogenic and lactogenic liver binding sites. Diabetes 1983; 32: 1060-1069.

25. Flyvbjerg A. The role of growth hormone, insulin-like growth factors (IGFs) and IGF-binding proteins in the renal complications of diabetes. Kidney Int 1997; 60: S12-S19.

26. Flyvbjerg A, Frystyk J, Østerby R, Ørskov H. Kidney IGF-I and renal hypertrophy in GH deficient dwarf rats. Am J Physiol 1992; 262: E956-E962.

393

27. Flyvbjerg A, Thorlacius-Ussing O, Næraa R, Ingerslev J, Ørskov H. Kidney tissue somatomedin C and initial renal growth in diabetic and uninephrectomized rats. Diabetologia 1988; 31: 310-314.

28. Flyvbjerg A, Frystyk J, Thorlacius-Ussing O, Ørskov H. Somatostatin analogue administration prevents increase in kidney somatomedin C and initial renal growth in diabetic and uninephrectomized rats. Diabetologia 1989; 32: 261-265.

29. Bach LA, Jerums G. Effect of puberty on initial kidney growth and rise in kidney IGF-I in diabetic rats. Diabetes 1990; 39: 557-562.

30. Segev Y, Landau D, Marbach M, Schadeh N, Flyvbjerg A, Phillip M. Renal hypertrophy in hyperglycemic nonobese diabetic (NOD) mice is associated with persistent renal accumulation of insulin-like growth factor (IGF) I. J Am Soc Nephrol 1997; 8: 436-444.

31. Charlton HM, Clark RG, Robinson ICAF, Goff AE, Cox BS, Bugnon C, Bloch BA. Growth hormone-deficient dwarfism in the rat: a new mutation. J Endocrinol 1988; 119: 51-58.

32. Grønbæk H, Volmers P, Bjørn SF, Østerby R, Ørskov H, Flyvbjerg A. Effect of isolated GH and IGF-I deficiency on long-term renal changes and urinary albumin excretion in streptozotocin diabetic dwarf rats. Am J Physiol 1997; 272: E918-E924.

33. Chen WY, Wight DC, Wagner TE, Kopchick JJ. Expression of a mutated bovine growth hormone gene suppresses growth of transgenic mice. Proc Natl Acad Sci USA 1990; 87: 5061-5065.

34. Chen WY, White ME, Wagner TE, Kopchick JJ. Functional antagonism between endogenous mouse growth hormone (GH) and a GH analog results in dwarf transgenic mice. Endocrinology 1991; 129: 1402-1408.

35. Chen N-Y, Chen WY, Bellush L, Yang C-W, Striker LJ, Striker GE, Kopchick JJ. Effects of streptozotocin treatment in growth hormone (GH) and GH antagonist transgenic mice. Endocrinology 1995; 136: 660-667.

36. Chen N-Y, Chen WY, Kopchick JJ. A growth hormone antagonist protects mice against streptozotocin induced glomerulosclerosis even in the presence of elevated levels of glucose and glycated hemoglobin. Endocrinology 1996; 137: 5163-5165.

37. Bellush LL, Doublier S, Holland AN, Striker LJ, Striker GE, Kopchick JJ. Protection against diabetes-induced nephropathy in growth hormone receptor/binding protein gene-disrupted mice. Endocrinology 2000; 141: 163-168.

38. Segev Y, Landau D, Rasch R, Flyvbjerg A, Phillip M. Growth hormone receptor antagonism prevents early renal changes in nonobese diabetic mice. J Am Soc Nephrol 1999; 10: 2374-2381.

39. Flyvbjerg A, Rasch R. Effect of growth hormone (GH) receptor antagonist (G120K-PEG) treatment on manifest renal changes in non obese diabetic (NOD) mice [Abstract]. J Am Soc Nephrol 1999; 10: A3443.

40. Neufeld G, Cohen T, Gengrinovitch S, Poltorak Z. Vascular endothelial growth factor (VEGF) and its receptors. FASEB J 1999; 13:9-22.

41. Ferrara N, Houck KA, Jakeman LB, Winer J, Leung DW. The vascular endothelial growth factor family of polypeptides. J Cell Biochem 1991; 47:211-218.

42. Senger DR, Connolly DT, Van de WL, Feder J, Dvorak HF. Purification and NH2-terminal amino acid sequence of guinea pig tumor- secreted vascular permeability factor. Cancer Res 1990; 50: 1774-1778.

43. Simon M, Röckl W, Horning C, Gröne EF, Theis H, Weich HA et al. Receptors of vascular endothelial growth factor/vascular permeability factor (VEGF/VPF) in fetal and adult human kidney: localization and [125I]-VEGF binding sites. J Am Soc Nephrol 1998; 9: 1032-1044.

44. Williams B, Gallacher B, Patel H, Orme C. Glucose-induced protein kinase C activation regulates vascular permeability factor mRNA expression and peptide production by human vascular smooth muscle cells in vitro. Diabetes 1997; 46:1497-1503.

45. Hood JD, Meininger CJ, Ziche M, Granger HJ. VEGF upregulates ecNOS message, protein and NO production in human endothelial cells. Am J Physiol 1998; 274: H1054-H1058.

46. Cooper ME, Vranes D, Youssef S, Stacker SA, Cox AJ, Rizkalla B et al. Increased renal expression of vascular endothelial growth factor (VEGF) and its receptor VEGFR-2 in experimental diabetes. Diabetes 1999; 48:2229-2239.

47. Tsuchida K, Makita Z, Yamagishi S, Atsumi T, Miyoshi H, Obara S et al. Suppression of transforming growth factor beta and vascular endothelial growth factor in diabetic nephropathy in rats by a novel advanced glycation end product inhibitor, OPB-9195. Diabetologia 1999; 42:579-588.

48. Hoshi S, Shu Y, Yoshida F, Inagaki T, Sonoda J, Watanabe T, Nomoto K, Nagata M. Podocyte injury promotes progressive nephropathy in zucker diabetic fatty rats. Lab Invest 2002; 82: 25-35.

49. Malamitsi-Puchner A, Sarandakou A, Tziotis J, Dafogianni C, Bartsocas CS. Serum levels of basic fibroblast growth factor and vascular endothelial growth factor in children and adolescents with type 1 diabetes mellitus. Pediatr Res 1998; 44:873-875.

50. Chiarelli F, Spagnoli A, Basciani F, Tumini S, Mezzetti A, Cipollone F, Cuccurullo F, Morgese G, Verrotti A. Vascular endothelial growth factor (VEGF) in children, adolescents and young adults with Type 1 diabetes mellitus: relation to glycaemic control and microvascular complications. Diabet Med 2000; 17: 650-656.

51. McLaren M, Elhadd TA, Greene SA, Belch JJ. Elevated plasma vascular endothelial cell growth factor and thrombomodulin in juvenile diabetic patients. Clin Appl Thromb Hemost 1999; 5: 21-24.

52. Hovind P, Tarnow L, Østergaard PB, Parving H-H. Elevated vascular endothelial growth factor in type 1 diabetic patients with diabetic nephropathy. Kidney Int 75: S56-S61.

53. Chaturvedi N, Fuller JH, Pokras F, Rottiers R, Papazoglou N, Aiello LP. Circulating plasma vascular endothelial growth factor and microvascular complications of type 1 diabetes mellitus: the influence of ACE inhibition. Diabet Med 2001; 18: 288-294.

54. Wasada T, Kawahara R, Katsumori K, Naruse M, Omori Y. Plasma concentration of immunoreactive vascular endothelial growth factor and its relation to smoking. Metabolism 1998; 47: 27-30.

55. Cha DR, Kim NH, Yoon JW, Jo SK, Cho Wy, Kim HK, Won NH. Role of vascular endothelial growth factor in diabetic nephropathy. Kidney Int 2000; 77: S104-S112.

56. Flyvbjerg A, Schrijvers BF, De Vriese AS, Tilton RG, Rasch R. Compensatory glomerular growth following unilateral nephrectomy is VEGF dependent. Am J Physiol Endocrinol Metab 2002; 283: E362-E366.

57. Schrijvers BF, Rasch R, Tilton RG, Flyvbjerg A. High protein-induced glomerular hypertrophy is vascular endothelial growth factor-dependent. Kidney Int 2002; 61:1600-1604.

58. De Vriese AS, Tilton RG, Elger M, Stephan CC, Kriz W, Lameire NH. Antibodies against vascular endothelial growth factor improve early renal dysfunction in experimental diabetes. J Am Soc Nephrol 2001; 12:993-1000.

59. Flyvbjerg A, Dagnaes-Hansen F, De Vriese AS, Schrijvers BF, Tilton RG, Rasch R. Amelioration of long-term renal changes by administration of a neutralizing VEGF-ab in obese type 2 diabetic mice. Diabetes 2002; 51: 3090-3094.

60.   Gilbert RE, Kelly DJ, Cox AJ, Wilkinson-Berka JL, Rumble JR, Osicka T, Panagiotopoulos S, Lee V, Hendrich EC, Jerums G, Cooper ME. Angiotensin converting enzyme inhibition reduces retinal overexpression of vascular endothelial growth factor and hyperpermeability in experimental diabetes. Diabetologia 2000; 43:1360-1367.

61.   Hogeboom van Buggenum IM, Polak BC, Reichert-Thoen JW, de Vries-Knoppert WA, van Hinsbergh VW, Tangelder GJ. Angiotensin converting enzyme inhibiting therapy is associated with lower vitreous vascular endothelial growth factor concentrations in patients with proliferative diabetic retinopathy. Diabetologia 2002; 45: 203-209.

62.   Chaturvedi N, Fuller JH, Pokras F, Rottiers R, Papazoglou N, Aiello LP; EUCLID Study Group. Circulating plasma vascular endothelial growth factor and microvascular complications of type 1 diabetes mellitus: the influence of ACE inhibition. Diabet Med 2001;18: 288-294.

63.   Ozaki H, Seo MS, Ozaki K, Yamada H, Yamada E, Okamoto N, Hofmann F, Wood JM, Campochiaro PA. Blockade of vascular endothelial cell growth factor receptor signaling is sufficient to completely prevent retinal neovascularization. Am J Pathol 2000; 156: 697-707.

64.   Benjamin LE. Glucose, VEGF-A and diabetic complications. Am J Pathol 2001; 158: 1181-1184

65.   Pal S, Claffey KP, Dvorak HF, Mukhopadhyay D. The von Hippel-Lindau gene product inhibits vascular permeability factor/vascular endothelial growth factor expression in renal cell carcinoma by blocking protein kinase C pathways. J Biol Chem 1997; 272: 27509-27512

66.   Ostendorf T, Kunter U, Eitner F, Loos A, Regele H, Kerjaschki D, Henninger DD, Janjic N, Floege J. VEGF(165) mediates glomerular endothelial repair. J Clin Invest 1999; 104: 913-923

67.   Lai YK, Shen WY, Brankov M, Lai CM, Constable IJ, Rakoczy PE. Potential long-term inhibition of ocular neovascularization by recombinant adeno-associated virus-mediated secretion gene therapy. Gene Ther 2002; 12: 804-813

24

TRANSFORMING GROWTH FACTOR-β AND OTHER CYTOKINES IN EXPERIMENTAL AND HUMAN DIABETIC NEPHROPATHY

Belinda Jim, Sheldon Chen, and Fuad N. Ziyadeh

Penn Center for Molecular Studies of Kidney Diseases, Renal-Electrolyte and Hypertension Division, Department of Medicine, University of Pennsylvania Philadelphia, PA, USA

Genetic, hemodynamic, and metabolic factors are important in the pathogenesis of diabetic nephropathy. This chapter, complementing the coverage of related chapters in this book, will focus on some of the metabolic mediators, especially the various cytokines and growth factors, with particular focus on the transforming growth factor-β (TGF-β) system. Various mediator factors and signal transduction pathways interact in an intricate circuitry of autocrine, paracrine, or even endocrine mechanisms when the kidney is chronically exposed to high ambient glucose concentrations. The effects of high glucose on renal cells may arise as a consequence of increased flux of glucose metabolism through the polyol pathway [1], increased *de novo* synthesis of diacylglycerol (DAG) with subsequent activation of protein kinase C (PKC) [2, 3], activation of the hexosamine pathway [4], and increased non-enzymatic glycation of proteins [5, 6]. Recent studies have demonstrated the importance of many soluble mediators in diabetic renal disease (reviewed in [7, 8]), including platelet-derived growth factor (PDGF), endothelin, angiotensin II (AngII), prostanoids, leptin, and vascular endothelial growth factor (VEGF). Some features of these mediators will be highlighted here, after providing a detailed account of the crucial role that TGF-β plays in the pathogenesis of diabetic nephropathy. Additionally, the discussion will summarize the evidence linking the diverse mediators to the overactivity of the TGF-β system in diabetic renal disease.

OVERVIEW OF THE TGF-β SYSTEM

The TGF-β superfamily comprises over 40 related proteins, including the three mammalian isoforms of TGF-β (-β1, -β2, and -β3), the activins, and the bone morphogenetic proteins [9]. The past decade has witnessed an expansive literature supporting important roles for the TGF-β family in several types of kidney diseases. In pathophysiological states, the renal TGF-β system plays a central role in cell growth and differentiation, chemotaxis (of fibroblasts, monocytes, and neutrophils), and stimulation of various extracellular matrix molecules [10, 11]. In particular, TGF-β promotes renal cell hypertrophy and stimulates glomerular and tubular production of a host of extracellular matrix molecules [12, 13].

The matrix-stimulating effects of TGF-β involve several key systems: 1) stimulation of gene expression of matrix molecules such as fibronectin, proteoglycans, and several collagen isotypes; 2) inhibition of matrix degradation via a dual-pronged pathway of suppressing the expression and activity of serine, thiol, and metalloproteinases (e.g., plasminogen activator, collagenase, elastase, stromelysin) as well as stimulating tissue inhibitors of metalloproteinases (TIMPs) and plasminogen activator inhibitor-1 (PAI-1) [14, 15]; and 3) upregulation of integrins (the cell receptors of extracellular matrix), thereby enhancing the ability of cells to interact with specific matrix proteins [16]. Additionally, excess TGF-β activity is important in mediating fibroproliferative disorders because of its potent chemotactic properties for macrophages and fibroblasts and its ability to stimulate proliferation of fibroblasts (including renal interstitial cells) under certain conditions.

The three mammalian isoforms of TGF-β share similar actions *in vitro* but not *in vivo* [9, 17]. This is partly due to differences in developmental regulation and tissue-specific expression. In the adult kidney, TGF-β1 has been described in tubular epithelial cells (both proximal and distal), in interstitial cells, and to a lesser extent in glomerular mesangial, endothelial, and epithelial cells. TGF-β3 follows a similar pattern of expression but in quantitatively lower amounts. The TGF-β2 protein is largely restricted to the juxtaglomerular apparatus where it may play an important role in renin metabolism (reviewed in [7, 18]). It should be kept in mind that non-renal cells like platelets, macrophages, and vascular smooth muscle cells can also contribute to the overall TGF-β activity in the kidney. Unless otherwise specified, the discussion in this chapter will focus on the ubiquitous TGF-β1 isoform.

The active form of TGF-β1 is a homodimer of two cysteine-rich 12.5-kDa polypeptide subunits derived from the C-terminal end of the gene product and linked by a single disulfide bond. This mature, active form is capable of binding to its receptor and propagating a signal [19]. TGF-β is initially secreted as latent complexes, and these in turn exist in soluble forms or insoluble forms bound to extracellular matrix constituents [20, 21]. The latent complex is composed of the mature TGF-β dimer linked non-covalently to a latency-associated peptide (LAP), which is also encoded by the TGF-β gene [22]. LAP imparts latency by blocking TGF-β binding to the signaling receptor. In certain tissues including the glomerulus, the latent complex exists in covalent association with the product of another gene, the latent TGF-β binding protein (LTBP) [23]. Its role in TGF-β activation will be discussed below. In the kidney, tubular epithelial cells secrete the small latent complex (mature TGF-β1 + LAP), whereas glomerular parenchymal and arteriolar cells secrete the large latent complex (mature TGF-β1 + LAP + LTBP) [24]. This pattern of tissue expression implies potentially important differences in activation and functional regulation of the TGF-β system between the glomerular/vascular compartment and the tubular compartment.

Activation of latent TGF-β *in vivo* is largely controlled by proteases (e.g., plasmin) that cleave the LAP from the bioactive TGF-β dimer [25]. Plasmin-mediated activation of TGF-β involves the binding of the latent form to a mannose-6-phosphate receptor on the cell surface and then the concerted action of transglutaminase and plasmin to remove LAP. A protease-independent conformational change of the latent complex can also occur when thrombospondin (TSP), derived from the alpha-granules of platelets, allows the active TGF-β moiety to bind to its cell surface receptor. As will be discussed later, the TSP system may partly explain how TGF-β1 can be activated in mesangial cells by high ambient glucose. Activation of TGF-β *in vitro* can be achieved by treatment with acid (pH 4), alkali, heat (80°C), or detergents.

The three TGF-β isoforms share a common receptor system and an intracellular signaling cascade [26]. Virtually all cell types produce one or more isoforms of

TGF-β and express TGF-β receptors. Three major types of TGF-β receptors have been identified: type I (also called Alk5), type II, and type III (also called betaglycan). Type III lacks an identifiable cytoplasmic signaling domain and may act to enhance the delivery of TGF-β on the cell surface to the signaling receptor. A molecule similar to betaglycan that is found on endothelial cells is called endoglin. Signaling begins when TGF-β engages the type II receptor, also called the primary receptor since it directly binds ligand. The ligand-bound type II receptor then binds to the type I receptor to form a heterotetramer. Within this complex, the type II receptor phosphorylates the type I receptor at a serine/glycine rich domain. This enables the type I receptor to phosphorylate further downstream signaling molecules and is thus considered the *sine qua non* event in TGF-β signaling [27]. The serine-threonine kinase activity of the TGF-β receptor complex is believed to be necessary for the profibrotic and antiproliferative actions of TGF-β [26, 28].

The TGF-β receptors transduce their signals through novel intracellular proteins called Smad proteins [29, 30]. Receptor-activated Smad2 and Smad3 are specific for the TGF-β isoforms [31, 32] (while Smad1 and Smad5 are specific for other ligands such as the bone morphogenetic proteins). Phosphorylation of Smad2 or Smad3 by the type I receptor allows them to interact with Smad4 (also called DPC4), a different member of the Smad family that does not get phosphorylated by the type I receptor. The Smad2-Smad4 or Smad3-Smad4 complex translocates into the nucleus and interacts with other transcription factors, including FAST-1, CBP (cyclic AMP-response element-βinding protein), and AP-1, to effect a coordinated transcriptional response from many different genes. Such target genes contain Smad-specific binding sequences in their promoter. A third type of Smad proteins is inhibitory in action; Smad6 and Smad7 can inhibit the binding of Smad2 or Smad3 to the type I receptor [33]. Experimental evidence indicates that the Smad pathway is directly involved in cell cycle regulation by TGF-β, but other intracellular signaling pathways such as the mitogen-activated protein (MAP) kinase cascades may also participate [34]. Likewise, Smad proteins and possibly other unrelated signaling molecules may mediate some of the other functions of TGF-β such as stimulation of extracellular matrix production [35, 36].

As will be discussed later in relation to diabetic kidney disease, TGF-β production is stimulated by high ambient glucose, glycated proteins, as well as a host of cytokines and growth factors such as the mitogen PDGF and the vasoactive agents AngII, thromboxane, and endothelin. Dysregulation of the

TGF-β system in profibrotic states often represents an unregulated degree of tissue repair that swings the balance toward excess scar deposition. This is exacerbated by the fact that TGF-β1 has the peculiar ability to induce its own production, thereby amplifying the fibroproliferative response in a positive feedback fashion.

EFFECTS OF HIGH AMBIENT GLUCOSE IN RENAL CELL CULTURE SYSTEMS

To mimic the effects of diabetes on the kidney, researchers have grown different renal cell types in tissue culture under high ambient glucose conditions. High glucose stimulates proximal tubular [37, 38] and mesangial cell hypertrophy [39-41] and it stimulates the production of matrix molecules such as fibronectin and collagens in proximal tubule cells and glomerular mesangial, epithelial, and endothelial cells [37, 42-50]. Cell culture studies have also demonstrated that renal cortical fibroblasts produce excess type I collagen under high glucose conditions [51]. In rat mesangial cell and human tubulointerstitial cell culture, periodically elevated glucose levels increase collagen production to a greater extent than persistently elevated glucose concentrations [52, 53]. This more closely mimics the fluctuation of blood glucose levels *in vivo* and may highlight the detrimental effects of labile hyperglycemia on the pathogenesis of diabetic glomerulosclerosis.

In most kidney cell types, high ambient glucose up-regulates the expression and bioactivity of TGF-β, which itself has been shown to mediate the hypertrophic and profibrotic effects of high glucose. Mesangial cells [45, 54], glomerular endothelial cells [55], proximal tubular cells [56], and interstitial fibroblasts [51] incubated in high glucose have increased expression of TGF-β1 and in some cases TGF-β type II receptor (TβRII) [50, 57], which directly binds to the TGF-β ligand. This enables TGF-β1 to act in an autocrine or paracrine fashion to effect significant changes in cellular behavior. For example, murine mesangial cells initially show increased proliferation in high glucose, but after 72 hours the cells demonstrate decreased proliferation due to high glucose-induced TGF-β, which has hypertrophic/growth inhibitory effects [39] that may be partially mediated by p27[Kip1] [41]. Even in the absence of high glucose, addition of exogenous TGF-β1 causes the mesangial cell and the interstitial fibroblast to increase their expression and production of collagen matrix proteins, showing that TGF-β can reproduce the effects of high glucose [45, 51,

57]. Finally, antagonism of TGF-β by specific neutralizing monoclonal antibodies [58] or by antisense oligonucleotides [59] significantly decreases and even completely abolishes the high glucose-induced rise in extracellular matrix expression, indicating that TGF-β predominantly mediates the profibrotic effect of high glucose on kidney cells.

Certainly, not all of the high glucose effects are mediated by the TGF-β system. High glucose stimulates the expression and production of type IV collagen by the cultured, differentiated podocyte, but rather than increasing all the alpha chains of collagen IV, exogenous TGF-β1 actually decreases certain alpha chains [50]. Specifically, high glucose increases the α1, α3, and α5 chains of collagen IV [50]. On the other hand, exogenous TGF-β1 stimulates α3 but inhibits the expression of α1 and α5(IV) collagen. Although it is unlikely that the high glucose effects on α1 and α5(IV) collagen would be mediated by TGF-β in the podocyte, the high glucose-induced production of α3(IV) collagen is completely prevented by an inhibitor of TGF-β signaling (SB-431542) [35, 50]. To ascertain the mechanism of this TGF-β-mediated effect on α3(IV) collagen, the effects of high glucose were studied on components of the TGF-β system. Contrary to other renal cell types, the podocyte did not respond to high glucose with a significant increase in TGF-β1 ligand [50]. Rather, it increased its cell surface expression of the TGF-β type II receptor. In this way, high glucose activates the TGF-β system in podocytes, adding a variation to the theme that high glucose stimulates TGF-β activity in renal cells.

TGF-β cooperates with hyperglycemia
TGF-β and high glucose can also interact by an insidious mechanism. High glucose increases the activity of TGF-β, but TGF-β in turn can augment the effect of high glucose. In both human and rat mesangial cells, TGF-β has been shown to up-regulate the mRNA expression and protein production of the insulin-independent, transmembrane glucose transporter, GLUT1 [60, 61], thus facilitating glucose uptake and increasing the flux of glucose through its biochemical pathways [62]. Intermediates in glucose metabolism can activate signaling pathways such as protein kinase C [63] and the hexosamine pathway [64] that then stimulate the TGF-β system even further. In deciphering the mechanism by which high glucose increases GLUT1, Inoki *et al.* found that the addition of neutralizing anti-TGF-β antibody prevented the stimulatory effects of high glucose on GLUT1 expression [60]. Interestingly, overexpression of

GLUT1 protein in cultured rat mesangial cells caused a marked increase in glucose uptake and the synthesis of extracellular matrix molecules, even when grown in normal ambient glucose concentrations [65, 66]. Thus, TGF-β and GLUT1 are both up-regulated by a hyperglycemic milieu, and each can influence the expression of the other.

Role of Smads in TGF-β signaling

Moving beyond high glucose to probing the mechanisms of TGF-β signaling, we investigated the role of the Smad pathway that transduces the TGF-β signal from the receptor complex to the nucleus. Our data suggest that high glucose may exert some of its effects on extracellular matrix expression through the system of intracellular Smad proteins. In mouse mesangial cells, high glucose stimulates the transcription of fibronectin and, furthermore, potentiates the transcriptional activation of fibronectin by TGF-β1 [36]. This particular effect of TGF-β1 appears to be mediated by the receptor-activated Smads (R-Smad), which include Smad2 and Smad3. Smad2 was not investigated, but overexpression of Smad3 alone was able to induce fibronectin promoter activity. In conjunction with exogenous TGF-β1, Smad3 overexpression synergistically increased fibronection expression, as if the extra Smad3 had increased the efficiency of TGF-β signaling. Finally, transfection of a Smad3-dominant-negative construct was able to inhibit TGF-β1 from stimulating the promoter activity of fibronectin [36]. However, part of the TGF-β1-induced fibronectin expression may also be mediated in parallel by the p38 mitogen-activated protein kinase (MAPK) pathway [35]. Finally, there is evidence to suggest that Smad3 predominantly mediates the effect of TGF-β1 to increase the mRNA expression of α1(I) collagen [35].

TGF-β IN EXPERIMENTAL DIABETIC KIDNEY DISEASE

In experimental animal models, TGF-β has been shown to play an important role in the pathogenesis of diabetic kidney disease. Several groups of investigators have demonstrated that the TGF-β level is elevated in the kidneys of insulin-dependent diabetic animals during both early and late stages of disease [67-75]. A progressive increase in the TGF-β1 mRNA and protein levels was noted in glomeruli isolated from the streptozotocin (STZ)-induced diabetic rat [67, 68] in association with an increased expression of extracellular matrix molecules [76]. Treatment of the STZ-diabetic rat with sufficient insulin to reduce hyperglycemia ameliorated the enhanced expression of TGF-β [73] and matrix components in the glomeruli [67, 68].

Increased TGF-β expression in the kidney may manifest very early after the onset of diabetes. In our study on the spontaneously diabetic Biobreeding (BB) rat and the non-obese diabetic (NOD) mouse, we found increased TGF-β1 mRNA and protein levels in the kidney cortex as early as a few days after the appearance of glycosuria and coincident with the development of renal hypertrophy [70]. In the STZ-diabetic rat and mouse, increased TGF-β1 expression in the renal cortex and glomeruli was noted as soon as one to three days after the onset of diabetes [73, 77]. Interestingly, up-regulation of the TGF-β type II receptor mRNA and protein also occurred early in the natural history of STZ-diabetic rodents [57, 75, 77].

The intrarenal TGF-β system is also activated in animal models of type 2 diabetes. The *db/db* mouse, characterized by hyperglycemia, obesity, and insulin resistance, develops increased amounts of TGF-β1 that are localized to the glomerular compartments [78]. In contrast, the mRNA and protein levels of the TGF-β type II receptor are significantly up-regulated in both the glomerular [78] and the tubulointerstitial compartments [78]. Overall, the increased glomerular TGF-β and the more widespread increases in TGF-β type II receptor result in activation of the renal TGF-β system and stimulation of the downstream Smad signaling cascade. By immunohistochemistry of the diabetic *db/db* mouse (compared with the *db/m* mouse), Smad3 was found to accumulate in the nuclei of glomerular and tubular cells where Smad proteins could influence the expression of genes that are regulated by TGF-β signaling [78]. More evidence of Smad nuclear translocation could be seen by Southwestern histochemistry in which labeled oligonucleotides comprising the Smad binding element (SBE) were increasingly localized to the nuclei of glomerular and tubular cells of diabetic mice [78], suggesting increased transcription of genes that are modulated by TGF-β. Thus, the net bioactivity of the renal TGF-β system is increased in the type 2 diabetic *db/db* mouse.

Intervention with anti-TGF-β therapies
The development of diabetic renal hypertrophy and glomerulosclerosis is likely caused by heightened activity of the TGF-β system. Short-term treatment of the STZ-diabetic mouse with a neutralizing monoclonal antibody against all three isoforms of TGF-β prevented glomerular hypertrophy, reduced the increment in kidney weight by 50%, and significantly attenuated the increase in TGF-β1,

$\alpha 1(IV)$ collagen, and fibronectin mRNAs without affecting glycemic control [77]. The results of this study suggested a cause-and-effect relationship between the renal TGF-β system and the development of early structural changes in diabetic nephropathy.

To expand upon these findings, we conducted a similar study, this time on the *db/db* mouse, to examine whether long-term anti-TGF-β antibody treatment would ameliorate the late structural changes and functional consequences of diabetic nephropathy [79]. We found that systemic anti-TGF-β therapy for eight weeks prevented the mesangial matrix expansion of diabetic glomerulosclerosis and, most important, the treatment preserved kidney function, showing for the first time that neutralization of TGF-β activity could prevent the progression of renal failure in diabetes. However, the anti-TGF-β antibody did not reduce albuminuria, which itself may promote the progression of renal insufficiency [80]. The paradox of preserved renal function in the face of persistent albuminuria may perhaps be explained by postulating that the deleterious effects of proteinuria are themselves mediated by the TGF-β system [81].

However, prevention of diabetic nephropathy in humans is not always feasible. More often than not, the physician has to treat diabetic kidney disease that is far advanced, with pathological lesions that are well established. It used to be thought that the structural damage of diabetic nephropathy was irreversible, so treatment recommendations focused on preventing further injury and slowing the rate of decline in renal function. More recently, however, physicians have contemplated the reality of 'curing' diabetic nephropathy. If diabetes could be optimally treated, then perhaps the kidney could heal itself. We reasoned that if TGF-β mediates most of the renal damage in diabetes, then neutralizing TGF-β overactivity might not only prevent but also reverse the structural lesions of diabetic nephropathy. We performed a study in *db/db* mice similar to the above with anti-TGF-β antibodies, but instead of starting treatment with the onset of diabetes (preventive trial), we started treatment after the establishment of diabetic kidney disease (therapeutic trial). Compared with the control diabetic mice, the treated *db/db* mice displayed significant improvements in the glomerular basement membrane thickening and in the index of mesangial matrix expansion [82]. These structural parameters approached the normal measurements of the nondiabetic *db/m* mice. Even at this late stage and even though the hyperglycemia was left untreated, antagonizing the intrarenal TGF-β system was able to at least partially reverse the histologic lesions of diabetic glomerulopathy.

Additional parts of the TGF-β system

In addition to TGF-β1, other members of the TGF-β family deserve mention. Though it is much less studied, TGF-β2 is believed to play a fibrogenic role [83]. Daily injections of human recombinant TGF-β2 to adult mice caused tissue levels of endothelin-1 and Angiotensin II to increase in the kidney and fibrosis to develop in the cortical tubular interstitium and vasculature [83]. TGF-β2 and other TGF-β system components have also been examined in the STZ-induced diabetic rat and the genetically prone Biobreeding (BB) rat [75]. Interestingly, though renal TGF-β1 mRNA levels were elevated in the first 30 days after STZ-induction, the corresponding TGF-β1 protein did not increase. TGF-β2, however, showed the opposite profile. Its mRNA expression did not significantly increase, but its protein content rose by two-fold after 30 days of diabetes. Finally, TGF-β type II receptor demonstrated a three-fold increase in protein by day 90 of STZ-induction, making this the most responsive of the TGF-β receptor subtypes. Because TGF-β2 seemed to correlate better with fibrogenesis in the diabetic kidney, the same research group used a human monoclonal anti-TGF-β2 antibody to treat STZ-diabetic rats [84]. Compared with non-diabetic controls, the untreated diabetic rats had increased kidney weights, urinary albumin excretion rates, and protein synthesis of collagen I. Therapy with an anti-TGF-β2 antibody, however, prevented diabetes from increasing these measures of disease. The authors conclude that the anti-TGF-β2 regimen had a renoprotective effect, and they extrapolate from the attenuation of collagen I that targeting TGF-β2 would suppress kidney fibrogenesis in diabetes [84]. Nevertheless, TGF-β1 remains the most abundant and most studied isoform in the kidney. The importance of TGF-β2 or TGF-β3 is not as well established. Future studies will need to address the specific role that each isoform plays in diabetic nephropathy.

HUMAN DIABETIC KIDNEY DISEASE AND TGF-B

Studies performed in diabetic patients with various degrees of nephropathy also implicate the renal TGF-β system in the development of human diabetic renal disease. All three isoforms of TGF-β have been discovered to be elevated in both the glomerular and the tubulointerstitial compartments of patients with established diabetic nephropathy [68, 85, 86]. Furthermore, glomerular TGF-β1 mRNA, measured by the reverse-transcription polymerase chain reaction method, was markedly increased in renal biopsy specimens from patients with proven diabetic kidney disease [87]. These investigations support the belief that increased renal TGF-β levels correlate closely with the degree of mesangial matrix expansion, interstitial fibrosis, and renal insufficiency.

Another study was designed to determine if diabetic patients have enhanced renal production of TGF-β [88]. Aortic, renal vein, and urinary levels of TGF-β were measured in fourteen type 2 diabetic and eleven non-diabetic control patients undergoing elective coronary artery catheterization. Both groups were roughly matched with regard to the range of renal function and the presence of hypertension and proteinuria. Renal blood flow was measured to calculate the net mass balance across the kidney. The gradient of TGF-β1 concentration across the renal vascular bed was negative in the non-diabetic patients indicating net renal extraction of TGF-β1, whereas the gradient was positive in the diabetic patients indicating net renal production of TGF-β1. When the renal TGF-β1 mass balance was calculated, a similar pattern was observed with the non-diabetic kidney removing approximately 3500 ng/min of TGF-β1 from the circulation, and the diabetic kidney adding approximately 1000 ng/min of TGF-β1 to the circulation. In addition, the level of bioassayable TGF-β was increased four-fold in the urine of diabetic *vs.* non-diabetic patients. The increased urinary TGF-β was not simply a function of enhanced glomerular permeability to protein since diabetic patients both with and without microalbuminuria displayed similarly high rates of urinary TGF-β excretion. These results support the conclusion that the kidneys of diabetic patients overproduce TGF-β1 protein. The details of this phenomenon and the exact contribution of the different renal cell types to TGF-β1 production need to be investigated.

TGF-β levels correlate with outcomes

An interesting *post-hoc* study [89] assessed whether captopril treatment would lower serum TGF-β1 levels in a small subset of patients with diabetic nephropathy who had been enrolled in the Collaborative Study Group [90]. After six months, the serum TGF-β1 level decreased significantly by 21% in the captopril-treated group, whereas it increased slightly by 11% in the placebo-treated group. Interestingly, the captopril-treated patients who had a decrease in the serum TGF-β1 level tended to have better preserved renal function over the ensuing two-year period. This association was even more pronounced in the subset of patients with an initial glomerular filtration rate of less than 75 ml/min. These results suggest that TGF-β1 plays a pivotal role in the progression of diabetic nephropathy and that angiotensin converting enzyme inhibitor therapy may protect the kidney by lowering TGF-β1 production.

More recently, the EURODIAB Prospective Complications Study examined the correlation between levels of TGF-β1, Amadori albumin, and the microvascular complications of type 1 diabetes [91]. An increased circulating TGF-β1 was associated with an increased prevalence of proliferative retinopathy. On the other hand, increased urinary TGF-β1 levels were highly correlated with the severity of albuminuria. Both of these parameters were largely accounted for in the multivariate model by the changes in blood pressure, glycemic control, and levels of Amadori albumin. Perhaps these features of the diabetic state, given their impact on urinary TGF-β1 levels, should be aggressively controlled to reduce the risk of progression to microalbuminuria, the incipient stage of diabetic nephropathy.

TGF-β regulation and propensity for diabetic nephropathy

Factors that regulate the bioavailability of TGF-β also influence the predisposition to diabetic kidney disease. One such factor is the family of latent TGF-β binding proteins (LTBP). These regulatory molecules covalently bind with the small latent forms of TGF-β, facilitating the efficient secretion of TGF-β [23] and targeting the TGF-β complex to the extracellular matrix [92]. The relevance of LTBP to human diabetic nephropathy can be seen in a study that tried to link expression levels of TGF-β components with the likelihood of developing diabetic nephropathy [93]. Type 1 diabetic patients were ranked according to their severity of mesangial expansion and their duration of diabetes and then were categorized into 'fast-track' and 'slow-track' risk groups for the development of diabetic nephropathy. From these two cohorts and normal control subjects, skin fibroblasts were cultured in high glucose and then assayed for mRNA levels (by real-time RT-PCR) of TGF-β1, type II receptor, thrombospondin-1, and LTBP-1. No differences were found in the mRNA expression of TGF-β1, type II receptor, or thrombospondin-1 between 'fast-track' and 'slow-track' patients. The only significant difference between the two groups was found with LTBP-1 [93]. 'Slow-track' patients had lower levels of LTBP-1 than normal or 'fast-track' patients, suggesting that the decreased LTBP-1 and presumably the decreased TGF-β bioavailability may have protected the 'slow-track' patients from developing diabetic nephropathy as quickly. Therefore, with regard to TGF-β regulation, genetic variability of LTBP levels seems to play an important role in the susceptibility to diabetic renal disease.

OTHER MEDIATORS IN DIABETIC RENAL DISEASE

AngII
An important concept that has emerged in diabetes research is the idea that AngII not only mediates intraglomerular hypertension but also behaves as a growth factor that causes some of the hypertrophy and fibrosis seen in diabetic renal disease (reviewed in [94]). Much of the latter effect of AngII appears to be mediated by TGF-β. Tissue culture studies have demonstrated that AngII stimulates TGF-β1 production in proximal tubular cells [95] and mesangial cells [96]. AngII also stimulates the biosynthesis of matrix by cultured renal cells [97-99]. This appears to be mediated by the TGF-β system because various anti-TGF-β regimens have abolished the AngII-induced increases in collagen I, collagen IV, and fibronectin [96, 99-101].

AngII has also been shown to cause hypertrophy in both proximal tubule cells and mesangial cells [97, 102-104]. This mechanism of action is most likely mediated by TGF-β since neutralizing anti-TGF-β antibodies ameliorates the hypertrophic effects [38, 105, 106]. Thus, the antifibrotic and anti-hypertrophic effects of angiotensin blockade are partly related to its ability to reduce TGF-β overexpression in the kidney. This viewpoint may help explain the renoprotective effects of the angiotensin converting enzyme (ACE) inhibitors or angiotensin receptor blockers (ARBs) [94, 107], in addition to their well-accepted hemodynamic benefits [108]. Indeed, ACE inhibitors or ARBs decrease the intrarenal levels of TGF-β1, both in animal models of diabetes and in human diabetes.[109-113] These data suggest that TGF-β can mediate the hypertrophic and sclerotic effects of AngII, offering angiotensin blockade as another modality to combat TGF-β associated disease.

Clinical conditions that are associated with upregulation of the renin-angiotensin system often upregulate TGF-β expression. For example, a high intraglomerular hydrostatic pressure secondary to efferent arteriolar constriction by AngII stretches the mesangial cell and stimulates it to produce TGF-β isoforms [114]. That AngII increases TGF-β can also be seen in the unilateral ureteral obstruction (UUO) model of tubulointerstitial fibrosis. UUO was performed in a group of transgenic mice that express different numbers of angiotensinogen genes (zero to four copies). As expected, the number of genes determined the tissue levels of AngII in a graded fashion. More remarkably, the number of angiotensinogen genes increased linearly with the levels of TGF-β mRNA in the obstructed kidney, and mice with no angiotensinogen genes had TGF-β expression levels similar to those of non-obstructed control animals [115]. This study supports the idea that angiotensin availability regulates the extent of TGF-β transcription.

Human studies further support the interaction of AngII and TGF-β. A subanalysis of The Collaborative Study Group Captopril Trial demonstrated that treatment with captopril correlated with the reduction of serum TGF-β1 levels [89]. There was a significant decrease of 21% in serum TGF-β1 levels in the captopril-treated group after 6 months, while there was a slight increase of 11% in the placebo group after the same period. The decrease in serum TGF-β1 levels in the captopril group correlated with stabilization of the glomerular filtration rate over the ensuing 2-year period, and this association was even more pronounced in the subset of patients with an initial glomerular filtration rate of less than 75 ml/min. Further, the addition of an ARB to maximal ACE inhibitor therapy was able to suppress urinary TGF-β1 levels even more than the ACE inhibitor alone, suggesting that more comprehensive blockade of the renin-angiotensin system would confer extra renoprotection [116].

Endothelins
The polypeptide endothelin-1 (ET-1) appears to have important links to AngII and TGF-β. When either AngII or ET-1 was injected into transgenic mice that express the reporter gene luciferase under the control of the collagen type I promoter, the mRNA expression of collagen I was increased in the aorta and renal cortex [100]. The increase in collagen I induced by AngII was inhibited by the administration of an endothelin receptor antagonist, bosentan. In addition, the AngII-stimulated collagen I was also blocked by a TGF-β scavenger, decorin. These data indicate that AngII can activate the collagen I gene in the renal cortex by a mechanism requiring the participation or cooperation of ET and TGF-β [100].

Studies on diabetic models showed that glomerular expression of ET-1 mRNA is increased in STZ-diabetic rats [117] and the urinary level of ET-1 is elevated in the diabetic BB rat [117]. Moreover, an endothelin receptor A antagonist,

FR139317, given to STZ-diabetic rats attenuated glomerular hyperfiltration and urinary protein excretion and decreased glomerular mRNA levels of collagens, laminins, tumor necrosis factor (TNF-α), PDGF-B, TGF-β1, and basic fibroblast growth factor (bFGF) [118].

In humans, studies show that type 2 diabetic patients exhibit higher endothelin levels than the general population [119]. Among the type 2 diabetic patients, those with retinopathy have even higher levels of endothelin. In another study of type 2 diabetes, treatment with captopril reduces circulating ET-1 levels [120], again suggesting a role for AngII in the upregulation of ET-1 in diabetes.

Thromboxane and prostaglandin

Studies in experimental animal models have demonstrated increased renal thromboxane expression [121] and urinary excretion of thromboxane B2 shortly after the onset of diabetes [122-124]. The source of increased thromboxane production may be the diabetic glomerulus [125] and/or infiltrating platelets [126]. Addition of thromboxane analogs to mesangial cells in culture results in stimulation of fibronectin production [127] that appears to be mediated by PKC activation [128]. Inhibitors of thromboxane synthesis and its receptor have been found to ameliorate diabetes-induced albuminuria [125, 129] and mesangial matrix expansion [125], but they may not prevent thickening of the GBM [125, 130]. Thromboxane may also exert a hemodynamic effect on the glomerulus via AngII. Thromboxane inhibitors administered to normoglycemic or STZ-induced diabetic Wistar Kyoto (WKY) rats reduced the AngII-induced increase in perfusion pressure [131].

It should be noted that exogenous prostaglandin E_2 (PGE$_2$) or drugs capable of increasing endogenous PGE$_2$ dose-dependently decrease the level of extracellular matrix protein and mRNA and also dampen TGF-β gene expression in cultured rat mesangial cells [132]. In streptozotocin-diabetic rats, an antagonist of the prostaglandin receptor EP1 inhibited TGF-β transcription and the expression of fibronectin. In terms of histologic and clinical benefits, the prostaglandin inhibitor ameliorated renal hypertrophy, decreased mesangial expansion, and completely suppressed proteinuria [133].

PDGF

Platelet-derived growth factor (PDGF) has a well-known role in mediating cellular proliferation and extracellular matrix (ECM) protein synthesis in glomerulonephritis. However, its role in the development of diabetic nephropathy has not been established. But recently, an increase in the mRNA expression of PDGF-B and PDGF Receptor has been demonstrated in rat mesangial cells exposed to high ambient glucose [134]. PDGF-B mRNA expression is also upregulated in glomeruli from diabetic rats [135]. The mechanism by which PDGF responds to high glucose may involve the mitogen-activated protein kinase (MAPK) p38 pathway [136]. Rats exposed to high glucose followed by stimulation with PDGF showed enhanced p38 activity and subsequent activation of the cAMP responsive element binding (CREB) transcription factor [136]. Given that MAPK p38 has also been strongly associated with the TGF-β Smad pathway [137], this may be another mechanism of action of PDGF in diabetic nephropathy.

Studies in human mesangial cells have found that antibodies to PDGF inhibited high glucose-stimulated TGF-β1 mRNA [138]. A study in human proximal tubular cells found that high ambient glucose was sufficient to increase TGF-β1 mRNA levels but that PDGF was required to cause secretion and activation of the TGF-β protein [139]. Of interest is that the expression of the PDGF-B receptor is increased in mesangial and other vascular cells (such as vascular smooth muscle and capillary endothelial cells) exposed to high ambient glucose [134]. An increase in immunostaining for PDGF-B and PDGF-B receptor was found in mesangial and visceral epithelial cells of STZ-diabetic rats [140]. Inhibiting PDGF with an antagonist, trapidil, prevented the increase in glomerular volume, a feature of diabetic kidney involvement. Thus, activation of the PDGF system in glomerular cells might play an important role in the development of early glomerular lesions in diabetes [140].

In addition, PDGF may be of great importance during the advanced stages of human diabetic nephropathy. Urinary levels of PDGF-BB were markedly increased in diabetic patients with microalbuminuria and macroalbuminuria but not in diabetic patients without albuminuria [141].

PDGF may also play a role in mediating glycation-stimulated matrix production in mesangial cells [142]. Neutralizing anti-PDGF antibody reduces the mRNA of the α1 chain of type IV collagen that is induced by advanced glycation end-products (AGEs) in cultured mouse mesangial cells [143].

VEGF
This growth factor is implicated in the microvascular complications of diabetes, especially retinopathy, but its role in nephropathy remains speculative. VEGF, also known as vascular permeability factor (VPF), is a homodimeric glycoprotein that exists in at least five different isoforms that are produced by

differential exon splicing [144]. Smaller isoforms are freely soluble and larger isoforms are locally bound to extracellular matrix [145]. Virtually all cell types produce VEGF; an increase in VEGF secretion occurs mostly in response to hypoxia which stimulates endothelial cell proliferation and new blood vessel formation (angiogenesis) [146].

VEGF and its receptors are widely expressed in the kidney. The glomerular visceral epithelial podocyte expresses VEGF constitutively [147], and the collecting duct epithelial cell expresses it at a lower level [148]. Under hypoxic conditions, proximal and distal tubular epithelial cells, interstitial cells, and vascular smooth muscle cells synthesize VEGF [149]. The mesangial cell can be stimulated to produce VEGF by AngII, an effect that is blocked by the AT_1 receptor antagonist losartan [150]. Although the endothelial cell is normally thought of as a target for VEGF, it too produces VEGF [151], creating an autocrine loop. The two high-affinity receptors for VEGF, fms-like tyrosine kinase-1 (flt-1 or VEGF-R1) and Kinase Domain Region/fetal liver kinase-1 (KDR/flk-1 or VEGF-R2), appear to be mostly restricted to the endothelial cell, being found on pre- and post-glomerular vessels and on glomerular capillaries [152]. Mesangial cells also possess at least one form of the VEGF receptor [153].

In the normal kidney, VEGF may function to maintain the integrity of the glomerular endothelium and its fenestrations [154, 155]. During an ischemic or hypoxic injury, VEGF may help to alleviate decreased blood flow and restore vascular integrity [149]. The importance of VEGF in normal kidney functioning can be seen when the VEGF system becomes dysregulated. When VEGF is selectively deleted (Cre-Lox) from the podocyte, the glomeruli fail to develop a filtration barrier. On the other hand, when VEGF is overexpressed in the podocyte, it results in a collapsing glomerulopathy, histologically similar to HIV-associated nephropathy [156]. Thus, tight regulation of VEGF signaling is crucial for the establishment and maintenance of the glomerular filtration barrier.

The possibility that diabetes can increase renal VEGF/VPF production has led to the theory that this factor is one of the causes of albuminuria. However, experimental and clinical evidence to support this reasoning are currently lacking. Infusion of VEGF into isolated perfused rat kidneys did not change the glomerular permeability to albumin [157]. Nevertheless, the diabetic state results in the upregulation of many mediators that can stimulate the production of VEGF. High glucose itself stimulates vascular smooth muscle cells to augment VEGF expression [158] perhaps via glucose-induced PKC activation [159]. Phorbol esters stimulate mesangial cell VEGF production [160] and inhibition of PKC blocks the signaling of VEGF [161]. Reactive oxygen species can induce VEGF in both endothelial cells [162] and vascular smooth muscle cells [163]. Various cytokines such as TGF-β [164], AngII [150], IGF-I [165], bFGF [166], PDGF [167], and platelet activating factor (PAF) [168] all raise VEGF production. Mechanical stretch, the *in vitro* correlate of intraglomerular hypertension, also increases mesangial VEGF production via an AngII-independent mechanism [169].

Several lines of evidence suggest that increased VEGF is associated with diabetes. In OLETF rats, an experimental model of type 2 diabetes, renal VEGF mRNA and glomerular VEGF immunoreactivity were found to be elevated over 9-68 weeks of diabetes [170]. Another study involving STZ-induced diabetic rats demonstrated an increase in renal VEGF mRNA and protein levels, mostly localized to the glomerular epithelial cells [171].

However, the association between increased VEGF and proteinuria has not been definitively established in diabetic kidney disease. In one study, type 1 diabetic children and adolescents were found to have similar serum VEGF levels as compared to healthy controls [172]. Even the patients with longer duration of diabetes and worse metabolic control did not have significantly increased serum VEGF levels. Another study examined VEGF expression in renal biopsy specimens with various diseases including diabetic nephropathy [173]. It found that five of the 47 cases had diabetes, and the glomeruli free of sclerosis displayed strong expression of VEGF, while those with extensive sclerosis showed markedly decreased expression of VEGF. This does not necessarily imply that VEGF is always decreased in diabetic nephropathy. It is possible that advanced diabetes, with loss of podocytes, is characterized by decreased VEGF, whereas early diabetes may be characterized by increased glomerular VEGF.

The role of VEGF in the etiology of non-diabetic proteinuria is equally inconclusive. VEGF levels are not elevated in either Finnish nephropathy [174] or steroid-sensitive nephrotic syndrome [175]. However, in a rat model of bovine serum albumin-induced nephritis [176], VEGF and VEGF receptor mRNA expression increased proportionally with the severity of proteinuria.

Interestingly, however, in a study on STZ-induced diabetic rats, infusion of a neutralizing murine VEGF antibody abolished diabetes-associated hyperfiltration and partially blocked the increase in urinary albumin excretion [177]. In the diabetic *db/db* mouse, a model of obese type 2 diabetes, administration of the same antibody attenuated the glomerular volume, basement membrane thickening, and urinary albumin excretion, as compared with diabetic controls [178]. These effects occurred independently of glycemic control, insulin levels, or body weight, suggesting that VEGF plays a causative role in the development of certain late changes in diabetic nephropathy, including the progression of albuminuria/proteinuria.

Leptin

Leptin, a circulating hormone abundant in obese patients with or without type 2 diabetes, has recently been implicated as a contributor to glomerulosclerosis [179]. Leptin is made primarily by adipose cells and acts on the hypothalamus to reduce food intake and to increase energy expenditure [180]. Thus, higher body fat results in increased leptin production which then participates in a negative feedback loop that regulates body weight. Indeed, a spontaneous mutation in the *ob* gene, which encodes leptin, results in massive obesity in the *ob/ob* mouse [181]. Exogenous leptin treatment in this mouse corrects the obesity.

The *db/db* mouse contains a mutation that confers leptin resistance [182]. Specifically, the long form of the leptin receptor, Ob-Rb, is defective in the hypothalamus [183]. Such mice exhibit hyperphagia and rapid weight gain. With development of obesity, the mice become insulin-resistant and hyperglycemic. After several months, the *db/db* mouse develops renal lesions that are indistinguishable from those of human diabetic glomerulopathy [184]. Because kidney cells contain shorter forms of the leptin receptor that may transduce a discrete signal, it has been postulated [179] that hyperleptinemia (in addition to hyperglycemia) [40] may mediate the renal fibrogenic process in this mouse model of type 2 diabetes. However, the predominant short form receptor in the kidney, Ob-Ra, has not yet been shown to activate the traditional signaling pathway of leptin [185-188].

Our group recently studied the effects of exogenous leptin on the production of TGF-β and type IV collagen by the kidney [179]. Recombinant leptin added to cultures of rat glomerular endothelial cells enhanced TGF-β mRNA and protein expression. These cells possess the short form Ob-Ra receptor and display activation of downstream signaling cascades in response to leptin binding. When leptin is infused into normal rats for 72 hours or 3 weeks, there is increased renal glomerular expression of TGF-β followed by increased type IV collagen expression, proteinuria, and segmental glomerulosclerosis.

Although leptin increases TGF-β1 levels in the glomerular endothelial cell, it does not enhance TGF-β1 production by the mesangial cell. Rather, leptin upregulates the expression of the TGF-β type II receptor [189]. Mesangial cells pretreated with leptin to increase the type II receptor responded briskly to a minuscule dose of exogenous TGF-β1, expressing more collagen I than in response to either leptin or TGF-β1 alone [189]. Thus, by increasing the type II receptor, leptin sensitizes the mesangial cell to the effects of TGF-β1, setting the stage for a paracrine interaction in which TGF-β1 produced in endothelial cells may induce mesangial cells to amplify its matrix production [189]. Leptin also stimulates glucose transport and type I collagen production through signal transduction pathways that involve phosphatidylinositol-3-kinase (PI-3K). In the end, both glomerular endothelial and mesangial cells increase their expression of extracellular matrix in response to leptin. Therefore, the kidney is not only a site of leptin metabolism but also a target organ for leptin action in pathophysiologic states.

MECHANISMS OF RENAL UPREGULATION OF THE TGF–β SYSTEM IN THE DIABETIC STATE IN RELATIONSHIP TO OTHER MEDIATORS

Vasoactive humoral factors such as AngII, endothelins, and altered prostaglandin metabolism have all been implicated in the pathogenesis of diabetic nephropathy, and all these factors may upregulate the TGF-β/TGF-β receptor system in the diabetic kidney (reviewed in [7, 18]). AngII is capable of stimulating TGF-β production in proximal tubular and mesangial cell cultures [95, 96]. Hyperglycemia acts in synergy with locally increased AngII to stimulate renal hypertrophy and synthesis of extracellular matrix proteins (reviewed in [13]). In return, AngII can potentiate the effects of high glucose by inhibiting proteinases responsible for protein turnover and stimulating TGF-β synthesis [13]. Moreover, hyperglycemia can enhance the expression of AngII-receptors and prolong the half-life of AngII itself by inhibiting the enzymes that would degrade AngII. The net effect, therefore, is increased bioactivity of AngII.

As reviewed above, endothelins may stimulate TGF-β production because endothelin receptor antagonists decrease the overexpression of glomerular TGF-β1 mRNA in diabetic rats [118]. Thromboxane has also been demonstrated to stimulate TGF-β production in mesangial cells [128].

The stimulus for chronic upregulation of TGF-β may be partly related to the presence of glycated proteins in long-standing diabetes [190, 191]. The early Amadori-glucose adducts of proteins such as serum albumin have been shown to stimulate TGF-β expression in mesangial cells and glomerular endothelial cells [191, 192]. Administration of AGE-modified proteins to normal mice elevates the mRNA levels of TGF-β1, a1(IV) collagen, and laminin B1. These increases are reversed by concomitant aminoguanidine therapy [193]. Exposure to glycated LDL increases TGF-β1 and fibronectin mRNA levels in cultured murine mesangial cells [194]. The increased fibronectin message is prevented by anti-TGF-β antibody treatment [194]. Finally, mesangial cells have specific receptors for AGE which may result in enhanced matrix and cytokine production [143, 195].

In addition to the metabolic factors listed above, hemodynamic and mechanical forces are operative in the diabetic state. The cyclical stretch/relaxation of mesangial cells in culture, which closely mimics increased glomerular pressure *in vivo* [114, 196, 197], has been associated with increased synthesis of TGF-β and extracellular matrix molecules. Fluid shear stress increases message expression and synthesis of the active form of TGF-β in cultured bovine aortic endothelial cells [198].

The link between oxidative stress and TGF-β is gaining increasing attention in mediating diabetic renal injury. Oxidative stress, generated by glucose metabolism and advanced glycation end-products (AGEs), can trigger a multitude of pathogenetic mechanisms that collectively contribute to the microvascular complications of diabetes [199]. A major component of oxidative stress, the reactive oxygen species (ROS), may act through the TGF-β pathway to exert a profibrotic effect. To generate ROS under experimental conditions, investigators have used glucose oxidase (GO), an enzyme that continuously catalyzes ambient glucose to hydrogen peroxide. The addition of GO to human mesangial cells in culture stimulates the promoter activity, mRNA level, bioactivity, and protein production of TGF-β1 [200]. GO also increases the gene expression of several extracellular matrix proteins, including collagen types I, III, and IV, and fibronectin. However, this GO-stimulated

417

expression of matrix was prevented by a panselective, neutralizing anti-TGF-β antibody [200]. Thus, the reactive oxygen species may exert their deleterious effects on kidney cells via the TGF-β system.

Oxidative stress has also been shown to activate the protein kinase C (PKC) pathway. Recent data have demonstrated that inhibition of high glucose-induced PKC activation effectively abrogates reactive oxygen species generation and nuclear factor-κB (NF-κB) activity, decreasing monocyte chemoattractant protein-1 secretion in mesangial cells [201]. Transcription factors such as NF-κB enhance the transactivation of genes encoding cytokines like TGF-β and the related Connective Tissue Growth Factor (CTGF) that up-regulate extracellular matrix expression [200, 202]. Taken together, evidence is accumulating to suggest that the different biochemical abnormalities produced by hyperglycemia can influence one another, since many of the glucose metabolites serve as important intermediates for the different metabolic pathways.

Upregulation of the renal type II TGF-β receptor in the diabetic state represents another major pathway for enhanced bioactivity of the TGF-β system. Type 1 diabetes in the STZ-induced mouse model increases the quantity of type II receptor at both the mRNA and protein levels [57]. In tissue culture, high ambient glucose [57] and Amadori glucose adducts of albumin [191] both increase the expression of the TGF-β type II receptor by mesangial cells. Interestingly, captopril inhibits high glucose-mediated hypertrophy of tubular LLC-PK$_1$ cells, perhaps by blunting the protein expression of the types I and II TGF-β receptors [203]. This illustrates that AngII can upregulate the TGF-β system, also at the receptor level.

CONCLUDING REMARKS

The characteristic lesions of diabetic nephropathy such as renal hypertrophy, increased glomerular hypertension, and altered extracellular matrix metabolism may be intimately related to the effects of high ambient glucose on various growth factors and cytokines that are increased locally or in the circulation. Recent studies using cell culture techniques and experimental animal models have provided important insights into the pathogenetic mechanisms of diabetic nephropathy (Table 1). Much attention has been devoted to clarifying the role of TGF-β as a mediator of kidney disease. The data we have reviewed strongly support the hypothesis that elevated renal production or activity of TGF-β predominantly mediates the renal hypertrophy and extracellular matrix expansion seen in experimental and human diabetic nephropathy. Ongoing genetic studies linking cytokines and growth factors, especially the TGF-β/TGF-β receptor system, may further shed light on the predictability of diabetic nephropathy in the population at risk.

In summary, TGF-β successfully fulfills all of Koch's postulates to qualify as a causative agent of diabetic nephropathy [204]. Although Koch's postulates were originally developed to identify agents of infectious diseases, the criteria can be modified to ascertain whether TGF-β mediates diabetic kidney disease.

Table 1: Mediators of Diabetic Renal Disease

I.	Genetic predisposition
II.	Glomerular hemodynamic stress*
III.	Metabolic Perturbations
	A. Non-enzymatic glycation of circulating or structural proteins
	Amadori-glucose adducts*
	Advanced glycosylation end-products (AGE)*
	B. Activation of pathways of glucose metabolism
	Polyol pathway (increased sorbitol)*
	Pentose phosphate shunt (increased UDP glucose)

De novo synthesis of diacylglycerol and stimulation of protein kinase C*
    Disordered *myo*-inositol metabolism
Altered cellular redox state (increased NADPH/NADP$^+$, NADH/NAD$^+$)
    Hexosamine pathway*
    Oxidant injury*
  C. Activation of cytokines and growth factor systems
    Transforming growth factor-β*
    Angiotensin II*
    Endothelins*
    Thromboxane*
    Platelet-derived growth factor*
    Insulin-like growth factor-I
    Vascular endothelial growth factor
    Leptin*

* Factors known to stimulate the transforming growth factor-β system

First, diabetes (or its surrogate) must increase TGF-β in the affected kidney or in cultured renal cells. For example, 1) Increased amounts of TGF-β are produced in renal cells when grown in high glucose (e.g., mesangial, proximal tubular, and renal interstitial cells). 2) Increased renal production and urinary levels of TGF-β1 are observed in diabetic animals and humans. 3) Upregulation of TGF-β receptors is observed in the glomerular and tubular compartments of experimental diabetic animals. 4) Features of the diabetic state such as high levels of vasoactive agents (thromboxane, AngII, and endothelin) in the glomerulus, increased levels of nonenzymatically-glycated proteins, and intraglomerular hypertension can all increase glomerular TGF-β1 production. 5) Patients with type 2 diabetes have increased renal production of TGF-β1 prior to established overt nephropathy, and the increased glomerular expression of TGF-β1 correlates with glycemic control.

Second, in the absence of diabetes, TGF-β alone can reproduce the disease phenotype. 1) High ambient glucose and recombinant TGF-β1 exert similar actions on renal cells (i.e., cell hypertrophy and increased extracellular matrix synthesis). 2) Genetic manipulation to overexpress TGF-β1 leads to glomerulosclerosis and tubulointerstitial fibrosis.

Third and most important, inhibition of TGF-β must prevent or reverse kidney disease, even in the face of active diabetes.

1) Inhibition of TGF-β bioactivity using neutralizing anti-TGF-β antibodies or antisense TGF-β1 oligodeoxynucleotides reverses the glucose-stimulated matrix production in cultured renal cells.
2) Systemic treatment with neutralizing panselective anti-TGF-β antibodies or antisense TGF-β1 oligodeoxynucleotides prevents the early manifestations of diabetic renal disease in STZ-diabetic mice and effectively prevents renal insufficiency and mesangial matrix expansion in type 2 diabetic *db/db* mice.
3) Finally, beyond prevention, reversal of diabetic glomerular lesions can be achieved by administration of the neutralizing anti-TGF-β antibodies in *db/db* mice.

Given the importance of the TGF-β system in the pathophysiology of diabetic renal disease, future methods that intercept the renal TGF-β axis to arrest the damaging effects of fibrosis will likely constitute the mainstays of therapy. It is hoped that future innovative treatments that rationally target the TGF-β system will vastly improve clinical outcomes beyond what is achievable with current practices [205].

ACKNOWLEDGMENTS

Dr. Belinda Jim is supported by the National Institutes of Health (NIH) training grant DK-07006. Dr. Sheldon Chen is supported by NIH grants DK-07006, DK-09993, and DK-61537. Dr. Fuad N. Ziyadeh is supported by NIH grants DK-45191, DK-54608, and DK-44513.

REFERENCES:

1. Goldfarb S, Ziyadeh FN, Kern EFO, Simmons DA: Effects of polyol-pathway inhibition and dietary myo-inositol on glomerular hemodynamic function in experimental diabetes mellitus in rats. *Diabetes* 40:465-471, 1991

2. DeRubertis FR, Craven PA: Activation of protein kinase C in glomerular cells in diabetes. Mechanisms and potential links to the pathogenesis of diabetic glomerulopathy. *Diabetes* 43:1-8, 1994

3. Fumo P, Kuncio GS, Ziyadeh FN: PKC and high glucose stimulate collagen a1(IV) transcriptional activity in a reporter mesangial cell line. *Am J Physiol* 267:F632-F638, 1994

4. Kolm-Litty V, Sauer U, Nerlich A, *et al*: High glucose-induced transforming growth factor b1 production is mediated by the hexosamine pathway in porcine glomerular mesangial cells. *J Clin Invest* 101:160-169, 1998

5. Brownlee M, Vlassara H, Cerami A: Nonenzymatic glycosylation and the pathogenesis of diabetic complications. *Ann Intern Med* 101:527-537, 1984

6. Cohen MP, Ziyadeh FN: Amadori glucose adducts modulate mesangial cell growth and collagen gene expression. *Kidney Int* 45:475-484, 1994

7. Hoffman BB, Ziyadeh FN: The role of growth factors in the development of diabetic nephropathy. *Curr Opin Endocrinol Diabetes* 3:322-329, 1996

8. Abboud HE: Growth factors and diabetic nephrology: An overview. *Kidney Int Suppl* 60:S3-S6, 1997

9. Roberts AB, Kim S-J, Noma T, *et al*: Multiple forms of TGF-β: Distinct promoters and differential expression, in *Clinical Applications of TGF-β*, edited by Sporn MB, Roberts AB, Chichester, UK, Ciba Foundation Symposium, 1991, pp 7-28

10. Cheng J, Grande JP: Transforming growth factor-β signal transduction and progressive renal disease. *Exp Biol Med (Maywood)* 227:943-956, 2002

11. Mozes MM, Bottinger EP, Jacot TA, Kopp JB: Renal expression of fibrotic matrix proteins and of transforming growth factor-β (TGF-β) isoforms in TGF-β transgenic mice. *J Am Soc Nephrol* 10:271-280, 1999

12. Ziyadeh FN: The extracellular matrix in diabetic nephropathy. *Am J Kidney Dis* 22:736-744, 1993

13. Wolf G, Ziyadeh FN: Molecular mechanisms of diabetic renal hypertrophy. *Kidney Int* 56:393-405, 1999

14. Laiho M, Saksela O, Andreasen PA, Keski-Oja J: Enhanced production and extracellular deposition of the endothelial-type plasminogen activator inhibitor in cultured human lung fibroblasts by transforming growth factor-β. *J Cell Biol* 103:2403-2410, 1986

15. Singh R, Song RH, Alavi N, *et al*: High glucose decreases matrix metalloproteinase-2 activity in rat mesangial cells via transforming growth factor-β1. *Exp Nephrol* 9:249-257, 2001

16. Thannickal VJ, Lee DY, White ES, *et al*: Myofibroblast differentiation by TGF-β1 is dependent on cell adhesion and integrin signaling via focal adhesion kinase. *J Biol Chem*, 2003

17. MacKay K, Kondaiah P, Danielpour D, *et al*: Expression of transforming growth factor-β1 and β2 in rat glomeruli. *Kidney Int* 38:1095-1100, 1990

18. Sharma K, Ziyadeh FN: Biochemical events and cytokine interactions linking glucose metabolism to the development of diabetic nephropathy. *Semin Nephrol* 17:80-92, 1997

19. Hoffman M: Researchers get a first look at the versatile TGF-β family. *Science* 257:332, 1992

20. Miyazono K, Heldin CH: Latent forms of TGF-β: Molecular structure and mechanisms of activation, in *Clinical Applications of TGF-β*, edited by Bock GR, Marsh J, Chichester, UK, Wiley, 1991, pp 81-92

21. Paralkar VM, Vukicevic S, Reddi AH: Transforming growth factor b type 1 binds to collagen IV of basement membrane matrix: Implications for development. *Dev Biol* 143:303-308, 1991

22. Wakefield LM, Winokur TS, Hollands RS, *et al*: Recombinant latent transforming growth factor β1 has a longer plasma half-life in rats than active transforming growth factor b1, and a different tissue distribution. *J Clin Invest* 86:1976-1984, 1990

23. Penttinen C, Saharinen J, Weikkolainen K, *et al*: Secretion of human latent TGF-β-βinding protein-3 (LTBP-3) is dependent on co-expression of TGF-β. *J Cell Sci* 115:3457-3468, 2002

24. Ando T, Okuda S, Tamaki K, *et al*: Localization of transforming growth factor-β and latent transforming growth factor-β binding protein in rat kidney. *Kidney Int* 47:733-739, 1995

25. Flaumenhaft R, Abe M, Mignatti P, Rifkin DB: Basic fibroblast growth factor-induced activation of latent transforming growth factor β in endothelial cells: Regulation of plasminogen activator activity. *J Cell Biol* 118:901-909, 1992

26. Massague J, Attisano L, Wrana JL: The TGF-β family and its composite receptors. *Trends Cell Biol* 4:172-178, 1994

27. Wrana JL, Attisano L, Wieser R, *et al*: Mechanism of activation of the TGF-β receptor. *Nature* 370:341-347, 1994

28. Wieser R, Attisano L, Wrana JL, Massague J: Signaling activity of transforming growth factor-β type II receptors lacking specific domains in the cytoplasmic region. *Mol Cell Biol* 13:7239-7247, 1993

29. Sekelsky JJ, Newfeld SJ, Raftery LA, *et al*: Genetic characterization and cloning of mothers against dpp, a gene required for decapentaplegic function in *Drosophila melanogaster*. *Genetics* 139:1347-1358, 1995

30. Liu F, Hata A, Baker JC, *et al*: A human Mad protein acting as a BMP-regulated transcriptional activator. *Nature* 381:620-623, 1996

31. Zhang Y, Feng X, We R, Derynck R: Receptor-associated Mad homologues synergize as effectors of the TGF-β response. *Nature* 383:168-172, 1996

32. Miyazawa K, Shinozaki M, Hara T, *et al*: Two major Smad pathways in TGF-β superfamily signalling. *Genes Cells* 7:1191-1204, 2002

33.   Hayashi H, Abdollah S, Qiu Y, *et al*: The MAD-related protein Smad7 associates with the TGF-β receptor and functions as an antagonist of TGF-β signaling. *Cell* 89:1165-1173, 1997

34.   Ungefroren H, Lenschow W, Chen WB, *et al*: Regulation of biglycan gene expression by TGF-β requires MKK6-p38 MAP kinase signaling downstream of Smad signaling. *J Biol Chem*, 2003

35.   Laping NJ, Grygielko E, Mathur A, *et al*: Inhibition of transforming growth factor (TGF)-β1-induced extracellular matrix with a novel inhibitor of the TGF-β type I receptor kinase activity: SB-431542. *Mol Pharmacol* 62:58-64, 2002

36.   Isono M, Chen S, Hong SW, *et al*: Smad pathway is activated in the diabetic mouse kidney and Smad3 mediates TGF-β-induced fibronectin in mesangial cells. *Biochem Biophys Res Commun* 296:1356-1365, 2002

37.   Ziyadeh FN, Snipes ER, Watanabe M, *et al*: High glucose induces cell hypertrophy and stimulates collagen gene transcription in proximal tubule. *Am J Physiol* 259:F704-F714, 1990

38.   Wolf G, Ziyadeh FN: Renal tubular hypertrophy induced by angiotensin II. *Semin Nephrol* 17:448-454, 1997

39.   Wolf G, Sharma K, Chen Y, *et al*: High glucose-induced proliferation in mesangial cells is reversed by autocrine TGF-β. *Kidney Int* 42:647-656, 1992

40.   Wolf G, Schroeder R, Thaiss F, *et al*: Glomerular expression of p27^{Kip1} in diabetic *db/db* mouse: Role of hyperglycemia. *Kidney Int* 53:869-879, 1998

41.   Wolf G, Schroder R, Ziyadeh FN, *et al*: High glucose stimulates expression of p27^{Kip1} in cultured mouse mesangial cells: relationship to hypertrophy. *Am J Physiol* 273:F348-F356, 1997

42.   Ayo SH, Radnik R, Garoni JA, *et al*: High glucose increases diacylglycerol mass and activates protein kinase C in mesangial cell cultures. *Am J Physiol* 261:F571-F577, 1991

43.   Ayo SH, Radnik RA, Glass WF, *et al*: Increased extracellular matrix synthesis and mRNA in mesangial cells grown in high-glucose medium. *Am J Physiol* 260:F185-F191, 1991

44.   Haneda M, Kikkawa R, Horide N, *et al*: Glucose enhances type IV collagen production in cultured rat glomerular mesangial cells. *Diabetologia* 34:198-200, 1991

45.   Ziyadeh FN, Sharma K, Ericksen M, Wolf G: Stimulation of collagen gene expression and protein synthesis in murine mesangial cells by high glucose is mediated by autocrine activation of transforming growth factor-β. *J Clin Invest* 93:536-542, 1994

46.   Wakisaka M, Spiro MJ, Spiro RG: Synthesis of type VI collagen by cultured glomerular cells and comparison of its regulation by glucose and other factors with that of type IV collagen. *Diabetes* 43:95-103, 1994

47.   Kolm V, Sauer U, Olgemooller B, Schleicher ED: High glucose-induced TGF-β1 regulates mesangial production of heparan sulfate proteoglycan. *Am J Physiol* 270:F812-F821, 1996

48.   van Det NF, Verhagen NA, Tamsma JT, *et al*: Regulation of glomerular epithelial cell production of fibronectin and transforming growth factor-β by high glucose, not by angiotensin II. *Diabetes* 46:834-840, 1997

49.   Isono M, Cruz MC, Chen S, *et al*: Extracellular signal-regulated kinase mediates stimulation of TGF-β1 and matrix by high glucose in mesangial cells. *J Am Soc Nephrol* 11:2222-2230, 2000

50.   Iglesias-de la Cruz MC, Ziyadeh FN, Isono M, *et al*: Effects of high glucose and TGF-β1 on the expression of collagen IV and vascular endothelial growth factor in mouse podocytes. *Kidney Int* 62:901-913, 2002

51. Han DC, Isono M, Hoffman BB, Ziyadeh FN: High glucose stimulates proliferation and collagen type I synthesis in renal cortical fibroblasts: mediation by autocrine activation of TGF-β. *J Am Soc Nephrol* 10:1891-1899, 1999

52. Takeuchi A, Throckmorton DC, Brogden AP, *et al*: Periodic high extracellular glucose enhances production of collagens III and IV by mesangial cells. *Am J Physiol* 268:F13-F19, 1995

53. Jones SC, Saunders HJ, Qi W, Pollock CA: Intermittent high glucose enhances cell growth and collagen synthesis in cultured human tubulointerstitial cells. *Diabetologia* 42:1113-1119, 1999

54. Hoffman BB, Sharma K, Zhu Y, Ziyadeh FN: Transcriptional activation of transforming growth factor-β1 in mesangial cell culture by high glucose concentration. *Kidney Int* 54:1107-1116, 1998

55. Montero A, Munger KA, Khan RZ, *et al*: F_2-isoprostanes mediate high glucose-induced TGF-β synthesis and glomerular proteinuria in experimental type I diabetes. *Kidney Int* 58:1963-1972, 2000

56. Rocco MV, Chen Y, Goldfarb S, Ziyadeh FN: Elevated glucose stimulates TGF-β gene expression and bioactivity in proximal tubule. *Kidney Int* 41:107-114, 1992

57. Isono M, Mogyorosi A, Han DC, *et al*: Stimulation of TGF-β type II receptor by high glucose in mouse mesangial cells and in diabetic kidney. *Am J Physiol Renal Physiol* 278:F830-F838, 2000

58. Arteaga CL, Hurd SD, Winnier AR, *et al*: Anti-transforming growth factor (TGF)-β antibodies inhibit breast cancer cell tumorigenicity and increase mouse spleen natural killer cell activity. Implications for a possible role of tumor cell/host TGF-β interactions in human breast cancer progression. *J Clin Invest* 92:2569-2576, 1993

59. Han DC, Hoffman BB, Hong SW, *et al*: Therapy with antisense TGF-β1 oligodeoxynucleotides reduces kidney weight and matrix mRNAs in diabetic mice. *Am J Physiol* 278:F628-F634, 2000

60. Inoki K, Haneda M, Maeda S, *et al*: TGF-β1 stimulates glucose uptake by enhancing GLUT1 expression in mesangial cells. *Kidney Int* 55:1704-1712, 1999

61. Liu ZH, Li YJ, Chen ZH, *et al*: Glucose transporter in human glomerular mesangial cells modulated by transforming growth factor-β and rhein. *Acta Pharmacol Sin* 22:169-175, 2001

62. Mogyorosi A, Ziyadeh FN: GLUT1 and TGF-β: the link between hyperglycaemia and diabetic nephropathy. *Nephrol Dial Transplant* 14:2827-2829, 1999

63. Lee TS, Saltsman KA, Ohashi H, King GL: Activation of protein kinase C by elevation of glucose concentration: Proposal for a mechanism in the development of diabetic vascular complications. *Proc Natl Acad Sci USA* 86:5141-5145, 1989

64. Du XL, Edelstein D, Rossetti L, *et al*: Hyperglycemia-induced mitochondrial superoxide overproduction activates the hexosamine pathway and induces plasminogen activator inhibitor-1 expression by increasing Sp1 glycosylation. *Proc Natl Acad Sci U S A* 97:12222-12226, 2000

65. Heilig CW, Concepcion LA, Riser BL, *et al*: Overexpression of glucose transporters in rat mesangial cells cultured in a normal glucose milieu mimics the diabetic phenotype. *J Clin Invest* 96:1802-1814, 1995

66. Henry DN, Busik JV, Brosius FC, 3rd, Heilig CW: Glucose transporters control gene expression of aldose reductase, PKCα, and GLUT1 in mesangial cells in vitro. *Am J Physiol* 277:F97-104, 1999

67. Nakamura T, Fukui M, Ebihara I, *et al*: mRNA expression of growth factors in glomeruli from diabetic rats. *Diabetes* 42:450-456, 1993

68. Yamamoto T, Nakamura T, Noble NA, *et al*: Expression of transforming growth factor β is elevated in human and experimental diabetic nephropathy. *Proc Natl Acad Sci USA* 90:1814-1818, 1993

69. Bollineni JS, Reddi AS: Transforming growth factor-β1 enhances glomerular collagen synthesis in diabetic rats. *Diabetes* 42:1673-1677, 1993

70. Sharma K, Ziyadeh FN: Renal hypertrophy is associated with upregulation of TGF-β1 gene expression in diabetic BB rat and NOD mouse. *Am J Physiol* 267:F1094-F1101, 1994

71. Yang C-W, Hattori M, Vlassara H, *et al*: Overexpression of transforming growth factor-β1 mRNA is associated with up-regulation of glomerular tenascin and laminin gene expression in nonobese diabetic mice. *J Am Soc Nephrol* 5:1610-1617, 1995

72. Pankewycz OG, Guan JX, Bolton WK, *et al*: Renal TGF-β regulation in spontaneously diabetic NOD mice with correlations in mesangial cells. *Kidney Int* 46:748-758, 1994

73. Shankland SJ, Scholey JW, Ly H, Thai K: Expression of transforming growth factor-β1 during diabetic renal hypertrophy. *Kidney Int* 46:430-442, 1994

74. Gilbert RE, Cox A, Wu LL, *et al*: Expression of transforming growth factor-β1 and type IV collagen in the renal tubulointerstitium in experimental diabetes: effects of ACE inhibition. *Diabetes* 47:414-422, 1998

75. Hill C, Flyvbjerg A, Gronbaek H, *et al*: The renal expression of transforming growth factor-β isoforms and their receptors in acute and chronic experimental diabetes in rats. *Endocrinology* 141:1196-1208, 2000

76. Fukui M, Nakamura T, Ebihara I, *et al*: ECM gene expression and its modulation by insulin in diabetic rats. *Diabetes* 41:1520-1527, 1992

77. Sharma K, Jin Y, Guo J, Ziyadeh FN: Neutralization of TGF-β by anti-TGF-β antibody attenuates kidney hypertrophy and the enhanced extracellular matrix gene expression in STZ-induced diabetic mice. *Diabetes* 45:522-530, 1996

78. Hong SW, Isono M, Chen S, *et al*: Increased glomerular and tubular expression of transforming growth factor-β1, its type II receptor, and activation of the Smad signaling pathway in the *db/db* mouse. *Am J Pathol* 158:1653-1663, 2001

79. Ziyadeh FN, Hoffman BB, Han DC, *et al*: Long-term prevention of renal insufficiency, excess matrix gene expression, and glomerular mesangial matrix expansion by treatment with monoclonal antitransforming growth factor-β antibody in *db/db* diabetic mice. *Proc Natl Acad Sci U S A* 97:8015-8020, 2000

80. Remuzzi G, Bertani T: Pathophysiology of progressive nephropathies. *N Engl J Med* 339:1448-1456, 1998

81. Reeves WB, Andreoli TE: Transforming growth factor β contributes to progressive diabetic nephropathy. *Proc Natl Acad Sci U S A* 97:7667-7669, 2000

82. Chen S, Carmen Iglesias-de la Cruz M, Jim B, *et al*: Reversibility of established diabetic glomerulopathy by anti-TGF-β antibodies in *db/db* mice. *Biochem Biophys Res Commun* 300:16-22, 2003

83. Ledbetter S, Kurtzberg L, Doyle S, Pratt BM: Renal fibrosis in mice treated with human recombinant transforming growth factor-β2. *Kidney Int* 58:2367-2376, 2000

84. Hill C, Flyvbjerg A, Rasch R, *et al*: Transforming growth factor-β2 antibody attenuates fibrosis in the experimental diabetic rat kidney. *J Endocrinol* 170:647-651, 2001

85. Yoshioka K, Takemura T, Murakami K, *et al*: Transforming growth factor-β protein and mRNA in glomeruli in normal and diseased human kidneys. *Lab Invest* 68:154-163, 1993

86. Yamamoto T, Noble NA, Cohen AH, *et al*: Expression of transforming growth factor-β isoforms in human glomerular diseases. *Kidney Int* 49:461-469, 1996

87. Iwano M, Kubo A, Nishino T, *et al*: Quantification of glomerular TGF-β1 mRNA in patients with diabetes mellitus. *Kidney Int* 49:1120-1126, 1996

88. Sharma K, Ziyadeh FN, Alzahabi B, *et al*: Increased renal production of transforming growth factor-β1 in patients with type II diabetes. *Diabetes* 46:854-859, 1997

89. Sharma K, Eltayeb BO, McGowan TA, *et al*: Captopril-induced reduction of serum levels of transforming growth factor-β1 correlates with long-term renoprotection in insulin-dependent diabetic patients. *Am J Kidney Dis* 34:818-823, 1999

90. Lewis EJ, Hunsicker LG, Bain RP, Rohde RD: The effect of angiotensin-converting-enzyme inhibition on diabetic nephropathy. The collaborative study group. *N Engl J Med* 329:1456-1462, 1993

91. Chaturvedi N, Schalkwijk CG, Abrahamian H, *et al*: Circulating and urinary transforming growth factor b1, Amadori albumin, and complications of type 1 diabetes: the EURODIAB prospective complications study. *Diabetes Care* 25:2320-2327, 2002

92. Dallas SL, Miyazono K, Skerry TM, *et al*: Dual role for the latent transforming growth factor-β binding protein in storage of latent TGF-β in the extracellular matrix and as a structural matrix protein. *J Cell Biol* 131:539-549, 1995

93. Huang C, Kim Y, Caramori ML, *et al*: Cellular basis of diabetic nephropathy: II. The transforming growth factor-β system and diabetic nephropathy lesions in type 1 diabetes. *Diabetes* 51:3577-3581, 2002

94. Wolf G, Ziyadeh FN: The role of angiotensin II in diabetic nephropathy: emphasis on nonhemodynamic mechanisms. *Am J Kidney Dis* 29:153-163, 1997

95. Wolf G, Mueller E, Stahl RAK, Ziyadeh FN: Angiotensin II-induced hypertrophy of cultured murine proximal tubular cells is mediated by endogenous transforming growth factor-β. *J Clin Invest* 92:1366-1372, 1993

96. Kagami S, Border WA, Miller DE, Noble NA: Angiotensin II stimulates extracellular matrix protein synthesis through induction of transforming growth factor-β expression in rat glomerular mesangial cells. *J Clin Invest* 93:2431-2437, 1994

97. Wolf G, Haberstroh U, Neilson EG: Angiotensin II stimulates the proliferation and biosynthesis of type I collagen in cultured murine mesangial cells. *Am J Pathol* 140:95-107, 1992

98. Wolf G, Killen PD, Neilson EG: Intracellular signaling of transcription and secretion of type IV collagen after angiotensin II-induced cellular hypertrophy in cultured proximal tubular cells. *Cell Regul* 2:219-227, 1991

99. Wolf G, Kalluri R, Ziyadeh FN, *et al*: Angiotensin II induces α3(IV) collagen expression in cultured murine proximal tubular cells. *Proc Assoc Am Physicians* 111:357-364, 1999

100. Fakhouri F, Placier S, Ardaillou R, *et al*: Angiotensin II activates collagen type I gene in the renal cortex and aorta of transgenic mice through interaction with endothelin and TGF-β. *J Am Soc Nephrol* 12:2701-2710, 2001

101. Tharaux PL, Chatziantoniou C, Fakhouri F, Dussaule JC: Angiotensin II activates collagen I gene through a mechanism involving the MAP/ER kinase pathway. *Hypertension* 36:330-336, 2000

102. Wolf G, Zahner G, Mondorf U, *et al*: Angiotensin II stimulates cellular hypertrophy of LLC-PK$_1$ cells through the AT$_1$ receptor. *Nephrol Dial Transplant* 8:128-133, 1993

103. Wolf G, Neilson EG: Angiotensin II induces cellular hypertrophy in cultured murine proximal tubular cells. *Am J Physiol* 259:F768-777, 1990

104. Anderson PW, Do YS, Hsueh WA: Angiotensin II causes mesangial cell hypertrophy. *Hypertension* 21:29-35, 1993

105. Wolf G, Mueller E, Stahl RA, Ziyadeh FN: Angiotensin II-induced hypertrophy of cultured murine proximal tubular cells is mediated by endogenous transforming growth factor-β. *J Clin Invest* 92:1366-1372, 1993

106. Wolf G, Ziyadeh FN, Zahner G, Stahl RA: Angiotensin II-stimulated expression of transforming growth factor β in renal proximal tubular cells: attenuation after stable transfection with the c-mas oncogene. *Kidney Int* 48:1818-1827, 1995

107. Mezzano SA, Ruiz-Ortega M, Egido J: Angiotensin II and renal fibrosis. *Hypertension* 38:635-638, 2001

108. Zatz R, Dunn BR, Meyer TW, *et al*: Prevention of diabetic glomerulopathy by pharmacological amelioration of glomerular capillary hypertension. *J Clin Invest* 77:1925-1930, 1986

109. Kalender B, Ozturk M, Tuncdemir M, *et al*: Renoprotective effects of valsartan and enalapril in STZ-induced diabetes in rats. *Acta Histochem* 104:123-130, 2002

110. Wong VY, Laping NJ, Contino LC, *et al*: Gene expression in rats with renal disease treated with the angiotensin II receptor antagonist, eprosartan. *Physiol Genomics* 4:35-42, 2000

111. Shin GT, Kim SJ, Ma KA, *et al*: ACE inhibitors attenuate expression of renal transforming growth factor-β1 in humans. *Am J Kidney Dis* 36:894-902, 2000

112. Cao Z, Cooper ME, Wu LL, *et al*: Blockade of the renin-angiotensin and endothelin systems on progressive renal injury. *Hypertension* 36:561-568, 2000

113. Peters H, Border WA, Noble NA: Targeting TGF-β overexpression in renal disease: maximizing the antifibrotic action of angiotensin II blockade. *Kidney Int* 54:1570-1580, 1998

114. Riser BL, Cortes P, Heilig C, *et al*: Cyclic stretching force selectively up-regulates transforming growth factor-β isoforms in cultured rat mesangial cells. *Am J Pathol* 148:1915-1923, 1996

115. Fern RJ, Yesko CM, Thornhill BA, *et al*: Reduced angiotensinogen expression attenuates renal interstitial fibrosis in obstructive nephropathy in mice. *J Clin Invest* 103:39-46, 1999

116. Agarwal R, Siva S, Dunn SR, Sharma K: Add-on angiotensin II receptor blockade lowers urinary transforming growth factor-β levels. *Am J Kidney Dis* 39:486-492, 2002

117. Morabito E, Corsico N, Arrigoni Martelli E: Endothelins urinary excretion is increased in spontaneously diabetic rats: BB/BB. *Life Sci* 56:PL13-PL18, 1995

118. Nakamura T, Ebihara I, Fukui M, *et al*: Effect of a specific endothelin receptor A antagonist on mRNA levels for extracellular matrix components and growth factors in diabetic glomeruli. *Diabetes* 44:895-899, 1995

119. Takahashi K, Ghatei MA, Lam HC, *et al*: Elevated plasma endothelin in patients with diabetes mellitus. *Diabetologia* 33:306-310, 1990

120. Ferri C, Laurenti O, Bellini C, *et al*: Circulating endothelin-1 levels in lean non-insulin-dependent diabetic patients. Influence of ACE inhibition. *Am J Hypertens* 8:40-47, 1995

121. Ledbetter S, Copeland EJ, Noonan D, *et al*: Altered steady-state mRNA levels of basement membrane proteins in diabetic mouse kidneys and thromboxane synthase inhibition. *Diabetes* 39:196-203, 1990

122. Craven PA, Caines MA, DeRubertis FR: Sequential alterations in glomerular prostaglandin and thromboxane synthesis in diabetic rats: Relationship to the hyperfiltration of early diabetes. *Metabolism* 36:95-103, 1987

123. Craven PA, DeRubertis FR: Protein kinase C is activated in glomeruli from streptozotocin diabetic rats. *J Clin Invest* 83:1667-1675, 1989
124. Gambardella S, Andreani D, Cancelli A, *et al*: Renal hemodynamics and urinary excretion of 6-keto-prostaglandin F1 alpha and thromboxane B2 in newly diagnosed type I diabetic patients. *Diabetes* 37:1044-1048, 1988
125. Craven PA, Melhem MF, DeRubertis FR: Thromboxane in the pathogenesis of glomerular injury in diabetes. *Kidney Int* 42:937-946, 1992
126. DeRubertis FR, Craven PA: Contribution of platelet thromboxane production to enhanced urinary excretion and glomerular production of thromboxane and to the pathogenesis of albuminuria in the streptozotocin-diabetic rat. *Metabolism* 41:90-96, 1992
127. Bruggeman LA, Horigan EA, Horikoshi S, *et al*: Thromboxane stimulates synthesis of extracellular matrix proteins *in vitro*. *Am J Physiol* 261:F488-F494, 1991
128. Studer RK, Negrete H, Craven PA, DeRubertis FR: Protein kinase C signals thromboxane induced increases in fibronectin synthesis and TGF-β bioactivity in mesangial cells. *Kidney Int* 48:422-430, 1995
129. Matsuo Y, Takagawa I, Koshida H, *et al*: Antiproteinuric effect of a thromboxane receptor antagonist, S-1452, on rat diabetic nephropathy and murine lupus nephritis. *Pharmacology* 50:1-8, 1995
130. Hora K, Oguchi H, Furukawa T, *et al*: Effects of a selective thromboxane synthetase inhibitor OKY-046 on experimental diabetic nephropathy. *Nephron* 56:297-305, 1990
131. Cediel E, Vazquez-Cruz B, Navarro-Cid J, *et al*: Role of endothelin-1 and thromboxane A2 in renal vasoconstriction induced by angiotensin II in diabetes and hypertension. *Kidney Int Suppl*:2-7, 2002
132. Pricci F, Pugliese G, Mene P, *et al*: Regulatory role of eicosanoids in extracellular matrix overproduction induced by long-term exposure to high glucose in cultured rat mesangial cells. *Diabetologia* 39:1055-1062, 1996
133. Makino H, Tanaka I, Mukoyama M, *et al*: Prevention of diabetic nephropathy in rats by prostaglandin E receptor EP1-selective antagonist. *J Am Soc Nephrol* 13:1757-1765, 2002
134. Inaba T, Ishibashi S, Gotoda T, *et al*: Enhanced expression of platelet-derived growth factor-β receptor by high glucose. Involvement of platelet-derived growth factor in diabetic angiopathy. *Diabetes* 45:507-512, 1996
135. Fukui M, Nakamura T, Ebihara I, *et al*: Effects of enalapril on endothelin-1 and growth factor gene expression in diabetic rat glomeruli. *J Lab Clin Med* 123:763-768, 1994
136. Tsiani E, Lekas P, Fantus IG, *et al*: High glucose-enhanced activation of mesangial cell p38 MAPK by ET-1, ANG II, and platelet-derived growth factor. *Am J Physiol Endocrinol Metab* 282:E161-169, 2002
137. Leivonen SK, Chantry A, Hakkinen L, *et al*: Smad3 mediates transforming growth factor-β-induced collagenase-3 (matrix metalloproteinase-13) expression in human gingival fibroblasts. Evidence for cross-talk between Smad3 and p38 signaling pathways. *J Biol Chem* 277:46338-46346, 2002
138. Di Paolo S, Gesualdo L, Ranieri E, *et al*: High glucose concentration induces the overexpression of transforming growth factor-β through the activation of a platelet-derived growth factor loop in human mesangial cells. *Am J Path* 149:2095-2106, 1996
139. Phillips AO, Steadman R, Topley N, Williams JD: Elevated D-glucose concentrations modulate TGF-β1 synthesis by human cultured renal proximal tubular cells. The permissive role of platelet-derived growth factor. *Am J Path* 147:362-374, 1995

140. Nakagawa H, Sasahara M, Haneda M, *et al*: Immunohistochemical characterization of glomerular PDGF B-chain and PDGF beta-receptor expression in diabetic rats. *Diabetes Res Clin Pract* 48:87-98, 2000

141. Fagerudd JA, Groop PH, Honkanen E, *et al*: Urinary excretion of TGF-β1, PDGF-BB and fibronectin in insulin-dependent diabetes mellitus patients. *Kidney Int Suppl* 63:S195-S197, 1997

142. Throckmorton DC, Brogden AP, Min B, *et al*: PDGF and TGF-β mediate collagen production by mesangial cells exposed to advanced glycosylation end products. *Kidney Int* 48:111-117, 1995

143. Doi T, Vlassara H, Kirstein M, *et al*: Receptor-specific increase in extracellular matrix production in mouse mesangial cells by advanced glycosylation end products is mediated via platelet-derived growth factor. *Proc Natl Acad Sci USA* 89:2873-2877, 1992

144. Tischer E, Mitchell R, Hartman T, *et al*: The human gene for vascular endothelial growth factor. Multiple protein forms are encoded through alternative exon splicing. *J Biol Chem* 266:11947-11954, 1991

145. Neufeld G, Cohen T, Gengrinovitch S, Poltorak Z: Vascular endothelial growth factor (VEGF) and its receptors. *FASEB J* 13:9-22, 1999

146. Shweiki D, Itin A, Soffer D, Keshet E: Vascular endothelial growth factor induced by hypoxia may mediate hypoxia-initiated angiogenesis. *Nature* 359:843-845, 1992

147. Brown LF, Berse B, Tognazzi K, *et al*: Vascular permeability factor mRNA and protein expression in human kidney. *Kidney Int* 42:1457-1461, 1992

148. Simon M, Grone HJ, Johren O, *et al*: Expression of vascular endothelial growth factor and its receptors in human renal ontogenesis and in adult kidney. *Am J Physiol* 268:F240-F250, 1995

149. Grone HJ, Simon M, Grone EF: Expression of vascular endothelial growth factor in renal vascular disease and renal allografts. *J Pathol* 177:259-267, 1995

150. Pupilli C, Lasagni L, Romagnani P, *et al*: Angiotensin II stimulates the synthesis and secretion of vascular permeability factor/vascular endothelial growth factor in human mesangial cells. *J Am Soc Nephrol* 10:245-255, 1999

151. Uchida K, Uchida S, Nitta K, *et al*: Glomerular endothelial cells in culture express and secrete vascular endothelial growth factor. *Am J Physiol* 266:F81-F88, 1994

152. Simon M, Rockl W, Hornig C, *et al*: Receptors of vascular endothelial growth factor/vascular permeability factor (VEGF/VPF) in fetal and adult human kidney: Localization and [125I]VEGF binding sites. *J Am Soc Nephrol* 9:1032-1044, 1998

153. Takahashi T, Shirasawa T, Miyake K, *et al*: Protein tyrosine kinases expressed in glomeruli and cultured glomerular cells: Flt-1 and VEGF expression in renal mesangial cells. *Biochem Biophys Res Commun* 209:218-226, 1995

154. Jakeman LB, Winer J, Bennett GL, *et al*: Binding sites for vascular endothelial growth factor are localized on endothelial cells in adult rat tissues. *J Clin Invest* 89:244-253, 1992

155. Risau W: Angiogenesis and endothelial cell function. *Arzneimittelforschung* 44:416-417, 1994

156. Eremina V, Sood M, Haigh J, *et al*: Glomerular-specific alterations of VEGF-A expression lead to distinct congenital and acquired renal diseases. *J Clin Invest* 111:707-716, 2003

157. Klanke B, Simon M, Rockl W, *et al*: Effects of vascular endothelial growth factor (VEGF)/vascular permeability factor (VPF) on haemodynamics and permselectivity of the isolated perfused rat kidney. *Nephrol Dial Transplant* 13:875-885, 1998

158. Natarajan R, Bai W, Lanting L, *et al*: Effects of high glucose on vascular endothelial growth factor expression in vascular smooth muscle cells. *Am J Physiol* 273:H2224-H2231, 1997

159. Williams B, Gallacher B, Patel H, Orme C: Glucose-induced protein kinase C activation regulates vascular permeability factor mRNA expression and peptide production by human vascular smooth muscle cells *in vitro*. *Diabetes* 46:1497-1503, 1997

160. Iijima K, Yoshikawa N, Connolly DT, Nakamura H: Human mesangial cells and peripheral blood mononuclear cells produce vascular permeability factor. *Kidney Int* 44:959-966, 1993

161. Pal S, Claffey KP, Dvorak HF, Mukhopadhyay D: The von Hippel-Lindau gene product inhibits vascular permeability factor/vascular endothelial growth factor expression in renal cell carcinoma by blocking protein kinase C pathways. *J Biol Chem* 272:27509-27512, 1997

162. Chua CC, Hamdy RC, Chua BH: Upregulation of vascular endothelial growth factor by H_2O_2 in rat heart endothelial cells. *Free Radic Biol Med* 25:891-897, 1998

163. Ruef J, Hu ZY, Yin LY, *et al*: Induction of vascular endothelial growth factor in balloon-injured baboon arteries. A novel role for reactive oxygen species in atherosclerosis. *Circ Res* 81:24-33, 1997

164. Pertovaara L, Kaipainen A, Mustonen T, *et al*: Vascular endothelial growth factor is induced in response to transforming growth factor-β in fibroblastic and epithelial cells. *J Biol Chem* 269:6271-6274, 1994

165. Goad DL, Rubin J, Wang H, *et al*: Enhanced expression of vascular endothelial growth factor in human SaOS-2 osteoblast-like cells and murine osteoblasts induced by insulin-like growth factor I. *Endocrinology* 137:2262-2268, 1996

166. Hata Y, Rook SL, Aiello LP: Basic fibroblast growth factor induces expression of VEGF receptor KDR through a protein kinase C and p44/p42 mitogen-activated protein kinase-dependent pathway. *Diabetes* 48:1145-1155, 1999

167. Nauck M, Roth M, Tamm M, *et al*: Induction of vascular endothelial growth factor by platelet-activating factor and platelet-derived growth factor is downregulated by corticosteroids. *Am J Respir Cell Mol Biol* 16:398-406, 1997

168. Ahmed A, Dearn S, Shams M, *et al*: Localization, quantification, and activation of platelet-activating factor receptor in human endometrium during the menstrual cycle: PAF stimulates NO, VEGF, and FAKpp125. *FASEB J* 12:831-843, 1998

169. Gruden G, Thomas S, Burt D, *et al*: Interaction of angiotensin II and mechanical stretch on vascular endothelial growth factor production by human mesangial cells. *J Am Soc Nephrol* 10:730-737, 1999

170. Tsuchida K, Makita Z, Yamagishi S, *et al*: Suppression of transforming growth factor b and vascular endothelial growth factor in diabetic nephropathy in rats by a novel advanced glycation end product inhibitor, OPB-9195. *Diabetologia* 42:579-588, 1999

171. Cooper ME, Vranes D, Youssef S, *et al*: Increased renal expression of vascular endothelial growth factor (VEGF) and its receptor VEGFR-2 in experimental diabetes. *Diabetes* 48:2229-2239, 1999

172. Malamitsi-Puchner A, Sarandakou A, Tziotis J, *et al*: Serum levels of basic fibroblast growth factor and vascular endothelial growth factor in children and adolescents with type 1 diabetes mellitus. *Pediatr Res* 44:873-875, 1998

173. Shulman K, Rosen S, Tognazzi K, *et al*: Expression of vascular permeability factor (VPF/VEGF) is altered in many glomerular diseases. *J Am Soc Nephrol* 7:661-666, 1996

174. Haltia A, Solin ML, Jalanko H, *et al*: Mechanisms of proteinuria: Vascular permeability factor in congenital nephrotic syndrome of the Finnish type. *Pediatr Res* 40:652-657, 1996

175. Webb NJ, Watson CJ, Roberts IS, *et al*: Circulating vascular endothelial growth factor is not increased during relapses of steroid-sensitive nephrotic syndrome. *Kidney Int* 55:1063-1071, 1999

176. Horita Y, Miyazaki M, Koji T, *et al*: Expression of vascular endothelial growth factor and its receptors in rats with protein-overload nephrosis. *Nephrol Dial Transplant* 13:2519-2528, 1998

177. de Vriese AS, Tilton RG, Elger M, *et al*: Antibodies against vascular endothelial growth factor improve early renal dysfunction in experimental diabetes. *J Am Soc Nephrol* 12:993-1000, 2001

178. Flyvbjerg A, Dagnaes-Hansen F, De Vriese AS, *et al*: Amelioration of long-term renal changes in obese type 2 diabetic mice by a neutralizing vascular endothelial growth factor antibody. *Diabetes* 51:3090-3094, 2002

179. Wolf G, Hamann A, Han DC, *et al*: Leptin stimulates proliferation and TGF-β expression in renal glomerular endothelial cells: Potential role in glomerulosclerosis. *Kidney Int* 56:860-872, 1999

180. Hamann A, Matthaei S: Regulation of energy balance by leptin. *Exp Clin Endocrinol Diabetes* 104:293-300, 1996

181. Halaas JL, Gajiwala KS, Maffei M, *et al*: Weight-reducing effects of the plasma protein encoded by the obese gene. *Science* 269:543-546, 1995

182. Maffei M, Fei H, Lee GH, *et al*: Increased expression in adipocytes of *ob* RNA in mice with lesions of the hypothalamus and with mutations at the *db* locus. *Proc Natl Acad Sci USA* 92:6957-6960, 1995

183. Chua SCJ, Chung WK, Wu-Peng XS, *et al*: Phenotypes of mouse diabetes and rat fatty due to mutations in the OB (leptin) receptor. *Science* 271:994-996, 1996

184. Cohen MP, Clements RS, Hud E, *et al*: Evolution of renal function abnormalities in the *db/db* mouse that parallels the development of human diabetic nephropathy. *Exp Nephrol* 4:166-171, 1996

185. Bjorbaek C, Uotani S, da Silva B, Flier JS: Divergent signaling capacities of the long and short isoforms of the leptin receptor. *J Biol Chem* 272:32686-32695, 1997

186. Bjorbaek C, Buchholz RM, Davis SM, *et al*: Divergent roles of SHP-2 in ERK activation by leptin receptors. *J Biol Chem* 276:4747-4755, 2001

187. Vaisse C, Halaas JL, Horvath CM, *et al*: Leptin activation of Stat3 in the hypothalamus of wild-type and *ob/ob* mice but not *db/db* mice. *Nat Genet* 14:95-97, 1996

188. Ghilardi N, Ziegler S, Wiestner A, *et al*: Defective STAT signaling by the leptin receptor in diabetic mice. *Proc Natl Acad Sci U S A* 93:6231-6235, 1996

189. Han DC, Isono M, Chen S, *et al*: Leptin stimulates type I collagen production in *db/db* mesangial cells: glucose uptake and TGF-β type II receptor expression. *Kidney Int* 59:1315-1323, 2001

190. Ziyadeh FN, Mogyorosi A, Kalluri R: Early and advanced non-enzymatic glycation products in the pathogenesis of diabetic kidney disease [editorial]. *Exp Nephrol* 5:2-9, 1997

191. Ziyadeh FN, Han DC, Cohen JA, *et al*: Glycated albumin stimulates fibronectin gene expression in glomerular mesangial cells: involvement of the transforming growth factor-β system. *Kidney Int* 53:631-638, 1998

192. Chen S, Cohen MP, Lautenslager GT, *et al*: Glycated albumin stimulates TGF-β1 production and protein kinase C activity in glomerular endothelial cells. *Kidney Int* 59:673-681, 2001

193. Yang C-W, Vlassara H, Peten EP, *et al*: Advanced glycation end products up-regulate gene expression found in diabetic glomerular disease. *Proc Natl Acad Sci USA* 91:9436-9440, 1994

194. Ha H, Kamanna VS, Kirschenbaum MA, Kim KH: Role of glycated low density lipoprotein in mesangial extracellular matrix synthesis. *Kidney Int Suppl* 60:S54-S59, 1997

195. Skolnik EY, Yang Z, Makita Z, *et al*: Human and rat mesangial cell receptors for glucose-modified proteins: Potential role in kidney tissue remodelling and diabetic nephropathy. *J Exp Med* 174:931-939, 1991

196. Riser BL, Cortes P, Zhao X, *et al*: Intraglomerular pressure and mesangial stretching stimulate extracellular matrix formation in the rat. *J Clin Invest* 90:1932-1943, 1992

197. Yasuda T, Kondo S, Homma T, Harris RC: Regulation of extracellular matrix by mechanical stress in rat glomerular mesangial cells. *J Clin Invest* 98:1991-2000, 1996

198. Ohno M, Cooke JP, Dzau VJ, Gibbons GH: Fluid shear stress induces endothelial transforming growth factor β-1 transcription and production. Modulation by potassium channel blockade. *J Clin Invest* 95:1363-1369, 1995

199. Brownlee M: Biochemistry and molecular cell biology of diabetic complications. *Nature* 414:813-820, 2001

200. Iglesias-de la Cruz MC, Ruiz-Torres P, Alcami J, *et al*: Hydrogen peroxide increases extracellular matrix mRNA through TGF-β in human mesangial cells. *Kidney Int* 59:87-95, 2001

201. Ha H, Yu MR, Choi YJ, *et al*: Role of high glucose-induced nuclear factor-κB activation in monocyte chemoattractant protein-1 expression by mesangial cells. *J Am Soc Nephrol* 13:894-902, 2002

202. Park SK, Kim J, Seomun Y, *et al*: Hydrogen peroxide is a novel inducer of connective tissue growth factor. *Biochem Biophys Res Commun* 284:966-971, 2001

203. Guh JY, Yang ML, Yang YL, *et al*: Captopril reverses high-glucose-induced growth effects on LLC-PK$_1$ cells partly by decreasing transforming growth factor-β receptor protein expressions. *J Am Soc Nephrol* 7:1207-1215, 1996

204. Ziyadeh FN: Evidence for the involvement of transforming growth factor-β in the pathogenesis of diabetic kidney disease: Are Koch's postulates fulfilled? *Curr Pract Med* 1:87-89, 1998

205. Mogensen CE, Christensen CK: Predicting diabetic nephropathy in insulin-dependent patients. *N Engl J Med* 311:89-93, 1984

25

BLOOD PRESSURE ELEVATION IN DIABETES: THE RESULTS FROM 24-h AMBULATORY BLOOD PRESSURE RECORDINGS

Klavs Würgler Hansen, [2]Per Løgstrup Poulsen, [2]Eva Ebbehøj, [2]Søren Tang Knudsen and [2]Carl Erik Mogensen

Medical dept., Silkeborg Centralsygehus, DK-8600 Silkeborg,, 2) Medical dept. M, Aarhus kommunehospital, DK-8000 Aarhus

Ambulatory blood pressure (BP) measurement permits assessment of BP in the patients' own surroundings, during normal daily activities on the job and in the night. Previously semiautomatic monitors were used, which required manually inflation of the cuff [1], or direct (intra-arterial) BP measurement [2]. The first true ambulatory 24-h report of indirectly measured BP obtained with a portable and fully automatic monitor was published in 1975 [3]

Rubler first reported the application of the technique to diabetic patients in 1982 using equipment weighing 3.07 kg [4]. The number of studies using ambulatory BP monitoring in diabetic patient in the eighties were moderate and with a few exceptions [4-7] focusing on autonomic neuropathy [8-13].

METHODOLOGICAL ASPECTS: A GUIDE TO THE CRITICAL READER

The two most popular ways of obtaining automatic indirect BP records are either by use of a microphone in the cuff or by oscillometric technique [14,15]. Some monitors offer both options. While the manufacturer of the monitor is always stated in papers dealing with ambulatory BP monitoring, the technique is not necessarily described.

No monitor is perfect and even in monitors, which have fulfilled national standards, major discrepancies between the monitors and values obtained by sphygmomanometry are observed in some of the patients. Some papers state that individually "calibration" of the monitor to each of the studied patients has been performed (by 3 to 5 simultaneous or sequential measurements). However, it is not possibly to calibrate a fully automatic monitor in strict terms (without returning to the manufacturer) and the word calibration is a misnomer in this context. The difference between auscultatory BP and the monitor can be evaluated in each patient (rather inaccurate) and this difference can either be accepted or not.

If the result of clinic BP measurement is provided it should be observed whether this is obtained by sphygmomanometry or by use of the same monitor as used for ambulatory measurements [16]. Only in the latter case are clinic and ambulatory values directly comparable.

Although more sophisticated methods exist [17,18], the diurnal variation of BP is usually reported as the night/day ratio. Obviously this must be based on individual information of the night period; otherwise the ratio is overestimated [19].

The term "non-dipper" has become a popular short term for a person who does not describe a normal reduction of BP at night. A commonly used definition of a "non-dipper" requires a relative reduction of night blood pressure less than 10 % of the day value for both systolic and diastolic BP [20]. Unfortunately no consensus exists. In addition the proportion of non-dippers also depends on the definition of night and day time which should be based on individual information of time for going to bed and rising rather than fixed periods. If individual information is not available the use of "short fixed intervals" have been proposed [21].

Patients who are hypertensive by clinic measurements but show a normal ambulatory BP are designated "white coat hypertensive" [22]. This term is well understood in literature although "isolated clinic hypertension" may be more precise [23]. The effect of the "white coat" was originally described as a transient (5 min) elevation of BP [23]. At present the "white coat effect" is usually calculated as the difference (clinic BP - day time BP) [24]. The proportion of white coat hypertensive subjects in a hypertensive population depends on:

i: The definition of hypertension (usually clinic BP > 140/90 mmHg)

ii: How carefully the hypertensive subjects are identified (if patients are labelled as hypertensive based on only one clinic BP the frequency of white coat hypertension is high, if a several clinic BP measurements -as recommended- are obtained at different occasions before diagnosis, the frequency is lower).

iii: The definition of a normal ambulatory BP (if the cut off limit for a normal ambulatory BP is defined as a day time BP < 131/86 mmHg the frequency of white coat hypertension is lower than for a cut off limit of BP < 140/90 mmHg).

iiii: The presence of other selection criteria related to clinic BP level or possible end organ signs. (The frequency of white coat hypertension is higher in a population with mild hypertension than in a population with moderate or severe hypertension even if the white coat effect is higher in the latter group [24]). If a hypertensive population are selected on the basis of criteria which may be related to elevated BP (i.e. albuminuria, retinopathy or left ventricular hypertrophy) the proportion of patients who fulfil the criteria for white coat hypertension is assumed to be low.

NIDDM AND AMBULATORY BP

The influence of changes in metabolic control
Shift from sulfonulurea to insulin in poorly controlled elderly NIDDM patient improved glycemic control but ambulatory BP after one year was unaffected perhaps due to weight gain [25]. Neither metformin nor glibenclamide affected ambulatory BP in a study of 1 month duration [26] Metformin for 12 weeks improved glycemic control while ambulatory BP was unaffected [27]. Glitazone therapy has reduced both HbA1c and ambulatory BP [28].

Comparison with healthy individuals
Some discrepancies exist. One study has reported an increase in 24-h systolic (but not diastolic) BP in normoalbuminuric diabetic patients [29]. Two studies did not found any difference in 24-h average BP, however the nocturnal reduction of systolic BP was impaired in normoalbuminuric patients [30,31].

If patients (UAE not specified) and healthy subjects were divided into groups with and without hypertension no statistical difference of 24-h BP have been reported [7,32].

The relation to abnormal albuminuria.

No difference in day-time or 24-h BP were noticed between normo- and microalbuminuric patients [29,31,33-36]. In contrast ambulatory BP was reported significantly higher in microalbuminuric patients (90 % males, 50 % non-Caucasians) than in normoalbuminuric patients (71 % males, 28 % non-Caucasians) [37]. In NIDDM both ambulatory and clinic BP correlates with UAE roughly to a similar extent [29,37] although one study using albumin/creatinin ratio reported no correlation [38]. Ambulatory BP is higher in patients with diabetic nephropathy than in normoalbuminuric patients [30,39].

Abnormal diurnal BP pattern (high night BP) are seen in patients with microalbuminuria [31,35,36,39-42] and overt diabetic nephropathy [30,39,41]. As in IDDM this abnormality seems closely linked to the presence of autonomic neuropathy [30,31,43,45].

The time course of ambulatory BP

In patients receiving standard clinical care including antihypertensive medication, 24-h BP was remarkable stable in both normo- and microalbuminuric patients during an observation period of 4.6 years. Individual changes in both systolic and diastolic 24-h BP were related to changes in UAE [45]. The evolution of UAE did not differ between patients with and without abnormal diurnal BP profile at baseline [45].

Non-dipper: Autonomic neuropathy, nephropathy and extra-cellular volume [ECV].

Numerous studies in mixed IDDM and NIDDM populations or unclassified diabetic patients have demonstrated a reduction or (in few patients) even a reversal of the normal nocturnal decline of BP [11-13,46-50] in patients with autonomic neuropathy. Also in homogenous NIDDM diabetic patients several studies demonstrate [30,34,43,51,52] the association between diabetic nephropathy, signs of autonomic neuropathy or both and a blunted diurnal variation of blood pressure. According to two studies increased nocturnal sympathetic activity (rather than expansion of ECV) seems to be involved in reduced nocturnal BP in NIDDM patients with nephropathy [30,51]. However, a physiological defence against nocturnal volume expansion may explain why a lower night level of aldosterone and a higher level of plasma atrial natriuretic peptide have been reported in "non-dippers", who also had more pronounced signs of autonomic neuropathy than "dippers" [51].

Postprandial hypotension is also a phenomenon observed in patients with autonomic neuropathy [53,54].

436

The relation to insulin resistance and sodium-lithium counter transport

Ambulatory systolic BP (and clinic systolic BP) correlated in one study with glucose disposal rate, but not with fasting insulin level [55]. However, this relation was not confirmed in another study (S Nielsen personal communication) [33]. No relation has been found between ambulatory BP and sodium-lithium counter transport [37].Insulin resistance has in one study been related to reduced nocturnal BP fall [56].

The relation to diabetic retinopathy and to ambulatory pulse pressure

A relation between "non-dipping" status and retinopathy has been suggested [45]. Ambulatory pulse pressure is related to macro- and microvascular complications including retinopathy [57]. Ambulatory BP is similar in patients with and without of macular oedema [58].

IDDM AND AMBULATORY BP

The influence of diabetes duration

Two cross sectional study reports a reduction of the nocturnal BP fall in long term normoalbuminuric diabetic patients [59,60].

The influence of gender

The well-known BP difference between healthy males and females seems attenuated in IDDM [60-62].

The influence of short term changes in metabolic control

This question has so far never been addressed by well designed intervention studies employing ambulatory BP. Clinic BP has been reported lower after short term improvement of diabetic control by insulin pumps (24-h insulin dose unchanged) [63]. Intra-arterial BP (10-h day time average) was also reduced after improved glycemic control achieved by increasing insulin dose in most patients [64]. No significant change in clinic BP was observed in a study where poor metabolic control was obtained by reducing insulin dose [65].

Recently it has been suggested that intensive insulin therapy by hyperinsulinemia (1.0 U/kg) is associated with high night blood pressure [66]. However, it has convincingly been demonstrated that tight blood glucose control obtained by normal insulin doses (0.6 U/kg) by no means affects the normal nocturnal blood pressure reduction [67].

The influence of smoking and type of day (work day/day-off)

We have compared ambulatory BP in 16 normoalbuminuric smokers and non-smokers without hypertension. Systolic BP was slightly higher (3mmHg day time, 5 mmHg night time) in smokers, but this failed to reach statistical significance [68]. In a larger study encompassing 24 normoalbuminuric smokers and non-smokers diastolic day and night BP was significantly higher (3.9 and 3.5 mmHg respectively) in smokers. In addition a dose response relationship was demonstrated [69]. Notably, this effect of smoking in diabetic individuals contrast the well known finding of a lower night BP in non-diabetic smokers [68,70]. Smoking does not affect the night/day ratio of BP in diabetes [68,69,71].

Day-time BP is significantly lower (5 mmHg) on a day off than on a work day [60].

Comparison with healthy individuals

Most studies [72-77], but not all [61,78,79] agree that day-time BP is comparable between normoalbuminuric diabetic patients and healthy subjects. Since ambulatory BP is higher in normoalbuminuric females than in healthy females [60,61], the result of a comparison between a diabetic and a control population depends on the sex distribution. Also the majority of investigators found no difference in the diurnal BP profile [72,73,76-79,80,81] In contrast two studies have reported a slightly reduced nocturnal BP fall [61,74,82] and one study has surprisingly described a much higher night/day ratio of BP in normoalbuminuric patients [75].

Recently ambulatory BP was compared in normoalbuminuric IDDM patients and healthy controls (n=55 in each group) [61]. In contrast to previous comparison [72] (n=34 in each group) a slightly but significantly higher ambulatory BP was observed in diabetic patients. This may be explained by a higher proportion of women (42% vs. 29% in the previous study) and partly by increased statistical power due to the larger number of patients. Ambulatory BP (24h and day) was higher in diabetic women than in control women but no difference (for 24h and day time) was observed between diabetic men and control men. The night dip in BP was similar in diabetic and control women but a reduced night dip was reported for diabetic men compared with control men. Diastolic night dip in BP correlated in the total diabetic population with indices of autonomic neuropathy [61].

With this exception, the diversities are minor and may be explained by varying diabetes duration or proportion of males/females. Thus, as a rule normoalbuminuric patients have a 24-h BP profile very similar to healthy control subjects (Fig 1).

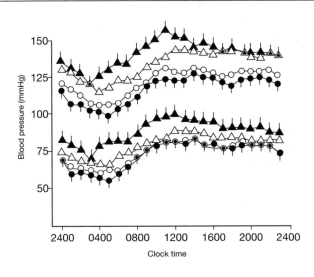

Figure 1. Twenty-four hour profile of mean systolic and diastolic BP for type 1 diabetic patients and healthy controls. Diabetic patients with nephropathy and without antihypertensive treatment (n=13, filled triangles), microalbuminuric patients (n=26, open triangles), normoalbuminuric patients (n=26, open circles) and healthy individuals (n=26, filled circles). From [90] with permission.

The relation to abnormal albuminuria
This subject has been reviewed [83]. Ambulatory BP is significantly higher and the diurnal BP pattern is abnormal in consecutively studied patients compared with healthy controls [84]. This largely depends on abnormal albuminuria present in some of the patients [84]. Ambulatory BP is significantly increased in microalbuminuric as compared with normoalbuminuric patients [72,85-87]. In some studies day-time BP were only numerically but not statistically significantly higher in microalbuminuric patients [81,82,88,89]. This is probably due to lower number of microalbuminuric patients in these studies. The night/day ratio of diastolic BP is significantly higher in microalbuminuric patients than in healthy individuals [90] and night/day ratio for normoalbuminuric patients is in between [19,90]. If the comparison between

micro- and normoalbuminuric patients is restricted to patients in good metabolic control and without any signs of autonomic neuropathy day time BP is still elevated in microalbuminuric patients [77]. Ambulatory BP correlates more closely with UAE than clinic BP [72,73,77,78,88](Table 1). This is probably due to the multiplicity of measurements rather than their quality as true ambulatory values.

Table 1 Correlations between blood pressure and urinary albumin excretion in combined normo- and microalbuminuric type 1 diabetic patients.

	A Hansen et al [72]	B Moore et al [78]	C Benhamou et al [73]	D Lurbe et al [88]
UAE	Three overnight collections	One 24h collection	Three overnight collections	Three 24h collections
Correlations:	Normo (n=34) Micro (n=34)	Normo (n=27) Micro (n=11)	Normo (n=23) Micro (n=12)	Normo (n=34) Micro (n=11)
UAE vs. clinic BP (auscultatory)	r=0.21, NS (systolic)	-	r=-0.01, NS (systolic)	r=0.19, NS (MAP)
UAE vs day time BP	r=0.45, p<0.05 (systolic)	-	r=0.17, NS (systolic)	r=0.035, p<0.05 (MAP)
UAE vs. night time BP	r=0.53, p<0.00001 (systolic)	-	r=0.38, p<0.05 (systolic)	r=0.60, p<0.01 (MAP)
UAE vs. 24h BP	r=0.49, p<0.0001 (systolic)	r=0.40, p<0.01 (systolic) r=0.60, p<0.01 (diastolic)	r=0.29, NS (systolic)	-

Ambulatory BP is further increased in patients with overt diabetic nephropathy [90] (Fig 1) and the circadian variation of BP is severely disturbed in patients with advanced diabetic nephropathy [82,90,91] (Fig 2).

The transition from normo- to microalbuminuria

In a recent study 40 initially normoalbuminuric patients were reinvestigated with ambulatory BP monitoring and measurement of UAE after a mean period of 3 years [92]. Six patients progressed to microalbuminuria and their baseline UAE (9.7 µg min^{-1}) was statistically significantly higher than baseline UAE in non-progressors (5.5 µg min^{-1}). Importantly, no difference was noticed between 24-h ambulatory BP at baseline in progressors (124/74 mmHg) and non-progressors (124/75 mmHg). However, the rise in UAE even to low microalbuminuria (31.7 µg min^{-1}) were accompanied with an increase in 24-h ambulatory BP (12/5 mmHg) which was statistically higher than the increase in non-progressors (4/2 mmHg). No statistically significant changes were seen if these changes were evaluated from the average of three clinic BP measurements at baseline and at follow up [92]. The diastolic night/day ratio at baseline was significantly higher in progressors (0.88) than in non-progressors (0.81), but no further increase was found in progressors during follow-up and the overlap between the two groups was large.

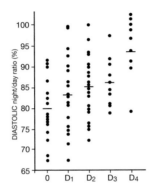

Figure 2. Individual night/day ratio for diastolic BP in healthy individuals and type 1 diabetic patients. C= control subjects (n=26), D_1= normoalbuminuric patients (n=26), D_2= microalbuminuric patients (n=26), D_3= patients with diabetic nephropathy without antihypertensive treatment (n=13), D_4= patients with diabetic nephropathy with antihypertensive treatment. From [90] with permission.

In a recent study Lurbe et al. argue that increased night BP in normoalbuminuric patients precedes progression to microalbuminuria [93]. The study has been debated [94]: Urinary albumin excretion measured at every 3 months visits was surprisingly stable during the period of 27 months from the first (11.6 ± 8.5 mg/24h) to the final (16.8 ± 10.3 mg/24h) evaluation in patients who developed microalbuminuria (> 30 mg/24h) at the following two visits. The night/day ratio of systolic BP was similar at the *first* evaluation in the group who developed microalbuminuria (0.89) and in the group who persisted normoalbuminuric (0.89). The frequency of microalbuminuria (21.9 %) in patients with an abnormal BP at the *first* evaluation did not differ significantly from the frequency of microalbuminuria (16.3 %) in patients with normal diurnal BP variation. This finding implies that ambulatory BP measured approximately two years before progression to microalbuminuria cannot foresee this event. The *final* ambulatory BP performed just (approx 6 months) before the patients fulfilled the criteria for microalbuminuria showed high night BP. This information is of limited in clinical practice. At this late stage of progression to microalbuminuria the demonstration of elevated night BP is compatible with a parallel progression of the kidney disease and increase in night BP.

In a cross sectional study of normoalbuminuric patients the 24-h BP were significantly higher in patients with "high" normal UAE than in patients with "low" normal UAE [95,96]. Similar results have been reported in a study comparing "high" normoalbuminuric patients with healthy individuals [97].

These results support the idea that rise in UAE and ambulatory BP cannot be separated even in the very early phase of diabetic nephropathy.

Non-dipper: Autonomic neuropathy, nephropathy and extracellular volume (ECV)

In IDDM the presence of autonomic neuropathy is clearly associated with impaired reduction of night BP [10,98,99]. Autonomic neuropathy and diabetic nephropathy are closely associated [100-103]. Their relative role for the abnormal diurnal variation in blood pressure is therefore difficult to ascertain. However, the literature gives no examples of a group of IDDM patients with blunted diurnal variation of BP without concomitant signs of autonomic neuropathy either by formal test [98,99] or by increased heart rate [72]. Indeed autonomic dysfunction can be documented even in "high" normoalbuminuric patients if refined test (spectral analysis of heart rate variability) is employed [96]. In contrast an impaired reduction of night BP and increased heart rate is seen in long term diabetic patients who are stricly normoalbuminuric [59,60].

Naturally the question of a possible causative role of autonomic neuropathy for the development of diabetic nephropathy has arisen [104,105]. The link could be a higher night BP, which is more readily transmitted to the glomeruli because of renal vasodilation. Alternatively early autonomic dysfunction may just be part of a syndrome indicative of later diabetic complications in patients with suboptimal glycemic control [96,106]. A retrospective study in patients with diabetic nephropathy has described a faster decline of renal function in patients with a "non-dipping" BP profile compared with "dippers" [107]. However there was no baseline or follow-up measurement of ambulatory BP,

442

which was measured at one time point only during a 6-year observation period. Since renal function was already reduced in "non-dippers" at the time when the ambulatory BP measurement was performed it is not possible to postulate a cause/effect relationship.

Expanded ECV has been described even in normoalbuminuric "non-dippers"[108]. Two lines of evidence suggest that homeostasis of ECV is associated with elevated night BP in particular in patients abnormal albuminuria. First plasma aldosteron is reported significantly lower in "non-dipping" patients with incipient diabetic nephropathy, which could be interpreted as a defence again fluid retention [109]. Second, in patients with overt diabetic nephropathy, elevated nocturnal BP is associated with expansion of ECV. This may reflect the result of a nocturnal shift of fluid from the interstitial to the intravascular space [110]. This view has been challenged by a study, which did not find any association between elevated night BP and ECV in IDDM patients with nephropathy [111].

Increased QTc dispersion is associated with high night BP in normoalbuminuric patients. The pathophysiological link is unclarified but may involve both autonomic dysfunction and left ventricular hypertrophy [112].

The relation to glomerular filtration rate (GFR) and renal strucure.
A negative correlation between ambulatory BP and GFR has been described in microalbuminuric patients [78,113]. Non dippers with microalbuminuria or overt nephropathy seems not to have a reduced GFR [109-111]. One study in normoalbuminuric patients reported a higher night BP and expanded ECV (23 litre) in patients with glomerular hyperfiltration compared with the group with normofiltration (19 litre) [108]. Despite similar methods (Cr EDTA single shot) ECV is found inexplicable high in this latter study [108] compared with the two previously mentioned studies dealing with nephropathy (14 litre) [108,111]. In adolescents who have had performed a kidney biopsy the nocturnal BP (and heart rate) correlated with basal membrane thickness. This is further indirect support for the hypothesis that early autonomic dysfunction and related high (night) BP could be causative related to ultrastructural renal damage [114].

The relation to diabetic retinopathy
Elevated night BP is reported in patients with more advanced signs of diabetic retinopathy. Importantly this association was described in strictly normoalbuminuric patients excluding the confounding effect of diabetic kidney disease [115].

Predisposition to hypertension and diabetic nephropathy

The controversy of predisposition to hypertension and development of diabetic nephropathy has recently been addressed by performing ambulatory BP in parents of IDDM patients with and without diabetic nephropathy [116]. The 24h BP was almost identical among the two groups of parents without antihypertensive medication (126/76 vs. 126/74 mmHg respectively, NS). The frequency of hypertension defined as use of antihypertensive medication or a 24h BP > 135/85 mmHg was significantly higher in parents of patients with nephropathy (57%) than in parents of patients without nephropathy (41%).

Relation to pregnancy

Ambulatory BP monitoring has been applied to both non-diabetic [117] (several publications) and diabetic pregnant women with purpose of early identification of patients at risk for developing preeclampsia [118]. So far only microalbuminuria can predict this event in diabetes [119].

AMBULATORY BLOOD PRESSURE AND INTERVENTION STUDIES

Due to the high reproducibility of ambulatory BP compared with clinic measurements it is an ideal tool for intervention studies [16,120]. The 24-h effectiveness of the intervention can be evaluated, the number of patients needed can be reduced without loosing power and small changes in BP, which would be overlooked by traditional measurements, can be recognised. Ambulatory BP is now a standard methodology for monitoring BP changes in intervention studies.So far there have been no confirmed reports of an altered circadian BP profile after antihypertensive treatment in diabetic patients.

AMBULATORY BLOOD PRESSURE AND CARDIAC MASS

An early study did not find any significant differences in either 24-h BP or cardiac mass NIDDM patients and healthy subjects [6]. Later, increased cardiac mass has been reported in diabetic patients (mixed IDDM and NIDDM) with autonomic neuropathy and associated reduced nocturnal decline of BP as compared with patients without autonomic neuropathy [121]. This may be an effect of autonomic dysfunction per se or the higher nocturnal BP. Similar results has been found in NIDDM patients with nephropathy, who have elevated 24h BP and higher night BP than patients with normoalbuminuria [122].

Left ventricular mass (LVM) and day-time diastolic BP were found higher in microalbuminuric than in normoalbuminuric IDDM patients [77]. We have found no significant differences in cardiac mass between microalbuminuric IDDM patients with and without a normal reduction of night BP [109]. In an other study LVM did not differ between white coat hypertensive and normotensive NIDDM patients and LVM was lower in dippers compared to non-dippers (no information about UAE) [123].

THE RELATION TO CLINIC BP

We have found a markedly lower day time BP (147/ 85 mmHg) than clinic BP (163/95 mmHg) in 102 consecutive NIDDM and IDDM patients referred to ambulatory BP measurement because of repeated clinic BP > 140/90 mmHg [124]. The frequency of white coat hypertension in normoalbuminuric diabetic patients is about 25 % [124,125]. If patients are selected for the presence of organ lesions related to hypertension (diabetic nephropathy) the proportion of white coat hypertension may be reduced [125]. One study reported a much higher frequency of white coat hypertension (41 %) probably due to a shorter observation period before labelling patients as hypertensive and because patients was designated as "true" normotensive on the basis of 24h BP (containing the lower night BP) rather than day time values [126]. Obviously the reported frequency of white coat hypertension also varies with the definition of a normal ambulatory BP [22,23]. An extremely high frequency of white coat hypertension (62 %) was reported in a study measuring clinic BP at one occasion only and using the same cut-off level for establishing the diagnosis of hypertension (clinic mean arterial BP > 100 mmHg) as for identifying those with apparent normal ambulatory BP (day time mean arterial BP < 100 mmHg) [127]. Also in adolescents a very high frequency of white coat hypertension has been disclosed [128]. A low frequency (11 %) was reported in NIDDM patients who was categorized as normotensive if day time BP was < 131/86 (women) and < 136/87 (men) [123]. For patients older than 60 years with isolated systolic hypertension the average systolic day time BP is reported much lower (about 20 mmHg) than clinic BP during the placebo run-in phase of the Syst-Eur trial also containing diabetic patients [129]. During a follow-up of 3.2 years the rate of cardiovascular events was comparable in normotensive and in white coat hypertensive diabetic subjects. Although the absolute number of events in the three groups were low the data suggest a benign clinical course of white coat hypertensive patients at least in the short term. The study showed a higher event rate in female "non-dippers" versus "dippers" [123]

Several international and national institutions now approve ambulatory BP monitoring in certain clinical circumstances [130-132]. The important problems about establishing a normal reference for ambulatory BP have been reviewed thoroughly [133]. Although large individual differences do exist, a clinic BP of 140/90 roughly corresponds to a day time average of 135/85 mmHg [133]. The present general recommendations (for non-diabetic patients) implies that a day time BP < 135/85, and a night BP < 125/75 mmHg is considered normal. Even lower cut off limits (< 125/80 mmHg) for a normal day-time BP has been suggested [131], however the background for this proposal can be questioned indeed [134]. A pertinent question is the optimal goal for ambulatory BP in diabetes. Clearly this depends on coexisting risk factors like microalbuminuria or previous cardiovascular events. While day-time BP usually is lower than clinic BP for (clinic) hypertensive patients, this is not true for patients with a normal clinic BP. The day-time ambulatory BP (125.5/ 77.2) was identical to the clinic BP (125.3/ 76.5) in 137 normoalbuminuric and normotensive (clinic BP< 149/90 mmHg) type 1 diabetic patients (Table 2) [135]. If the goal for clinic BP in a normoalbuminuric diabetic patients without end organ damage is < 130/85 or < 130/80 mmHg, a similar value can be proposed as a goal for the day time ambulatory BP. The recommendations of the British Hypertension Society [132] that a clinic BP goal < 140/80 mmHg corresponds to day time BP goal < 130/75 mmHg is not scientifically based and leads to unjustified statements concerning the usefulness of ambulatory monitoring [136,137].

Table 2: BP for 137 normotensive and normoalbuminuric type 1 diabetic patients [135]

	Mean BP ± SD (systolic/diastolic)	90, 95 percentile (systolic/diastolic)
Clinic BP (auscultatory, Hawskley, mmHg)	117.4 ± 10.0/ 77.8 ± 7.2	132/87, 135/89
Clinic BP (oscillometric, Spacelabs, mmHg)	125.3 ± 9.6/ 76.5 ± 7.0	139/85, 144/86
Day-time AMBP (oscillometric, Spacelabs, mmHg)	125.7 ± 8.1/ 77.2 ± 5.7	137/85, 140/87
Night-time AMBP (oscillometric, Spacelabs mmHg)	110.8 ± 8.2/ 63.1 ± 6.2	122/71, 125/74
Night/day ratio	0.88 ±0.05/ 0.82 ±0.07	0.95/0.90, 0.97/0.94
24-hour AMBP (oscillometric, Spacelabs mmHg)	120.8 ± 7.5/ 72.6 ± 5.4	131/80, 134/82

The guidelines will doubtless need corrections based on future studies, which ideally should relate ambulatory BP to end organ damage and to clinical events in antihypertensive drug trials. The clinical value of large-scale implementation of ambulatory BP monitoring has never been investigated. However, it seems wise to hesitate with respect to antihypertensive drug treatment of normoalbuminuric diabetic patients (without any other signs of organ damage) with white coat hypertension. The value of targeting antihypertensive drug regimen towards high night BP is unexplored.

DIPPERS AND NON-DIPPERS

Non-dipping status has been associated with progression of diabetic nephropathy [107] and increased mortality rate [138,139]. In these studies important risk factors may be present in the non-dipper group at baseline, leaving the question open whether non-dipping per se is a sign of poor prognosis or merely reflects clustering of risk factors (reduced GFR, old age, high clinic BP, autonomic neuropathy etc.) Importantly the superiority of ambulatory BP (mainly night BP) versus clinic BP as a predictor of cardiovascular risk has recently been documented in the placebo arm of the Syst-Eur study [129].

CONCLUSION

Ambulatory BP is increased in NIDDM and IDDM patients with abnormal albuminuria even in the absence of a detectable difference in clinic BP. An association exist in both NIDDM and IDDM patients between impaired reduction of night BP and the two complications, autonomic neuropathy and diabetic nephropathy. This also counts for the very early phases of diabetic nephropathy in IDDM patients. It remains to be eluciated if the abnormal BP variation independently contributes to development of microalbumimuria or to the progression of diabetic nephropathy, or whether this abnormality is merely a co-phenomenon found in patients with poor glycemic control and diabetic complications including autonomic neuropathy [104,105]

The high reproducibility of ambulatory BP permits registration of small changes in BP, which are overlooked by conventional measurement. Large-scale longitudinal studies of ambulatory BP and UAE are necessary to characterize the important transition phase from normo- to microalbuminuria. Simultaneous continuous indirect registration of both the sympathovagal balance [140] and BP [141] are perspectives for the future, which probably will add to the understanding of BP variation in diabetes.

Ambulatory BP monitoring is now a well-established and valuable procedure [142,143] also in the diabetes clinic. It seems wise to hesitate with respect to antihypertensive drug treatment in patients with white coat hypertension, if there are no signs of organ damage including microalbuminuria. The number of these patients who ultimately will become hypertensive by ambulatory BP is unknown and careful observation of BP is essential. There is still a need for more secure guidelines for the use of ambulatory BP including the consequences of specifically addressing antihypertensive treatment towards nocturnal hypertension [144].

REFERENCES

1   Sokolow M, Werdegar D, Kain HK, Hinman AT. Relationship between level of blood pressure measured casually and by portable recorders and severity of complications in essential hypertension. Circulation 1966; 34: 279-298

2   Bevan AT, Honour AJ, Stott FH. Direct arterial pressure recording in unrestricted man. Clin Sci 1969; 36: 329-344

3   Schneider RA, Costiloe JP. Twenty-four hour automatic monitoring of blood pressure and heart rate at work and at home. Am Heart J 1975; 90: 695-702

4   Rubler S, Abenavoli T, Greenblatt HA, Dixon JF, Cieslik CJ. Ambulatory blood pressure monitoring in diabetic males: A method for detecting blood pressure elevations undisclosed by conventional methods. Clin Cardiol 1982; 5: 447-454

5   Osei K. Ambulatory and exercise-induced blood pressure responses in type I diabetic patients and normal subjects. Diabetes Research and Clinical Practice 1987; 3: 125-134

6   Porcellati C, Gatteschi C, Benemio G, Guerrieri M, Boldrini F, Verdecchia P. Analisi ecocardiografica del ventriculo sinistro in pazienti con diabete mellito di tipo II. G Ital Cardiol 1989; 19: 128-135

7   Verdecchia P, Gatteschi C, Benemio G, Porcellati C. Ambulatory blood pressure monitoring in normotensive and hypertensive patients with diabetes (abstract). J Hypertension 1988; 6 (suppl 4): S692-S693

8   Rubler S, Chu DA, Bruzzone CL. Blood pressure and heart rate responses during 24-h ambulatory monitoring and exercise in men with diabetes mellitus. Am J Cardiol 1985; 55: 801-806

9   Guilleminault C, Mondini S, Hayes B. Diabetic autonomic dysfunction, blood pressure and sleep. Ann Neurol 1985; 18: 670-675

10   Reeves RA, Shapiro AP, Thompson ME, Johnsen A-M. Loss of nocturnal decline in blood pressure after cardiac transplantation. Circulation 1986; 73: 401-408

11   Liniger C, Favre L, Adamec R, Pernet A, Assal J-Ph. Profil nyctémeral de la pression artérielle et de la fréquence cardiaque dans la neuropathie diabétique autonome. Schweiz med Wschr 1987; 117: 1949-1953

12   Hornung RS, Mahler RF, Raftery EB. Ambulatory blood pressure and heart rate in diabetic patients: an assessment of autonomic function. Diabetic Med 1989; 6: 579-585

13   Chanudet X, Bauduceau B, Ritz P, Jolibois P, Garcin JM, Larroque P, Gautier D. Neuropathie végétative et régulation tensionelle chez le diabétique. Arch Mal Coer 1989; 82: 1147-1151

14 Staessen JA, Fagard R, Thijs L, Amery A. A consensus view of the technique of ambulatory blood pressure monitoring. Hypertens 1995; [part 1]: 912-918

15 Hansen KW, Christiansen JS. Research methodologies for recording blood pressure in diabetic patients. In: Mogensen CE, Standl E (eds). Diabetes Forum Series volume V (part 2). Research methodologies in human diabetes. Berlin, New York: Walter de Gruyter; 1994; pp. 113-124

16 Coats AJS, Radaelli A, Clark SJ, Conway J, Sleight P. The influence of ambulatory blood pressure monitoring on the design and interpretation of trials in hypertension. J Hypertens 1992; 10: 385-391

17 Coats AJS, Clark SJ, Conway J. Analysis of ambulatory blood pressure data. J Hypertens 1991; 9 (suppl 8): S19-S21

18 Germano G, Damiani S, Caparra A, Cassone-Faldetta M, Germano U, Coia F, De Mattia G, Santucci A, Balsano F. Ambulatory blood pressure recording in diabetic patients with abnormal responses to cardiovascular autonomic tests. Acta Diabetol 1992; 28: 221-228

19 Hansen KW, Poulsen PL, Mogensen CE. Ambulatory blood pressure and abnormal albuminuria in type 1 diabetic patients. Kidney Int 1994; 45 (suppl.45): S134-S140 (Correction. Kidney Int 45: 1799-1800, 1994)

20 Verdecchia P, Schillaci G, Guerrieri M, Gatteschi C, Benemio G, Boldrini F, Porcellati C. Circadian blood pressure changes and left ventricular hypertrophy in essential hypertension. Circulation 1990; 81: 528-536

21 Fagard R, Brguljan J, Lutgarde T, Staessen J. Prediction of the actual awake and asleep blood pressure by various methods of 24 h pressure analysis. J Hypertens 1996; 14: 557-563

22 Pickering TG. White coat hypertension. Curr Opin Nephrol Hypertens 1996; 5: 192-198

23 Mancia G, Zanchetti A. White-coat hypertension: misnomers, misconceptions and misunderstandings. What should we do next ?. J Hypertens 1996; 14: 1049-1052

24 Verdecchia P, Schillaci G, Borgioni C, Ciucci A, Zampi I, Gattobigio R, Sacchi N, Porcellati C. White coat hypertension and white coat effect. Similarities and differences. Am J Hypertens 1995; 8: 790-798

25 Tovi J, Theobald H, Engfeldt P. Effect of metabolic control on 24-h ambulatory blood pressure in elderly non-insulin-dependent diabetic patients. J Hum Hypertens 1996; 10: 589-594

26 Sundaresan P, Lykos D, Daher A, Diamond T, Morris R, Howes LG. Comparative effects of glibenclamide and metformin on ambulatory blood pressure and cardiovascular reactivity in NIDDM. Diabetes Care 1997; 692-697

27 Uehara, MH, Kohlmann NEB, Zanella MT, Ferreira SRG. Metabolic and haemodynamic effects of metformin in patients with tye 2 diabetes and hypertension. Diabetes, Obesity and Metabolism 2001; 3: 319-325

28 Sutton SJ, Rendell M, Dandona P, Dole JF, Murphy K, Patwardhan R, Patel J, Freed M. A comparison of the effects of rosiglitazone and glyburide on cardiovascular function with type 2 diabetes. Diabetes Care 2002; 25: 2058-2064

29 Schmitz A, Mau Pedersen M, Hansen KW. Blood pressure by 24 h ambulatory recordings in type 2 (non-insulin-dependent) diabetics. Relationship to urinary albumin excretion. Diabete Metab (Paris) 1991; 17: 301-307

30 Nielsen FS, Rossing P, Bang Lia E, Svendsen TL, Gall M-A, Smidt UM, Parving H-H. On the mechanism of blunted nocturnal decline in arterial blood pressure in NIDDM patients with diabetic nephropathy. Diabetes 1995; 44: 783-789

31   Mitchell TH, Nolan B, Henry M, Cronin C, Baker H, Greely G. Microalbuminuria in patients with non-insulin-dependent diabetes mellitus relates to nocturnal systolic blood pressure. Am J Med 1997; 102: 531-535.

32   Fogari R, Zoppi A, Malamani GD, Lazzari P, Destro M, Corradi L. Ambulatory blood pressure monitoring in normotensive and hypertensive type 2 diabetics. Prevalence of impaired diurnal blood pressure patterns. Am J Hypertens 1993; 6: 1-7

33   Nielsen S, Schmitz O, Ørskov H, Mogensen CE. Similar insulin sensivity in NIDDM patients with normo- and microalbuminuria. Diabetes Care 1995; 18: 834-842

34   Jermendy G, Ferenzi J, Hernandez E, Farkas K, Nadas J. Day-night blood pressure variations in normotensive and hypertensive NIDDM patients with asymptomatic autonomic neuropathy. Diabetes Res Clin Pract 1996; 34: 107-114

35   Berrut G, Fabbri P, Bouhanick B, Lalanne P, Guilloteau G, Marre M, Fressinaud P. Loss of nocturnal blood pressure decrease in non-insulin dependent diabetis subjects with microalbuminuria. Arch Mal Coeur 1996; 89: 1041-1044

36   Lindsay RS, Stewart MJ, Nairn IM, Baird JD, Padfield PL. Reduced diurnal variation of blood pressure in non-insulin-dependent diabetic patients with microalbumnuria. J Hum Hypertens 1995; 9: 223-227

37   Pinkney JH, Foyle W-J, Denver AE, Mohamed-Ali V, McKinlay S, Yudkin JS. The relationship of urinary albumin excretion rate to ambulatory blood pressure and erythrocyte sodium-lithium countertransport in NIDDM. Diabetologia 1995; 38: 356-362

38   Waeber B, Weidmann P, Wohler D, Le Bloch Y. Albuminuria in diabetes mellitus. Relation to ambulatory versus office blood pressure and effects of cilazapril. Am J Hypertens 1996; 9: 1220-1227

39   Iwase M, Kaseda S, Iino K, Fukuhura M, Yamamoto M, Fukudome Y, Yoshizumi H, Abe I, Yoshinari M, Fujishima M. Circadian blood pressure variation in non-insulin-dependent diabetes mellitus with diabetic nephropathy. Diabetes Research and Clinical Practice 1994; 26: 43-50

40   Fogari R, Zoppi A, Malamani GD, Lazzari P, Albonico B, Corradi L. Urinary albumin excretion and nocturnal blood pressure in hypertensive patients with type II diabetes. Am J Hyp 1994; 7: 808-813

41   Equiluz-Bruck S, Schnack C, Schernthaner G. Nondipping of nocturnal blood pressure is related to urinary albumin excretion in patients with type 2 diabetes mellitus. Am J Hypertens 1996; 9: 1139-1143

42   Inaba M, Negishi K, Takashi M, Serizawa N, Maruno Y, Takahashi K, Katayama S. Increased night:day blood pressure ratio in microalbuminuric normotensive NIDDM subjects. Diabetes Res Clin Pract 1998; 40: 161-161

43   Nakano S, Uchida K, Kigoshi T, Azukizawa S, Iwasaki R, Kaneko M, Morimoto S. Circadian rhytm of blood pressure in normotensive NIDDM subjects. Its relation to microvascular complications. Diabetes Care 1991; 14: 707-711

44   Nielsen FS Hansen HP, Jacobsen P, Rossing P, Smidt UM, Christensen NJ, Pevett P, Vivien-Roels B, Parving H-H. Increased sympathetic activity during sleep and nocturnal hypertension in type 2 diabetic patients with diabetic nephropathy. Diabetic Med 1999; 16: 555-562

45   Nielsen S, Schmitz A, Poulsen PL, Hansen KW, Mogensen CE. Albuminuria and 24-h ambulatory blood pressure in normoalbuminuric and microalbuminuric NIDDM patients. Diabetes Care 1995; 18: 1434-1441

46   Chamontin B, Barbe P, Begasse F, Ghisolfi A, Amar J, Louvet JP, Salvador M. Presion artérielle ambulatoire au cours de l'hypertension arterielle avec dysautonomie. Arch Mal Coer 1990; 83: 1103-1106

47 Felici MG, Spallone V, Maillo MR, Gatta R, Civetta E, Frontoni S, Gambardella S, Menzinger G. Twenty-four hours blood pressure and heart rate profiles in diabetics with and without autonomic neuropathy. Funct Neurol 1991; 6: 299-304

48 Liniger C, Favre L, Assal J-Ph. Twenty-four hour blood pressure and heart rate profiles of diabetic patients with abnormal cardiovascular reflexes. Diabetic Med 1991; 8: 420-427

49 Spallone V, Bernardi L, Ricordi L, Soldà P, Maillo MR, Calciati A, Gambardella S, Fratino P, Menzinger G. Relationship between the circadian rhytms of blood pressure and sympathovagal balance in diabetic autonomic neuropathy. Diabetes 1993; 42: 1745-1752

50 Ikeda T, Matsubara T, Sato Y, Sakamoto N. Circadian variation in diabetic patients with autonomic neuropathy. J Hypertens 1993: 11: 581-587

51 Nakano S, Uchida K, Ishii T, Takeuchi M, Azukizawa S, Kigoshi T, Morimoto S. Association of a nocturnal rise in plasma "-atrial natriuretic peptide and reversed diurnal rhytm in hospitalized normotensive subjects with non-insulin dependent diabetes mellitus. Eur J Endocrinol 1994; 131: 184-190

52 Kondo K, Matsubara T, Nakamura J, Hotta N. Characteristic pattern of circadian variation in plasma catecholamine levels, blood pressure and heart rate variability in type 2 diabetic patients. Diabet Med 2002; 19: 359-365

53 Sasaki E, Kitaoka H, Ohsawa N. Postprandial hypotension in patients with non-insulin-dependent diabetes mellitus. Diabetes Research and Clinical Practice 1992; 18: 113-121

54 Nakajima S, Otsuka K, Yamanaka T, Omori K, Kubo Y, Toyoshima T, Watanabe Y, Watanabe H. Ambulatory blood pressure and postprandial hypotension. Am Heart J 1992; 124: 1669-1671

55 Pinkney JH, Mohamed-Ali V, Denver AE, Foster C, Sampson MJ, Yudkin JS. Insulin resistance, insulin, proinsulin, and ambulatory blood pressure in type II diabetes. Hypertension 1994; 24: 362-367

56 Nakano S, Kitazawa M, Tsuda S, Himeno M, Makiishi H, Nakagawa A, Kigoshi T, Uchida K. Insulin resistance is associated with reduced nocturnal falls of blood pressure in normotensive, nonobese type 2 diabetic subjects. Clin Exp Hypertens 2002; 24: 65-73

57 Knudsen ST, Poulsen PL, Hansen KW, Ebbehøj E, Bek T, Mogensen CE. Pulse pressure and diurnal blood pressure variation: association with micro-and macrovascular complications in type 2 diabetes. Am J Hypertens 2002; 15: 244-250

58 Knudsen ST, Bek T, Poulsen PL, Hove MN, Rehling M, Mogensen CE. Macular edema reflects generalized vascular hyperpermeability in type 2 diabetic patients with retinopathy. Diabetes Care 2002; 25: 2328-2334

59 Rynkiewicz A, Furmanski J, Narkiewicz K, Semetkowska E, Bieniaszewski L, Horoszek-Maziarz S, Krupa-Wojciechowska B. Influence of duration of type 1 (insulin-dependent) diabetes mellitus on 24-h ambulatory blood pressure and heart rate profile (letter). Diabetologia 1993; 36: 577

60 Hansen KW, Poulsen PL, Christiansen JS, Mogensen CE. Determinants of 24-h blood pressure in IDDM patients. Diabetes Care 1995; 18: 529-535

61 van Ittersum FJ, Spek JJ, Praet IJA, Lambert J, Ijzerman RG, Fischer HRA, Nikkels RE, Van Bortel LMAB, Donker AJM, Stehouwer CDA. Ambulatory blood pressure and autonomic function in normoalbuminuric type 1 diabetic patients. Nephrol Dial Transplant 1998; 13: 326-332

62 Donaldson DL, Moore WV, Chonko AM, Shipman JJ, Wiegmann T. Incipient hypertension precedes incipient nephropathy in adolescents and young adults with type I diabetes (abstract). Diabetes 1992; 42 (suppl 1): 97A

63   Mathiesen ER, Hilsted J, Feldt-Rasmussen B, Bonde-Petersen F, Christensen NJ, Parving H-H. The effect of metabolic control on hemodynamics in short-term insulin-dependent diabetic patients. Diabetes 1985; 34: 1301-1305

64   Richards AM, Donelly T, Nicholls MG, Ikram H, Hamilton EJ, Espiner EA. Blood pressure and vasoactive hormones with improved glycemic control in patients with diabetes mellitus. Clin Exp Hypertens [A] 1989; A11:391-406

65   Mathiesen ER, Gall M-A. Hommel E, Skøtt P, Parving H-H. Effects of short term strict metabolic control on kidney function and extracellular volume in incipient diabetic nephropathy. Diabetic Med 1989; 6: 595-600

66   Azar ST, Birbari A. Nocturnal blood pressure elevation in patients with type 1 diabetes receiving intensive insulin therapy compared with that in patients receiving conventional insulin therapy. J Clin Endocrinol Metab 1998; 83: 3190-3193

67   Poulsen PL, Hansen KW, Ebbehøj E, Knudsen ST, Mogensen CE. No deleterious effects of tight blood glucose control on 24-hour ambulatory blood pressure in normoalbuminuric insulin-dependent diabetes mellitus patients. J Clin Endocrinol Metab 2000; 85: 155-158

68   Hansen KW, Pedersen MM, Christiansen JS, Mogensen CE. Night blood pressure and cigarette smoking: disparate associations in healthy subjects and diabetic patients. Blood Pressure 1994; 3: 381-388

69   Poulsen PL, Ebbehøj E, Hansen KW, Mogensen CE. Effects of smoking on 24-h ambulatory blood pressure and autonomic function in normoalbuminuric insulin-dependent diabetes mellitus patients. Am J Hypertens 1998; 11: 1093-1099

70   Mikkelsen KL, Wiinberg N, Høegholm A, Christensen HR, Bang LE, Nielsen PE, Svendsen TL, Kampmann JP, Madsen NH, Bentzon MW. Smoking related to 24.h ambulatory blood pressure and heart rate. A study in 352 normotensive danish subjects. Am J ypertens 1997; 10: 483-491

71   Sinha RN, Patrick AW, Richardson L, MacFarlane IA. Diurnal variation in blood pressure in insulin-dependent diabetic smokers and non-smokers with and without microalbuminuria. Diabetic Med 1997; 14: 291-295.

72   Hansen KW, Christensen CK, Andersen PH, Mau Pedersen M, Christiansen JS, Mogensen CE. Ambulatory blood pressure in microalbuminuric type 1 diabetic patients. Kidney Int 1992; 41: 847-854

73   Benhamou PY, Halimi S, De Gaudemaris R, Boizel R, Pitiot M, Siche JP, Bachelot I, Mallion JM. Early disturbances of ambulatory blood pressure load in normotensive type 1 diabetic patients with microalbuminuria. Diabetes Care 1992; 15: 1614-1619

74   Peters A, Gromeier S, Kohlmann T, Look D, Kerner W. Nocturnal blood pressure elevation is related to adrenomedullary hyperactivity, but not to hyperinsulinemia, in nonobese normoalbuminuric type 1 diabetic patients. J Clin Endocrinol Metab 1996; 81: 507-512

75   Gilbert R, Philips P, Clarke C, Jerums G. Day-night blood pressure variation in normotensive normoalbuminuric type I diabetic subjects. Diabetes Care 1994; 17: 824-827

76   Khan N, Couper J, Dixit M, Couper R. Ambulatory blood pressure and heart rate in adolescents with insulin-dependent diabetes mellitus. Am J Hyp 1994; 7: 937-940

77   Guglielmi MD, Pierdomenico SD, Salvatore L, Romano R, Tascione E, Pupillo M, Porreca E, Imbastaro T, Cuccurullo F, Mezzetti A. Impaired left ventricular diastolic function and vascular postischemic vasodilation associated with microalbuminuria in IDDM patients. Diabetes Care 1995; 18: 353-360

78   Moore WV, Donaldson DL, Chonko AM, Ideus P, Wiegmann TB, Wiegmann. Ambulatory blood pressure in type I diabetes mellitus. Comparison to presence of incipient nephropathy in adolescents and young adults. Diabetes 41; 1992: 1035-1041

79   Sivieri R, Deandrea M, Gai V, Cavallo-Perin P. Circadian blood pressure levels in normotensive normoalbuminuric type 1 diabetic patients. Diabetic Med 1994; 11; 357-361

80   Laferty AR, Werther GA, Clarke CF. Ambulatory blood pressure, microalbuminuria, and autonomic neuropathy in adolescents with type 1 diabetes. Diabetes Care 2000; 23: 533-538

81   Lurbe E, Redon J, Pascual JM, Tacons J, Alvarez V. The spectrum of circadian blood pressure changes in type I diabetic patients. J Hypertens 2001; 19: 1421-1428

82   Cohen CN, Filho FM, de Fatima Goncalves M, de Brito Gomes M. Early alterations of blood pressure in normotensive and normoalbuminuric type 1 diabetic patients. Diabetes Res Clin Pract 2001; 53: 85-90

83   Hansen KW. Ambulatory blood pressure in insulin-dependent diabetes; the relation to stages of diabetic kidney disease. J Diabetes Complications 1996; 10:331-351

84   Wiegmann TB, Herron KG, Chonko AM, Macdougall ML, Moore WV. Recognition og hypertension and abnormal blood pressure burden with ambulatory blood pressure recordings in type I diabetes mellitus. Diabetes 1990; 39: 1556-1560

85   Yip J, Mattock MB, Morocutti A, Sethi M, Trevisan R, Viberti G. Insulin resistance in insulin-dependent diabetic patients with microalbuminuria. Lancet 1993; 342: 883-887

86   Voros P, Lengyel Z, Nagy V, Nemeth C, Rosivall L, Kammerer L. Diurnal blood pressure variation and albuminuria in normotensive patients with insulin-dependent diabetes mellitus. Nephrol Dial Transplant 1998; 13: 2257-2260

87   Sochett EB, Poon I, Balfe W, Daneman D. Ambulatory blood pressure monitoring in insulin-dependent diabetes mellitus with and without microalbuminuria. J Diab Comp 1998; 12;1: 18-23

88   Lurbe A, Redón J, Pascual JM, Tacons J, Alvarez V, Batlle DC. Altered blood pressure during sleep in normotensive subjects with type I diabetes. Hypertension 1993; 21: 227-235

89   Berrut G, Hallab M, Bouhanick B, Chameau A-M, Marre M, Fressinaud Ph. Value of ambulatory blood pressure in type I (insulin-dependent) diabetic patients with incipient diabetic nephropathy. Am J Hyp 1994; 7: 222-227

90   Hansen KW, Mau Pedersen M, Marshall SM, Christiansen JS, Mogensen CE. Circadian variation of blood pressure in patients with diabetic nephropathy. Diabetologia 1992; 35: 1074-1079

91   Torffvit O, Agardh C-D. Day and night variations in ambulatory blood pressure in type 1 diabetes mellitus with nephropathy and autonomic neuropathy. J Intern Med 1993; 233: 131-137

92   Poulsen PL, Hansen KW, Mogensen CE. Ambulatory blood pressure in the transition from normo- to microalbuminuria. A longitudinal study in IDDM patients. Diabetes 1994; 43; 1248-1253

93   Lurbe E, Redon J, Kesani A, Pascual JM, Tacons J, Alvarez V, Batlle D. Increase in nocturnal blood pressure and progression to microalbuminuria in type 1 diabetes. N Eng J Med 2002; 347: 797-805

94   Brotman DJ, Girod JP, Thomas S. Increase in nocturnal blood pressure and progression to microalbuminuria in type 1 diabetes (letters and reply). N Eng J Med 2003; 348: 260-264

95   Hansen KW, Pedersen MM, Christiansen, Mogensen CE. Diurnal blood pressure variations in normoalbuminuric type 1 diabetic patients. J Int Med 1993; 234: 175-180

96   Poulsen PL, Ebbehøj E, Hansen KW, Mogensen CE. 24-h blood pressure and autonomic function is related to albumin excretion within the normoalbuminuric range in IDDM patients. Diabetologia 1997; 40: 718-725

97   Page SR, Manning G, Ingle AR, Hill P, Millar-Craig MW, Peacock I. Raised ambulatory blood pressure in type 1 diabetes with incipient microalbuminuria. Diabetic Med 1994; 11; 877-882

98   Spallone V, Gambardella S, Maiello MR, Barini A, Frontoni S, Menzinger G. Relationship between autonomic neuropathy, 24-h blood pressure, and nephropathy in normotensive IDDM patients. Diabetes Care 1994; 17: 578-584

99   Monteagudo PT, Nóbrega JC, Cazarini PR, Ferreira SRG, Kohlmann O, Ribeiro AB, Zanella M-T. Altered blood pressure profile, autonomic neuropathy and nephropathy in insulin-dependent diabetic patients. European J of Endocrinology 1996; 135: 683-688.

100   Dyrberg T, Benn J, Sandahl Christiansen J, Hilsted J, Nerup J. Prevalence of diabetic autonomic neuropathy measured by simple bedside test. Diabetologia 1981; 20: 190-194

101   Zander E, Schulz, Heinke P, Grimmberger E, Zander G, Gottschling HD. Importance of cardiovascular autonomic dysfunction in IDDM subjects with diabetic nephropathy. Diabetes Care 1989; 12: 259-264

102   Mølgaard H, Christensen PD, Sørensen KE, Christensen CK, Mogensen CE. Association of 24-h cardiac parasympathetic activity and degree of nephropathy in IDDM patients. Diabetes 1992; 41: 812-817

103   Mølgaard H, Christensen PD, Hermansen K, Sørensen KE, Christensen CK, Mogensen CE. Early recognition of autonomic dysfunction in microalbuminuria: significance for cardiovascular mortality in diabetes mellitus. Diabetologia 1994; 37; 788-796

104   Hansen KW. Diurnal blood pressure profile, autonomic neuropathy and nephropathy in diabetes. European J of Endocrinology 1997; 136: 35-36

105   Poulsen PL, Ebbehøj E, Hansen KW, Mogensen CE. Characteristics and prognosis of normoalbuminuric type 1 diabetic patients. Diabetes Care 1999; 22(suppl.2); B72-B75

106   Schernthaner G, Ritz E, Philipp T, Bretzel RG. Night time blood pressure in diabetic patients-the submerged portion of the iceberg? Nephrol Dial Transplant 1999; 14: 1061-1064

107   Farmer CKT, Goldsmith DJA, Quin JD, Dallyn P, Cox J, Kingswood JC, Sharpstone P. Progression of diabetic nephropathy-is diurnal blood pressure rhythm as important as absolute blood pressure level ? Nephrol Dial Transplant 1998; 13: 635-639

108   Pecis M, Azevedo MJ, Gross JL. Glomerular hyperfiltration is associated with blood pressure abnormalities in normotensive normoalbuminuric IDDM patients. Diabetes Care 1997; 20: 1329-1333

109   Hansen KW, Sørensen K, Christensen PD, Pedersen EB, Christiansen JS, Mogensen CE. Night blood pressure: relation to organ lesions in microalbuminuric type 1 diabetic patients. Diabetic Med 1995; 12: 42-45

110   Mulec H, Blohmé G, Kullenberg K, Nyberg G, Bjørck S. Latent overhydration and nocturnal hypertension in diabetic nephropathy. Diabetologia 1995; 38; 216-229

111   Hansen HP, Rossing P, Tarnow L, Nielsen FS, Jensen BR, Parving H-H. Circadian rhythm of arterial blood pressure and albuminuria in diabetic nephropathy. Kidney Int 1996; 50; 579-585

112   Poulsen PL, Ebbehøj E, Arildsen A, Knudsen ST, Hansen KW, Mølgaard H, Mogensen CE. Increased QTc dispersion is related to blunted circadian blood pressure variation in normoalbuminuric type 1 diabetic patients. Diabetes 2002; 50: 837-842

113   Poulsen PL, Juhl B, Ebbehøj E, Klein F, Christiansen C, Mogensen CE. Elevated ambulatory blood pressure in microalbuminuric IDDM patients is inversely associated with renal plasma flow. A compensatory mechanism ? Diabetes Care 1997; 20: 429-432

114 Torbjörnsdotter TB, Jaremko GA, Berg UB. Ambulatory blood pressure and heart rate in relation to kidney structure and metabolic control in adolescents with type I diabetes.. Diabetologia 2001; 44: 865-873

115 Poulsen PL, Bek T, Ebbehøj E, Hansen KW, Mogensen CE. 24-h ambulatory blood pressure and retinopathy in normoalbuminuric IDDM patients. Diabetologia 1998; 41: 105-110

116 Fagerudd JA, Tarnow L, Jacobsen P, Stenman S, Nielsen FS, Petterson-Fernholm KJ, Grönhagen-Riska C, Parving H-H, Groop P-H. Predisposition to essential hypertension and development of diabetic nephropathy in IDDM patients. Diabetes 1998; 47: 439-444

117 Bellomo G, Narducci PL, Rondoni F, Pastorelli G, Stangoni G, Angeli G, Verdecchia P. Prognostic value of 24-hour blood pressure in pregnancy. JAMA 1999; 282: 1447-1452

118 Flores L, Levy I, Aguilera E, Martinez S, Gomis R, Esmatjes E. Usefulness of ambulatory blood pressure monitoring in pregnant women type 1 diabetes. Diabetes Care 1999; 22: 1507-1501

119 Ekbom P, Damm P, Nørgaard K, Clausen P, Feldt-Rasmussen U, Feldt-Rasmussen B, Nielsen LH, Mølsted-Pedersen L, Mathiesen ER. Urinary albumin excretion and 24-hour blood pressure as predictors of pre-eclampsia in type I diabetes. Diabetologia 2000; 43: 927-931

120 Hansen KW, Schmitz A, Mau Pedersen M. Ambulatory blood pressure measurement in type 2 diabetic patients: Methodological aspects. Diabetic Med 1991; 8: 567-572

121 Gambardella S, Frontoni S, Spallone V, Maiello MR, Civetta E, Lanza G, Sandric S, Menzinger G. Increased left ventricular mass in normotensive diabetic patients with autonomic neuropathy. Am J Hyp 1993; 6: 97-102

122 Nielsen FS, Ali S, Rossing P, Bang LE, Svendsen TL, Gall M-A, Smidt UM, Kastrup J, Parving H-H. Left ventricular hypertrophy in non-insulin dependent diabetic patients with and without diabetic nephropathy. Diabetic Med 1997; 538-546

123 Verdecchia P, Porcellati C, Schillaci G, Borgioni, Ciucci A, Gatteschi C, Zampi I, Santucci A, Santucci C, Reboldi G. Ambulatory blood pressure and risk of cardiovascular disease in type II diabetes mellitus. Diab Nutr Metab 1994; 7: 223-231

124 Ebbehøj E, Poulsen PL, Hansen KW, Mogensen CE. White coat effect in diabetes: ambulatory blood pressure in relation to clinic based measurement (abstract). Diabetologia 1997; 40 (suppl 1): A12

125 Nielsen FS, Gæde P, Vedel P, Pedersen O, Parving H-H. White coat hypertension in NIDDM patients with and without incipient and over diabetic nephropathy. Diabetes Care 1997; 20: 859-863

126 Puig JG, Ruilope LM, Ortega R. Antihypertensive treatment efficacy in type II diabetes mellitus. Dissociation between casual and 24-hour ambulatory blood pressure. Hypertension 1995; 26 (part 2): 1093-1099

127 Burgess E, Mather K, Ross S, Josefsberg Z. Office hypertension in Type 2 (non-insulin-dependent) diabetic patients (letter). Diabetologia 1991; 34: 684

128 Holl RW, Pavlovic M, Heinze E, Thon A. Circadian blood pressure during the early course of type 1 diabetes. Analysis of 1,011 ambulatory blood pressure recordings in 354 adolescents and young adults. Diabetes Care 1999; 22: 1151-1157

129 Staessen JA, Thijs L, Fagard R, O`Brien E, Clement D, de Leeuw PW, Mancia G, Nachev C, Palatini P, Parati G, Tuomilehto J, Webster J. Predicting cardiovascular risk using conventional vs ambulatory blood pressure in older patients with systolic hypertension. JAMA 1999; 282: 539-546

130 The Joint National Committee on Detection, Evaluation, and Treatment of High Blood Pressure. The sixth report of the joint national committee on detection, evaluation, and treatment of high blood pressure. Arch Intern Med 1997; 157: 2413-2446

131 Guidelines Subcommittee. 1999 World Health Organization-International Society of Hypertension guidelines for the management of hypertension. J Hypertens 1999; 17: 151-183

132 Ramsay LE, Williams B, Johnston GD, MacGregor GA, Poston L, Potter JF, Poulter NR, Russel G. Guidelines for management of hypertension: report of the third working party of the British Hypertension Society. J Hum Hypertens 1999; 13: 569-592

133 O'Brien E, Staessen J. Normotension and hypertension as defined by 24-hour ambulatory blood pressure monitoring. Blood Pressure 1995; 4; 266-282

134 O´Brien E, Staessen JA. What is "hypertension"? Lancet 1999; 353: 1541-1543

135 Hansen KW, Ebbehøj E, Poulsen PL, Mogensen CE. What is hypertension in diabetes ? Ambulatory blood pressure in 137 normoalbuminuric and normotensive type 1 diabetic patients. Diabet Med 2001; 18: 370-373

136 Strachan MWJ, Gough K, McKnight JA, Padfield PL. Ambulatory blood pressure monitoring: is it necessary for the routine assessment of hypertension in people with diabetes ? Diabet Med 2002; 19: 787-789

137 Hansen KW, Poulsen PL, Mogensen CE. Ambulatory blood pressure monitoring in patients with diabetes (letter). Diabet Med 2003 (in press)

138 Nakano S. Fukuda M, Hotta F, Ito T, Ishii T, Kitazawa M, Nishizawa M, Kigoshi T, Uchida K. Reversed circadian blood pressure rhythm is associated with occurrences of both fatal and nonfatal vascular events in NIDDM subjects. Diabetes 1998; 47: 1501-1506

139 Sturrock NDC, George E, Pound N, Stevenson J, Peck GM, Sowter H. Non-dipping circadian blood pressure and renal impairment are associated with increased mortality in diabetes mellitus. Diabet Med 2000, 17: 360-364

140 Mølgaard H, Hermansen K. Evaluation of cardiac autonomic neuropathy by heart rate variability. In: Mogensen CE, Standl E (eds). Diabetes Forum Series volume V (part 1). Research methodologies in human diabetes. Berlin, New York: Walter de Gruyter; 1994, pp 219-240

141 Imholz BPM, Langewouters GJ, van Montfrans A, Parati G, van Goudoever J, Wesseling KH, Wieling W, Mancia G. Feasibility of ambulatory, continous 24-hour finger arterial pressure recording. Hypertens 1993; 21: 65-73

142 Staessen JA, Beilin L, Parati G, Waeber B, White W. Task Force IV: Clinical use of ambulatory blood pressure monitoring. Blood Press Monit 1999; 4: 319-331

143 Staessen JA, O'Brien E, Lutgarde Thijs, Fagard RH. Modern approaches to blood pressure measurement. Occup Environ Med 2000; 57:510-520

144 Weir MR, Blantz RC. Blood pressure and cardiovascular risks: implications of the presence or absence of a nocturnal dip in blood pressure. Current Opinion in Nephrology and hypertension 2003; 12:57-60

26

MICROALBUMINURIA IN YOUNG PATIENTS WITH TYPE 1 DIABETES

Henrik Bindesbøl Mortensen
Pediatric Department, Glostrup Hospital, DK 2600 Glostrup

Diabetic nephropathy is the main cause of the increased morbidity and mortality among patients with Type 1 diabetes [1,2,3]. In recent years, it has been shown that a slightly elevated urinary albumin excretion rate (microalbuminuria) is an early predictor for later development of overt diabetic nephropathy [4,5,6,7] and is associated with elevated arterial blood pressure [8,9,10,11,12]. Based on recent literature, the reported prevalence of microalbuminuria in paediatric populations varies from 4.3 to 21% (Table 1a+b). Consequently, microalbuminuria is the first easily identifiable sign of risk of incipient diabetic nephropathy and other vascular complications of the disease. Treatment and intervention consensus guidelines have already been developed for adults [13] and it is equally important to set up a uniform intervention programme for treatment of microalbuminuria in adolescents with Type 1 diabetes [93].

MEASURING ALBUMIN EXCRETION

There are several different ways of measuring albumin excretion. Timed overnight urine collection was used to assess the prevalence of microalbuminuria in a nation-wide screening for microalbuminuria in Denmark in 1989 [14]. This urine fraction avoids the effect of posture, physical exercise, major blood pressure variations and the acute effect of diet on albuminuria and it is a convenient and practical method for most children. Two samples were taken from each patient, on separate occasions, and if the urinary albumin excretion rate (AER) was over 20 μg min⁻¹ in one of the two samples, a third sample was taken to confirm whether the child had elevated albumin excretion – microalbuminuria. This limit was chosen as the lowest AER that is predictive of diabetic nephropathy – on the basis of investigations of the upper 95th percentile for albumin excretion in the control group of 209 healthy children [14]. The AER was determined by an immunoturbidimetric method which on average gave 13% higher results than those measured by radioimmunoassay.

Various workers have reported upper 95% confidence limits for the different methods of measuring albumin excretion. Rowe et al. [15] established an upper 95% confidence limit for overnight urine of 12.2 μg min⁻¹ in normal children, while Davies et al. [16] reported a value related to surface area of 10 μg min⁻¹ 1.73m⁻². In another study, Gibb et al. [17] estimated the upper 95th centile for overnight albumin excretion rate in healthy children as being 8.2 μg min⁻¹ 1.73m⁻².

Table 1a. Cross-sectional studies on prevalence of microalbuminuria in paediatric populations.

Author	Screening procedure	Population	Micro-albuminuria (%)	Mean duration of diabetes(yrs)
Mathiesen et al. 1986 [31]	AER Overnight	97	20	10
Dahlquist and Rudberg 1987 [38]	AER Overnight	129	20%	10
Mortensen et al 1990 [14]	AER Overnight	957	4%	6
Joner et al 1992 [34]	AER Overnight	371	12%	10.5
Olsen et al 1995 [35]	AER Overnight	339	9.0	13.2
Moore and Shield 2000 [94]	AER Overnight	1007	9.7%	>1

Table 1b Longitudinal studies on prevalence of microalbuminuria in paediatric populations

Author	Screening procedure	Population	Follow-up (yrs)	Microalbuminuria (%)
Nørgaard et al 1989 [32]	AER 24-h urine	113	2	15
Jones CA et al 1998 [95]	AER Morning spot urine	233	8	Intermittent: 9 Persistent: 14
D'Antonio et al. 1989 [33]	AER 24-h urine	62	5	21
Janner et al. 1994 [37]	AER 12h urine 3 monthly	164	8	20
Barkai et al. 1998 [96]	AER 24-h urine 6 monthly	74 (20 prepubertal,28 pubertal, 26 postpubertal	3	Prepubertal:0 Pubertal:21 Postpubertal: 8
Rudberg et al. 1993 [39]	AER 3 monthly	156	3-9	4.8%
Danne et al. 1997 [97]	AER Overnight	249	9	Intermittent:3% Persistent:5%
Schultz et al. 1999 [98]	AER Overnight or morning	514	10	Persistent:4.8%

DEFINITION OF MICROALBUMINURIA

Microalbuminuria has been defined using a variety of screening procedures for urine sampling [18-26]:

- Urinary albumin excretion rate (UAE) 20–200 μg/min (overnight urine collection) or 30–300 mg/24 h (24 h urine collection).
- Albumin/creatinine ratio (A/C ratio) 2.5–25 mg/mmol (spot urine) (Europe). Note that a lower limit of 3.5 mg/mmol has been proposed in females because of lower creatinine excretion.
- Albumin/creatinine ratio (A/C ratio) 30–300 mg/g (spot urine). (North America).
- Albumin concentration (AC) 30–300 mg/l (early morning urine).

When screening for microalbuminuria, a spot urine albumin/creatinine ratio or albumin concentration (Micraltest or other bedside test) can be used. However, timed urine collection is more accurate. If the result is positive, microalbuminuria should be confirmed by UAE. Incipient diabetic nephropathy is suspected when microalbuminuria is found in at least two out of three urine samples, preferably within a 1 to 6 month period [13]. The within-individual variation in observations of AER can vary by as much as 40% due to natural fluctuations, and there are several other confounding factors that can affect AER (Table 2) [14,27]. Therefore, a minimum of two estimations is necessary per individual to determine the true mean value of urine albumin excretion with reasonable confidence.

Table 2. Confounding factors for microalbuminuria.

- Variability in albumin excretion (about 40%)
- Posture or diurnal variation
- Strenuous exercise
- Urinary tract infection
- Acute febrile illness
- Menstrual bleeding
- Vaginal discharge

ALBUMIN EXCRETION RATE AMONG CHILDREN WITH AND WITHOUT DIABETES

The ranges for AER in urine samples collected overnight in both non-diabetic and diabetic children aged 12 years or less and adolescents from 12 to 19 years are given in Table 3. The geometric mean for albumin excretion was significantly higher (p<0.001) in adolescents than in children under 12 years independent of diabetes. There were no significant differences (p>0.05) in albumin excretion rates between the sexes.

Table 3. Timed overnight urinary albumin excretion in children and adolescents with and without Type 1 diabetes.

| | Children ≤12 years | | Adolescents >12-19 years | |
	Boys	Girls	Boys	Girls
Normal children				
N	47	30	58	74
AER (μg min^{-1})	1.28x/÷2.75	1.27x/÷1.97	2.73x/÷2.18[a]	2.23x/÷2.14[a]
Diabetic children				
N	154	124	334	297
AER (μg min^{-1})	1.70x/÷2.11	1.72x/÷2.07	2.94x/÷2.38[a]	3.16x/÷2.23[a]

Geometric mean x/÷ SD factor.

P<0.001 compared with younger age groups. Boys vs. girls all NS [ref. 14, with permission]

These findings are consistent with recent results reported on overnight collections of urine [15,16]. In non-diabetic adolescents, the relationship between AER, body surface area and level of maturity was fairly constant, which is in accordance with the results of Gibb et al. [17]. By contrast, in diabetic adolescents, AER was positively correlated with body surface area and age. This correlation was independent of the current HbA_{1c} level, suggesting that specific metabolic changes other than poor blood glucose control might affect AER, particularly in diabetic subjects during the pubertal period. Hypersecretion of growth hormone (GH) as a result of altered feedback drive from reduced insulin-like growth factor I (IGF-1) levels and IGF-1 bioactivity have been demonstrated in adolescents with Type 1 diabetes [28], which may lead to glomerular hyperfiltration [29] and an increased risk of developing microalbuminuria [30].

TYPE 1 DIABETIC CHILDREN WITH ELEVATED ALBUMIN EXCRETION RATE

The prevalence of persistent microalbuminuria was 4.3% in the Danish nation-wide screening study in 1989 (which involved 957 Danish children and adolescents aged 2–19 years with Type 1 diabetes and mean diabetes duration of 6 years) [14]. However, the reported prevalence of microalbuminuria in cross-sectional and longitudinal studies varies from 4.3 to 21% (see Tables 1a+b) [14,31,32,33,34,35,37,38, 94,95,96,97,98]. The wide variation in persistent microalbuminuria between these studies may partly be explained by differences in age, diabetes duration, blood glucose control, the populations investigated and the screening procedure. However, a decrease in the incidence of nephropathy in Type 1 diabetes mellitus during the period that these studies were conducted may also have contributed to the variable results [36]. In children and adolescents, the natural history of microalbuminuria is not necessarily the progression to frank proteinuria and overt nephropathy. In fact, there is increasing evidence that microalbuminuria can be non-progressive or even transient [99]. Some longitudinal studies even suggest that as many as 50% of subjects might revert to normoalbuminuria at the end of the pubertal years [98,100,101].

The prevalence of persistent microalbuminuria in different age groups and in groups with different durations of diabetes, from 909 children and adolescents with Type 1 diabetes [14], is shown in figures 1 and 2. In this study, the prevalence of microalbuminuria in adolescent patients (over 16 years) was 13–14%, which is similar to previous investigations. The occurrence of microalbuminuria is extremely rare before puberty. Two prepubertal children were diagnosed with microalbuminuria in a study by Nørgaard et al. [32], while Joner et al. [34] and Janner et al. [37] each reported one case. In our study [14], two children (both girls) were diagnosed with microalbuminuria, while none were detected in the studies by Mathiesen et al. [31] and Dahlquist et al. [38].

It remains controversial whether diabetes duration *per se* is associated with raised urinary albumin. Some studies have shown a possible association [14,39], while others dispute this [40]. Nonetheless, it seems reasonable that young people should be screened for microalbuminuria regardless of diabetes duration, beginning at the very first stage of puberty [14,37].

OVERNIGHT ALBUMIN EXCRETION RATE AND BLOOD GLUCOSE CONTROL

Several previous reports have suggested a relationship between poor blood glucose control and increased urinary albumin excretion [39,41,42,43]. In our study [14] we found that only females with microalbuminuria had significantly elevated HbA_{1c} values compared with diabetic patients with normoalbuminuria. Blood glucose control tends to be poorer during puberty, particularly in girls, which may be explained by changes in hormonal and/or lifestyle factors [44,45,46,47,48]. In recent studies [49,50,102], urinary albumin excretion correlated significantly and independently with prepubertal diabetes duration, prepubertal hyperglycaemia, female sex and poor long-term metabolic control. Thus, good metabolic control should be the goal from the onset of diabetes. However in a recent longitudinal study by Schultz et al. [103] HbA$_{1c}$ was a determinant of risk for microalbuminuria, but in their cohort. pubertal factors had a greater effect on the rates of progression of urine albumin excretion during adolescence.

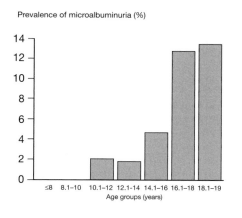

Prevalence of microalbuminuria (%)

Figure 1. The prevalence of microalbuminuria in different age groups in 909 children and adolescents with type 1 diabetes. [ref. 14, with permission]

An impaired linear growth observed in females with microalbuminuria may also be associated with long-term poor blood glucose. However, recent studies [51,52] have suggested an association between short stature and diabetic nephropathy, particularly in males. Furthermore, in males who have had diabetes for 10 to 25 years, there is a threefold increase in the prevalence of micro/macroalbuminuria compared with females [53]. The DCCT study [54] demonstrated that improved metabolic control could retard but not prevent the progression of incipient diabetic kidney disease. Recently, Krolewski et al. [55] reported that the risk of microalbuminuria in patients with Type 1 diabetes increases abruptly above an HbA$_{1c}$ level of 8.1%, suggesting that efforts to reduce the frequency of diabetic nephropathy should be focused on the patients with HbA$_{1c}$ values above this threshold. In their study Warram et al. (104)

463

found that in patients with microalbuminuria the risk of progression to overt poroteinuria could be reduced by improved glycaemic control only if the HbA_{1c} is maintained below 8.5%. Moreover, below that value, the risk declines as the level of HbA_{1c} decreases.

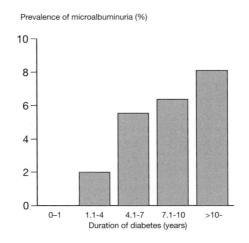

Figure 2. The relationship between duration of diabetes and prevalence of microalbuminuria in 909 children and adolescents with type 1 diabetes [ref. 14, with permission]

CLINICAL OUTCOME INDICATORS/TARGETS FOR GLYCAEMIC CONTROL

In view of the importance of good blood glucose control in preventing microvascular complications, we have defined specific outcome indicators to be measured and audited annually:

- 90% of all patients with HbA_{1c} values of 10 % or above should achieve a 1% reduction of this value within a year.
- More than 50% of children aged 0–6 years should have HbA_{1c} values below 9%, or in patients aged 7–18 years, below 8.5%, within at least 2

years and below 8% within 4 years in all age groups.
- The rate of severe hypoglycaemic events (loss of consciousness/seizures) in all our patients should be less than 20/100 patient years.

We use the HbA_{1c} level of 8% as a treatment target in patients aged 7–18 years on the basis of previous evidence [56,57,58,59]. In children under 6 years with Type 1 diabetes, the HbA_{1c} target is a little higher (about 8–9%) because of the greater risk of severe hypoglycaemia [60,61,62,63,64,65], which in this age group may have potentially harmful effects on neuropsychological and intellectual functions in the developing brain [65,66,67,68]. However, we try (carefully) to reduce the HbA_{1c} level to 8% in these children too, if this is achievable without increasing the number of severe hypoglycaemic events.

OVERNIGHT ALBUMIN EXCRETION RATE AND ARTERIAL BLOOD PRESSURE

The normal range for diastolic blood pressure in diabetic boys (Figure 3) and girls (Figure 4) aged 8 to 18 years with normoalbuminuria was determined in a study of the relationship between blood pressure and urinary albumin excretion in young Danish Type 1 diabetic patients [69]. Figures 3 and 4 also include data from patients diagnosed with micro- and macroalbuminuria [69]. Ten out of 16 boys with microalbuminuria had diastolic blood pressure above the upper quartile while eight out of 14 girls with microalbuminuria had diastolic blood pressure above this quartile [69]. Three of four boys with macroalbuminuria had diastolic blood pressure below the upper quartile while two of three girls with macroalbuminuria had values above [69]. Overall, 60% of adolescents with microalbuminuria had diastolic blood pressure in the upper quartile for normoalbuminuria [69]. In keeping with this, Kordonouri et al. [70] reported a relationship between diastolic blood pressure and albumin excretion rate in juvenile Type 1 diabetic patients. This excess prevalence of raised blood pressure in Type 1 diabetic patients could, therefore, be explained by the presence of elevated blood pressure in adolescents with micro- and macroalbuminuria [32]

Re-examination of 15 of the adolescents with microalbuminuria, 2 years after identification, revealed that two of these (13%) had developed overt proteinuria during this period. They had initially an overnight albumin excretion rate of

465

62.0 and 115.7 µg.min^{-1}, respectively, increasing to 184.4 and 448.3 µg.min^{-1}, respectively (unpublished data). Gorman et al. [71] showed that microalbuminuria detected in the first decade of disease will persist or progress in the second decade in around two-thirds of patients, while a third of those initially normoalbuminuric will develop microalbuminuria. Thus, without treatment, a marked increase in the progression to overt diabetic nephropathy is seen in many individuals. In a study of young diabetic patients all diagnosed before 15 years of age, Bojestig et al. [72] found no relationship between the level of microalbuminuria at the initial investigation and the development of nephropathy. They conclude that, even in the upper range of AER, excellent glycaemic control seems to be effective in preventing macroalbuminuria and reversing AER to normal.

Altered glomerular haemodynamics with increased glomerular plasma flow and transcapillary pressures are considered key factors in the initiation and progression of diabetic nephropathy [73,74,75,76]. Therapy with an angiotensin converting enzyme (ACE) inhibitor has been shown to lower albumin excretion rate and mean arterial blood pressure in normotensive adolescents [77,78] and adults [79] with Type 1 diabetes and microalbuminuria, in the short term at least. Recently, long-term studies have demonstrated that ACE-inhibition delays progression to diabetic nephropathy in normotensive Type 1 diabetic patients with persistent microalbuminuria [80,81,82,83]. Rudberg et al. [84] found less progression of early diabetic glomerulopathy in Type 1 diabetic young microalbuminuric patients who were treated with either ACE-inhibitors or beta blockers (for an average of 3 years) than in patients who did not receive antihypertensive treatment and that this effect possibly was due to maintenance of a normal or low blood pressure. Thus, ACE inhibitors have beneficial effects in nephropathy [85], a microvascular complication of Type 1 diabetes that shares many of the risk factors of retinopathy. Interestingly, The EUCLID Study Group [86] recently reported that the ACE inhibitor, lisinopril, both reduced the progression and incidence of retinopathy and that this is not fully accounted for by effects on blood pressure. The EUCLID study investigators suggest that ACE inhibitor therapy should be considered for all patients with Type 1 diabetes who have some degree of retinopathy.

Previous investigations in adults with Type 1 diabetes have shown that, at the time of recognition of microalbuminuria, blood pressure is often within the normal range [87] and tends to increase in parallel with the extent of albuminuria. However some studies have shown a progressive elevation of blood pressure, even in the normotensive range, before the occurrence of persistent microalbuminuria (105). This was particularly true for patients with a family history of hypertension (106). However, in a recent matched case-control study it was reported that a rise in systemic blood pressure could not be detected before the first appearance of microalbuminuria in children. Blood pressure rose concurrently with the onset of microalbuminuria and was also closely related to BMI (107). However, higher levels of albumin-to-creatinine ratio within the first 2 years after diagnosis and a significantly higher rate of increase of the albumin-to-creatinine ratio within the first 5 years from diagnosis could be detected in subjects who subsequently developed microalbuminuria (103).

Only two out of five adolescents with macroalbuminuria had elevated blood pressure in our study of blood pressure and AER (Figures 3 and 4) [69]. This may be a selection bias because two patients with macroalbuminuria were excluded due to antihypertensive treatment. However, shorter duration of diabetes and lower body mass index compared to an adult population could explain the observed discrepancies.

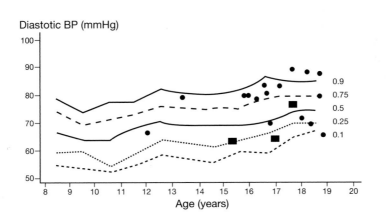

Figure 3. Percentile distribution of diastolic blood pressure in 487 boys aged 8 to 18 years with type 1 diabetes. The dots represent diastolic blood pressure for the 16 boys with microalbuminuria, the squares the three boys with macroalbuminuria [ref. 69, with permission].

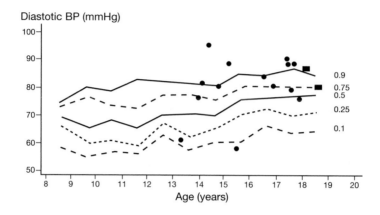

Figure 4. Percentile distribution of diastolic blood pressure in 425 girls aged 8 to 18 years with type 1 diabetes. The dots represent diastolic blood pressure of the 14 girls with microalbuminuria, the squares the two girls with macroalbuminuria [69, with permission].

These findings suggest that elevated arterial blood pressure may be related to the increased prevalence of elevated albumin excretion rate observed in adolescents with Type 1 diabetes and it suggests that hypertension plays an important role for the initiation and the progression of diabetic nephropathy in keeping with previous reports [4,7,10]

AT WHAT AGE SHOULD ROUTINE SCREENING FOR MICROALBUMINURIA BEGIN?

Young people should be screened for microalbuminuria regardless of diabetes duration [40] beginning at the very first stage of puberty [37]. Subsequently, annual screening should be carried out particularly if the metabolic control is unsatisfactory or abnormalities are found. Arterial blood pressure should be measured at least annually.

INTERVENTION PROGRAMME FOR TREATMENT OF PERSISTENT MICROALBUMINURIA (20-200 µg/min)

In children with microalbuminuria (>20–200 µg/min) blood glucose control should be improved over a period of 6 months and the status of microalbuminuria should be monitored closely. If microalbuminuria disappears or improves there is no indication for pharmacological intervention. However, if the microalbuminuria deteriorates, whether or not blood glucose control improves and blood pressure is within the normal limits, antihypertensive treatment by an ACE-inhibitor should be instituted.

The ACE inhibitors have potential therapeutic advantages over other antihypertensive drugs because they may selectively reduce efferent arteriolar pressures, and thereby glomerular capillary pressures, by lowering angiotensin II levels [88,89]. There has been extensive experience with ACE inhibitor use in children and therapy has been associated with very few side effects at low doses in the presence of normal renal function [78,84,90,91]. However, long-term follow up studies in children are required to evaluate whether intervention at an early stage with ACE inhibitors will prevent or only slow down progression to established diabetic nephropathy [92].

As well as starting ACE inhibitor treatment, the following measures should be taken over a 6-month period:

- Improvement of blood glucose control, HbA_{1c} to below 8.0% (normal HbA_{1c} range 4.3–5.8%).
- Frequent home blood glucose determination (4 times a day) and adjustment of insulin, diet and physical activity according to measured values.
- Monitor the status of microalbuminuria every other month (overnight urine collections).
- Monthly monitoring of arterial blood pressure and comparison of the readings to age appropriate values, if available.
- Discourage smoking and encourage exercise and reduction in overweight.
- Reduce daily protein intake to 1.0 –1.2 g /kg body weight.

Blood pressure should be monitored under standard conditions, after at least 5 min rest, with the adolescent sitting. The measurement should be taken on the right arm with an inflatable cuff size of 140 mm. A diagnosis of hypertension should be based on several readings and home monitored BP values. If 'white coat' hypertension is suspected, 24 h ambulatory BP may be used.

If microalbuminuria disappears or improves, there is no indication for pharmacological intervention. If the status of microalbuminuria deteriorates, even if the blood glucose control improves, the intervention programme for management of microalbuminuria shown in Table 4 should be implemented. The target of treatment is to achieve a blood pressure of 120–130/80–85 mmHg or less. The ideal is to achieve a reduction in microalbuminuria of 20–30% per year or at least to stabilise the AER.

Table 4 Intervention programme for microalbuminuria

Microalbuminuria in normotensive and hypertensive patients	What to monitor
☐ ACE-inhibitor should be initiated (pregnancy contraindication) ☐ Antihypertensive treatment: adolescents > 40 kg, capoten 50 mg, b.d. ☐ Increase the dose gradually from 12.5 mg	☐ Microalbuminuria: 1–3 months using A/C ratio or UAE (depending on the child's ability to comply with the collection method) ☐ Blood pressure: 1–3 months ☐ Serum creatinine: 1/2 yearly ☐ Serum potassium: 1/2 yearly ☐ Retinopathy yearly ☐ Neuropathy yearly

PRECAUTIONS WITH ACE-INHIBITOR TREATMENT

It should be noted that treatment with ACE inhibitors should be discontinued in the case of pregnancy and other antihypertensive treatment may be indicated. If serum potassium increases or the patients show sodium retention, low dose diuretic agents should be added.

CONCLUSION

The prevalence of persistent microalbuminuria was only 4.3% in a study consisting of a large proportion of all Danish children and adolescents with Type 1 diabetes. Elevated AER occurs mainly during the very first stage of puberty, and screening for microalbuminuria is recommended in children at the age of 9,

12, 15 and 18 years at least. However, yearly examinations are recommended if the metabolic control is unsatisfactory or abnormalities are found. Sixty percent of adolescents with microalbuminuria had diastolic blood pressure above the upper quartile for normoalbuminuric patients. Therefore, elevated blood pressure in childhood should lead to careful observation of the blood pressure level in the long term and examination of the urinary albumin excretion rate to prevent development of end-organ damage.

REFERENCES

1. Dorman JS, Laporte RE, Kuller LH, Cruickshanks KJ, Orchard TJ, Wagener DK, Becker DJ, Cavender DE, Drash AL. The Pittsburgh insulin-dependent diabetes mellitus (IDDM). Morbidity and mortality study. Mortality results. Diabetes 1984;33:271–276.
2. Borch-Johnsen K, Andersen PK, Deckert T. The effect of proteinuria on relative mortality in Type 1 (insulin dependent) diabetes mellitus. Diabetologia 1985;28:590–596.
3. Borch-Johnsen K, Kreiner S. Proteinuria: value as predictor of cardiovascular mortality in insulin dependent diabetes mellitus. Br Med J 1987;294:1651–1654.
4. Mogensen CE, Damsgaard EM, Frøland A, Hansen KW, Nielsen S, Pedersen MM, Schmitz A, Thuesen L, Østerby R. Reduced glomerular filtration rate and cardiovascular damage in diabetes: a key role for abnormal albuminuria. Acta Diabetologia 1992;29:201–213.
5. Bangstad H-J, Østerby R, Dahl-Jørgensen K, Berg KJ, Hartmann A, Nyberg G, Frahm Bjørn S, Hanssen KF. Early glomerulopathy is present in young, Type 1 (insulin-dependent) diabetic patients with microalbuminuria. Diabetologia 1993;36:523–529.
6. Ellis EN, Pysher TJ. Renal disease in adolescents with Type 1 diabetes mellitus: A report of the southwest pediatric nephrology study group. Am J Kidney Dis 1993;22:783–790.
7. Viberti GC. Prognostic significance of microalbuminuria. Am J Hypertens 1994;7:69–72.
8. Epstein M, Sowers JR. Diabetes mellitus and hypertension. Hypertension 1992;19:403–418.
9. Microalbuminuria Collaborative Study Group, United Kingdom. Risk factors for development of microalbuminuria in insulin dependent diabetic patients: a cohort study. BMJ 1993;306:1235–1239.
10. Mathiesen ER, Rønn B, Storm B, Foght H, Deckert T. The natural course of microalbuminuria in insulin-dependent diabetes: A 10-year prospective study. Diabetic Med 1995;12:482–487.
11. Mangili R, Deferrari G, Di Mario U, Giampietro O, Navalesi R, Nosadini R, Rigamonti G, Spezia R, Crepaldi G, for the Italian Microalbuminuria Study Group. Arterial hypertension and microalbuminuria IDDM: The Italian microalbuminuria study. Diabetologia 1994;37:1015–1024.
12. Parving H-H. Renoprotection in diabetes: Renoprotection in diabetes: genetic and non-genetic risk factors and treatment. Diabetologia 1998;41:745–759.
13. Mogensen CE, Keane WF, Bennett PH, Jerums G, Parving H-H, Passa P, Steffes MW, Striker GE, Viberti GC. Prevention of diabetic renal disease with special reference to microalbuminuria. Lancet 1995;346:1080-84.

14. Mortensen HB, Marinelli K, Nørgaard K, Main K, Kastrup KW, Ibsen KK et al. A nation-wide cross-sectional study of urinary albumin excretion rate, arterial blood pressure and blood glucose control in Danish children with Type 1 diabetes. Diabetic Med 1990;7:887–897.

15. Rowe DJF, Hayward M, Bagga H, Betts P. Effect of glycaemic control and duration of disease on overnight albumin excretion in diabetic children. BMJ 1984;289:957–959.

16. Davies AG, Postlethwaite RJ, Price DA, Burn JL, Houlton CA, Fielding BA. Urinary albumin excretion in school children. Arch Dis Child 1984;59:625–630.

17. Gibb DM, Dunger D, Levin M, Shah V, Smith C, Barratt TM. Early markers of the renal complications of insulin dependent diabetes mellitus. Arch Dis Child 1989;64:984–991.

18. Mogensen CE, Chachati A, Christensen CK, Close CF, Deckert T, Hommel E, Kastrup J, Lefebvre P, Mathiesen ER, Feldt-Rasmussen B, Schmitz A, Viberti GC. Microalbuminuria: An early marker of renal involvement in diabetes. Uremia Invest 1985–86;9:85–95.

19. Feldt-Rasmussen B, Microalbuminuria and clinical nephropathy in Type 1 (insulin-dependent) diabetes mellitus: Pathophysiological mechanisms and intervention studies. Dan Med Bull 1989;36:405–415.

20. Eshøj O, Feldt-Rasmussen B, Larsen ML, Mogensen EF. Comparison of overnight, morning and 24h urine collections in assessment of diabetic microalbuminuria. Diabetic Med 1987;4:531–533.

21. Viberti GC, Mogensen CE, Passa P, Bilous R, Mangili R. St Vincent declaration, 1994: guidelines for the prevention of diabetic renal failure. In: Mogensen CE, ed. The kidney and hypertension in diabetes mellitus, 2nd ed. Boston/Dordrecht/London: Kluwer, 1994: 515–527.

22. Anon. Prevention of diabetes mellitus: report of a WHO study group. WHO Technical Report Series 844. Geneva: WHO, 1994:55–59

23. Jerums G, Cooper M, Gilbert R, O'Brian R, TaftJ. Microalbuminuria in Diabetes. Med J Aust 1994;161:265–268.

24. Consensus development conference on the diagnosis and management of nephropathy in patients with diabetes mellitus. Diabetes Care 1994;17:1357–1361.

25. Bennett PH, Haffner S, Kasiske BL et al. Screening and management of microalbuminuria in patients with diabetes mellitus: recommendations to the scientific advisory board of the National Kidney Foundation from an ad hoc committee of the council on diabetes mellitus of the National Kidney Foundation. Am J Kidney Dis 1995;25:107–112.

26. Striker GE. Report on a workshop to develop management recommendations for the prevention of progression in chronic renal disease (Bethesda, April, 1994). Nephrol Dial Transplant 1995;10:290–292.

27. Gibb DM, Shah V, Preece M, Barratt TM. Variability of urine albumin excretion in normal and diabetic children. Pediatr Nephrol 1989; 3:414–419.

28. Taylor AM, Dunger DB, Preece MA, Holly JMP, Smith CP, Wass JAH, Patel S, Tate VE. The growth hormone independent insulin-like growth factor-I binding protein BP-28 is associated with serum insulin-like growth factor-I inhibitory bioactivity in adolescent insulin-dependent diabetics. Clin Endocrinol 1990;32: 229–239.

29. Blankestijn PJ, Derkx FHM, Birkenhäger JC, Lamberts SWJ, Mulder P, Verschoor L, Schalekamp MADH, Weber RFA. Glomerular hyperfiltration in insulin-dependent diabetes mellitus is correlated with enhanced growth hormone secretion. J Clin Endocrinol Metab 1993;77:498–502.

30. Chiarelli F, Verrotti A, Morgese G. Glomerular hyperfiltration increases the risk of developing microalbuminuria in diabetic children. Pediatr Nephrol 1995; 9:154–158.

31. Mathiesen ER, Saurbrey N, Hommel E, Parving H.-H. Prevalence of microalbuminuria in children with Type 1 (insulin-dependent) diabetes mellitus. Diabetologia 1986;29:640–643.

32. Nørgaard N, Storm B, Graa M, Feldt-Rasmussen B. Elevated albumin excretion and retinal changes in children with Type 1 diabetes are related to long-term poor blood glucose control. Diabetic Med 1989;6:325–328.

33. D`Antonio JA, Ellis D, Doft BH, Becker DJ, Drash AL, Kuller LH, Orchard TJ. Diabetic complications and glycemic control. The Pittsburgh prospective insulin-dependent diabetes cohort study status report after 5 yr of IDDM. Diabetes Care 1989;12:694–700.

34. Joner G, Brinchmann-Hansen O, Torres CG, Hanssen KF. A nationwide cross-sectional study of retinopathy and microalbuminuria in young Norwegian Type 1 (insulin-dependent) diabetic patients. Diabetologia 1992;35:1049–1054.

35. Olsen BS, Johannesen J, Sjølie AK, Borch-Johnsen K, Hougaard P, Thorsteinsson B, Prammning S, Marinelli K, Mortensen HB and the Danish Study Group of Diabetes in Childhood. Metabolic control and prevalence of microvascular complications in young Danish patients with Type 1 diabetes mellitus. Diabet. Med 1999;16:79–85.

36. Bojestig M, Arnqvist HJ, Hermansson G, Karlberg BE, Ludvigsson J. Declining incidence of nephropathy in insulin-dependent diabetes mellitus. N Engl J Med 1994;330:15–18.

37. Janner M, Eberhard Knill SE, Diem P, Zuppinger KA, Mullis PE. Persistent microalbuminuria in adolescents with Type 1 (insulin-dependent) diabetes mellitus is associated to early rather than late puberty. Eur J Pediatr 1994;153:403–408.

38. Dahlquist G, Rudberg S. The prevalence of microalbuminuria in diabetic children and adolescents and its relation to puberty. Acta Pædiatr Scand 1987;76:795–800.

39. Rudberg S, Ullman E, Dahlquist G. Relationship between early metabolic control and the development of microalbuminuria – a longitudinal study in children with Type 1 (insulin-dependent) diabetes mellitus. Diabetologia 1993;36:1309–1314.

40. Stephenson JM, Fuller JH, the EURODIAB IDDM Complications Study Group and the WHO Multinational Study of Vascular Disease in Diabetes Study Group. Microalbuminuria is not rare before 5 years of IDDM. J Diab Comp 1994;8:166–173.

41. Bangstad H-J, Østerby R, Dahl-Jørgensen K, Berg KJ, Hartmann A, Hanssen KF. Improvement of blood glucose control in IDDM patients retards the progression of morphological changes in early diabetic nephropathy. Diabetologia 1994;37:483–490.

42. Powrie JK, Watts GF, Ingham JN, Taub NA, Talmud PJ, Shaw KM. Role of glycaemic control in development of microalbuminuria in patients with insulin dependent diabetes. BMJ 1994;309:1608–1612.

43. Klein R, Klein BEK, Moss SE, Cruickshanks KJ. Ten-year incidence of gross proteinuria in people with diabetes. Diabetes 1995;44:916–923.

44. Mortensen HB, Hartling SG, Petersen KE, and the Danish study group of diabetes in childhood. A nation-wide cross-sectional study of glycosylated haemoglobin in Danish children with Type 1 diabetes. Diabetic Med 1988;5:871–876.

45. Mortensen HB, Villumsen J, Vølund Aa, Petersen KE, Nerup J and The Danish Study Group of Diabetes in Childhood. Relationship between insulin injection regimen and metabolic control in young Danish Type 1 diabetic patients. Diabetic Med 1992;9:834–839.

46. Mortensen HB, Hougaard P, for the Hvidøre Study Group on Childhood Diabetes. Comparison of metabolic control in a cross-sectional study of 2873 children and adolescents with IDDM from 18 countries. Diabetes Care 1997; 20:714–720.

47. Mortensen HB, Hougaard P, for the Hvidøre Study Group on Childhood Diabetes. International perspectives in childhood and adolescent diabetes: A review. J Pediatr Endocrinol Metab 1997;10:261–264.

48. Mortensen HB , Robertson KJ et al., for the Hvidøre Study Group on Childhood Diabetes.Insulin management and metabolic control of Type 1 diabetes in childhood and adolescence in 18 countries. Diabetic Med 1998;15:752–759.

49. Holl RW, Grabert M, Thon A, Heinze E. Urinary excretion of albumin in adolescents with type 1 diabetes. Persistent versus intermittent microalbuminuria and relationship to duration of diabetes, sex, and metabolic control. Diabetes Care 1999;22:1555–1560.

50. Schultz CJ, Konopelska-Bamu T, Carroll TA, Stratton I, Gale EAM, Neil A, Dunger D for the Oxford Regional Prospective Study Group. Microalbuminuria prevalence varies with age, sex and puberty in children with type 1 diabetes followed from diagnosis in a longitudinal study. Diabetes Care 1999;22:495–502.

51. Brenner BM, Chertow GM. Congenital oligonephropathy and the etiology of adult hypertension and progressive renal injury. Am J Kidney Dis 1994;23:171–175.

52. Rossing P, Tarnow L, Nielsen FS, Boelskifte S, Brenner BM, Parving H-H. Short stature and diabetic nephropathy. BMJ 1995;310:296–297.

53. Orchard TJ, Dorman JS, Maser RE, Becker DJ, Drash AL, Ellis D, LaPorte RE, Kuller LH. Prevalence of complications in IDDM by sex and duration. Pittsburgh epidemiology of diabetes complications study II. Diabetes 1990;39:1116–1124.

54. The Diabetes Control and Complications Trial Research Group. The effect of intensive treatment of diabetes on the development and progression of long-term complications in insulin-dependent diabetes mellitus. N Engl J Med 1993;329:977–986.

55. Krolewski AS, Laffel LBM, Krolewski M, Quinn M, Warram JH. Glycosylated hemoglobin and the risk of microalbuminuria in patients with insulin-dependent diabetes mellitus. N Engl J Med 1995;332:1251–1255.

56. The Diabetes Control and Complications Trial Research Group. Effect of intensive diabetes treatment on the development and progression of long-term complications in adolescents with insulin-dependent diabetes mellitus. J Pediatr 1994;125:177–188.

57. Danne T, Weber B, Hartmann R, Enders I, Burger W, Hovener G. Long-term glycemic control has a nonlinear association to the frequency of background retinopathy in adolescents with diabetes. Diabetes Care 1994;17:1390–1396.

58. Danne T, Dinesen B, Weber B, Mortensen HB: Threshold of HbA1c for the effect of hypergycaemia on the risk of diabetic micrangiopathy (letter). Diabetes Care 1996;19:183.

59. Lobefalo L, Verrotti A, Della Loggia G, Morgese G, Mastropasqua L, Chiarelli F, Gallenga PE. Diabetic retinopathy in childhood and adolescence. Effects of puberty. Diab Nutr Metab 1997;10:193–197.

60. Davis EA, Keating B, Byrne GC, Russell M, Jones TW. Hypoglycemia: incidence and clinical predictors in a large population-based sample of children and adolescents with IDDM. Diabetes Care 1997;20:22–25.

61. The Diabetes Control and Complications Trial Research Group. Hypoglycemia in the diabetes control and complications trial. Diabetes 1997;46:271–286.

62. Bognetti E, Brunelli A, Meschi F, Viscardi M, Bonfanti R, Chiumello G. Frequency and correlates of severe hypoglycaemia in children and adolescents with diabetes mellitus. Eur J Pediatr 1997:156:589–591.

63. Davis EA, Keating B, Byrne GC, Russell M, Jones TW. Impact of improved glycaemic control on rates of hypoglycaemia in insulin dependent diabetes mellitus. Arch Dis Child 1998;78:111–115.

64. Tupola S, Rajantie J. Documented symptomatic hypoglycemia in children and adolescents using multiple daily insulin injection therapy. Diabetic Med 1998;15:492–496.

65. Rovet JF, Ehrlich RM. The effect of hypoglycemic seizures on cognitive function in children with diabetes: a 7-year prospective study. J Pediatr 1999;134:503–506.

66. Becker DJ, Ryan CM. Intensive diabetes therapy in childhood: Is it achievable? Is it desirable? Is it safe? Editorial. J Pediatr 1999;134:392–394.

67. Hershey T, Bhargva N, Sadler M, White NH, Craft S. Conventional versus intensive diabetes therapy in children with type 1 diabetes. Diabetes Care 1999; 22:1318–1324.

68. Ryan CM. Memory and metabolic control in children (editorial). Diabetes Care 1999;22:1239–1241.

69. Mortensen HB, Hougaard P, Ibsen KK, Parving H-H and The Danish Study Group of Diabetes in Childhood. Relationship between blood pressure and urinary albumin excretion rate in young Danish Type 1 diabetic patients: Comparison to non-diabetic children. Diabetic Med 1994;11:155–161.

70. Kordonouri O, Danne T, Hopfenmüller W, Enders I, Hövener G, Weber B. Lipid profiles and blood pressure: are they risk factors for the development of early background retinopathy and incipient nephropathy in children with insulin-dependent diabetes mellitus. Acta Paediatr 1996;85:43–48.

71. Gorman D, Sochett E, Daneman D. The natural history of microalbuminuria in adolescents with type 1 diabetes. J Pediatr 1999;134:333–337.

72. Bojestig M, Arnqvist HJ, Karlberg BE, Ludvigsson J. Glycemic control and prognosis in Type 1 diabetic patients with microalbuminuria. Diabetes Care 1996; 19:313–317.

73. Mogensen CE. Microalbuminuria as a predictor of clinical diabetic nephropathy. Kidney Int 1987;31:673–689.

74. Mogensen CE, Christensen CK, Christiansen JS, Boyle N, Pederson MM, Schmitz A. Early hyperfiltration and late renal damage in insulin-dependent diabetes. Pediatr Adolesc Endocrinol 1988;17:197–205.

75. Feldt-Rasmussen B, Mathiesen ER, Deckert T, Giese J, Christensen NJ, Bent-Hansen L, Damkjær Nielsen M. Central role for sodium in the pathogenesis of blood pressure changes independent of angiotensin, aldosterone and catecholamines in Type 1 (insulin-dependent) diabetes mellitus. Diabetologia 1987;30:610–617.

76. Deckert T, Kofoed-Enevoldsen A, Nørgaard K, Borch-Johnsen K, Feldt-Rasmussen B, Jensen T. Microalbuminuria: implications for micro- and macrovascular disease. Diabetes Care 1992;15:1181–1191.

77. Cook J, Daneman D, Spino M, Sochett E, Perlman K, Balfe JW. Angiotensin converting enzyme inhibitor therapy to decrease microalbuminuria in normotensive children with insulin-dependent diabetes mellitus. J. Pediatr 1990;117:39–45.

78. Rudberg S, Aperia A, Freyschuss U, Persson B. Enalapril reduces microalbuminuria in young normotensive Type 1 (insulin-dependent) diabetic patients irrespective of its hypotensive effect. Diabetologia 1990;33:470–476.

79. Marre M, Chatellier G, Leblanc H, Guyene TT, Menard J, Passa P. Prevention of diabetic nephropathy with enalapril in normotensive diabetics with microalbuminuria. BMJ 1988;297:1092–1095.

80. Mathiesen ER, Hommel E, Giese J, Parving H-H. Efficacy of captopril in postponing nephropathy in normotensive insulin dependent diabetic patients with microalbuminuria. BMJ 1991;303:81–87.

81. Hallab M, Gallois Y, Chatellier G, Rohmer V, Fressinaud P, Marre M. Comparison of reduction in microalbuminuria by enalapril and hydrochlorothiazide in normotensive patients with insulin dependent diabetes. BMJ 1993;306:175–182.

82. Viberti GC, Mogensen CE, Groop LC, Pauls JF, for the European Microalbuminuria Captopril Study Group. Effect of captopril on progression to clinical proteinuria in patients with insulin-dependent diabetes mellitus and microalbuminuria. JAMA 1994;271:275–279.

83. Breyer JA, Hunsicker LG, Bain RP, Lewis EJ, and The Collaborative Study Group. Angiotensin converting enzyme inhibition in diabetic nephropathy. Kidney Int 1994;45:156–160.

84. Rudberg S, Østerby R, Bangstad H.-J, Dahlquist G, Persson B. Effect of angiotensin converting enzyme inhibitor or beta blocker on glomerular structural changes in young microalbuminuric patients with type 1 (insulin-dependent) diabetes mellitus. Diabetologia 1999;42:589–595.

85. The Microalbuminuria Captopril Study Group (Barnes DJ, Cooper M, Gans DJ, Laffel L, Mogensen CE, Viberti GC. Captopril reduces the risk of nephropathy in insulin-dependent diabetic patients with microalbuminuria. Diabetologia 1996; 39:587–593.

86. Chaturvedi N, Sjolie A-K, Stephenson JM, Abrahamian H, Keipes M, Castellarin A, Rogulja-Pepeonik Z, Fuller JH, and the EUCLID Study Group. Effect of lisinopril on progression of retinopathy in normotensive people with Type 1 diabetes. Lancet 1998;351:28–31.

87. Mathiesen ER, Rønn B, Jensen T, Storm B, Deckert T. Relation between blood pressure and urinary albumin excretion in development of microalbuminuria. Diabetes 1990;39:245–249.

88. Zusman RM. Renin- and non-renin-mediated antihypertensive actions of converting enzyme inhibitors. Kidney Int 1984;25:969–83.

89. Anderson S, Brenner BM. Pathogenesis of diabetic glomerulopathy: Hemodynamic considerations: Diabetes Metab Rev 1988;4:163–177.

90. Frohlich ED, Cooper RA, Lewis EJ. Review of the overall experience of captopril in hypertension. Arch Intern Med 1984;144:1441–1444.

91. Mirkin BL, Newman TJ. Efficacy and safety of captopril in the treatment of severe childhood hypertension: report of the International Collaborative Study Group. Pediatrics 1985;75:1091–1100.

92. Shield JPH. Microalbuminuria and nephropathy in childhood diabetes. Practical Diabetes 1994;11:146–149.

93. Chiarelli F, Trotta D, Verrotti A, Mohn A. Treatment of hypertension and microalbuminuria in children and adolescents with type 1 diabetes (Review). Pediatric Diabetes 2002:3:113-124

94. Moore THM, Shield JPH. Prevalence of abnormal urinary albumin excretion in adolescents and children with insulin dependent diabetes : The MIDAC study. Arch Dis Child 2000:83:239-243

95. Jones CA, Leese QP, KerrS, Bestwick K, Isherwood DI. Development and progression of microalbuminuria in a clinic sample of patients with insulin dependent diabetes mellitus. Arch Dis Child 1995:78:518-523.

96. Barkai L, Vamosi I, Lukacs K. Enhanced progression of urinary albumin excretion in IDDM during puberty. Diabetes Care 1998:21:1019-1023

97. Danne T, Kordonouri O, Hovener G, Weber B. Diabetic angiopathy in children. Diabet Med 1997:14:1012-1025

98. Schultz CJ, Konopelska-Bahu T, Dalton RN etal. Microalbuminuria prevalence varies with age, sex and puberty in children with type 1 diabetes followed from diagnosis in a longitudinal study. Oxford Regional Prospective Study Group. Diabetes Care 1999:22:495-502

99   Gorman D, Sochett E, Daneman. The natural history of microalbuminuria in adolescents with type 1 diabetes. J Pediatr 1999:134:333-337

100 Rudberg S, Østerby R. Diabetic glomerulopathy in young IDDM patients. Preventive and diagnostic aspects. Horm Res 1998:50 (Suppl 1) :17-22.

101 Rudberg S, Dahlquist G. Determinants of progression of microalbuminuria in adolescents with IDDM. Diabetes Care 1996:19:369-371.

102. Olsen BS, Sjølie AK, Hougaard P, Johannesen J, Borch-Johnsen K, Marinelli K, Thorsteinsson B, Pramming S, Mortensen HB and the Danish Study Group of Diabetes in Childhood. A 6 year nation-wide cohort study of glycemic control in young people with type 1 diabetes. Risk markers for the development of retinopathy, nephropathy and neuropathy. Journal of Diabetes and its Complications 2000; 14:295-300

103. Schultz CJ, Neil HAW, Dalton RN, Dunger DB. Risk of nephropathy can be detected before the onset of microalbuminuria during the early years after diagnosis of type 1 diabetes. Diabetes Care 2000:23:1811-1815,

104 Warram JH, Scott LJ, Hanna LS, Wantman M, Cohen SE, Laffel LMB, Ryan L, Krolewski AS. Progression of microalbuminuria to proteinuria in type 1 diabetes. Diabetes 2000:49:94-1000

105. Lafferty AR, Werther GA, Clarke CF. Ambulatory blood pressure, microalbuminuria, and autonomic neuropathy in adolescents with type 1 diabetes. Diabetes Care 2000,23:533-538.

106. Collado-Mesa F, Colhoun HM, Stevens LK et al. Prevalence and management of hypertension in type 1 diabetes mellitus in Europe: The EUROPEAN IDDM Complications study. Diabet Med 1999:16:41-48.

107. Schultz CJ, Neil HAW, Dalton RN, Bahu TK, Dunger DB. Blood pressure does not rise before the onset of microalbuminuria in children followed from diagnosis of type 1 diabetes. Diabetes Care 2001:24:555-560

27

EARLY RENAL HYPERFUNCTION AND HYPERTROPHY IN IDDM, INCLUDING COMMENTS ON EARLY INTERVENTION

Margrethe Mau Pedersen
Department of Internal Medicine and Cardiology, Aarhus University Hospital, Denmark

Diabetic nephropathy is the main cause of reduced survival in insulin-dependent diabetes. Much interest is paid to early alterations in kidney function and structure, since a relationship may exist between such early abnormalities and later development of diabetic nephropathy. A modest increase in urinary albumin excretion, microalbuminuria, has been identified as an early marker of diabetic nephropathy, and therapeutical intervention postponing the onset of overt nephropathy has been introduced. Characteristic renal changes before the onset of microalbuminuria are glomerular hyperfunction and renal hypertrophy, and in this chapter these abnormalities will be addressed.

GLOMERULAR HYPERFUNCTION

From the onset of IDDM, kidney function is characterised by elevation of glomerular filtration rate (GFR) and renal plasma flow (RPF) [for reviews see 1,2]. Using precise measurements e.g. renal clearance of inulin or iothalamate, it has been found, that mean GFR in groups of short-term IDDM patients is increased by 15-25% - to approximately 135-140 ml/min/1.73m^2 during 'usual metabolic control' [3-7]. Before start of insulin treatment, but in the absence of ketoacidosis, glomerular hyperfiltration is even more pronounced, often showing elevations of approximately 40% [8,9]. RPF is elevated synchronously with the increase in GFR, but less pronounced [3,5]. Estimation of RPF from renal clearance of hippuran appears to be a reliable measure also in the diabetic state [10].

During the first one or two decades of diabetes glomerular hyperfunction remains a characteristic feature of kidney function. In cross-sectional studies patients with microalbuminuria - typically developed after 10 to 15 years of diabetes - show more pronounced hyperfiltration than normoalbuminuric patients [7,11]. However, no prospective studies have described the individual course in GFR during transmission from normo- to microalbuminuria. With further increase in albumin excretion and development of nephropathy, GFR and RPF start to decline, whereas in patients with persistent normoalbuminuria a moderate degree of glomerular hyperfunction persists [12].

Early renal changes in experimental diabetes in some degree parallel the characteristic glomerular hyperfunction in early stages of human diabetes. As described elsewhere in this book, besides hyperperfusion, increased intraglomerular hydraulic pressure is an important factor in hyperfiltration in diabetic animals. In humans the larger increase in GFR than RPF (increased filtration fraction) suggests similar intraglomerular hypertension. However, elevation of the ultrafiltration coefficient due to increased filtration surface may also represent a mechanism for the increased filtration fraction [13].

RENAL HYPERTROPHY

Kidney volume estimated from ultrasonic techniques or roentgenographically, like GFR is markedly increased from the debut of diabetes. During initial insulin-treatment, kidney hypertrophy is somewhat reduced. The relative reduction in kidney volume is apparently delayed and smaller than the relative lowering of GFR [14]. The mean size remains elevated by approximately 20-30% during short-term IDDM [5,15-17]. At this stage, kidney volume is strongly correlated to GFR, corresponding to the state in non-diabetic subjects, and in most forms of non-diabetic renal hypertrophy [18]. Later in the course of diabetes this association cannot be found and possibly kidney volume increases further in the microalbuminuric state [19]. Hypertrophy persists also after the onset of overt nephropathy. Morphologically, studies concerning the initial renal enlargement show glomerular and tubular hypertrophy [20,21]. Subsequently PAS-positive material is deposited in the glomerular tuft and further enlargement of open glomeruli occurs, however, without influencing total kidney volume.

DETERMINANTS FOR GLOMERULAR HYPERFUNCTION AND HYPERTROPHY

The pathophysiological mechanisms behind the increased glomerular filtration rate and renal plasma flow are still not fully clarified. Several intervention studies in human and experimental diabetes have suggested various substances of specific importance. Such factors with a possible involvement in glomerular hyperfunction are listed in table 1. Many factors, however, may represent normal modulators of kidney function influenced by an abnormal metabolic milieu and changes in fluid homeostasis. Furthermore, many of these factors are interrelated and represent different steps in regulatory mechanisms.

The abnormal carbohydrate metabolism no doubt plays a key-role in development of glomerular hyperfunction. An increase in blood glucose concentration is associated with vasodilation in a number of tissues including the glomerular capillaries [22,23]. Suggested mechanisms for this vasodilation include an osmotic effect on cells lining small vessels [24], an increase in production of kallikrein and endothelium-derived-relaxing-factor (EDRF) [25,26], and increased production of vasodilator prostaglandins [27]. Furthermore, the increased amount of filtered and reabsorbed glucose coupled to increased tubular sodium reabsorption may suppress the tubuloglomerular feedback system and thereby contribute to hyperfiltration [25,28]. In human IDDM the influence of elevated blood glucose on GFR and RPF has been investigated through intervention studies with glucose administration, through studies with intensified insulin treatment, and through cross-sectional studies analysing correlations between metabolic status and kidney function. In IDDM patients a rise in blood glucose by glucose infusion or an oral glucose load increases GFR and RPF in some studies [29-31]. Results, however, have not been completely uniform [32-34], maybe due to different responses in different subgroups of diabetic patients [33,34]. In studies with intensified insulin treatment, a few days of strict metabolic control has not been found to reduce GFR [35], whereas a reduction in GFR was observed during long-term (2 years) insulin pump treatment [36]. In cross sectional studies a correlation between GFR and HbA_{1c} and between intra-individual variation in blood glucose and in RPF has been reported [37,38,86]. Taken together these studies suggest that the 'acute' glucose level is associated mainly to RPF, whereas long-term metabolic control (e.g. represented by HbA_{1c}) shows a closer correlation to GFR. It may be that e.g. biochemical membrane properties are important to the long-term influence of glycemic control of GFR.

Another aspect of hyperglycaemia is enhanced glucose metabolism through the polyol pathway in tissues with insulin-independent glucose uptake. High activity of the enzyme aldose reductase leads to sorbitol accumulation and probably to changes in the redox state. These alterations, which appear to be rather closely linked to depletion of myoinositol [39], have been related to development of late diabetic complications in different tissues and recently also to glomerular hyperfiltration [40-42]. In normoalbuminuric diabetic patients we found that acute ($\leq$ 3 days) and long-term (6 months) aldose reductase inhibition markedly reduced hyperfiltration [40,41].

An increase in blood concentration of ketone bodies also accompanies fairly well-regulated diabetes and intervention studies have suggested this to be of significance for hyperfiltration and hyperperfusion [43]. However, no statistical correlation has been demonstrated between the concentration of ketone bodies and GFR or RPF.

Besides the indirect effect of insulin deficiency on renal hemodynamics through the blood glucose level, it has been suggested that inadequate delivery of insulin to the liver is associated with increased production of renal vasoregulatory factors [44]. In diabetic patients conventional insulin treatment with subcutaneous injections give rise to such portal hypoinsulinaemia, while hyperinsulinaemia is found in the systemic circulation [44]. No influence of insulin per se on GFR and RPF has been found [45].

A consequence of hyperglycaemia and peripheral hyperinsulinaemia appears to be an increase in total exchangeable body sodium and extracellular volume expansion [4,46]. Apart from an influence on the tubuloglomerular feedback system, this condition might induce hyperfiltration through a reflectoric increase in atrial natriuretic peptide (ANP).

ANP has been shown to increase GFR and FF in microalbuminuric IDDM patients [87]. A significant role for ANP in hyperfiltration is also suggested by experimental studies in animals showing marked reductions in GFR during treatment with anti-ANP serum [27,47] or an ANP-receptor antagonist [48]. In our study on intra-individual variation in kidney function [38] an involvement of ANP in the mechanisms behind human diabetic hyperfiltration was indicated by the finding of a close co-variation between GFR and ANP (figure 1).

Table 1. Factors with possible involvement in early diabetic glomerular hyperfunction including suggested intermediary steps (indicated in brackets).

Metabolic factors:	Blood glucose Long-term glycemic control (HbA$_{1c}$) Activity of polyol pathway Ketone bodies	[bradykinin, EDRF, prostaglandins]
Hormonal/peptide substances:	GH, IGF-I Glucagon Insulin (peripheral hyperinsulinemia, hepatic insulinpenia) Atrial natriuretic peptide Kallikrein, bradykinin, kinin Catecholamines (abnormal response) Arginine vasopressin C-peptide (lack of)	[prostaglandins] [restraining effect from adenosine] [nitric oxide]
Other vasoactive substances:	Vasodilatory prostaglandins Endothelial derived relaxing factor (EDRF) Nitric oxide	
Dietary factors other than carbohydrates	Protein intake kallikrein, adenosine, Fat intake Vitamin E	[glucagon, prostaglandins, dopamine, nitric oxide] [reduced oxidative stress]
Genetic factors	Angiotensin converting enzyme gene polymorphism	

References : 22-27,29-44,47-54,56-60,64-70, 86-91, 96-97, 100-102

Growth hormone (GH) and glucagon represent possible mediators of diabetic hyperfiltration. Both hormones induce elevation in GFR when injected (through GH not acutely) [49,50]; increased plasma levels of the hormones may be brought about by the diabetic state, and a statistical correlation between plasma levels and GFR has been reported for both hormones [51]. The influence of GH is apparently indirect - acting through insulin-like growth factor I (IGF-I) [52]. Glucagon seems mainly to be of significance for hyperfiltration in poorly regulated diabetic patients [50].

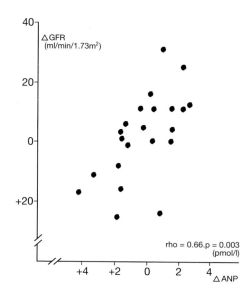

Fig. 1 Intra-individual variation in glomerular filtration rate (ΔGFR) in relation to variation in plasma concentration of atrial natriuretic peptide (ΔANP) in 22 patients with IDDM. 0.66 , p=0.003. From Mau Pedersen et al [38, with permission].

Protein intake plays a special role in diabetic hyperfiltration in the sense that it represents a iatrogenic stimulator of GFR. It is well-know that protein meals and infusion of aminoacids increases GFR [53]. Typically, diabetic diets have a higher protein content than non-diabetic diets [54,55]. By lowering protein intake from 19 to 12% we observed a decrease in mean GFR from 146 to 132 ml/min/1.73m^2 in a group of normoalbuminuric IDDM patients [54]. The type of protein ingested seems to be of importance to the magnitude of influence on GFR [56,57] Furthermore, the content of phosphate may be relevant [58].

Lately, attention has been paid to a possible beneficial effect of antioxidants, especially vitamin E, on diabetic complications. In early, uncomplicated diabetes, it has been reported that vitamin E reduces glomerular hyperfiltration [88]. However, in this study creatinine clearance from overnight urine collections was used as a measure for GFR. To solve the issue, further investigations with more precise measurements of GFR, will be needed.

Polymorphism in the angiotensin converting enzyme (ACE) gene has been suggested as a genetic factor that may influence the risk of developing nephropathy. It has been found that an insertion/deletion (I/D) polymorphism is important for the plasma ACE level, and that the allele D is associated with high plasma ACE-concentration and with increased risk of developing nephropathy [89]. With respect to glomerular hyperfiltration, no final conclusion on a possible association between the ACE-gene polymorphism and GFR can be drawn from available studies [90-92]. It has been indicated, however, that the genotype may be important by influencing the way renal hemodynamics respond to increases in blood glucose [92]. Thus, in patients with the DD genotype a rise in GFR and RPF has been observed when blood glucose is changed from normo- to hyperglycemia as opposed to findings for the II genotype.

With respect to renal hypertrophy glycemic control is a determinant for kidney volume during the early stage of IDDM, as described above. It is unclarified whether kidney volume may still be modulated by alterations in glycemic control after years of diabetes and during the microalbuminuric state [19,59,60]. Knowledge on other pathogenetic factors in renal hypertrophy in human diabetes is limited. Experimental studies points towards GH/IGF-1 as contributors to very early kidney growth [52] (see also chapter 23), and also a cross-sectional study in human diabetes suggest a role for growth factor in kidney hypertrophy [93]. Furthermore, studies in experimental diabetes indicate that renal hypertrophy is associated with increased activity of the transforming growth factor-beta (TGF-β) system [63, 94,95] and with a depressed protein degradation due to reduced proteinase activity in both glomeruli and tubuli [61,62]. In experimental diabetes the lack of C-peptide has also been suggested to contribute to renal hypertrophy and enlargement of glomeruli. Thus C-peptide replacement in diabetic rats has prevented these abnormalities (D)

POSSIBLE ROLE OF HYPERFILTRATION AS A RISK MARKER FOR DIABETIC NEPHROPATHY

In certain IDDM patients, glomerular hyperfiltration is especially marked and sustained during many years, and it has been suggested that such hyperfiltration represents a pathogenetic factor for later development of diabetic nephropathy. This suspicion is supported by the apparent analogy between the characteristic early renal hemodynamic changes in human IDDM and in animal models of diabetes. Thus, in experimental diabetes a normalisation of the high GFR or the high intraglomerular hydraulic pressure by pharmacological or dietary means, has attenuated progression of renal disease [71]. In human diabetes retrospective data has suggested that marked hyperfiltration is associated with later nephropathy [12,72]. Two studies later questioned these early observations (75,76), but long-term prospective studies have confirmed an associations between glomerular hyperfiltration and later development of nephropathy. In a swedish cohort of normoalbuminuric adolescent patients multiple regression analysis after 8 years identified glomerular hyperfiltration as a strong independent predictor for nephropathy (73). The same cohort of diabetic patients has recently been studied after another 8-10 years ie. 16-18 years after baseline examination (diabetes duration 29 ± 3 years) [103]. Of 75 patients included at baseline, 60 patients participated in the recent follow-up study. It was found that 32% of the patients had developed either persistent micro- or macroalbuminuria. It is noteworthy that 6 out of 7 patients with persistent macroalbuminuria and 10 of 12 with persistent microalbuminuria had an increased GFR at baseline. Approximately half of the patients with initial glomerular hyperfiltration showed progression to micro- or macroalbuminuria. When adjusted for duration of diabetes increased baseline GFR represented a risk factor for later development of micro- or macroalbuminuria with odds ratio 5.44. Also in a group of diabetic children, studied during 10 years, hyperfiltration was found to predict later development of microalbuminuria [74].

Concerning a possible association between hyperfiltration and development of morphological renal abnormalities, this was recently investigated in a follow-up study in adolescent IDDM patients before the stage of microalbuminuria [98]. This biopsy study reported a positive correlation between mesangial matrix volume fraction and the filtration fraction measured repeatedly during years before the biopsy. Filtration fraction also correlated to basement membrane thickness.

486

Indirect evidence for a pathogenetic role of abnormal renal hemodynamics is found in the marked slowing of early renal disease observed during antihypertensive treatment. This especially applies for ACE-inhibitors, which are considered to reduce intraglomerular pressure more specifically than other antihypertensives [78]. In a pilot study treatment with an ACE-inhibitor reduced both albumin excretion and kidney volume in microalbuminuric, normotensive IDDM patients [79].

Addressing kidney hypertrophy rather than hemodynamic parameters, a recent sonographic study in IDDM patients has indicated that large kidneys may be a morphological marker for later diabetic nephropathy [99].

POSSIBILITIES FOR INTERVENTIONS

An obvious goal for therapeutic intervention is to optimize glycemic control in order to decrease the risk of late complications. Such therapy will tend to reduce hyperfiltration as discussed above. However, since the pathogenetic basis for the association between glomerular hyperfiltration and later nephropathy is still not clarified, non-glycemic therapy against glomerular hyperfiltration is not presently indicated. It seems rational though, not to prescribe higher protein content in diabetic than in non-diabetic diets to avoid inducing additional hyperfiltration.

Future possibilities for non-glycemic pharmacological intervention include aldose reductase inhibitors, aiming at normalization of the polyol pathway activity [40-42], and treatment with somatostatin analogues [80-82], which may act on GFR through a lowering of GH (or IGF-I) and a suppression of glucagon secretion. Until now these interventions have been tested only in rather short term or small scale studies and the possible long-term benefits await further investigation.

Also ACE-inhibitors may represent candidates for early interventions. Although these agents have not generally been found to reduce GFR, their ability to reduce filtration fraction and probably intraglomerular pressure [83] may prove valuable also before the onset of microalbuminuria [84]. In addition to the hemodynamic effects of ACE-inhibitors, these drugs may also be valuable through attenuation of the growth stimulating effect of ANG II [85].

REFERENCES

1. Mogensen CE. Glomerular hyperfiltration in human diabetes. Diabetes Care 1994; 17: 770-775.
2. Bank N. Mechanisms of diabetic hyperfiltration. Nephrology Forum. Kidney Int 1991; 40: 792-807.
3. Mogensen CE. Glomerular filtration rate and renal plasma flow in short-term and long-term juvenile diabetes mellitus. Scand J Clin Lab Invest 1971; 28: 91-100.
4. Ditzel J, Schwartz M. Abnormally increased glomerular filtration rate in short-term insulin-treated diabetic subjects. Diabetes 1976; 16: 264-267.
5. Christensen JS, Gammelgaard J, Frandsen M, Parving H-H. Increased kidney size, glomerular filtration rate and renal plasma flow in short-term insulin-dependent diabetics. Diabetologia 1981; 20: 451-456.
6. Brøchner-Mortensen J, Ditzel J. Glomerular filtration rate and extracellular fluid volume in insulin-dependent patients with diabetes mellitus. Kidney Int 1982; 21: 696-698.
7. Hansen KW, Mau Pedersen M, Christensen CK, Schmitz A, Christiansen JS, Mogensen CE. Normoalbuminuria ensures no reduction of renal function in type 1 (insulin-dependent) diabetic patients. J Intern Med 1992; 232: 161-167.
8. Mogensen CE. Kidney function and glomerular permeability to macromolecules in juvenile diabetes. Dan Med Bull 1972; 19: 1-36.
9. Christiansen JS, Gammelgaard J, Tronier B, Svendsen PA, Parving H-H. Kidney function and size in diabetics before and during initial insulin treatment. Kidney Int 1982; 21: 683-688.
10. Nyberg G, Granerus G, Aurell M. Renal extraction ratios for ^{51}Cr-EDTA, PAH, and glucose in early insulin-dependent diabetic patients. Kidney Int 1982; 21: 706-708.
11. Christensen CK, Mogensen CE. The course of incipient diabetic nephropathy: studies of albumin excretion and blood pressure. Diabetic Med 1985; 2: 97-102.
12. Mogensen CE, Christensen CK. Predicting diabetic nephropathy in insulin-dependent patients. N Engl J Med 1984; 311: 89-93.
13. Ellis EN, Steffes MW, Coetz FC, Sutherland DER, Mauer SM. Glomerular filtration surface in type 1 diabetes mellitus. Kidney Int 1986; 29: 889-894.
14. Christiansen JS, Frandsen M, Parving H-H. The effect of intravenous insulin infusion on kidney function in insulin-dependent diabetes mellitus. Diabetologia 1981; 20: 199-204.
15. Mogensen CE, Andersen MJF. Increased kidney size and glomerular filtration rate in early juvenile diabetes. Diabetes 1973; 22: 706-713.
16. Mogensen CE, Andersen MJF. Increased kidney size and glomerular filtration rate in untreated juvenile diabetes: Normalization by insulin-treatment. Diabetologia 1975; 11: 221-224.
17. Puig JG, Antón FM, Grande C, Pallardo LF, Arnalich F, Gil A, Vázquez JJ, García AM. Relation on kidney size to kidney function in early insulin-dependent diabetes. Diabetologia 1981; 21: 363-367.
18. Schwieger J, Fine LG. Renal hypertrophy, growth factors, and nephropathy in diabetes mellitus. Semin Nephrol 1990; 10: 242-253.
19. Feldt-Rasmussen B, Hegedüs L, Mathiesen ER, Deckert T. Kidney volume in type 1 (insulin-dependent) diabetic patients with normal or increased urinary albumin excretion: effect of long-term improved metabolic control. Scand J Lab Invest 1991; 51: 31-36.
20. Østerby R, Gundersen HJG. Glomerular size and structure in diabetes mellitus: I. Early abnormalities. Diabetologia 1975; 11: 225-229.

21. Seyer-Hansen K, Hansen J, Gundersen HJG. Renal hypertrophy in experimental diabetes: a morphometric study. Diabetologia 1980; 18: 501-505.

22. Mathiesen ER, Hilsted J, Feldt-Rasmussen B, Bonde-Petersen F, Christensen NJ, Parving H-H. The effect of metabolic control on hemodynamics in short-term insulin-dependent diabetic patients. Diabetes 1985; 34: 1301-1305.

23. Wolpert HA, Kinsley BT, Clermont AC, Wald H, Bursell S-E. Hyperglycaemia modulates retinal hemodynamics in IDDM. Diabetes 1993; 42: A489.

24. Gray SD. Effect of hypertonicity on vascular dimensions in skeletal muscle. Microvasc Res 1971; 3: 117-124.

25. Bank N. Mechanisms of diabetic hyperfiltration. Kidney Int 1991; 40: 792-807.

26. Harvey JN, Edmundson AW, Jaffa AA, Martin LL, Mayfield RK. Renal excretion of kallikrein and eicosanoids in patients with Type 1 (insulin-dependent) diabetes mellitus. Relationship to glomerular and tubular function. Diabetologia 1992; 35: 857-862.

27. Perico N, Benigni A, Gabanelli M, Piccinelli A, Rog M, De-Riva C, Remuzzi G. Atrial natriuretide peptide and prostacyclin synergistically mediate hyperfiltration and hyperperfusion of diabetic rats. Diabetes 1992; 41: 533-538.

28. Blantz RC, Peterson OW, Gushwa L, Tucker BJ. Effect of modest hyperglycaemia on tubuloglomerular feedback activity. Kidney Int 1982; 22: S206-S212.

29. Christiansen JS, Christensen CK, Hermansen K, Pedersen EB, Mogensen CE. Enhancement of glomerular filtration rate and renal plasma flow by oral glucose load in well controlled insulin-dependent diabetics. Scand J Clin Lab Invest 1986; 46: 265-272.

30. Christiansen JS, Frandsen M, Parving H-H. Effect of intravenous glucose infusion on renal function in normal man and in insulin-dependent diabetics. Diabetologia 1981; 21: 368-373.

31. Wiseman MJ, Mangili R, Alberetto M, Keen H, Viberti GC. Glomerular response mechanisms to glycemic changes in insulin-dependent diabetics. Kidney Int 1987; 31: 1012-1018.

32. Mogensen CE. Glomerular filtration rate and renal plasma flow in normal and diabetic man during elevation of blood sugar levels. Scand J Clin Lab Invest 1971; 28: 177-182.

33. Marre M, Dubin T, Hallab M, Berrut G, Bouhanick B, Lejeune J-J, Fressinaud P. Different renal response to hyperglycaemia in insulin-dependent diabetics at risk for, or protected against diabetic nephropathy. Diabetes 1993; 42: A423.

34. Skøtt P, Vaag A, Hother-Nielsen O, Andersen P, Bruun NE, Giese J, Beck-Nielsen H, Parving H-H. Effects of hyperglycaemia on kidney function, atrial natriuretic factor and plasma renin in patients with insulin-dependent diabetes mellitus. Scand J Clin Lab Invest 1991; 51: 715-727.

35. Mathiesen ER, Gall M-A, Hommel E, Skøtt P, Parving H-H. Effects of short-term strict metabolic control on kidney function and extracellular fluid volume in incipient diabetic nephropathy. Diabetic Med 1989; 6: 595-600.

36. Christensen CK, Christiansen JS, Schmitz A, Christensen T, Hermansen K, Mogensen CE. Effect of continuous subcutaneous insulin infusion on kidney function and size in IDDM patients - a two years controlled study. J Diabetes and Its Complications 1987; 1: 91-95.

37. Mogensen CE, Christensen CK, Mau Pedersen M, Alberti KGMM, Boye N, Christensen T, Christiansen JS, Flyvbjerg A, Ingerslev J, Schmitz A, Ørskov H. Renal and glycemic determinants of glomerular hyperfiltration in normoalbuminuric diabetics. J Diabetic Compl 1990; 4: 159-165.

38. Mau Pedersen M, Christiansen JS, Pedersen EB, Mogensen CE. Determinants of intra-individual variation in kidney function in normoalbuminuric insulin-dependent diabetic patients: importance of atrial natriuretic peptide and glycemic control. Clin Sci 1992; 83: 445-451.

39. Greene DA, Lattimer SA, Sima AAF. Sorbitol, phosphoinositides, and sodium-potassium-ATPase in the pathogenesis of diabetic complications. N Engl J Med 1987; 316: 599-606.

40. Mau Pedersen M, Christiansen JS, Mogensen CE. Reduction of glomerular hyperfiltration in normoalbuminuric IDDM patients by 6 mo of aldose reductase inhibition. Diabetes 1991; 40: 527-531.

41. Mau Pedersen M, Mogensen CE, Christiansen JS. Reduction of glomerular hyperfunction during short-term aldose reductase inhibition in normoalbuminuric, insulin-dependent diabetic patients. Endocrinol Metab 1995; 2: 55-62.

42. Passariello N, Sepe J, Marrazzo G, De Cicco A, Peluso A, Pisano MCA, Sgambato S, Tesauro P, D'Onofrio F. Effect of aldose reductase inhibitor (tolrestat) on urinary albumin excretion rate in IDDM subjects with nephropathy. Diabetes Care 1993; 16: 789-795.

43. Trevisan R, Nosadini R, Fioretto P, Avogaro A, Duner E, Iori E, Valerio A, Doria A, Crepaldi G. Ketone bodies increase glomerular filtration rate in normal man and in patients with type 1 (insulin dependent) diabetes. Diabetologia 1987; 30: 214-221.

44. Gwinup G, Elias AN. Hypothesis. Insulin is responsible for the vascular complications of diabetes. Med Hypotheses 1991; 34: 1-6.

45. Christiansen JS, Frandsen M, Parving H-H. The effect of intravenous insulin infusion on kidney function in insulin-dependent diabetes mellitus. Diabetologia 1981; 20: 199-204.

46. Skøtt P, Hother-Nielsen O, Bruun NE, Giese J, Nielsen MD, Beck-Nielsen H, Parving H-H. Effects of insulin on kidney function and sodium excretion in healthy subjects. Diabetologia 1989; 32: 694-699.

47. Ortola FV, Ballermann BJ, Anderson S, Mendez RE, Brenner BM. Elevated plasma atrial natriuretic peptide levels in diabetic rats. Potential mediator of hyperfiltration. J Clin Invest 1987; 80: 670-674.

48. Kikkawa R, Haneda M, Sakamoto K, Koya D, Shikano T, Nakanishi S, Matsuda Y, Shigeta Y. Antagonist for atrial natriuretic peptide receptors ameliorates glomerular hyperfiltration in diabetic rats. Biochem Biophys Res Commun 1993; 193: 700-705.

49. Christiansen JS, Gammelgaard J, Frandsen M, Ørskov H, Parving H-H. Kidney function and size in normal subjects before and during growth hormone administration for one week. Eur J Clin Invest 1981; 11: 487-490.

50. Parving H-H, Christiansen JS, Noer I, Tronier B, Mogensen CE. The effect of glucagon infusion on kidney function in short-term insulin-dependent juvenile diabetics. Diabetologia 1980; 19: 350-354.

51. Hoogenberg K, Dullaart RPF, Freling NJM, Meijer S, Sluiter WJ. Contributory roles of circulatory glucagon and growth hormone to increased renal haemodynamics in type 1 (insulin-dependent) diabetes mellitus. Scand J Clin Lab Invest 1993; 53: 821-828.

52. Flyvbjerg A. »The role of insulin-like growth factor I in initial renal hypertrophy in experimental diabetes.« In *Growth Hormone and Insulin-Like Growth Factor I*. Flyvbjerg A, Ørskov H, Alberti KGMM, eds. John Wiley & Sons Ltd., 1993; pp 271-306.

53. Castellino P, Hunt W, DeFronzo RA. Regulation of renal hemodynamics by plasma amino acid and hormone concentrations. Kidney Int 1987; 32: S-15-S-20.

54. Mau Pedersen M, Mogensen CE, Schönau Jørgensen F, Møller B, Lykke G, Pedersen O. Renal effects from limitation of high dietary protein in normoalbuminuric diabetic patients. Kidney Int 1989; 36: S-115-S-121.

55.   Mau Pedersen M, Winther E, Mogensen CE. Reducing protein in the diabetic diet. Diabete Metab (Paris) 1990; 16: 454-459.
56.   Jones MG, Lee K, Swaminathan R. The effect of dietary protein on glomerular filtration rate in normal subjects. Clin Nephrol 1987; 27: 71-75.
57.   Pecis M, de Azevedo MJ, Gross JL. Chicken and fish diet reduces glomerular hyperfiltration in IDDM patients. Diabetes Care 1994; 17: 665-672.
58.   Kraus ES, Cheng L, Sikorski I, Spector DA. Effects of phosphorus restriction on renal response to oral and intravenous protein loads in rats. Am J Physiol 1993; 264: F752-F759.
59.   Tuttle KR, Bruto JL, Perusek MC, Lancaster JL, Kopp DT, DeFronzo RA. Effect of strict glycemic control on renal hemodynamic response to amino acids and renal enlargement in insulin-dependent diabetes mellitus. N Engl J Med 1991; 324: 1626-1632.
60.   Wisemann MJ, Saunders AJ, Keen H, Viberti GC. Effect of blood glucose control on increased glomerular filtration rate and kidney size in insulin-dependent diabetes. N Engl J Med 1985; 312: 617-621.
61.   Shechter P, Boner G, Rabkin R. Tubular cell protein degradation in early diabetic renal hypertrophy. J Am Soc Nephrol 1994; 4: 1582-1587.
62.   Schaefer L, Schaefer RM, Ling, Teschner M, Heidland A. Renal proteinases and kidney hypertrophy in experimental diabetes. Diabetologia 1994; 37: 567-571.
63.   Shankland SJ, Scholey JW, Ly H, Thai K. Expression of transforming growth factor-ß1 during diabetic renal hypertrophy. Kidney Int 1994; 46: 430-442.
64.   Wang YX, Brooks DP. The role of adenosine in glycine-induced glomerular hyperfiltration in rats. J Pharmacol Exp Ther 1992; 263: 1188-1194.
65.   Angielski S, Redlak M, Szczepanska KM. Intrarenal adenosine prevents hyperfiltration induced by atrial natriuretic factor. Miner Electrolyte Metab 1990; 16: 57-60.
66.   Wang YX, Gellai M, Brooks DP. Dopamine DA1 receptor agonist, fenoldopam, reverses glycine-induced hyperfiltration in rats. Am J Physiol 1992; 262: F1055-F1060.
67.   Jaffa AA, Vio CP, Silva RH, Vavrek RJ, Stewart JM, Rust PF, Mayfield RK. Evidence for renal kinins as mediators of amino acid-induced hyperfusion and hyperfiltration in the rat. J Clin Invest 1992; 89: 1460-1468.
68.   Friedlander G, Blanchet BF, Nitenberg A, Laborie C, Assan R, Amiel C. Glucagon secretion is essential for aminoacid-induced hyperfiltration in man. Nephrol Dial Transplant 1990; 5: 110-117.
69.   Johansson BL, Kernell A, Sjöberg S, Wahren J. Influence of combined C-peptide and insulin administration on renal function and metabolic control in diabetes type 1. J Clin Endocrinol Metab 1993; 77: 976-981.
70.   Bouhanick B, Suraniti S, Berrut G, Bled F, Simard G, Lejeune JJ, Fressinaud P, Marre M. Relationship between fat intake and glomerular filtration rate in normotensive insulin-dependent diabetic patients. Diabete Metab (Paris) 1995; 21: 168-172.
71.   Hostetter TH. Diabetic nephropathy. Metabolic versus hemodynamic considerations. Diabetes Care 1992; 15: 1205-1215.
72.   Mogensen CE. Early glomerular hyperfiltration in insulin-dependent diabetics and late nephropathy. Scand J Clin Lab Invest 1986; 46: 201-206.
73.   Rudberg S, Persson B, Dalqvist G. Increased glomerular filtration rate predicts diabetic nephropathy-results form an 8 year prospective study. Kidney Int 1992; 41: 822-828.
74.   Chirelli F, Verrotti A, Morgese G. Glomerular hyperfiltration increases the risk of developing microalbuminuria in diabetic children. Pediatr Nephrol 1995; 9: 154-158.

75. Lervang H-H, Jensen S, Brøchner-Mortensen J, Ditzel J. Does increased glomerular filtration rate or disturbed tubular function early in the course of childhood type 1 diabetes predict the development of nephropathy? Diabetic Med 1992; 9: 635-640.

76. Yip WJ, Jones LS, Wiseman JM, Hill C, Viberti GC. Glomerular hyperfiltration in the prediction of nephropahty in IDDM. Diabetes vol. 45, dec. 1996; 1729-1733.

77. Anderson S. Renal effects of converting enzyme inhibitors in hypertension and diabetes. J Cardiovasc Pharmacol 1990; 15: Suppl. 3: S11-S15.

78. Mau Pedersen M, Christensen CK, Hansen KW, Christiansen JS, Mogensen CE. ACE-inhibition and renoprotection in early diabetic nephropathy. Response to enalapril acutely and in long-term combination with conventional antihypertensive treatment. Clin Invest Med 1991; 14: 642-651.

79. Bakris GL, Slataper R, Vicknair N, Sadler R. ACE inhibitor mediated reductions in renal size and microalbuminuria in normotensive, diabetic subjects. J Diabetic Compl 1994; 8: 2-6.

80. Mau Pedersen M, Christensen SE, Christiansen JS, Pedersen EB, Mogensen CE, Ørskov H. Acute effects of a somatostatin analogue on kidney function in type i diabetic patients. Diabetic Med 1990; 7: 304-309.

81. Serri O, Beauregard H, Brazeau P, Abribat T, Lamber J, Harris A, Vachon L. Somatostatin analogue, octreotide, reduces increased glomerular filtration rate and kidney size in insulin-dependent diabetes. JAMA 1991; 265; 888-892.

82. Jacobs ML, Derkx FH, Stijnen T, Lamberts SW, Weber RF. Effect of long-acting somatostatin analog (Somatolin) on renal hyperfiltration in patients with IDDM. Diabetes Care 1997; 20 (4): 632-636.

83. Mau Pedersen M, Schmitz A, Pedersen EB, Danielsen H, Christiansen JS. Acute and long-term renal effects of angiotensin converting enzyme inhibition in normotensive, normoalbuminuric insulin-dependent diabetic patients. Diabetic Med 1988; 5: 562-569.

84. Pecis M, Azevedo JM, Gross LJ. Glomerular Hyperfiltration is associated with blood pressure abnormalities in normotensive normoalbuminuric IDDM patients. Diabetes Care, vol. 20, no. 8, 1997; 1329-1333.

85. Ichikawa I, Harris RC. Angiotensin actions in the kidney: Renewed insight into the old hormone (Editorial Review). Kidney Int 1991; 40: 583-596.

86. Soper CP, Barron JL, Hyer SL. Long-term glycaemic control directly correlates with glomerular filtration rate in early Type 1 diabetes mellitus before the onset of microalbuminuria. Diabet Med, 1998; 15: 1012-4.

87. Jacobs EM, Vervoort G, Branten AJ, Klasen I, Smits P, Wetzels JF. Atrial natriuretic peptide increases albuminuria in type I diabetic patients: evidence for blockade of tubular protein reabsorption. Eur J Clin Invest, 1999; 2: 109-15.

88. Bursell S-E, Clermont AC, Aiello LP, Aiello LM, Schlossman DK, Feener EP, Laffel L, King GL. High-dose vitamin E supplementation normalizes retinal blood flow and creatinine clearance in patients with type 1 diabetes. Diabetes Care, 1999; 22: 1245-1251.

89. Fujisawa T, Ikegami H, Kawaguchi Y, Hamada Y, Ueda H, Shintani M, Fukuda M, Ogihara T. Meta-analysis of association of insertion/deletion polymorphism of angiotensin I-converting enzyme gene with diabetic nephropathy and retinopathy. Diabetologia, 1998; 41: 47-53.

90. Miller JA, Scholey JW, Thaik K, Pei YP. Angiotensin converting enzyme gene polymorphism and renal hemodynamic function in early diabetes. Kidney Int, 1997; 51:119-24.

91. Bouhanick B, Gallois Y, Hadjadj S, Boux de Casson F, Limal JM, Marre M. Relationship between glomerular hyperfiltration and ACE insertion/deletion polymorphism in type 1 diabetic children and adolescents. Diabetes Care, 1999; 22: 618-22.

92. Marre M, Bouhanick B, Berrut G, Gallois Y, Le Jeune J-J, Chatellier G, Menard J, Alhenc-Gelas F. Renal changes on hyperglycemia and angiotensin-converting enzyme in type 1 diabetes. Hypertension, 1999; 33: 775-780.

93. Cummings EA, Sochett EB, Dekker MG, Lawson ML, Daneman D. Contribution of growth hormone and IGF-I to early diabetic nephropathy in type 1 diabetes. Diabetes, 1998; 47: 1341-6.

94. Wolf G, Ziyadeh FN. Molecular mechanisms of diabetic renal hypertrophy. Kidney Int, 1999; 56: 393-405.

95. Sharma K, Jin Y, Guo J, Ziyadeh FN. Neutralization of TGF-beta by anti-TGF-beta antibody attenuates kidney hypertrophy and the enhanced extracellular matrix gene expression in STZ-induced diabetic mice.Diabetes, 1996; 45: 522-30.

96. Bardoux P, Martin H, Ahloulay M, Schmitt F, Bouby N, Trinh-Trang-Tan MM, Bakir L. Vasopressin contributes to hyperfiltration, albuminuria and renal hypertrophy in diabetes mellitus: study in vasopressin-deficient Brattleboro rats. Proc Natl Acad Sci USA, 1999; 96:10397-402.

97. Forst T, Kunt T, Pfutzner A, Beyer J, Wahren J. New aspects on biological activity of C-peptide in IDDM patients. Exp Clin Endocrinol Diabetes, 1998; 106: 270-6.

98. Berg UB, Torbjornsdotter TB, Jaremko G, Thalme B. Kidney morphological changes in relation to long-term renal function and metabolic control in adolescents with IDDM. Diabetologia, 1998; 41: 1047-56.

99. Baumgartl H-J, Sigl G, Banholzer P, Haslbeck M, Standl E. On the prognosis of IDDM patients with large kidneys. Nephrol Dial Transplant, 1998; 13: 630-634.

100. Bankir l, Bardoux P, Ahloulay M. Vasopressin and diabetes mellitus. Nephron 2001; 87: 8-18.

101. Wahren J, Ekberg K, Johansson J, Henriksson M, Pramanik A, Johansson BL, Rigler R, Jörnvall H. Role of C-peptide in human physiology. Am J Physiol Endocrinol Metab 2000; 278: E759-E768.

102. Samnegård B, Jacobson SH, Jaremko G, Johansson BL, Sjöquist M. Effects of C-peptide on glomerular and renal size and renal function in diabetic rats. Kidney International 2001; 60: 1258-1265.

103. Dahlquist G, Stattin E-L, Rudberg S. Urinary albumin excretion rate and glomerular filtration rate in the prediction of diabetic nephropathy; a long-term follow-up study of childhood onset type-1 diabetic patients. Nephrol Dial Transplant 2001; 16: 1382-1386.

28

AUTOREGULATION OF GLOMERULAR FILTRATION RATE IN PATIENTS WITH DIABETES

Per K. Christensen and Hans-Henrik Parving
Steno Diabetes Center, Copenhagen, Denmark.

INTRODUCTION

The close relationship between elevated blood pressure (BP) and diabetic nephropathy are documented both in Type 1 and Type 2 diabetic patients. Approximately 75-85% of diabetic patients with nephropathy are hypertensive [1-3].

Arterial BP and albuminuria are strong predictors for a faster decline in glomerular filtration rate (GFR). Conversely, antihypertensive treatment reduces the rate of decline in GFR and postponed ESRD in diabetic nephropathy [4-11]. Antihypertensive treatment induces a faster initial and slower subsequent decline in GFR, in hypertensive Type 1 and Type 2 diabetic patients with incipient or overt diabetic nephropathy [7,12,13]. This biphasic phenomenon may be due to a functional (haemodynamic) effect of antihypertensive treatment and/or impaired in autoregulation of GFR in patients with diabetic nephropathy [14,15]. Understanding the pathogenesis of abnormal renal haemodynamic in the diabetic state seems important, because it has been suggested, that abnormal haemodynamics plays a major role in the development and progression of diabetic nephropathy [16-22].

AUTOREGULATION OF THE NORMAL KIDNEY

Regulation of renal haemodynamics is a vital component in the overall control of renal function [23]. The ability of the kidney to maintain constancy of renal function (GFR) over a wide range of renal perfusion pressures is termed autoregulation [24] figure 1. Experimental studies suggests that autoregulation of GFR is due to autoregulation of two of the main GFR determinants, i.e. renal plasma flow and glomerular capillary pressure [25,26].

Both human [27] and animal [28] studies evaluating renal autoregulation in pharmacological and surgical denervated kidneys have made it possible to conclude that renal blood flow (RBF) is determined by an autonomous intrinsic activity of the renal arterioles, which is not dependent upon tonic activity in the sympathetic pathways. The consequence of this statement was that intrinsic mechanisms could respond to extrinsic changes to ensure stability and efficiency of renal haemodynamic control.

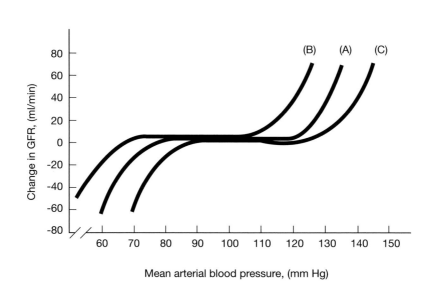

Fig. 1.
    A) Change in glomerular filtration rate (GFR) induced by change in mean arterial blood pressure in the normal kidney
    B) Shift in autoregulation interval to the left
    C) Shift in autoregulation interval to the right

Mechanisms

The intrinsic autoregulation of renal function is complex and involves several systems, which modulate the vascular smooth muscle tone and diameter of the afferent and efferent arterioles. The three major mechanisms involved in renal autoregulation are: myogenic factors intrinsic to the pre- and postglomerular arterioles [29], the tubuloglomerular feedback (TGF) mechanism [30], and various vasoactive hormones produced in and out side the kidney acting on the smooth muscle cells in the arterioles.

The myogenic response: The myogenic mechanism is probably the most important component of renal autoregulation and refers to the active contraction of vascular smooth muscle elicited by an increased in intravascular pressure. An increase in wall tension, e.g. caused by increased arterial blood pressure, leads to an activation of the vascular smooth muscle cells and a decrease in vascular diameter and wall tension. The myogenic response probably represents one of the principle means by which many organs and tissue autoregulate blood flow. The phenomenon is well known and was described already in 1902 by Bayliss [31].

Tubuloglomerular feedback: TGF is a phenomenon unique to the kidney, by which a change in GFR induce a change in flow and/or pressure [32-34] and/or composition of tubular fluid flowing past the macula densa region of the nephrons [23,35]. The structural basis for the TGF is located in the juxtaglomerular apparatus, where the contact between the thick ascending limb of Henle and the vascular pole of the glomerulus are located.

It is thought that macula dense is a sensor, which is able to send at signal to the afferent and efferent arteriole, which leads to a change in the wall tension in the arterioles, when the flow and/or pressure and/or NaCl concentration and/or osmolality in the thick ascending limb of Henle change [26] and, thus, correct the initial changes in GFR.

Intra- extrarenale vasoactive hormones: Even though studies indicate that vasodilatation and vasoconstricting intrarenal hormones such as prostaglandin's and hormones in the renin-angiotensin system contribute to autoregulation of GFR [36,37], information is as yet inconclusive [38-40]. However, The setting of the above-mentioned intrinsic systems is believed to be under influence from the sympathetic nervous system [41] and various systemic and local hormones (long-term regulation of GFR and shift in autoregulation interval (fig. 1)) [42].

There are advocates for a singular mechanism mediating autoregulation by the myogenic response [43,44], whereas others suggest that TGF is the most important mechanism [45]. However, there is emerging consensus that a complicated interplay between both myogenic and TGF mechanisms best explains the efficient autoregulatory response typical of the renal vasculature [30,32,46]. Difference in response time to change in perfusion pressure [33] and to location of the two components [47,48] may be part of the dispute.

Regardless of the precise mechanisms, the arteriole ability to change the diameter is the key to autoregulation of GFR when perfusion pressure change. Autoregulation of flow requires that resistance increase or decrease in parallel with changes in perfusion pressure. If efferent arteriolar resistance declined significantly when perfusion pressure is reduced, glomerular capillary pressure and GFR would also fall. Consequently, it is the afferent arteriole, which plays a pivotal role in regulating glomerular capillary pressure, renal plasma flow and consequently GFR [26,49-52].

The range of renal autoregulation in animal studies is from 75-95 mm Hg [28,46,53,54] to 180 mm Hg [55] of renal arterial pressure. The range of systemic BP for normal renal autoregulation in healthy humans is partly unknown. But a mean arterial blood pressure (MABP) of 80 mm Hg is usually suggested as the lower limit for normal autoregulation of GFR [56,57]

ANIMAL STUDIES OF RENAL AUTOREGULATION IN DIABETES MELLITUS

Several studies in streptozotocin diabetic rats and dogs have suggested that hyperglycaemia induces impaired autoregulation of RBF and GFR [52,58-60]. Changes in vasoactive hormone activities have been suggested to contribute to impaired renal autoregulation [61,62]. Furthermore, a rise in growth hormones in diabetic patients induces glomerular structural changes, which may change the regulation of GFR [63]. Diabetic autoregulation impairment develops over time [58,59], but impaired afferent arteriolar contraction during increased renal arterial pressure can occur in the early course of experimental diabetes [52,64]. Furthermore diabetes has been shown to impair TGF response [60,65]. Other investigators have however shown preserved [66] or even enhanced autoregulatory ability (shift of the autoregulation range to the left (fig. 1)) in rats with short time diabetes [67].

RENAL AUTOREGULATION IN PATIENTS WITH DIABETES

In the first human study of renal autoregulation Parving et al. [68] studied Type 1 diabetic patients with and without diabetic nephropathy. They found no significant change in GFR during acute lowering of BP with clonidine in patients without clinical signs of microangiopathy. The patients had mean blood glucose less than 13 mmol/l during the investigation [68]. In the first study of Type 2 diabetic patients with and without diabetic nephropathy [69] no significant change in GFR during acute lowering of BP in normoalbuminuric Type 2 diabetic patients was revealed. Mean blood glucose was less than 10 mmol/l during this investigation. The above-mentioned studies were not designed to evaluate the potential effect of acute changes in blood glucose on autoregulation of GFR. In a randomised crossover study of GFR autoregulation, in normoalbuminuric type 2 diabetic patients during blood glucose < 10 mmol/l ("normoglycaemia") and during acute blood glucose > 15 mmol/l (hyperglycaemia) [70]. Acute reduction in systemic BP induced a mean (SE) reduction in GFR from 92 (3.1) to 86 (3.7) ml/min/1.73 m^2 during "normoglycaemia" (p<0.05), whereas the reduction in GFR during hyperglycaemia was from 102 (4.1) to 98 (4.2) ml/min/1.73 m^2, NS). Mean difference between the mean reductions in GFR during the two examinations was 2.3 (95% CI, -1.3 to 5.9) ml/min/1.73 m^2, NS. The significant reduction in GFR during "normoglycaemia" might be explained by a more profound reduction in MABP compared to the examination during hyperglycaemia. However, it is possible that hyperglycaemia enhances renal autoregulation (shift the autoregulation range to the left (fig 1.)) as described by Mauer et al. [67].

STRUCTURAL CHANGES THAT MAY IMPAIR AUTOREGULATION OF GFR

The most characteristic glomerular lesion in patients with incipient or overt nephropathy is mesangial expansion. Biopsies from patients with hypertension and/or diabetic nephropathy have furthermore revealed arteriolar hyalinosis [71,72].

Arteriolar hyalinosis may impair the afferent arteriole capacity to constrict, and can thereby lead to enhanced transmission of the systemic BP into the glomerular capillary network, and lead to glomerular hypertension [19,73,74]. This haemodynamic alteration is associated with increase wall tension causing distension of the elastic glomerulus. Studies have shown that mechanical stretch of vascular smooth muscle cells, vascular endothelial cells and mesangial cells leads to an overproduction of extracellular matrix [75,76]. Mesangial expansion is closely associated with renal function in diabetic nephropathy [77]. This relationship probably results from the expanding mesangium compromising the structure of contiguous glomerular capillaries and from a reduction in filtration surface, which may per se lead to increased intraglomerular pressure, and creating a vicious circle.

However, impaired autoregulation have been demonstrated in remnant kidney models in rats and in humans with non-diabetic nephropathies in the absence of arteriolar hyalinosis [37,78-80]. Consequently, autoregulation can be impaired before structural changes are detectable and thereby contribute to the progression of nephropathy, by creating glomrular hypertension [16].

IMPAIRED AUTOREGULATION OF GFR IN PATIENTS WITH DIABETIC NEPHROPATHY

Animal studies have demonstrated impaired renal autoregulation in models of glomerulosclerosis [81], glomerulonephritis [74], nephrosclerosis [82,83] and nephrosis [84,85]. In humans Parving et al [68] demonstrated a wide variation in response to clonidine induced acute BP reduction ranging from normal to severely impaired GFR autoregulation in long-term Type 1 diabetic patients with nephropathy. A similar clonidine induced reduction in MABP had no impact on autoregulation in short-term normoalbuminuric Type 1 diabetic patients and in the nondiabetic control group. The reduction in arterial BP induced a reduction in albuminuria in the Type 1 diabetic patients with nephropathy, suggesting diminished glomerular capillary pressure.

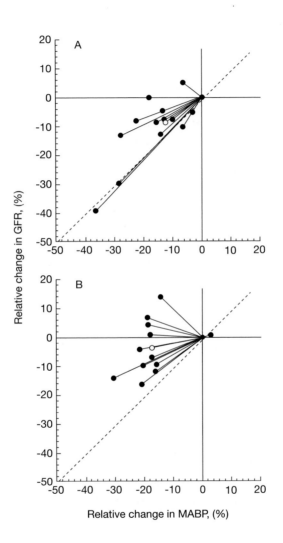

Fig. 2. Relative change in glomerular filtration rate (GFR) (percentage change of control GFR) and relative change in MABP (percentage change of control MABP) induced by intravenous injection of clonidine. (A). Fourteen Type 2 diabetic patients with nephropathy (●), *Mean response* *(○)* (B) Twelve Type 2 diabetic patients with normoalbuminuria (●), *Mean response (○)*

501

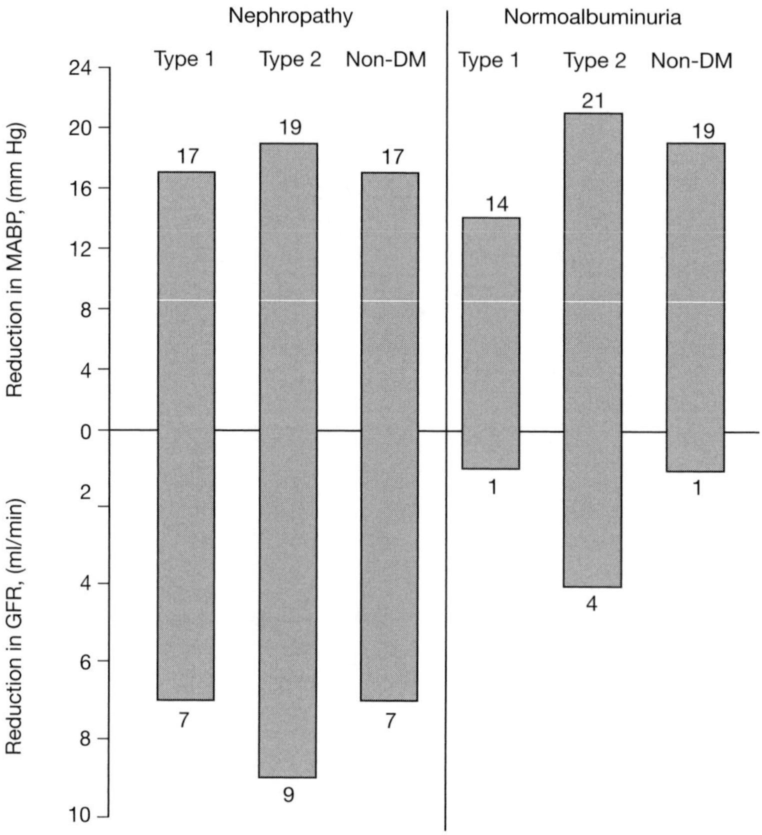

Figure 3. Reduction in mean arterial blood pressure (MABP) and glomerular filtration rate (GFR) induced by intravenous injection of clonidine in Type 1 and Type 2 diabetic patients with or without nephropathy, and in non-diabetic (Non-DM) subjects with or without nephropathy.

In a randomised single blinded case-control study comparing the effect of acute lowering of BP on GFR autoregulation in 26 hypertensive Type 2 diabetic patients with (n=14) and without (n=12) diabetic nephropathy [69], it was demonstrated that autoregulation of GFR was impaired to abolished in the hypertensive Type 2 diabetic patient with nephropathy, whereas the hypertensive Type 2 patients without nephropathy only showed moderate signs of altered renal autoregulation, and none of these patients had abolished autoregulation.

Furthermore, the study revealed a significant correlation between the relative changes in MABP and GFR, and a significant reduction of fractional renal clearance of albumin in patients with nephropathy. These data indicate that Type 2 diabetic patients with nephropathy frequently have enhanced transmission of systemic BP into the capillary network, whereas the glomerular arterioles in Type 2 diabetic patients without nephropathy respond adequately to changes in systemic BP

In addition, a study investigated the autoregulation of GFR in non-diabetic patients with nephropathy using the same methods as mention in the above studies [80], also suggested that albuminuric non-diabetic patients with different nephropathies suffer from impaired autoregulation of GFR. The main results from the above mention 3 studies [80] are shown in fig. 3.

ANTIHYPERTENSIVE TREATMENT AND RENAL AUTOREGULATION

Changes in cytosolic Ca^{2+} is recognized as a pivotal step in mediating smooth muscle contraction. Myogenic control of renal autoregulation is primarily regulated by afferent arteriolar smooth muscle permeability to Ca^{2+} [86,87]. In accordance, data have revealed that the major vasoconstrictive effect of raised extracellular ionised Ca^{2+} is a pressure dependent alteration in membrane Ca^{2+} permeability [88]. The efferent arteriole seems to be less responsive to changes in membrane Ca^{2+} permeability [87,89], and respond to angiotensin II with a major component of intracellular calcium release. The different signalling mechanisms in afferent and efferent arterioles indicate that the overall autoregulatory response to pressure changes is characterized by a combination of calcium entry and mobilization pathways [90].

Since calcium channel blockers (CCB's) interfere with the influx of Ca^{2+} they may affect normal renal autoregulation. Studies of dogs [91,92], isolated perfused rat kidneys [88,93], normal rat kidneys [94], hydronephrotic rat kidneys [50,95], remnant rat models [96], models of spontaneously hypertensive rats

[30,97-99] and rat models of diabetes [66] have all shown that CCB′s impair renal autoregulation. The effect of CCB′s on autoregulation seems to be a dose-dependent inhibition of the vasoconstriction [50,100], which at high doses make the system pressure-passive (abolish autoregulation) [91] and not influenced by renin secretion [93].

In a placebo controlled cross-over study of hypertensive Type 2 diabetic patients without overt nephropathy, therapy with dihydropyridine CCB induced a variable response ranging from no impact to impaired or abolished GFR autoregulation [101]. In fact 38% of these patients showed complete pressure passive vasculature during CCB treatment. The patients with abolished autoregulation of GFR had an increase in GFR during CCB treatment. The enhanced GFR probably reflects a more pronounced vasodilatation of the afferent arteriole during isradipine treatment as compared to patients without this response. The CCB therapy induced vasodilatation enhances the transmission of the systemic BP into the glomerular capillary network resulting in increased glomerular capillary hydraulic pressure (P_{GC}) and GFR.

Animal studies have revealed that angiotensin II receptor antagonists (AIIA) do not change whole kidney autoregulation. In hypertensive Type 2 diabetic patients without overt nephropathy treatment with candesartan cilexetil16 mg o.d does not interfere with normal GFR autoregulation [102].

In animal studies the effect of Alpha 1-receptor blockade on renal autoregulation have been investigated, and no impact on whole kidney autoregulation has been demonstrated [103,104].

Only one study has investigated the effect of beta-adrenergic blockade on renal autoreguation. The results suggested that autoregulation of both GFR and RBF are maintained during propranolol-treatment[105].

Thiazide diuretics decrease systemic vascular resistance, whereas the opposite effect has been demonstrated in the renal vasculature [106]. This results in a decrease in RBF and GFR [106,107]. However there are disagreements on the effect of thiazide diuretics on TGF [108].

Whereas amilorid have no effect on TGF, the acute effects of loop diuretics have been shown to be a dose dependent impairment of both TGF [109] and the myogenic response to changes in renal perfusion pressure [46,110]. However, if loop diuretic is given as a continuous infusion both autoregulation of RBF and GFR are maintained [111,112].

CONSEQUENCES OF DEFECTIVE AUTOREGULATION

The interplay between impaired renal autoregulation on one hand, and systemic BP [20,78,113-116], glomerular mechanical strain [75,76,117-120], different growth hormones [121-124], glomerular permselective properties [125,126], diabetes [69,127,128], albuminuria [81,82,85] on the other hand, and the development/progression of renal histological changes has been studied [84,113,129]. Although the pathogenesis in the different models differs in several aspects, impairment of renal autoregulation might induce the following pathological events: Enhanced transmission of systemic BP into the capillary network, induces wide swings and increased glomerular volume [119,130]. These alterations are further magnified by hypertension [119]. The pressure induced wide swings induces capillary distension and mesangial stretch [131]. Capillary distension induces glomerular epithelial cell hypertrophy with epithelial cell protein droplets, increase in lysosomes, vacuolisation [132], focal and segmental detachment of endothelial and epithelial cells from the basement membrane [85,126], segmental capillary collapse with adhesion to Bowman's capsule [132] and fusion of foot processes [129,130]. These changes combined with increased in P_{GC} [85,125] lead to changes in size- and charge-selective properties of the glomerular capillaries, and results in increase urinary albumin excretion rate [85,126].

Cultured mesangial cells undergoing cyclic stretching demonstrates increased synthesis of extracellular matrix components (collagen, laminin, fibronectin) [75], this synthesis is further increased in the presence of high glucose concentration [117]. Furthermore mechanical stretching increases the synthesis and activation of the prosclerotic molecule transforming growth factor-ß [118]. Transforming growth factor-ß is found to be a critical mediator in the net accumulation of extracellular matrix especially in cell culture exposed to high glucose [120,124]. The above-mentioned changes are ultimately leading to albuminuria and glomerulosclerosis with hyalinosis [81,116,128].

The importance of glomerular capillary hypertension in the development/progression of renal disease is supported by the fact that normotension [82,84, 113,114] and reduction of glomerular capillary pressure with antihypertensive treatment [132,134,135] or low protein diet [79,116,126,129,136] protects against the development and progression in renal disease in animals.

The clinical significance of impaired autoregulation of GFR in hypertensive diabetic patients with nephropathy is lack or diminished protection against hyper- or hypoperfusion induced by alteration in blood pressure. In other words, there is increased vulnerability to hypertension or ischemic injuries of glomerular capillaries in diabetic patients with nephropathy.

REFERENCES

1. Mogensen CE, Christensen CK: Predicting diabetic nephropathy in insulin-dependent patients. N Engl J Med. 1984; 311:89-93.
2. Andersen AR, Christiansen JS, Andersen JK, Kreiner S, Deckert T: Diabetic nephropathy in Type 1 (insulin-dependent) diabetes: an epidemiological study. Diabetologia. 1983; 25:496-501.
3. Tarnow L, Rossing P, Gall M-A, Nielsen FS, Parving H-H: Prevalence of arterial hypertension in diabetic patients before and after the JNC-V. Diabetes Care. 1994; 17 (11):1247-1251.
4. Rossing P, Hommel E, Smidt UM, Parving H-H: Impact of arterial blood pressure and albuminuria on the progression of diabetic nephropathy in IDDM patients. Diabetes . 1993; 42:715-719.
5. Parving H-H, Smidt UM, Hommel E, Mathiesen ER, Rossing P, Nielsen FS, Gall M-A: Effective Antihypertensive Treatment Postpones Renal Insufficiency in Diabetic Nephropathy. Am J Kidney Dis. 1993; 22:188-195.
6. Parving H-H, Rossing P, Hommel E, Smidt UM: Angiotensin converting enzyme inhibition in diabetic nephropathy: ten years experience. Am J Kidney Dis. 1995; 26:99-107.
7. Bjôrck S, Mulec H, Johnsen SA, Nordén G, Aurell M: Renal protective effect of enalapril in diabetic nephropathy. Br Med J. 1992; 304:339-343.
8. Breyer JA, Bain P, Evans JK, Nahman NS, Lewis E, Cooper ME, McGill JB, Berl T, THE COLLABORATIVE STUDY GROUP: Predictors of the progression of renal insufficiency in patients with insulin-dependent diabetes and overt diabetic nephropathy. Kidney Int. 1996; 50:1651-1658.
9. Walker WG, Hermann J, Murphy RP, Russell RP: Prospective study of the impact of hypertension upon kidney function in diabetes mellitus. Nephron. 1990; 55(suppl 1):21-26.
10. Yokoyama H, Tomanaga O, Hirayama M, Ishii A, Takeda M, Babazono T, Ujihara U, Takahashi C, Omori Y: Predictors of the progression of diabetic nephropathy and the beneficial effect of angiotensin-converting enzyme inhibitors in NIDDM patients. Diabetologia. 1997; 40:405-411.
11. Peterson JC, Adler S, Burkart JM, Greene T, Herbert LA, Hunsicker LG, King AJ, Klahr S, Massry SG, Seifter JL: Blood pressure control, proteinuria, and the progression of renal disease. The modification of diet in renal disease study. Ann Intern Med . 1995; 123:754-762.

12. Parving H-H, Andersen AR, Smidt UM, Hommel E, Mathiesen ER, Svendsen PA: Effect of antihypertensive treatment on kidney function in diabetic nephropathy. Br Med J. 1987; 294:1443-1447.

13. Lebovitz HE, Wiegmann TB, Cnaan A, Shahinfar S, Sica D, Broadstone V, Schwartz SL, Mengel MC, Segal R, Versaggi JA, Bolten WK: Renal protective effects of enalapril in hypertensive NIDDM: Role of baseline albuminuria. Kidney Int. 1994; 45 (suppl. 45):S150-S155.

14. Hansen HP, Rossing P, Tarnow L, Nielsen FS, Jensen BR, Parving H-H: Increased glomerular filtration rate after withdrawal of long-term antihypertensive treatment in diabetic nephropathy. Kidney Int. 1995; 47:1726-1731.

15. Hansen HP, Nielsen FS, Rossing P, Jacobsen P, Jensen BR, Parving H-H: Kidney function after withdrawal of long-term antihypertensive treatment in diabetic nephropathy. Kidney Int. 1997; 52:S49-S53.

16. Hostetter TH, Rennke HG, Brenner BM: The case for intrarenal hypertension in the initiation and progression of diabetic and other glomerulopathies. Am. J. Med. 1982; 72:375-380.

17. Hostetter TH, Troy JL, Brenner BM: Glomerular hemodynamics in experimental diabetes mellitus. Kidney Int. 1981; 19:410-415.

18. Steffes MW, Brown DM, Mauer SM: Diabetic glomerulopathy following unilateral nephrectomy in the rat. Diabetes. 1978; 27:35-41.

19. Zatz R, Dunn BR, Meyer TW, Anderson S, Rennke HG, Brenner BM: Prevention of diabetic glomerulopathy by pharmacological amelioration of glomerular capillary hypertension. J.Clin.Invest. 1986; 77:1925-1930.

20. Zatz R, Meyer TW, Rennke HG, Brenner BM: Predominance of hemodynamic rather than metabolic factors in the pathogenesis of diabetic glomerulopathy. Proc.Natl.Acad.Sci.USA. 1985; 82:5963-5967.

21. Cortes P, Riser BL, Yee J, Narins RG: Mechanical strain of glomerular mesangial cells in the pathogenesis of glomerulosclerosis: clinical implications. Nephrol.Dial.Transplant. 1999; 14:1351-1354.

22. Mogensen CE: Renal function changes in diabetes. Diabetes. 1976; 25:872-879.

23. Navar LG: Renal autoregulation: perspectives from whole kidney and single nephron studies. Am.J.Physiol. 1978; 234:F357-F370.

24. Thurau K: Renal Hemodynamics. Am.J.Med. 1964; 36:698-719.

25. Anderson S: Relevance of single nephron studies to human glomerular function. Kidney Int. 1994; 45:384-389.

26. Maddox DA, Brenner BM: Glomerular ultrafiltration, in The Kidney, edited by Brenner BM, Philidelphia, Saunders, 1996, p. 286

27. Smith HW, Rovenstein EA, Goldring W, Chasis H, Ranges HA: The effects of spinal anesthesia on the circulation in normal, unoperated man with reference to the autonomy of the arterioles and especially those of renal circulation J.Clin.Invest. 1939; 18:319-341.

28. Forster RP, Maes JP: Effect of experimental neurogenic hypertension on renal blood flow and glomerular filtration rates in intact denervated kidneys of unanesthetized rabbits with adrenal glands demedullated. Am.J.Physiol. 1947; 150:534-540.

29. Ush DJ, Fray JCS: Steady-state autoregulation of renal blood flow: a myogenic model. Am.J.Physiol. 1984; 247:R89-R99.

30. Aukland K, Öien AH: Renal autoregulation: models combining tubuloglomerular feedback and myogenic response. Am.J.Physiol. 1987; 252:F768-F783.

31. Bayliss WM: On the local reaction of the arterial wall to changes of internal pressure. Journal of Physiology London. 1902; 28:220-231.

32. Moore LC, Casellas D: Tubuloglomerular feedback dependence of autoregulation in rat juxtamedullary afferent arterioles. Kidney Int. 1990; 37:1402-1408.

33. Holstein-Rathlou NH, Wagner AJ, Marsh DJ: Tubuloglomerular feedback dynamics and renal blood flow autoregulation in rats. Am.J.Physiol. 1991; 260:F53-F68.

34. Daniels FH, Arendshorst WJ, Roberds RG: Tubuloglomerular feedback and autoregulation in spontaneously hypertensive rats. Am.J.Physiol. 1990; 258:F1479-F1489.

35. Karlsen FM, Holstein-Rathlou NH, Leyssac PP: A re-evaluation of the determinants of glomerular filtration rate. Acta.Physiol.Scand. 1995; 155:335-350.

36. Wang X, Aukland K, Iversen BM: Acute effects of angiotensin II receptor antagonist on autoregulation of zonal glomerular filtration rate in renovascular hypertensive rats. Kidney Blood Pressure Research. 1997; 20:225-232.

37. Iversen BM, Kvam FI, Mørkrid L, Sekse I, Ofstad J: Effect of cyclooxygenase inhibition on renal blood flow autoregulation in SHR. Am J Physiol. 1992; 32:F534-F539.

38. Pelayo JC, Westcott JY: Impaired autoregulation of glomerular capillary hydrostatic pressure in the rat remnant nephron. J Clin Invest. 1991; 88:101-105.

39. Iversen BM, Kvam FI, Matre K, Ofstad J: Resetting of renal blood autoregulation during acute blood pressure reduction in hypertensive rats. Am J Physiol. 1998; 44:R343-R349.

40. Dworkin LD, Brenner BM: The renal circulations, in The Kidney, edited by Brenner BM, Philadelphia, Saunders, 1996, p. 247

41. DiBona GF: Neural control of renal function in health and disease. Clin.Auton.Res. 1994; 4:69-74.

42. Ito S, Abe K: Contractile properties of afferent and efferent arterioles. Clin.Exp.Pharmacol.Physiol. 1997; 24:532-535.

43. Maddox DA, Troy JL, Brenner BM: Autoregulation of filtration rate in the absence of macula densa- glomerulus feedback. Am.J.Physiol. 1974; 227:123-131.

44. Knox FG, Ott C, Cuche JL, Gasser J, Haas J: Autoregulation of single nephron filtration rate in the presence and the absence of flow to the macula densa. Circ.Res. 1974; 34:836-842.

45. Sakai T, Hallman E, Marsh DJ: Frequency domain analysis of renal autoregulation in the rat. Am.J.Physiol. 1986; 250:F364-F373.

46. Takenaka T, Harrison-Bernard LM, Inscho EW, Carmines PK, Navar LG: Autoregulation of afferent arteriolar blood flow in juxtamedullary nephrons. Am.J.Physiol. 1994; 267:F879-F887.

47. Casellas D, Moore LC: Autoregulation of intravascular pressure in preglomerular juxtamedullary vessels. Am.J.Physiol. 1993, 264:F315-F321.

48. Ofstad J, Iversen BM: The interlobular artery: its possible role in preventing and mediating renal disorders. Nephrol.Dial.Transplant. 1988; 3:123-129.

49. Lush DJ, Fray JCS: Steady-state autoregulation of renal blood flow: a myogenic model. Am J Physiol 1984; 247:R89-R99.

50. Hayashi K, Epstein M, Loutzenhiser R: Determinants of the renal actions of atrial natriuretic peptide (ANP): lack of effect of ANP on pressure-induced vasocontriction. Circ Res. 1990; 67:1-10.

51. Hayashi K, Epstein M, Loutzenhiser R: Pressure-induced vasocontriction of renal microvessels in normotensive and hypertensive rats: studies in the isolated perfused hydronephrotic kidney. Circ Res. 1989; 65:1475-1484.

52. Hayashi K, Epstein M, Loutzenhiser R, Forster H: Impaired myogenic responsiveness of the afferent arteriole in streptozotocin-induced diabetic rats: Role of eicosanoid derangements. J Am Soc Nephrol. 1992; 2:1578-1586.

53. Shipley RE, Study RS: Changes in renal blood flow, extraction of insulin, glomerular filtration rate, tissue pressure and urine flow with acute alteration of renal artery blood pressure. Am.J.Physiol. 1951; 167:676-688.

54. Selkurt EE, Hall PW, Spencer MP: Influence of graded arterial pressure decrement on renal clearance of creatinine, p-amino-hippurate and sodium. Am.J.Physiol. 1949; 159:369-378.

55. Forster HG, ter Wee PM, Hohman TC, Epstein M: Impairment of afferent arteriolar myogenic responsiveness in the galactose-fed rat is prevented by tolrestat. Diabetologia. 1996; 39:907-914.

56. Pollock DM, Banks RO: Perspectives on renal blood flow autoregulation. Proc.Soc.Exp.Biol.Med. 1991; 198:800-805.

57. Holechek MJ: Renal physiology series: Part 2 of 8. Glomerular filtration and renal hemodynamics. ANNA.J. 1992; 19:237-245.

58. Hashimoto Y, Ideura T, Yoshimura A, Koshikawa S: Autoregulation of renal blood flow in streptozocin-induced diabetic rats. Diabetes. 1989; 38:1109-1113.

59. Tolins JP, Shultz PJ, Raij L, Brown DM, Mauer M: Abnormal renal hemodynamic response to reduced renal perfusion pressure in diabetic rats: role of NO. Am.J.Physiol. 1993; 265:F866-F895.

60. Woods LL, Mizelle HL, Hall JG: Control of renal hemodynamics in hyperglycemia. Am.J.Physiol. 1987; 252:F65-F73.

61. Ortola FV, Ballermann BJ, Anderson S, Mendez RE, Brenner BM: Elevated plasma arterial natriuretic peptide levels in diabetic rats. Potential mediators of hyperfiltration. J.Clin.Invest. 1987; 80:670-674.

62. Ballermann BJ, Skorecki KL, Brenner BM: Reduced glomerular angiotensin II receptor density in early untreated diabetes mellitus in the rat. Am.J.Physiol. 1984; 247:F110-F115.

63. Christiansen JS, Gammelgaard J, Frandsen M, Ørskov H, Parving H-H: Kidney function and size in type I diabetic patients before and during growth hormone administration for one week. Diabetologia. 1982; 22:333-337.

64. Wee PM, Forster H, Epstein M: Rapid initiation of attenuated pressure- and angiotensin II (AII)-induced vasoconstriction of rat afferent arterioles (AA) in untreated diabetes mellitus (DM). (abstract) J.Am.Soc.Nephrol. 1992; 3:767.

65. Blantz RC, Peterson OW, Gushwa L, Tucker BJ: Effect of modest hyperglycemia on tubuloglomerular feedback activity. Kidney Int. 1982; 22 (suppl. 12):S206-S212.

66. Sarubbi D, Quilley J: Evidence against a role of arachidonic acid metabolites in autoregulatory responses of the isolated perfused kidney of the rat. Eur.J.Pharmacol. 1991; 197:27-31.

67. Mauer SM, Brown DM, Steffes MW, Azar S: Studies of renal autoregulation in pancreatectomized and streptozotocin diabetic rats. Kidney Int. 1990; 37:909-917.

68. Parving H-H, Kastrup J, Smidt UM, Andersen AR, Feldt-Rasmussen B, Christiansen JS: Impaired autoregulation of glomerular filtration rate in Type 1 (insulin-dependent) diabetic patients with nephropathy. Diabetologia. 1984; 27:547-552.

69. Christensen PK, Hansen HP, Parving H-H: Impaired autoregulation of GFR in hypertensive non-insulin dependent diabetic patients. Kidney Int. 1997; 52:1369-1374.

70. Christensen PK, Lund S, Parving H-H: The impact of glyceamic control on autoregulation of glomerular filtration rate in non-insulin dependent diabetes mellitus. Scand.J.Clin.Lab.Invest. 2001; 61:43-50.

71. Dustin P: Arteriolar hyalinosis. Int Rev Exp Pathol 1962; 1:73-138.

72. Østerby R, Gall M-A, Schmitz A, Nielsen FS, Nyberg G, Parving H-H: Glomerular structure and function in proteinuric Type 2 (non-insulin-dependent) diabetic patients. Diabetologia. 1993; 36:1064-1070.

73. Hill GS, Heptinstall RH: Steorid-induced hypertension in the rat. Am J Pathol. 1968; 52:1-39.

74. Iversen BM, Ofstad J: Loss of renal blood flow autoregulation in chronic glomerulonephritic rats. Am J Physiol. 1988; 254:F284-F290.

75. Riser BL, Cortes P, Zhao X, Bernstein J, Dumler F, Narins RG: Intraglomerular pressure and mesangial stretchning stimulate extracellular matrix formation in the rat. J Clin Invest. 1992; 90:1932-1943.

76. Kollros PR, Bates SR, Mathews MB, Horwitz AL, Glagov S: Cyclic AMP inhibits increased collagen production by cyclically stretched smooth muscle cells. Lab Invest. 1987; 56:410-417.

77. Mauer SM: Structural-functional correlations of diabetic nephropathy. Kidney Int . 1994; 45:612-622.

78. Griffin KA, Picken MM, Bidani AK: Method of renal mass reduction is a critical modulator of subsequent hypertension and glomerular injury. J Am Soc Nephrol. 1994; 4:2023-2031.

79. Bidani AK, Schwartz M, Lewis E: Renal autoregulation and vulnerability to hypertensive injury in remnant kidney. Am J Physiol. 1987; 252:F1003-F1010.

80. Christensen PK, Hommel E, Clausen P, Feldt-Rasmussen B, Parving H: Impaired autoregulation of the glomerular filtration rate in patients with non-diabetic nephropathies. Kidney Int. 1999; 56:1517-1523.

81. Fries JW, Sandstrom DJ, Meyer TW, Rennke HG: Glomerular hypertrophy and epithelial cell injury modulate progressive glomerulosclerosis in the rat. Lab. Invest. 1989; 60:205-218.

82. Meyer TW, Rennke HG: Progressive glomerular injury after limited renal infarction in the rat. Am.J.Physiol. 1988; 254:F856-F862.

83. Miller PL, Rennke HG, Meyer TW: Hypertension and progressive glomerular injury caused by focal glomerular ischemia. Am.J.Physiol. 1990; 259:F239-F245.

84. Amato D, Tapia E, Bobadilla NA, Franco M, Calleja C, Garcia-Torres R, Lopez P, Alvarado JA, Herrera-Acosta J: Mechanisms involved in the progression to glomerular sclerosis induced by systemic hypertension during mild puromycin aminonucleoside nephrosis. Am.J.Hypertens. 1992; 5:629-636.

85. Miller PL, Scholey JW, Rennke HG, Meyer TW: Glomerular hypertrophy aggravates epithelial cell injury in nephrotic rats. J.Clin.Invest. 1990; 85:1119-1126.

86. Ogawa N: Effect of nicardipine on the relationship of renal blood flow and of renal vascular resistance to perfusion pressure in dog kidney. J.Pharm.Pharmacol. 1990; 42:138-140.

87. Fleming JT, Parekh N, Steinhausen M: Calcium antagonists preferentially dilate preglomerular vessels of hydronephrotic kidney. Am.J.Physiol. 1987; 253:F1157-F1163.

88. Heller J, Horacek V: The effect of two different calcium antagonists on the glomerular haemodynamics in the dog. Pflugers Arch. 1990; 415:751-755.

89. Ruan X, Arendshorst WJ: Calcium entry and mobilization signaling pathways in ANG II-induced renal vasoconstriction in vivo. Am.J.Physiol. 1996; 270:F398-F405.

90. Cohen AJ, Fray JC: Calcium ion dependence of myogenic renal plasma flow autoregulation: evidence from the isolated perfused rat kidney. J.Physiol. 1982; 330:449-460.

91. Navar LG, Champion WJ, Thomas CE: Effects of calcium channel blockade on renal vascular resistance responses to changes in perfusion pressure and angiotensin-converting enzyme inhibition in dogs. Circ.Res. 1986; 58:874-881.

92. Ono H, Kokubun H, Hashimoto K: Abolition by calcium antagonists of the autoregulation of renal blood flow. Naunyn Schmiedebergs Arch.Pharmacol. 1974; 285:201-207.

93. Scholz H, Kurtz A: Disparate effects of calcium channel blockers on pressure dependence of renin secretion and flow in the isolated perfused rat kidney. Pflugers Arch. 1992; 421:155-162.

94. Loutzenhiser R, Epstein M, Horton C: Inhibition by diltiazem of pressure-induced afferent vasoconstriction in the isolated perfused rat kidney. Am.J.Cardiol. 1987; 59:72A-75A.

95. Ozawa Y, Hayashi K, Nagahama T, Fujiwara K, Wakino S, Saruta T: Renal afferent and efferent arteriolar dilation by nilvadipine: studies in the isolated perfused hydronephrotic kidney. J.Cardiovasc.Pharmacol. 1999; 33:243-247.

96. Griffin KA, Picken MM, Bidani AK: Deleterious effects of calcium channel blockade on pressure transmission and glomerular injury in rat remnant kidneys. J.Clin.Invest. 1995; 96:793-800.

97. Huang C, Davis G, Johns EJ: Effect of nitrendipine on autoregulation of perfusion in the cortex and papilla of kidneys from Wistar and stroke prone spontaneously hypertensive rats. Br.J.Pharmacol. 1994; 111:111-116.

98. Wang X, Aukland K, Iversen BM: Autoregulation of total and zonal glomerular filtration rate in spontaneously hypertensive rats during antihypertensive therapy. J.Cardiovasc.Pharmacol. 1996; 28:833-841.

99. Kawata T, Hashimoto S, Koike T: Diversity in the renal hemodynamic effects of dihydropyridine calcium blockers in spontaneously hypertensive rats. J.Cardiovasc.Pharmacol. 1997; 30:431-436.

100. Hayashi K, Nagahama T, Oka K, Epstein M, Saruta T: Disparate effects of calcium antagonists on renal microcirculation. Hypertens.Res. 1996; 19:31-36.

101. Christensen PK, Akram K, Kønig KB, Parving, H-H. Autoregulation of glomerular filtration rate in type 2 diabetic patients during isradipine therapy. Diabetes care 2003. In Press

102. Christensen PK, Lund S, Parving, H-H. Autoregulated glomerular filtration rate during candesartan treatment in hypertensive type 2 diabetic patients. Kidney Int. 2001; 60:1435-1442.

103. Kvam FI, Ofstad J, Iversen BM: Effects of antihypertensive drugs on autoregulation of RBF and glomerular capillary pressure in SHR. Am.J.Physiol. 1998; 275:F576-F584.

104. Numabe A, Komatsu K, Frohlich ED: Effects of ANG-converting enzyme and alpha 1-adrenoceptor inhibition on intrarenal hemodynamics in SHR. Am.J.Physiol. 1994; 266:R1437-R1442.

105. Anderson RJ, Taher MS, Cronin RE, McDonald KM, Schrier RW: Effect of beta-adrenergic blockade and inhibitors of angiotensin II and prostaglandins on renal autoregulation. Am.J.Physiol. 1975; 229:731-736.

106. Aperia AC: Tubular sodium reabsorption and the regulation of renal hemodynamics. The effect of chlorothiazide on renal vascular resistance. Acta.Physiol.Scand. 1969; 75:360-369.

107. Okusa MD, Persson AE, Wright FS: Chlorothiazide effect on feedback-mediated control of glomerular filtration rate. Am.J.Physiol. 1989; 257:F137-F144.

108. Gutsche HU, Brunkhorst R, Muller-Ott K, Franke H, Niedermayer W: Effect of diuretics on the tubuloglomerular feedback response. Can.J.Physiol. Pharmacol. 1984; 62:412-417.

109. Brunkhorst R, Muller-Ott K, Gutsche HU, Niedermayer W: Effect of furosemide, bumetanide and piretanide on the sensor of the tubuloglomerular feedback mechanism. Proc.Eur.Dial.Transplant.Assoc. 1978; 15:613-616.

110. Sanchez-Ferrer CF, Roman RJ, Harder DR: Pressure-dependent contraction of rat juxtamedullary afferent arterioles. Circ.Res. 1989; 64:790-798.

111. Duchin KL, Peterson LN, Burke TJ: Effect of furosemide on renal autoregulation. Kidney Int. 1977; 12:379-386.

112. Loon NR, Wilcox XS, Unwin RJ: Mechanism of impaired natriuretic responce to furosemide during prolonged therapy. Kidney Int. 1989; 36:682-689.

113. Bidani AK, Griffin KA, Picken M, Lansky DM: Continuous telemetric blood pressure monitoring and glomerular injury in the rat remnant kidney model. Am.J.Physiol. 1993; 265:F391-F398.

114. Bidani AK, Mitchell KD, Schwartz MM, Navar LG, Lewis EJ: Absence of glomerular injury or nephron loss in a normotensive rat remnant kidney model. Kidney Int. 1990; 38:28-38.

115. Yoshida Y, Fogo A, Ichikawa I: Glomerular hemodynamic changes vs hypertrophy in experimental glomerular sclerosis. Kidney Int. 1989; 35:654-660.

116. Dworkin LD, Feiner HD: Glomerular injury in uninephrectomized spontaneously hypertensive rats. A consequence of glomerular capillary hypertension. J.Clin.Invest. 1986; 77:797-809.

117. Cortes P, Zhao X, Riser BL, Narins RG: Role fo glomerular mechanical strain in the pathogenesis of diabetic nephropathy. Kidney Int. 1997; 51:57-68.

118. Riser BL, Cortes P, Heilig C, Grondin J, Ladson-Wofford S, Patterson D, Narins RG: Cyclic stretching force selectively up-regulates transforming growth factor-beta isoforms in cultured rat mesangial cells. Am.J.Pathol. 1996; 148:1915-1923.

119. Cortes P, Zhao X, Riser BL, Narins RG: Regulation of glomerular volume in normal and partially nephrectomized rats. Am.J.Physiol. 1996; 270:F356-F370.

120. Riser BL, Cortes P, Yee J, Sharba AK, Asano K, Rodriguez-Barbero A, Narins RG: Mechanical st. J.Am.Soc.Nephrol. 1998; 9:827-836.

121. El Nahas AM, Bassett AH, Cope GH, Le Carpentier JE: Role of growth hormone in the development of experimental renal scarring. Kidney Int. 1991; 40:29-34.

122. Doi T, Striker LJ, Quaife C, Conti FG, Palmiter R, Behringer R, Brinster R, Striker GE: Progressive glomerulosclerosis develops in transgenic mice chronically expressing growth hormone and growth hormone releasing factor but not in those expressing insulinlike growth factor-1. Am.J.Pathol. 1988; 131:398-403.

123. Schnermann J, Gokel M, Weber PC, Schubert G, Briggs JP: Tubuloglomerular feedback and glomerular morphology in Goldblatt hypertensive rats on varying protein diets. Kidney Int. 1986; 29:520-529.

124. Riser BL, Ladson-Wofford S, Sharba A, Cortes P, Drake K, Guerin CJ, Yee J, Choi ME, Segarini PR, Narins RG: TGF-? receptor expression and binding in rat mesangial cells: modulation by glucose and cyclic mechanical strain. Kidney Int. 1999; 56:428-439.

125. Johnsson E, Rippe B, Haraldsson B: Reduced permselectivity in isolated perfused rat kidneys following small elevations of glomerular capillary pressure. Acta.Physiol.Scand. 1994; 150:201-209.

126. Olson JL, Hostetter TH, Rennke HG, Brenner BM, Venkatachalam MA: Altered glomerular permselectivity and progressive sclerosis following extreme ablation of renal mass. Kidney Int. 1982; 22:112-126.

127. Parving H-H, Viberti GC, Keen H, Christiansen JS, Lassen NA: Hemodynamic factors in the genesis of diabetic microangiopathy. Metabolism. 1983; 32:943-949.

128. Mauer SM, Steffes MW, Azar S, Sandberg SK, Brown DM: The effects of Goldblatt hypertension on development of the glomerular lesions of diabetes mellitus in the rat. Diabetes. 1978; 27:738-744.

129. Hostetter TH, Olson JL, Rennke HG, Venkatachalam MA, Brenner BM: Hyperfiltration in remnant nephrons: a potentially adverse response to renal ablation. Am.J.Physiol. 1981; 241:F85-F93.

130. Jenkins AJ, Steele JS, Janus ED, Best JD: Increased plasma apolipoprotein(a) levels in IDDM patients with microalbuminuria. Diabetes. 1991; 40:787-790.

131. Cortes P, Riser BL, Zhao X, Narins RG: Glomerular volume expansion and mesangial cell mechanical strain: mediators of glomerular pressure injury. Kidney Int. Suppl. 1994; 45:S11-S16.

132. Anderson S, Meyer TW, Rennke HG, Brenner BM: Control of glomerular hypertension limits glomerular injury in rats with reduced renal mass. J.Clin.Invest. 1985; 76:612-619.

133. Bank N, Alterman L, Aynedjian HS: Selective deep nephron hyperfiltration in uninephrectomized spontaneously hypertensive rats. Kidney Int. 1983; 24:185-191.

134. Anderson S, Rennke HG, Brenner BM: Therapeutic advantage of converting enzyme inhibitors in arresting progressive renal disease associated with systemic hypertension in the rat. J.Clin.Invest. 1986; 77:1993-2000.

135. Dworkin LD, Benstein JA, Parker M, Tolbert E, Feiner HD: Calcium antagonists and converting enzyme inhibitors reduce renal injury by different mechanisms. Kidney Int. 1993; 43:808-814.

136. Hostetter TH, Meyer TW, Rennke HG, Brenner BM: Chronic effects of dietary protein in the rat with intact and reduced renal mass. Kidney Int. 1986; 30:509-517.

29

THE ROLE OF RENAL BIOPSY IN THE CLINIC

Satishkumar A Jayawardene and Neil S Sheerin
Department of Nephrology and Transplantation, Guy's Hospital, King's College London, UK

The introduction of renal biopsy in the early 1950s [1] and its increasing use in the late 1960s and 1970s has had a major impact on our understanding and management of renal disease. Its use has become widespread and is now a routine investigation in most renal units. Nevertheless, it is an invasive intervention that has a small but definite risk of morbidity and mortality. Therefore it is not an investigation performed on all diabetic patients with suspected renal disease. There is considerable, often heated, debate as to what criteria we should use to decide which diabetic patients should have a renal biopsy.

Those in favour of a more conservative approach to biopsy would argue that biopsy should only be performed if it is likely to influence choice of treatment and therefore prognosis of the patient. A more expansionist view would be that our current understanding of many elements of renal pathology is limited and therefore every opportunity should be taken to examine renal histology, irrespective of whether it is likely to result in a specific treatment. This chapter will try and explore these approaches as they apply to the diabetic patient and discuss the evidence available that should influence a decision to biopsy a diabetic patient. Specific questions that will be addressed are:

- Is there a higher incidence of non-diabetic renal disease in diabetics compared to non-diabetics
- What are the indications to biopsy a diabetic patient

- Is there any clinical benefit in knowing the nature of the histological lesion in a diabetic patient

NON-DIABETIC RENAL DISEASE IN THE DIABETIC PATIENT

Many authors have reported their experience of non-diabetic glomerular disease in patients with diabetes (summarised in table 1).

Table 1. Summary of the studies quoting rates of non-diabetic renal disease diagnosed on renal biopsy in diabetic patients

	N° of biopsies	Biopsy criteria		Non-diabetic disease
Type 1 diabetes				
Amoah et al 1988 [10]	49	Clinical suspicion of non-diabetic disease	6	12%
Type 2 diabetes – Unselected				
Schwartz et al 1998 [11]	36	Proteinuria 0.5g/day	2	5.6%
Brocco et al 1997 [4]	53	Microalbuminuria (20-200μg/min)	0	0%
Mak et al 1997 [12]	51	Proteinuria >1g/24 hours	17	33%
Fioretto et al 1996 [5]	34	Microalbuminuria (20-200μg/min)	0	0%
Parving et al 1992 [3]	35	Albuminuria >300mg/24hrs	8	23%
Type 2 diabetes – Selected				
Mazzucco et al 2002 [2]	393	Variable	177	45%
Serra et al 2002 [13]	35	Clinical suspicion of non-diabetic disease	4	11.4%
Suzuki et al 2001 [14]	109	Not stated	29	26.6%
Prakash et al 2001 [15]	260	Not stated	32	12.3%
Christensen et al 2000 [16]	52	Microalbuminuria and absence of retinopathy	7	13%
Olsen and Mogensen 1996 [17]	33	Clinical suspicion of non-diabetic disease	4	12%
John et al 1994[8]	80	Clinical suspicion of non-diabetic disease	65	81%
Gambara et al 1993 [18]	52	Not stated	17	32.7%

Table 1. (cont.)

Richards et al 1992 [19]	46	Not stated	22	48%
Amoah et al 1988 [10]	60	Clinical suspicion of non-diabetic disease	17	28%
Yum et al 1984 [20]	18	Not stated	8	44%
Type 1 and type 2 Diabetes				
Taft et al 1990 [21]	136*	Proteinuric patients referred for biopsy	38	27.9%
Chihara et al 1986 [9]	164	Not stated	36	22%
Kasinath et al 1983 [22]	122	Clinical suspicion of non-diabetic disease	12	8.2%

* All patients demonstrated diabetic changes on biopsy

These frequently report that glomerular diseases, other than that relating to diabetes, are more common in the diabetic patients. This is particularly true of patients with type 2 diabetes. The largest series of 393 biopsies from three Italian centres reported a rate of non-diabetic disease of 45% in type 2 diabetics who underwent renal biopsy [2]. Even in the centre with a relatively unselective biopsy policy 33% of patients had evidence of non-diabetic disease.

However, the evidence for an increased incidence of non-diabetic disease is clouded by several factors. The first and most important factor is that of patient selection. Most series reported in the literature are retrospective analyses of patients who have undergone renal biopsy because of a suspicion that they have non-diabetic renal disease. This is based on clinical and laboratory assessment by both diabetologists and nephrologists. These studies are therefore heavily weighted towards detecting high rates of non-diabetic disease and consequently tell us little about the rate of non-diabetic disease in the diabetic population as a whole. The denominator for any calculation of this sort should be the total number of diabetics in the population studied rather than the number of biopsies performed. This information is rarely used in the studies reported.

This problem can be addressed by studying the prevalence of non-diabetic renal disease in an unselected diabetic population, although in reality this is difficult to achieve. Parving et al studied all type 2 diabetics <66 yrs of age (n=370) with macroalbuminuria (n=50) [3]. All patients fitting this criterion were studied and 35 underwent biopsy. Eight patients (23%) had non-diabetic disease, although of note, 4 of these had minimal change lesions that could be compatible with early diabetic nephropathy. Importantly, in no case did the finding of non-

517

diabetic disease lead to a change in management. Although this study does suggest a higher rate of non-diabetic disease in an unselected diabetic population, even this study cannot exclude a referral bias. In contrast, Brocco et al and Fioreto et al reported the biopsy findings respectively of 53 and 35 consecutive microalbuminuric type 2 diabetic patients none of whom had non-diabetic disease [4,5]. The low rate of non-diabetic renal suggested by the later 2 studies is also supported by 2 post mortem studies [6,7]. Waldherr et al found only 1 case of non-diabetic renal disease in over 200 post mortems on diabetic patients, half of whom had documented abnormal renal function [7]. This suggests that the incidence of non-diabetic disease is no higher in diabetic patients than in the general population.

The marked variability in the reported rates on non-diabetic disease may also reflect ethnic and geographical patterns of disease. For example the high rates of non-diabetic disease reported in India could reflect high rates of proliferative disease and the biopsy of patients with an acute decline in renal function [8]. One other factor that may affect the rates of diagnosis of non-diabetic disease is the increasing recognition of atypical lesions, such as focal tubulointerstitial scarring, particularly in type 2 diabetes. These may have been classified as non-diabetic lesions in older studies. One other confounding factor is that of publication bias toward series that report a higher incidence of non-diabetic glomerular diseases.

A separate question is whether knowledge of non-diabetic disease allows an alteration in therapy and therefore prognosis. This is certainly the case for rapidly progressive diseases that are clearly responsive to immunosuppression. However, for other diseases such as membranous nephropathy and focal segmental glomerulosclerosis the treatment benefit is less clear and for IgA nephropathy there is no specific treatment. The evidence we do have often involves high dose steroid based regimes, the benefits of which in a diabetic patient group has not been explored. Chihara et al were unable to demonstrate a prognostic benefit in diagnosing non-diabetic renal disease [9].

Rather than a general increase in the rate of non-diabetic renal disease, several authors have suggested an increase rate of specific glomerular diseases in the diabetic patient. The evidence for this is discussed below.

Membranous nephropathy
From the literature, membranous nephropathy is the most likely glomerular disease to have an excess incidence in diabetic patients. Membranous

nephropathy, although a common cause of adult nephrotic syndrome, is nevertheless a relatively rare disease with an incidence of 1-2 per 100000 adults per year [23]. The co-existence of membranous nephropathy and diabetic renal disease has been extensively reported [24-26]. and several series have suggested a relatively high rate of membranous nephropathy on biopsy of proteinuric diabetic patients [2,21]. Again these reports suffer from selection bias and a failure to refer to the number of at risk patients. Cahen et al looked at 82 consecutive patients with membranous nephropathy and found that only 1 of them had diabetes [27]. Nevertheless the rarity of membranous nephropathy in the general population raises the possibility an association with diabetes.

IgA nephropathy

Prior to 1992 only 6 cases of IgA nephropathy had been reported in diabetic patients. In 1992 Gans et al described 5 patients with diabetes and biopsy proven IgA nephropathy [28] and suggested that this may represent more than coincidence. However, the proportion of biopsies showing IgA nephropathy was similar in both diabetics and non-diabetics and the diabetic patients biopsied were highly selected. Other studies have supported an association between diabetes and IgA nephropathy [2]. Mak et al found an incidence of non-diabetic renal disease greater than 30% and over half of these had IgA nephropathy [12]. Geographical factors may influence this result as IgA nephropathy is common in Hong Kong, accounting for 30% of all biopsies performed. However, caution is necessary when suggesting an association between diabetes and a common glomerular disease, the prevalence of which in the general population (worldwide) is not accurately known.

Rapidly progressive (crescentic) glomerulonephritis

There are numerous reports of rapidly progressive glomerulonephritis occurring in diabetics, often superimposed on diabetic lesions [29,30]. However there is no evidence that the rate of crescentic glomerulonephritis is increased in diabetics.

PREDICTING PATIENTS WITH NON-DIABETIC RENAL DISEASE

Obviously some diabetic patients will develop non-diabetic renal disease. Therefore, are there any clinical parameters that clinicians can use to predict non-diabetic renal disease in a population that has high rates of renal insufficiency and abnormal urinary sediment? Several clinical parameters have been reported to predict a high rate of non-diabetic renal disease.

Haematuria

Haematuria occurs in diabetic nephropathy in over 50% of cases. Nevertheless some authors have suggested that its presence predicts non-diabetic disease. For example, in a Chinese population, in whom rates of IgA nephropathy were predictably high, the presence of haematuria was useful in predicting non-diabetic disease [12]. In contrast, in the series of 136 proteinuric diabetic patients who underwent biopsy described by Taft et al [21], 66% had microscopic haematuria. The presence or absence of microscopic haematuria did not help to predict whether the patient had non-diabetic renal disease.

Generally haematuria is not a strong predictor of non-diabetic glomerular disease but it may be a sign of lower tract disease. In older patients without associated proteinuria, the presence of haematuria warrants imaging of the renal tract and cystoureteroscopy, as indicated for non-diabetic patients.

Absence of retinopathy

The absence of retinopathy has different implications in type 1 and type 2 diabetes. In type 1 diabetes there is a very close association between retinopathy and nephropathy. The absence of retinopathy, assessed formally by photography or angiography, in a type 1 diabetic with abnormal renal function or proteinuria would be an indication to biopsy the patient if no other cause of renal disease was evident.

The situation is less clear in type 2 diabetes. Many patients with type 2 diabetes do not have classical histological changes of diabetes but nevertheless their renal disease is related to their diabetes. The presence of retinopathy strongly predicts the presence of typical diabetic glomerular changes [4,5,31], in particular Kimmelsteil-Wilson nodules [11]. What is less clear is how useful is its absence in predicting non-diabetic disease. Parving et al suggested that the absence of retinopathy strongly predicted non-diabetic renal disease in macroalbuminaemic type 2 diabetics [3]. Christensen et al described the biopsy findings from 52 type 2 diabetics with microalbuminuria but absent retinopathy (defined by fundal photography) [16]. Most patients had diabetic nephropathy but non-diabetic disease was found in 7 patients (13%) and normal glomerular structure in a further 9 patients (18%). Therefore although the presence of retinopathy indicates diabetic nephropathy, even in its absence the patient is likely to have diabetic kidney disease.

Rapid decline in renal function

The course of diabetic nephropathy has been extensively described. A rapid decline in renal function (perhaps >10% of residual function per month) in a normotensive diabetic is inconsistent with diabetic disease and is an indication for further assessment and biopsy.

Nephrotic syndrome

The course of diabetic nephropathy, with microalbuminuria preceding heavier proteinuria and nephrotic syndrome, is well documented, particularly in type 1 diabetes [32]. Patients who develop significant, nephrotic range proteinuria without preceding microalbuminuria despite appropriate testing should be considered for biopsy. For patients who develop lesser degrees of proteinuria (for example <1g/24 hours) the case for biopsy is less clear. In the absence of positive serology, reduced GFR or hypertension there is no consensus as to whether biopsy is indicated for any patient with this level of proteinuria irrespective of whether they are diabetic.

Short duration of diabetes

The clinical course of type 1 diabetes is usually predictable with diabetes diagnosed many years before the onset of diabetic nephropathy. In contrast, type 2 diabetics may present with established microvascular complications. Therefore a short duration of diabetes prior to the development of abnormal renal functional parameters is highly predictive of non-diabetic renal disease in type 1 diabetes. This is not the case in type 2 diabetes where, in general, studies show no correlation between duration of diabetes and the presence of non-diabetic renal disease [2,3,12,16,18].

THE ROLE OF THE BIOPSY IN ASSESSING DIABETIC KIDNEY DISEASE

This is an issue that has prompted much discussion in the literature with some authors arguing in favour of an increasing use of biopsy. There is certainly a role for renal biopsy in clinical studies of diabetic nephropathy. However, the routine clinical use of biopsy in these patients is less clear and may vary according to the stage of the disease. We have not differentiated between type 1 and type 2 diabetes as the same issues apply to both groups.

Early stages of disease

Once overt nephropathy has developed histological lesions are predictably advanced. In contrast, patients with lower levels of microalbuminuria can have very variable light microscopic appearances, from normal structure to well established diabetic lesions [33]. Structural changes can also be apparent even in the absence of functional changes. The lack of correlation between functional measurements and histological changes has been suggested as a reason to biopsy patients with low levels of microalbuminuria [34,35]. This is justifiable within the context of a clinical study. Whether or not it is justified in normal clinical practice depends on whether it will provide important diagnostic or prognostic information or guide therapeutic decision-making.

This will depend on whether biopsy offers any advantage over functional assessment in early disease. Biopsy could identify a group of patients with normal functional parameters but established histological disease, thereby identifying a group likely to progress to overt nephropathy. To identify this group of patients biopsy would need to be considered even in the absence of functional abnormalities [35]. Would these patients be treated more aggressively in terms of glycaemic and blood pressure control? There is insufficient evidence to suggest that treatment would be significantly altered and any evidence provided would need to be very convincing to justify biopsying all diabetics with no functional abnormality. In addition biopsying this large group of patients is not a feasible option for most renal units. Although a normal biopsy may reassure a patient it is difficult to justify a biopsy on these grounds alone.

Therefore, should patients be biopsied once a functional abnormality is detected? The major recent studies in the treatment of microalbuminuric diabetics have not included renal biopsy as an entry criteria [36]. It is likely that the same glycaemic and blood pressure control targets would be adopted in a microalbuminuric diabetic patient irrespective of the biopsy result. Admittedly the co-existence of more severe glomerular lesions may predict a worse prognosis but careful functional monitoring would identify this group of patients.

Later stages of disease

Many studies in type 1 diabetes have demonstrated a close correlation between renal histology and loss of function once overt nephropathy has developed. In particular mesangial expansion and loss of capillary wall area correlate closely with GFR [34,37]. The strong predictive value of functional parameters at this stage means that biopsy is of little prognostic value.

THE RISKS INVOLVED IN RENAL BIOPSY

Renal biopsy is an invasive procedure and is not without risk. Clinically evident complications have been reported in 7-13% of biopsies [38,39]. Many of these are self-limiting, for example macroscopic haematuria or perirenal haematoma. These are historical reports and the rate of complication should be reduced with improved imaging techniques and biopsy needles. Nevertheless serious potential complications can arise and death has been reported in up to 0.2% of biopsies [40]. This factor needs to be considered when deciding whether or not to biopsy a diabetic patient.

CONCLUSION

We feel that at the moment the literature does not support the conclusion that there is an increased rate of non-diabetic glomerular disease in either type 1 or type 2 diabetes. Most studies suffer from selection bias, making any suggestion of an association between diabetes and other diseases such as membranous nephropathy difficult to interpret. Clearly some diabetic patients will develop non-diabetic glomerular disease and therefore benefit from biopsy. Unfortunately we have no reliable way of identifying this group of patients. Certainly no single observation is useful in isolation, but careful clinical assessment of the patients will increase the rate of detection of non-diabetic disease. This is demonstrated by the high rates of non-diabetic disease found in the reported series of selected patients. Examples of clinical findings that warrant biopsy include:

- Renal disease in the presence of features of systemic disease or positive serology
- Abrupt onset of proteinuria without previous microalbuminuria
- Rapidly declining renal function in a normotensive patient

This list is not exhaustive and each patient needs to be assessed carefully.

There is no evidence that use of renal biopsy to assess the nature or severity of diabetic nephropathy has any role in routine clinical practice. It would not be possible to biopsy all diabetics with functional abnormalities nor is there evidence that therapy or prognosis would be altered by such practice. Despite this, whilst our understanding of the pathogenesis of this common renal disease remains incomplete, there is an undoubted role for renal biopsy in the context of clinical research.

REFERENCES

1. Iversen P, Brun C: Aspiration biopsy of the kidney. American Journal of Medicine 11:324-330, 1951
2. Mazzucco G, Bertani T, Fortunato M, Bernardi M, Leutner M, Boldorini R, Monga G: Different patterns of renal damage in type 2 diabetes mellitus: A multicentric study on 393 biopsies. American Journal of Kidney Diseases 39:713-720, 2002
3. Parving HH, Gall MA, Skott P, Jorgensen HE, Lokkegaard H, Jorgensen F, Nielson B, Larsen S: Prevalence and causes of albuminuria in non-insulin-dependent diabetic patients. Kidney International 41:758-762, 1992
4. Brocco E, Fioretto P, Mauer M, Saller A, Carraro A, Frigato F, Chiesura-Corona M, Bianchi L, Baggio B, Maioli M, Abaterusso C, Velussi M, Sambataro M, Virgili F, Ossi E, Nosadini R: Renal structure and function in non-insulin dependent diabetic patients with microalbuminuria. Kidney International - Supplement 63:S40-S44, 1997
5. Fioretto P, Mauer M, Brocco E, Velussi M, Frigato F, Muollo B, Sambataro M, Abaterusso C, Baggio B, Crepaldi G, Nosadini R: Patterns of renal injury in NIDDM patients with microalbuminuria. Diabetologia 39:1569-1576, 1996
6. Ditscherlein G: Pathomorphology of the diabetic kidney. Clinical Nephrology 46:256-258, 1996
7. Waldherr R, Ilkenhans C, Ritz E: How Frequent Is Glomerulonephritis in Diabetes-Mellitus Type-II. Clinical Nephrology 37:271-273, 1992
8. John GT, Date A, Korula A, Jeyaseelan L, Shastry JC, Jacob CK: Nondiabetic renal disease in noninsulin-dependent diabetics in a south Indian Hospital. Nephron 67:441-443, 1994
9. Chihara J, Takebayashi S, Taguchi T, Yokoyama K, Harada T, Naito S: Glomerulonephritis in diabetic-patients and its effect on the prognosis. Nephron 43:45-49, 1986
10. Amoah E, Glickman JL, Malchoff CD, Sturgill BC, Kaiser DL, Bolton WK: Cinical-identification of nondiabetic renal-disease in diabetic patients with type-I and type-II disease presenting with renal dysfunction. American Journal of Nephrology 8:204-211, 1988
11. Schwartz MM, Lewis EJ, Leonard-Martin T, Lewis JB, Batlle D: Renal pathology patterns in type II diabetes mellitus: relationship with retinopathy. Nephrology Dialysis Transplantation 13:2547-2552, 1998
12. Mak SK, Gwi E, Chan KW, Wong PN, Lo KY, Lee KF, Wong AKM: Clinical predictors of non-diabetic renal disease in patients with non-insulin dependent diabetes mellitus. Nephrology Dialysis Transplantation 12:2588-2591, 1997
13. Serra A, Romero R, Bayes B, Lopez D, Bonet J: Is there a need for changes in renal biopsy criteria in proteinuria in type 2 diabetes. Diabetes Research & Clinical Practice 58:149-153, 2002

14. Suzuki Y, Ueno M, Hayashi H, Nishi S, Satou H, Karasawa R, Inn H, Suzuki S, Maruyama Y, Arakawa M: A light-microscopic study of glomerulosclerosis in Japanese patients with noninsulin-dependent diabetes mellitus - the relationship between clinical and histological features. Clinical Nephrology 42:155-162, 1994

15. Prakash J, Sen D, Usha, Kumar NS: Non-diabetic renal disease in patients with type 2 diabetes mellitus. Journal of the Association of Physicians of India 49:415-20, 2001

16. Christensen PK, Larsen S, Horn T, Olsen S, Parving HH: Causes of albuminuria in patients with type 2 diabetes without diabetic retinopathy. Kidney International 58:1719-1731, 2000

17. Olsen S, Mogensen CE: How often is NIDDM complicated with non-diabetic renal disease? An analysis of renal biopsies and the literature. Diabetologia 39:1638-1645, 1996

18. Gambara V, Mecca G, Remuzzi G, Bertani T: Heterogenous nature of renal lesions in type II diabetes. Journal of the American Society of Nephrology 3:1458-1466, 1993

19. Richards NT, Greaves I, Lee SJ, Howie AJ, Adu D, Michael J: Increased prevalence of renal biopsy findings other than diabetic glomerulopathy in type II diabetes mellitus.[comment]. Nephrology Dialysis Transplantation 7:397-399, 1992

20. Yum MN, Maxwell DR, Hamburger R, Kleit SA: Primary glomerulonephritis complicating diabetic nephropathy - Report of 7 cases and review of the literature. Human Pathology 15:921-927, 1984

21. Taft JL, Billson VR, Nankervis A, Kincaidsmith P, Martin FIR: A clinical-histological study of individuals with diabetes mellitus and proteinuria. Diabetic Medicine 7:215-221, 1990

22. Kasinath BS, Mujais SK, Spargo BH, Katz AI: Non-diabetic renal disease in patients with diabetes mellitus. American Journal of Medicine 75:613-617, 1983

23. Simon P, Ramee MP, Autuly V, Laruelle E, Charasse C, Cam G, Ang KS: Epidemiology of primary glomerular diseases in a French region. Variations according to period and age. Kidney International 46:1192-1198, 1994

24. Warms PC, Rosenbaum BJ, Michelis MF, Haas JE: Idiopathic membranous glomerulonephritis occurring with diabetes mellitus. Archives of Internal Medicine 132:735-738, 1973

25. Rao KV, Crosson JT: Idiopathic membranous glomerulonephritis in diabetic patients. Archives of Internal Medicine 140:624-627, 1980

26. Premalatha G, Vidhya K, Deepa R, Ravikumar R, Rema M, Mohan V: Prevalence of non-diabetic renal disease in type 2 diabetic patients in a diabetes centre in Southern India. Journal of the Association of Physicians of India 50:1135-1139, 2002

27. Cahen R, Francois B, Trolliet P, Gilly J, Parchoux B: Aetiology of membranous glomerulonephritis: a prospective study of 82 adult patients. Nephrology Dialysis Transplantation 4:172-180, 1989

28. Gans ROB, Ueda Y, Ito S, Kohli R, Min I, Shafi M, Brentjens JR: The occurrence of IgA-Nephropathy in patients with diabetesmellitus may not be coincidental - A report of 5 cases. American Journal of Kidney Diseases 20:255-260, 1992

29. Carstens SA, Hebert LA, Garancis JC, Piering WF, Lemann J: Rapidly progressive glomerulonephritis superimposed on diabetic glomerulosclerosis - recognition and treatment. Journal of the American Medical Association 247:1453-1457, 1982

30. Lui SL, Chan KW, Yip PS, Chan TM, Lai KN, Lo WK: Simultaneous occurence of diabetic glomerulosclerosis, IgA nephropathy, crescentic nephropathy, and myeloperoxidase-antineutrophil cytoplasmic antibody seropositivity in a Chinese patient. American Journal of Kidney Diseases 40:E14, 2002

31.   Kanauchi M, Dohi K: Predictors of diabetic renal lesions in type 2 diabetes associated with microalbuminuria. European Journal of Clinical Investigation 31:110-112, 2001

32.   Mogensen CE: Urinary albumin excretion in early and long-term juvenile diabetes. Scandinavian Journal of Clinical & Laboratory Investigation 28:183-193, 1971

33.   Chavers BM, Bilous RW, Ellis EN, Steffes MW, Mauer SM: Glomerular lesions and urinary albumin excretion in type-I diabetes without overt proteinuria. New England Journal of Medicine 320:966-970, 1989

34.   Mauer SM, Steffes MW, Ellis EN, Sutherland DER, Brown DM, Goetz FC: Structural-functional relationships in diabetic nephropathy. Journal of Clinical Investigation 74:1143-1155, 1984

35.   Mauer SM, Chavers BM, Steffes MW: Should there be an expanded role for kidney biopsy in the management of patients with type-I diabetes. American Journal of Kidney Diseases 16:96-100, 1990

36.   Parving HH, Lehnert H, Brochner-Mortensen J, Gomis R, Andersen S, Arner P. Irbesartan in Patients with Type: The effect of irbesartan on the development of diabetic nephropathy in patients with type 2 diabetes. New England Journal of Medicine 345(12):870-8, 2001

37.   Ellis EN, Steffes MW, Goetz FC, Sutherland DER, Mauer SM: Glomerular filtration surface in type-I diabetes mellitus. Kidney International 29:889-894, 1986

38.   Burstein DM, Schwartz MM, Korbet SM: Percutaneous renal biopsy with the use of real-time ultrasound. American Journal of Nephrology 11:195-200, 1991

39.   Diaz-Buxo JA, Donadio JV, Jr.: Complications of percutaneous renal biopsy: an analysis of 1,000 consecutive biopsies. Clinical Nephrology 4:223-227, 1975

40.   Parrish AE: Complications of percutaneous renal biopsy: a review of 37 years' experience. Clinical Nephrology 38:135-141, 1992

30

INHIBITION OF THE RENIN ANGIOTENSIN ALDOSTERONE SYSTEM, WITH PARTICULAR REFERENCE TO THE DUAL BLOCKADE PRINCIPLE

Niels Holmark Andersen

Department of internal medicine, Aarhus Kommunehospital, Aarhus University Hospital, Aarhus, Denmark.

INTRODUCTION

The dual blockade principle can possibly provide the broadest and most efficient blockade of circulating Angiotensin II, by using the combination of an ACE-inhibitor and an Angiotensin II receptor blocker.

The following chapter will provide a selection of results from studies using dual blockade therapy in hypertension, nephropathy and cardiovascular disease, and give an overview of how far we have come with this new treatment principle.

ACTIONS OF ANGIOTENSIN II

Inhibition of Angiotensin II might be the main issue in the diabetes patient with hypertension, nephropathy or both conditions in coexistence. The effects of this active metabolite are potentially damaging to an extent superior to many other peptides and metabolites. This makes inhibition and control of Angiotensin II essential.

The renin-Angiotensin system can be stimulated by stress, high sodium intake, or an increase in sympathetic activity. This stimulation results in increased renin levels, leading to increased levels of Angiotensin I. This inactive decapeptide is then chemically modified by Angiotensin-converting enzyme (ACE) in the lungs and in other tissues to the active octapeptide, Angiotensin II, finally leading to increased levels of Angiotensin II. Action of this substance causes an increase in blood pressure by direct vasoconstriction and increases aldosterone synthesis, which additionally results in sodium retention, increased extracellular volume and higher blood pressure.

Several non-hemodynamic effects of Angiotensin II may also be of importance. Experimental studies have revealed increasing mesangial cell proliferation and induction of transforming growth factor beta (TGF-β) expression in chronic renal disease [1]. This results in the increased synthesis of extracellular matrix and stimulation of plasminogen activator inhibitor-1 production by endothelial cells and vascular smooth muscle cells. Angiotensin II also mediates macrophage activation and increases phagocytosis in failing organs, like chronic heart or renal failure and is believed to be one of the major determinants in left ventricular remodelling and induction of hypertrophy, fibrosis and apoptosis in the failing heart [2;3].

Angiotensin II has the potential to influence key aspects of the endothelial function via disturbance of vasodilator substances like bradykinin, nitric oxide (NO) and vasoendothelial growth factor VEGF. This can aggravate diabetic microvascular disease and result in the development of a prothrombotic surface in small and large vessels.

Finally the superimposed adrenal production of aldosterone is recently recognized as a potent contributor to renal or myocardial injury [4].

All these factors are essential to the subsequent pathogenesis of renal and cardiovascular disease in patients with diabetes and hypertension.

INCOMPLETE ACE-INHIBITION

By use of an ACE-inhibitor this cascade of tissue alterations and blood pressure elevation can be altered. ACE inhibitors improve survival in nephropathy and heart failure, but as an antihypertensive drug it is well known that blood pressure levels can rise to pre-treatment values after long term ACE-inhibitor treatment. This could be due to the phenomenon termed "ACE-Escape". This is a mechanism where levels of plasma Angiotensin II and aldosterone somehow return to pre-treatment levels despite continues treatment with an ACE-inhibitor. This is due to bypassing of the Angiotensin converting enzyme and conversion of Angiotensin I to Angiotensin II by alternative enzymatic pathways [5]. Non- ACE dependant conversions of Angiotensin I to Angiotensin II are enhanced, especially in the failing heart, in the kidneys and in large resistance vessels [6]. Both Chymase and Cathepsin and other enzymes are able to contribute to the conversion of Angiotensin I to Angiotensin II and are found activated in disorders where, high levels of oxidative stress are present such as vascular pro-inflammatory processes, atherogenesis and especially diabetes mellitus [7].

Up to 60-70 % of circulating Angiotensin II may be produced by alternative pathways [8].

Secondary high levels of tissue ACE-activity mediating local Angiotensin I conversion, found in the lung, the blood vessels, myocardium and in the kidneys [9], have also been proposed to mediate a more long-term tissue damage like glomerular hypertrophy and left ventricular remodeling [10;11].

This is essential, since tissue ACE activity is not always sufficiently blocked by regular doses of ACE-1 inhibitor, so even though circulating levels of Angiotensin II are reduced, incessant tissue damage is ongoing.

The Angiotensin II receptor blockers should block circulating Angiotensin II, but other loopholes in the blockade of the RAS-system might also influence these agents. By blocking the receptor, circulating levels of Angiotensin II will rise and obviously compete with the AT_1 receptor blocker at the receptor site. This requires use of a long acting ARB agents, since otherwise the AT_1 receptor is totally exposed in long intervals during the day [12-14].

Furthermore, we do not know very much about the harmful effects of activating the other subgroups of the Angiotensin II receptors. At present 4 subgroups of receptors are known AT_{1-4}.

The effects of subclass 3 and 4 are unknown and in adult tissues the AT_2 receptors are present only at low levels, mainly in the uterus, the adrenal gland, the central nervous system, the heart (cardiomyocytes and fibroblasts), and the kidney. But the AT_2 receptors seem to be re-expressed or up regulated in experimental cardiac hypertrophy, myocardial infarction, and wound healing [15-17]. In humans all the known clinical effects of Angiotensin II are mediated by the AT_1 receptor, but since AT_1 antagonists do not block the AT_2 receptor, exaggerated stimulation of the AT_2 receptor occurs. This receptor could play an important role in apoptosis and fibrosis in the glomerulus and the myocardium, and could mediate vasoconstriction and elevated aldosterone production despite, Angiotensin II receptor blocker treatment.

We do not have detailed information about these mechanisms at present, but the role of unopposed stimulation of AT_2 receptor will have a major bearing on the question of whether combined therapy with an Angiotensin II receptor blocker and an ACE inhibitor will exert additive benefit [18].

RATIONALE BEHIND DUAL BLOCKADE TREATMENT

The mentioned factors support our clinical experiences that neither the ACE-inhibitor nor the Angiotensin II receptor blocker is always able to achieve the requested blood pressure reduction or reduce proteinuria even in maximum recommended doses, so the seek for a more superior renin Angiotensin system blockade is ongoing.

Dual blockade treatment is based on a principle of obtaining the broadest and most efficient blockade of the effects of Angiotensin II, by using the combination of an ACE-inhibitor and an Angiotensin II receptor blocker.

By combining the 2 different pharmacological principles and inhibiting both the Angiotensin converting enzyme and the Angiotensin II receptor, it seems possible to block both the production and the action of Angiotensin II, and serve as excellent anti hypertensive therapy. Additionally, it may be possible to increase the beneficial effects of bradykinin on blood pressure and renal function, because of reduced degrading of this metabolite. Figure 1 displays the principle behind dual blockade.

Several experimental studies have supported the idea of beneficial effects of dual blockade therapy since 1995 where Michel Azizi, from the Joel Menard group was the first to demonstrate an additive effect on blood pressure and a significant rise in circulating renin-levels from single doses of losartan combined with captopril in a group of sodium-depleted normotensive volunteers [19].

The following will provide a selection of the present available studies with dual blockade treatment in hypertension, nephropathy and heart failure and thoughts of how to explore this new treatment principle in the future.

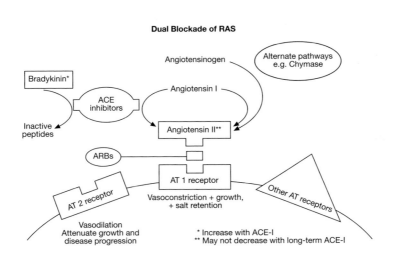

Dual Blockade of RAS

Figure 1. Schematic display of the mechanisms behind the dual blockade treatment. [From Andersen NH et al. Curr. Hypertens Rep, 2003; Oct. 4(5): 394-402]

DUAL BLOCKADE IN DIABETES MELLITUS

Only few studies are published using the dual blockade treatment principle to treat hypertension and nephropathy in patients with diabetes mellitus, even though the indication seems obvious. Hebert et al. were among the first to apply dual blockade to diabetic patients in a small series of only 7 patients with diabetes, hypertension and macroalbuminuria. They found arterial blood pressure significantly lowered, when adding 50 mg's of Losartan to concomitant ACE-inhibition treatment, but proteinuria was not significantly reduced [20].This was obtained in another small trial including Type 2 diabetes patients with nephropathy. Rossing et al conducted a trial of 18 patients with Type 2 diabetes, severe proteinuria (>1g/day) and hypertension, who where all treated with recommended doses of long acting ACE inhibitors among a wide variety of other antihypertensive drugs. By adding 8 mg candesartan cilexetil both blood pressure and proteinuria were significantly reduced [21]. This was also found in a second trial from the same group using the Angiotensin II receptor blocker Irbesartan in combination with concomitant ACE-inhibitor treatment in Type 1 diabetes patients with severe nephropathy and concomitant hypertension. Dual blockade was again able to significantly reduce both blood pressure and albuminuria compared to monotherapy [22].

These findings have recently been confirmed by the same study group in two small short term studies in Type 1 diabetes patients with nephropathy[23;24].

For the sake of completeness, a small trial on nephropathy should be mentioned. It included 12 patients with diabetes, out of a total number of 16 severely obese patients with nephropathy. In one period, patients received lisinopril 40 mg once daily along with other antihypertensive therapy, and in the other period, losartan 50 mg was added to the previously mentioned regimen. The study failed to show any effects of dual blockade treatment over one month treatment, with a two-week washout between periods [25]. In a companion paper Agarwal and colleagues were able to find significant reduction in TGF-beta 1 levels among patients in dual blockade treatment, and the authors postulated that some renoprotection might be present, due to these findings [26]. The lack of solid evidence in these 2 trials could partially be explained by study design and size. The CALM study still stands as the largest dual blockade trial concerning diabetes patients. This randomized, double blind study was performed on 197 patients between 30 and 75 years of age who were previously diagnosed with Type 2 diabetes mellitus, hypertension and microalbuminuria. The included patients were treated with 20 mg lisinopril, or16 mg candesartan cilexetil daily, or both drugs in combination. After 4 weeks of placebo treatment, patients were treated with lisinopril or candesartan for 12 weeks. Thereafter, patients continued with either monotherapy or the combination of lisinopril and candesartan for an additional 12 weeks. All three treatments significantly reduced blood pressure from baseline to 24 weeks, with dual blockade being the most effective. There was also a significant blood pressure reduction obtained with dual blockade as compared to either lisinopril or candesartan alone. The trial also found greater reductions in the urine albumin-creatinine ratio with combination treatment (50%) compared to lisinopril alone (39%) and candesartan alone (24%). But when adjusting for diastolic blood pressure, baseline values, and weight, the differences were not significant [27]. Table 1 provides an overview of the mentioned trials.

Table 1. Selected dual blockade-trials

Study	Study drugs	N	Follow-up	Results
Hebert et al [20]	Losartan 50 mg ACE-inhibitor	7	1 week	Significant blood pressure reduction. No effects on proteinuria.
Rossing et al. [21]	Candesartan 8 mg ACE-inhibitor	18	9 weeks	Significant blood pressure reduction Significant reduction in albuminuria
Jacobsen et al. [22]	Irbesartan 300 mg ACE-inhibitor	21	8 weeks	Significant blood pressure reduction Significant reduction in albuminuria
Jacobsen et al. [23]	Irbesartan 300 mg Enalapril 40 mg	24	8 weeks	Significant blood pressure reduction Significant reduction in albuminuria
Jacobsen et al. [24]	Benazepril 20 mg Valsartan 80 mg	18	8 weeks	Significant blood pressure reduction Significant reduction in albuminuria
Agarwal * [25;26]	Losartan 50mg Lisinopril 40 mg	12	1 month	No effects on blood pressure or proteinuria. Improvement in GFR significant TGF-β 1 reduction.
CALM [27]	Candesartan 16 mg Lisinopril 20 mg	199	12 weeks	Significant blood pressure reduction Significant reduction in albuminuria
COOPERATE [38]†	Losartan 100 mg Trandolapril 3 mg	245	4 yrs	Significant reduction in both end-stage renal disease and doubling of serum creatinine

*] *Two Studies*
†]*Patients with non-diabetic nephropathy*

CONGESTIVE HEART FAILURE

The ACE-inhibitor is well established as a fundamental part of heart failure treatment, but the role of the Angiotensin II receptor blocker in heart failure treatment has not yet been fully established.

The ELITE-II, OPTIMAAL and VALHEFT trials all failed to show benefits from the Angiotensin II receptor blocker compared with ACE-inhibition in heart failure patients.

Retrospectively some might suggest that this was mostly due to inferior study design, and it is worthwhile noticing that these studies were planned in the early nineties where knowledge was different.

It was surprising, however, that the VALHEFT trial, which was a comprehensive heart failure study using the Angiotensin receptor blocker Valsartan added to concomitant heart failure medication showed that patients treated with both an ACE-inhibitor and an Angiotensin II receptor blocker did not benefit from this treatment, and it was indeed unexpected that patients treated with both ACE-inhibitor ß-blocker and Valsartan had a 10 per cent increase in the combined endpoint of all-cause mortality and morbidity [28].

The study was not designed to investigate dual blockade in heart failure and the mentioned results were based on subgroup analysis and should be interpreted with caution, but one must question whether some precautions should be taken in this specific group of patients.

The VALHEFT trial results stand in clear contrast to several small dual blockade studies in heart failure patients which all have shown promising results.

Several small experimental studies have found beneficial effects on the neurohumeral activation in the failing heart [29-31]. Clinical trials support these observations. The smaller V-heft trail found beneficial effect on both blood pressure, hormonal and haemodynamic factors in a small short-term placebo-controlled study in 83 heart failure patients treated with varying dosages of Valsartan added to concomitant ACE-inhibitor treatment [32].

Hamroff and colleges found exercise capacity in a treadmill exercise significantly improved over a 6 months follow-up period, when 50 mg of Losartan was added to the maximal recommended or tolerated doses of ACE-I inhibitor in a placebo-controlled study including 33 patients with heart failure [33].

Also the RESOLVD pilot trial found positive results, randomising 768 heart failure patients (NYHA II to IV) to either candesartan (up to 8 mg) or enalapril or candesartan and enalapril in combination. The combination of candesartan and enalapril was more effective in preventing left ventricular remodelling than both candesartan and enalapril alone. Levels of brain-natriuretic-peptide were also significantly reduced during the 43 week follow-up period [34].

The issue of using ARBs combined with ACE inhibitors will probably not be resolved until the results of the next major trials are reported. This could be the CHARM trial with candesartan.

The [CHARM] trial (Candesartan in Heart Failure-Assessment of Reduction in Mortality and Morbidity), will include approximately 6,500 patients with heart failure. The CHARM program consists of 3 independent, parallel, placebo-controlled studies in patients with 1) LVEF less than or equal to 40%, ACE-inhibitor treated (n = 2,300); 2) LVEF less than or equal to 40%, ACE-inhibitor intolerant (n = 1,700); 3) LVEF greater than 40%, not treated with ACE inhibitors (n = 2,500). The 3 studies will be combined to evaluate the effect of candesartan on all-cause mortality in the broad spectre of symptomatic heart failure.

Another study of great interest is also directed towards the Valiant trial (Valsartan in Acute Myocardial Infarction Trial) including 14,500 patients with prior MI and heart failure. The trial is designed with 3 arms, giving equal statistical consideration to survival comparisons of captopril versus the Angiotensin II receptor blocker valsartan, as well as the combination of captopril plus valsartan, compared with a proven effective dose of captopril. Patients will be randomised to either Captopril 50mg o.d, Valsartan 160 mg o.d or the combination of Captopril 50 mg plus Valsartan 80 mg o.d. Results are due in 2005 [35].

TOLERABILITY

It seems likely that efficient blockage of this essential enzymatic system would be associated with high complication rates, but this is not the case. Angiotensin II receptor blockers are generally well tolerated even in maximum dosage and the ACE-inhibitors exert the side-effects well know by all clinicians like cough and angio-oedema. Dual blockade seems as safe as monotherapy with either drug alone, and only reversible side effects have yet been reported. Typical side effects are cough, feeling weak, hypotension and hyperkaliaemia.

In a previously published overview of dual blockade trials incidences of side effects were between 0.6-10.9 per cent [36].

FUTURE ASPECTS

Dual blockade therapy efficiently reduces blood pressure and proteinuria in diabetes patients with hypertension and nephropathy compared to treatment with either drug alone but many of the mentioned trials include very few patients and treatment periods have only been short term. So an overall conclusion is difficult to give.

Many new studies are under way including the CALM II study, which will be finished in 2004. The study aims to investigate the effects of dual blockade on blood pressure, albuminuria, and left ventricular mass and function. The study investigates 75 hypertensive patients with diabetes mellitus over a 12 months follow-up period [37].

FUTURE DUAL BLOCKADE TRIALS

Large clinical trials need to be conducted before general recommendations can be given. We do not have any information on long-term effects, risk reduction in mortality, end-stage renal disease, stroke, myocardial infarction etc. and we do not have valid information whether it is possible to "escape" dual blockade like seen in ACE-inhibition.

Only one larger end-point trial (COOPERATE) is currently available. In this study 245 non-diabetic patients with proteinuria by various ethiologies were treated with monotheraphy of Trandolapril, Losartan or both drugs in combination, over a 4-year period. The investigators found significant endpoint reduction (end stage renal disease) with dual blockade therapy compared to monotherapy of either drug [38].

The ON-TARGET trial will further clarify if dual blockade has any influence on hard end-points. This is a large, long-term study (23,400 patients, 5.5 years). It will compare the benefits of ACE inhibitor treatment, ARB treatment, and treatment with an ACE inhibitor and ARB together, in a study population with established coronary artery disease, stroke, peripheral vascular disease, or diabetes with end-organ damage [39].

CONCLUSION

Dual blockade therapy efficiently reduces blood pressure and proteinuria in diabetes patients with hypertension and nephropathy compared to either drug alone. Until further investigations are available in diabetes patients, dual blockade should be kept for patients with uncontrollable blood pressure, or incessant nephropathy.

REFERENCES

1. Kagami S, Border WA, Miller DE, Noble NA. Angiotensin II Stimulates Extracellular Matrix Protein Synthesis Through Induction of Transforming Growth Factor-Beta Expression in Rat Glomerular Mesangial Cells. J Clin.Invest 1994;93(6):2431-7.
2. Ruzicka M, Yuan B, Harmsen E, Leenen FH. The Renin-Angiotensin System and Volume Overload-Induced Cardiac Hypertrophy in Rats. Effects of Angiotensin Converting Enzyme Inhibitor Versus Angiotensin II Receptor Blocker. Circulation 1993;87(3):921-30.
3. Sadoshima J. Izumo. S. Molecular Characterization of Angiotensin II—Induced Hypertrophy of Cardiac Myocytes and Hyperplasia of Cardiac Fibroblasts. Critical Role of the AT1 Receptor Subtype. Circ.Res. 1993;73(3):413-23.
4. Greene EL, Kren S, Hostetter TH. Role of Aldosterone in the Remnant Kidney Model in the Rat. J Clin.Invest 15-8-1996;98(4):1063-8.
5. van den Meiracker AH, Man in 't Veld AJ, Admiraal PJ, et al. Partial Escape of Angiotensin Converting Enzyme (ACE) Inhibition During Prolonged ACE Inhibitor Treatment: Does It Exist and Does It Affect the Antihypertensive Response? J Hypertens. 1992;10(8):803-12.
6. Balcells, E., Meng, Q. C., Johnson, W. H., Jr., Oparil, S., and Dell'Italia, L. J. Angiotensin II Formation From ACE and Chymase in Human and Animal Hearts: Methods and Species Considerations. Am.J Physiol 1997;273(4 Pt 2):H1769-H1774.
7. Ihara M, Urata H, Kinoshita A et al. Increased Chymase-Dependent Angiotensin II Formation in Human Atherosclerotic Aorta. Hypertension 1999;33(6):1399-405.
8. Hollenberg NK, Fisher ND, Price DA. Pathways for Angiotensin II Generation in Intact Human Tissue: Evidence From Comparative Pharmacological Interruption of the Renin System. Hypertension 1998;32(3):387-92.
9. MacFadyen RJ, Lees KR, Reid JL. Tissue and Plasma Angiotensin Converting Enzyme and the Response to ACE Inhibitor Drugs. Br.J Clin.Pharmacol. 1991;31(1):1-13.
10. Dzau VJ. Re R. Tissue Angiotensin System in Cardiovascular Medicine. A Paradigm Shift? Circulation 1994;89(1):493-8.
11. Rakugi H, Wang DS, Dzau VJ, Pratt RE. Potential Importance of Tissue Angiotensin-Converting Enzyme Inhibition in Preventing Neointima Formation. Circulation 1994;90(1):449-55.
12. Burnier M, Maillard M. The Comparative Pharmacology of Angiotensin II Receptor Antagonists. Blood Press 2001;10 Suppl 1:6-11.

13. Burnier, M. and Brunner, H. R. Angiotensin II Receptor Antagonists. Lancet 19-2-2000;355(9204):637-45.

14. Burnier, M. Angiotensin II Type 1 Receptor Blockers. Circulation 13-2-2001;103(6):904-12.

15. Nio, Y., Matsubara, H., Murasawa, S., Kanasaki, M., and Inada, M. Regulation of Gene Transcription of Angiotensin II Receptor Subtypes in Myocardial Infarction. J Clin.Invest 1995;95(1):46-54.

16. Ohkubo N, Matsubara H, Nozawa Y et al. Angiotensin Type 2 Receptors Are Reexpressed by Cardiac Fibroblasts From Failing Myopathic Hamster Hearts and Inhibit Cell Growth and Fibrillar Collagen Metabolism. Circulation 2-12-1997;96(11):3954-62.

17. Janiak P, Pillon A, Prost JF, Vilaine JP. Role of Angiotensin Subtype 2 Receptor in Neointima Formation After Vascular Injury. Hypertension 1992;20(6):737-45.

18. Hilgers K F, Mann JF. ACE Inhibitors Versus AT(1) Receptor Antagonists in Patients With Chronic Renal Disease. J Am.Soc.Nephrol. 2002;13(4):1100-8.

19. Azizi M, Chatellier G, Guyene TT, Murieta-Geoffroy D, Menard J. Additive Effects of Combined Angiotensin-Converting Enzyme Inhibition and Angiotensin II Antagonism on Blood Pressure and Renin Release in Sodium-Depleted Normotensives. Circulation 15-8-1995;92(4):825-34.

20. Hebert LA, Falkenhain ME, Nahman NS, Jr, Cosio FG, O'Dorisio T. M. Combination ACE Inhibitor and Angiotensin II Receptor Antagonist Therapy in Diabetic Nephropathy. Am.J Nephrol. 1999;19(1):1-6.

21. Rossing K, Christensen PK, Jensen BR, Parving HH. Dual Blockade of the Renin-Angiotensin System in Diabetic Nephropathy: a Randomized Double-Blind Crossover Study. Diabetes Care 2002;25(1):95-100.

22. Jacobsen P, Andersen S, Rossing K, Hansen BV, Parving, HH. Dual Blockade of the Renin-Angiotensin System in Type 1 Patients With Diabetic Nephropathy. Nephrol.Dial.Transplant. 2002;17(6):1019-24.

23. Jacobsen P, Andersen S, Jensen BR, Parving HH. Additive Effect of ACE Inhibition and Angiotensin II Receptor Blockade in Type I Diabetic Patients With Diabetic Nephropathy. J Am.Soc.Nephrol. 2003;14(4):992-9.

24. Jacobsen P, Andersen S, Rossing K, Jensen BR, Parving HH. Dual Blockade of the Renin-Angiotensin System Versus Maximal Recommended Dose of ACE Inhibition in Diabetic Nephropathy. Kidney Int. 2003;63(5):1874-80.

25. Agarwal R. Add-on Angiotensin Receptor Blockade With Maximized ACE Inhibition. Kidney Int. 2001;59(6):2282-9.

26. Agarwal R, Siva S, Dunn SR, Sharma K. Add-on Angiotensin II Receptor Blockade Lowers Urinary Transforming Growth Factor-Beta Levels. Am.J Kidney Dis. 2002;39(3):486-92.

27. Mogensen CE, Nelda, S, Tikkanen I, et al. Randomised Controlled Trial of Dual Blockade of Renin-Angiotensin System in Patients With Hypertension, Microalbuminuria, and Non-Insulin Dependent Diabetes: the Candesartan and Lisinopril Microalbuminuria (CALM) Study. BMJ 9-12-2000;321(7274):1440-4.

28. Cohn JN, Tognoni GA. Randomized Trial of the Angiotensin-Receptor Blocker Valsartan in Chronic Heart Failure. N.Engl.J Med. 6-12-2001;345(23):1667-75.

29. Koji T, Onishi K et al. Addition of Angiotensin II Receptor Antagonist to an ACE Inhibitor in Heart Failure Improves Cardiovascular Function by a Bradykinin-Mediated Mechanism. J Cardiovasc.Pharmacol. 2003;41(4):632-9.

30. Nakamura Y, Yoshiyama M, Omura T et al. Beneficial Effects of Combination of ACE Inhibitor and Angiotensin II Type 1 Receptor Blocker on Cardiac Remodeling in Rat Myocardial Infarction. Cardiovasc.Res. 2003;57(1):48-54.

31. Krombach RS, Clair MJ, Hendrick JW et al. Angiotensin Converting Enzyme Inhibition, AT1 Receptor Inhibition, and Combination Therapy With Pacing Induced Heart Failure: Effects on Left Ventricular Performance and Regional Blood Flow Patterns. Cardiovasc.Res. 1998;38(3):631-45.

32. Baruch L, Anand I, Cohen IS, Ziesche S, Judd D, Cohn JN. Augmented short- and long-term hemodynamic and hormonal effects of an Angiotensin receptor blocker added to Angiotensin converting enzyme inhibitor therapy in patients with heart failure. Vasodilator Heart Failure Trial (V-HeFT) Study Group.. Circulation 25-5-1999;99(20):2658-64.

33. Hamroff G, Katz SD, Mancini D, et al. Addition of Angiotensin II Receptor Blockade to Maximal Angiotensin-Converting Enzyme Inhibition Improves Exercise Capacity in Patients With Severe Congestive Heart Failure. Circulation 2-3-1999;99(8):990-2.

34. McKelvie RS, Yusuf S, Pericak D, et al.. Comparison of Candesartan, Enalapril, and Their Combination in Congestive Heart Failure: Randomized Evaluation of Strategies for Left Ventricular Dysfunction (RESOLVD) Pilot Study. The RESOLVD Pilot Study Investigators. Circulation 7-9-1999;100(10):1056-64.

35. Pfeffer MA, McMurray J, Leizorovicz et al. Valsartan in Acute Myocardial Infarction Trial (VALIANT): Rationale and Design. Am.Heart J 2000;140(5):727-50.

36. Andersen NH, Mogensen CE. Inhibition of the Renin-Angiotensin System, With Particular Reference to Dual Blockade Treatment. J Renin.Angiotensin.Aldosterone.Syst. 2001;2(3):146-52.

37. Andersen, N. H., Poulsen, S. H., Eiskjaer, H., Poulsen, P. L., and Mogensen, C. E. Dual blockade with Candesartan Cilexetil and Lisinopril in Hypertensive patients with Diabetes Mellitus and hypertension. Rationale and design of the CALM II study. J Renin.Angiotensin.Aldosterone.Syst. In press. 2003

38. Nakao N, Yoshimura A, Morita H, Takada M, Kayano T, Ideura T. Combination Treatment of Angiotensin-II Receptor Blocker and Angiotensin-Converting-Enzyme Inhibitor in Non-Diabetic Renal Disease (COOPERATE): a Randomised Controlled Trial. Lancet 11-1-2003;361[9352]:117-24.

39. Yusuf S. From the HOPE to the ONTARGET and the TRANSCEND Studies: Challenges in Improving Prognosis. Am.J Cardiol. 24-1-2002;89(2A):18A-25A.

31

THE CONCEPT OF INCIPIENT DIABETIC NEPHROPATHY AND THE EFFECT OF EARLY ANTIHYPERTENSIVE INTERVENTION

Per Løgstrup Poulsen
Medical Dept. M, Aarhus Kommunehospital, Aarhus, Denmark

INTRODUCTION

Twenty-seven years ago it was described that the rate of decline in glomerular filtration rate (GFR) correlated with clinic blood pressure (BP) in patients with overt diabetic nephropathy [1]. This observation, which was in remarkable contrast to the prevailing concepts, subsequently formed the part of the basis for antihypertensive treatment in patients with diabetic nephropathy, one of the most clinically significant interventions in modern diabetology, documented to preserve GFR [2-5] and reduce mortality [6-8]. However, although these beneficial effects are of immense importance, evaluation of all available studies document that despite antihypertensive treatment a significant proportion of patients still develop end-stage renal disease - "acquiring the goal" has not yet been fully accomplished [9].

The concept of microalbuminuria is another important step forward. Microalbuminuria not only predicts later development of nephropathy in diabetic subjects [10] but may also guide the detection or prediction of other complications e.g. proliferative retinopathy. In addition, microalbuminuria is also strongly associated with cardiovascular risk factors and coronary heart disease in diabetic as well as non-diabetic patients. At present, microalbuminuria is the first abnormality, which clearly allows an early identification of the subgroup of patients at increased risk of developing clinical kidney disease [11]. Clearly additional early disease identifiers should be searched for [12], but so far in vain as e.g. the case for genetic markers [13].

The clinical value of the versatile and strong predictive power of microalbuminuria has been further augmented as it has now been shown that effective intervention modalities exist. Several studies have shown that antihypertensive treatment of normotensive (maybe a questionable concept) microalbuminuric diabetic patients reduces urinary albumin excretion rate considerably and postpones or prevents clinical nephropathy. Furthermore, it is now established that achievement of good glycemic control has similar beneficial effects. Microalbuminuria is an important cardiovascular risk factor in type 2 diabetes along with hypertension, hypercholesterolaemia, and smoking, in addition to predicting nephropathy. The strong predictive power in combination with effective treatment modalities clearly indicates that screening for microalbuminuria should be an essential part of the care for diabetic patients [14].

MICROALBUMINURIA: TECHNIQUES OF MEASUREMENT AND MONITORING

In Fig 1 the different methods and cut off points for the detection of microalbuminuria are depicted. For large scale screening, we find the use of albumin:creatinine ratio in early morning urine a convenient and reliable screening method. In other settings, office tests such as microalbuminuria test-strips [15] and microalbumin/creatinine assays seem to fulfil the requirements of adequate sensitivity, specificity and reproducibility. It is important to consider potential confounders in the detection of microalbuminuria such as exercise, urinary tract infection, menstruation, and severe dysregulation. In addition, there is considerable intra-individual variation in urinary albumin excretion, up to 40-50% when measuring albumin concentrations or albumin:creatinine ratios under routine clinical conditions. Thus, several samples should be taken in order to avoid misclassification of patients and screening should be a continuous process. Detection of microalbuminuria facilitates the identification of high-risk patients and should lead to a thorough screening for other diabetic complications such as retinopathy, silent ischemia etc. as well as a high level of attention regarding the general risk profile of the patient (including glycemic control, lipids, and smoking).

Microalbuminuria: Definition and detection

Abnormal urinary albumin excretion without clinical proteinuria

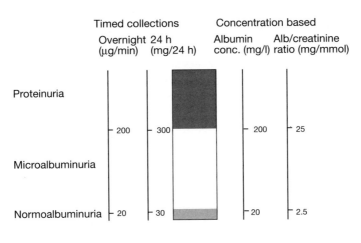

Figure 1.

WHEN TO INTERVENE IN TYPE 1 DIABETIC PATIENTS

Based on several clinical trials [16] ACE inhibitors are now being advised for all type 1 diabetic patients with microalbuminuria, regardless of BP [10;14]. There are, however, some caveats: Firstly, the range of renal disease included in studies of patients with microalbuminuria is quite broad, from those with relatively high UAE associated with advanced renal pathology, to those with only mild elevations of UAE and presumably relatively normal glomerular structure. Relatively young people may be started on ACE inhibitors based upon this indication alone, and would be expected to continue with these drugs for a lifetime. Furthermore, change in UAE is used as a surrogate endpoint, with the implicit assumption that this is an indicator of risk of progressive nephropathy.

Identification of at-risk subjects

Three early studies observed a risk of progression from microalbuminuria (slightly different UAE criteriae) to proteinuria of approximately 80% over the subsequent 6-14 years [17-19]. Later studies confirmed the initial observations and demonstrated that microalbuminuria in addition was strongly predictive of C-V mortality [20;21]. Mauer et al. [12] recently challenged the use of microalbuminuria for clinical decision making, mainly based on two assertions:

I) The predictive power of microalbuminuria is far below the originally estimated, and

II) There is a wide range of glomerular lesions in longstanding type 1 diabetic patients and normoalbuminuric patients may have reduced GFR (creatinine clearance) and advanced glomerular lesions [22].

Regarding assertion I), the lack of predictive power of microalbuminuria, it is important to recognize methodological problems, such as selection bias: In a study by Forsblom et al [23] progression of microalbuminuria to proteinuria ten years later was found in only 25%. However, by selecting patients with over 15 years of duration [mean duration 26 years] the study was biased towards patients less likely to progress. This was demonstrated by Rossing et al. who reported progression to proteinuria in 45% of microalbuminuric patients with duration <15 years vs 26% in patients with duration >15 years [24]. Also changes in treatment strategies over time must be taken into consideration; the reduction in progression to proteinuria in some recent series of patients may reflect the increased use of antihypertensive treatment especially in microalbuminuric patients and the effectiveness of this intervention in postponing overt nephropathy. In the largest double-blind randomized trial of 235 normotensive type 1 diabetic patients with microalbuminuria, 21% of patients treated with placebo developed proteinuria over two years while 7% regressed to normoalbuminuria [25]. The recent follow-up study on the DCCT [26] showed that 31% of 64 microalbuminuric patients developed proteinuria after further four years of conventional treatment compared to only 2% of 573 initially normoalbuminuric patients.

Regarding assertion ii) concerning lack of concordance between UAE staging and GFR/glomerular lesions, Hansen et al. found normal GFR (constant-infusion-technique) in all of 134 normoalbuminuric patients [27]. Østerby found similar mesangial fractional volume in control subjects and normoalbuminuric patients [28]. Thus, as albuminuria and glomerulopathy are continuous

544

parameters a certain overlap is to be expected, but in general GFR and structural parameters are consistent with levels of diabetic nephropathy as defined by UAE.

The above mentioned studies show differences in risk of progression to proteinuria that may be explained by factors such as definition of microalbuminuria (one vs. multiple samples, level of UAE), characteristics of the population studied (duration of diabetes, glycemic control, antihypertensive treatment, etc.), and length of follow-up, but it can be concluded that microalbuminuria is a strong predictor of subsequent development of overt nephropathy.

Many other possible predictors have been proposed, amongst these prorenin [29-32] and von Willebrand factor [33;34]. Elevated plasma lipids (LDL cholesterol [35], triglycerides [36], apolipoprotein B [37]) have been described in patients at risk of subsequent microalbuminuria. Interestingly, hyperlipidemia apparently also promotes progression of established nephropathy [38;39]. At present, however there are no alternatives to microalbuminuria in the prediction of diabetic nephropathy.

ACE-i intervention: Effects on UAE

In a recent metaanalysis by Chaturvedi et al. *[40]* the effect of ACE inhibition in 698 normotensive type 1 diabetic patients with microalbuminuria was evaluated. The risk of progression to macroalbuminuria on ACE inhibitor treatment was reduced to approximately one third compared to the placebo treated patients. Conversely, regression to normoalbuminuria was three times greater in the ACE-i group compared with the placebo group. The estimated treatment effect did not vary by factors such as age, glycemic control and sex. However, the trials encompassed a broad spectrum of patients, including patients with severe albuminuria. New trials have disclosed a long list of pathophysiological abnormalities in patients with microalbuminuria compared to patients with normoalbuminuria: Blood pressure elevation, autonomic abnormalities, and ultrastructural findings indicate the presence of glomerular and arteriolar abnormalities in diabetic patients with incipient nephropathy. Thus, early intervention has attracted interest. In a recent trial patients with type 1 diabetic and low-grade microalbuminuria (AE between 20-70 µgr/min)were examined [41]. Two years ACE inhibitor treatment reduced both overnight and exercise UAE significantly. In the intervention group approximately two thirds reversed to normoalbuminuria. Thus, the UAE lowering effect of ACE inhibitor treatment seems to apply also to patients with low-grade microalbuminuria. In a study concerning two different doses of ramipril (1.25 and 5 mg) versus placebo in 55 microalbuminuric type 1 diabetic patients Bojestig et al. [42] found a correlation between change in systolic BP and change in UAE and concluded, that the UAE lowering effect of ACE-i was dependent on the BP reduction.

This conclusion is somewhat hampered by the fact that neither UAE lowering nor BP reduction was detected in the ACE-i treated patients. This leads the authors to question the clinical use of ACE-i in normotensive patients that do not demonstrate a concomitant reduction in BP. Apart from the practical difficulties associated with this strategy, their negative findings may at least in part be explained by the study size, and the long duration of diabetes in the participants. In addition, the good glycemic control (mean HbA1c below 7.5%) may have defined patients with an a priori good prognosis. The effect of ramipril 1.25 and 5 mg versus placebo was also tested in the ATLANTIS study [43], encompassing a total of 140 microalbuminuric patients with type 1 diabetes. Both ACE-i doses reduced microalbuminuria as well as clinic BP significantly, and the authors conclude that a separation between proteinuria-lowering and BP-lowering effects is unattainable.

The question whether ACE inhibitor treatment should be introduced in normoalbuminuric type 1 diabetic patients has arisen. The EUCLID study [44] considered a mixed population of normo- and microalbuminuric patients and confirmed the effect of ACE-inhibition on microalbuminuric patients but found no significant difference in albumin excretion rate between normoalbuminuric (<20 µg/min) placebo and ACE inhibitor treated patients and could not demonstrate a significant reduction in incidence of microalbuminuria in ACE inhibitor treated normoalbuminuric patients.

At present, the consensus calls for antihypertensive treatment in most patients with microalbuminuria regardless of BP but preventive treatment of normoalbuminuric patients is not warranted. Aggressive antihypertensive treatment frequently leads to normalization of albumin excretion in patients with established microalbuminuria. Reduction or normalization of microalbuminuria can be considered as an indicator of effective antihypertensive treatment. It is important to consider that in almost all studies evaluating the effect of ACE inhibitors or angiotensin II blockers, the vast majority of patients receiving one of these agents has received a diuretic in addition. In the recently published PREMIER study [45] the positive effects of the combination of ACE inhibition and diuretics treatment was documented.

546

ACE-i intervention: Effects on GFR and glomerulopathy

Data on preservation of kidney function are very limited. Mathiesen et al. have performed an eight year prospective, randomised study comprising forty four normotensive, microalbuminuric patients [46]. The decline in GFR was 11.8 ml/min in the control group (p<0.03) and 1.4 (ns) in the captopril group (after pause in treatment). The difference between groups was not statistically significant (p=0.09).

Rudberg et al. investigated the influence of ACE-i and beta blockers on the progression of early diabetic glomerulopathy [47]. Thirteen patients with type 1 diabetes mellitus and microalbuminuria were treated with either enalapril or metoprolol. Renal biopsies were taken before and after 38 months of treatment. Data from nine patients (from another study) served as a reference material. The groups were comparable regarding age, diabetes duration and degree of microalbuminuria, but glycemic control was poorer (although not statistically significant) and diastolic BP higher in the reference group during the study period. Contrary to findings in the group without antihypertensive treatment, no progression of glomerulopathy was seen in those treated with enalapril or metoprolol. There were no detectable differences in glomerular structure between the two groups, but the study was not powered to answer whether ACE-i carry special reno-protective properties independent of BP reduction. In the recently published ESPRIT study [48], encompassing 54 type 1 diabetic patients with micro- or macroalbuminuria, there was no detectable effect of enalapril 10 mg once daily compared with either nifedipine or placebo on renal structure over 3 years.

ACE-i intervention: Effects on other diabetic complications

The HOPE study [49] confirmed that ACE-i lower the risk of overt diabetic nephropathy. More importantly, ramipril significantly reduced the risk of major C-V outcomes by 25-30% in high risk (previous C-V disease or at least one other risk factor) people with diabetes (the vast majority type 2 diabetes). These results, consistent with results from other trials [50], may have important therapeutic implications, but it is important to stress that the HOPE study included a broad population of patients with different risk profiles; in the subgroup of diabetic patients without prior manifest C-V disease (1119 patients), the risk reduction did not reach the level of statistical significance as discussed by Jensen [51].

In the HOPE study, ramipril also reduced the risk of (self reported) retinal laser therapy by 22%, although this reduction was not significant. Retinal photographs were not taken.

In the former mentioned Euclid study [52] treatment with lisinopril apparently decreased retinopathy progression. Retinopathy was, however, not a primary endpoint, and after adjustment for differences in glycemic control and baseline retinopathy the results were barely statistically significant. Other smaller studies have shown non-significant benefits with other ACE inhibitors [53-55]. In newly diagnosed hypertensive type 2 diabetic patients the UKPDS [56] clearly demonstrated that tight BP control reduced risk of progression of diabetic retinopathy. Progression was similar in those allocated to captopril and atenolol [57].

Data regarding possible effects of ACE-i treatment on diabetic neuropathy are scarce, despite the fact that hypertension has been identified as a risk factor for the development of neuropathy [58]: one short-term open-label study [59] and one randomised double-blind placebo-controlled study [60] have shown modest improvement in peripheral nerve function with ACE-i. Data on the effect on autonomic function are conflicting, with some studies describing improvement in parameters reflecting parasympathetic function [61;62], whereas other find no change [60;63;64].

24-H AMBULATORY BLOOD PRESSURE AND DIABETIC NEPHROPATHY

The implementation of 24-h ambulatory BP (24-h AMBP) in the study of diabetic nephropathy has underscored the role of blood pressure elevation even in the earliest phases of diabetic nephropathy. Higher 24-AMBP characterizes type 1 diabetic patients with high normal urinary albumin excretion [65] and a close association between increases in UAE and blood pressure was found in the transition from normo- to microalbuminuria [66]. In the above mentioned study of patients with low-grade microalbuminuria[41] differences in BP were undetectable with clinic BP (mean of three random zero measurements) but using 24-h AMBP, statistically highly significant differences between the two groups were demonstrated. Likewise, in a substudy of the HOPE study, highly significant reductions in night blood pressure were detected by 24-h AMBP [67], - reductions that could account for a substantial part of the beneficial effects obtained. A critical appraisal of the insensitivity of clinical BP measurement is important [68], - especially regarding conclusions, which from a statistical point of view are negations. Although trivial, it is still pertinent that "absence of evidence is not evidence of absence".

CONCLUSIONS

Recent studies emphasize the importance of screening diabetic patients for microalbuminuria and the importance of treating these patients as early as possible in order to prevent both renal and cardiovascular complications. Prevention of the development of microalbuminuria in normoalbuminuric patients by ACE-i has not yet been demonstrated. Data on harder endpoints such as GFR and glomerulopathy as well as C-V events and other diabetic complications are limited but currently available data suggest beneficial effects. The implementation of 24 h ambulatory blood pressure measurements has emphasized the role of blood pressure elevation even in the earliest phases of diabetic nephropathy. Glycemic control should be optimised and aggressive antihypertensive treatment e.g. with ACE inhibitors or angiotensin II blockers in combination with diuretics is important.

REFERENCES

1. Mogensen,CE: Progression of nephropathy in long-term diabetics with proteinuria and effect of initial anti-hypertensive treatment. *Scand.J.Clin.Lab Invest* 36:383-388, 1976
2. Mogensen,CE: Long-term antihypertensive treatment inhibiting progression of diabetic nephropathy. *BMJ* 285:685-688, 1982
3. Parving,H-H, Andersen,AR, Smidt,UM, Svendsen,PA: Early aggressive antihypertensive treatment reduces rate of decline in kidney function in diabetic nephropathy. *Lancet* 1:1175-1179, 1983
4. Anderson,S, Brenner,BM: Influence of antihypertensive therapy on development and progression of diabetic glomerulopathy. *Diabetes Care* 11:846-849, 1988
5. Parving,H-H, Smidt,UM, Hommel,E, Mathiesen,ER, Rossing,P, Nielsen,F, Gall,MA: Effective antihypertensive treatment postpones renal insufficiency in diabetic nephropathy. *Am.J.Kidney Dis.* 22:188-195, 1993
6. Parving,H-H, Hommel,E: Prognosis in diabetic nephropathy. *BMJ.* 299:230-233, 1989
7. Mathiesen,ER, Borch Johnsen,K, Jensen,DV, Deckert,T: Improved survival in patients with diabetic nephropathy. *Diabetologia* 32:884-886, 1989
8. Hasslacher,C, Borgholte,G, Ritz,E, Wahl,P: Impact of hypertension on prognosis in IDDM. *Diabete.Metab.* 15:338-342, 1989
9. Brenner,BM: Remission of renal disease: recounting the challenge, acquiring the goal. *J.Clin.Invest* 110:1753-1758, 2002
10. Cooper,ME: Pathogenesis, prevention, and treatment of diabetic nephropathy. *Lancet* 352:213-219, 1998

11. Mogensen,CE: Microalbuminuria, blood pressure and diabetic renal disease: origin and development of ideas. *Diabetologia* 42:263-285, 1999

12. Caramori,ML, Fioretto,P, Mauer,M: The need for early predictors of diabetic nephropathy risk: is albumin excretion rate sufficient? *Diabetes* 49:1399-1408, 2000

13. Mogensen,CE: Genetics and Diabetic renal disease. Still a big black hole [editorial]. *Diabetes Care,* In press, 2003

14. Mogensen,CE, Keane,WF, Bennett,PH, Jerums,G, Parving,HH, Passa,P, Steffes,MW, Striker,GE, Viberti,GC: Prevention of diabetic renal disease with special reference to microalbuminuria. *Lancet* 346:1080-1084, 1995

15. Mogensen,CE, Viberti,GC, Peheim,E, Kutter,D, Hasslacher,C, Hofmann,W, Renner,R, Bojestig,M, Poulsen,PL, Scott,G, Thoma,J, Kuefer,J, Nilsson,B, Gambke,B, Mueller,P, Steinbiss,J, Willamovski,KD: Multicenter evaluation of the Micral-testII test-strip, an immunological rapid test for the detection of microalbuminuria. *Diabetes Care* 20:1642 1646, 1997

16. Kasiske,BL, Kalil,RS, Ma,JZ, Liao,M, Keane,WF: Effect of antihypertensive therapy on the kidney in patients with diabetes: a meta-regression analysis. *Ann.Intern.Med.* 118:129-138, 1993

17. Parving,H-H, Oxenboll,B, Johansen,K, Svendsen,PA, Christiansen,JS, Andersen,AR: Early detection of patients at risk of developing diabetic nephropathy: a longitudinal study of urinary albumin excretion. *Acta Endocrinol.Copenh.* 100:500-505, 1982

18. Viberti,GC, Hill,RD, Jarrett,RJ, Argyropoulos,A, Mahmud,U, Keen,H: Microalbuminuria as a predictor of clinical nephropathy in insulin-dependent diabetes mellitus. *Lancet* I:1430-1432, 1982

19. Mogensen,CE, Christensen,CK: Predicting diabetic nephropathy in insulin-dependent patients. *N.Engl.J.Med.* 311:89-93, 1984

20. Messent,JW, Elliott,TG, Hill,RD, Jarrett,RJ, Keen,H, Viberti,GC: Prognostic significance of microalbuminuria in insulin-dependent diabetes mellitus: a twenty-three year follow-up study. *Kidney Int.* 41:836-839, 1992

21. Rossing,P, Hougaard,P, Borch-Johnsen,K, Parving,HH: Predictors of mortality in insulin dependent diabetes: 10 year observational follow up study. *BMJ* 313:779-784, 1996

22. Fioretto,P, Steffes,MW, Mauer,M: Glomerular structure in nonproteinuric IDDM patients with various levels of albuminuria. *Diabetes* 43:1358-1364, 1994

23. Forsblom,CM, Groop,PH, Ekstrand,A, Groop,LC: Predictive value of microalbuminuria in patients with insulin- dependent diabetes of long duration. *BMJ.* 305:1051-1053, 1992

24. Rossing P, Hougaard P, Borch-Johnsen K, Parving H-H: Progression from microalbuminuria to diabetic nephropathy in IDDM [Abstract]. *J.Am.Soc.Nephrol.* 8, 1997

25. Captopril reduces the risk of nephropathy in IDDM patients with microalbuminuria. The Microalbuminuria Captopril Study Group. *Diabetologia* 39:587-593, 1996

26. Retinopathy and nephropathy in patients with type 1 diabetes four years after a trial of intensive therapy. The Diabetes Control and Complications Trial/Epidemiology of Diabetes Interventions and Complications Research Group. *N.Engl.J.Med.* 342:381-389, 2000

27. Hansen,KW, Mau Pedersen,M, Christensen,CK, Schmitz,A, Christiansen,JS, Mogensen,CE: Normoalbuminuria ensures no reduction of renal function in type 1 [insulin-dependent] diabetic patients. *J.Intern.Med.* 232:161-167, 1992

28. Osterby,R: Glomerular structural changes in type 1 [insulin-dependent] diabetes mellitus: causes, consequences, and prevention. *Diabetologia* 35:803-812, 1992

29. Franken,AA, Derkx,FH, Blankestijn,PJ, Janssen,JA, Mannesse,CK, Hop,W, Boomsma,F, Weber,R, Peperkamp,E, De Jong,PT, et al: Plasma prorenin as an early marker of microvascular disease in patients with diabetes mellitus. *Diabete.Metab.* 18:137-143, 1992

30. Daneman,D, Crompton,CH, Balfe,JW, Sochett,EB, Chatzilias,A, Cotter,BR, Osmond,DH: Plasma prorenin as an early marker of nephropathy in diabetic [IDDM] adolescents. *Kidney Int.* 46:1154-1159, 1994

31. Allen,TJ, Cooper,ME, Gilbert,RE, Winikoff,J, Skinni,SL, Jerums,G: Serum total renin is increased before microalbuminuria in diabetes. *Kidney Int.* 50:902-907, 1996

32. Deinum,J, Ronn,B, Mathiesen,E, Derkx,FH, Hop,WC, Schalekamp,MA: Increase in serum prorenin precedes onset of microalbuminuria in patients with insulin-dependent diabetes mellitus. *Diabetologia* 42:1006-1010, 1999

33. Jensen,T: Increased plasma concentration of von Willebrand factor in insulin dependent diabetics with incipient nephropathy. *BMJ.* 298:27-28, 1989

34. Stehouwer,CD, Stroes,ES, Hackeng,WH, Mulder,PG, den Ottolander,GJ: von Willebrand factor and development of diabetic nephropathy in IDDM [published erratum appears in Diabetes 1991 Dec;40[12]:1746]. *Diabetes* 40:971-976, 1991

35. Coonrod,BA, Ellis,D, Becker,DJ, Bunker,CH, Kelsey,SF, Lloyd,CE, Drash,AL, Kuller,LH, Orchard,TJ: Predictors of Microalbuminuria in Individuals with IDDM. Pittsburg Epidemiology of Diabetes Complication Study. *Diabetes Care* 16:1376-1383, 1993

36. Chaturvedi,N, Bandinelli,S, Mangili,R, Penno,G, Rottiers,R, Fuller,JH: Microalbuminuria in type 1 diabetes: Rates, risk factors, and glycemic threshold. *Kidney Int.* 60:219-227, 2001

37. Watts,GF, Powrie,JK, O'Brien,SF, Shaw,KM: Apolipoprotein B independently predicts progression of very-low- level albuminuria in insulin-dependent diabetes mellitus. *.Metabolism* 45:1101-1107, 1996

38. Moorhead,JF, Chan,MK, El Nahas,M, Varghese,Z: Lipid nephrotoxicity in chronic progressive glomerular and tubulo-interstitial disease. *Lancet* 2:1309-1311, 1982

39. Hovind,P, Rossing,P, Tarnow,L, Smidt,UM, Parving,H-H: Progression of diabetic nephropathy. *Kidney Int.* 59:702-709, 2001

40. The ACE Inhibitors in Diabetic Nephropathy Trialist Group*: Should all patients with type 1 diabetes mellitus and microalbuminuria receive Angiotensin-Converting Enzyme Inhibitors? A meta-analysis of individual patient data. *Ann.Intern.Med.* 134:340-379, 2001

41. Poulsen,PL, Ebbehoj,E, Nosadini,R, Crepaldi,G, Mogensen,CE: Early ACE-i intervention in microalbuminuric patients with type 1 diabetes: Effects on albumin excretion, 24 h ambulatory blood pressure, and renal function. *Diabetes Metab* 27:123-128, 2001

42. Bojestig,M, Karlberg,B, Lindström,T, Nystrom,F: Reduction of ACE activity is insufficient to decrease microalbuminuria in normotensive patients with type 1 diabetes. *Diabetes Care* 24[5]:919-924, 2001

43. Low-dose ramipril reduces microalbuminuria in type 1 diabetic patients without hypertension: results of a randomized controlled trial. The ATLANTIS Study Group. *Diabetes Care* 23:1823-1829, 2000

44. The EUCLID Study Group: Randomised placebo-controlled trial of lisinopril in normotensive patients with insulin-dependent diabetes and normoalbuminuria or microalbuminuria. *Lancet* 349:1787-1792, 1997

45. Mogensen,CE, Viberti,G, Halimi,S, Ritz,E, Ruilope,L, Jermendy,G, Widimsky,J, Sareli,P, Taton,J, Rull,J, Erdogan,G, de Leeuw,PW, Ribeiro,A, Sanchez,R, Mechmeche,R, Nolan,J, Sirotiakova,J, Hamani,A, Scheen,A, Hess,B, Luger,A, Thomas,SM: Effect of Low-Dose Perindopril/Indapamide on Albuminuria in Diabetes. Preterax in Albuminuria Regression: PREMIER. *Hypertension .:* 2003

46. Mathiesen,ER, Hommel,E, Hansen,HP, Smidt,UM, Parving,HH: Randomised controlled trial of long term efficacy of captopril on preservation of kidney function in normotensive patients with insulin dependent diabetes and microalbuminuria. *BMJ* 319:24-25, 1999

47. Rudberg,S, Osterby,R, Bangstad,HJ, Dahlquist,G, Persson,B: Effect of angiotensin converting enzyme inhibitor or beta blocker on glomerular structural changes in young microalbuminuric patients with Type I [insulin-dependent] diabetes mellitus. *Diabetologia* 42:589-595, 1999

48. Effect of 3 years of antihypertensive therapy on renal structure in type 1 diabetic patients with albuminuria: the European Study for the Prevention of Renal Disease in Type 1 Diabetes [ESPRIT]. *Diabetes* 50:843-850, 2001

49. Effects of ramipril on cardiovascular and microvascular outcomes in people with diabetes mellitus: results of the HOPE study and MICRO-HOPE substudy. Heart Outcomes Prevention Evaluation Study Investigators. *Lancet* 355:253-259, 2000

50. Hansson,L, Lindholm,LH, Niskanen,L, Lanke,J, Hedner,T, Niklason,A, Luomanmaki,K, Dahlof,B, de Faire,U, Morlin,C, Karlberg,BE, Wester,PO, Bjorck,JE: Effect of angiotensin-converting-enzyme inhibition compared with conventional therapy on cardiovascular morbidity and mortality in hypertension: the Captopril Prevention Project [CAPPP] randomised trial. *Lancet* 353:611-616, 1999

51. Jensen,T: The HOPE study and diabetes. Heart Outcomes Prevention Evaluation. *Lancet* 355:1181-1184, 2000

52. Chaturvedi,N, Sjolie,AK, Stephenson,JM, Abrahamian,H, Keipes,M, Castellarin,A, Rogulja-Pepeonik,Z, Fuller,JH: Effect of lisinopril on progression of retinopathy in normotensive people with type 1 diabetes. The EUCLID Study Group. EURODIAB Controlled Trial of Lisinopril in Insulin-Dependent Diabetes Mellitus. *Lancet* 351:28-31, 1998

53. Chase,HP, Satish,K, Harris,S, Hoops,S, Jackson,WE, Holmes,DL: Angiotensin-converting enzyme inhibitor treatment for young normotensive diabetic subjects: A two-year trial. *Ann Opthalmol* 25:284-289, 1993

54. Larsen,M, Hommel,E, Parving,HH, Lund-Andersen,H: Protective effect of captopril on the blood-retina barrier in normotensive insulin-dependent diabetic patients with nephropathy and background retinopathy. *Graefes Arch.Clin.Exp.Ophthalmol.* 228:505-509, 1990

55. Jackson,WE, Holmes,DL, Garg,SK, Harris,S, Chase,HP: Angiotensin-converting enzyme inhibitor therapy and diabetic retinopathy. *Ann.Ophthalmol.* 24:99-103, 1992

56. Tight blood pressure control and risk of macrovascular and microvascular complications in type 2 diabetes: UKPDS 38. UK Prospective Diabetes Study Group [published erratum appears in BMJ 1999 Jan 2;318[7175]:29]. *BMJ* 317:703-713, 1998

57. Efficacy of atenolol and captopril in reducing risk of macrovascular and microvascular complications in type 2 diabetes: UKPDS 39. UK Prospective Diabetes Study Group. *BMJ* 317:713-720, 1998

58. Forrest,KY, Maser,RE, Pambianco,G, Becker,DJ, Orchard,TJ: Hypertension as a risk factor for diabetic neuropathy: a prospective study. *Diabetes* 46:665-670, 1997

59. Reja,A, Tesfaye,S, Harris,ND, Ward,JD: Is ACE inhibition with lisinopril helpful in diabetic neuropathy? *Diabet.Med.* 12:307-309, 1995

60. Malik,RA, Williamson,S, Abbott,C, Carrington,AL, Iqbal,J, Schady,W, Boulton,AJ: Effect of angiotensin-converting-enzyme [ACE] inhibitor trandolapril on human diabetic neuropathy: randomised double-blind controlled trial. *Lancet* 352:1978-1981, 1998

61. Moore,MV, Jeffcoate,WJ, Macdonald,IA: Apparent improvement in diabetic autonomic neuropathy induced by captopril. *J.Hum.Hypertens.* 1:161-165, 1987

62. Athyros,VG, Didangelos,TP, Karamitsos,DT, Papageorgiou,AA, Boudoulas,H, Kontopoulos,AG: Long-term effect of converting enzyme inhibition on circadian sympathetic and parasympathetic modulation in patients with diabetic autonomic neuropathy. *Acta Cardiol.* 53:201-209, 1998

63. Salo,TM, Viikari,JS, Antila,KJ, Voipio-Pulkki,LM, Jalonen,JO, Valimaki,IA: Antihypertensive treatment and heart rate variability in diabetic patients: role of cardiac autonomic neuropathy. *J.Auton.Nerv.Syst.* 60:61-70, 1996

64. Malik,RA: Can diabetic neuropathy be prevented by angiotensin-converting enzyme inhibitors? *Ann.Med.* 32:1-5, 2000

65. Poulsen,PL, Ebbehøj,E, Hansen,KW, Mogensen,CE: 24-h blood pressure and autonomic function is related to albumin excretion within the normoalbuminuric range in IDDM patients. *Diabetologia* 40:718-725, 1997

66. Poulsen,PL, Hansen,KW, Mogensen,CE: Ambulatory blood pressure in the transition from normo- to microalbuminuria. A longitudinal study in IDDM patients. *Diabetes* 43:1248-1253, 1994

67. Svensson,P, de Faire,U, Sleight,P, Yusuf,S, Ostergren,J: Comparative effects of ramipril on ambulatory and office blood pressures: a HOPE Substudy. *Hypertension* 38:E28-E32, 2001

68. Kurtz,TW: False claims of blood pressure-independent protection by blockade of the renin angiotensin aldosterone system? *Hypertension* 41:193-196, 2003

32

THE ROLE OF PROTEINURIA IN THE DIAGNOSIS AND TREATMENT OF TYPE 2 DIABETES

William F. Keane and Paulette A. Lyle
Merck & Co., Inc. Whitehouse Station, New Jersey, USA

Renal and cardiovascular diseases associated with type 2 diabetes present significant burdens to patients and health care systems, and are increasing at epidemic proportions. The prevalence of type 2 diabetes and the concurrent end-organ diseases are increasing at an alarming rate in world populations. The 1997 prevalence of type 2 diabetes is predicted to nearly double by the year 2010 [1]. The microvascular complications of diabetes are currently estimated to be responsible for over 40% of newly diagnosed cases of nephropathy [2,3].

Diabetic nephropathy as a sequela to type 2 diabetes has become the leading cause of end-stage renal disease. Diabetic nephropathy is approximately twice as common a cause of end-stage renal disease than is nephropathy caused by hypertension or primary glomerular diseases. Mortality among patients receiving chronic hemodialysis is estimated to be 21-25% per year, with the majority of deaths secondary to cardiovascular causes. Even though current recommendations for diabetics include the need for early screening for microalbuminuria, these patients who are at high risk for the development of nephropathy often go unidentified. At the time of diagnosis of type 2 diabetes, approximately 30% of the patients will already have albumin or protein in the urine: 75% will have microalbuminuria (30-300 mg/24 hr), and 25% will have overt proteinuria (> 300 mg/24 hr). Persistent albuminuria indicates underlying structural changes in the kidney consistent with diabetic nephropathy [4-8]. Microalbuminuria *per se* may be a silent harbinger of future vascular disease.

Prevention of albuminuria and delaying the progression of nephropathy must be major goals of any treatment strategy developed for the diabetic patient – a treatment strategy that must include lowering of blood pressure and glucose, as well as the prevention or reduction of proteinuria [9-12].

CLASSIFICATION OF PROTEINURIA

Measurement of urinary albumin:creatinine ratio is most commonly used for diagnosing and tracking urine albumin excretion. Although collection of a 24-hour urine sample might be desirable, the use of an early-morning (first voided) sample is common practice. Early-morning urine is more concentrated, which facilitates detection of albumin. Inclusion of the urinary creatinine factor adjusts for variation in urine volume. Use of the urinary albumin:creatinine ratio has been made increasingly feasible by the commercial availability of reliable, sensitive assays. A sensitive assay is important because renal disease prediction and progression is optimally tracked as urinary albumin:creatinine ratio progresses from the "normal" range, which is not detectable by urine dipstick (15-30 mg/24 hour or <200 mg/g [spot urine albumin:creatinine ratio]) [13-19], to microalbuminuria (30-300 mg/24 hour or > 3 mg/dL [dipstick]), to proteinuria (urinary protein excretion >300 mg/24 hr) [10, 20-23]. Because urinary albumin excretion is known to be higher in men and older patients [24, 25], some researchers advocate gender- and age-specific ranges for spot urine albumin:creatinine ratio, e.g., microalbuminuria 17-250 mg/g and proteinuria >250 mg/g for males and microalbuminuria 25-355 mg/g and proteinuria > 355 mg/g for females [26, 27].

The terms primary prevention (preventing microalbuminuria), secondary prevention (preventing the progression of microalbuminuria to macroalbuminuria), and tertiary prevention (preventing the progression of macroalbuminuria to end-stage renal disease) are sometimes used for 3 stages of the goals of the management of diabetic renal disease [28]. The National Kidney Foundation (NKF) recently published it's Kidney Disease Outcomes Quality Initiative (K/DOQI), which included a recommendation that a new classification system, similar to classifications used in other disciplines in medicine, be used to designate stages of severity of chronic renal disease (Table 1). This classification is based on five levels of glomerular filtration rate (mL/min/1.73 m^2): Stage 1 is >90, Stage 2 is 60-89, Stage 3 is 30-59, Stage 4 is 15-29, and Stage 5 is <15 or dialysis. The NKF advocates adoption of this classification system to minimize ambiguity and overlap of terms in the medical literature, to facilitate communication between patients and health care providers, to enhance public education, to promote communication of research results, and to enhance conduct of clinical research [29].

Table 1. Stages of renal disease according to the National Kidney Foundation Kidney Disease Outcomes Quality Initiative (K/DOQI)

Stage	GFR (mL/min/1.73 m^2)	Description
1	> 90	Normal or increased GFR or with early renal damage
2	60-89	Early renal insufficiency
3	30-59	Moderate renal failure (chronic renal failure)
4	15-29	Severe renal failure (pre-end stage renal disease)
5	<15 (or dialysis)	End stage renal disease (uremia)

GFR = glomerular filtration rate
Adapted from National Kidney Foundation-K/DOQI. Clinical practice guidelines for chronic kidney disease: evaluation, classification and stratification. Am J Kidney Dis 2002;39(Suppl 1):S1-S266.

BLOOD PRESSURE AND PROTEINURIA

It is incontrovertible that controlling blood pressure is an extremely important intervention to slow renal disease progression [30-40]. Current treatment guidelines specify a goal blood pressure of < 130/80 mm Hg [41-43] or < 130/85 mm Hg [44]. In patients with > 1 g protein/24 hours, a goal blood pressure of <125/75 mm Hg has been suggested [39]. No clinical trial has provided evidence of increased cardiovascular risk at low blood pressures.

HYPERGLYCEMIA AND PROTEINURIA

The onset of microalbuminuria in patients with type 2 diabetes may be transient and related to increases in glomerular filtration rate in association with hyperglycemia. Albuminuria has been shown to decrease with decreases in glucose levels in patients with newly diagnosed type 1 or type 2 diabetes [45-47]. However, other researchers reported no decline in albumin excretion with control of hyperglycemia in patients with newly diagnosed type 2 diabetes [48]. The United Kingdom Prospective Diabetes Study showed that the risk for microalbuminuria was proportional to the level and duration of glucose elevation [49]. Furthermore, in type 1 diabetes the level of glycosylated hemoglobin correlates with glomerular disease [50]. In type 1 diabetic patients in the Diabetes Control and Complications Trial, rigorous control of blood glucose reduced the development of microalbuminuria and the progression from microalbuminuria to overt proteinuria [51]. The United Kingdom Prospective Diabetes Study in type 2 diabetic subjects showed that well-controlled blood glucose reduced the risk of diabetic nephropathy and other microvascular, but not macrovascular, sequelae [49]. Glycemic control must be optimized to prevent or retard the development of diabetic nephropathy.

ENDOTHELIAL DYSFUNCTION AND PROTEINURIA

There is substantial support for the view that microalbuminuria is a marker of a generalized arterial endothelial dysfunction — a process that involves the glomerli, retina, and intima of large arteries, and that microalbuminuria may be a marker of preclinical atherosclerosis [52-56]. It is now recognized that appropriate treatment of type 2 diabetes, with or without concurrent hypertension, must address the numerous components of the metabolic syndrome – consequences of generalized endothelial dysfunction and vascular inflammation – in order to prevent or optimally retard renal and cardiovascular consequences of this disease. In the Steno-2 study, Gaede et al reported that an intensive 7.8-year disease management program of patients with type 2 diabetes that included treatment of hyperglycemia, hypertension, dyslipidemia, and microalbuminuria; secondary prevention of cardiovascular disease with aspirin; and behavior modification decreased the risk of the primary composite of endpoint of cardiovascular death, nonfatal myocardial infarction, nonfatal stroke, revascularization, and amputation by 50% versus a treatment strategy based on less-intensive guidelines that were current at the time of the study. Glycosylated hemoglobin levels, systolic and diastolic blood pressure, and serum cholesterol and triglyceride levels were significantly lower, and urinary albumin excretion rate was significantly higher in the intensive versus the conventional treatment groups. Patients on the intensive therapy also had a significantly lower risk of cardiovascular disease, nephropathy, retinopathy, and autonomic neuropathy [57].

PROTEINURIA

In the Third National Health and Nutrition Examination Survey (NHANES III), 8.3% and 1.0% of the 14,622 general-population participants had microalbuminuria and macroalbuminuria, respectively. Also, 37% of the participants with glomerular filtration rate less than 30 mL/min/1.73 m^2 did not have albuminuria [58]. Other research supports the possibility that abnormal urinary albumin excretion can precede, and be a risk factor for, diabetes [59, 60]. Angiotensin converting enzyme inhibitors have been shown to improve glomerular permeability in patients with type 1, but not type 2, diabetic nephropathy [61]. In addition to the incontrovertible requirements that blood pressure and blood glucose levels be controlled in patients with type 2 diabetes, urine protein excretion must be prevented or reduced [62-64].

Microalbuminuria is a strong predictor of progressive renal failure and cardiovascular morbidity and mortality in patients with diabetes [65, 66] or hypertension [67-69]. Urinary protein excretion is the most important predictor of renal disease progression in both diabetic and non diabetic forms of kidney disease. The mechanism(s) for this are still unclear but may include a direct toxic effect of urinary protein on various kidney cells [70-72]. The level of pre-treatment albuminuria predicts the risk of progression of renal disease and influences the response to treatment: higher baseline urine protein excretion may predict a greater response to therapy. Bos et al showed in a rat study that the severity of systemic abnormalities caused by proteinuria could predict response to angiotensin converting enzyme inhibitor therapy, and used serum cholesterol as a marker of systemic alterations. Increased cholesterol levels reduced the efficacy of angiotensin converting enzyme inhibition in reducing proteinuria [73]. On the other hand, in a study of the effect of an angiotensin converting enzyme inhibitor on the progression of non-diabetic renal disease, it was found that the current level of urine protein excretion (baseline level minus the change from baseline during treatment) was a better predictor of the risk of renal disease progression than the baseline level of urine protein excretion alone [70].

Proteinuria may contribute to renal damage. The toxic effects of proteinuria are thought to be due to a variety of mechanisms: direct mesangial toxicity, tubular overload, toxicity from specific filtered proteins, and induction of proinflammatory molecules. Proteinuria can be the cause of sodium retention, volume expansion, hypoalbuminemia, coagulation abnormalities, and hyperlipidemia [74, 75]. There is a correlation between the degree of proteinuria, interstitial fibrosis, and rate of progression of nephropathy [76, 77].

The Reduction of Endpoints in NIDDM with the Angiotensin II Antagonist Losartan (RENAAL) study provided an opportunity to evaluate the risk predictors for progression of renal disease measured by doubling of serum creatinine or the occurrence of end-stage renal disease in patients with type 2 diabetes. Univariate analyses demonstrated a group of 23 clinical or laboratory risk factors that significantly predicted doubling of serum creatinine or occurrence of end-stage renal disease. From these univariate analyses, a multivariate model was developed that demonstrated four independent risk factors: proteinuria, serum creatinine, serum albumin, and hemoglobin level. The level of proteinuria was the most important modifiable risk for progressive kidney injury in these diabetic patients. Because blood pressure was aggressively treated to a goal level, the impact of hypertension on development of a renal endpoint was probably blunted. Interestingly, glycemic control did not appear to differentiate those patients at increased risk for progression of kidney disease [78]. The reduction of proteinuria in the RENAAL study accounted for approximately one-half of the effect of losartan on the reduction of risk of end-stage renal disease: when proteinuria was adjusted as a time-varying covariant, the risk reduction for end-stage renal disease was reduced from 28.1 to 14.1%. The benefits of angiotensin receptor blockade on end-stage renal disease are not yet fully understood; however, reduction of proteinuria and delay of end-stage renal disease must remain as treatment goals in patients with type 2 diabetic nephropathy [79].

How far should urinary protein excretion be lowered? No clinical studies have been performed that examined titrating renin-angiotensin-aldosterone system therapy, the current gold standard for reducing the risk of end-stage renal disease in type 2 diabetic nephropathy, against protein excretion; however, de Jong and others have advocated the conduct of such trials [63].

THE RENIN-ANGIOTENSIN-ALDOSTERONE SYSTEM AND PROTEINURIA

It is recognized that many patients, including those with type 2 diabetes, require multiple drug therapy in order to achieve optimal blood pressure control [80]. In order to reduce the risk of progression to end-stage renal disease, this treatment regimen should include an agent that inhibits the angiotensin II type 1 receptor.

While the angiotensin converting enzyme inhibitor captopril has been shown to reduce the incidence of end-stage renal disease or death in patients with type 1 diabetes [81], similar beneficial results of angiotensin converting enzyme inhibitor therapy have not been replicated in type 2 diabetes. Studies of the effect of angiotensin converting enzyme inhibitors on proteinuria beyond blood pressure control have been relatively small and inconsistent, with some trials demonstrating a reduction in proteinuria [82-85], while others, including United Kingdom Prospective Diabetes Study (UKPDS) [80] and Appropriate Blood pressure Control in Diabetes study (ABCD) [86], failing to demonstrate these benefits beyond blood pressure control. Data in support of prevention of end-stage renal disease with the use of angiotensin converting enzyme inhibitors in patients with type 2 diabetes do not exist [80, 82-86]. When renoprotection is a goal, patients with type 2 diabetes should have an angiotensin receptor antagonist as part of their antihypertension regimen. Angiotensin receptor blockers have been efficacious in overt hypertensive type 2 diabetic nephropathy (RENAAL and IDNT), and diabetic microalbuminuria with [87] and without hypertension [88]. Agents that provide angiotensin II type-1 receptor blockade are more effective that other antihypertensive agents, even for comparable levels of blood pressure control, in reducing proteinuria and slowing progression to end-stage renal disease. In patients with type 2 diabetes, strict blood pressure control is not sufficient for maximal reduction of the decline in glomerular filtration rate. The antiproteinuric action of renin-angiotensin-aldosterone system blockade cannot be completely attributed to reduction in blood pressure [88-90]. It is common to use diuretics to potentiate the antihypertensive and antiproteinuric effect of renin-angiotensin-aldosterone system agents [91, 92].

Angiotensin II can cause endothelial dysfunction and promote vascular disease [93, 94]. Angiotensin II has receptor-mediated effects on renal hemodynamics and glomerular permeselectivity [81, 95]. Other actions are on transforming growth factor-beta-1 and plasminogen activator inhibitor (PAI) synthesis, and on inflammation via protein kinase C in mesangial and proximal tubular renal cells [96, 97]. Hyperglycemia may activate the intrarenal renin system [98] and stimulate angiotensin II production in mesangial cells [99]. It also contributes to endothelial dysfunction, probably due to decreased nitric oxide generation [100] and protein kinase C and reactive oxygen species [101].

The Reduction of Endpoints in NIDDM with the Angiotensin II Antagonist Losartan (RENAAL) study was a multinational, double-blind, randomized, placebo-controlled study that evaluated the renoprotective effects of losartan in 1513 patients with type 2 diabetes and nephropathy [89]. The primary efficacy measure was the time to first event of the composite endpoint of a doubling of serum creatinine, the onset of end-stage renal disease, or death. End-stage renal disease was defined as the need for chronic dialysis or renal transplantation. The three secondary endpoints included 1) the time to first event of cardiovascular morbidity and mortality (a composite of myocardial infarction, stroke, cardiovascular-related death, coronary or peripheral revascularization procedures, or first hospitalization for heart failure or unstable angina); 2) changes in the level of proteinuria; and 3) progression of renal disease (slope of the reciprocal of serum creatinine). The effects of losartan on proteinuria were evident at Month 3 (-29.1%, p<0.001) and persisted throughout the remainder of the mean 3.4-year follow-up: Year 1 35% and end-of study 39% (both p<0.001) [79]. Treatment with losartan resulted in a significant risk reduction of 16% in risk of the primary composite endpoint; P=0.02. The decrease in risk remained essentially unchanged after correction for blood pressure. For the components of the primary endpoint, losartan significantly reduced the risk of progression to end-stage renal disease by 29% (P=0.002), and significantly reduced the risk of doubling of serum creatinine by 25% (P=0.006). The risk of death was not significantly different between study groups. Losartan significantly reduced the risk of end-stage renal disease or death by 20%; P=0.01. There was no significant difference in the secondary composite endpoint of cardiovascular morbidity and mortality between the two treatment groups. An exception was first hospitalization for heart failure, a component of the cardiovascular composite endpoint, which was significantly reduced by 32% in the group treated with losartan; P=0.005.

The study also showed that losartan compared to the placebo significantly reduced proteinuria (the urinary albumin:creatinine ratio) by 34.3% (P<0.001), and reduced the rate of decline in renal function (as measured by the reciprocal of the serum creatinine concentration over time) by 18.5%; P=0.01. As an element of its prospective design, the RENAAL study included populations in whom the prevalence of type 2 diabetes is high, including Asian, Black, and Hispanic patients. There were no interactions between ethnicity/race and treatment benefit in the RENAAL study, indicating that the beneficial effects of treatment with losartan were applicable to the racial groups studied. The reduction of proteinuria in the RENAAL study accounted for approximately one-half of the effect of losartan on the reduction of risk of end-stage renal disease: when proteinuria was adjusted as a time-varying covariant, the risk reduction for end-stage renal disease was reduced from 28.1 to 14.1%.

Thus, reduction of proteinuria does not completely explain the impact of intervention on outcomes such as end-stage renal disease. However, reduction of proteinuria must remain an important consideration when treating patients with type 2 diabetes and nephropathy. Furthermore, future studies in this patient group should include reduction of risk for end-stage renal disease or death as the treatment goal [79].

The Irbesartan Diabetic Nephropathy Trial (IDNT) was a multinational, randomized, double-blind, placebo-controlled study that evaluated the renoprotective effects of irbesartan compared to amlodipine or conventional antihypertensive therapy in 1715 hypertensive patients with type 2 diabetes and nephropathy [90]. The primary efficacy measure was the time to first event of the composite endpoint of a doubling of serum creatinine, end-stage renal disease, or death. End-stage renal disease was defined as the need for chronic dialysis, renal transplantation, or a serum creatinine of $\geq$ 6 mg/dL. The secondary efficacy measure was the time to first event of the composite endpoint of death from cardiovascular causes, non-fatal myocardial infarction, hospitalization for heart failure, a permanent neurologic deficit caused by cerebrovascular event, or lower limb amputation above the ankle. Treatment with irbesartan significantly reduced the risk of reaching the composite primary endpoint by 20% compared to placebo (P=0.02), and by 23% compared to amlodipine (P=0.006); the effect was independent of blood pressure. Irbesartan significantly reduced the risk of doubling of serum creatinine by 33% compared to placebo (P=0.003), and by 37% compared to amlodipine (P<0.001). The risk of end-stage renal disease and death were not significantly different between study groups. There were no significant differences among the treatment groups in the secondary composite cardiovascular outcome.

Some researchers believe that doses of angiotensin converting enzyme inhibitors or angiotensin receptor blockers higher than those needed for blood pressure optimization should be employed to achieve additional reduction of urine protein excretion [102]. In the Irbesartan in Patients with Type 2 Diabetes and Microalbuminuria (IRMA-2) study, the 300-mg (70%, p <0.001), but not the 150-mg (39%, P=ns) dose of irbesartan was associated with a statistically significant risk reduction in progression from incipient to overt diabetic nephropathy (urinary albumin excretion rate > 200 microg/min and at least 30% higher than baseline) [87].

Combination angiotensin converting enzyme inhibitor - angiotensin receptor blocker therapy has been suggested, on the theory that it is advantageous to reduce the amount of angiotensin II available for binding to the angiotensin type 1 receptor, and to block the binding of available angiotensin II (e.g., what has escaped angiotensin converting enzyme inhibition by being produced by alternative pathways such as chymase) to the receptor site. Concomitant use of an angiotensin type 1-selective angiotensin receptor blocker might completely block the reduced level of angiotensin II that reaches receptor [97, 103-106]. For example, in a study of 199 patients with hypertension and type 2 diabetes who received 12 weeks of monotherapy with candesartan 16 mg daily or lisinopril 20 mg daily followed by 12 weeks of monotherapy or combination treatment, mean (95% confidence interval) reductions in diastolic blood pressure were 9.5 mm Hg (7.7-11.2 mm Hg, p<0.001) and 9.7 mm Hg (7.9-11.5, p<0.001), respectively, and in urinary albumin:creatinine ratio were 30% (15-42, p<0.001) and 46% (35-56, p<0.001) for candesartan and lisinopril, respectively. At 24 weeks the mean reduction in diastolic blood pressure with combination treatment (mean 16.3 mm Hg, 13.6-18.9, p<0. 001) was significantly greater than that with candesartan (10.4 mm Hg, 7.7-13.1, p<0.001) or lisinopril (mean 10.7 mm Hg, 8.0 mm Hg to 13.5 mm Hg, p<0.001). Furthermore, the reduction in urinary albumin:creatinine ratio with combination treatment (50%, 36-61, p<0.001) was greater than with candesartan (24%, 0-43, P=0.05) or lisinopril (39%, 20-54, p<0.001) monotherapy [107].

It remains unclear whether the demonstrated effects of combined angiotensin receptor antagonists and angiotensin converting enzyme inhibitors are a result of greater blood pressure reduction and or the effect of combined therapy on the renin-angiotensin-aldosterone system [108]. More studies are necessary before conclusions can be reached.

Although one might postulate that there would be an advantage to inhibiting renin [109], current renin inhibitors are large molecules and are limited by their poor bioavailability.

CARDIOVASCULAR DISEASE AND PROTEINURIA

Urinary albumin excretion has been linked to all-cause and, especially, cardiovascular mortality in patients with diabetes and in the general population [56, 66, 110-119]. The Framingham Heart Study identified the direct correlation between diabetes and the morbidity and mortality associated with coronary heart disease. The total number of deaths from cardiac causes in diabetic patients is greater than that from the next five most common causes of death combined. The net effect of diabetes increases the risk of coronary death and coronary events approximately two fold, regardless of whether or not coronary disease is a pre-existing condition in these populations. Studies in diabetic patients with proteinuria at all levels have demonstrated an increased risk of cardiovascular events in these patients, and this risk increases with the severity of the underlying nephropathy. In fact, proteinuria might be considered to be a marker for generalized endothelial damage and atherosclerosis [100, 120-123]. Cardiovascular complications can occur with proteinuria even at levels that are currently considered to be low normal in the general population, in patients with diabetes, and in patients with diabetic or non-diabetic renal disease [119]. The presence of microalbuminuria in otherwise healthy individuals is probably associated with increased risk of cardiovascular disease but perhaps the association is stronger in the presence of other risk factors for cardiovascular disease [124].

The Heart Outcomes Prevention Evaluation (HOPE) trial demonstrated the benefit of angiotensin converting enzyme inhibition with ramipril when compared with the routine standard of care in reducing cardiac events in patients at increased risk of cardiovascular disease. The inclusion criteria for HOPE required either a history of vascular disease or diabetes, and the mean duration of follow-up was 4.5 years. The ramipril treatment group experienced a significant benefit in the reduction of cardiovascular events and mortality [125]. In the diabetic HOPE subgroup, the magnitude of benefits were more pronounced. The HOPE investigators also analyzed a sub-population of patients with pre-existing nephropathy, and found that the presence of nephropathy conferred an increased risk of cardiac events when compared to patients with normal renal function [126]. The HOPE study was designed as a cardiovascular outcome trial and did not demonstrate a benefit of therapy on renal outcome of end-stage renal disease.

The Losartan Intervention For Endpoint reduction in hypertension (LIFE) trial provided an opportunity to study the effects of treatment with the angiotensin II receptor antagonist losartan versus the beta-blocker atenolol in hypertensive patients with diabetes. This study investigated the effects of losartan- versus atenolol-based therapy in 9193 patients with hypertension and left ventricular hypertrophy followed for a mean of 4.8 years [127]. Lindholm *et al* analyzed the LIFE subgroup of 1195 patients with diabetes, hypertension, and left ventricular hypertrophy, and reported that in this subgroup of patients losartan reduced the risk of the primary composite endpoint of cardiovascular morbidity and mortality by 24%; P=0.031. The risk of cardiovascular mortality was 37% lower in the losartan group than in the atenolol group (P=0.028). Total mortality was 39% lower in the losartan group (P=0.002) [128].

The Reduction of Endpoints in NIDDM with the Angiotensin II Antagonist Losartan (RENAAL) study included three secondary cardiovascular endpoints: 1) the time to first event of cardiovascular morbidity and mortality (a composite of myocardial infarction, stroke, cardiovascular-related death, coronary or peripheral revascularization procedures, or first hospitalization for heart failure or unstable angina); 2) changes in the level of proteinuria; and 3) progression of renal disease. The RENAAL trial was not powered to detect differences in cardiovascular endpoints, and found no difference between treatment groups in cardiovascular events and mortality. There was, however, an observed trend towards a reduction in myocardial infarction (risk reduction 28%, P=0.08), and a statistically significant reduction in the time to first hospitalization for heart failure in the losartan group (risk reduction 32%, P=0.005) [89].

In IDNT, the secondary efficacy measure was the time to first event of the composite endpoint of death from cardiovascular causes, non-fatal myocardial infarction, hospitalization for heart failure, a permanent neurologic deficit caused by cerebrovascular event, or lower limb amputation above the ankle. There were no significant differences among the treatment groups in the secondary composite cardiovascular outcomes.

RENAAL and IDNT were designed as renal protective studies, not cardiovascular outcome trials. With regard to heart failure, the blockade of angiotensin II's effect on transforming growth factor-beta (TGF-beta-1) in the heart may retard the formation of fibrosis and the preservation of cardiac function [129, 130]. However, further studies are needed in this area.

NON-RENIN-ANGIOTENSIN-ALDOSTERONE SYSTEM THERAPIES AND PROTEINURIA

In addition to therapy with drugs that affect the renin-angiotensin-aldosterone system, other interventions reduce urine protein excretion.

The benefits of a low-protein diet in patients with type 2 diabetes have not been definitively proven in patients with type 2 diabetic nephropathy A number of studies have suggested that urinary protein is reduced and this might have a potential beneficial effect on progression of kidney disease but this remains to be evaluated [131-133].

Non-steroidal anti-inflammatory drugs (NSAIDs) that are prostaglandin inhibitors (e.g., indomethacin) lower urine protein excretion at relatively high doses and especially in conjunction with a low-sodium diet [92, 134-146]. However these drugs reduce glomerular filtration rate and reduce renal potassium excretion as well as having considerable gastrointestinal intolerability in patients with severe kidney dysfunction [147]. In patients treated with angiotensin converting enzyme inhibitors, use of NSAIDS may be associated with hyperkalemia or acute renal failure.

Recently, COX-2 inhibitors have been shown to reduce proteinuria and preserve renal structure in animal models of renal disease [148, 149]. Human studies in patients with proteinuria have only recently been initiated and definitive results are not yet available. Rossat et al reported similarities in magnitude of improvements in renal hemodynamics and sodium handling for an NSAID compared to a COX-2 inhibitor [150].

Fried et al performed a meta-analysis of 13 statin trials that showed decreased in proteinuria and preservation of glomerular filtration rate in patients with renal disease. These effects were not completely explained by reductions in cholesterol [151].

Recent studies have suggested that anemia may contribute to both cardiovascular and kidney disease progression. At this time, there are no reliable clinical trial data demonstrating a clinical benefit of treatment of anemia on cardiovascular or renal end points. Nonetheless, based on early data, current guidelines recommend maintenance of hemoglobin > 11 g/dL [152, 153].

CONCLUSIONS

The presence of persistent urinary protein excretion is associated with impending or existing renal and vascular disease. High-risk patients, such as those with or at high-risk for type 2 diabetes, should be screened for microalbuminuria, and treated with angiotensin receptor antagonists with or without additional antihypertensive therapies, as needed. Hyperglycemia should be intensively treated. The current gold standard drug class for the reduction of risk for type 2 diabetic nephropathy and end-stage renal disease is the angiotensin receptor antagonists. Because not all of their beneficial effects are due to their known benefits on hypertension and proteinuria, additional research with these agents would be highly desirable.

REFERENCES

1. Amos AF, McCarty DJ, Zimmet P. The rising global burden of diabetes and its complications: estimates and projections to the year 2010. Diabet Med 1997;14 Suppl 5:S1-S85.
2. US Renal Data System. USRDS 1998 Annual Data Report. Bethesda, National Institutes of Health National Institute of Diabetes, 1998.
3. Pastan S, Bailey J. Dialysis therapy. N Engl J Med 1998;338:1428-1437.
4. Delcourt C, Vauzelle-Kervroedan F, Cathelineau G, Papoz L. Low prevalence of long-term complications in non-insulin-dependent diabetes mellitus in France: a multicenter study. CODIAB-INSERM-ZENECA Pharma Study Group. J Diabet Complications 1998;12:88-95.
5. Passa P, Chatellier G. The DIAB-HYCAR Study. Diabetologia 1996;39:1662-1667.
6. Krolewski AS, Warram JH, Freire MB. Epidemiology of late diabetic complications. A basis for the development and evaluation of preventive programs. Endocrinol Metab Clin North Am 1996;25:217-42.
7. Esmatjes E, Castell C, Gonzalez T, Tresserras R, Lloveras G. Epidemiology of renal involvement in type II diabetics (NIDDM) in Catalonia. The Catalan Diabetic Nephropathy Study Group. Diabetes Res Clin Pract 1996;32:157-163.
8. Lievre M, Marre M, Chatellier G, Plouin P, Reglier J, Richardson L, Bugnard F, Vasmant D. The non-insulin-dependent diabetes, hypertension, microalbuminuria or proteinuria, cardiovascular events, and ramipril (DIABHYCAR) study: design, organization, and patient recruitment. DIABHYCAR Study Group. Control Clin Trials 2000;21:383-396.
9. Campbell RC, Ruggenenti P, Remuzzi G. Halting the progression of chronic nephropathy. J Am Soc Nephrol 2002;13:S190-S195.
10. Mogensen CE. Microalbuminuria predicts clinical proteinuria and early mortality in maturity-onset diabetes. N Engl J Med 1984;310:356-360.
11. Esmail ZN, Loewen PS. Losartan as an alternative to ACE inhibitors in patients with renal dysfunction. Ann Pharmacother 1998;32:1096-1098.
12. Parving HH. Diabetic nephropathy: Prevention and treatment. Kidney Int 2001;60:2041-2055.
13. Mogensen CE, Hansen KW, Nielsen S, Pedersen MM, Rehling M, Schmitz A. Monitoring diabetic nephropathy: glomerular filtration rate and abnormal albuminuria in diabetic renal disease—reproducibility, progression, and efficacy of antihypertensive intervention. Am J Kidney Dis 1993;22:174-187.
14. Parving HH, Kastrup H, Smidt UM, Andersen AR, Feldt-Rasmussen B, Christiansen JS. Impaired autoregulation of glomerular filtration rate in type 1 (insulin-dependent) diabetic patients with nephropathy. Diabetologia 1984;27:547-552.
15. Mogensen CD. Early glomerular hyperfiltration in insulin-dependent diabetes and late nephropathy. Scan J Clin Lab Invest 1986;46:201-206.
16. Rudberg S, Persson B, Dahlquist G. Increased glomerular filtration rate as a predictor of diabetic nephropathy—an 8-year prospective study. Kidney Int 1992;41:822-828.
17. Vora JP, Dolben J, Dean JD, Thomas D, Williams JD, Owens DR, Peters JR. Renal hemodynamics in newly presenting non-insulin dependent diabetes mellitus. Kidney Int 1992;41:829-835.

18. Schmitz A, Hansen HH, Christensen T. Kidney function in newly diagnosed type 2 (non-insulin-dependent) diabetic patients before and during treatment. Diabetologia 1989;32:434-439.

19. Hostetter TH, Rennke HG, Brenner BM. The case for intrarenal hypertension in the initiation and progression of diabetic and other glomerulopathies. Am J Med 1982;72:375-380.

20. Viberti GC, Hill RD, Jarrett RJ, Argyropoulos A, Mahmud U, Keen H. Microalbuminuria as a predictor of clinical nephropathy in insulin-dependent diabetes mellitus. Lancet 1982;1:1430-1432.

21. Mogensen CE, Christensen CK, Vittinghus E. The stages in diabetic renal disease. With emphasis on the stage of incipient diabetic nephropathy. Diabetes 1983;32(Suppl 2):64-78.

22. Fioretto P, Mauer M, Brocco E, Velussi M, Frigato F, Muollo B, Sambataro M, Abaterusso C, Baggio B, Crepaldi G, Nosadini R. Patterns of renal injury in NIDDM patients with microalbuminuria. Diabetologia 1996;39:1569-1576.

23. Pinto-Siestma SJ, Janssen WMT, Hillege HL, Navis G, de Zeeuw D, de Jong PE. Urinary albumin excretion is associated with renal functional abnormalities in a nondiabetic population. J Am Soc Nephrol 2000;11:1882-1888.

24. Gould MM, Mohamed-Ali V, Goubet SA, Yudkin JS, Haines AP. Microalbuminuria: associations with height and sex in non-diabetic subjects. BMJ 1993;306:240-242.

25. Metcalf P, Baker J, Scott A, Wild C, Scragg R, Dryson E. Albuminuria in people at least 40 years old: effect of obesity, hypertension, and hyperlipidemia. Clin Chem 1992;38:1802-1808.

26. Mattix HJ, Hsu CY, Shaykevich S, Curhan G. Use of the albumin/creatinine ratio to detect microalbuminuria: implications of sex and race. J Am Soc Nephrol 2002;13:1034-1039.

27. Verhave JC, Hillege HL, de Zeeuw D, de Jong PE. How to measure the prevalence of microalbuminuria in relation to age and gender? Am J Kidney Dis 2002;40:436-437.

28. Tobe SW, McFarlane PA, Naimark DM. Microalbuminuria in diabetes mellitus. Canadian Med Assoc J 2002;167:499-503.

29. National Kidney Foundation-K/DOQI. Clinical practice guidelines for chronic kidney disease: evaluation, classification and stratification. Am J Kidney Dis 2002;39(Suppl 2):S1-S246.

30. Zanchetti A, Ruilope LM. Antihypertensive treatment in patients with type-2 diabetes mellitus: what guidance from recent controlled randomized trials? J Hypertens 2002;20:2099-2110.

31. Klag MJ, Whelton PK, Randall BL, Neaton JD, Brancati FL, Ford CE, Shulman NB, Stamler J. Blood pressure and end-stage renal disease in men. N Engl J Med 1996;334:13-18.

32. Parving HH, Andersen AR, Smidt UM, Hommel E, Mathiesen ER, Svendsen PA. Effect of antihypertensive treatment on kidney function in diabetic nephropathy. Br Med J (Clin Res Ed) 1987;294:1443-1447.

33. Mogensen CE. Long-term antihypertensive treatment inhibiting progression of diabetic nephropathy. Br Med J (Clin Res Ed) 1982;285:685-688.

34. Mehler PS, Jeffers BW, Estacio R, Schrier RW. Associations of hypertension and complications in non-insulin-dependent diabetes mellitus. Am J Hypertens 1997;10:152-161.

35. Estacio RO, Jeffers BW, Gifford N, Schrier RW. Effect of blood pressure control on diabetic microvascular complications in patients with hypertension and type 2 diabetes. Diabetes Care 2000;23(Suppl 2):B54-B64.

36. Schrier RW, Estacio RO, Esler A, Mehler P. Effects of aggressive blood pressure control in normotensive type 2 diabetic patients on albuminuria, retinopathy, and strokes. Kidney Int 2002;61:1086-1097.

37. Alvestrand A, Gutierrez A, Bucht H, Bergstrom J. Reduction of blood pressure retards the progression of chronic renal failure in man. Nephrol Dial Transplant 1988;3:624-631.

38. Hannedouche T, Albouze G, Chauveau P, Lacour B, Jungers P. Effects of blood pressure and antihypertensive treatment on progression of advanced chronic renal failure. Am J Kidney Dis 1993;21:131-137.

39. Peterson JC, Adler S, Burkart JM, Greene T, Hebert LA, Hunsicker LG, King AJ, Klahr S, Massry SG, Seifter JL. Blood pressure control, proteinuria, and the progression of renal disease. The Modification of Diet in Renal Disease Study. Ann Intern Med 1995;123:754-762.

40. Bakris GL, Williams M, Dworkin L, Elliott WJ, Epstein M, Toto R, Tuttle K, Douglas J, Hsueh W, Sowers J. Preserving renal function in adults with hypertension and diabetes: a consensus approach. Am J Kidney Dis 2000;36:646-661.

41. Joint National Committee on Prevention, Detection, Evaluation, and Treatment of High Blood Pressure. The Sixth Report of the Joint National Committee on Prevention, Detection, Evaluation, and Treatment of High Blood Pressure. Arch Intern Med 1997;157:2413-2448.

42. American Diabetes Association. Standards of medical care for patients with diabetes mellitus. Diabetes Care 2003;26(Suppl 1):S33-S50.

43. Bakris GL, Williams M, Dworkin L, Elliott WJ, Epstein M, Toto R, Tuttle K, Douglas J, Hsueh W, Sowers J for the National Kidney Foundation Hypertension and Diabetes Executive Committees Working Group. Am J Kidney Dis 2000;36:646-661.

44. Guidelines Subcommittee. 1999 World Health Organization and International Society of Hypertension guidelines for the management of hypertension. J Hypertens 1999;17:151-183.

45. Mogensen CD, Damsgaard EM, Froland A, Nielsen S, de Fine Olivarius N, Schmitz A. Microalbuminuria in non-insulin-dependent diabetes. Clin Nephrol 1992;38(Suppl 1):S28-S39.

46. Viberti GC, Pickup RJ, Jarrett RJ, Keen H. Effect of control of blood glucose on urinary excretion of albumin and B2-microglobin in insulin-dependent diabetes. N Engl J Med 1979;300:638-641.

47. Nelson RG, Bennett PH, Beck GJ, Tan M, Knowler WC, Mitch WE, Hirschman GH, Myers BD. Development and progression of renal disease in Pima Indians with non-insulin-dependent diabetes mellitus. Diabetes Renal Disease Study Group. N Engl J Med 1996;335:1636-1642.

48. Cathelineau G, de Champvallins M, Bouallouche A, Lesobre B. Management of newly diagnosed non-insulin-dependent diabetes mellitus in the primary care setting. Effects of 2 years of gliclazide treatment – the Diadem Study. Metabolism 1997;46:31-34.

49. UK Prospective Diabetes Study Group. Intensive blood-glucose control with sulfonylureas or insulin compared with conventional treatment and risk of complications in patients with type 2 diabetes (UKPDS 33). Lancet 1998;352:837-853.

50. Mulec H, Blohme G, Grande B, Bjorck S. The effect of metabolic control on rate of decline in renal function in insulin-dependent diabetes mellitus with overt diabetic nephropathy. Nephrol Dial Transplant 1998;13:651-655.

51. The Diabetes Control and Complications Trial Research Group. The effect of intensive treatment of diabetes on the development and progression of long-term complications in insulin-dependent diabetes mellitus. N Eng J Med 1993;14:977-987.

52. Deckert T, Feldt-Rasmussen G, Borch-Johnsen K, Jensen T, Kofoed-Enevoldsen A. Albuminuria reflects widespread vascular damage. The Steno hypothesis. Diabetologia 1989;32:219-226.

53. Stern MP. Diabetes and cardiovascular disease. The "common soil" hypothesis. Diabetes 1995;44:369-374.

54. Mogensen CD. Systemic blood pressure and glomerular leakage with particular reference to diabetes and hypertension. J Intern Med 1994;235:297-316.

55. Jensen JS. Renal and systemic transvascular albumin leakage in severe atherosclerosis. Arterioscler Thromb Vasc Biol 1995;15:1324-1329.

56. Yudkin JS, Forrest RD, Jackson CA. Microalbuminuria as a predictor of vascular disease in non-diabetic subjects: Islington Diabetes Survey. Lancet 1988;2:530-533.

57. Gaede P, Vedel P, Larsen N, Jensen GVH, Parving HH, Pedersen O. Multifactorial intervention and cardiovascular disease in patients with type 2 diabetes. N Engl J Med 2003;348:383-393.

58. Garg AX, Kiberd BA, Clark WF, Haynes RB, Clase CM. Albuminuria and renal insufficiency prevalence guides population screening: Results from the NHANES III. Kidney Int 2002;61:2165-2175.

59. Mykkanen L, Haffner SM, Kuusisto J, Pyorala K, Laakso M. Microalbuminuria precedes the development of NIDDM. Diabetes 1994;43:552-557.

60. Robbins DC, Hu D, Howard BV, Sosenko JM. Elevated urinary albumin excretion is an independent risk factor for type 2 DM: The Strong Heart Study (Abstract) Diabetes 2000;49(Suppl 1):A24.

61. Ruggenenti P, Mosconi L, Sangalli F, Casiraghi F, Gambara V, Remuzzi G, Remuzzi A. Glomerular size-selective dysfunction in NIDDM is not ameliorated by ACE inhibition or by calcium channel blockade. Kidney Int 1999;55:984-994.

62. Vogt L, Navis G, de Zeeuw D. Renoprotection: a matter of blood pressure reduction or agent-characteristics? J Am Soc Nephrol 2002;13:S202-S207.

63. De Jong PE, Navis G, de Zeeuw D. Renoprotective therapy: titration against urinary protein excretion. Lancet 1999;354:352-353.

64. Peters H, Ritz E. Dosing angiotensin II blockers—beyond blood pressure. Nephrol Dial Transplant 1999;14:2568-2570.

65. Mogensen CE. Microalbuminuria, blood pressure and diabetic renal disease: origin and development of ideas. Diabetologia 1999;42:263-285.

66. Dinneen SF, Gerstein HC. The association of microalbuminuria and mortality in non-insulin-dependent diabetes mellitus. A systematic overview of the literature. Arch Intern Med 1997;157:1413-1418.

67. Cerasola G, Cottone S, Mule G, Nardi E, Mangano MT, Andronico G, Contorno A, Li Vecchi M, Galione P, Renda F, Piazza G, Volpe V, Lisi A, Ferrara L, Panepinto N, Riccobene R. Microalbuminuria, renal dysfunction and cardiovascular complication in essential hypertension. J Hypertens 1996;14:915-920.

68. Pontremoli R, Nicolella C, Viazzi F, Ravera M, Sofia A, Berruti V, Bezante GP, Del Sette M, Martinoli C, Sacchi G, Deferrari G. Microalbuminuria is an early marker of target organ damage in essential hypertension. Am J Hypertens 1998;11:430-438.

69. Bigazzi R, Bianchi S, Baldari D, Campese VM. Microalbuminuria predicts cardiovascular events and renal insufficiency in patients with essential hypertension. J Hypertens 1998;16:1325-1333.

70. Jafar TH, Stark PC, Schmid CH, Landa M, Maschio G, Marcantoni C, de Jong PE, de Zeeuw D, Shahinfar S, Ruggenenti P, Remuzzi G, Levey AS for the AIPRD Study Group. Proteinuria as a modifiable risk factor for the progression of non-diabetic renal disease. Kidney Int 2001;60:1131-1140.

71. Williams PS, Fass G, Bone JM. Renal pathology and proteinuria determine progression in untreated mild/moderate chronic renal failure. Q J Med 1988;67:343-354.

72. Remuzzi G, Bertani T. Is glomerulosclerosis a consequence of altered glomerular permeability to macromolecules? Kidney Int 1990;38:384-394.

73. Bos H, Henning RH, de Jong PE, de Zeeuw D, Navis G. Do severe systemic sequelae of proteinuria modulate the antiproteinuric response to chronic ACE inhibition? Nephrol Dial Transplant 2002;17:793-797.

74. Burton C, Harris KP. The role of proteinuria in the progression of chronic renal failure. Am J Kidney Dis 1996;27:765-775.

75. Wang Y, Rangan GK, Tay YC, Wang Y, Harris DCH. Induction of monocyte chemoattractant protein-1 by albumin is mediated by nuclear factor kappaB in proximal tubule cells. J Am Soc Nephrol 1999;10:1204-1213.

76. Remuzzi G, Bertani T. Pathophysiology of progressive nephropathies. N Engl J Med 1998;339:1448-1456.

77. Hebert LA, Wilmer WA, Falkenhain ME, Ladson-Wofford SE, Nahman NS Jr, Rovin BH. Renoprotection: one or many therapies? Kidney Int 2001;59:1211-1226.

78. Keane WF, Brenner BM, De Zeeuw D, Grunfeld JP, McGill J, Mitch WE, Ribeiro AB, Shahinfar S, Simpson RL, Snapinn S, Toto R. The risk of developing end-stage renal disease in patients with type 2 diabetes and nephropathy: lessons from the RENAAL study. Kidney Int 2003;63:1499-1507.

79. Shahinfar S, Dickson TZ, Ahmed T, Zhang Z, Ramjit D, Smith RD, Brenner BM. Losartan in patients with type 2 diabetes and proteinuria: observations from the RENAAL study. Kidney Int 2002;62:S64-S67.

80. UK Prospective Diabetes Study group. Tight blood pressure control and risk of macrovascular and microvascular complications in type 2 diabetes: UKPDS 38. BMJ 1998;317:703-713.

81. Lewis EJ, Hunsicker LB, Bain RP, Rohde RD. The effect of angiotensin-converting-enzyme inhibition on diabetic nephropathy. The Collaborative Study Group. N Engl J Med 1993;329:1456-1462.

82. Ravid M, Savin H, Jutrin I, Bental T, Katz B, Lishner M. Long-term stabilizing effect of angiotensin-converting enzyme inhibition on plasma creatinine and on proteinuria in normotensive type 2 diabetic patients. Ann Intern Med 1993;118:577-581.

83. Lebovitz HE, Wiegmann TB, Cnaan A, Shahinfar S, Sica DA, Broadstone V, Schwartz SL, Mengel MC, Segal R, Versaggi JA, et al. Renal protection effects of enalapril in hypertensive NIDDM: role of baseline albuminuria. Kidney Int Suppl 1994;45:S150-S155.

84. Bakris GL, Copley JB, Vicknair N, Sadler R, Leurgans S. Calcium channel blockers versus other antihypertensive therapies on progression of NIDDM associated nephropathy. Kidney Int 1996;50:1641-1650.

85. Taguma Y, Kitamoto Y, Futaki G, Ueda H, Monma H, Ishizaki M, Takahashi H, Sekino H, Sasaki Y. Effect of captopril on heavy proteinuria in azotemic diabetics. N Engl J Med 1985;313:1617-1620.

86. Estacio RO, Jeffers BW, Hiatt WR, Biggerstaff SL, Gifford N, Schrier RW. The effect of nisoldipine as compared with enalapril on cardiovascular outcomes in patients with non-insulin-dependent diabetes and hypertension. N Engl J Med 1998;338:645-652.

87. Parving HH, Lehnert H, Brochner-Mortensen J, Gomis R, Andersen S, Arner P; Irbesartan in Patients with Type 2 Diabetes and Microalbuminuria Study Group. The effect of irbesartan on the development of diabetic nephropathy in patients with type 2 diabetes. N Engl J Med. 2001;345:870-878.

88. Viberti G, Wheeldon NM, for the MicroAlbuminuria Reduction With VALsartan (MARVAL) Study Investigators. Microalbuminuria reduction with valsartan in patients with type 2 diabetes mellitus. A blood pressure-independent effect. Circulation 2002;106:672-678.

89. Brenner BM, Cooper ME, de Zeeuw D, Keane WF, Mitch WE, Parving HH, Remuzzi G, Snapinn SM, Zhang Z, Shahinfar S; RENAAL Study Investigators. Effects of losartan on renal and cardiovascular outcomes in patients with type 2 diabetes and nephropathy. N Engl J Med 2001;345:861-869.

90. Lewis EJ, Hunsicker LG, Clarke WR, Berl T, Pohl MA, Lewis JB, Ritz E, Atkins RC, Rohde R, Raz I; Collaborative Study Group. Renoprotective effect of the angiotensin-receptor antagonist irbesartan in patients with nephropathy due to type 2 diabetes. N Engl J Med 2001;345:851-860.

91. Buter H, Hemmelder MH, Navis G, de Jong PE, de Zeeuw D. The blunting of the antiproteinuric efficacy of ACE inhibition by high sodium intake can be restored by hydrochlorothiazide. Nephrol Dial Transplant 1998;13:1682-1685.

92. Heeg JE, de Jong PE, van der Hem GK, de Zeeuw D. Efficacy and variability of the antiproteinuric effect of ACE inhibition by lisinopril. Kidney Int 1989;36:272-279.

93. Schiffrin EL, Park JB, Intengan HD, Touyz RM. Correction of arterial structure and endothelial dysfunction in human essential hypertension by the angiotensin receptor antagonist losartan. Circulation 2000;101:1653-1659.

94. Strawn WB, Chappell MC, Dean RH, Kivlighn S, Ferrario CM. Inhibition of early atherogenesis by losartan in monkeys with diet-induced hypercholesterolemia. Circulation 2000;101:1586-1593.

95. Andersen S, Blouch K, Bialek J, Deckert M, Parving HH, Myers BD. Glomerular permselectivity in early stages of overt diabetic nephropathy. Kidney Int 2000;58:2129-2137.

96. Benigni A, Remuzzi G. How renal cytokines and growth factors contribute to renal disease progression. Am J Kidney Dis 2001;37:S21-S24.

97. Taal MW, Brenner BM. Renoprotective benefits of RAS inhibition: From ACEI to angiotensin II antagonists. Kidney Int 2000;57:1803-1817.

98. Hollenberg NK. ACE inhibition, angiotensin II receptor blockade and diabetic nephropathy. In: Mogensen CE, ed. The Kidney and Hypertension in Diabetes Mellitus. Boston: Kluwer Academic Publishers;2000:417-422.

99. Singh R, Alavi N, Singh AK, Leehey DJ. Role of angiotensin II in glucose-induced inhibition of mesangial matrix degradation. Diabetes 1999;48:2066-2073.

100. Goligorsky MS, Chen J, Brodsky S. Endothelial cell dysfunction leading to diabetic nephropathy: focus on nitric oxide. Hypertension 2001;37:744-748.

101. Gutterman DD. Vascular dysfunction in hyperglycemia. Is protein kinase C the culprit? Circ Res 2002;90:5-7.

102. Gansevoort RT, de Zeeuw D, de Jong PE. Is the antiproteinuric effect of ACE inhibition mediated by interference in the renin-angiotensin system? Kidney Int 1994;45:861-867.

103. Komine N, Khang S, Wead LM, Blantz RC, Gabbai FB. Effect of combining an ACE inhibitor and an angiotensin II receptor blocker on plasma and kidney tissue angiotensin II levels. Am J Kidney Dis 2002;39:159-164.

104. Hilgers KF, Mann JF. ACE inhibitors versus AT(1) receptor antagonists in patients with chronic renal disease. J Am Soc Nephrol 2002;13:1100-1108.

105. Boner G, Cao Z, Cooper ME. Combination antihypertensive therapy in the treatment of diabetic nephropathy. Diab Tech Thera 2002;4:313-321.

106. Laverman GD, Navis G, Henning RH, de Jong PE, de Zeeuw D. Dual rennin-angiotensin system blockade at optimal doses for proteinuria. Kidney Int 2002;62:1020-1025.

107. Mogensen CE, Neldam S, Tikkanen I, Oren S, Viskoper R, Watts RW, Cooper ME. Randomised controlled trial of dual blockade of renin-angiotensin-aldosterone system in patients with hypertension, microalbuminuria, and non-insulin dependent diabetes: the candesartan and lisinopril microalbuminuria (CALM) study. BMJ 2000;321:1440-1444.

108. Campbell R, Sangalli F, Perticucci E, Aros C, Viscarra C, Perna A, Remuzzi A, Bertocchi F, Fagiani L, Remuzzi G, Ruggenenti P. Effects of combined ACE inhibitor and angiotensin II antagonist treatment in human chronic nephropathies. Kidney Int 2003;63:1094-1103.

109. van Paassen P, de Zeeuw D, Navis G, de Jong PE. Renal and systemic effects of continued treatment with renin inhibitor remikiren in hypertensive patients with normal and impaired renal function. Nephrol Dial Transplant 2000;15:637-643.

110. Gerstein HC, Mann JF, Yi Q, Zinman B, Dinneen SF, Hoogwerf B, Halle JP, Young J, Rashkow A, Joyce C, Nawaz S, Yusuf S; HOPE Study Investigators. Albuminuria and risk of cardiovascular events, death, and heart failure in diabetic and nondiabetic individuals. JAMA 2001;286:421-426.

111. Hillege HL, Fidler V, Diercks GF, van Gilst WH, de Zeeuw D, van Veldhuisen DJ, Gans RO, Janssen WM, Grobbee DE, de Jong PE; Prevention of Renal and Vascular End Stage Disease (PREVEND) Study Group. Urinary albumin excretion predicts cardiovascular and noncardiovascular mortality in general population. Circulation 2002;106:1777-1782.

112. Rossing P, Hougaard P, Borch-Johnsen K, Parving HH. Predictors of mortality in insulin dependent diabetes: 10 year observational follow up study. BMJ 1996;313:779-784.

113. Jager A, Kostense PJ, Ruhe HG, Heine RJ, Nijpels G, Dekker JM, Bouter LM, Stehouwer CD. Microalbuminuria and peripheral arterial disease are independent predictors of cardiovascular and all-cause mortality, especially among hypertensive subjects: five-year follow-up of the Hoorn Study. Arterioscler Thromb Vasc Biol 1999;19:617-624.

114. Damsgaard EM, Froland A, Jorgensen OD, Mogensen CE. Microalbuminuria as predictor of increased mortality in elderly people. BMJ 1990;300:297-300.

115. Roest M, Banga JD, Janssen WM, Grobbee DE, Sixma JJ, de Jong PE, de Zeeuw D, van Der Schouw YT. Excessive urinary albumin levels are associated with future cardiovascular mortality in postmenopausal women. Circulation 2001;103:3057-3061.

116. Borch-Johnsen K, Feldt-Rasmussen B, Strandgaard S, Schroll M, Jensen JS. Urinary albumin excretion: an independent predictor of ischemic heart disease. Arterioscler Thromb Vasc Biol 1999;19:1992-1997.

117. Gerstein HC, Mann JF, Pogue J, Dinneen SF, Halle JP, Hoogwerf B, Joyce C, Rashkow A, Young J, Zinman B, Yusuf S. Prevalence and determinants of microalbuminuria in high-risk diabetic and nondiabetic patients in the Heart Outcomes Evaluation Study. The HOPE Study Investigators. Diabetes Care 2000;23(Suppl 2):B35-B39.

118. Winocour PH, Harland JO, Millar JP, Laker MF, Alberti KG. Microalbuminuria and associated cardiovascular risk factors in the community. Atherosclerosis 1992;93:71-81.

119. Hillege HL, Janssen WM, Bak AA, Diercks GF, Grobbee DE, Crijns HJ, Van Gilst WH, De Zeeuw D, De Jong PE; The PREVEND Study Group. Microalbuminuria is common, also in a nondiabetic, nonhypertensive population, and an independent indicator of cardiovascular risk factors and cardiovascular morbidity. J Int Med 2001;249:519-526.

120. Grimm RH Jr, Svendsen KH, Kasiske B, Keane WF, Wahi MM. Proteinuria is a risk factor for mortality over 10 years of follow-up. MRFIT Research Group. Multiple Risk Factor Intervention Trial. Kidney Int Suppl 1997;52:S10-S14.

121. Nelson RG, Pettitt DJ, Carraher MJ, Baird HR, Knowler WC. Effect of proteinuria on mortality in NIDDM. Diabetes 1988;37:1499-1504.

122. Ballard DJ, Humphrey LL, Melton LJ 3rd, Frohnert PP, Chu PC, O'Fallon WM, Palumbo PJ. Epidemiology of persistent proteinuria in type II diabetes mellitus. Population-based study in Rochester, Minnesota. Diabetes 1988;37:405-412.

123. Stephenson JM, Kenny S, Stevens LK, Fuller JH, Lee E. Proteinuria and mortality in diabetes: the WHO Multinational Study of Vascular Disease in Diabetes. Diabet Med 1995;12:149-155.

124. Romundstad S, Holmen J, Hallan H, Kvenild K, Kruger O, Midthjell K. Microalbuminuria, cardiovascular disease and risk factors in a nondiabetic/nonhypertensive population. The Nord-Trondelag Health Study (HUNT, 1995-97), Norway. J Int Med 2002;252:164-172.

125. Heart Outcomes Prevention Evaluation (HOPE) Study Investigators. Effects of an angiotensin-converting-enzyme inhibitor, ramipril, on cardiovascular events in high-risk patients. N Engl J Med 2000;342:145-153.

126. Heart Outcomes Prevention Evaluation (HOPE) Study Investigators. Effects of ramipril on cardiovascular and microvascular outcomes in people with diabetes mellitus: results of the HOPE study and MICRO-HOPE substudy. Lancet 2000;355:253-259.

127. Dahlof B, Devereux RB, Kjeldsen SE, Julius S, Beevers G, de Faire U, Fyhrquist F, Ibsen H, Kristiansson K, Lederballe-Pedersen O, Lindholm LH, Nieminen MS, Omvik P, Oparil S, Wedel H. Cardiovascular morbidity and mortality in the Losartan Intervention For Endpoint reduction in hypertension study (LIFE): a randomised trial against atenolol. Lancet 2002;359:995-1003.

128. Lindholm LH, Ibsen H, Dahlof B, Devereux RB, Beevers G, de Faire U, Fyhrquist F, Julius S, Kjeldsen SE, Kristiansson K, Lederballe-Pedersen O, Nieminen MS, Omvik P, Oparil S, Wedel H, Aurup P, Edelman J, Snapinn S. Cardiovascular morbidity and mortality in patients with diabetes in the Losartan Intervention For Endpoint reduction in hypertension study (LIFE): a randomised trial against atenolol. Lancet 2002;359:1004-1010.

129. Zanella MT, Ribeiro AB. The role of angiotensin II antagonism in type 2 diabetes mellitus: a review of renoprotection studies. Clin Ther 2002;24:1019-1034.

130. Williams B. The renin angiotensin system in the pathogenesis of diabetic complications. In: Mogensen CE, ed. The Kidney and Hypertension in Diabetes Mellitus. Boston: Kluwer Academic Publishers;2000:645-654.

131. El Nahas AM, Masters-Thomas A, Brady SA, Farrington K, Wilkinson V, Hilson AJ, Varghese Z, Moorhead JF. Selective effect of low protein diets in chronic renal diseases. BMJ (Clin Res Ed) 1984;289:1337-1341.

132. Gansevoort RT, de Zeeuw D, de Jong PE. Additive antiproteinuric effect of ACE inhibition and a low protein diet in human renal disease. Nephrol Dial Transplant 1995;10:497-504.

133. Modification of Diet in Renal Disease Study Group. Effects of diet and antihypertensive therapy on creatinine clearance and serum creatinine in the Modification of Diet in Renal Disease Study. J Am Soc Nephrol 1996;7:556-566.

134. Idelson BA, Smithline N, Smith GW, Harrington JT. Prognosis in steroid-treated idiopathic nephrotic syndrome in adults. Analysis of major predictive factors after ten-year follow-up. Arch Intern Med 1977;137:891-896.

135. Donker AJ, Brentjens JR, van der Hem GK, Arisz L. Treatment of the nephrotic syndrome with indomethacin. Nephron 1978;22:374-381.

136. Arisz L, Donker AJ, Brentjens JR, van der Hem GK. The effect of indomethacin on proteinuria and kidney function in the nephrotic syndrome. Acta Med Scand 1976;199:121-125.

137. Conte J, Suc JM, Mignon-Conte M. Anti-proteinuric effect of indomethacin in glomerulopathies (nephrotic syndrome, acute glomerulonephritis and chronic glomerulonephritis). J Urol Nephrol 1967;73:850-856.

138. Michielsen P, Verberckmoes R, Desmet V, Hermerijckx W. Histological course of diffuse proliferative glomerulonephritis treated with indomethacin. J Urol Nephrol 1969;75:315-318.

139. Hommel E, Mathiesen E, Arnold-Larsen S, Edsberg B, Olsen UB, Parving HH. Effects of indomethacin on kidney function in type 1 (insulin-dependent) diabetic patients with nephropathy. Diabetologia 1987;30:78-81.

140. Vriesendorp R, de Zeeuw D, de Jong PE, Donker AJ, Pratt JJ, van der Hem GK. Reduction of urinary protein and prostaglandin E2 excretion in the nephrotic syndrome by non-steroidal anti-inflammatory drugs. Clin Nephrol 1986;25:105-110.

141. Shehadeh IH, Demers LM, Abt AB, Schoolwerth AC. Indomethacin and the nephrotic syndrome. JAMA 1979;241:1264-1266.

142. Garini G, Mazzi A, Buzio C, Mutti A, Allegri L, Savazzi G, Borghetti A. Renal effects of captopril, indomethacin and nifedipine in nephrotic patients after an oral protein load. Nephrol Dial Transplant 1996;11:628-634.

143. Heeg JE, de Jong PE, Vriesendorp R, de Zeeuw D. Additive antiproteinuric effect of the NSAID indomethacin and the ACE inhibitor lisinopril. Am J Nephrol 1990;10(Suppl 1):94-97.

144. Perico N, Remuzzi A, Sangalli F, Azzollini N, Mister M, Ruggenenti P, Remuzzi G. The antiproteinuric effect of angiotensin antagonism in human IgA nephropathy is potentiated by indomethacin. J Am Soc Nephrol 1998;9:2308-2317.

145. Vriesendorp R, Donker AJM, de Zeeuw D, de Jong PE, van der Hem GK, Brentjens JRH. Effects of nonsteroidal anti-inflammatory drugs on proteinuria. Am J Med 1986;81(Suppl 2B):84-94.

146. Vriesendorp R, Donker AJM, de Zeeuw D, de Jong PE, van der Hem GK. Antiproteinuric effect of naproxen and indomethacin. A double-blind crossover study. Am J Nephrol 1985;5:236-242.

147. Stosic Z, Sedlak V, Felle D, Curic S, Ubavic M, Vodopivec S. Anti-proteinuria effects of nonsteroidal anti-inflammatory drugs in patients with nephrotic syndrome: an illusion or a real improvement? Med Pregl 1995;48:155-158.

148. Harris RC. Cyclooxygenase-2 in the kidney. J Am Soc Nephrol 2000;11:2387-2394.

149. Wang JL, Cheng HF, Shappell S, Harris RC. A selective cyclooxygenase-2 inhibitor decreases proteinuria and retards progressive renal injury in rats. Kidney Int 2000;57:2334-2342.

150. Rossat J, Maillard M, Nussberger J, Brunner HR, Burnier M. Renal effects of selective cyclooxygenase-2 inhibition in normotensive salt-depleted subjects. Clin Pharmacol Ther 1999;66:76-84.

151. Fried LF, Orchard TJ, Kasiske BL. Effect of lipid reduction on the progression of renal disease: a meta-analysis. Kidney Int 2001;59:260-269.

152. National Kidney Foundation – Dialysis Outcomes Quality Initiative. Clinical practice guidelines for the treatment of anemia of chronic renal failure. Am J Kidney Dis 1997;30(Suppl 3):S150-S191.

153. European best practice guidelines for the management of anaemia in patients with chronic renal failure. Nephrol Dial Transplant 1999;14(Suppl 5):1-50.

33

ANTIHYPERTENSIVE TREATMENT IN TYPE 2 DIABETES, WITH SPECIAL REFERENCE TO ABNORMAL ALBUMINURIA: A FOCUS ON THE NEW TRIALS

Geoffrey Boner, Paul G McNally, Mark Cooper

Diabetic complications Group, Baker Heart Research Institute, Commercial Rd, Prahran 3181, VIC Australia

The deleterious effects of systemic blood pressure on glomerular structure were reported thirty years ago in a patient with type 2 diabetes mellitus (DM2) and unilateral renal artery stenosis, in which characteristic nodular diabetic glomerulosclerosis was present in the non-ischemic kidney only [1]. It is only over the past few years that attention has been paid to the impact of antihypertensive treatment on renal injury in patients with DM2 [2-6]. This is despite the fact that the cumulative incidence of persistent proteinuria and microalbuminuria in DM2 patients is very similar to that in type 1 diabetes mellitus (DM1) patients [7]. The clinical relevance of these figures is reflected by statistics, which show that more than 30% of patients entering dialysis programs in most developed nations have diabetic nephropathy, with most of them having DM2 [8]. The data from the United Kingdom Prospective Diabetes Study (UKPDS) have been analyzed in order to delineate the progression of nephropathy in DM2 [9]. The authors have shown that there is a steady progression of renal involvement in patients with DM2, so that 10 years after diagnosis, 24.9% of patients have microalbuminuria, 5.3% have macroalbuminuria and 0.8% have developed an elevated serum creatinine or were on renal replacement therapy.

There appears to be an association between generalized and abdominal obesity and increased risk for hypertension-diabetes comorbidity in most ethnic groups [10]. Furthermore, in DM2 the relationship between nephropathy and hypertension is more complex than in DM1, since hypertension is not necessarily linked to the presence of renal disease, and often precedes the diagnosis of diabetes. There also seems to be a trend for increasing risk of cardiovascular death with increasing nephropathy [9]. In fact, macroalbuminuria was associated with a risk of death, which was greater than that of developing renal failure in any one year. Sowers et al have reviewed the relationships among hypertension, diabetes and cardiovascular disease and have stated that up to 75% of cardiovascular disease in diabetic subjects may be attributable to hypertension [11]. It has also been shown recently that cigarette smoking and increased urinary albumin excretion are interrelated predictors of progressive renal involvement and that cigarette smoking is associated with increased albuminuria even in the presence of improved blood pressure control and treatment with ACE inhibitors [12].

This review focuses on the role of antihypertensive agents in DM2 subjects with abnormal albuminuria (microalbuminuria and macroalbuminuria), the significance of albuminuria in DM2 and the consequences of treatment with these agents.

THE USE OF ANTIHYPERTENSIVE AGENTS IN DM2 SUBJECTS WITH ESTABLISHED DIABETIC NEPHROPATHY

The impact of angiotensin converting enzyme inhibitors (ACEI), angiotensin II receptor blockers (ARB), calcium channel blockers (CCB) and conventional antihypertensive agents on renal function has been evaluated in both normotensive and hypertensive DM2 subjects with persistent proteinuria and variable degrees of renal impairment. In hypertensive DM2 subjects with persistent proteinuria studied for periods of greater than 6 months, ACEI [13-21], ARB [4, 6] and certain CCB [19, 21-23] reduced albuminuria. In general, the earlier reports showed that ACEI were very effective in reducing blood pressure and urinary albumin excretion [13-15, 17-21]. The decrease in blood pressure and albuminuria was usually associated with a slowing of the progression of renal failure. Parving's group has reported a disparity in effects on albuminuria and renal function [15]. Whereas lisinopril was more effective than atenolol in reducing albuminuria, both agents were similar in efficacy in terms of rate of decline in GFR. A number of studies have confirmed that ACE inhibitors are superior to other antihypertensive agents including dihydropyridine CCB [16-19] as well as the vasodilator, hydralazine [20], in reducing albuminuria in hypertensive DM2 subjects with macroproteinuria. Veelken et al have described the use of ACEI in an unselected group of patients [24].

In their group of 2504 DM2 patients, 328 had nephropathy, as defined as a serum creatinine concentration >1.3 mg/dl. The addition of 2.5 mg of cilazapril to their usual treatment resulted in improved blood pressure control, improved renal function and a reduction in urinary albumin excretion (UAE) as assessed at one year. That study showed that even in an unselected group of patients one is able to achieve results similar to those obtained in the randomized controlled studies.

The past two years have seen the publication of the results of major studies using ARB (See Tables 1 and 2).

In the RENAAL study [4] 1513 patients with DM2 and nephropathy (albuminuria in the range of macroalbuminuria) were randomized to receive losartan (n=751) or placebo (n=762) in addition to their usual antihypertensive therapy (excluding ACEI or ARB). Over 90% of patients in both groups were receiving antihypertensive therapy and a high percentage had additional co-morbid conditions.

These patients were followed for a mean period of 3.4 years. Blood pressure was significantly reduced to a similar degree in both groups, the only difference between the two groups being at one year. Treatment with losartan led to an average reduction of 35% in UAE, whereas in the placebo group there was no change. Analysis of the primary composite outcome (doubling of serum creatinine concentration, end-stage renal failure or death), according to an intention to treat analysis showed a 16% reduction in the patients receiving losartan. Analyzing for the individual end-points, losartan treatment was associated with a 25% reduction in doubling of serum creatinine and a 28% reduction in end-stage renal failure, whereas the risk for death was similar in both groups.

An additional finding was a 32% decrease in the risk for first hospitalization for heart failure in the losartan group.

Table 1. The effect of antihypertensive agents in albuminuria, renal function and blood pressure in hypertensive DM2 subjects with established nephropathy

Agent	Duration	n	AER(%)*	RF	BP	Reference
Lisinopril (L)	5 years	18	↓(−25)	↓	↓	Bakris et al [13]
Atenolol V		16	→	↓↓	↓	
or Diltiazem		16	↓(−18)	↓	↓	
Verapamil	>4 years	18	↓(−60)	↓	↓	Bakris et al [22]
Atenolol		16	↓(−20)	↓↓	↓	
Lisinopril	12 months	16	↓ (−45)	↓	↓	Nielsen et al [15]
Atenolol		19	→	↓	↓	
Enalapril	5 years	11	→	→	↓	Chan et al [17]
Nifedipine		14	→	↓	↓	
Ramipril	2 years	26	↓ (−32)	→	↓	Fogari et al [19]
Nitrendipine		25	↓ (−19)	→	↓	
Enalapril	12 months	18	↓ (−87)	→	↓	Ferder et al [18]
Nifendipine		12	→	→	↓	
Captopril	18 months	24	↓(−27)	→	↓	Liou et al [20]
Hydralazine		18	→	↓	↓	
Lisinopril	18 months	10	↓ (−42)	→	↓	Slataper et al [21]
Diltiazem		10	↓ (−45)	→	↓	
Frus & Atenolol		10	↓	↓	↓	
V	12 months	14	↓(−30)	→	↓	Bakris et al [14]
Trandolapril		12	↓(−35)	→	↓	
(T)		11	↓(−63)	→	↓	
T + V						
Losartan	3.4 years	751	↓ (−35)	↓	↓	Brenner et al [4]
Placebo		762	→	↓	↓	
Irbesartan	2.6 years	579	↓ (−33)	↓	↓	Lewis et al. [6]
Amlodipine		567	↓ (−6)	↓	↓	
Placebo		569	↓ (−10)	↓	↓	

Abbreviations: AER, Albumin excretion rate. RF, renal function. BP, Blood pressure.
V, Verapamil, Frus, Frusemide. * In some of these studies proteinuria rather than AER was measured.

Table 2. Comparison of the results in the RENAAL and IDNT studies

Composite and individual end-points	Losartan vs placebo* RR (%)	Irbesartan vs placebo# RR (%)	Irbesartan vs amlodipine# RR (%)	Amlodipine vs placebo# RR (%)
DsCr, ESRD or death	16 p=0.024	20 p=0.024	23 p=0.006	-4 NS
DsCr	25 p=0.006	33 p=0.003	37 p=0.001	-6 NS
ESRD	28 p=0.002	23 NS (p=0.074)	23 NS (p=0.074)	0 NS
Death	NS	NS	NS	NS
ESRD or death	20 p=0.01	N/A	N/A	N/A

Abbreviations: RR = risk reduction, DsCr = doubling of serum creatinine. ESRD = end-stage renal disease. NS = not significant. N/A = not analyzed. * RENAAL [4] # IDNT [6]

Lewis et al reported the results of a similar study (IDNT) comparing treatment with either irbesartan, amlodipine or placebo [6]. In that study 1715 hypertensive patients with DM2 and proteinuria in excess of 900 mg/day were randomized to receive irbesartan (n=579), amlodipine (n=567) or placebo (n=569) in addition to their usual antihypertensive therapy (excluding ACEI, ARB or CCB). Similar to the RENAAL study, these patients had a high percentage of comorbid conditions. The participants were followed for a mean period of 2.6 years. The mean blood pressure decreased significantly in all three groups, the mean arterial pressure being slightly, but significantly higher in the placebo group than in the two treatment groups. Treatment with irbesartan led to an average reduction of 33% in proteinuria, whereas there was a small decrease in the amlodipine and placebo groups. Analysis of the primary composite outcome (doubling of serum creatinine concentration, end-stage renal failure or death), according to an intention to treat analysis, showed a 20% reduction in this endpoint in the patients receiving irbesartan as compared to placebo and a 23% reduction as compared to amlodipine. Analysis of the individual end-points showed a 33% reduction in risk for doubling of serum creatinine as compared to placebo and 37% as compared to amlodipine and a 23% reduction in risk for end-stage renal failure in the irbesartan group as compared to both the placebo and amlodipine groups. However, the risk of death was similar in all the three groups. These two studies in DM2 patients with overt nephropathy have demonstrated that treatment with ARB in addition to other antihypertensive agents significantly reduces blood pressure and proteinuria. Moreover both studies showed that ARB treatment has a beneficial effect on progression of diabetic renal disease as measured by a doubling of serum creatinine and the percentage of patients reaching end-stage renal failure. This beneficial effect seemed to be partly independent of blood pressure reduction. Moreover, in the IDNT study the reduction in blood pressure in those patients receiving amlodipine was similar to that of patients receiving irbesartan, yet there was no improvement in proteinuria or progression of renal disease in the CCB treated cohort. The results of the RENAAL study have been used to estimate the possible savings of treating suitable patients in the European Union with losartan [25]. The authors came to the conclusion that this treatment could potentially lead to a decrease in 44100 patients with end-stage renal failure and a saving of Euro2.6 billion over 3.5 years.

There have been significant differences in the effect on albuminuria obtained with various CCB, which has been attributed by Bakris and others to the particular class of CCB [21, 26, 27]. Bakris [27] initially demonstrated in hypertensive, nephrotic NIDDM subjects that diltiazem, a benzothiazepine CCB, had a comparable affect to lisinopril in decreasing albuminuria. This author has also reported an anti-proteinuric effect with the CCB, verapamil [23]. In contrast, nifedipine, a dihydropyridine CCB, given for 6 weeks to 14 hypertensive NIDDM patients with baseline renal impairment, led to an increase in albuminuria and deterioration in renal function, despite equivalent blood pressure reduction to diltiazem [28]. Other groups have also reported this lack of efficacy, particularly on proteinuria, of the dihydropyridine class of CCB [17, 18]. In a study in African American NIDDM subjects with hypertension and macroproteinuria, isradipine was associated with an increase in proteinuria whereas captopril reduced proteinuria [29]. Finally the study by Lewis et al showed that the addition of amlodipine to other antihypertensive agents did not reduce proteinuria and had no additional effect on renal function decline or kidney survival [6].

Bakris et al have reported the findings of 2 studies in hypertensive NIDDM subjects with overt proteinuria followed for at least 4 years [13, 22]. In both studies, the beta blocker atenolol was associated with a more rapid decline in GFR and less efficacy in terms of reduction in albuminuria than the non-dihydropyridine CCBs, verapamil and diltiazem [13, 22] or the ACEI, lisinopril [22].

The role of alpha blockers in macroproteinuric DM2 patients has not been as well documented. Nevertheless, Rachmani et al reported in a cross-over study which included predominantly macroproteinuric but also microalbuminuric

584

NIDDM subjects, that the alpha blocker doxazosin tended to reduce albuminuria, although possibly to a lesser extent than the ACEI, cilazapril [30].

THE USE OF ANTIHYPERTENSIVE AGENTS IN HYPERTENSIVE DM2 PATIENTS WITH NORMOALBUMINURIA AND MICROALBUMINURIA

Comparison of the use of ACEI versus placebo in DM2 subjects with hypertension and normoalbuminuria or microalbuminuria has not been well studied A double blind study compared captopril with conventional therapy (metoprolol and hydrochlorothiazide) in normoalbuminuric and microalbuminuric hypertensive DM2 subjects over a 3 year period [31]. Both regimens reduced blood pressure without altering UAE in the normoalbuminuric DM2 subjects. However, their findings in hypertensive DM2 patients with microalbuminuria indicated that despite a comparable reduction in blood pressure, only the ACEI induced a persistent decline in albuminuria during the 36 months of therapy. Sano et al found in a small number of normotensive and well controlled hypertensive patients with microalbuminuria, treated with enalapril for a period of four years, that there was a 47% decrease in albuminuria, whereas in the placebo group there was no change [32]. Trevisan et al reported similar findings when comparing ramipril to placebo over a period of 6 months [33]. Veelken et al treated a large unselected group of hypertensive, diabetic patients (2176 patients) with normal renal function, with cilazapril for 52 weeks [24]. Treatment resulted in a significant decrease in blood pressure in 75% of patients, with 56.4% of them achieving the target value of less than or equal to 140/90 mmHg. Renal function and urine protein excretion remained stable during the treatment period.

The emphasis in the more recent studies has been to analyze the effects of treatment with ARB. Lacourciere et al compared the effects of enalapril to losartan in 103 hypertensive patients. Both these medications, given alone or in combination with other antihypertensive agents (the study medications and CCB were excluded) resulted in a significant but similar decrease in albuminuria and a similar decrease in renal function, which had stabilized by 52 weeks [34]. In a similar study, Muirhead et al, compared the effects of valsartan (dosages of 80 mg and 160 mg daily) to captopril and placebo over a period of 12 months [35].

Table 3. The effect of antihypertensive agents on albuminuria, renal function and blood pressure in DM2 with normo- and microalbuminuria

Patients	Agent	Duration of study	N	Δ in AER (%)	Δ in GFR	Δ in BP	Reference
Normo HT	Enalapril (E) Nifedipine (N)	5 yrs	18 25	→ →	→ →	↓ ↓	Chan et al [17]
Micro HT	Enalapril Nifedipine		21 13	↓ (−13) ↑ (+13)	→ →	↓ ↓	
Normo HT	Captopril M or HCTZ	36 mths	25 28	→ →	→ →	↓ ↓	Lacourcière et al [31]
Micro HT	Captopril M or HCTZ		9 12	↓ (−65) →	→ →	↓ ↓	
Micro NT	Nifedipine Perindopril	12 mths	13 11	→ →	→ →	→ →	MDNSG [43]
Micro HT	E + N Nifedipine Enalapril	48 mths	11 13 12	↓ (−42) ↑ (+29) ↓ (−47)	→ → →	↓ ↓ ↓	Sano et al [32]
Micro NT	Untreated		12	→	→	→	
Micro HT	Enalapril Nitrendipine	12 mths	8 8	↓ (−28) ↓ (−17)	↑ ↑	↓ ↓	Ruggenenti et al [39]
Micro HT	Cilazipril Amlodipine	3 years	9 9	↓ (−27) ↓ (−31)	↓ ↓	↓ ↓	Velussi et al [40]
Micro HT	Lisinopril Nifedipine	12 mths	156 158	↓ (−37) →	→ →	↓ ↓	Agardh et al [41]
Micro HT	R ± Felodipine At ± HCTZ	12 mths	46 45	→ ↑	→ ↓	↓ ↓	Schnack et al [38]
Micro NT	Enalapril Placebo	5 years	49 45	→ ↑(+152)	→ ↓	→ →	Ravid et al [52]
Micro NT	Enalapril Placebo	5 years	52 51	↓ (−64) ↑(+60)	→ →	→ →	Ahmad et al [54]
Normo NT	Enalapril Placebo	6 years	97 97	↑(+36) ↑ (+144)	↓ ↓	→ →	Ravid et al [55]
Normo, micro, HT	Nifedipine Enalapril	2 years	228 208	↑ ↑	↓ ↓		Baba et al [45]
Micro, NT, HT	Valsartan Amlodipine	24 weeks	169 163	↓ (−44) ↓ (−8)		↓ ↓	Viberti et al [48]
HT, micro	Losartan Enalapril	52 weeks	52 51	↓ (−35) ↓ (−55)	↓ ↓	↓ ↓	Lacourciere et al. [34]

Table 3. (cont.)

HT, micro	Amlodipine Fosinopril (F) Amlodipine + F	4 years	103 102 104	↓ (−35) ↓ (−54) ↓ (−65)	→ → →	↓ ↓ ↓↓	Fogari et al. [44]
HT, micro	Irbesartan 150 Irbesartan 300 Placebo	2 years	195 194 201	↓ (−24) ↓ (−38) ↓ (−2)	↓ ↓ ↓	↓ ↓ ↓	Parving et al. [37]
HT, NT, micro	Valsartan 80 Valsartan 160 Captopril Placebo	52 weeks	31 31 29 31	↓ (−24) ↓ (−24) ↓ (−24) ↑(+18)	→ → → →	→ → → →	Muirhead et al [35]

Abbreviations: Normo, Normoalbuminuria. Micro, Microalbuminuria. HT, Hypertensive.
NT, Normotensive. N/D, not done. AER, Albumin excretion rate. GFR, glomerular filtration rate.
BP, Blood pressure. HCTZ, hydrochlorothiazide. M, metoprolol. At, atenolol.

The patients were normotensive or receiving treatment for hypertension. All three-treatment groups showed a significant decrease in albuminuria, when compared to the placebo group. There was no difference in the anti-albuminuric effect between the ACEI and ARB treated groups. However, treatment with captopril was associated with the most side effects. In a small crossover study involving 64 hypertensive patients, receiving irbesartan (150 mg/day) or placebo for 60 days, treatment was associated with a significant decrease both in UAE and blood pressure as compared to placebo [36].

These studies of the efficacy of ARB have been complemented by a large randomized study (IRMA-2), in which Parving et al compared the effects of irbesartan, 150 mg and 300 mg to placebo, given over a period of two years to 590 hypertensive patients with type 2 diabetes and microalbuminuria [37]. Significantly fewer patients receiving 300 mg irbesartan per day reached the primary end-point (overt nephropathy, defined as macroalbuminuria), than in the placebo group (See fig 1). However, in the patients receiving 150 mg daily, the difference between the placebo and irbesartan treated groups, did not reach statistical significance, but was intermediate between the two other groups. The decrease in systolic blood pressure was also significantly greater in the patients receiving 300 mg irbesartan daily than in the placebo group. These studies have shown that both ACEI and ARB have significant beneficial effects in hypertensive type 2 diabetic patients with normo- or microalbuminuria. However, only the study of Parving et al had the power to demonstrate that the optimal dose of a therapeutic agent, an ARB in this case, could delay progression to overt nephropathy [37].

587

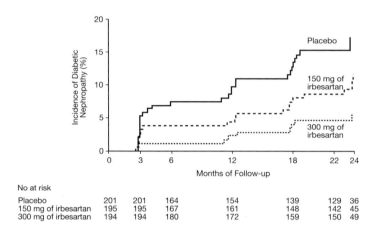

Fig. 1. The effects of treatment with irbesartan in DM2 patients with microalbuminuria. [37].

Most other studies have reported on the use of CCB, usually in comparison to placebo or ACEI. Schnack et al have reported that ramipril with/without felodipine stabilised albuminuria. By contrast, atenolol with/without diuretic treatment was associated with an increase in UAE [38]. Furthermore, the ramipril treated group had stable renal function whereas the group receiving beta blockers had a decline in GFR. A reduction in albuminuria by ACE inhibition has also been observed by a number of other investigators in studies of patients receiving ACEI or CCB [17, 39-42]. In general, effects of CCB in reducing albuminuria were not as readily evident as seen in the ACEI treated groups.

In the Melbourne Diabetic Nephropathy Study, nifedipine was shown to produce a similar response to perindopril in decreasing albuminuria over 12 months in the DM2 subjects with microalbuminuria [43]. It has been reported by Chan et al that the ACEI, enalapril, was more effective than nifedipine over a median of 5 years in reducing albuminuria in a group of hypertensive microalbuminuric subjects [17]. Several studies have been reported which have compared calcium channel blockade with ACE inhibition in hypertensive microalbuminuric DM2 subjects [39-41, 44, 45]. In a study over 3 years, in a relatively small number of subjects, amlodipine was as effective as the ACEI, cilazapril in reducing albuminuria with both treatment groups having similar declines in renal function [40]. Fogari et al reported similar efficacy of enalapril and amlodipine in 50 hypertensive DM2 subjects with microalbuminuria [42]. The same group have recently reported on a large group of patients, who received fosinopril, amlodipine or a combination of both for a period of 4 years. Fosinopril treatment resulted in a significant reduction in albuminuria, starting from the third month of treatment [44]. The patients receiving amlodipine showed a decrease in albuminuria starting after 18 months of treatment. At the end of the treatment phase albuminuria was significantly decreased in both groups, the mean decrease being greater in the fosinopril group, but not statistically significant. Baba et al have also shown that there is no difference between an ACEI (enalapril) and CCB (nifedipine) in preventing progression of normoalbuminuria and microalbuminuria [45]. A similar study was performed by Kopf et al, comparing perindopril to nitrendipine [46]. There was no difference between the groups in UAE and renal function at one year.

The ABCD trial was designed to study the effect of intensive versus moderate blood pressure control on progression of nephropathy [47]. Hypertensive DM2 subjects, of whom less than 20% had overt nephropathy, were randomized to an intensive treatment group (diastolic blood pressure goal of 75 mmHg – 237 patients) and a moderate blood pressure group (diastolic blood pressure goal 80-89 mmHg – 233 patients) and were followed for five years. The patients in each group were also randomized to receive either nisoldipine or enalapril as the primary antihypertensive medication. Treatment was associated with a decrease in renal function in the first year of treatment and stabilization thereafter in the patients with normoalbuminuria or microalbuminuria, whereas there was a steady decline in renal function in those patients who had overt nephropathy at initial examination. There was no difference in results between those patients, randomized to intensive or moderate blood pressure control. Moreover, there was no difference between patients receiving nisoldipine or enalapril. UAE was less in the patients receiving enalapril than in those receiving nisoldipine up till 3.5 years but no difference was detected by the end of the study.

In a large multi-centre study of over 300 subjects, the ACEI, lisinopril, reduced albuminuria over 12 months whereas nifedipine failed to significantly influence UAE [41]. In a more recent study comparing the use of valsartan to amlodipine in normotensive and hypertensive subjects treated for 24 weeks Viberti et al were able to detect a significantly greater decrease in UAE in the valsartan group despite no difference was achieved in blood pressure [48]. Therefore, in the larger studies, which may have greater power to detect differences, dihydropyridine CCB were clearly less anti-albuminuric than agents, which interrupt the renin-angiotensin system (RAS) [41, 48].

Other groups of medications have been investigated in DM2 patients with microalbuminuria. Gambardella and coworkers [49] showed that indapamide 2.5 mg daily did not alter UAE or glomerular filtration rate over a 24 month period in hypertensive normoalbuminuric patients despite a significant reduction in blood pressure. In contrast, in the microalbuminuric patients indapamide reduced albuminuria after 6 months and this effect was sustained at 36 months [49].

THE USE OF ANTIHYPERTENSIVE AGENTS IN NORMOTENSIVE DM2 WITH MICROALBUMINURIA

The possibility that early therapy will postpone or retard progression of renal injury in diabetes has led to the use of antihypertensive agents in normotensive subjects. UAE has been shown to be reduced in a group of normotensive DM2 patients with microalbuminuria treated with captopril over a period of 6 months, whereas the untreated group had no change in albuminuria [50]. In the Melbourne study [43] there was no change in albuminuria after 12 months treatment with either nifedipine or perindopril in normotensive microalbuminuric patients, despite a small but significant reduction in blood pressure (4 mmHg). Nonetheless, on stopping therapy at 12 months a dramatic increase in albuminuria was detected in the DM2 but not in the DM1 subjects, which was independent of mode of treatment [51]. The inability of either agent to reduce albuminuria in the normotensive cohort coupled with the rapid rise after stopping therapy needs to be considered in the setting of the natural history of microalbuminuria. Albuminuria would be anticipated to rise by an average of 20 to 50 per cent if left untreated for 12 months in microalbuminuric DM2 subjects. This phenomenon of a rapid rise in albuminuria was not apparent in the DM1 patients and may indicate a difference in the underlying etiology and pathogenesis of albuminuria in DM2 as compared to DM1 It is possible that there are differences in the sensitivity to structural damage incurred from blood pressure between DM1 and DM2.

The first long-term (5 years) placebo controlled double blind randomized study to evaluate the effect of an antihypertensive agent in normotensive microalbuminuric DM2 with normal renal function (as assessed by a serum creatinine < 123 μmol/l) was reported by Ravid et al [52]. These investigators reported an initial decrease of 15% in UAE during the first year of treatment in the enalapril treated group and a slow return to baseline levels at 5 years. Conversely, in the placebo treated patients there was an increase of 144% over the five years. Renal function, as assessed by the reciprocal of serum creatinine, decreased less in patients receiving enalapril than placebo. A follow up report after 7 years of treatment confirmed a renoprotective effect of ACE inhibition in this cohort [53]. Sano et al have observed in a 4 year study that enalapril treatment reduced albuminuria whereas placebo treatment was associated with no change in albuminuria in a group of normotensive, microalbuminuric DM2 patients [32]. Similar effects on albuminuria have been observed in a 6 month study by an Italian multi-centre group using the ACEI, ramipril [33]. Ahmad et al have reported similar effects on albuminuria after 5 years of ACEI therapy in a group of Indian normotensive DM2 subjects with microalbuminuria [54]. Enalapril treatment was associated with a reduction in albuminuria whereas in the placebo group there was a progressive rise in urinary albumin excretion. Of particular interest was the finding that these effects were observed in the absence of a discernible difference in blood pressure between the two groups. Muirhead et al, as described in the previous section, showed that both valsartan and captopril slow the progressive rise in albuminuria in DM2 normotensive and treated hypertensive patients with microalbuminuria [35].

The exciting results obtained with antihypertensive drugs including ACEI in hypertensive and macroalbuminuric diabetic subjects stimulated investigators to explore the possible role of these agents in the prevention of diabetic nephropathy. Ravid et al reported that treatment with enalapril for 6 years in a group of normotensive, normoalbuminuric DM2 subjects was associated with a retardation in the increase in AER and in the decrease in renal function [55]. Schrier et compared the effects of moderate control of blood pressure (diastolic blood pressure goal 80 – 90 mmHg, 243 patients) to intensive control (diastolic blood pressure less than 10 mmHg below the diastolic blood pressure at randomization, 237 patients) in normotensive DM2 patients, with only approximately 30% having microalbuminuria or overt albuminuria [56]. The patients in the intensive care group were randomized to receive either nisoldipine or enalapril, whereas those in the moderate group, received placebo and were only randomized to one of the two treatment drugs, if an increase in blood pressure was observed during the time-course of the study. The mean follow-up was over 5 years. In the patients with either normoalbuminuria or microalbuminuria at randomization, there was an initial fall in renal function (creatinine clearance), but this stabilized within the first year. Subsequently there was no difference between the moderate and intensive groups nor any difference between those receiving nisoldipine and enalapril. These findings contrast with those observed in the patients with macroalbuminuria at randomization, who showed a steady fall in renal function throughout the follow-up period, which was independent of intensity of treatment or therapeutic regimen.

ROLE OF COMBINATION THERAPY

It has been proposed that the combination of two or more antihypertensive agents may be beneficial in the treatment of hypertension in the diabetic patient with or without evidence of renal involvement. The various combinations have been reviewed recently [57].

Brown et al postulated in 1993, that the combination of a calcium antagonist with a converting enzyme inhibitor should result in a greater reduction in urinary protein excretion and slow progression of nephropathy, as assessed morphologically [58]. Bakris et al have compared the renal hemodynamic and antiproteinuric effects of a calcium antagonist, verapamil, and an ACEI, lisinopril, alone and in combination in three groups of DM2 subjects with documented nephrotic range proteinuria, hypertension, and renal insufficiency [23]. Patients treated with the combination of a calcium antagonist and an ACEI manifested the greatest reduction in albuminuria. In addition, the decline in GFR was the lowest in that group. Similar findings are suggested by another study performed in microalbuminuric subjects using the combination of verapamil and cilazapril [59]. Sano et al have shown that the addition of enalapril to nifedipine conferred an additional effect in decreasing albuminuria in a group of microalbuminuric DM2 subjects [32]. Bakris et al have suggested that the combination of verapamil and trandolapril, administered in a fixed dose combination, is more effective at reducing proteinuria than either drug alone, despite similar effects on blood pressure [14, 60]. Fogari et al have also shown that ACEI (benazepril) plus CCB (amlodipine) tends to be more effective than benazepril alone in reducing albuminuria in microalbuminuric, hypertensive DM2 patients [61]. Shigihara et al also compared the effects of the combination of different ACEI drugs and CCB (amlodipine) and found that in DM2 the combination resulted in a greater decrease in diastolic blood pressure and in a greater reduction in UAE [62]. In a study comparing the use of a combination of verapamil and trandolapril to a combination of enalapril and a thiazide diuretic,

Fernandez et al were able to show a similar decrease in blood pressure and albuminuria, whereas metabolic control was better in the CCB-ACEI group [63]. In a recent study, designed to study the effects of an ACEI-CCB (benazapril-amlodopine) combination on lipid subfractions, Bakris et al showed that this combination had the greatest effect on systolic blood pressure, while the effect on albuminuria was similar to that in patients receiving only an ACE-I [64]. Fogari et al also showed that the ACEI-CCB (fosinopril-amlodipine) combination had a greater effect on blood pressure and albuminuria than either of the drugs alone [44]. In summary these studies show that the addition of either a non-dihydropyrdine CCB or dihydropyridine CCB to an ACEI or ARB result in a substantial improvement in control of hypertension with a concomitant reduction in albuminuria. Rachmani et al have explored the combination of cilazapril and doxazosin and shown this regimen to be effective at reducing blood pressure and albuminuria [30].

Mogensen et al showed in a relatively short-term study that 3 months of dual blockade of the RAS with a combination of ACEI (lisinopril) and ARB (candesartan) was superior to each of the individual agents in reducing blood pressure and superior to candesartan in reducing albuminuria [65]. In an acute study, in which DM1 and DM2 patients, who received their regular ACEI treatment for one week, followed by the addition of losartan for another week, Hebert et al were able to show that the combination of ACEI and ARB produced a more complete blockade of the RAS as shown by a sharp rise in serum renin [66]. Kuriyama et al added candesartan to a group of diabetic patients with overt nephropathy, who had previously received either temocapril or amlodipine for a period of 12 weeks [67]. These subjects were followed for an additional 12 weeks. The combination ARB-CCB reduced albuminuria significantly more than CCB alone, but the greatest decrease was achieved with the combination of ARB-ACEI. Rossing et al performed a crossover study in 18 DM2 hypertensive subjects with overt albuminuria, where the patients received candesartan or placebo in addition to regular treatment [68]. All patients were receiving ACEI and most were receiving a diuretic and CCB. Addition of the ARB resulted in a 10 mmHg drop in the 24 hour systolic blood pressure and 25% reduction in albuminuria. This was accompanied by a 5 ml/min decrease in GFR. In another randomized crossover study, where candesartan was added to patients with chronic renal disease and proteinuria who were receiving an ACEI, there was no change in albuminuria in the diabetic patients despite a decrease in blood pressure [69]. These studies show that the combination of ACEI-ARB has a superior effect on blood pressure control than either agent as

593

monotherapy alone or in another combination. The effect of the combination on albuminuria is not yet fully clarified and requires more long-term studies.

The above findings with combination therapy provide an exciting approach for optimizing antihypertensive therapy in diabetic patients with renal disease. Indeed, the recent criteria for blood pressure control in diabetes as proposed by JNC-VI [70] and WHO-ISH [71, 72] will require the use of multiple antihypertensive agents. This has also been stressed in recent review articles [73, 74].

THE USE OF ANTIHYPERTENSIVE AGENTS IN DM2 PATIENTS

The choice of an antihypertensive agent in the management of abnormal albuminuria in DM2 depends not only on its potential renoprotective effect but must also take into consideration other factors, which could be deleterious to the patient. Microalbuminuria in the DM2 patient is more closely linked to subsequent death from cardiovascular disease than from nephropathy [75-78], although this association has not been substantiated in all populations [77, 79]. It has also been shown that rapid progression of albuminuria is an independent predictor of cardiovascular mortality in DM2 with microalbuminuira [80]. Therefore it is important that any antihypertensive intervention in the DM2 patient, especially those with albuminuria does not exacerbate existing lipid abnormalities such as further reducing HDL-cholesterol [81]. Furthermore, reduced sensitivity to insulin after administration of thiazides and various beta-blockers may be detrimental [82]. However, subsequent studies suggest that low dose diuretics do not have deleterious effects on plasma glucose or lipid levels [83]. In contrast, improved insulin sensitivity is seen after captopril and other ACEI [82, 84, 85], doxazocin [82, 84-86] and minimal or neutral effects are observed with CCB [87]. The effect of CCB may be dependent on the duration of action. The short-acting CCB tend to have a detrimental effect, whereas the long-acting CCB improve insulin sensitivity [85]. Also, in contrast to beta-blockers and thiazide diuretics, neither CCB nor ACEI affect glucose tolerance deleteriously [87]. The effects of the AII receptor antagonists such as losartan and candesartan have not been as extensively studied but they appear to have no or a beneficial effect on insulin sensitivity. [84, 85, 88].

ANTIHYPERTENSIVE THERAPY IN DM2 MORE THAN JUST REDUCING ALBUMINURIA

Since microalbuminuria is also is a strong predictor of all-cause and in particular cardiovascular mortality [75, 76, 78], the effects of these antihypertensive agents must include assessment of cardiovascular endpoints. In the ABCD study it was suggested that ACEI therapy was superior to dihydropyridine CCBs in conferring cardiovascular protection [89]. Similar findings were reported from the FACET study which suggested that fosinopril was associated with less cardiovascular events than amlodipine [90]. However, It was not clear from those small studies whether ACEI confer cardioprotective effects while the dihydropyridine CCB have a deleterious effect. It is likely that the ACEI may confer in certain contexts an additional beneficial effect rather than the CCBs having a deleterious effect on cardiovascular events in the DM2 population. For example, in the Syst-EUR study, a subgroup analysis of the diabetic cohort with systolic hypertension revealed a beneficial effect of nitrendipine on cardiovascular outcomes [91]. In the HOT study which involved randomisation of subjects to 3 different target blood pressures with a felodipine based regimen, analysis of the diabetic subgroup showed that the lowest blood pressure target group had the lowest incidence of cardiovascular morbidity and mortality [92].

This would suggest that blood pressure reduction *per se* is a major determinant of cardioprotection in this diabetic population. However, it must be appreciated that the group randomized to the lowest blood pressure group required the most concomitant antihypertensive agents, including ACE inhibitors and beta-blockers, which may have conferred additional cardioprotection. Within the diabetic subgroup in the CAPPP study, captopril was superior to conventional treatment (diuretic/beta blocker) despite similar blood pressure reduction [93, 94]. There was an approximately 40% decrease in the risk ratio for the primary end-point, combination of fatal and non-fatal myocardial infarction, stroke and other cardiovascular deaths, in patients receiving captopril compared to conventional therapy. In the UKPDS blood pressure reduction was clearly shown to reduce vascular events [95]. Further analysis revealed no difference between the group treated with captopril or atenolol [96]. However, in this study there was a very high level of non-compliance (20-40%) and over 60% of subjects were on 2 or more drugs.

The importance of ACE inhibitors in conferring macrovascular in addition to renal protection has been demonstrated in the HOPE study. In the diabetic subgroup, despite the fact that ramipril treatment was reported to reduce blood pressure by only 2/1 mmHg more than the control group, there was a 25%

decrease in cardiovascular death, myocardial infarction and stroke and a 24% decrease in total mortality [97]. This decrease in blood pressure with high dose ramipril as an add on treatment remains controversial with ambulatory blood pressure data obtained in a small subgroup from that study suggested greater reduction in blood pressure with active treatment [98]. In an early report on the hypertensive cohort in the ABCD study, Estacio et al demonstrated a reduction in overall mortality in those patients, which received intensive treatment [47]. Yet, they were unable to demonstrate a significant difference in cardiovascular events. However, in a recent report of the same study, including an analysis of both the hypertensive and normotensive cohorts, the investigators were able to show that intensive blood pressure control reduced the risk for a cardiovascular event in those patients, who had peripheral arterial disease [99]. The LIFE study was designed to determine the most suitable antihypertensive drug to reduce the risk of cardiovascular disease in patients with hypertension and left ventricular hypertrophy [100, 101]. This study included a diabetic cohort and within this group, the subjects were randomized to either losartan (586 patients) or atenolol (609 patients). The patients in both groups received non-trial antihypertensive drugs (excluding ACEI) in order to reduce blood pressure and were followed for a mean of 4.7 years. There was a difference of 2 mmHg mean systolic pressure between the groups. The risk reduction for the primary endpoint (cardiovascular morbidity or death) in the losartan group was 0.76 and for cardiovascular death was 0.63. However, that study did not include a significant number of patients with renal disease. A separate detailed analysis of the microalbuminuric subjects both diabetic and non-diabetic, in the LIFE study is eagerly awaited. In the RENAAL study, there was a significant decrease in first time admission to hospital for cardiac failure, amongst those subjects receiving losartan [4]. A similar, albeit non-statistical, benefit on hospitalization for heart failure was also reported in the IDNT study [6]. These studies showed that both ACEI and ARB have a substantial beneficial effect of the development of cardiovascular complications in DM2 patients.

Treatment with ACEI has also been shown in the CAPPP and HOPE study to reduce the number of patients developing de novo diabetes [94, 102]. Furthermore, in the LIFE study losartan treatment was associated with less development of diabetes than atenolol [100]. It still remains to be determined if these effects on the development of diabetes are linked to the deleterious effects of agents such as thiazide diuretics and beta blockers on glucose tolerance or the beneficial effects of agents, which interrupt the RAS, on insulin sensitivity. This issue remains controversial with Gress et al having reported in a large study of non-diabetic hypertensive subjects that treatment with thiazide diuretics, ACEI

596

or CCB was not associated with an increased risk for the development of diabetes, whereas beta-blockers increased the risk [103].

Nosadini and Tonolo have recently analyzed the effect of CCBs on cardiovascular complications [104]. They summarized the results of four trials, where patients were randomized to either CCB (dihydropyridine). ACEI or ARB [6, 89, 90, 105]. These authors reached the conclusion that CCB compared with conventional therapy resulted in an average of 25% fewer strokes and an average of 18% more non-fatal acute myocardial infarctions. Thus the ACEI and ARB drugs seem to be superior to CCB in reducing cardiovascular but not cerebrovascular risk. However, CCB do seem to reduce the risk for stroke. Indeed, such a pattern is further suggested by the ALLHAT study [106]. However, one must be cautious in over-interpreting the findings of the ALLHAT study to the diabetic population. Although 40% of participants had diabetes, there was a very high drop out rate, significant compliance issues and a much higher proportion of Afro-American subjects than seen in trials performed outside the United States.

WHICH AGENT TO USE?

A large body of evidence has been collected as to the beneficial effects of various antihypertensive agents in DM1 and DM2 patients with abnormal albuminuria [4, 6, 37, 53, 107, 108]. It has been postulated that ACEI and ARB may possess beneficial effects over and above simple blood pressure control, although till recently most studies have involved small numbers of subjects and thereby introduced a potential Type II statistical error. Several meta-analyses of trials involving patients with either DM1 or DM2 have demonstrated the salutary effects of ACEI on proteinuria and renal function compared to other classes of antihypertensive agent, whether or not the patients had DM1 or DM2, hypertension, normoalbuminuria, microalbuminuria or macroproteinuria [109, 110]. These analyses have suggested that ACE inhibitors have an ability to reduce proteinuria independent of their hypotensive effects. However, an recent update of one of these meta-analyses has suggested that at maximal hypotensive doses there is no significant difference in the anti-proteinuric effects of ACE inhibitors and other antihypertensive drugs [111]. In another study in African American with hypertensive renal disease it was shown that lowering blood pressure to a lower level (goal MAP$\leq$92 mmHg versus MAP 102-107 mmHg) had no additional effect on progression of renal disease [112]. However, the recent large randomized studies patients with microalbuminuria or macroalbuminuria have reduced the need to rely on meta-analyses with all their deficiencies to determine the potential renoprotective effects of the various classes of antihypertensive agents. Specifically the RENAAL, IDNT and IRMA2 studies have demonstrated a significant delay in progression of the renal disease in patients receiving ARB [4, 6, 37]. It does seem that there may be an optimal dose for ARB in treating diabetic patients. It has been suggested for instance that the optimal dose of irbesartan is 300 mg, for losartan 100 mg and for candesartan 16mg [37, 113, 114]. In order to try and define the clinical outcome differences, if any, between treatment with an ACEI and ARB a study (DETAIL) has been initiated to compare the effects of telmisartan to enalapril and a combination of both of them in DM2 patients with hypertension and diabetic nephropathy [115, 116].

Following the guidelines for treatment of hypertension [70, 71], Bakris et al published a consensus report on the treatment of hypertension in the diabetic subject [73]. These authors suggested that the blood pressure goal should be 130/80 mmHg and that initial treatment should be an ACE-I and/or a diuretic, followed by CCB and other agents in order to achieve the goal. They also stressed the necessity for the combination of several drugs. Kaplan supported these suggestions adding that lifestyle changes, control of hyperglycemia, dyslipidemia, and proteinuria should be an essential part of the treatment regimen [74]. Bakris has provided a practical approach using the above criteria [117]. Other recent reviews have offered similar suggestions and have also included the use of ARB [118-120].

Thus, hypertensive DM2 patients with normoalbuminuria, microalbuminuria or overt proteinuria and normotensive patients with microalbuminuria or overt proteinuria should receive antihypertensive therapy. In fact it has been suggested that it may be cost-effective to treat all middle-aged DM2 patients with ACEI, irrespective of blood pressure or presence of albuminuria [121, 122]. The treatment goal should be a reduction in the average blood pressure to ≤130/80 mmHg. Most patients will require several drugs in order to achieve this goal. The first drug to be used should be either an ACEI or ARB. This is based on the extensive experience using ACEI in DM1 and DM2 over many years and the latest trials using ARB in DM2. Theoretically, ACEI may be superior to ARB in that these agents by blocking ACE not only inhibit formation of angiotensin II (AII) but also inhibit the degradation of the vasodilator bradykinin. However, ARB block the action of AII at the AT1 receptor subtype without affecting AII's interaction with the AT2 receptor subtype [123]. Indeed, if the AT2 receptor subtype is protective as suggested by some investigators, unopposed action of AII on the AT2 receptor may be highly desirable [124]. However, this view of the AT2 receptor remains controversial with several investigators proposing a deleterious role of the AT2 receptor on the kidney [125, 126]. Additional medications, which should be added to achieve the target blood pressure, include low-dose diuretics, CCB, beta-blockers or alpha-blockers. The combinations of ACEI-CCB, ARB-CCB and ACEI-ARB may be particularly useful regimens in this context.

It is important to emphasize that antihypertensive treatment should only be considered one part of the regimen and needs to include improved control of hyperglycemia and hyperlipidemia. It is important to note that cigarette smoking has been implicated as an important factor in promoting progresion of diabetic nephropathy even in the presence of controlled blood pressure and treatment with ACEI [12, 127]. Therefore, cessation of smoking should also be part of the therapeutic strategy. It has recently been reported that pravastatin may reduce proteinuria in non-diabetic normo-lipemic patients with well-controlled blood pressure [128] and several groups have reported antialbuminuric and renoprotective affects of various statins in DM2 patients with microalbuminuria and overt nephropathy, although these findings have not been universal [129-131]. Until more evidence becomes available it is suggested that treatment with lipid-lowering agents should be restricted to patients with hyperlipidemia and/or cardiovascular disease rather than renal disease. Increasingly, cost analyses are consistent with this view.

ALBUMINURIA AND RENAL STRUCTURE IN NIDDM

Although the principal endpoint in evaluating the influence of an antihypertensive agent on renal function in diabetes is its ability to alter the progression of the disease, it is clear that abnormally elevated albuminuria is also associated with progressive renal injury [132]. Nevertheless, many of the short-term trials that have been performed in DM2 subjects only document a reduction in albuminuria in the absence of a change in glomerular filtration rate. Long-term studies in both DM1 and DM2 subjects suggest that the severity of proteinuria also correlates with the rate of progression of renal disease [4, 6, 133]. Nonetheless, studies involving renal structural assessment are warranted to more accurately determine the response to antihypertensive agents. Fioretto et al have investigated the underlying renal pathology which occurs in DM2 patients with various stages of nephropathy [134]. There appears to be a marked variation in the degree of glomerulosclerosis and tubulointerstitial fibrosis in this population with only about one third having the typical histology of diabetic nephropathy. Recently it has been demonstrated in a small study that the ACEI, perindopril, can attenuate the development of renal injury and in particular tubulointerstitial expansion [135, 136]. The utility of detailed histomorphometric studies in this content remain to be validated and this morphological approach may be more relevant for research purposes, particularly if they incorporate studies to delineate the importance of various cellular and molecular processes implicated in progressive diabetes related renal injury.

CONCLUDING REMARKS

Finally, although the focus of treatment of DM2 subjects with early and overt renal disease has been on antihypertensive therapy one cannot ignore the role of glycaemic control. In natural history studies, it has been shown that glycaemic control is a major determinant of the rate of progression of albuminuria, not only in DM1 but also in DM2 subjects [137]. Furthermore, the Kumamoto study in Japanese DM2 subjects demonstrated that intensified insulin therapy over a 6 year period prevented the progression of diabetic microvascular complications including nephropathy [138]. These findings are similar to those reported from the DCCT study, which was performed in DM1 subjects [139]. The recent findings from the UKPDS confirm a pivotal role for glycaemic control in the progression of vascular complications including nephropathy [140]. Ravid et al have shown in a cross-sectional analysis of recently diagnosed DM2 patients that multiple factors are involved in the increase in albuminuria and the decrease in renal function [141]. These include glycated hemoglobin, mean blood pressure and total cholesterol. Indeed, the Steno 2 study has emphasized in a group of DM2 patients with microalbuminuria, the role of multifactorial intervention (strict control of hypertension, strict control of blood glucose levels, strict control of serum lipids, treatment with ACEI, aspirin and antioxidants, increased exercise and cessation of smoking). They compared the effects of this intensive approach to conventional treatment [142, 143]. In the initial analysis after 4 years of intensified treatment, benefits on microvascular complications including nephropathy were already detected [142]. Of particular interest are the recent updated findings in the patients receiving intensive therapy for a mean period of 7.8 years [143]. In this group there was a significantly reduced risk ratio for nephropathy, retinopathy and autonomic neuropathy and of particular clinical significance for cardiovascular disease. Thus the treatment of DM2 patients with normo- or hypertension and different degrees of UAE requires a varied and intensive treatment program.

REFERENCES

1.   Berkman J R.H., Unilateral nodular diabetic glomerulosclerosis (Kimmelstiel-Wilson). Report of a case. Metabolism Clin Exp, 1973. 22. 715-722.
2.   Mehler P.S. and Schrier R.W., Antihypertensive drugs and diabetic nephropathy. Curr Hypertens Rep, 1999. 1(2). 170-7.
3.   Schrier R.W., Treating high-risk diabetic hypertensive patients with comorbid conditions. Am J Kidney Dis, 2000. 36(3 Suppl 1). S10-7.
4.   Brenner B.M., Cooper M.E., de Zeeuw D., Keane W.F., Mitch W.E., Parving H.H., Remuzzi G., Snapinn S.M., Zhang Z., and Shahinfar S., Effects of losartan on renal and cardiovascular outcomes in patients with type 2 diabetes and nephropathy. N Engl J Med, 2001. 345(12). 861-9.
5.   Schrier R.W. and Estacio R.O., Additional follow-up from the ABCD trial in patients with type 2 diabetes and hypertension. N Engl J Med. 2000, 2000. 343(26). 645-652.
6.   Lewis E.J., Hunsicker L.G., Clarke W.R., Berl T., Pohl M.A., Lewis J.B., Ritz E., Atkins R.C., Rohde R., and Raz I., Renoprotective effect of the angiotensin-receptor antagonist irbesartan in patients with nephropathy due to type 2 diabetes. N Engl J Med, 2001. 345(12). 851-60.
7.   Ritz E. and Stefanski A., Diabetic nephropathy in type II diabetes. Am J Kidney Dis, 1996. 27. 167-194.
8.   USRDS, U.S. Renal Data System, USRDS 2002 Annual Data Report: Atlas of End-Stage Renal Disease in the United States, National Institutes of Health, National Institute of Diabetes and Digestive and Kidney Diseases, Bethesda, MD, 2002. 2002.
9.   Adler A.I., Stevens R.J., Manley S.E., Bilous R.W., Cull C.A., and Holman R.R., Development and progression of nephropathy in type 2 diabetes: The United Kingdom Prospective Diabetes Study (UKPDS 64). Kidney Int, 2003. 63(1). 225-232.
10. Okosun I.S., Chandra K.M.D., Choi S., Christman J., Dever G.E.D., and Prewitt T.E., Hypertension and type 2 diabetes comorbidity in sdults in the United States: risk of overall and regional adiposity. Obesity Research, 2001. 9. 1-9.
11. Sowers J.R., Epstein M., and Frohlich E.D., Diabetes, hypertension and cardiovascular disease. An update. Hypertension, 2001. 37. 1053-1059.
12. Chuahirun T., Khanna A., Kimball K., and Wesson D.E., Cigarette smoking and increased urine albumin excretion are interrelated predictors of nephropathy progression in type 2 diabetes. Am J Kidney Dis, 2003. 41(1). 13-21.
13. Bakris G.L., Copley J.B., Vicknair N., Sadler R., and Leurgans S., Calcium channel blockers versus other antihypertensive therapies on progression on NIDDM associated nephropathy. Kidney Int, 1996. 50. 1641-1650.
14. Bakris G.L., Weir M.R., Dequattro V., and McMahon F.G., Effects of an ACE inhibitor calcium antagonist combination on proteinuria in diabetic nephropathy. Kidney Int, 1998. 54. 1283-1289.
15. Nielsen F.S., Rossing K., Gall M.A., Skott P., Smidt U.M., and Parving H.H., Impact of lisinopril and atenolol on kidney function in hypertensive NIDDM subjects with diabetic nephropathy. Diabetes, 1994. 43. 1108-1113.

16. Chan J.C., Cockram C.S., Nicholls M.G., Cheung C.K., and Swaminathan R., Comparison of enalapril and nifedipine in treating non-insulin dependent diabetes associated with hypertension: one year analysis. BMJ, 1992. 305. 981-985.

17. Chan J.C.N., Ko G.T.C., Leung D.H.Y., Cheung R.C.K., Cheung M.Y.F., So W.Y., Swaminathan R., Nicholls M.G., Critchley J., and Cockram C.S., Long-term effects of angiotensin-converting enzyme inhibition and metabolic control in hypertensive type 2 diabetic patients. Kidney International, 2000. 57(2). 590-600.

18. Ferder L., Daccordi H., Martello M., Panzalis M., and Inserra F., Angiotensin converting enzyme inhibitors versus calcium antagonists in the treatment of diabetic hypertensive patients. Hypertension, 1992. 19. II237-II242.

19. Fogari R., Zoppi A., Corradi L., Mugellini A., Lazzari P., Preti P., and Lusardi P., Long-term effects of ramipril and nitrendipine on albuminuria in hypertensive patients with type II diabetes and impaired renal function. J Hum Hypertens, 1999. 13. 47-53.

20. Liou H.H., Huang T.P., and Campese V.M., Effect of long-term therapy with captopril on proteinuria and renal function in patients with non-insulin-dependent diabetes and with non-diabetic renal diseases. Nephron, 1995. 69. 41-48.

21. Slataper R., Vicknair N., Sadler R., and Bakris G.L., Comparative effects of different antihypertensive treatments on progression of diabetic renal disease. Arch Intern Med, 1993. 153. 973-980.

22. Bakris G.L., Mangrum A., Copley J.B., Vicknair N., and Sadler R., Effect of calcium channel or beta-blockade on the progression of diabetic nephropathy in African Americans. Hypertension, 1997. 29. 744-750.

23. Bakris G.L., Barnhill B.W., and Sadler R., Treatment of arterial hypertension in diabetic humans: importance of therapeutic selection. Kidney Int, 1992. 41. 912-919.

24. Veelken R., Delles C., Hilgers K.F., and Schmieder R.E., Outcome survey in unselected hypertensive patients with type 2 diabetes mellitus: effects of ACE inhibition. Am J Hypertens, 2001. 14(7 Pt 1). 672-8.

25. Gerth W.C., Remuzzi G., Viberti G., Hannedouche T., Martinez Castelao A., Shahinfar S., Carides G.W., and Brenner B.M., Losartan reduces the burden and cost of ESRD: public health implications from the RENAAL study for the European Union. Kidney Int, 2002. 62(Supplement 82). S68-S72.

26. Salako B.L., Finomo F.O., Kadiri S., Arije A., and Olatosin A.O., Comparative effect of lisinopril and lacidipine on urinary albumin excretion in patients with type 11 diabetic nephropathy. Afr J Med Med Sci, 2002. 31(1). 53-7.

27. Bakris G.L., Effects of diltiazem or lisinopril on massive proteinuria associated with diabetes mellitus. Ann Intern Med, 1990. 112. 707-708.

28. Demarie D.K. and Bakris G.L., Effects of different calcium antagonists on proteinuria associated with diabetes mellitus. Ann Intern Med, 1990. 113. 987-988.

29. Guasch A., Parham M., Zayas C.F., Campbell O., Nzerue C., and Macon E., Contrasting effects of calcium channel blockade versus converting enzyme inhibition on proteinuria in African Americans with non-insulin-dependent diabetes mellitus and nephropathy. J Am Soc Nephrol, 1997. 8. 793-798.

30. Rachmani R., Levi Z., Slavachevsky I., Half-Onn E., and Ravid M., Effect of an alpha-adrenergic blocker, and ACE inhibitor and hydrochlorothiazide on blood pressure and on renal function in type 2 diabetic patients with hypertension and albuminuria. A randomized cross-over study. Nephron, 1998. 80. 175-182.

31. Lacourciere Y., Nadeau A., Poirier L., and Tancrede G., Captopril or conventional therapy in hypertensive type II diabetics. Three-year analysis. Hypertension, 1993. 21. 786-94.

32. Sano T., Kawamura T., Matsumae H., Sasaki H., Nakayama M., Hara T., Matsuo S., Hotta N., and Sakamoto N., Effects of long-term enalapril treatment on persistent microalbuminuria in well-controlled hypertensive and normotensive NIDDM patients. Diabetes Care, 1994. 17. 420-4.

33. Trevisan R. and Tiengo A., Effect of low-dose ramipril on microalbuminuria in normotensive or mild hypertensive non-insulin-dependent diabetic patients. North-East Italy Microalbuminuria Study Group. Am J Hypertens, 1995. 8. 876-83.

34. Lacourciere Y., Belanger A., Godin C., Halle J.P., Ross S., Wright N., and Marion J., Long-term comparison of losartan and enalapril on kidney function in hypertensive type 2 diabetics with early nephropathy. Kidney Int, 2000. 58(2). 762-9.

35. Muirhead N., Feagan B.F., Mahon J., Lewanczuk R.Z., Rodger N.W., Botteri F., Oddou-Stock P., Pecher E., and Cheung R., The effects of valsartan and captopril on reducing microalbuminuria in patients with type 2 diabetes mellitus: a placebo-controlled trial. Curr Therapeutic Res, 1999. 60(12). 650-660.

36. Sasso F.C., Carbonara O., Persico M., Iafusco D., Salvatore T., D'Ambrosio R., Torella R., and Cozzolino D., Irbesartan reduces the albumin excretion rate in microalbuminuric type 2 diabetic patients independently of hypertension: a randomized double-blind placebo-controlled crossover study. Diabetes Care, 2002. 25(11). 1909-13.

37. Parving H.H., Lehnert H., Brochner-Mortensen J., Gomis R., Andersen S., and Arner P., The effect of irbesartan on the development of diabetic nephropathy in patients with type 2 diabetes. N Engl J Med, 2001. 345(12). 870-8.

38. Schnack C., Hoffmann W., Hopmeier P., and Schernthaner G., Renal and metabolic effects of 1-year treatment with ramipril or atenolol in NIDDM patients with microalbuminuria. Diabetologia, 1996. 39(12). 1611-1616.

39. Ruggenenti P., Mosconi L., Bianchi L., Cortesi L., Campana M., Pagani G., Mecca G., and Remuzzi G., Long-term treatment with either enalapril or nitrendipine stabilizes albuminuria and increases glomerular filtration rate in non-insulin-dependent diabetic patients. American Journal of Kidney Diseases, 1994. 24(5). 753-761.

40. Velussi M., Brocco E., Frogato F., Zolli M., Muollo B., Maioli M., Carraro A., Tonolo G., Fresu P., Cernigoi A.M., Fioretto P., and Nosadini R., Effects of cilazapril and amlodipine on kidney function in hypertensive NIDDM patients. Diabetes, 1996. 45. 216-222.

41. Agardh C.D., Garcia Puig J., Charbonnel B., Angelkort B., and Barnett A.H., Greater reduction of urinary albumin excretion in hypertensive type II diabetic patients with incipient nephropathy by lisinopril than by nifedipine. J Hum Hypertens, 1996. 10. 185-92.

42. Fogari R., Zoppi A., Malamani G.D., Lusardi P., Destro M., and Corradi L., Effects of amlodipine vs enalapril on microalbuminuria in hypertensive patients with type II diabetes. Clinical Drug Investigation, 1997. 13(Suppl 1). 42-49.

43. Melbourne Diabetic Nephropathy Study Group, Comparison between perindopril and nifedipine in hypertensive and normotensive diabetic patients with microalbuminuria. Br Med J, 1991. 302. 210-6.

44. Fogari R., Preti P., Zoppi A., Rinaldi A., Corradi L., Pasotti C., Poletti L., Marasi G., Derosa G., Mugellini A., Voglini C., and Lazarri P., Effects of amlodipine fosinopril combination on microalbuminuria in hypertensive type 2 diabetic patients. Am J Hypertens, 2002. 15. 1042-1049.

45. Baba S., Nifedipine and enalapril equally reduce the progression of nephropathy in hypertensive type 2 diabetics. Diabetes Res Clin Pract, 2001. 54(3). 191-201.

46. Kopf D., Schmitz H., Beyer J., Frank M., Bockisch A., and Lehnert H., A double-blind trial of perindopril and nitrendipine in incipient diabetic nephropathy. Diabetes Nutr Metab, 2001. 14(5). 245-52.

47. Estacio R.O., Jeffers B.W., Gifford N., and Schrier R.W., Effect of blood pressure control on diabetic microvascular complications in patients with hypertension and type 2 diabetes. Diabetes Care, 2000. 23(Suppl 2). B54-B64.

48. Viberti G. and Wheeldon N.M., Microalbuminuria reduction with valsartan in patients with type 2 diabetes mellitus: a blood pressure-independent effect. Circulation, 2002. 106(6). 672-8.

49. Gambardella S., Frontoni S., Lala A., Felici M.G., Spallone V., Scoppola A., Jacoangeli F., and Menzinger G., Regression of microalbuminuria in type II diabetic, hypertensive patients after long-term indapamide treatment. Am Heart J, 1991. 122. 1232-8.

50. Romero R., Salinas I., Lucas A., Abad E., Reverter J.L., Johnston S., and Sanmarti A., Renal function changes in microalbuminuric normotensive type II diabetic patients treated with angiotensin-converting enzyme inhibitors. Diabetes Care, 1993. 16. 597-600.

51. Jerums G., Allen T.J., Tsalamandris C., Cooper M.E., and Melbourne Diabetic Nephropathy Study Group, Angiotensin Converting Enzyme inhibition and Calcium Channel Blockade in incipient diabetic nephropathy. Kidney Int, 1992. 41. 904-911.

52. Ravid M., Savin H., Jutrin I., Bental T., Katz B., and Lishner M., Long-term stabilizing effect of angiotensin-converting enzyme inhibition on plasma creatinine and on proteinuria in normotensive type II diabetic patients. Ann Intern Med, 1993. 118(8). 577-81.

53. Ravid M., Lang R., Rachmani R., and Lishner M., Long-term renoprotective effect of angiotensin-converting enzyme inhibition in non-insulin-dependent diabetes mellitus. A 7-year follow-up study. Arch Intern Med, 1996. 156. 286-9.

54. Ahmad J., Siddiqui M.A., and Ahmad H., Effective postponement of diabetic nephropathy with enalapril in normotensive type 2 diabetic patients with microalbuminuria. Diabetes Care, 1997. 20(10). 1576-1581.

55. Ravid M., Brosh D., Levi Z., Bardayan Y., Ravid D., and Rachmani R., Use of enalapril to attenuate decline in renal function in normotensive, normoalbuminuric patients with type 2 diabetes mellitus - a randomized, controlled trial. Annals of Internal Medicine, 1998. 128(12 Part 1). 982-8.

56. Schrier R.W., Estacio R.O., Esler A., and Mehler P., Effects of aggressive blood pressure control in normotensive type 2 diabetic patients on albuminuria, retinopathy and strokes. Kidney Int, 2002. 61(3). 1086-97.

57. Boner G., Cao Z., and Cooper M.E., Combination antihypertensive therapy in the treatment of diabetic nephropathy. Diabetes Technol Ther, 2002. 4(3). 313-21.

58. Brown S.A., Walton C.L., Crawford P., and Bakris G.L., Long-term effects of antihypertensive regimens on renal hemodynamics and proteinuria. Kidney Int, 1993. 43. 1210-8.

59. Fioretto P., Frigato F., Velussi M., Riva F., Muollo B., Carraro A., Brocco E., Cipollina M.R., Abaterusso C., Trevisan M., Crepaldi G., and Nosadini R., Effects of angiotensin converting enzyme inhibitors and calcium antagonists on atrial natriuretic peptide release and action and on albumin excretion rate in hypertensive insulin-dependent diabetic patients. Am J Hypertens, 1992. 5. 837-46.

60. Bakris G., Weir M., De Quattro V., Rosendorff C., and McMahon G., Renal effects of a long acting ACE inhibitor, trandolapril (T) or nondihydropyridine calcium blocker, verapamil (V) or in a fixed dose combination in diabetic nephropathy: A randomized double blind placebo controlled multicenter study. Nephrology, 1997. 3 (Suppl 1). S271.

61. Fogari R., Zoppi A., Mugellini A., Lusardi P., Destro M., and Corradi L., Effect of benazepril plus amlodipine vs benazepril alone on urinary albumin excretion in hypertensive patients with type ii diabetes and microalbuminuria. Clinical Drug Investigation, 1997. 13(Suppl 1). 50-55.

62. Shigihara T., Sato A., Hayashi K., and Saruta T., Effect of combination therapy of angiotensin-converting enzyme inhibitor plus calcium channel blocker on urinary albumin excretion in hypertensive microalbuminuric patients with type II diabetes. Hypertens Res, 2000. 23(3). 219-26.

63. Fernandez R., Puig J.G., Rodriguez-Perez J.C., Garrido J., and Redon J., Effect of two antihypertensive combinations on metabolic control in type-2 diabetic hypertensive patients with albuminuria: a randomised, double-blind study. J Hum Hypertens, 2001. 15(12). 849-56.

64. Bakris G.L., Smith A.C., Richardson D.J., Hung E., Preston R., Goldberg R., and Epstein M., Impact of an ACE inhibitor and calcium antagonist on microalbuminuria and lipid subfractions in type 2 diabetes: a randomised, multi-centre pilot study. J Hum Hypertens, 2002. 16(3). 185-91.

65. Mogensen C.E., Neldam S., Tikkanen I., Oren S., Viskoper R., Watts R.W., and Cooper M.E., Randomised controlled trial of dual blockade of renin-angiotensin system in patients with hypertension, microalbuminuria, and non-insulin dependent diabetes: the candesartan and Lisinopril microalbuminuria (CALM) study. British Medical Journal, 2000. 321(7274). 1440-1444.

66. Hebert L.A., Falkenhain M.E., Nahman N.S., Jr., Cosio F.G., and O'Dorisio T.M., Combination ACE inhibitor and angiotensin II receptor antagonist therapy in diabetic nephropathy. Am J Nephrol, 1999. 19(1). 1-6.

67. Kuriyama S., Tomonari H., Tokudome G., Horiguchi M., Hayashi H., Kobayashi H., Ishikawa M., and Hosoya T., Antiproteinuric effects of combined antihypertensive therapies in patients with overt type 2 diabetic nephropathy. Hypertens Res, 2002. 25(6). 849-55.

68. Rossing K., Christensen P.K., Jensen B.R., and Parving H.-H., Dual blockade of the renin-angiotensin system in diabetic nephropathy : a randomized double blind crossover study. Diabetes Care, 2002. 25. 95-100.

69. Kincaid-Smith P., Fairley K., and Packham D., Randomized controlled crossover study of the effect on proteinuria and blood pressure of adding an angiotensin II receptor antagonist to an angiotensin converting enzyme inhibitor in normotensive patients with chronic renal disease and proteinuria. Nephrol Dial Transplant, 2002. 17(4). 597-601.

70. Joint National Committee on Prevention, Detection, Evaluation, and and Treatment of High Blood Pressure, The sixth report of the Joint National Committee on Prevention, Detection, Evaluation, and Treatment of High Blood Pressure. Arch Intern Med, 1997. 157. 2413-2445.

71. Guidelines Subcommittee, 1999 World Health Organization - International Society of Hypertension guidelines for the management of hypertension. J Hypertens, 1999. 17. 151-183.

72. Kjeldsen S.E., Farsang C., Sleigh P., and Mancia G., 1999 WHO/ISH hypertension guidelines—highlights and esh update. J Hypertens, 2001. 19(12). 2285-8.

73. Bakris G.L., Williams M., Dworkin L., Elliott W.J., Epstein M., Toto R., Tuttle K., Douglas J., Hsueh W., and Sowers J., Preserving renal function in adults with hypertension and diabetes: a consensus approach. National Kidney Foundation Hypertension and Diabetes Executive Committees Working Group. Am J Kidney Dis, 2000. 36(3). 646-61.

74. Kaplan N.M., Management of hypertension in patients with type 2 diabetes mellitus: guidelines based on current evidence. Ann Intern Med, 2001. 135(12). 1079-83.

75. Mogensen C.E., Microalbuminuria predicts clinical proteinuria and early mortality in maturity-onset diabetes. N Engl J Med, 1984. 310. 356-60.

76. Wilson P.W., Diabetes mellitus and coronary heart disease. Am J Kidney Dis, 1998. 32(5 Suppl 3). S89-100.

77. Wirta O., Pasternack A., Mustonen J., and Laippala P., Renal and cardiovascular predictors of 9-year total and sudden cardiac mortality in non-insulin-dependent diabetic subjects. Nephrol Dial Transplant, 1997. 12(12). 2612-7.

78. Molgaard H., Christensen P.D., Hermansen K., Sorensen K.E., Christensen C.K., and Mogensen C.E., Early recognition of autonomic dysfunction in microalbuminuria: significance for cardiovascular mortality in diabetes mellitus? Diabetologia, 1994. 37(8). 788-96.

79. Araki S., Haneda M., Togawa M., Sugimoto T., Shikano T., Nakagawa T., Isono M., Hidaka H., and Kikkawa R., Microalbuminuria is not associated with cardiovascular death in Japanese NIDDM. Diabetes Res Clin Pract, 1997. 35(1). 35-40.

80. Spoelstra-de Man A.M., Brouwer C.B., Stehouwer C.D., and Smulders Y.M., Rapid progression of albumin excretion is an independent predictor of cardiovascular mortality in patients with type 2 diabetes and microalbuminuria. Diabetes Care, 2001. 24(12). 2097-101.

81. Garber A.J., Vinik A.I., and Crespin S.R., Detection and management of lipid disorders in diabetic patients. A commentary for clinicians. Diabetes Care, 1992. 15. 1068-74.

82. Lind L., Pollare T., Berne C., and Lithell H., Long-term metabolic effects of antihypertensive drugs. Am Heart J, 1994. 128. 1177-83.

83. Harper R., Ennis C.N., Heaney A.P., Sheridan B., Gormley M., Atkinson A.B., Johnston G.D., and Bell P.M., A comparison of the effects of low- and conventional-dose thiazide diuretic on insulin action in hypertensive patients with NIDDM. Diabetologia, 1995. 38. 853-9.

84. Laakso M., Karjalainen L., and Lempiainenkuosa P., Effects of losartan on insulin sensitivity in hypertensive subjects. Hypertension, 1996. 28(3). 392-396.

85. Imazu M., Hypertension and insulin disorders. Curr Hypertens Rep, 2002. 4(6). 477-82.

86. Giordano M., Matsuda M., Sanders L., Canessa M.L., and DeFronzo R.A., Effects of angiotensin-converting enzyme inhibitors, Ca2+ channel antagonists, and alpha-adrenergic blockers on glucose and lipid metabolism in NIDDM patients with hypertension. Diabetes, 1995. 44. 665-71.

87. Stein P. and Black H., Drug treatment of hypertension in patients with diabetes mellitus. Diabetes Care, 1991. 14. 425-448.

88. McClellan K.J. and Goa K.L., Candesartan cilexetil. A review of its use in essential hypertension. Drugs, 1998. 56(5). 847-69.

89. Estacio R.O., Jeffers B.W., Hiatt W.R., Biggerstaff S.L., Gifford N., and Schrier R.W., The effect of nisoldipine as compared with enalapril on cardiovascular outcomes in patients with non-insulin-dependent diabetes and hypertension. N Engl J Med, 1998. 338. 645-652.

90. Tatti P., Pahor M., Byington R.P., DiMauro P., Guarisco R., Strollo G., and Strollo F., Outcome results of the Fosinopril versus Amlodipine Cardiovascular Events randomised Trial (FACET) in patients with hypertension and non-insulin dependent diabetes mellitus. Diabetes Care, 1998. 21. 597-603.

91. Tuomilehto J., Rastenyte D., Birkenhager W.H., Thijs L., Antikainen R., Bulpitt C.J., Fletcher A.E., Forette F., Goldhaber A., Palatini P., Sarti C., Fagard R., Staessen J.A., Arabidze G.G., Carrageta M., Celis H., Kocemba J., Leonetti G., Nachev C., O'Brien E.T., Ritz E., Rodicio J.L., Rosenfeld J., Heyrman J., Stibbe G., and et al., Effects of calcium-channel blockade in older patients with diabetes and systolic hypertension. New England Journal of Medicine, 1999. 340(9). 677-684.

92. Hansson L., Zanchetti A., Carruthers S.G., Dahlof B., Elmfeldt D., Julius S., Ménard J., Rahn K.H., Wedel H., Westerling S., and for the HOT Study Group, Effects of intensive blood-pressure lowering and low-dose aspirin in patients with hypertension: principal results of the Hypertension Optimal treatment (HOT) randomised trial. Lancet, 1998. 351. 1755-62.

93. Niskanen L., Hedner T., Hansson L., Lanke J., and Niklason A., Reduced cardiovascular morbidity and mortality in hypertensive diabetic patients on first-line therapy with an ACE inhibitor compared with a diuretic/beta-blocker-based treatment regimen: a subanalysis of the Captopril Prevention Project. Diabetes Care, 2001. 24(12). 2091-6.

94. Hansson L., Lindholm L.H., Niskanen L., Lanke J., Hedner T., Niklason A., Luomanmaki K., Dahlof B., de Faire U., Morlin C., Karlberg B.E., Wester P.O., and Bjorck J.E., Effect of angiotensin-converting-enzyme inhibition compared with conventional therapy on cardiovascular morbidity and mortality in hypertension: the Captopril Prevention Project (CAPPP) randomised trial. Lancet, 1999. 353(9153). 611-616.

95. UK Prospective Diabetes Study (UKPDS) Group, Tight blood pressure control and risk of macrovascular and microvascular complications in type 2 diabetes - UKPDS 38. British Medical Journal, 1998. 317(7160). 703-713.

96. UK Prospective Diabetes Study (UKPDS) Group, Efficacy of atenolol and captopril in reducing risk of macrovascular and microvascular complications in type 2 diabetes - UKPDS 39. British Medical Journal, 1998. 317(7160). 713-720.

97. MICRO-HOPE, Effects of ramipril on cardiovascular and microvascular outcomes in people with diabetes mellitus: results of the HOPE study and MICRO-HOPE substudy. Heart Outcomes Prevention Evaluation Study Investigators. Lancet, 2000. 355(9200). 253-9.

98. Svensson P., de Faire U., Sleight P., Yusuf S., and Ostergren J., Comparative effects of ramipril on ambulatory and office blood pressures: a HOPE Substudy. Hypertension, 2001. 38(6). E28-32.

99. Mehler P.S., Coll J.R., Estacio R., Esler A., Schrier R.W., and Hiatt W.R., Intensive blood pressure control reduces the risk of cardiovascular events in patients with peripheral arterial disease and type 2 diabetes. Circulation, 2003. 107(5). 753-6.

100. Dahlof B., Devereux R.B., Kjeldsen S.E., Julius S., Beevers G., Faire U., Fyhrquist F., Ibsen H., Kristiansson K., Lederballe-Pedersen O., Lindholm L.H., Nieminen M.S., Omvik P., Oparil S., and Wedel H., Cardiovascular morbidity and mortality in the Losartan Intervention For Endpoint reduction in hypertension study (LIFE): a randomised trial against atenolol. Lancet, 2002. 359(9311). 995-1003.

101. Lindholm L.H., Ibsen H., Dahlof B., Devereux R.B., Beevers G., de Faire U., Fyhrquist F., Julius S., Kjeldsen S.E., Kristiansson K., Lederballe-Pedersen O., Nieminen M.S., Omvik P., Oparil S., Wedel H., Aurup P., Edelman J., and Snapinn S., Cardiovascular morbidity and mortality in patients with diabetes in the Losartan Intervention For Endpoint reduction in hypertension study (LIFE): a randomised trial against atenolol. Lancet, 2002. 359(9311). 1004-10.

102. Yusuf S., Sleight P., Pogue J., Bosch J., Davies R., and Dagenais G., Effects of an angiotensin-converting-enzyme inhibitor, ramipril, on cardiovascular events in high-risk patients. The Heart Outcomes Prevention Evaluation Study Investigators. N Engl J Med, 2000. 342(3). 145-53.

103. Gress T.W., Nieto F.J., Shahar E., Wofford M.R., and Brancati F.L., Hypertension and antihypertensive therapy as risk factors for type 2 diabetes mellitus. Atherosclerosis Risk in Communities Study. N Engl J Med, 2000. 342(13). 905-12.

104. Nosadini R. and Tonolo G., Cardiovascular and renal protection in type 2 diabetes mellitus: the role of calcium channel blockers. J Am Soc Nephrol, 2002. 13 Suppl 3. S216-23.

105. Hansson L., Lindholm L.H., Ekbom T., Dahlof B., Lanke J., Schersten B., Wester P.O., Hedner T., and de Faire U., Randomised trial of old and new antihypertensive drugs in elderly patients: cardiovascular mortality and morbidity the Swedish Trial in Old Patients with Hypertension-2 study. Lancet, 1999. 354(9192). 1751-6.

106. ALLHAT, Major outcomes in high-risk hypertensive patients randomized to angiotensin-converting enzyme inhibitor or calcium channel blocker vs diuretic: The Antihypertensive and Lipid-Lowering Treatment to Prevent Heart Attack Trial (ALLHAT). Jama, 2002. 288(23). 2981-97.

107. Lewis E.J., Hunsicker L.G., Bain R.P., and Rohde R.D., The effect of angiotensin converting enzyme inhibition on diabetic nephropathy. N Engl J Med, 1993. 329. 1456-62.

108. Parving H.H., Diabetic hypertensive patients. Is this a group in need of particular care and attention? Diabetes Care, 1999. 22 Suppl 2. B76-9.

109. Kasiske B.L., Kalil R.S., Ma J.Z., Liao M., and Keane W.F., Effect of antihypertensive therapy on the kidney in patients with diabetes: a meta-regression analysis. Ann Intern Med, 1993. 118. 129-38.

110. Bohlen L., de Courten M., and Weidmann P., Comparative study of the effect of ACE-inhibitors and other antihypertensive agents on proteinuria in diabetic patients. Am J Hypertens, 1994. 7. 84s-92s.

111. Weidmann P., Schneider M., and Bohlen L., Therapeutic efficacy of different antihypertensive drugs in human diabetic nephropathy: an updated meta-analysis. Nephrol Dial Transpl, 1995. 10(suppl). 39-45.

112. Wright J.T., Jr., Bakris G., Greene T., Agodoa L.Y., Appel L.J., Charleston J., Cheek D., Douglas-Baltimore J.G., Gassman J., Glassock R., Hebert L., Jamerson K., Lewis J., Phillips R.A., Toto R.D., Middleton J.P., and Rostand S.G., Effect of blood pressure lowering and antihypertensive drug class on progression of hypertensive kidney disease: results from the AASK trial. Jama, 2002. 288(19). 2421-31.

113. Andersen S., Rossing P., Juhl T.R., Deinum J., and Parving H.H., Optimal dose of losartan for renoprotection in diabetic nephropathy. Nephrol Dial Transplant, 2002. 17(8). 1413-8.

114. Rossing K., Christensen P.K., Hansen B.V., Carstensen B., and Parving H.H., Optimal Dose of Candesartan for Renoprotection in Type 2 Diabetic Patients With Nephropathy: A double-blind randomized cross-over study. Diabetes Care, 2003. 26(1). 150-5.

115. Barnett A.H., The role of angiotensin II receptor antagonists in the management of diabetes. Blood Press, 2001. 10 Suppl 1. 21-6.

116. Rippin J., Bain S.C., and Barnett A.H., Rationale and design of diabetics exposed to telmisartan and enalapril (DETAIL) study. J Diabetes Complications, 2002. 16(3). 195-200.

117. Bakris G.L., A practical approach to achieving recommended blood pressure goals in diabetic patients. Arch Intern Med, 2001. 161(22). 2661-7.

118. Arauz-Pacheco C., Parrott M.A., and Raskin P., The treatment of hypertension in adult patients with diabetes. Diabetes Care, 2002. 25(1). 134-47.

119. Zanchetti A. and Ruilope L.M., Antihypertensive treatment in patients with type-2 diabetes mellitus: what guidance from recent controlled randomized trials? J Hypertens, 2002. 20(11). 2099-110.

120. American Diabetes Association, Diabetic Nephropathy. Diabetes Care, 2002. 25(90001). S85-S89.

121. Brenner L., Finkelstein S., and Brenner B.M., Clinical and economic benefits of angiotensin-converting enzyme inhibitors in diabetic nephropathy. Curr Opin Nephrol Hypertens, 1999. 8. 243-249.

122. Golan L., Birkmeyer J.D., and Welch H.G., The cost-effectiveness of treating all patients with type 2 diabetes with angiotensin-converting enzyme inhibitors. Ann Intern Med, 1999. 131(9). 660-7.

123. Johnston C.I., Angiotensin receptor antagonists: focus on losartan. Lancet, 1995. 346(8987). 1403-7.

124. Nakajima M., Hutchinson H.G., Fujinaga M., Hayashida W., Morishita R., Zhang L., Horiuchi M., Pratt R.E., and Dzau V.J., The angiotensin II type 2 (AT2) receptor antagonizes the growth effects of the AT1 receptor: gain-of-function study using gene transfer. Proc Natl Acad Sci U S A, 1995. 92(23). 10663-7.

125. Cao Z., Bonnet F., Candido R., Nesteroff S.P., Burns W.C., Kawachi H., Shimizu F., Carey R.M., De Gasparo M., and Cooper M.E., Angiotensin type 2 receptor antagonism confers renal protection in a rat model of progressive renal injury. J Am Soc Nephrol, 2002. 13(7). 1773-87.

126. Wolf G., "The road not taken": role of angiotensin II type 2 receptor in pathophysiology. Nephrol Dial Transpl, 2002. 17. 195-198.

127. Chuahirun T. and Wesson D.E., Cigarette smoking predicts faster progression of type 2 established diabetic nephropathy despite ACE inhibition. Am J Kidney Dis, 2002. 39(2). 376-82.

128. Lee T.M., Su S.F., and Tsai C.H., Effect of pravastatin on proteinuria in patients with well-controlled hypertension. Hypertension, 2002. 40(1). 67-73.

129. Tonolo G., Ciccarese M., Brizzi P., Puddu L., Secchi G., Calvia P., Atzeni M.M., Melis M.G., and Maioli M., Reduction of albumin excretion rate in normotensive microalbuminuric type 2 diabetic patients during long-term simvastatin treatment. Diabetes Care, 1997. 20(12). 1891-5.

130. Lam K.S., Cheng I.K., Janus E.D., and Pang R.W., Cholesterol-lowering therapy may retard the progression of diabetic nephropathy. Diabetologia, 1995. 38(5). 604-9.

131. Jandeleit-Dahm K., Cao Z.M., Cox A.J., Kelly D.J., Gilbert R.E., and Cooper M.E., Role of hyperlipidemia in progressive renal disease: Focus on diabetic nephropathy. Kidney International, 1999. 56(Suppl 71). S31-S36.

132. Remuzzi G. and Bertani T., Is glomerulosclerosis a consequence of altered glomerular permeability to macromolecules? Kidney Int, 1990. 38. 384-394.

133. Rossing P., Hommel E., Smidt U.M., and Parving H.H., Impact of arterial blood pressure and albuminuria on the progression of diabetic nephropathy in IDDM patients. Diabetes, 1993. 42. 715-9.

134. Fioretto P., Stehouwer C.D., Mauer M., Chiesura-Corona M., Brocco E., Carraro A., Bortoloso E., van Hinsbergh V.W., Crepaldi G., and Nosadini R., Heterogeneous nature of microalbuminuria in NIDDM: studies of endothelial function and renal structure. Diabetologia, 1998. 41(2). 233-6.

135. Cordonnier D.J., Pinel N., Barro C., Maynard M., Zaoui P., Halimi S., de Ligny B.H., Reznic Y., Simon D., and Bilous R.W., Expansion of cortical interstitium is limited by converting enzyme inhibition in type 2 diabetic patients with glomerulosclerosis. The Diabiopsies Group. J Am Soc Nephrol, 1999. 10(6). 1253-63.

136. White K.E., Pinel N., Cordonnier D.J., and Bilous R.W., Does ACE inhibition slow progression of glomerulopathy in patients with Type 2 diabetes mellitus? Diabet Med, 2001. 18(11). 933-6.

137. Gilbert R.E., Tsalamandris C., Bach L., Panagiotopoulos S., O'Brien R.C., Allen T.J., Goodall I., Young V., Seeman E., Murray R.M.L., Cooper M.E., and Jerums G., Glycemic control and the rate of progression of early diabetic kidney disease: a nine year longitudinal study. Kidney Int, 1993. 44. 855-859.

138. Ohkubo Y., Kishikawa H., Araki E., Miyata T., Isami S., Motoyoshi S., Kojima Y., Furyoshi N., and Shichiri M., Intensive insulin therapy prevents the progression of diabetic microvascular complications in Japanese patients with non-insulin-dependent diabetes mellitus: a randomized prospective 6-year study. Diabetes Res Clin Pract, 1995. 28. 103-117.

139. Diabetes Control and Complications Trial Research Group, The effect of intensive treatment on the development and progression of long-term complications in insulin-dependent diabetes mellitus. N Engl J Med, 1993. 329. 977-86.

140. UK Prospective Diabetes Study (UKPDS) Group, Intensive blood-glucose control with sulphonylureas or insulin compared with conventional treatment and risk of complications in patients with type 2 diabetes (UKPDS 33). Lancet, 1998. 352(9131). 837-53.

141. Ravid M., Brosh D., Ravid-Safran D., Levy Z., and Rachmani R., Main risk factors for nephropathy in type 2 diabetes mellitus are plasma cholesterol levels, mean blood pressure, and hyperglycemia. Arch Intern Med, 1998. 158(9). 998-1004.

142. Gaede P., Vedel P., Parving H.H., and Pedersen O., Intensified multifactorial intervention in patients with type 2 diabetes mellitus and microalbuminuria: the Steno type 2 randomised study. Lancet, 1999. 353(9153). 617-622.

143. Gæde P., Vedel P., Larsen N., Jensen G.V.H., Parving H.-H., and Pedersen O., Multifactorial intervention and cardiovascular disease in patients with type 2 diabetes. N Engl J Med, 2003. 348. 383-93.

34

BLOOD PRESSURE LOWERING TREATMENT AND THE PREVENTION OF STROKE IN THE DIABETIC PATIENT

John Chalmers* & Neil Chapman[†]

*Institute for International Health, University of Sydney, Sydney, Australia, [†]St Mary's Hospital, Paddington, London, UK

INTRODUCTION

Individuals with diabetes are at substantially greater risk of cardiovascular diseases than those without. Prospective observational studies suggest that the risk of fatal or non-fatal stroke is 2-3 fold greater among diabetics than non-diabetics [1-3], findings that cannot be explained by relative hyperglycaemia alone. However, raised blood pressure is common among individuals with diabetes [4,5] and blood pressure is a strong independent risk factor for cardiovascular diseases, particularly stroke [6]. In this chapter, we examine evidence of the benefits of blood pressure lowering therapy in preventing stroke among diabetics with or without hypertension.

BLOOD PRESSURE AND STROKE RISK AMONG DIABETICS

Among the general population, usual levels of both systolic and diastolic blood pressure are positively and continuously associated with the risk of stroke and there appears to be no threshold of blood pressure below, which this relationship fails to hold [6,7]. Overviews of prospective observational studies have shown that each 10mmHg lower level of usual systolic blood pressure and each 5mmHg lower level of usual diastolic blood pressure is associated with approximately 35-40% lower risk of fatal and non-fatal stroke [6,7]. While the majority of participants in the epidemiological studies included in these overviews did not have diabetes, where data do exist, the association between blood pressure and the risk of stroke appears to be similar among diabetics to that among non-diabetics (Figure 1). Similar continuous relationships have been observed among diabetic participants in clinical trials [8].

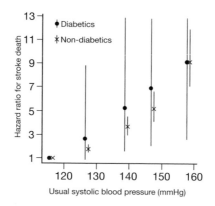

Figure 1. Association between usual systolic blood pressure and fatal stroke among individuals with and without diabetes.

Previously unpublished data from the first round of overview analyses of the Asia Pacific Cohort Studies Collaboration demonstrating similar associations between usual systolic blood pressure and the risk of fatal stroke among participants with and without diabetes (Personal Communication: Woodward M, 2003). Data are included from 24 prospective cohort studies that involved 4,873 participants with diabetes (72 fatal strokes) and 156,341 without (1,082 fatal strokes) [3].

OBSERVATIONAL STUDIES OF BLOOD PRESSURE LOWERING THERAPY AND THE PREVENTION OF STROKE

Early observational studies raised the possibility that blood pressure lowering treatment, particularly with diuretics, might be associated with a worsening of prognosis among hypertensive individuals with diabetes [9,10]. More recently, based on the results of case-control studies, cohort studies and some relatively small randomised trials, there had been concern that the use of calcium antagonists rather than other antihypertensive agents may result in greater cardiovascular morbidity and mortality among diabetics [11-13]. Such observational data, however, are prone to confounding [14] and in this instance they have not been confirmed by the results of clinical trials.

RANDOMISED CONTROLLED TRIALS OF BLOOD PRESSURE LOWERING THERAPY AND THE PREVENTION OF STROKE

There is now clear evidence from randomised clinical trials that treatment with the major classes of blood pressure lowering drugs is beneficial among hypertensive individuals with diabetes. The following sections summarise the effects of lowering blood pressure on the risk of stroke among diabetic participants in major clinical trials of blood pressure lowering therapy. Details of the trials that are discussed are summarised in Tables 1-3.

PLACEBO-CONTROLLED TRIALS OF BLOOD PRESSURE LOWERING THERAPY

Placebo-controlled trials of diuretic-based and beta-blocker-based therapy
By 1990, the benefits of blood pressure lowering on the risk of initial stroke among hypertensives had been clearly established from an overview of 14 randomised controlled trials that principally used regimens based on diuretics and beta-blockers [15]. The findings of these trials, which were mainly conducted among middle-aged subjects with mild-moderate essential hypertension, were subsequently extended by results of trials in older subjects with both essential hypertension and systolic hypertension. In combination, these trials demonstrated that net reductions of 10-12mmHg in usual systolic blood pressure and of 5-6 mm Hg in usual diastolic blood pressure were associated with a 38% reduction in the risk of stroke within just a few years of starting treatment [16], matching the benefit predicted from epidemiological studies [6,7].

Table 1. Characteristics of placebo-controlled trials of antihypertensive therapy that included participants with diabetes

Trial	Entry criteria	N		Mean age (years)		Entry BP (mmHg)		Difference in BP (active − placebo) during follow-up (mmHg)		Duration of follow-up (years)
		Overall	Diabetic (%)	Overall	Diabetic	Overall	Diabetic	Overall	Diabetic	
Diuretics vs. placebo										
SHEP [19, 22]	≥60 years, ISH	4,736	583 (12.3)	72	70	170/77	170/76	-12/4	-10/-2	4.5
PATS [23]	Stroke/TIA	5,665	NA	60	NA	154/93	NA	-5/-2	NA	2
ACE inhibitors vs. placebo										
HOPE [24,25]	CHD, CVD or DM+CVD RF	9,297	3,577 (38.5)	66	65	139/79	142/80	-3/-1	-2/-1	4.5
PROGRESS [26]	Stroke/TIA	6,105	762 (12.5)	64	NA	147/86	NA	-9/-4	NA	4
Calcium antagonists vs. placebo										
Syst-Eur [27, 28]	≥60 years, ISH	4,695	492 (10.5)	70	NA	174/85	175/84	-10/-5	-9/-4	2
Syst-China [29]	≥60 years, ISH	2,394	98 (4.1)	67	NA	170/86	NA	-9/-3	-6/-5	3
Angiotensin receptor blockers vs. placebo										
IDNT [30]	DM + HBP + nephropathy	1,715	1,715 (100%)	59	–	159/87	–	-4/-3	–	2.6
IRMA2 [31]	DM + HBP + microalbuminuria	590	590 (100%)	58	–	153/90	–	-2/0	–	2
RENAAL [32]	DM + nephropathy	1,513	1,513 (100%)	60	–	152/82	–	-2/0	–	3.4

Trial acronyms listed at end of chapter.
BP, blood pressure; CHD, coronary heart disease; CVD, cardiovascular disease; DM, diabetes mellitus; HBP, high blood pressure; ISH, isolated systolic hypertension; NA, data not available; RF, risk factor; TIA, transient ischaemic attack.

Table 2. Characteristics of trials comparing blood pressure lowering regimens based on different drug classes

Trial	Primary treatments compared	Entry criteria	n		Diabetic (%)	Mean age (years)		Entry BP (mmHg)		Duration of follow-up (years)
			Overall	Diabetic		Overall	Diabetic	Overall	Diabetic	
ABCD hypertensive [46]	CA vs. ACE-I	HBP + DM	470	470	(100%)	57	–	155/98	–	5
ABCD normotensive [47]	CA vs. ACE-I	DM + BP<140/90mmHg	480	480	(100%)	59	–	136/84	–	5.3
ALLHAT [33]	CA vs. ACE-I vs. D	HBP + CVD RF	33,357	12,063	(36.2%)	67	NA	146/84	NA	4.9
ALLHAT [45]	AB vs. D	HBP + CVD RF	24,335	NA	(35.6%)	67	NA	145/83	NA	3.3
ANBP2 [34]	ACE-I vs. D	>65 years + HBP	6,083	NA	(7%)	72	NA	168/91	NA	4.1
CAPP [35, 36]	ACE-I vs. D or BB	HBP	10,985	572	(4.9%)	53	55	161/99	163/97	6.1
FACET [48]	CA vs. ACE-I	DM + HBP	380	380	(100%)	63	–	170/95	–	2.5
INSIGHT [40]	CA vs. D	HBP + CVD RF	6,321	1,302	(20.6%)	65	NA	173/99	NA	4
LIFE [43, 44]	ARB vs. BB	HBP + LVH	9,193	1,195	(13.0%)	67	67	174/98	177/96	4.8
NORDIL [41]	CA vs. BB or D	HBP	10,881	727	(6.7%)	60	NA	173/106	NA	4.5
STOP-2 [37, 38]	CA vs. ACE-I vs. D or BB	≥70 years + HBP	6,614	719	(10.9%)	76	76	194/98	195/96	5
UKPDS [39]	ACE-I vs. BB	HBP + DM	758	758	(100%)	56	–	160/94	–	8.4

Trial acronyms listed at end of chapter.
AB, alpha-blocker; ACE-I, angiotensin converting enzyme inhibitor; ARB, angiotensin receptor blocker; BB, beta-blocker; CA, calcium antagonist; CVD, cardiovascular disease; D, diuretic; DM, diabetes mellitus; HBP, high blood pressure; LVH, left ventricular hypertrophy; NA, data not available; RF, risk factor.

Table 3. Characteristics of trials comparing blood pressure lowering strategies of different intensity

Trial	Target BP compared (mmHg)	Entry criteria	n		Mean age (years)		Entry BP (mmHg)		Achieved BP (mmHg)	Duration of follow-up (years)
			Overall	Diabetic (%)	Overall	Diabetic	Overall	Diabetic		
ABCD hypertensive [46]	DBP ≤75 mmHg vs. 80–89 mmHg	HBP + DM	470	470 (100%)	57	–	155/98	–	132/78 vs. 138/86	5
ABCD normotensive [47]	DBP 10 mmHG <baseline vs. 80–89 mmHg	DM + BP<140/90 mmHg	480	480 (480%)	59	–	136/84	–	137/81	5.3
HOT [49]	DBP ≤80 mmHg vs. ≤85 mmHg vs. ≤90 mmHg	HBP	18,790	1501 (8.0%)	61	NA	170/105	NA	140/81 vs. 141/83 vs. 144/85	3.8
UKPDS [53]	BP <150/85 mmHg vs. <180/105 mmHg	HBP + DM	1,148	1148 (100%)	56	–	160/94	–	144/82 vs. 154/87	8.4

Trial acronyms listed at end of chapter.
BP, blood pressure; DBP, diastolic blood pressure; DM, diabetes mellitus; HBP, high blood pressure; NA, data not available.

Despite the fact that raised blood pressure is frequent among individuals with diabetes [4,5], many of the earliest randomised trials either excluded diabetic patients or failed to report their inclusion. This may have been due to concerns about possible adverse metabolic effects of diuretics and beta-blockers [17] or concern that diuretics might increase mortality among hypertensive subjects with diabetes [9,10]. The INDANA Collaborative Group conducted a meta-analysis of individual participant data from three trials (HDFP, STOP-Hypertension and SHEP [18-20]) that did include diabetic participants, that used mainly diuretics as first-line therapy (with some use of beta-blockers), and that collected data on fatal and non-fatal stroke [21]. In combination, among 2,162 diabetic participants with hypertension, active treatment lowered blood pressure by 11/4mmHg more than placebo. The relative risk of stroke was reduced by 36% (95%CI 10-55) (Figure 2), a result virtually identical to that observed among non-diabetics (37% reduction [95%CI 24-47]). The results of SHEP, the only trial to have published results separately in diabetic and non-diabetic subgroups, were consistent with these overall findings (Figure 2) [22].

However, despite the similar *relative* benefits of treatment, the *absolute* benefit was almost twice as great among those with diabetes (29 vs. 15 strokes avoided for every 1,000 patients treated for 5 years), due to their greater absolute risk of stroke [21].

A single large-scale study, PATS, has compared a diuretic with placebo among individuals with prior stroke. The study was not adequately randomised and the preliminary published results provide no information about diabetic participants [23]. Overall, however, active treatment lowered blood pressure by 5/2mmHg and the relative risk of stroke by 29% (95%CI 12-42) compared with placebo.

Placebo-controlled trials of ACE-inhibitor-based therapy
More recently, two large placebo-controlled trials (HOPE and PROGRESS) have reported on the use of ACE-inhibitor-based drug regimens in different patient groups (Table 1).

The HOPE trial was conducted among high-risk hypertensive and normotensive patients, many of who had coronary artery disease at baseline [24]. Among diabetics, ACE inhibitor treatment lowered clinic blood pressure by 2/1mmHg more than placebo and the relative risk of stroke by 33% (95%CI 10-50) (Figure 2), results similar to those observed among the study population as a whole [24,25]. PROGRESS was conducted among normotensive and hypertensive participants with a history of cerebrovascular disease (stroke or transient ischaemic attack) [26]. Compared with placebo, ACE inhibitor-based treatment (with the addition of a diuretic if neither indicated nor contraindicated) lowered blood pressure by 9/4mmHg and the risk of stroke by 28% (95%CI 17-38). The benefits observed were similar among participants with and without diabetes (unpublished data), and among those with and without hypertension at baseline.

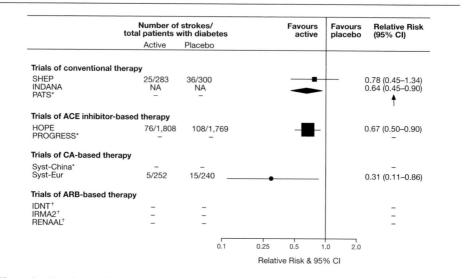

Figure 2: Results of placebo-controlled trials of blood pressure lowering therapy that included participants with diabetes

Relative risks of fatal and non-fatal stroke among diabetic participants in placebo-controlled trials of blood pressure lowering therapy. The size of each box is proportional to the number of strokes that occurred and horizontal lines represent 95% confidence intervals. The diamond represents the pooled estimate of treatment effect in three trials (HDFP, STOP-Hypertension and SHEP) included in the INDANA meta-analysis [21]. *Complete data in diabetic subgroup not published separately. †Data for the outcome of stroke not published.
(ACE, angiotensin converting enzyme; ARB, angiotensin receptor blocker; CA, calcium antagonist; CI, confidence interval; NA, data not available)

Placebo-controlled trials of calcium antagonist-based therapy
Although observational evidence led to concerns about the safety of calcium antagonist use among hypertensive diabetics [11-13], this has not been supported by evidence from clinical trials (Table 1).

Syst-Eur compared a dihydropyridine calcium antagonist with placebo among elderly subjects with systolic hypertension [27,28]. Among diabetic participants, active treatment lowered blood pressure by 9/4mmHg more than placebo and was associated with a 69% (95%CI 14-89) lower relative risk of stroke (Figure 2) [28]. These reductions were not significantly different from those observed among non-diabetics [27]. However, as in trials of diuretic therapy, the absolute treatment benefits were substantially greater among diabetics due to their greater absolute risk of stroke [28]. Similar, though non-significant, trends were observed in the smaller non-randomised Syst-China trial [29].

Placebo-controlled trials of angiotensin receptor blocker-based therapy

Three published trials (IDNT, IRMA2 and RENAAL) have assessed the effects of angiotensin receptor blockers among populations with diabetes (Table 1) [30-32]. In each case, active treatment was associated with a reduction in the primary endpoint, progression of renal disease. However, none had sufficient power to detect reductions in the risks of individual cardiovascular endpoints, and no results have so far been reported separately for the outcome of stroke.

In summary, placebo-controlled trials of blood pressure lowering therapy demonstrate that diuretics, beta-blockers, ACE inhibitors and calcium antagonists all substantially reduce the risk of stroke among individuals with diabetes. There is insufficient evidence from placebo-controlled trials of angiotensin receptor blockers to determine whether they confer similar benefits.

TRIALS COMPARING REGIMENS BASED ON DIFFERENT DRUG CLASSES

In the following trials that compared blood pressure lowering regimens based on different drug classes (Table 2), randomised groups were generally well matched in terms of blood pressure at study entry, and differences in blood pressure achieved during follow-up were generally small. Where differences in blood pressure achieved between randomised groups may have affected the results, this has been highlighted in the text.

Trials comparing ACE inhibitors with conventional therapy

Five major trials (ALLHAT, ANBP2, CAPPP, STOP-2 and UKPDS) that compared ACE inhibitor-based regimens with those based on conventional therapy (diuretics and/or beta-blockers) have contained substantial numbers of diabetic participants (Table 2) [33-39].

Among participants with diabetes in the ALLHAT, CAPPP, STOP-2 and UKPDS studies, no significant differences between the effects of each regimen were observed (Figure 3) [33,36,38,39]. In the recently published ANBP2 study, no difference in the risk of stroke was observed in the study population as a whole, although the results have not yet been published separately among diabetic participants [34].

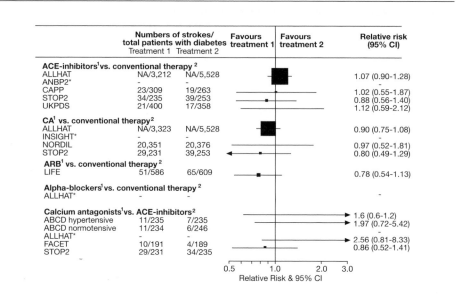

Figure 3: Results of trials that compared different classes of blood pressure lowering drug and included participants with diabetes

Relative risks of fatal and non-fatal stroke among diabetic participants in trials that compared different active blood pressure lowering regimens. The size of each box is proportional to the number of strokes that occurred and horizontal lines represent 95% confidence intervals. *Data in diabetic subgroup not published separately.
CI, confidence interval; NA, data not available.

In STOP-2 the result among diabetics was similar to that obtained overall [37]. In CAPPP, while there was an apparent benefit in favour of conventional therapy in the study population as a whole [35], differences in blood pressure between the randomised groups make the result difficult to interpret. ALLHAT is the largest trial of blood pressure lowering therapy to be completed to date. In the study population as a whole, the risk of stroke was significantly greater in those taking the ACE inhibitor than among those assigned the diuretic (relative risk [RR] 1.15 [95%CI 1.02-1.30]) [33]. However, this may be due, at least in part, to a 2mmHg difference in systolic blood pressure between the two groups during follow-up. The apparent benefit conferred by diuretic therapy appeared to be predominantly among black participants, among whom the blood pressure difference between the randomised groups was even greater.

When the results of all these studies are taken into consideration therefore, it seems unlikely that any substantial difference exists between the effects of diuretics and ACE inhibitors on the risk of stroke, independently of their effects on blood pressure.

Trials comparing calcium antagonists with conventional therapy

Four major trials (ALLHAT, INSIGHT, NORDIL and STOP-2) that compared calcium antagonist-based regimens with those based on conventional therapy have contained substantial numbers of diabetic participants (Table 2) [33,37,38,40,41]. Of these, one used a non-dihydropyridine [41] and the remainder used dihydropyridine agents. A further study, VHAS, excluded patients with uncontrolled diabetes and did not report numbers of participants with diabetes at study entry [42].

The INSIGHT study did not report results separately in subgroups with and without diabetes, but observed no difference between the regimens in the study group as a whole [40]. Among diabetic participants in the remaining three trials (ALLHAT, NORDIL and STOP-2), no significant differences between regimens were observed (Figure 3) [33,37,38,41]. In each case, the results in diabetics were not materially different from those observed among non-diabetics or the study population as a whole.

Trials comparing angiotensin receptor blockers with conventional therapy

Only one completed trial to date, the LIFE study, has compared an angiotensin receptor blocker with conventional therapy (a beta-blocker) (Table 2) [43,44]. Among diabetic participants, the risk of stroke did not differ significantly between the randomised groups (Figure 3) [44]. However, the magnitude of this result was similar to that observed in the whole study population, among whom angiotensin receptor blocker treatment was associated with marginally lower systolic blood pressure during follow-up and a significantly greater reduction in the relative risk of stroke (hazard ratio 0.74 [95%CI 0.63-0.88]) [43].

Thus, although placebo-controlled trials failed to demonstrate any reduction in the risk of stroke among participants treated with angiotensin receptor blockers [30-32], this result, albeit from a single trial, supports the use of this class of drug as they appear to be at least as effective as conventional therapy. Further randomised trials are required to confirm this finding.

Trials comparing alpha-blockers with diuretics and/or beta-blockers
Only one large trial, ALLHAT, has included a randomised comparison between an alpha-blocker and conventional therapy (a diuretic) (Table 2). The alpha-blocker arm of the trial was discontinued early due to significantly higher risks of heart failure and of stroke among those randomised to doxazosin (RR for stroke 1.19 [95%CI 1.01-1.40]) [45], findings that may be explained at least partially by the 2mmHg lower systolic blood pressure achieved during follow-up among participants assigned the diuretic. The result has not been published separately in subgroups with and without diabetes.

Trials comparing calcium antagonists with ACE inhibitors
Three major trials (ABCD, ALLHAT and STOP-2) have compared dihydropyridine calcium antagonist-based regimens with those based on ACE inhibitors (Table 2) [33,37,38,46,47]. A fourth, smaller, trial (FACET) compared a non-dihydropyridine agent with an ACE inhibitor [48].

The ABCD study was stopped early in a hypertensive subgroup due to an apparent extreme excess of cardiovascular (mainly coronary heart disease) events among participants randomised to the calcium antagonist [46]. No such difference between treatments was observed for the outcome of stroke. Likewise, no difference in stroke risk was observed in a normotensive subgroup of ABCD [47] or among diabetic participants in STOP-2 or FACET (Figure 3) [38,48]. All participants in ABCD and FACET were diabetic [46-48], and in STOP-2 the result in diabetic subjects was similar to that observed in the study population overall [37]. The results of the comparison between a calcium antagonist and an ACE inhibitor in ALLHAT have not yet been published. While examination of the published data suggests that there was a modest benefit in favour of calcium antagonist therapy in the study population as a whole (unadjusted relative risk 0.83 [95%CI 0.72-0.94]), once again, this may be partly related to the marginally lower blood pressure achieved in this group [33].

Overall, trials that have compared blood pressure lowering regimens based on different drug classes suggest that differences in their effects on the risk of stroke are modest, both among diabetics and among populations with hypertension. Where such differences have been found, they may be at least partially explained by differences in blood pressure between randomised groups, and their magnitude has tended to be less than that observed in placebo-controlled trials of blood pressure lowering therapy.

Trials comparing blood pressure lowering strategies of different intensity
Three trials (ABCD, HOT and UKPDS) have compared blood pressure lowering strategies of different intensity (Table 3) [46,47,49,50].

The ABCD and UKPDS trials were both conducted solely among diabetics and each compared groups randomised to one of two blood pressure targets [46,47,50]. More intensive blood pressure lowering reduced the risks of stroke in the UKPDS (RR 0.56 [95%CI 0.35-0.89]) [50] and in a normotensive subgroup of ABCD (RR 0.30 [95%CI 0.10-0.94]) (Figure 4) [47]. No such benefit was observed in the hypertensive subgroup of ABCD [46,51]. In the HOT study, diabetic and non-diabetic participants were randomised to one of three target blood pressures [49]. However, differences between the blood pressures achieved in each group were small and there was no significant trend in the risk of stroke with differing intensity of blood pressure control, either overall or in the subgroup of participants with diabetes.

Overall, the two studies in diabetic populations suggest that more intensive blood pressure lowering strategies lower the risk of stroke. While no such benefit was observed in HOT, this is likely to result from the close similarity between the blood pressures achieved in each randomised group.

GUIDELINES AND RECOMMENDATIONS

Current national and international guidelines on the management of hypertension emphasise the need for effective lowering of blood pressure in diabetic subjects to reduce the high risk of cardiovascular complications such as stroke and myocardial infarction. Both JNC-VI and WHO-ISH 1999 specifically recommend a lower threshold for institution of blood pressure lowering treatment, and a lower target blood pressure for such treatment, in diabetics than in hypertensive patients without diabetes [52,53]; both recommend that drug treatment be initiated for diabetic subjects with blood pressure in the "high normal range" (systolic blood pressure 130-139mmHg and diastolic blood pressure 85-89mmHg) and both emphasise the need to normalise blood pressure in these subjects to levels below 130/85mmHg.

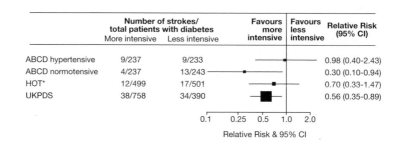

	Number of strokes/ total patients with diabetes		Favours more intensive	Favours less intensive	Relative Risk (95% CI)
	More intensive	Less intensive			
ABCD hypertensive	9/237	9/233			0.98 (0.40-2.43)
ABCD normotensive	4/237	13/243			0.30 (0.10-0.94)
HOT*	12/499	17/501			0.70 (0.33-1.47)
UKPDS	38/758	34/390			0.56 (0.35-0.89)

0.1   0.25   0.5   1.0   2.0

Relative Risk & 95% CI

Figure 4: Results of trials that compared blood pressure lowering strategies of different intensity and included participants with diabetes

Relative risks of fatal and non-fatal stroke among diabetic participants in trials that compared blood pressure lowering strategies of different intensities. The size of each box is proportional to the number of strokes that occurred and horizontal lines represent 95% confidence intervals. *For HOT, the risk of stroke in the most intensive group (target diastolic BP ≤80mmHg) is compared with that in the least intensive group (target ≤90mmHg) [49].
CI, confidence interval

As a result of these recommendations, one of the major challenges facing clinicians responsible for the care of diabetic patients will be to achieve adequate blood pressure control at a time when blood pressure is lowered to below 140/90mmHg in less than one quarter of the hypertensive population [54,55]. Given that the target blood pressure is even more stringent in the diabetic patient, it is clear that therapy with combinations of blood pressure lowering drugs will be needed in the majority of diabetic patients [49,50].

While there has been extensive debate about the merits of different classes of blood pressure lowering drug, there is now substantial evidence that any of five major classes of drug (diuretics, beta-blockers, ACE inhibitors, calcium antagonists and angiotensin receptor blockers) is effective in the primary prevention of stroke (i.e. the prevention of initial stroke) in hypertensive subjects. While there is less direct evidence in individuals with diabetes, with or without hypertension, the available evidence supports the use of each class of drug to lower blood pressure in such patients.

There is even less evidence that particular drug classes have specific advantages over one another in the primary prevention of stroke among diabetics. Randomised trials that have compared different classes of drug suggest that any differences are likely to be less important than lowering blood pressure with any effective agent rather than none. Furthermore, the evidence from comparative studies of blood pressure lowering drugs confirms that diuretics are at least as effective in preventing stroke as newer agents. This is likely to be confirmed in the next round of prospectively designed overview analyses conducted by the Blood Pressure Lowering Treatment Trialists' Collaboration [51], publication of which is anticipated in 2003. In the light of this evidence, and of their cost advantage over newer and more expensive drugs, it seems reasonable to recommend that diuretics should be included in any blood pressure lowering regimen in diabetic subjects, unless coexistent conditions in particular patients favour the use of other classes of drugs [52,53].

As documented in an ISH Statement on Blood Pressure Lowering and Stroke Prevention [56], recent evidence also confirms the value of reducing blood pressure for the prevention of recurrent stroke, though data are currently limited to diuretics and ACE inhibitors [23,25,26]. These studies demonstrated similar relative reductions in the risk of recurrent stroke in patients with and without hypertension, and in those with and without diabetes. There is currently little evidence regarding differential effects across drug classes and, once again, such differences as might exist are likely to be less important than the benefits conferred by any treatment compared with none [56].

Finally, while lifestyle measures for lowering blood pressure are beyond the scope of this chapter, it must be emphasised that attention to non-drug factors such as weight control, restriction of alcohol consumption, and adequate physical activity are even more important in diabetics than in hypertensive subjects without diabetes, and form an indispensable foundation for drug treatment.

CONCLUSIONS

Usual levels of blood pressure are positively and continuously associated with the risk of stroke among diabetics as well as the general population, and diabetics are at increased risk of stroke compared with non-diabetics. Randomised controlled trials have shown that lowering blood pressure reduces the risk of both primary and secondary stroke, as well as other forms of cardiovascular disease, and most trials suggest that the relative benefits of blood pressure lowering are similar among those with and without diabetes. However, due to the greater risk of stroke among those with diabetes, the absolute benefits of treatment tend to be substantially greater than among non-diabetics.

Both the threshold above which blood pressure lowering therapy is recommended, and the target blood pressure below which it should be reduced, are lower in those with diabetes than in those without. Measures to lower blood pressure should include lifestyle factors as well as drug treatment and most patients will require more than a single agent in order to achieve currently recommended levels of control. All five major classes of blood pressure lowering drug reduce the risk of stroke and the initial choice of drug is probably of less importance than the choice of any drug rather than none.

ACKNOWLEDGEMENTS

We would like to thank Mark Woodward of the Institute for International Health for providing previously unpublished data from the Asia Pacific Cohort Studies Collaboration and Sam Colman from the same Institute for assistance with the preparation of figures.

Trial acronyms:
ABCD – Appropriate Blood Pressure Control in Diabetes Study
ALLHAT – Antihypertensive and Lipid-Lowering Treatment to Prevent Heart Attack Trial
ANBP2 – Second Australian National Blood Pressure Study
CAPPP – Captopril Prevention Project
FACET – Fosinopril versus Amlodipine Cardiovascular Events Randomized Trial
HDFP – Hypertension Detection and Follow-up Program
HOPE – Heart Outcomes Prevention Evaluation Study
IDNT – Irbesartan Diabetic Nephropathy Trial
INDANA – Individual Data Analysis of Antihypertensive Drug Interventions
INSIGHT – International Nifedipine GITS Study: Intervention as a Goal in Hypertension Study

IRMA2 – Irbesartan in Patients with Type 2 Diabetes and Microalbuminuria Study

LIFE – Losartan Intervention for Endpoint Reduction in Hypertension Study

NORDIL – Nordic Diltiazem Study

PATS – Post-Stroke Antihypertensive Treatment Study

PROGRESS – Perindopril Protection Against Recurrent Stroke Study

RENAAL – Reduction of Endpoints in NIDDM with the Angiotensin II Antagonist Losartan Study

SHEP – Systolic Hypertension in the Elderly Program

STOP-Hypertension – Swedish Trial in Old Patients with Hypertension

STOP-2 – Swedish Trial in Old Patients with Hypertension-2

Syst-Eur – Systolic Hypertension in Europe Trial

Syst-China – Systolic Hypertension in China Trial

UKPDS – United Kingdom Prospective Diabetes Study

VHAS – Verapamil in Hypertension and Atherosclerosis Study

REFERENCES

1. Stamler J, Vaccaro O, Neaton J, Wentworth D. Diabetes, other risk factors, and 12-year cardiovascular mortality for men screened in the Multiple Risk Factor Intervention Trial. *Diabetes Care* 1993; 16: 434-444.

2. Abbott R, Donahue R, MacMahon S. Diabetes and the risk of stroke: the Honolulu Heart Project. *JAMA* 1987; 257: 949-52.

3. Asia Pacific Cohort Studies Collaboration. The effects of diabetes on the risks of major cardiovascular diseases and death in the Asia-Pacific region. *Diabetes Care* 2003; 26: 360-6.

4. World Health Organization Multinational Study of Vascular Disease in Diabetics: Prevalence of small vessel and large vessel disease in diabetic patients from 14 centres. *Diabetologia* 1985; 28: 615-40.

5. Hypertension in Diabetes Study (HDS). I. Prevalence of hypertension in newly presenting type 2 diabetic patients and the association with risk factors for cardiovascular and diabetic complications. *J Hypertens* 1993; 11: 309-17.

6. MacMahon S, Peto R, Cutler J, *et al.* Blood pressure, stroke, and coronary heart disease. Part 1, prolonged differences in blood pressure: prospective observational studies corrected for the regression dilution bias. *Lancet* 1990; 335: 765-774.

7. Eastern Stroke and Coronary Heart Disease Collaborative Research Group. Blood pressure, cholesterol, and stroke in eastern Asia. *Lancet* 1998; 352: 1801-7.

8. Adler A, Stratton I, Neil H, *et al.* Association of systolic blood pressure with macrovascular and microvascular complications of type 2 diabetes (UKPDS 36): prospective observational study. *Brit Med J* 2000; 321: 412-9.

9. Klein R, Moss S, Klein B, DeMets D. Relation of ocular and systemic factors to survival in diabetes. *Arch Int Med* 1989; 149: 266-72.

10. Warram J, Laffel L, Valsania P, Christlieb A, Krolewski A. Excess mortality associated with diuretic therapy in diabetes mellitus. *Arch Int Med* 1991; 151: 1350-6.

11. Alderman M, Madhaven S, Cohen H. Calcium antagonists and cardiovascular events in patients with hypertension and diabetes. *Lancet* 1998; 351: 216-7.

12. Pahor M, Psaty B, Furberg C. Treatment of hypertensive patients with diabetes. *Lancet* 1998; 351: 689-90.

13. Pahor M, Psaty B, Furberg C. New evidence on the prevention of cardiovascular events in hypertensive patients with type 2 diabetes. *J Cardiovasc Pharmacol* 1998; 32 (Suppl 2): S18-S23.

14. MacMahon S, Collins R. Reliable assessment of the effects of treatment on mortality and major morbidity, II: observational studies. *Lancet* 2001; 357: 455-62.

15. Collins R, Peto R, MacMahon S, *et al.* Blood pressure, stroke, and coronary heart disease. Part 2, short-term reductions in blood pressure: overview of randomised drug trials in their epidemiological context. *Lancet* 1990; 335: 827-39.

16. MacMahon S, Rodgers A. Hypertension and the prevention of stroke. *J Hypertens* 1994; 12 (Suppl. 10): S5-14.

17. Flamenbaum W. Metabolic consequences of antihypertensive therapy. *Ann Int Med* 1983; 98: 875-80.

18. Hypertension Detection and Follow-up Program Cooperative Group. Five-year findings of the Hypertension Detection and Follow-up Program. III. Reduction in stroke incidence among persons with high blood pressure. *JAMA* 1982; 247: 633-8.

19. SHEP Cooperative Research Group. Prevention of stroke by antihypertensive drug treatment in older persons with isolated systolic hypertension: Final results of the Systolic Hypertension in the Elderly Program (SHEP). *JAMA* 1991; 265: 3255-64.

20. Dahlof B, Lindholm LH, Hansson L, *et al.* Morbidity and mortality in the Swedish trial in old patients with hypertension (STOP-Hypertension). *Lancet* 1991; 338: 1281-4.

21. Lievre M, Gueyffier F, Ekbom T, *et al.* Efficacy of diuretics and beta-blockers in diabetic hypertensive patients: results from a meta-analysis. *Diabetes Care* 2000; 23 (Suppl 2): B65-B71.

22. Curb J, Pressel S, Cuttler J, *et al.* Effect of diuretic-based antihypertensive treatment on cardiovascular disease risk in older diabetic patients with isolated systolic hypertension. *J Am Med assoc* 1996; 276: 1886-1892.

23. PATS Collaborating Group. Post-stroke antihypertensive treatment study. A preliminary result. *Chin Med J* 1995; 108: 710-7.

24. Heart Outcomes Prevention Evaluation (HOPE) Study Investigators. Effects of ramipril on cardiovascular and microvascular outcomes in people with diabetes mellitus: results of the HOPE and MICRO-HOPE substudy. *Lancet* 2000; 355: 253-9.

25. Bosch J, Yusuf S, Pogue J, *et al.* Use of ramipril in preventing stroke: double blind randomised trial. *Br Med J* 2002; 324: 1-5.

26. PROGRESS Collaborative Group. Randomised trial of a perindopril-based blood pressure lowering regimen among 6,105 individuals with previous stroke or transient ischaemic attack. *Lancet* 2001; 358: 1033-41.

27. Staessen J, Fagard R, Thijs L, *et al.* Randomised double-blind comparison of placebo and active treatment for older patients with isolated systolic hypertension. *Lancet* 1997; 350: 757-764.

28. Tuomilehto J, Rastenyte D, Birkenhager W, *et al.* Effects of calcium-channel blockade in older patients with diabetes and systolic hypertension. *N Engl J Med* 1999; 340: 677-684.

29. Wang J-G, Staessen J, Gong L, Liu L, for the Systolic Hypertension in China (Syst-China) Collaborative Group. Chinese trial on isolated systolic hypertension in the elderly. *Arch Int Med* 2000; 160: 211-20.

30. Lewis E, Hunsicker L, Clarke W, *et al.* Renoprotective effect of the angiotensin-receptor antagonist irbesartan in patients with nephropathy due to type 2 diabetes. *N Engl J Med* 2001; 345: 851-60.

31. Parving H, Lehnert H, Brochner-Mortensen J, *et al.* The effect of irbesartan on the development of diabetic nephropathy in patients with type 2 diabetes. *N Engl J Med* 2001; 345: 870-8.

32. Brenner B, Cooper M, de Zeeuw D, *et al.* Effects of losartan on renal and cardiovascular outcomes in patients with type 2 diabetes and nephropathy. *N Eng J Med* 2001; 345: 861-9.

33. The ALLHAT Officers and Coordinators for the ALLHAT Collaborative Research Group. Major outcomes in high-risk hypertensive patients randomized to angiotensin-converting enzyme inhibitor or calcium channel blocker vs diuretic. *JAMA* 2002; 288: 2981-97.

34. Wing L, Reid C, Ryan P, *et al.* A comparison of outcomes with angiotensin-converting-enzyme inhibitors and diuretics for hypertension in the elderly. *N Engl J Med* 2003; 348: 583-92.

35. Hansson L, Lindholm L, Niskanen L, *et al.* Effect of angiotensin converting enzyme inhibition compared with conventional therapy on cardiovascular morbidity and mortality in hypertension: the Captopril Prevention Project (CAPPP) randomised trial. *Lancet* 1999; 353: 611-616.

36. Niskanen L, Lanke J, Hedner T, *et al.* Reduced cardiovascular morbidity and mortality in hypertensive diabetic patients on first-line therapy with an ACE inhibitor compared with a diuretic/beta-blocker-based treatment regimen. *Diabetes Care* 2001; 24: 2091-6.

37. Hansson L, Lindholm L, Ekbom T, *et al.* Randomised trial of old and new antihypertensive drugs in elderly patients: cardiovascular mortality and morbidity in the Swedish Trial in Old Patients with Hypertension-2 study. *Lancet* 1999; 354: 1751-56.

38. Lindholm L, Hansson L, Ekbom T, *et al.* Comparison of antihypertensive treatments in preventing cardiovascular events in elderly diabetic patients: results from the Swedish Trial in Old Patients with Hypertension-2. *J Hypertens* 2000; 18: 1671-5.

39. UK Prospective Diabetes Study Group. Efficacy of atenolol and captopril in reducing risk of macrovascular and microvascular complications in type 2 diabetes. *Br Med J* 1998; 317: 713-720.

40. Brown M, Palmer C, Castaigne A, *et al.* Morbidity and mortality in patients randomised to double-blind treatment with a long-acting calcium-channel blocker or diuretic in the International Nifedipine GITS study: Intervention as a Goal in Hypertension Treatment. *Lancet* 2000; 356: 366-72.

41. Hansson L, Hedner T, Lund-Johansen P, *et al.* Randomised trial of effects of calcium antagonists compared with diuretics and beta-blockers on cardiovascular morbidity and mortality in hypertension: the Nordic Diltiazem (NORDIL) study. *Lancet* 2000; 356: 359-65.

42. Agabiti-Rosei E, Dal Palu C, Leonetti G, *et al.* Clinical results of the Verapamil in Hypertension and Atherosclerosis Study. *J Hypertens* 1997; 15: 1337-44.

43. Dahlof B, Devereux R, Kjeldsen S, *et al.* Cardiovascular morbidity and mortality in the Losartan Intervention For Endpoint reduction in hypertension study (LIFE): a randomised trial against atenolol. *Lancet* 2002; 359: 995-1003.

44. Lindholm L, Ibsen H, Dahlof B, *et al.* Cardiovascular morbidity and mortality in patients with diabetes in the Losartan Intervention For Endpoint reduction in hypertension study (LIFE): a randomised trial against atenolol. *Lancet* 2002; 359: 1004-10.

45. The ALLHAT Officers and Coordinators for the ALLHAT Collaborative Research Group. Major cardiovascular events in hypertensive patients randomized to doxazosin vs chlorthalidone. *JAMA* 2000; 283: 1967-75.

46. Estacio R, Jeffers B, Hiatt W, *et al.* The effect of nisoldipine as compared with enalapril on cardiovascular outcomes in patients with non-insulin dependant diabetes and hypertension. *N Engl J Med* 1998; 338: 645-652.

47. Schrier R, Estacio R, Esler A, Mehler P. Effects of aggressive blood pressure control in normotensive type 2 diabetic patients on albuminuria, retinopathy and strokes. *Kidney Int* 2002; 61: 1086-97.

48. Tatti P, Pahor M, Byington R, *et al.* Outcome results of the fosinopril versus amlodipine cardiovascular events randomised trial (FACET) in patients with hypertension and NIDDM. *Diabetes Care* 1998; 21: 597-603.

49. Hansson L, Zanchetti A, Carruthers S, *et al.* Effects of intensive blood pressure lowering and low-dose aspirin in patients with hypertension: principal results of the hypertension optimal treatment (HOT) randomised trial. *Lancet* 1998; 351: 1755-1762.

50. UK Prospective Diabetes Study Group. Tight blood pressure control and risk of macrovascular and microvascular complications in type 2 diabetes. *Br Med J* 1998; 317: 703-713.

51. Blood Pressure Lowering Treatment Trialists' Collaboration. Effects of ACE inhibitors, calcium antagonists, and other blood-pressure-lowering drugs: results of prospectively designed overviews of randomised trials. *Lancet* 2000; 356: 1955-64.

52. The Sixth Report of the Joint National Committee on Prevention, Detection, Evaluation and Treatment of High Blood Pressure. *Arch Int Med* 1997; 157: 2413-46.

53. 1999 World Health Organization - International Society of Hypertension Guidelines for the Management of Hypertension. *J Hypertens* 1999; 17: 151-83.

54. Burt V, Cutler J, Higgins M, *et al.* Trends in the prevalence, awareness, treatment, and control of hypertension in the adult US population. Data from the health examination surveys, 1960 to 1991. *Hypertension* 1995; 26(1): 60-9.

55. EUROASPIRE II Study Group. Lifestyle and risk factor management and use of drug therapies in coronary patients from 15 countries; principal results from EUROASPIRE II Euro Heart Survey Programme. *Eur Heart J* 2001; 22: 554-72.

56. International Society of Hypertension (ISH) Statement on blood pressure lowering and stroke prevention. *J Hypertens* 2003; In Press.

35

NON-GLYCAEMIC INTERVENTION IN DIABETIC NEPHROPATHY: THE ROLE OF DIETARY PROTEIN AND SALT INTAKE

Henrik Post Hansen
Steno Diabetes Center, Copenhagen, Denmark

INTRODUCTION

Although long-term antihypertensive treatment has proved to reduce the average rate of decline in glomerular filtration rate (GFR) to approximately 5 ml/min/year [1] and improve survival in patients with diabetic nephropathy [2-7], the variation in rate of decline between individuals is still large, and these patients still have an increased mortality due to end-stage renal disease [ESRD] and cardio-vascular disease (CVD) as compared to patients without diabetic nephropathy [8]. New strategies for delaying the progression of renal failure and improving survival in patients with diabetic nephropathy are needed. Dietary protein restriction has long been advocated as a method for relieving symptoms in patients with advanced renal failure [9]. All major observational studies in type 1 and type 2 diabetic patients with diabetic nephropathy have failed to show an impact of dietary protein intake on the rate of decline in GFR [10-12]. However, since numerous experimental studies in animals [13-16] have suggested a beneficial effect of dietary protein restriction on survival and development of ESRD, new interest in dietary protein restriction as a strategy to retard the progression of chronic renal disease in man has been reawakened during the last 2 to 3 decades [17].

This chapter discusses the short-term impact of dietary protein intake on renal function and examines the long-term effects of the therapeutic manoeuvre of

Mogensen CE (ed.) THE KIDNEY AND HYPERTENSION IN DIABETES MELLITUS. Copyright©
2004 by Martin Dunitz, a member of the Taylor & Francis Group, plc. All rights reserved.

restricting dietary protein in diabetic nephropathy. The implication of dietary salt restriction will further be commented.

SHORT-TERM RENAL EFFECTS OF DIETARY PROTEIN INTAKE

Healthy subjects

For more than half a century it has been recognised that short-term changes in dietary protein intake is followed by significant alterations in GFR and renal plasma flow (RPF) in healthy subjects. Originally, Nielsen et al. [18] in 1948 demonstrated a decline in GFR of 7% in 8 healthy women during a low-protein, low caloric diet of two weeks. Subsequently, Pullman et al. [19] in 1954 extended this observation and documented a decline in GFR of 9% and RPF of 6 % in 20 healthy subjects after two weeks treatment with a low protein diet (average 0.3 g/kg/day), compared to a usual-protein diet (average 1.0 g/kg/day). It was further demonstrated that a short-term high-protein diet (average 2.6 g/kg/day) increased GFR and RPF, 13 % and 12 %, respectively, compared to a usual protein diet. Several investigators have since verified these findings [20-25].

Patients with diabetes mellitus

During a short-term high protein diet an increase in GFR and RPF has been demonstrated in most studies of type 1 diabetic patients with normo- and microalbuminuria [26-29], while a short-term low protein diet induces a decline in GFR of 10 % in these patients, although RPF remains unchanged [30-33].

In patients with diabetic nephropathy, however, no change in GFR in response to a high protein diet has been observed [34]. The setting of severe renal injury with maximal perfusion of residual renal tissue has been suggested in this setting. Three studies, using valid markers of GFR, have previously investigated the short-term impact of dietary protein restriction in diabetic nephropathy [35-37]. However, in two randomised crossover trials, neither Bending et al. [35] nor Pinto et al. [37] demonstrated any significant changes in GFR, measured by a continuous infusion technique with timed urine collections, during 3 weeks of dietary protein restriction [achieved 0.64 g/kg/day] in 10 type 1 diabetic patients with diabetic nephropathy. Nevertheless, diabetic cystopathy, a common feature in patients with diabetic nephropathy, often leads to major errors in urine collections [38], and may have blurred the results in these two studies.

In a prospective controlled trial with concealed randomisation, Hansen et al. [36] demonstrated a reversible decline in GFR (^{51}Cr-EDTA plasma clearance) and albuminuria in 14 type 1 diabetic patients with diabetic nephropathy during short-term (3-5 weeks) treatment with a low protein diet (recommended 0.6 g/kg/day). Correspondingly with a decrease in dietary protein intake of 0.4 g/kg/day, there was a reversible decline in GFR and albuminuria of approximately 8 % and 29 %, respectively. These changes were independent of glycaemic control, energy intake and blood pressure. The initial decline in GFR during dietary protein restriction was greater in patients with elevated GFR, as demonstrated in the MDRD study [39]. Interestingly, the antiproteinuric effect of dietary protein restriction was obtained during antihypertensive treatment [mostly with ACE-inhibitors] and was associated to the degree of dietary protein restriction, suggesting at least partly independent but additive effects of these two treatment modalities on albuminuria (see below).

In conclusion, short-term dietary protein restriction induces a parallel reduction in GFR in both healthy subjects and diabetic patients with normo- and microalbuminuria. Although controversial, recent data highly suggests an equivalent decline in GFR and albuminuria during dietary protein restriction in type 1 diabetic patients with diabetic nephropathy. Studies in patients with non-diabetic nephropathies have similarly demonstrated an acute decline in GFR and proteinuria after the initiation of dietary protein restriction [40], and further suggested an additive effect of dietary protein restriction and ACE inhibition [enalapril] on proteinuria [41;42], independently of the action on GFR.

Implications of short-term renal effects of dietary protein restriction

The short-term renal effects of dietary protein restriction may have considerable implications in clinical practice and trials. The short-term renal effects of dietary protein restriction theoretically may offset the potential long-term beneficial effect of this treatment on the progression of kidney disease, especially if the trial is of short duration (less than two to three years) and the rate of progression in kidney disease is slow [39].

Renal mechanisms of dietary protein intake

The exact mechanisms by which dietary protein restriction modulates kidney function are unclear, but both haemodynamic and non-haemodynamic factors seem to be modified by dietary protein restriction in chronic renal diseases.

The majority of animal studies have demonstrated a decline in glomerular capillary hydraulic pressure and renal plasma flow during dietary protein restriction due to renal vasoconstriction, located primarily at the site of the afferent arteriole [43-45]. Recently, it has been hypothesised that short-term dietary protein restriction may contribute to an improvement of impaired autoregulation of GFR [36] seen in patients with diabetic nephropathy [46;47]. However, although changes in the tubuloglomerular feedback system, renal synthesis of prostaglandin's, hormonal factors, endothelium-derived relaxing factor and the renin-angiotensin system [48], have been suggested as mediators of the haemodynamic response to protein intake, data are still controversial.

A considerable number of non-haemodynamic effects of dietary protein restriction have been identified [49]. Diminished proteinase activity in glomeruli and tubules, associated with renal hypertrophy characterised by accumulation of cellular protein and extracellular matrix, seen in several models of glomerulosclerosis [49-51], is stimulated during dietary protein restriction [52], while renal overproduction of TGF-β, a key mediator of progressive matrix accumulation and tissue fibrosis [53;54] is reduced during dietary protein restriction in several models of renal disease [55-57]. Recent data by Peters et al. [16] demonstrated that single therapy with maximal effective doses of enalapril, losartan, and dietary protein restriction significantly reduced glomerular TGF-β production to a similar degree (45 %) in experimental glomerulonephritis. However, when either maximal doses of enalapril or losartan were combined with low-protein feeding a further reduction in TGF-β production of approximately 15 % was demonstrated. The reduction in TGF-β over-expression was associated with a decrease in proteinuria and glomerular matrix accumulation. These data highly suggest that dietary protein restriction acts on pathways in addition to blocking of the renin-angiotensin system as mentioned above. Previous studies in experimental renal failure support these findings [15;58].

LONG-TERM RENAL EFFECTS OF DIETARY PROTEIN RESTRICTION

Progression of diabetic nephropathy

A valid determination of the rate of decline in GFR in patients with chronic renal disease requires a reliable method for the determination of GFR, repeated measurements of the GFR, and a follow-up of at least 2 years [59]. However, when short-term effects of intervention are likely, rate of decline in GFR is slow, and the hypothesised benefit of the intervention is proportional to the rate of decline in GFR without intervention, a time-to-event (ESRD/death) approach is favoured compared to a slope-based analysis [60]. If not accounted for in the design of the study, it would be expected that patients receiving a low protein diet would start dialysis later than patients with higher protein intake [61].

An ideal marker for the determination of GFR should be freely filtered through the glomerular capillary wall, biological inert, and neither secreted nor reabsorbed by the kidney tubules. ^{51}Cr-EDTA or ^{125}I-iothalamate has proved to be valid markers for the determination of the GFR [62], compared to serum creatinine and creatinine clearance. Creatinine clearance progressively overestimates GFR during deterioration of kidney function [63]. Furthermore, the generation of creatinine is influenced by muscle mass and dietary protein intake [64]. In studies dealing with the impact of dietary protein restriction, the effect of the intervention on renal creatinine handling invalidates serum creatinine as a measurement of renal function, as demonstrated in the MDRD study [65].

Impact of dietary protein restriction on the development of diabetic nephropathy

Persistent microalbuminuria precedes and predicts the development of diabetic nephropathy in both type 1 [66] and type 2 [67] diabetic patients. Two randomised and controlled trials have evaluated the beneficial effect of long-term dietary protein restriction on the course of urinary albumin excretion in type 1 [68] and type 2 [69] diabetic patients without diabetic nephropathy.

Dullaart et al. [68] performed a 2-year prospective and controlled trial with concealed randomisation in 30 type 1 diabetic patients with a mean urinary albumin excretion between 10 and 200 µg/min. Fourteen patients were assigned to a low protein diet [pre-scribed 0.6 g/kg/day] and 16 patients were assigned to continue their usual protein diet. The average protein intake during the study was 0.79 g/kg/day in the low protein diet group and 1.09 g/kg/day in the usual protein diet group [p<0.001, between groups]. Although urinary albumin excretion decreased by 16 % in the low protein diet group during the study, this was not significantly different from the decrease of 5 % in the usual protein diet group. After adjustment for blood pressure and diabetes duration the low protein diet group had a decrease in urinary albumin excretion of 26 % during follow-up, compared to 5 % in the usual protein diet group [p<0.005, between groups]. Glomerular filtration rate [measured with ^{125}I-iothalamate] decreased significantly in both diet groups during follow-up (non-significantly between groups).

Pijls et al. [69] performed a 1-year randomised, controlled and physician-blinded trial in type 2 diabetic patients with microalbuminuria or urinary albumin excretion >20 mg/24 h or diabetes duration of ≥5 years. Originally 160 patients were randomised, but due to loss to follow-up only data from 121 patients were analysed. Fifty-eight patients received a low protein diet [prescribed 0.8 g/kg] and 63 patients received their usual protein diet during follow-up. After 6 months, dietary protein intake slightly but significantly decreased by 0.05 g/kg in the low protein diet group, while an increase of 0.03 g/kg was demonstrated in the usual protein diet group (p<0.02, between groups). No significant change in dietary protein intake was seen between diet regimens after 12 months. Correspondingly, after 6 and 12 months, urinary albumin excretion was found to be 22 % (p<0.01) and 12 % (NS) lower in the low protein diet group compared to the usual protein diet group. After adjustment for diastolic blood pressure, urinary albumin excretion was 25 % (p<0.004) and 15 % (NS) lower in the low protein diet group after 6 and 12 months, respectively. Glomerular filtration rate, measured by creatinine clearance, remained unchanged in both diet groups during follow-up.

In conclusion, it is suggested by the studies of Dullaart et al. [68] and Pijls et al. [69] that dietary protein restriction may have a beneficial effect on the development of diabetic nephropathy in both type 1 and type 2 diabetic patients. However, adherence to a low protein diet was especially difficult to obtain in type 2 diabetic patients. Future studies have to confirm a beneficial impact of dietary protein restriction in these patients during treatment with blockers of the renin-angiotensin-system [70;71], now widely recommended.

Impact of dietary protein restriction on the progression of diabetic nephropathy

Three larger, long-term and controlled trials using valid markers of GFR (^{51}Cr-EDTA [61;72] or ^{125}I-iothalamate [73]) have evaluated the impact of dietary protein restriction on the progression of diabetic nephropathy in type 1 diabetic patients. Unfortunately, no similar studies have been performed in type 2 diabetic patients with diabetic nephropathy. However, in the Modification of Diet in Renal Disease (MDRD) study [40] 3 % of the patients had type 2 diabetes mellitus. This study tested the efficacy of dietary protein restriction upon the progression of various chronic renal diseases.

Walker et al. [72] performed a non-randomised, self-controlled trial in 19 type 1 diabetic patients with diabetic nephropathy. A period on a normal protein diet [achieved 1.13 g/kg/day] of 29 months was followed by a period on a low protein diet (achieved 0.67 g/kg/day) of 33 months. The rate of decline in GFR was 7.3 ml/min/year during a normal protein diet and 1.7 ml/min/year during a low protein diet (p<0.001). Similarly, there was a significant decline in urinary albumin excretion from 467 mg/24 h during a normal protein diet to 340 mg/24 h during a low protein diet (p=0.01). However, at baseline 9 patients were treated with antihypertensive drugs. In 9 of 19 patients, antihypertensive treatment was initiated or intensified during protein restriction, leading to a reduction in mean blood pressure from 106 to 102 mm Hg [72]. Blood pressure is a well-known progression promoter in diabetic nephropathy [74]. Previous studies in both diabetic and non-diabetic nephropathies have demonstrated a progressive, time dependent reduction in the rate of decline in GFR during long-term antihypertensive treatment [4;75;76] of unknown mechanism. This phenomenon may, in part, explain the findings in this self-controlled trial.

Zeller et al. [73] performed a prospective, controlled trial in 35 type 1 diabetic patients with diabetic nephropathy. Twenty patients were assigned to a low protein diet (pre-scribed 0.6 g/kg/day; achieved 0.72 g/kg/day) and followed for an average of 37 months, while 15 patients were assigned to continue their usual protein diet (achieved 1.08 g/kg/day; p<0.001, between groups) and were followed for 31 months. The rate of decline in GFR was 3.1 ml/min/year in the low protein diet group, while the decline in GFR was 12.1 ml/min/year in the usual protein diet group despite antihypertensive treatment, similar to what has been demonstrated during the natural course of diabetic nephropathy in patients not receiving antihypertensive treatment [77]. Approximately 25 percent of these patients, but none of the patients in the low protein diet group, had a follow-up of less than 10 months. Baseline proteinuria and mean blood pressure during follow-up were higher in the usual protein diet group (4.3 g/24-h and 106 mm Hg, respectively) as compared to the low protein diet group (3.1 g/24-h and 102 mm Hg, respectively), which could indeed have contributed to the accelerated decline in GFR in the usual protein diet group.

Recently, Hansen et al. [61] performed a 4-year prospective, controlled trial with concealed randomisation in 82 type 1 diabetic patients with progressive diabetic nephropathy (pre-study rate of decline in GFR >2 ml/min/year). Forty-one patients were assigned to a low protein diet (pre-scribed 0.6 g/kg/day) and 41 patients were assigned to continue their usual protein diet. The average dietary protein intake during protein restriction was 0.89 g/kg/day, compared to 1.02 g/kg/day in the control group (p=0.005, between groups). At entry and during follow-up, an equally number of patients in each diet group received antihypertensive treatment (≥80 %), predominantly with ACE-inhibitors.

During follow-up blood pressure was similar in the two diet groups. An intention-to-treat analysis demonstrated that the rate of decline in GFR slowed equally in both diet groups during follow-up (3.9 ml/min/year in the usual group versus 3.8 in the low protein diet group). Although comparable in both diet groups during follow-up, blood pressure, albuminuria and haemoglobin A_{1c} were independent risk factors for the deterioration of GFR. ESRD and death occurred in 27 % of patients in the control group as compared with only 10 % in the low protein diet group (p=0.042). The relative risk of ESRD or death was 0.23 (p=0.01) for patients assigned to dietary protein restriction, compared with those assigned to the usual protein diet, after adjustment for the presence of cardiovascular disease at baseline. This finding is comparable to what has been previously demonstrated in patients with non-diabetic nephropathies [78;79]. The widespread use of ACE inhibitors and lack of adherence to the prescribed level of protein intake in the low protein diet group, may explain the lack of impact of diet intervention upon the rate of decline in GFR in this study, compared to the studies of Walker et al. [72] and Zeller et al. [73].

In the MDRD study [40] 585 patients with chronic renal diseases were randomly assigned to a low protein diet (pre-scribed 0.58 g/kg/day; achieved 0.77 g/kg/day) or an usual protein diet (pre-scribed 1.3 g/kg/day; achieved 1.1 g/kg/day) for two years. At entry and during follow-up, an equally number of patients in each diet group received antihypertensive treatment (80 %), mainly with ACE-inhibitors. In the intention-to-treat analysis the projected decline in GFR was 1.2 ml/min/year less (NS) in the low protein diet group compared to the usual protein diet group. However, dietary protein restriction induced a biphasic decline in GFR, with a faster initial and a slower subsequent decline in GFR. The subsequent decline in GFR was 28 % less in the low protein diet group compared to the usual protein diet group (p=0.009).

In a meta-analysis by Pedrini et al. [78], it was suggested that dietary protein restriction slows the progression of diabetic nephropathy, since a low protein diet [<0.8 g/kg/day] significantly slowed the increase in urinary albumin excretion or the decline in GFR [relative risk 0.56]. This analysis was based on 5 previously published studies [68;72;73;80;81] in type 1 diabetic patients, including 30 patients with normo- and microalbuminuria [68]. However, the validity of this meta-analysis has been questioned [82].

In conclusion, these findings suggest that dietary protein restriction improves prognosis in type 1 diabetic patients with diabetic nephropathy independently of antihypertensive therapy. Whether a similar beneficial effect of dietary protein restriction is present in type 2 diabetic patients with diabetic nephropathy urgently needs to be elucidated.

Problems with long-term dietary protein restriction

Protein-caloric nutrition deficiency and adherence to the pre-scribed diet is two of the major problems during long-term dietary protein restriction.

Dietary protein regimens containing an iso-caloric protein intake of at least 0.6 g/kg/day have proved to attain nitrogen balance and maintain normal indices of nutrition during long-term therapy [83;84]. The recommended level of energy intake of 30 to 35 Kcal/kg/day [85] seems to be required to obtain the most sufficient use of the dietary protein in chronic renal disease [86]. Since mean values for various indices of nutritional status (body weight, serum albumin levels and mid-arm muscle circumference) remained within normal ranges during dietary protein restriction in the quoted long-term intervention studies [40;61;72;73], the obtained level of protein restriction appears to be save over a period of 2 to 4 years. However, during low protein diet in the MDRD study [40], small but significant declines in energy intake and various indices of nutritional status were observed throughout the study. Nevertheless, no difference in the rates of death or first hospitalisation was seen between diet groups.

Whether calorie deficiency *per se* has a beneficial effect on GFR is controversial [87-89]. Similarly, it has recently been suggested that vegetable proteins (regardless of their quantity) has a beneficial effect on renal haemodynamics compared to animal proteins [90]. At present, no data are yet available concerning the effects of vegetable proteins on the progression of chronic renal disease.

In a secondary analysis of the MDRD study a close association between achieved dietary protein intake and the rate of decline in GFR has been demonstrated [91]. A 0.2 g/kg/day lower achieved protein intake was associated with a 1.15 ml/min/year slower mean decline in GFR. However, as demonstrated above, it is difficult to obtain the prescribed level of long-term dietary protein restriction in chronic renal disease [40;61;72;73]. It has proved to be difficult to lower dietary protein intake to less than 0.8 g/kg/day over extended periods of time [90] and patients with advanced non-diabetic renal disease is only able to lower their protein intake by 0.1 to 0.2 g/kg/day despite intensive nutritional counseling [92].

DIETARY SALT INTAKE AND DIABETIC NEPHROPATHY

Systemic blood pressure elevation accelerates the progression of diabetic nephropathy in both type 1 and type 2 diabetic patients [93], and effective antihypertensive treatment reduces albuminuria and the rate of decline in GFR in these patients. Extracellular fluid volume expansion due to impaired renal sodium excretion is the most clinically important mechanism that leads to the development of secondary hypertension in diabetic and non-diabetic patients with chronic renal disease [94;95]. Regardless of which specific antihypertensive agent is used, sodium restriction and treatment with loop diuretics is of major importance for the management of hypertension in these patients [95]. Recent short-term studies have demonstrated that the antiproteinuric effect of blockers of the renin-angiotensin-system [RAS] and nondihydropyridine calcium channel blockers is enhanced during dietary salt restriction [independently of the blood pressure reduction] in both diabetic and non-diabetic renal diseases [96;97]. This additive effect of dietary salt restriction may have important implications for the treatment of diabetic nephropathy since proteinuria per se may contribute to the deterioration of kidney function in chronic renal disease [98].

Only a few short-term intervention studies in man have investigated the impact of dietary salt restriction upon kidney function in patients with diabetic nephropathy [99;100].

Mühlhauser et al. [99] performed a 4 weeks double-blind, randomised and placebo-controlled trial in type 1 diabetic patients with elevated urinary albumin excretion rate [>60 mg/day] and untreated mild hypertension. The major objective was to assess the effect of moderate sodium restriction on blood pressure. Eight patients were assigned to a low sodium diet [achieved 92 mmol/day] and 8 patients were assigned to a high sodium diet [achieved 199 mmol/day]. During follow-up there was a significant decline in clinic diastolic blood pressure of 3.1 mm Hg in the low sodium diet group, while blood pressure remained unchanged in the high sodium diet group. However, there were no significant differences in blood pressure, proteinuria or GFR [clearance of inulin] between groups at follow-up.

Yoshioka et al. [100] performed a 1-week randomised, cross-over trial in 19 lean type 2 diabetic patients with normo-, micro- or macroalbuminuria. Medication other than insulin and hyperglycaemic agents was not administered. The major objective was to evaluate glomerular size and charge selectivity in these patients, by comparing the effect of two diets with different salt contents (85 and 255 mEq of sodium/day, respectively) on the fractional clearance of IgG and albumin. Compared to normoalbuminuric patients, charge selectivity was worse in patients with microalbuminuria, while charge and size selectivity were completely lacking in macroalbuminuric patients. Interestingly, GFR (creatinine clearance) was significantly lower during a low-salt diet as compared to a high-salt diet in all three groups of patients. Although not significant, blood pressure was correspondingly lower during the low-salt diet compared to the high-salt diet.

In conclusion, dietary salt restriction is of major importance for the management of hypertension in chronic renal disease. However, future long-term studies may clarify whether dietary salt restriction has a beneficial effect in addition to antihypertensive treatment on the progression of diabetic nephropathy.

REFERENCES

1. Mogensen CE. How to protect the kidney in diabetic patients - With special reference to IDDM. Diab 1997;46:S104-S111.
2. Mogensen CE. Long-term antihypertensive treatment inhibiting progression of diabetic nephropathy. Br.Med.J. 1982;285:685-8.
3. Parving H-H, Hommel E, Smidt UM. Protection of kidney function and decrease in albuminuria by captopril in insulin dependent diabetics with nephropathy. Br.Med.J. 1988;297:1086-91.
4. Parving H-H, Andersen AR, Smidt UM, Hommel E, Mathiesen ER, Svendsen PA. Effect of antihypertensive treatment on kidney function in diabetic nephropathy. Br.Med.J. 1987;294:1443-7.
5. Björck S, Mulec H, Johnsen SAa, Nordén G, Aurell M. Renal protective effect of enalapril in diabetic nephropathy. Br.Med.J. 1992;304:339-43.
6. Lewis E, Hunsicker L, Bain R, Rhode R. The effect of angiotensin-converting-enzyme inhibition on diabetic nephropathy. N.Engl.J.Med. 1993;329:1456-62.
7. Parving H-H, Jacobsen P, Rossing K, Smidt UM, Hommel E, Rossing P. Benefits of long-term antihypertensive treatment on prognosis in diabetic nephropathy. Kidney Int. 1996;49:1778-82.
8. Rossing P, Hougaard P, Borch-Johnsen K, Parving H-H. Predictors of mortality in insulin dependent diabetes: 10 year follow-up study. Br.Med.J. 1996;313:779-84.
9. Bergström J. Discovery and rediscovery of low-protein diet. Clin.Nephrol. 1984;21:29-35.

10. Parving H-H, Rossing P, Hommel E, Smidt UM. Angiotensin converting enzyme inhibition in diabetic nephropathy: ten years experience. Am.J.Kidney Dis. 1995;26:99-107.

11. Breyer JA, Bain P, Evans JK, Nahman NS, Lewis E, Cooper ME et al. Predictors of the progression of renal insufficiency in patients with insulin-dependent diabetes and overt diabetic nephropathy. Kidney Int. 1996;50:1651-8.

12. Gall M-A, Nielsen FS, Smidt UM, Parving H-H. The course of kidney function in type 2 [non-insulin-dependent] diabetic patients with diabetic nephropathy. Diabetologia 1993;36:1071-8.

13. Schmidt-Nielsen B, Barrett JM, Graves B, Crossley B. Physiological and morphological responses of the rat kidney to reduced dietary protein. Am.J.Physiol. 1985:F31-F42.

14. Wen S-F, Huang T-P, Moorthy AV. Effects of low-protein diet on experimental diabetic nephropathy in the rat. J.Lab.Clin.Med. 1985;106:589-97.

15. Kliem V, Brunkhorst R, Ehlerding G, Kühn K, Neumann KH, Koch KM. Prevention of glomerular hypertrophy and glomerulosclerosis in milan normotensive rats by low-protein diet, but not by low-dose captopril treatment. Nephron 1995;71:208-12.

16. Peters H, Border WA, Noble NA. Angiotensin II blockade and low-protein diet produce additive therapeutic effects in experimental glomerulonephritis. Kidney Int. 2000;57:1493-501.

17. Brenner BM, Meyer TW, Hostetter TH. Dietary protein intake and the progressive nature of renal disease: the role of hemodynamically mediated glomerular injury in the pathogenesis of progressive glomerular sclerosis in aging, renal ablation, and intrinsic renal disease. N.Engl.J.Med. 1982;307:652-9.

18. Nielsen AL, Bang HO. The influence of diet on the renal function in healthy persons. Acta Med.Scand. 1948;CXXX:382-8.

19. Pullman TN, Alving AS, Dern RJ, Landowne M. The influence of dietary protein intake on specifik renal functions in normal man. J.Lab.Clin.Med. 1954;44:320-32.

20. Bosch JP, Saccaggi A, Lauer A, Ronco C, Belledonne M, Glabman S. Renal functional reserve in humans. Effect of protein intake on glomerular filtration rate. Am.J.Med. 1983;75:943-50.

21. Bergström J, Ahlberg M, Alvestrand A. Influence of protein intake on renal hemodynamics and plasma hormone concentration in normal subjects. Acta Med.Scand. 1985;217:189-96.

22. Hostetter TH. Human renal response to meat meal. Am.J.Physiol. 1986;250:F613.

23. Sølling K, Christensen CK, Sølling J, Christiansen JS, Mogensen CE. Effect on renal haemodynamics, glomerular filtration rate and albumin excretion of high oral protein load. Scand.J.Clin.Lab.Invest. 1986;46:351-7.

24. Viberti GC, Bognetti E, Wiseman MJ, Dodds R, Gross JL, Keen H. Effect of protein-restricted diet on renal response to a meat meal in humans. Am J Physiol 1987;253:F388-F393.

25. Chan AYM, Cheng M-LL, Keil LC, Myers BD. Functional response of healthy and diseased glomeruli to a large, protein-rich meal. J.Clin.Invest. 1988;81:245-54.

26. Brouhard BH, LaGrone LF, Richards GE, Travis LB. Short-term protein loading in diabetics with a ten-year duration of disease. AJDC 1986;140:473-6.

27. Kupin WL, Cortes P, Dumler F, Feldkamp CS, Kilates MC, Levin NW. Effect on renal function of change from high to moderate protein intake in type I diabetic patients. Diab 1987;36:73-9.

28. de Faria JBL, Friedman R, de Cosmo S, Dodds RA, Mortton JJ, Viberti GC. Renal functional response to protein loading in type 1 [insulin-dependent] diabetic patients on normal or high salt intake. Nephron 1997;76:411-7.

29. Fioretto P, Trevisan R, Giorato C, De Riva C, Doria A, Valerio A et al. Type 1 insulin-dependent diabetic patients show an impaired renal haemodynamic response to protein intake. J.Diabet.Complications 1988;2:27-9.

30. Cohen D, Dodds RA, Viberti GC. Effect of protein restriction in insulin-dependent diabetics at risk of nephropathy. Br.Med.J. 1987;294:795-8.

31. Wiseman MJ, Bognetti E, Dodds RA, Viberti GC. Changes in renal function in response to protein-restricted diet in type 1 [insulin-dependent] diabetic patients. Diabetologia 1987;30:154-9.

32. Rudberg S, Dahlquist G, Aperia A, Persson B. Reduction of protein intake decreases glomerular filtration rate in young type 1 [insulin-dependent] diabetic patients mainly in hyperfiltrating patients. Diabetologia 1988;31:878-83.

33. Pedersen MM, Mogensen CE, Jørgensen FS, Møller B, Lykke G, Pedersen O. Renal effects from limitation of high dietary protein in normoalbuminuric diabetic patients. Kidney Int. 1989;Suppl. 27:S115-S121.

34. Bosch JP, Lew S, Glabman S, Laver A. Renal haemodynamic changes in humans. Am.J.Med. 1986;81:809-15.

35. Bending JJ, Dodds RA, Keen H, Viberti GC. Renal response to restricted protein intake in diabetic nephropathy. Diab 1988;37:1641-6.

36. Hansen HP, Christensen PK, Tauber-Lassen E, Klausen A, Jensen BR, Parving H-H. Low-protein diet and kidney function in insulin-dependent diabetic patients with diabetic nephropathy. Kidney Int. 1999;55:621-8.

37. Pinto JR, Bending JJ, Dodds RA, Viberti GC. Effect of low protein diet on the renal response to meat ingestion in diabetic nephropathy. Eur.J.Clin.Invest. 1991;21:175-83.

38. Frimondt-Møller C. Diabetic cystopathy. Dan.Med.Bull. 1978;25:49-60.

39. Levey AS, Beck GJ, Bosch JP, Caggiula AW, Greene T, Hunsicker LG et al. Short-term effects of protein intake, blood pressure, and antihypertensive therapy on glomerular filtration rate in the modification on diet in renal disease study. J.Am.Soc.Nephrol. 1996;7:2097-109.

40. Klahr S, Levey AS, Beck GJ, Caggiula AW, Hunsicker L, Kusek JW et al. The effects of dietary protein restriction and blood-pressure control on the progression of chronic renal disease. N.Engl.J.Med. 1994;330:877-84.

41. Ruilope LM, Casal MC, Praga M, Alcazar JM, Decap G, Lahera V et al. Additive antiproteinuric effect of converting enzyme inhibition and low protein intake. J.Am.Soc.Nephrol. 1992;3:1307-11.

42. Gansevoort RT, de Zeeuw D, de Jong PE. Additive antiproteinuric effect of ACE inhibition and a low-protein diet in human renal disease. Nephrol.Dial.Transplant. 1995;10:497-504.

43. Hostetter TH, Olson JL, Rennke HG, Venkatachalam MA, Brenner BM. Hyperfiltration in remnant nephrons: a potentially adverse response to renal ablation. Am.J.Physiol. 1981;241:F85-F93.

44. Zatz R, Meyer TW, Rennke HG, Brenner BM. Predominance of hemodynamic rather than metabolic factors in the pathogenesis of diabetic glomerulopathy. Proc.Natl.Acad.Sci.USA 1985;82:5963-7.

45. Meyer TW, Anderson S, Rennke HG, Brenner BM. Reversing glomerular hypertension stabilizes established glomerular injury. Kidney Int. 1987;31:752-9.

643

46. Parving H-H, Kastrup J, Smidt UM, Andersen AR, Feldt-Rasmussen B, Christiansen JS. Impaired autoregulation of glomerular filtration rate in Type 1 [insulin-dependent] diabetic patients with nephropathy. Diabetologia 1984;27:547-52.

47. Christensen PK, Hansen HP, Parving H-H. Impaired autoregulation of GFR in hypertensive non-insulin dependent diabetic patients. Kidney Int. 1997;52:1369-74.

48. Navar LG, Inscho EW, Majid DSA, Imig JD, Harrison-Bernard LM, Mitchell KD. Paracrine Regulation of the Renal Microcirculation. Physiol.Rev. 1996;76:425-536.

49. Heidland A, Sebekova K, Ling H. Effects of low-protein diets on renal disease: are non-haemodynamic factors involved. Nephrol.Dial.Transplant 1995;10[9]:1512-4.

50. Paczek L, Teschner M, Schaefer RM, Kovar J, Romen W, Heidland A. Proteinase activity in isolated glomeruli of Goldblatt hypertensive rats. Clinical and Experimental Hypertension 1991;A13:339-56.

51. Schaefer L, Schaefer RM, Ling H, Teschner M, Heidland A. Renal proteinases and kidney hypertrophy in experimental diabetes. Diabetologia 1994;37:567-71.

52. Huang S, Reisch S, Schaefer L, Teschner M, Heidland A, Schaefer RM. Effect of dietary protein on glomerular proteinase activities. Miner Electrolyte Metab 1992;18:84-8.

53. Border WA, Noble NA. Transforming growth factor-β in tissue fibrosis. N.Engl.J.Med. 1994;331:1286-92.

54. Noble NA, Border WA. Angiotensin II in renal fibrosis: Should TGF-β rather than blood pressure be the therapeutic target? Semin.Nephrol. 1997;17:455-66.

55. Okuda S, Nakamichi T, Yamamoto T, Ruoslahti E, Border WA. Dietary protein restriction rapidly reduces transforming growth factor β1 expression in experimental glomerulonephritis. Proc.Natl.Acad.Sci.USA 1991;88:9765-9.

56. Eddy AA. Protein restriction reduces transforming growth factor-beta and interstitiel fibrosis in nephrotic syndrome. Am.J.Physiol. 1994;266:F884-F893.

57. Nakayama M, Okuda S, Tamaki K, Fujishima M. Short- and long-term effects of low protein diet on fibronectin and transforming growth factor-beta synthesis in ariamycin-induced nephropathy. J.Lab.Clin.Med. 1996;127:29-39.

58. Liu DT, Turner SW, Wen C, Whitworth JA. Angiotensin converting enzyme inhibition and protein restriction in progression of experimental chronic renal failure. Pathology 1996;28:156-60.

59. Levey AS, Gassman J, Hall PM, Walker WG. Assessing the progression of renal disease in clinical studies: effects of duration of follow-up and regression to the mean. J.Am.Soc.Nephrol 1991;1:1087-94.

60. Greene T, Beck GJ, Gassman JJ, Kutner MH, Paranandi L, Wang S-R et al. Comparison of time-to-event and slope-based analyses in nephrology clinical trials. Controlled Clinical Trials 1995;16:65S.

61. Hansen HP, Tauber-Lassen E, Jensen BR, Parving H-H. Effect of dietary protein restriction on prognosis in patients with diabetic nephropathy. Kidney Int. 2002;62:220-8.

62. Bröchner-Mortensen J, Giese J, Rossing N. Renal inulin clearance versus total plasma clearance of ^{51}Cr-EDTA. Scand.J.Clin.Lab.Invest. 1969;23:301-5.

63. Shemesh O, Golbetz HV, Kriss JP, Myers BD. Limitations of creatinine as a filtration marker in glomerulopathic patients. Kidney Int. 1985;28:830-8.

64. Maroni BJ, Mitch WE. Role of nutrition in preservation of the progression of renal disease. Annu.Rev.Nutr. 1997;17:435-55.

65. Levey AS, Bosch JP, Coggins CH, Greene T, Mitch WE, Schluchter MD et al. Effects of diet and antihypertensive therapy on creatinine clearance and serum creatinine concentration in the modification of diet in renal disease study. J.Am.Soc.Nephrol 1996;7:556-65.

66. Parving H-H, Oxenbøll B, Svendsen PAa, Christiansen JS, Andersen AR. Early detection of patients at risk of developing diabetic nephropathy. Acta Endocrinol. 1982;100:550-5.

67. Mogensen CE. Microalbuminuria predicts clinical proteinuria and early mortality in maturity onset diabetes. N.Engl.J.Med. 1984;310:356-60.

68. Dullaart RP, Beusekamp BJ, Meijer S, van Doormaal JJ, Sluiter WJ. Long-term effects of protein-restricted diet on albuminuria and renal function in IDDM patients without clinical nephropathy and hypertension. Diabetes Care 1993;16,2:483-92.

69. Pijls LTJ, de Vries H, Donker AJM, van Eijk JTM. The effect of protein restriction on albuminuria in patients with type 2 diabetes mellitus: a randomized trial. Nephrol.Dial.Transplant 1999;14:1445-53.

70. Chaturvedi N. Should all type 1 diabetic patients with microalbuminuria receive ACE inhibitors? A meta regression analysis. Ann.Intern.Med. 2001[In press].

71. Parving H-H, Lehnert H, Bröchner-Mortensen J, Gomis R, Andersen S, Arner P. The effect of irbesartan on the development of diabetic nephropathy in patients with type 2 diabetes. N.Engl.J.Med. 2001;345:870-8.

72. Walker JD, Bending JJ, Dodds RA, Mattock MB, Murrells TJ, Keen H et al. Restriction of dietary protein and progression of renal failure in diabetic nephropathy. Lancet 1989;ii:1411-5.

73. Zeller KR, Whittaker E, Sullivan L, Raskin P, Jacobson HR. Effect of restricting dietary protein on the progression of renal failure in patients with insulin-dependent diabetes melitus. N.Engl.J.Med. 1991;324:78-84.

74. Hovind P, Rossing P, Tarnow L, Smidt UM, Parving H-H. Progression of diabetic nephropathy. Kidney Int. 2001;59:702-9.

75. Björck S, Nyberg G, Mulec H, Granerus G, Herlitz H, Aurell M. Beneficial effect of angiotensin converting enzyme inhibition on renal function in patients with diabetic nephropathy. Br.Med.J. 1986;293:471-4.

76. Ruggenenti P, Perna A, Gheradi G, Gaspari F, Benini R, Remuzzi G. Renal function and requirement for dialysis in chronic nephropathy patients on long-term ramipril: REIN follow-up trial. Lancet 1998;352:1252-6.

77. Parving H-H, Smidt UM, Friisberg B, Bonnevie-Nielsen V, Andersen AR. A prospective study of glomerular filtration rate and arterial blood pressure in insulin-dependent diabetics with diabetic nephropathy. Diabetologia 1981;20:457-61.

78. Pedrini MT, Levey AS, Lau J, Chalmers TC, Wang PH. The effect of dietary protein restriction on the progression of diabetic and nondiabetic renal diseases: meta-analysis. Ann.Intern.Med. 1996;124:627-32.

79. Fouque D, Wang P, Laville M, Boissel J-P. Low protein diets delay end-stage renal disease in non-diabetic adults with chronic renal failure. Nephrology Dialysis Transplantation 2000;15:1986-92.

80. Ciavarella A, Di Mizio G, Stefani S, Borgnina LC, Vannini P. Reduced albuminuria after dietary protein restriction in insulin-dependent diabetic patients with clinical nephropathy. Diabetes Care 1987;10:407-13.

81. Barsotti G, Ciardella F, Morelli E, Cupisti A, Mantovanelli A, Giovanetti S. Nutritional treatment of renal failure in type 1 diabetic nephropathy. Clin.Nephrol. 1988;29:280-7.

82. Parving H-H. Effects of dietary protein on renal disease. Ann.Intern.Med. 1997;126[4]:330-1.

83. Goodship TH, Mitch WE, Hoerr RA, Wagner DA, Steinman TI, Young VR. Adaption to low-protein diets in renal failure: leucine turnover and nitrogen balance. J.Am.Soc.Nephrol 1990;1:66-75.

84. Tom K, Young VR, Chapman T, Masud T, Akpele L, Maroni BJ. Long-term adaptive responses to dietary protein restriction in chronic renal failure. Am J Physiol 1995;268:E668-E677.

85. Kopple JD. National Kidney Foundation K/DOQl Clinical Practice Guidelines for Nutrition in Chronic Renal Failure. Am J Kidney Disease 2001;37 Suppl 2.

86. Kopple JD, Monteon FJ, Shaib JK. Effect of energy intake on nitrogen metabolism in nondialysed patients with chronic renal failure. Kidney Int. 1986;29:734-42.

87. Ichikawa I, Purkerson ML, Klahr S, Troy JL, Martinez-Maldonado M, Brenner BM. Mechanism of reduced glomerular filtration rate in chronic malnutrition. J.Clin.Invest. 1980;65:982-8.

88. Tapp DC, Wortham WG, Addison JF, Hammonds DN, Barnes JL, Venkatachalam MA. Food restriction retards body growth and prevents end-stage renal pathology in remnant kidneys of rats regardless of protein intake. Lab.Invest. 1989;60 [2]:184-94.

89. Kobayashi S, Venkatachalam MA. Differential effects of caloric restriction on glomeruli and tubules of the remnant kidney. Kidney Int. 1992;42:710-7.

90. Locatelli F. Is the type of protein in the diet more important than its quantity for slowing progression of chronic renal insufficiency? Nephrology Dialysis Transplantation 1997;12:391-3.

91. Levey AS, Adler S, Caggiula AW, England BK, Greene T, Hunsicker LG et al. Effects of dietary protein restriction on the progression of advanced renal disease in the modification of diet in renal disease study. Am J Kidney Disease 1996;27:652-63.

92. Mehrotra R, Nolph KD. Treatment of advanced renal failure: Low-protein diets or timely initiation of dialysis. Kidney Int. 2000;58:1381-8.

93. Parving H-H. Renoprotection in diabetes: genetic and non-genetic risk factors and treatment. Diabetologia 1998;41:745-59.

94. Hommel E, Mathiesen ER, Giese J, Nielsen MD, Schütten HJ, Parving H-H. On the pathogenesis of arterial blood pressure elevation early in the course of diabetic nephropathy. Scand.J.Clin.Lab.Invest. 1989;49:537-44.

95. Preston RA. Renoprotective effects of antihypertensive drugs. Am.J.Hypertens. 1999;12:19S-32S.

96. Bakris GL, Smith A. Effects of sodium intake on albumin excretion in patients with diabetic nephropathy treated with long-acting calcium antagonists. Ann Intern Med 1996;125:201-4.

97. Heeg JE, de Jong PE, van der Hem GK, de Zeeuw D. Efficacy and variability of the antiproteinuric effect of ACE inhibition by lisinopril. Kidney Int. 1989;36:272-9.

98. Remuzzi G, Bertani T. Is glomerulosclerosis a consequence of altered glomerular permeability to macromolecules? Kidney Int. 1990;38:384-94.

99. Mühlhauser I, Prange K, Sawicki P, Bender R, Dworschak A, Schaden W et al. Effects of dietary sodium on blood pressure in IDDM patients with nephropathy. Diabetologia 1996;39:212-9.

100. Yoshioka K, Imanishi M, Konishi Y, Sato T, Tanaka S, Kimura G et al. Glomerular charge and size selectivity assessed by changes in salt intake in type 2 diabetic patients. Diabetes Care 1998;21:482-6.

36

DIABETIC NEPHROPATHY AND PREGNANCY

John L. Kitzmiller, MD
Regional Diabetes and Pregnancy Program, Good Samaritan Hospital, San Jose, California, USA

The potential problems of diabetic nephropathy (DN) and pregnancy require the anticipation of preconception care. Clinicians who care for adolescent and adult diabetic women need to recognize that they may become pregnant, that most of the risks to mother and offspring are related to poor control of hyperglycemia and hypertension, and that the risks may be reduced through intensified multifactorial interventions before conception and throughout pregnancy.

In recent years the most common cause of perinatal mortality in type 1 or type 2 diabetes is major congenital malformations [1]. A major advance is the demonstration that most malformations can be prevented by institution of strict metabolic control before conception in women with diabetic vascular complications [2-5]. Patients should have instruction in contraception [6-9] and should be intensively treated or referred to a specialized center when pregnancy is considered. Encouragement by diabetes care providers is a major factor in preventing unplanned pregnancies [10-11].

In the past, women with DN were generally advised to avoid pregnancy because there was a low probability of a healthy infant and a chance that nephropathy would worsen. Although advances in obstetrical and neonatal care have improved the outlook, nephropathy in pregnancy still presents a challenging situation requiring coordination between the patient and providers from many specialties. As reviewed in this chapter, women with nephropathy remain at high risk for many pregnancy complications, including superimposed preeclamptic toxemia (PET) or accelerated hypertension, preterm delivery, fetal growth restriction, and cesarean delivery. Excellent metabolic balance and control of hypertension are necessary to reduce these complications and prevent decline in renal and retinal function during and after pregnancy.

EVALUATION BEFORE CONCEPTION

An outline of preconception management of women with established diabetes is included in table 1.

Table 1. Management of DN before and during pregnancy

At all times
Prevent hyperglycaemia without untoward hypoglycemia
Control hypertension; angiotensin inhibition prior to pregnancy; other agents during pregnancy
Controlled carbohydrate, fat, and protein diet
Adequate rest
Prior to pregnancy
Measure renal function
Ophthalmologic exam
Cardiovascular evaluation
(history, exam, EKG, echocardiogram)
Thyroid evaluation
Hepatitis B surface antigen
Serologic testing for syphilis
Counseling and education
First prenatal visit
Measure renal function
Ophthalmologic exam
Sonogram for dating
Second trimester
Measure renal function (12, 24 weeks)
Maternal serum alphafetoprotein (15-18 weeks)
Detailed sonogram with fetal echocardiogram (18-20 weeks)
Third trimester
Monthly sonogram
Weekly nonstress test (26 weeks)
Ophthalmologic exam
Measure renal function (36 weeks); Delivery planning

Evaluation for diabetic microvascular disease and hypertension are critical. Creatinine clearance (CrCl) as an estimate of glomerular filtration rate (GFR), and the degree of microalbuminuria (*incipient DN*, urinary albumin excretion {UAE} 30-299 mg/24 hrs, >20 μg/min) or urinary total protein excretion {TPE} (*overt DN*, >500 mg/24 hrs total protein *or* >300 mg/24 hrs albumin, >200 μg/min albumin,) [12] should be quantified, preferably with a 24-hour specimen [13-20]. If overt DN is diagnosed, the patient should be thoroughly counseled regarding measures used to improve outcomes of pregnancy and the possible vascular complications and life expectancy. Hopefully then the decision on whether to attempt pregnancy will be more informed.

Current research is evaluating the use of plasma or serum cystatin C as an alternate indicator of GFR, since this positively charged cysteine protease inhibitor is produced at a constant rate in nucleated cells, freely filtered in the glomerulus and completely degraded in the tubules [21-26]. In a study of patients with type 1 diabetes and albuminuria, filtration of cystatin C was reduced along with mean podocyte filtration slit size, although GFR by iothalamate clearance was normal [27].

Renoprotective or *antihypertensive therapy* is indicated for patients with microalbuminuria or overt nephropathy [28] and agents used should be effective and safe in early pregnancy [29-31]. Although probably not teratogenic [32-33], *angiotensin converting-enzyme (ACE) inhibitors or Ang-II receptor blockers are contraindicated during pregnancy* because they are associated with neonatal renal failure [31,34]. This is unfortunate because there are extensive data, reviewed elsewhere in this volume, indicating that these drugs retard the development and progression of nephropathy, perhaps via direct effects on intrarenal cellular actions of angiotensin (AngII). On the other hand, control of blood pressure and renal hemodynamics with other anti-hypertensive agents is also effective [35]. The hypothesis that use of ACE-inhibitors in the preconception period will also decrease complications during pregnancy [36,37] should be tested in controlled trials in women with excellent glycemic control. In a study of 8 women with presumed DN, Jovanovic found that normoglycemia achieved by early pregnancy also resulted in stable renal function and low complication rates [38]. Diltiazem and other calcium-entry blockers are possibly best avoided during the first trimester since some data indicate an association with fetal limb defects (possibly related to reduced uteroplacental blood flow [39]), but not confirmed as teratogenic in a larger survey [40]. Diltiazem may have benefits for glomerular function not possessed by dihydropyridine calcium channel blockers [35,41-46]. Agents believed to be relatively safe for early pregnancy include alpha-methyldopa, clonidine, and beta-adrenergic antagonists with low lipid solubility [29-31].

Ophthalmologic examination is especially important for women with nephropathy because most also have *diabetic retinopathy*. Hyperglycemia induces retinal ischemia, and relatively rapid insulinization and normalization of blood glucose may elevate growth factor levels (IGF-1, VEGF, FGF) associated with worsening of retinopathy [47-53]. In the presence of background (BDR) or proliferative retinopathy (PDR) allow a few months to normalize blood glucose in the preconception period. PDR should be in remission or laser treated before pregnancy is attempted. In women with BDR at the beginning of pregnancy, the risk of development of neovascularization during gestation is 7-10% in hyperglycemic [54-56] or hypertensive women [57].

The *association of DN with cardiovascular disease* [58-64] gives concern in evaluating patients for pregnancy, since formerly there was a high mortality in pregnant diabetic women with coronary artery disease [65,66]. There are no cross-sectional or prospective studies of the coronary vessels in diabetic women preparing for pregnancy. However, Manske et al found little coronary disease by angiography in non-smoking diabetic patients <45 years old with end-stage renal disease if diabetes duration was less than 25 years, and there were no ST-T wave changes on ECG [67]. Therefore, pregnancy should be safe if these conditions are met. Otherwise, coronary angiography should be considered, since maternal-fetal outcome after the few reported coronary artery bypass grafts has been good [68-72]. Data are inadequate on pregnancy after percutaneous coronary revascularization procedures in diabetic women [73-76]. Stress echocardiography is also important in pre-conception screening [77], and a restricted left ventricular diastolic filling pattern during pregnancy may be associated with ventricular arrhythmias or dysfunction during delivery in type 1 diabetic women [Schannwell03*]. This impairment of early diastolic filling velocity can be "an early sign of cardiac dysfunction even before there is a systolic disturbance along with a loss of contractility" [78], and may reflect diabetic cardiomyopathy [79-82].

Regarding *treatment of diabetes prior to pregnancy*, glycemic control is achieved with a meal plan, monitoring the food intake and blood glucose levels, and intensive insulin therapy. The diet prescription for pregnancy is 25-35 kcal/kg ideal body weight. With nephropathy, protein intake should be controlled, but 60 g/day is probably required for fetal development. The preferred insulin regimen includes a mix of short and intermediate-acting human insulins or continuous subcutaneous insulin infusion therapy. The optimal doses and timing are determined by self-monitored capillary blood glucose determinations before and after each meal. The targets for capillary blood glucose control before and during pregnancy are premeal values of 3.9-5.6 mM (70-100 mg/dL) and peak postprandial values of 5.6-7.2 mM (100-129 mg/dL) [1,3].

COURSE OF NEPHROPATHY DURING PREGNANCY

GFR rises by 40-80% in normal and uncomplicated diabetic pregnancy, as reflected by increasing CrCl and decreasing serum creatinine (Cr) [83,84]. The increase in GFR occurs in the first weeks of pregnancy [85] in advance of the expansion of plasma volume [86], and reaches an increment of 40-50% by the end of the first trimester [83]. The *glomerular hyperfiltration* and increase in renal plasma flow (RPF) is maximal at 26-30 weeks gestation [87], then RPF declines significantly by term pregnancy (but not to control levels) in subjects lying on their sides, while GFR by inulin clearance does not [84,88]. Therefore, filtration fraction (GFR/RPF) must increase in late normal pregnancy as osmotic pressure declines [84]. Since there is a slight decline in endogenous CrCl from 29 to 37 weeks (141 to 126 ml/min), it is possible there is reduced tubular secretion of Cr in late pregnancy, at the same time there is enhanced net tubular reabsorption of uric acid and slight decrease in uric acid clearance [88,89].

Studies in pregnant women and rat models indicate that increased GFR is due to elevated RPF and vasodilation of afferent and efferent arterioles without evidence of increased glomerular capillary pressure (Pgc) [86], with some contribution from both decreased afferent and efferent osmotic pressure and increased Kf [84,90]. Based on studies in chronically instrumented rats, it is unlikely that vasodilatory prostaglandins mediate the renal hemodynamic changes of pregnancy [86,91]. Nitric oxide is the prime candidate for causing glomerular vasodilation in pregnancy [92], as acute selective blockade of both iNO and nNO reduce the gestational levels of RPF and GFR without effect on systemic arterial pressure [93,94]. Extensive studies in various pregnant rat models of experimental nephropathy never showed increased Pgc [86], which is reassuring since hyperfiltration and hypertension in the glomerulus is considered a prerequisite for human DN.

With DN in pregnancy, the expected rise in CrCl is seen in only about one-third of patients, as summarized in table 2 [38,95,96]. In another one-third of DN patients, CrCl actually decreases, probably reflecting the underlying natural progression of nephropathy or accelerating hypertension. In a recent analysis, initial elevated Cr of 109-163 μM (1.0-1.5 mg/dL) was associated with a decline in CrCl during pregnancy in 12 women with DN, whereas in 9 patients with initial Cr >163 μM (1.5 mg/dL), CrCl remained stable but low at 41-65 ml/min [97]. When inverse serum Cr levels are used as an indicator of GFR, about one third of DN patients show a rise in Cr by the third trimester, related to reduced renal function at baseline and/or superimposed PET [98-102]. A rise in Cr was associated with "cross-over" from a hyperdynamic cardiac output to a vasoconstricted state in a preliminary report on a large number of pregnant women with DN [103]. Jovanovic found that prevention of hyperglycaemia and hypertension allowed a normal rise in CrCl during pregnancy in 8 diabetic women with sub-par values prior to conception [38]. On the other hand, Biesenbach et al observed that mean CrCl declined by 16% during the first two trimesters in 7 proteinuric diabetic women with subnormal CrCl prior to pregnancy (37-73 ml/min/1.73m^2), in spite of intensified glycemic control and anthypertensive therapy during pregnancy [104]. These data illustrat the potential difficulty of pregnancy in DN patients with azotemia prior to pregnancy.

Table 2. Changes in creatinine clearance in 44 women with diabetic nephropathy with measurements in both first and third trimester of pregnancy[a]

CrCl	First trimester		Third trimester	
	n (%)	Increased >25%	Stable	Decreased>15%
>90 ml/min	14 (32%)	3 (21%)	5 (36%)	6 (43%)
60-89 ml/min	20 (45.5%)	9 (45%)	6 (30%)	5 (25%)
<60 ml/min	10 (22.5%)	2 (20%)	6 (60%)	2 (20%)
Total	44 (100%)	14 (32%)	17 (39%)	13 (29%)

Data stratified by CrCl in first trimester: normal, moderate reduction, and severe reduction. Data pooled from Kitzmiller et al [95], Jovanovic and Jovanovic [38], and Reece et al [96].

In streptozotocin (STZ)-treated pregnant rats with acute hyperglycemia from the onset of pregnancy, the diabetes leads to enhanced RPF and GFR dependent on increased renal synthesis of NO [105]. Increased NO production and changes in renal hemodynamics in pregnant rats are dependent on differential expression of renal NO synthase isoforms, with eNOS down-regulated and iNOS and nNOS upregulated [106]. STZ given at day 8 of pregnant rats produced hypertension, proteinuria , and reduced fetal size [107]. It is of interest that chronic nonselective inhibition of NO synthase in the pregnant rat reduces GFR accompanied by proteinuria and hypertension [108].

Data are few on use of serum cystatin C as a reciprocal indicator of GFR [24] during pregnancy. The mean serum concentration of cystatin C was found to be paradoxically higher for pregnant than healthy non-pregnant women, in spite of increased GFR, while mean serum creatinine levels were lower in normal pregnancy [26]. Since the serum level of a substance is inversely related to its clearance, reciprocals of cystatin C concentrations were correlated (r 0.76) with a reference method for GFR during pregnancy; perhaps there is increased production of cycstatin C during gestation [26]. Maternal cystatin C levels did not correlate with neonatal concentrations [109], nor with fetal or placental weight, although the highest serum levels were found in twin gestations [26]. Women with PET had higher serum levels of cystatin C and lower GFR (113 vs 153 ml/min) than healthy pregnant women [26], and the group in Sweden believes serum cystatin C to be a better marker for PET than serum urate [110]. I am not aware of published measurements in pregnant diabetic women with albuminuria.

An increase in *kidney volume* can be measured by ultrasound in pregnancies in normal controls [111] and in insulin-dependent diabetic women [112]. In the latter group the expansion occurs in spite of strict glycaemic control, and the increase correlates with CrCl but not with albuminuria or BP levels. Renal expansion is less in pregnant women withDN, but renal volume did not decline as expected 4 months postpartum in this group in one study [112]. Interestingly, development of persistent microalbuminuria was most likely in the group of diabetic women with normoalbuminuria and relatively small renal volumes in early pregnancy.

The urinary excretion of albumin (UAE) increases only slightly in*normal pregnancy* [84,113-117], while total urinary protein excretion (TPE) increases by 40-200 %, albeit to <300 mg/24hrs (table 3) [118,119]. Albumin represents a small fraction of TPE. The increase in TPE is presumably due to increased GFR and limited tubular reabsorption [18,119]. Low molecular weight proteins like μ2-microglobulin, retinol binding protein, and immunoglobulin light chains are freely filtered by the glomerulus and increased load to the proximal tubules in pregnancy must exceed reabsorptive capacity as there is increased urinary excretion [113,117]. This may be similar to the proximal tubular dysfunction seen in non-pregnant type 1 and type 2 diabetic patients ± microalbuminuria [120]. Glomerular permselectivity for the heart-shaped albumin [121] (radius 3.6 nm) remains relatively intact in normal pregnancy [122], or else specific tubular albumin uptake is stable or enhanced. I know of no studies of urinary albumin fragments (as a marker of tubular processing of albumin) [123] in pregnancy.

Table 3. Albuminuria and proteinuria before, during and after normal and type 1 diabetic pregnancies without clinical nephropathy.

	Before	3rd trimester	4*-6**mo PP
11 nl controls *			
UAE (mg/d)	9	12	13
TPE (mg/d)	117*	262	174
7 normoalb type 1**			
UAE	12	71	13
TPE	73	4	7
microalb type 1**			
UAE	80	478	114
TPE	233	2350	239

* Roberts et al 1996 [122]   UAE, urinary albumin excretion
** Biesenbach, Zasgornik 1989 [130]   TPE, total protein excretion

Glomerular permeability involves charge-, shape-, and size-selectivity for the filtered macromolecules [124], although the concept of charge-selectivity has become controversial [125]. Sieving studies with dextran particles of 3.5-6.0 nm radius are most consistent with an isoporous + shunt model of glomerular ultrafiltration in normal pregnant women, with a decrease in small pores of 3.0-4.9 nm [84,90]. This model assumes that the glomerular wall "is perforated by a series of restrictive pores of identical radius and has a parallel shunt pathway that fails to restrict the passage of large molecules" [90]. There are technical problems with dextran sieving due to changes in conformation during passage, and studies using the more rigid spherical Ficoll particles [126] are needed for normal and proteinuric pregnancies. The current general model of the structural determinants of glomerular permeability emphasizes the cellular layers (fenestrated endothelium, epithelial {podocyte} filtration slits) rather than the glomerular basement membrane (GBM) as determining the size selectivity for macromolecules [127]. The central size-selective filtration barriers are the slit diaphragms bridging the podocyte foot processes on the epithelial side of the GBM [128].

In *diabetic women without microalbuminuria* in early pregnancy (<30 mg/24 hrs), UAE increases slightly in the second trimester and sometimes greatly in the third trimester, while urinary TPE can rise to >300 mg/24hrs [129-131]. Of course, some cases of this proteinuria may be explained by mild PET, which always muddles the view of changes in renal function in pregnant diabetic women. The glomerulo-tubular functional/structural determinants of this diabetes-associated progression in albuminuria in pregnancy have not been adequately studied. Assuming analogous processes to those in non-pregnant women may be misleading. In the setting of the DCCT, only 10 of 180 type 1 diabetic women in either treatment group developed microalbuminuria (>40mg/24hr) during pregnancy [53]. With *microalbuminuria before pregnancy in diabetic women*, the increase in UAE and TPE during gestation is even greater (table 3) [132-134]. Most investigators have observed that diabetic microalbuminuria in early pregnancy predicts a risk of superimposed PET of 35-60% compared to 6-14 % in diabetic women without microalbuminuria [132, 133,135-137]. Similar findings are reported for non-diabetic pregnant women with microalbuminuria measured in mid-pregnancy [138-141], suggesting that this is a marker for a subtle generalized vascular disorder, related to insulin resistance or inflammation [142-147].

The gestational changes in *total proteinuria* mean that most clinical studies of DN in pregnancy have probably included women with undetected microalbuminuria prior to conception who happened to progress to mild macroproteinuria (400-600 mg total protein/24hrs) in early pregnancy, and thus were inappropriately selected as patients with mild DN. With definite *clinical diabetic nephropathy* diagnosed prior to pregnancy, albuminuria and total proteinuria often increase dramatically during gestation, even without associated hypertension, frequently exceeding 10 g/24 hours in the third trimester. Though some of this increase may reflect the underlying progression of nephropathy, protein excretion usually subsides after delivery, but not necessarily to preconception levels [95,96, 104,148]. It is unknown whether the heavy proteinuria is due to effacement of the podocyte foot processes and changes in the slit diaphragms with overload to the tubules, and the mechanisms of postpartum repair are also unclear. There is concern that temporary heavy overload proteinuria in pregnancy exceeding maximal proximal tubular reabsorption could contribute to later tubulo-interstitial fibrosis via upregulation of vasoactive and inflammatory genes [149]. Follow-up studies of women with DN are discussed in the next section.

Prior to pregnancy the subtle rise in daytime *blood pressure* (BP) observed in most diabetic women and adolescents with persistent microalbuminuria [150-152] has been considered secondary [153] or perhaps compensatory [154] to early renovascular pathology [155-157]. On the other hand, several studies of ambulatory BP monitoring suggest that subtly higher daytime or nocturnal systolic pressure precedes or predicts the development of microalbuminuria in type 1 and type2 diabetic women [158-163]. It is important to note that 24-hr ambulatory BP monitoring of non-diabetic controls showed that females have significantly lower daytime and nightime systolic and diastolic levels than males, but that this gender differential is minimized with type 1 diabetes for unknown reasons [164]. Diabetic microalbuminuria is associated with (1) enhanced BP responsiveness to norepinephrine and angiotensin II infusion and sodium intake [165-167], (2) increased $Na+/Li+$ countertransport activity [168], and (3) an increased peripheral transcapillary escape rate of albumin [169], suggesting linkage of renal and vascular pathogenic processes. These studies and many others raise the question of genetic susceptibility to hypertension and nephropathy [170] which is perhaps linked to PET [171].

During pregnancy ambulatory BP monitoring of non-diabetic women has been used to predict hypertensive complications in the third trimester with fairly low sensitivity and specificity [172,173]. In type 1 diabetic pregnant women, mid-pregnancy cutoffs of >105 nighttime systolic [174] or >122 daytime systolic [136] provided the best sensitivity-specificity for third trimester hypertension. However, a careful study in Denmark showed that UAE 30-299 mg/24hr was a better predictor of PET in type 1 diabetes than diurnal BP (patients with treated hypertension were excluded) [135]. In a study of early pregnancy TPE in American diabetic women (mixed type 1 and type 2), 27% of 45 women with microproteinuria (190-499 mg/24hr) were treated for chronic hypertension compared to 39% in 62 patients with 500 mg/24hr and only 6% in 204 women with TPE <190 mg/24hr [133]. Patients with both early pregnancy microproteinuria and chronic hypertension had the highest frequency (~50%) of superimposed PET.

In a New Zealand study of pooled groups of 100 each of type 1 and 2 diabetes, significant factors *predicting the development of hypertension in pregnancy* included nulliparity (RR 1.5), smoking (RR 0.39), duration diabetes ≥10 years (RR 1.87), earliest HbA1c ≥9.0 (RR 1.9), retinopathy (RR 1.8), earliest UAE 30-300 mg/24hr (RR 1.8), earliest systolic BP 116-129 mmHg or higher (RR 2.1), and earliest diastolic BP ≥80 mmHg (RR 2.5) [175]. Many of these parameters are interelated. Primary PET was more common in type 1 (19%) than in type 2 (7%) diabetes, while the latter cases had more chronic hypertension and micro- and macroalbuminuria. Similar predictors of hypertensive disorders in pregnant women with type 1 diabetes were identified in large Swedish and North American multicenter studies [176-178]. Initial hypertension in women with DN is a strong predictor of "cross-over" from a hyperdynamic hemodynamic state with increased cardiac output to vasoconstriction associated with PET and decline in renal function [103]. A combined family history for hypertension and type 2 diabetes is a strong predictor of risk of hypertension [171], perhaps related to insulin resistance as a risk factor for PET [179-180]. Prediction of risks for development of PET and understanding of its pathogenesis [181-183] is important to find means of preventing this syndrome [184], which is a major cause of maternal-fetal mortality and morbidity. Trials of supplementation of fish oil, calcium, magnesium, and zinc, and use of low-dose aspirin have generally been disappointing [185-186]. Trials of antihypertensive drugs for prevention of PET have been inadequately powered and choice of agents limited by concerns for fetal injury [185]. Supplementation with antioxidant vitamins in pregnant women at high risk holds some promise [187]. Undoubtedly studies will be designed to test the hypothesis (see below) that normalization of circulating free vascular endothelial growth factor (VEGF) and placental growth factor (PlGF) levels will halt progression of PET [188], which would certainly improve the outcome of DN in pregnancy if the pathogenesis is the same as in "pure" PET.

Maternal characteristics identified in early pregnancy in 225 cases of *clinical DN* reported in 1981-1996 include ~50% frequencies of proliferative retinopathy, anemia, and hypertension. Reduced CrCl (<80 ml/min) was recorded in 45% of cases and 15% of the total had serum creatinine (Cr) >134uM (table 4) [38,95,96,98,100,101,148,189-192]. Low-level proteinuria (<1 gm total protein/24 hrs before 20 weeks gestation) was detected in many of the women, so these cases are suspected not to be "true" DN, therefore the frequencies of anemia, hypertension, PDR, and impaired glomerular filtration probably should be higher. Of 146 diabetic women with >1 gm total protein/24 hrs in early pregnancy, 57 had impaired renal function at that stage of gestation (Cr>134 uM or CrCl <80 ml/min), and 37% showed a further decline of >15% during later pregnancy. Three series of pregnant women with DN reported since 1996 show similar proportions of these maternal complications [102, 104,193]. Pregnancy is probably contraindicated in patients with DN if the Cr is above 206 µM or CrCl is below 50 ml/min before or in early pregnancy, because of the high rate of maternal and fetal complications, until renal transplantation can be performed 2 years prior to conception.

Table 4. Course of renal parameters during and after pregnancy in women with diabetic nephropathy. Data pooled from references 95,96,100,101,148,190,191,192

	Hypertension	Ur Prot ≥ 5 gm/d	Decr CrC1 Incr Cr	Renal Failure	Death
Early preg	42%	9%	34%	0	0
Late preg	71%	26%	26%	0	0
Follow-up	60%	17%	43%	23%**	5.6%

* 195 women x 1-10 yrs, median 2.6 yrs

Maternal *anemia* results from both decreased erythropoietin production by damaged kidneys and the physiologic hemodilution of pregnancy. The degree of anemia is related to the severity of nephropathy as reflected in lower creatinine clearance and is not usually associated with abnormal iron studies [95]. Exogenous erythropoietin can be used to treat anemia unresponsive to iron and folate replacement [194-197]. Asymptomatic *bacteriuria* is more common in diabetic than non-diabetic women, leading to a greater risk of UTI [198-201], but there is controversy over screening and treatment outside of pregnancy [202,203]. During pregnancy screening and preventive treatment of women with hypertension or DN is justified due to the deleterious effects of pyelonephritis [95]. Although paradoxically PET in the third trimester may be less common in non-diabetic women who smoke cigarettes [175,177,204], *smoking* should be strongly discouraged in diabetic women due to impaired fetal oxygenation in mid-pregnancy and hazardous effects on progression of DN [206-209].

Diabetic nephropathy can progress to *end-stage renal disease (ESRD) during pregnancy*, although this is unusual. Of 195 women followed after pregnancy and summarized in table 4, none progressed to end-stage disease during pregnancy. There is experience with both hemodialysis and continuous ambulatory peritoneal dialysis in pregnancy, but analyzed cases include few diabetic women [210-216]. In about one-fourth of reported cases of dialysis in pregnancy the patients conceived prior to starting dialysis – they either were close to needing dialysis prior to the unplanned gestation or had a rapid decline in renal function during pregnancy [213]. In this group termination of pregnancy rarely rescues the kidneys [217,218], and "unless transplant is a certainty, the pregnancy may be the woman's last chance to have a child" [213]. In women using dialysis prior to conception treatment of anemia with erythropoietin and/or blood transfusion is usually required [195]. In a US national registry survey of pregnancy in dialysis patients with ESRD of various causes (36.6% primary glomerular diseases, 26.3% lupus or other vasculitis, 7.4% diabetes, 6.6% interstitial diseases, 14.2% other) , BP was normal in only 21%, and severe hypertension (BP >170/110) was noted at some time during pregnancy or postpartum in 48% [213]. There were 5 episodes of peritonitis in 59 pregnancies in women treated with peritoneal dialysis; there were 245 pregnancies in women using hemodialysis, and 2 maternal deaths in the entire group, which is "lower than the average for dialysis patients of child-bearing age as a whole" [213]. Therefore the risk of death for a dialysis patient who becomes pregnant is not increased by the pregnancy, but "the severity of the illness in the women with hypertensive crisis is evidence that pregnancy is a dangerous undertaking for a pregnant patient" [213].

EFFECT OF PREGNANCY ON THE SUBSEQUENT PROGRESSION OF DIABETIC NEPHROPATHY

For years, there has been concern that the hyperfiltration, hypertension, or heavy proteinuria of pregnancy might damage glomeruli, tubules, and interstitium and accelerate the postpartum progression of DN to end-stage renal disease. In a pooled series of 195 women experiencing pregnancies with DN and having renal function assessed 1-10 years afterwards, 23% were in renal failure and 5.6% had died (table 4). Not surprisingly, the frequency of progression to renal failure after pregnancy was 49% in the group of women with impaired renal function in early pregnancy, compared to 7% if Cr was <134 uM or CrCl was >80 ml/min in early gestation (table 5) [38,95,96, 98,100,101,148,189-192]. A similar risk of post-pregnancy decline of renal function based on pre- or early pregnancy CrCl was also reported by Biesenbach, and he speculated that inadequate antihypertensive therapy may have contributed to the original and further decline in renal function [104].

Table 5. Course of diabetic nephropathy during and after pregnancy comparing patients with preserved vs impaired renal function in early pregnancy. Data pooled from references 95,96,190, 192,192 . Note the limited number of cases with severe azotemia in early pregnancy.

| | Initial renal function | | |
	Preserved	Impaired*	Cr >177
Number	70	57	(6)
Decline during pregnancy	12 (17%)	21 (37%)	(1)
Renal failure after preg**	4 of 57 (7%)	37 of 55 (49%)	(3)
Died	2 (3.5%)	5 (9.1%)	(0)

* Cr >100 uM, CrCl < 80 ml/min
** 1-10 yrs.

Three early studies assessed renal function after pregnancy in women with nephropathy [95,99,192]. All found that Cr Cl declined an average of about 10 ml/min per year, similar to the average rate in men and women with DN at that time [219-221]. More recently the annual decline in GFR in DN has improved to 2-5 ml/min/yr [222,223] due to advances in renoprotection [28]. Rossing and colleagues at the Steno Diabetes Center in Denmark conducted an observational study of female patients who developed DN in 1984-89 and were followed until death or the year 2000 [224]. Decline in Cr Cl over a median of 10 years postpartum was 3.2 ± 3.4 ml/min/yr in 17 parous patients vs 3.2 ± 5.1 ml/min/yr in 42 women never pregnant.

Other approaches have been used to examine the question of whether experiencing pregnancy hastens the progression of DN. With impaired renal function, the speed of progression to end-stage disease is little or no different whether a pregnancy is terminated in the first trimester or carried into the third trimester [95]. Miodovnik observed that increasing parity did not increase the risk of renal failure after pregnancy [192], and the EURODIAB Type 1

Complications Survey [225] and the Pittsburgh Epidemiology of Diabetes Complications case control study [226] found that parity did not increase the incidence of micro- or macroalbuminuria. In the Diabetes Control and Complications Trial, pregnancy had no effect on the end-of-study prevalence of albuminuria [53]. Purdy et al thought that 5 of 11 women with DN and moderate renal insufficiency had an accelerated rate of decline in renal function during pregnancy, but in follow-up for a mean of 2 years postpartum the group of 11 had slightly less decline in inverse Cr than 11 similar patients without pregnancy [101]. Mackie and colleagues [100] and Kaaja et al [227] also found no evidence for accelerated decline of renal function after pregnancy compared to non-pregnant patients. Therefore the medical practice of discouraging pregnancy in women with DN with mild-to-moderate impairment of renal function based on presumed increased risks of renal failure has no basis in published experience.

DIABETIC NEPHROPATHY AND PERINATAL OUTCOME

In spite of the dramatic improvements in perinatal outcome over the last 25 years in pregnancies of diabetic women [228], complications remain more frequent when DN is present. Examining the pooled results of 13 clinical series published in 1981-96 (table 6) [36,38, 95,96, 98, 100,101,148, 189-192,229], of 265 infants born to women with DN, nearly 2/3 were preterm deliveries prior to 37 weeks gestation, 72.5% were delivered by cesarean section, and respiratory distress syndrome was diagnosed in 24.5% of liveborn infants. Fetal growth restriction was noted in 14.3%, and the major correlates of small size for dates were the degree of maternal hypertension and impaired renal function [95,96,191]. Major congenital malformations were diagnosed in 7.6% of the 265 infants. The frequencies of these perinatal complication were similar in 90 pregnancies reported in 1981-88 compared to 175 reported in 1992-96 (table 6), and in the subsequent reports of Reece et al [193] and Biesenbach and colleagues [230]. *Perinatal mortality* rates were 55.5/1000 and 34.3/1000 in the earlier and later group, respectively. Overall, 95.8% of infants survived to leave the neonatal intensive care unit. These clinical results would probably be somewhat worse in women with "true" clinical DN diagnosed prior to pregnancy. At least 16% of the pooled cases probably had only microalbuminuria preconception, as they were included in the DN reports based on <1 gm/day total protein excretion in the first trimester. Limiting the analysis of perinatal mortality to 223 cases with >1 gm/day total urinary protein excretion in the first trimester, perinatal mortality rates were 54.8/1000 in

1982-88 compared to 71.4/1000 in 1992-96 (table 6). Major congenital malformations and severe fetal growth restriction were responsible for most of the perinatal deaths.

Table 6. Diabetic nephropathy and perinatal outcome in two eras in which perinatal technology was utilized. Data pooled from references 38,95,96,98,100,101,148,189-192.

Year of report	1981-88	1992-96
Infants	90	275
Perinatal survival	94.4%	96.6%
Foetal growth restriction	13.3%	14.9%
Preterm delivery	57.8%	64.6%
Caesarean delivery	68.9%	74.3%
Respiratory distress syndrome	25.6%	24.2%
Major congenital malformations	7.8%	7.7%

The relationship of *perinatal morbidity* to the severity of diabetic nephropathy is illustrated in table 7. Selecting out cases from the pooled series with sufficient detail for analysis [95,96, 190,191], 19 women had >1 gm/day total urinary protein with preserved renal function in early pregnancy, compared to 41 proteinuric diabetic women with CrCl <80 ml/min. or serum Cr >134 uM. Not surprisingly, the latter group had much higher rates of fetal growth restriction, PET, fetal distress causing delivery, and serious prematurity (table 7). In a later analysis of 60 pregnancies with DN at the Cincinnati regional program, Khoury et al confirmed high rates of fetal growth restriction, preterm birth <32 weeks gestation, and attendant neonatal complications in 9 women with initial Cr levels above 163 μM (1.5 mg/dL), even though superimposed PET (44.4%) was no higher than in 39 women with Cr <109 μM (1.0 mg/dL) [97]. All of these data can be used for counseling women with DN prior to pregnancy. Very similar results and clinical relationships are reported for pregnancies in women with other chronic glomerular or tubulointerstitial diseases [194,217,218,231-236]. It is controversial whether fetal outcome is determined by type of glomerulopathy (eg, focal and segmental glomerulosclerosis being worse) [237] or primarily by risk factors associated with nephropathy, such as degree of hypertension and/or level of renal impairment [232,235,236].

Table 7. Perinatal outcome related to renal status in early pregnancy in women with diabetic nephropathy. Data combined from cases reported in references 95,96,190,191.

	Initial Renal Function with TPE >1 gm/d		
	Prot 0.3-0.9gm/d	Preserved	Impaired*
Number	18	19	41
Fetal growth restriction	1 (6%)	1 (5%)	11 (27%)
PET**	2 (11%)	4 (21%)	15 (37%)
Fetal distress	1 (6%)	4 (21%)	12 (29%)
Fetal death	1	1	1
Deliv 24-33 w	4 (22%)	5 (26%)	18 (38%)
Uncomplicated	10 (56%)	6 (32%)	9 (24%)

*Cr >130 uM (1.2 mg/dL) or CrCl <80 ml/min   **PET, preeclamptic toxemia

Perinatal outcome in women with *ESRD on dialysis* is expectedly poor, with few pregnancies reaching term or normal birth weight; published series include patients with all forms of renal failure, including diabetes [210,213-216,218, 238]. In the largest national registry series only 42% of 320 pregnancies resulted in surviving infants, but survival was better at 73.6% in women who conceived before starting dialysis [213]. The same differential regarding perinatal survival was seen in a smaller national survey in Belgium [215]. In women becoming pregnant already on dialysis, there is a continuum of mid-trimester fetal loss (21%) (often with severe growth restriction) and pre-term delivery before 28 weeks gestation in 18% [213,214]. Obstetric complications include polyhydramnios and placental abruption [210,212,214-216]. Pregnancy outcome does not seem to differ between women using hemodialysis vs. continuous ambulatory peritoneal dialysis, but is worse with severe hypertension in either group [213,216]. The high rate of congenital malformations of 14.7% reported in the US registry [213] was not observed in 3 smaller contemporary reports (none in 49 pregnancies) [214-216]. Susan Hou has published useful guidelines for the management of dialysis and pregnancy [239].

Superimposed *preeclamptic toxemia* (PET) is a leading cause of prematurity in pregnant women with diabetes [176,178,240,241] and diabetic nephropathy [95,96,190, 191]. This syndrome with variable features [242,243] is suspected when there is an increase in blood pressure and proteinuria in the third trimester. Albuminuria is often evident before hypertension. The hypertension is attributed to excess of vasoconstrictive or lack of vasodilator factors [244], and current research focuses on insufficient free VEGF activity [245,246] and NO action [247], excess sympathetic nervous activity [248-250], and excess reactive oxygen species [251-255] and endothelial dysfunction [256-259]. Physiologic renal measurements in diabetic [83] or non-diabetic women with PET demonstrate impaired GFR in the third trimester compared to hyperfiltering normal pregnant controls (105 vs 158 ml/min), with or without slightly reduced RPF [84]. It is doubtful the relative glomerular hypofiltration in PET is due to decreased plasma flow or glomerular transcapillary pressure. Physio-morphometric studies of the kidneys suggest impaired hydraulic permeability of the glomerular capillary walls curtailing water flow [84,260], secondary to reduced endothelial fenestration density and size, plus subendothelial fibrinoid deposits and loss of capillary patency due to mesangio-endotheliosis with inflammatory cell exudation [260]. Mesangio-endotheliosis progresses to focal or segmental glomeulosclerosis in a subset of patients [261,262]. In spite of diminished ulrafiltration, in PET there is a marked increase in excretion of albumin and total proteins. Competing explanations of the proteinuria include loss of charge-selectivity of the glomerular capillary wall [263], loss of size-selectivity due to increased shunt pathway [84], or perhaps to changes in the tubular lysosome-mediated degradation of albumin during renal passage [264].

An intriguing unifying hypothesis linking the placental, renal, and vascular pathology has emerged [188,265], in which PET my be an antiangiogenic state due to excess placental soluble VEGF1 receptor (sVEGF1R) (sFlt1) [266-268]. This tyrosine kinase-family ligand for VEGF that is expressed by human cytotrophoblasts [267,269-271] (1) captures free VEGF-A and PlGF needed for endothelial function [188], (2) inhibits VEGF-induced dilation of renal arterioles, (3) causes hypertension and proteinuria in pregnant and non-pregnant rats, and (4) causes glomerular endotheliosis (glomerular enlargement with occlusion of capillary loops by swelling and hypertrophy of endocapillary cells, fibrinoid deposits, protein-resorption droplets within podocytes with only focal foot-process effacement) [268]. In rodents and man VEGF is expressed by podocytes, distal duct epithelia, and activated mesangial cells, and VEGF1R by glomerular and peritubular capillaries and pre- and postglomerular vessels [272,273]. A separate study showed that glomeruli in mice with 50% VEGF signaling develop endotheliosis with hyaline deposits and then lose endothelial fenestrations and podocyte foot processes as they develop nephrosis [273].

With preexisting DN, it may not be possible to clinically distinguish "true" PET from a "simple" worsening of hypertension and proteinuria. The distinction is important because the former is best treated by delivery whereas the latter is treated with bed rest and antihypertensive agents. Edema and hyperuricemia are common in patients with both renal disease and PET and therefore are not useful in the differential diagnosis. Hypo-albuminemia commonly results from excessive proteinuria in PET and leads to generalized edema. Occasionally, thrombocytopenia or elevated transaminases are found and these support a diagnosis of superimposed PET in women with DN. As a practical matter, it is generally necessary to observe the patient at hospital bed rest, with or without anti-hypertensive therapy. We lack controlled studies of the timing of delivery in women with DN with or without PET. The decision to deliver the infant must balance the gestational age, the severity of the maternal condition, and indicators of fetal well-being.

Unfortunately no controlled trials of treatment of hypertensive pregnant women with DN have been reported. The Canadian Hypertension Society Consensus Conference recommended a threshold of 140/90 to start antihypertensive treatment during pregnancy [274]. An Australasian consensus group recommended maintaining BP between 110-140 systolic and 80-90 diastolic for pregnant women with chronic or gestational hypertension [275]. A U.S. National Heart, Lung, and Blood Institute consensus group recommended that antihypertensive treatment be used during pregnancy only for BP levels $\geq$150-160 mm Hg systolic and/or $\geq$100-110 mm Hg diastolic to protect the gravida, based on inconclusive effects on perinatal outcome at lower levels in controlled trials in non-diabetic hypertensive women [276]. The group reasoned that untreated women would be at low risk for cardiovascular complications within the short time frame of pregnancy. On the other hand, there is increasing focus on the potential implications of hypertension in pregnancy on long-term cardiovascular and renal risk in women [104,277,278]. Many investigators follow evidence-based guidelines recommending treatment for non-pregnant diabetic women with hypertension or micro—macroalbuminuria [279-282] and continue during pregnancy with agents that are safe for the fetus [30,283]. Such agents include methyldopa, beta-adrenergic blockers other than atenolol, calcium channel blockers, clonidine, and perhaps prazocin [274,284]. There is concern about impaired fetal growth with atenolol [285-287], although one controlled trial demonstrated less superimposed preeclampsia using atenolol in hypertensive women with elevated cardiac output [288]. Suggested BP targets to guide therapy outside of pregnancy are <140/90 for non-diabetic patients [279] and <130/80 for diabetic subjects [282]. Some believe use of the latter target during non-diabetic pregnancy may contribute to fetal growth restriction [283], but this concept has not been examined in controlled trials in diabetic pregnant women.

As noted, fetal growth delay is related to placental pathology, maternal hypertension or its treatment. Serial sonography is indicated to evaluate fetal growth. In addition, fetal heart rate monitoring or biophysical assessment should be employed because growth restriction or fetal hyperglycemia-hypoxia-acidosis [289] is frequently associated with evidence of fetal distress. For women with clinical DN, begin weekly nonstress testing at 26 weeks' gestation, move to twice-weekly testing at 34 weeks, but earlier if there is growth delay. Vaginal delivery is preferred if there is no evidence of fetal distress and no obstetric contraindication. However, as noted in table 6, there was a remarkably high cesarean rate with DN, the reasons for which are not entirely elucidated.

PREGNANCY AFTER RENAL TRANSPLANTATION

Ogburn et al. compiled the experience of 9 diabetic women from several centers who had pregnancy after renal transplantation for DN [290]. All were managed with prednisone and azathioprine; no transplant rejections occurred during pregnancy. Complications were frequent, including PET in 6, fetal distress in 6, and preterm delivery in all. Armenti and the US National Transplant Pregnancy Registry (NTPR) reported 28 pregnancies in diabetic renal transplant recipients after cyclosporine A (CsA) was added to the immunosuppression regimen to decrease acute rejection [291]. Rejection was observed in 4% and graft dysfunction in 11%. Preeclampsia was diagnosed in 17% although 59% had hypertension - 47% of the infants had neonatal complications.

Most studies of pregnancy after renal transplant included limited numbers of diabetic women among patients with other renal diseases [292,293]. GFR increases ~30% during pregnancy in women with renal allografts, but not to the extent of normal controls, and the gradual decline in CrCl the last 6 weeks of gestation is similar to controls [292,294]. The extent of increase in CrCl is dependent on preconception levels [294]. Early reports of fetal growth delay with CsA [295,296] were not confirmed in other small studies [297,298] and are difficult to compare with results in larger surveys. These report a prevalence of low birth weight of 23-63% and delivery <37 weeks in 38-75%, but most do not provide data on size-for-dates, so the contribution from prematurity to low birth weight is unclear [218, 292,293, 299,300]. Perinatal mortality ranges 30-270/1000 in pregnancies after renal allografts across several decades, but the high figures are in earlier pregnancies without recent improvements in perinatal management and antihypertensive-immunosuppressive therapy [292,293,299,301]. Many of the perinatal losses were in poorly controlled diabetic women. Prevention of infection is especially important in these immunosuppressed diabetic patients, and monthly urine cultures are recommended [218].

Predictors of increased risk for premature delivery in renal transplant patients include increased Cr level, hypertension before 28 weeks gestation [292,293,299], and graft dysfunction in the peripartum period [302]. Azathioprine is not associated with excess congenital malformations [218], and the prevalence rate with CsA was 4.1%, but the odds ratio of 3.83 vs other agents was not significant [300]. The NTPR also found no excess fetal malformations in 154 pregnancies [303]. Concern for toxic effects of maternal CsA treatment on fetal-placental function was not borne out in a study of nitric oxide synthase, endothelin-1 and tissue factor in human placentas [304]. There is limited information on outcomes with use of the newer immunosuppressants tacrolimus [301], the potentially reprotoxic mycophenolate mofetil [304], or the immunoglobulin G muromonab-CD3 (OKT3) [306] during pregnancy.

These studies of immuno-suppressive agents on perinatal outcome are not well controlled for confounders such as degree of hypertension and renal failure prior to pregnancy. CsA is associated with more hypertension in pregnancy [218,293] and later cardiovascular disease, which might be related to impaired basal and stimulated endothelial production of nitric oxide [307] or increased production of endothelin and thromboxane [218]. One wonders if there is more PET with CsA treatment than other agents – Hou gives a frequency of 29% [218]. A preliminary registry study of pregnancy outcomes with the newer immunosuppressive agents Neoral and tacrolimus showed similar high rates of hypertension, PET, and prematurity [308]. In a survey of 175 children exposed to CsA *in utero* and followed to preschool and early school age, 16% were noted to have delays or need educational support [309]. This may not be significantly greater than for premature infants in the general population. Continuous fetal exposure to CsA seemingly impairs development or maturation of lymphocytes, with effects still apparent at one year of age, but none of 6 infants had clinical evidence of an immunodeficient state [310]. There is also concern about possible remote effects of maternal immunosuppression causing auto-immune or reproductive disorders in daughters of treated mothers [311,312], but long-term followup studies are still inadequate. Finally, the impact and potential mechanisms for effects of female gender on many aspects of renal transplantation have been reviewed [313,314].

Combined kidney-pancreas transplants prior to pregnancy have been reported several times [315-318], and the NTPR also reported 23 pregnancies after combined transplants [319]. In this group 25% had PET while 91% were hypertensive; 70% of deliveries were premature. Two-thirds of these gravidas were treated for some type of infections. Barrou et al reviewed 19 cases of pregnancy after simultaneous pancreas-kidney transplants reported to the International Pancreas Transplant Registry in the CsA era [320]. There were 19 live births with average birth weight 2150 ± 680 gm and two major congenital malformations. Only one pancreas graft and one kidney graft were lost after pregnancy in two different recipients. Pancreas-kidney transplantation may reduce risk factors for the development of macroangiopathy but fails to halt progression of macrovascular diseases [321].

Beyond these studies, there has been hypothetical concern that pregnancy may adversely affect renal graft survival [294,297]. The NTPR reported an 11% frequency of rejection episodes during pregnancy or within 3 months postpartum in 197 CsA treated pregnancies [293]. CsA blood levels declined during pregnancy in groups with and without rejection. In a series of 29 women in southern Spain renal function remained stable during pregnancy in 72%, postpartum renal allograft deterioration was detected in 8 patients (28%), and 5 required reinitiation of dialysis at 4 months to 5 years after pregnancy [298]. Studies with long-term follow-up found no difference in graft survival or function between women who became pregnant and matched controls who did not [302,322,323]. Maternal and neonatal factors did not predict pancreas-kidney graft loss over two years postpartum in 6 of 37 diabetic women [324].On the other hand, renal graft failure seems to be greater after 2 or more pregnancies [325], an effect possibly related to pregnancy-induced anti-HLA immunization detected only by flow cytometric evaluation [326].

Lindheimer and Katz [327] and Susan Hou [218] provide guidelines on preconception counseling of women with renal transplants. Women should wait 2 years post-transplant with immunosuppression at maintenance levels (prednisone <15 mg/day, azathioprine <2 mg/kg/day, CsA <5 mg/kg/day) and no evidence of active graft rejection. This requires effective contraception. Renal function should show serum Cr <130 uM (<1.5 mg/dL) [327] or <163 uM (<2.0 mg/dl) [218] with 24-hr urine TPE <500 mg. Blood pressure and glycemic levels should be well controlled with medication, and post-transplant hyperglycemia should be ruled out in previously non-diabetic women [328,329].

REFERENCES

1. Kitzmiller JL, Buchanan TA, Kjos S, et al. Pre-conception care of diabetes, congenital malformations, and spontaneous abortions. Technical Review. Diab Care 1996; 19:514-41.

2. Damm P, Molsted-Pedersen L. Significant decrease in congenital malformations in newborn infants of an unselected population of diabetic women. Am J Obst Gynec 1989; 161:1163-7.

3. Kitzmiller JL, Gavin LA, Gin GD, et al. Preconception care of diabetes. Glycemic control prevents congenital anomalies. JAMA 1991; 265: 731-6.

4. McElvy SS, Miodovnik M, Rosenn B, et al: A focused preconceptional and early pregnancy program in women with type 1 diabetes reduces perinatal mortality and malformation rates to general population levels. J Mat Fetal Med 2000; 9:14-20.

5. Ray JG, O'Brien, Chan WS: Preconception care and the risk of congenital anomalies in the offspring of women with diabetes mellitus: a meta-analysis. Q J M 2001; 94:435-44.

6. StJames PJ, Younger MD, Hamilton BD, Waisbren SE. Unplanned pregnancies in diabetic women. Diab Care 1993; 16:1572-8.

7. Garg SK, Chase HP, Marshall G, et al: Oral contraceptives and renal and retinal complications in young women with insulin-dependent diabetes mellitus. JAMA 1994; 271:1099-1102.

8. Petersen KR, Skouby SO, Sidelmann J, et al: Effects of contraceptive steroids on cardiovascular risk factors in women with insulin-dependent diabetes mellitus. Am J Obst Gynecol 1994; 171:400-5.

9. Kjos SL: Contraception in diabetic women. Obst Gynecol Clinics North Amer 1996; 23:243-57

10. Janz NK, Herman WH, Becker MP, et al. Diabetes and pregnancy: factors associated with seeking pre-conception care. Diab Care 1995; 18: 157-65.

11. Holing E, Beyer CS. Why don't women with diabetes plan their pregnancies? Diabetes Care 1998;21:889-895.

12. Mogensen CE, Vestbo E, Poulsen PL, et al: Microalbuminuria and potential confounders. A review and some observations on variability of urinary albumin collection. Diabetes Care 1995; 18:572-581

13. Tomaselli L, Trischitta V, Vinci C, et al: Evaluation of albumin excretion rate in overnight versus 24-h urine. Diabetes Care 1989;12:585-87.

14. Stehouwer CDA, Fischer HRA, Hackeng WHL, den Ottolander GJH: Identifying patients with incipient diabetic nephropathy. Should 24-hour collections be used? Arch Int Med 1990;150:373-5.

15. Combs CA, Wheeler BC, Kitzmiller JL. Urinary protein/creatinine ratio before and during pregnancy in women with diabetes mellitus. Am J Obstet Gynecol 1991; 165: 920-923.

16. Stehouwer CDA, Fischer HRA, Hackeng WHL, et al. Diurnal variation in urinary protein excretion in diabetic nephropathy. Nephrol Dial Transplant 1991; 6: 238-243.

17. Lindow SW, Davey DA: The variability of urinary protein and creatinine excretion in patients with gestational proteinuric hypertension. Brit J Obst Gynecol 1992;99:869-72.

18. Quadri KHM, Bernardini J, Greenberg MD, et al. Assessment of renal function during pregnancy using a random urine protein to creatinine ratio and Cockcroft-Gault ratio. Amer J Kid Dis 1994;:416-420.

19. Houlihan CA, Tsalamandris C, Akdeniz A, Jerums G: Albumin to creatinine ratio: a screening test with limitations. Am J Kidney Dis 2002;39:1183-9.

20. Comper WD, Osicka TM, Jerums G: High prevalence of immuno-unreactive intact albumin in urine of diabetic patients. Am J Kidney Dis 2003;41:336-342.

21. Keevil BG, Kilpatrick ES, Nichols SP, Maylor PW: Biological variation of cystatin C: implications for the assessment of glomerular filtration rate. Clin Chem 1998; 44:1535-9.

22. Randers E, Erlandsen EJ: Serum cystatin c as an endogenous marker of the renal function – a review. Clin Chem Lab Med 1999; 37:389-95.

23. Harmoinen APT, Kouri TT, Wirta OR, et al: Evaluation of plasma cystatin C as a marker for glomerular filtration rate in patients with type 2 diabetes. Clin Nephrol 1999; 52:363-70.

24. Dworkin LD: Serum cystatin C as a marker of glomerular filtration rate. Curr Opin Nephrol Hypert 2001; 10:551-63.

25. Leach TD, Kitiyakara C, Price CP, et al: Prognostic significance of serum cystatin C concentrations in renal transplant recipients: 5-year follow-up. Transplant Proc 2002; 34:1152-8.

26. Strevens H, Wide-Swensson D, Torffvit O, Grubb A: Serum cystatin C for assessment of glomerular filtration rate in pregnant and non-pregnant women. Indications of altered filtration process in pregnancy. Scand J Clin Lab Invest 2002; 62:141-8.

27. Oberbauer R, Nenov V, Weidekamm C,et al: Reduction in mean glomerular pore size coincides with the development of large shunt pores in patients with diabetic nephropathy. Exp Nephrol 2001; 9:49-53.

28. Parving H-H, Hovind P, Rossing K, Andersen S: Evolving strategies for renoprotection: diabetic nephropathy. Curr Opin Nephrol Hypertens 2001;10,515-522

29. Conway DL, Langer O: Selecting antihypertensive therapy in the pregnant woman with diabetes mellitus. J Mat-Fetal Med 2000;9:66-9.

30. Magee LA: Treating hypertension in women of child-bearing age and during pregnancy. Drug Safety 2001;24:457-474.

31. Rosenthal T, Oparil S: The effect of antihypertensive drugs on the fetus. J Hum Hypertens 2002;16:293-8

32. Lip GYH, Churchill D, Beevers M, et al: Angiotensin-converting enzyme inhibitors in early pregnancy. Lancet 1997;350:1446-7

33. Burrows RF, Burrows EA: Assessing the teratogenic potential of angiotensin-converting enzyme inhibitors in pregnancy. Aust NZ J Obst Gynaecol 1998;38,306-311

34. Saji H, Yamanaka M, Hagiwara A, Iijri R: Losartan and fetal toxic effects. Lancet 2001,357:36319.

35. Kurz TW: False claims of blood pressure-independent protection by blockade of the renin angiotensin aldosterone system? Hypertens 2003; 41:193-6.

36. Hod M, van Dijk DJ, Karp M, et al. Diabetic nephropathy and pregnancy: the effect of ACE inhibitors prior to pregnancy on maternal outcome. Neph Dial Transpl 1995; 10: 2328-33

37. Bar JB, Schoenfeld A, Orvieto R, et al: Pregnancy outcome in patients with insulin dependent diabetes mellitus and diabetic nephropathy treated with ACE inhibitors before pregnancy. J Ped Endocrin Metab 1999;12:659-665

38. Jovanovic R, Jovanovic L. Obstetric management when normoglycemia is maintained in diabetic pregnant women with vascular compromise. Am J Obstet Gynecol 1984; 149: 617-623.

39. Danielsson BR, Reiland S, Rundqvist E, Danielson M: Digital defects induced by vasodilating agents: relationship to reduction in uteroplacental blood flow. Teratology 1989; 40:351-8.

40. Magee LA, Conover B, Schick B, et al. Exposure to calcium channel blockers in human pregnancy: a prospective, controlled, multicentre cohort study. Teratol 1994; 49:372-6.

41. Demarie BK, Bakris GL: Effects of different classes of calcium antagonists on proteinuria in diabetic subjects. Ann Int Med 1990; 113:987-8.

42. Bakris GL: Effects of diltiazem or lisinopril on massive proteinuria associated with diabetes mellitus. Ann Int Med 1990; 112:701-2.

43. Bakris G, Copley J, Vicknair N, et al: Calcium channel blockers versus other antohypertensive therapies on progression of NIDDM associated nephropathy. Kidney Intl 1996; 1641-50.

44. Podjarny E, Haskiah A, Pomeranz A, et al: Effect of diltiazem and methyldopa on gestastion-related renal complications in rats with adriamycin nephrosis. Relationship to glomerular prostanoid synthesis. Nephrol Dial Transplant 1995; 10:1598-1602.

45. Griffin KA, Picken MM, Bidani AK: Deleterious effects of calcium channel blockade on pressure transmission and glomerular injury in rat remnant kidneys. J Clin Invest 1995; 96:793-800.

46. Griffin KA, Picken MM, Bakris GL, Bidani AK: Comparative effects of selective T- and L-type calcium channel blockers in the remnant kidney model. Hypertension 2001; 37:1268-72.

47. Brinchmann-Hansen O, Dahl-Jørgensen K, Hanssen KF, et al. Effects of intensified insulin treatment on various lesions of diabetic retinopathy. Am J Ophthalmol 1985; 100: 644-9

48. Bereket A, Lang CH, Blethen SL, et al: Effect of insulin on the insulin-like growth factor system in children with new-onset insulin-dependent diabetes mellitus.J Clin Endocrinol Metab 1995;80:1312-7.

49. Attia N, Caprio S, Jones TW: Changes in free insulin-like growth factor-1 and leptin concentrations during acute metabolic decompensation in insulin withdrawn patients with type 1 diabetes. J Clin Endocrinol Metab 1999; 84:2324-8.

50. Lauszus FF, Klebe JG, Bek T, Flyvbjerg A: Increased serum IGF-I during pregnancy is associated with progression of diabetic retinopathy. Diabetes 2003;52:852-6.

51. Pfeiffer A, Spranger J, Meyer-Schwickerath R, Schatz H: Growth factor alterations in advanced diabetic retinopatrhy: a possible role of blood retina breakdown. Diabetes 1997; 46(Suppl2):S26-30.

52. Hill DJ, Flyvberg A, Arany E, et al: Increased serum levels of serum fibroblast growth factor-2 in diabetic pregnant women with retinopathy. J Clin Endocrinol Metab 1997; 82:1452-7.

53. DCCT Research Group: Effect of pregnancy on microvascular complications in the Diabetes Control and Complications Trial. Diabetes Care 2000; 23:1084-91.

54. Klein BEK, Moss SE, Klein R. Effect of pregnancy on progression of diabetic retinopathy. Diabetes Care 1990;13:34-40.

55. Chew EY, Mills JL, Metzger BE, et al. The diabetes and early pregnancy study. Metabolic control and progression of retinopathy. Diab Care 1995;18:631-7.

56. Axer-Siegel R, Hod M,Fink-Cohen S, et al: Diabetic retinopathy during pregnancy. Ophthalmology 1996;103:1815-9.

57. Rosenn B, Miodovnik M,Kranias G, et al: Progression of diabetic retinopathy in pregnancy: association with hypertension in pregnancy. Am J Obst Gynecol 1992;166:1214-8.

58. Jensen T, Borch-Johnson K, Kofoed-Enevoldsen A, Deckert T. Coronary heart disease in young type 1 (insulin dependent) diabetic patients with and without diabetic nephropathy: incidence and risk factors. Diabetologia 1987; 30: 144-8.

59. Krowlewski A, Kosinski EJ, Warram JH, et al: Magnitude and determinants of coronary artery disease in juvenile-onset, insulin-dependent diabetes mellitus. Am J Cardiol 1987; 59:750-5.

60. Abbott RD, Donahue RP, Kannel WB, Wilson PWF: The impact of diabetes on survival following myocardial infarction in men versus women. JAMA 1998; 260:3456-60.

61. Adler AI, Stratton IR, Neil AW, et al: Association of systolic blood pressure with macrovascular and microvascular complications of type 2 diabetes (UKPDS 36): prospective observational study. BMJ 2000; 321:412-9.

62. Hu FB, Stampfer MJ, Solomon CG, et al: The impact of diabetes mellitus on mortality from all causesand coronary heart disease in women. 20 years of follow-up. Arch Int Med 2001; 161:1717-23.

63. Goraya TY, Leibson CL, Palumbo PJ, et al: Coronary atherosclerosis in diabetes mellitus. A population-based study. J Am Coll Cardiol 2002; 40:946-53.

64. Grundy SM, Howard B, Smith S, et al: Prevention Conference VI: Diabetes and Cardiovascular Disease. Executive Summary. Conference proceeding for healthcare professionals from a special writing group of the American heart Association. Circulation 2002;105:2231-9.

65. Reece EA, Egan JFX, Coustan DR, et al. Coronary artery disease in diabetic pregnancies. Amer J Obst Gynec 1986; 154: 150-1.

66. Gordon MC, Landon MB, Boyle J,et al: Coronary artery disease in insulin-dependent diabetes mellitus of pregnancy (class H): a review of the literature. Obst Gynecil Surv 1996;51:437-444.

67. Manske CL, Thomas W, Wang Y, Wilson RF. Screening diabetic transplant candidates for coronary artery disease: identification of a low risk subgroup. Kidney Intl 1993; 44: 617-21

68. Pombar X, Strassner HT, Fenner PC: Pregnancy in a woman with class H diabetes mellitus and previous coronary artery bypass graft; a case report and review of the literature. Obst Gynecol 1995;85:825-9.

69. Weintraub WS, Kosinski A, Culler S: Comparison of outcome after coronary angioplasty and coronary surgery for multivessel coronary artery disease in persons with diabetes. Am Heart J 1999;138:S394-9

70. Detre KM, Lombardero MS, Brooks MM, et al: The effect of previous coronary-artery bypass surgery on the prognosis of patients with diabetes who have acute myocardial infarction. N Engl J Med 2000;342:989-97.

71. Majdan J, Walinsky P, Cowchock SF, et al: Coronary artery bypass surgery during pregnancy. Am J Cardiol 1983; 52:1145-6.

72. Silberman S, Fink D, Berko RS, et al: Coronary artery bypass surgery during pregnancy. Eur J Cardiothoracic Surg 1996; 10:925-6.

73. Ascarelli MH, Grider AR, Hsu HW: Acute myocardial infarction during pregnancy managed with immediate percutaneous transluminal coronary angioplasty. Obst Gynecol 1996; 88:655-7.

74. Craig S, Ilton M: Treatment of acute myocardial infarction in pregnancy with coronary artery balloon angioplasty and stenting. Austral NZ J Obst Gynecol 1999; 39:194-6.

75. Mathew V, Holmes DR: Outcomes in diabetics undergoing revascularization. J Am Coll Cardiol 2002;40:424-7.

76. Van Belle E, Parie M, Braune D, et al: Effects of coronary stenting on vessel patency and long-term clinical outcome after percutaneous coronary revascularization in diabetic patients. J Am Coll Cardiol 2002; 40:410-7.

77. Collins JS, Bossone E, Eagle KA, Mehta RJ: Asymptomatic coronary artery disease in a pregnant [diabetic] patient. A case report and review of literature. Herz 2002; 27:548-54.

78. Schannwell CM, Schneppenheim M, Perings SM, et al: Alterations of left ventricular function in women with insulin-dependent diabetes mellitus during pregnancy. Diabetologia 2003; 46:267-75.

79. Shapiro LM, Howat AP, Calter MM: Left ventricular function in diabetes mellitus. Br Heart J 1981; 45:122-32.

80. Airaksinen J, Ikaheimo M, Kaila J, et al: Impaired left ventricular filling in young female diabetics. An echocardiographic study. Acta Med Scand 1984; 216:509-16.

81. Airaksinen KEJ, Koistinen MJ, Ikaheimo MJ: Augmentation of atrial contribution to left ventricular filling in IDDM subjects as assessed by pulsed Doppler ecocardiography. Diabetes Care 1989;12:159-61.

82. Pinamonti B, DiLenarda A, Sinagra   G, et al: The Heart Muscle Disease Study Group: restrictive left ventricular filling pattern in dilated cardiomyopathy assessed by doppler echocardiography: clinical, echocardiographic and hemodynamic correlations and prognostic implications. J Am Coll Cardiol 1993; 22:808-15.

83. Krutzen E, Olofsson P, Back SE, Nilsson-Ehle P. Glomerular filtration rate in pregnancy: a study in normal subjects and in patients with hypertension, preeclampsia and diabetes. Scand J Clin Lab Invest 1992; 52: 387-392.

84. Moran P, Baylis PH, Lindheimer MD, Davison JM: Glomerular ultrafiltration in normal and preeclamptic pregnancies. J Am Soc Nephrol 2003;14:648-52.

85. Davison JM, Noble MCB: Serial changes in 24-hour creatinine clearance during normal menstrual cycles and the first trimester of pregnancy. Br J Obst Gynaec 1981;88:10-17

86. Baylis C: Glomerular filtration rate in normal and abnormal pregnancies. Sem Nephrol 1999; 19:133-9.

87. Davison JM, Dunlop W: Renal hemodynamics and tubular function in normal human pregnancy. Kidney Intl 1980; 18:152-61.

88. Ezimokhai M, Davison JM, Philips PR, Dunlop W: Non-postural serial changes in renal function during the third trimester of normal human pregnancy. Br J Obst Gynaecol 1981;88:465-471.

89. Dunlop W, Davison JM: The effect of normal pregnancy upon the renal handling of uric acid. Br J Obst Gynaecol 1977;84:13-21.

90. Milne JEC, Lindheimer MD, Davison JM: Glomerular heteroporous membrane modeling in third trimester and postpartum before and during amino acid infusion. Am J Physiol 2002;282:F170-5.

91. Conrad KP, Colpoys MC: Evidence against the hypothesis that prostaglandins are the vasodepressor agents of pregnancy. J Clin Invest 1986;77:236-45.

92. Danielson LA, Conrad KP: Acute blockade of nitric oxide synthase inhibits renal vasodilation and hyperfiltration during pregnancy in chronically instrumented conscious rats. J Clin Invest 1995; 96:482-90.

93. Abram SR, Alexander BT, Bennett WA, Granger JP: Role of neuronal nitric oxide synthase in mediating renal hemodynamic changes during pregnancy. Am J Physiol 2001;281:R1390-3.

94.   Alexander BT, Cockrell K, Cline FD, Granger JP; Inducible nitric oxide synthase inhibition attenuates renal hemodynamics during pregnancy. Hypertens 2002;36(part2):586-90.

95.   Kitzmiller JL, Brown ER, Phillippe M, et al. Diabetic nephropathy and perinatal outcome. Am J Obstet Gynecol 1981; 141:741-751.

96.   Reece EA, Coustan DR, Hayslett JP, et al. Diabetic nephropathy: pregnancy performance and fetomaternal outcome. Am J Obstet Gynecol 1988; 159: 56-66.

97.   Khoury JC, Miodovnik M, LeMasters G, Sibai B: Pregnancy outcome and progression of diabetic nephropathy. What's next? J Mat Fetal Neonat Med 2002; 11:238-44.

98.   Grenfell A, Brudenell JM, Doddridge MC, Watkins PJ. Pregnancy in diabetic women who have proteinuria. Quart J Med 1986; 59: 379-386

99.   Reece EA, Winn HN, Hayslett JP, et al. Does pregnancy alter the rate of progression of diabetic nephropathy? Am J Perinat 1990; 7: 193-7.

100. Mackie ADR, Doddridge MC, Gamsu HR, et al. Outcome of pregnancy in patients with insulin-dependent diabetes mellitus and nephropathy with moderate renal impairment. Diabetic Med 1996; 13:90-96.

101. Purdy LP, Hantsch CE, Molitsch ME, et al. Effect of pregnancy on renal function in patients with moderate-to-severe diabetic renal insufficiency. Diabetes Care 1996; 19:1067-74

102. Dunne FP, Chowdhury TA, Hartland A, et al: Pregnancy outcome in women with insulin-dependent diabetes mellitus complicated by nephropathy. Q J Med 1999; 92:451-4.

103. Carr D, Binney G, Brown Z, et al: Relationship between hemodynamics, renal function, and pregnancy outcome in class F diabetes. Am J Obst Gynecol 2002; 187(Suppl):S152

104. Biesenbach G, Grafinger P, Stoger H, Zasgornik J. How pregnancy influences renal function in nephropathic type 1 diabetic women depends on their pre-conception creatinine clearance. J Nephrol. 1999; 12:41-46.

105. Omer S, Shan J, Varma , Mulay S: Augmentation of diabetes-associated renal hyperfiltration and nitric oxide production by pregnancy in rats. J Endocrinol 1999;161:15-23.

106. Alexander BT, Miller MT, Kassab S, et al: Differential expression of renal nitric oxide synthase isoforms during pregnancy in rats. Hypertens 1999; 33(part 2):435-9.

107. Ishihara G, Hiramatsu Y, Masayuma H, Kudo T: Stretozotocin-induced diabetic pregnant rats exhibit signs and symptoms mimicking preeclampsia. Metab 2000; 49:853-7.

108. Deng A, Engels K, Baylis C: Impact of nitric oxide deficiency on blood pressure and glomerular hemodynamic adaptions to pregnancy in the rat. Kidney Intl 1996;50:1132-8.

109. Cataldi L, Mussap M, Bertelli L, et al: Cystatin C in healthy women at term pregnancy and in their infant newborns: relationship between maternal and neonatal serum levels and reference values. Am J perinatol 1999; 16:287-95.

110. Strevens H, Wide-Swensson D, Grubb A: Serum cystatin C is a better marker for preeclampsia than serum creatinine or serum urate. Scand J Clin Lab Invest 2001; 61:575-80.

111. Christensen T, Klebe JG, Berthelsen V, Hansen HE. Changes in renal volume during normal pregnancy. Acta Obst Gynec Scand 1989; 68:541-3.

112. Lauszas FF, Klebe JG, Rasmussen OW, et al. Renal growth during pregnancy in insulin-dependent diabetic women. A prospective study of renal volume and clinical variables. Acta Diabetol 1995; 32:225-9.

113. Pedersen EB, Rasmussen AB, Johannsen P, et al. Urinary excretion of albumin, beta-2-microglobulin and light chains in preeclampsia, essential hypertension in pregnancy, and

normotensive pregnant and non-pregnant control subjects. Scand J Clin Lab Invest 1981; 41:777-84.

114   Lopez-Espinoza I, Humphreys S, Redman CWG. Urinary albumin excretion in pregnancy. Br J Obst Gynec 1986; 93:176-81.

115.   Wright A, Steele P, Bennett JR, et al. The urinary excretion of albumin in normal pregnancy. Br J Obstet Gynaecol 1987; 94: 408-412.

116.   Misiani R, Marchesi D, Tiraboschi G, et al: Urinary albumin excretion in normal pregnancy and pregnancy-induced hypertension. Nephron 1991;59:416-22.

117.   Bernard A, Thielemans N, Lauwerys R, Van Lierde M: Selective increase in the urinary excretion of protein 1 (Clara cell protein) and other low molecular weight proteins during normal pregnancy. Scand J Clin Lab Invest 1992;52:871-8.

118.   Cheung CK, Lao T, Swaminathan R. Urinary excretion of some proteins and enzymes during normal pregnancy. Clin Chem 1989; 35: 1978-1980.

119.   Higby K, Suiter CR, Phelps JY, et al. Normal values of urinary albumin and total protein excretion during pregnancy. Am J Obst Gynec 1994; 171: 984-9.

120.   Holm J, Hemmingsen L, Nielsen: Low-molecular-mass proteinuria as a marker of proximal renal tubular dysfunction in norm- and microalbuminuric non-insulin-dependent diabetic subjects. Clin Chem 1993;39:517-9.

121.   Carter DC, He XM, Munson SH, et al: Three dimensional structure of human serum albumin. Science 1999; 244:1995-7.

122.   Roberts M, Lindheimer MD, Davison JM. Altered glomerular permselectivity to neutral dextrans and heteroporous membrane modeling in human pregnancy. Am J Physiol 1996; 270: F338-43.

123.   Osicka TM, Houlihan CA, Chan JG, et al: Albuminuria in patients with type 1 diabetes is directly linked to changes in the lysosome-mediated degradation of albumin during renal passage. Diabetes 2000; 49:1579-84

124.   Ohlson M, Sorensson J, Haraldsson B: Glomerular size and charge selectivity in the rat as revealed by FITC-Ficoll and albumin. Am J Physiol 2000;279:F84-91.

125.   Russo LM, Bakris GL, Comper WD: Renal handling of albumin: a critical review of basic concepts and perspective. Am J Kid Dis 2002;39:899-915.

126.   Blouch K, Deen WM, Fauvel J-P, Bialek J, et al: Molecular configuration and glomerular size selectivity in healthy and nephrotic humans. Am J Physiol 1997;273:F430-7.

127.   Deen WM, Lazzara MJ, Myers BD: Structural determinants of glomerular permeability. Am J Physiol 2001;281:F579-96.

128.   Tryggvason K, Wartiovaara J: Molecular basis of glomerular permselectivity. Curr Opin Nephrol Hypert 2001;10:543-9.

129.   McCance DR, Traub AI, Harley JMG, et al. Urinary albumin excretion in diabetic pregnancy. Diabetologia 1989; 32:236-9.

130.   Biesenbach G, Zasgornik J. Incidence of transient nephrotic syndrome during pregnancy in diabetic women with and without pre-existing microalbuminuria. Br Med J 1989; 299: 366-7.

131.   MacRury SM, Pinion S, Quin JD, et al. Blood rheology and albumin excretion in diabetic pregnancy. Diabetic Med 1995; 12: 51-5.

132.   Winocour PH, Taylor RJ. Early alterations of renal function in insulin-dependent diabetic pregnancies and their importance in predicting preeclamptic toxaemia. Diabetes Res 1989; 10: 159-164.

133.   Combs CA, Rosenn B, Kitzmiller JL, et al. Early-pregnancy proteinuria in diabetes related to preeclampsia. Obstet Gynecol 1993; 82: 802-7.

134. Biesenbach G, Zasgornik J, Stoger H, et al. Abnormal increases in urinary albumin excretion during pregnancy in IDDM women with preexisting albuminuria. Diabetologia 1994; 37: 905-10.

135. Ekbom P, Damm P, Norgaard K, et al: Urinary albumin excretion and 24-hour blood pressure as predictors of pre-eclampsia in Type I diabetes. Diabetologia 2000;43:927-31.

136. Schroder W, Heyl W, Hill-Grasshof B, Rath W: Clinical value of detecting microalbuminuria as a risk factor for pregnancy-induced hypertension in insulin-treated diabetic pregnancies. Eur J Obst Gynecol Reprod Biol 2000;94:155-8.

136. Lauszus FF, Rasmussen OW, Lousen T, et al: Ambulatory blood pressure as predictor of preeclampsia in diabetic pregnancies with respect to urinary albumin excretion rate and glycemic regulation. Acta Obst Gynecol Scand 2001;80:1096-1103.

137. Ekbom P, Damm P, Feldt-Rasmussen, et al: Pregnancy outcome in type 1 diabetic women with microalbuminuria. Diabetes Care 2001;24:1739-44.

138. Rodriguez MH, Masaki DI, Mestman J, et al: Calcium/creatinine ratio and microalbuminuria in the prediction of preeclampsia. Am J Obst Gynecol 1988;159:1452-5.

139. Konstantin-Hansen KF, Hesseldahl H, Moller Pedersen S. Microalbuminuria as a predictor of preeclampsia. Acta Obst Gynec Scand 1992; 71: 341-6.

140. Bar J, Hod M, Erman A, et al. Microalbuminuria as an early predictor of hypertensive complications in pregnant women at high risk. Am J Kidney Dis 1996; 28: 220-5.

141. Das V, Bhargava T, Das SK, Pandey S. Microalbuminuria: a predictor of pregnancy-induced hypertension. Br J Obst Gynec 1996; 103: 928-30.

142. Deckert T, Feldt-Rasmussen B, Borch-Johnsen K, et al: Albuminuria reflects widespread vascular damage: the Steno hypothesis. Diabetologia 1989;32:219-226.

143. Haffner SM, Stern MP, Kozlowski-Gruber MK, et al: Microalbuminuria. Potential marker for increased cardiovascular risk factors in non-diabetic subjects? Arteriosclerosis 1990; 10:727-31.

144. Groop L, Ekstrand A, Forsbloom C, et al: Insulin resistance, hypertension and microalbuminuria in patients with Type 2 (non-insulin-dependent) diabetes mellitus. Diabetologia 1993; 36:642-7.

145. Mykkanen L, Zaccaro DJ, Wagenknecht LE, et al: Microalbuminuria is associated with insulin resistance in diabetic subjects. The Insulin Resistance Atherosclerosis Study. Diabetes 1998; 47:793-800.

146. Cirillo M, Stellato D, Laurenzi M, et al: Pulse pressure and isolated systolic hypertension: association with microalbuminuria. Kidney Intl 2000; 58:1211-8.

147. Festa A, D'Agostino R, Howard G, et al: Inflammation and microalbuminuria in nondiabetic and type 2 diabetic subjects: The Insulin Resistance Atherosclerosis Study. Kidney Intl 2000; 58:1703-10.

148. Gordon M, Landon MB, Samuels P, et al: Perinatal outcome and long-term follow-up associated with modern management of diabetic nephropathy. Obst Gynecol 1996; 87:401-9.

149. Remuzzi G: Nephropathic nature of proteinuria. Curr Opin Nephrol Hypert 1999; 8:655-63.

150. Poulsen PL, Hansen KW, Mogensen CE: Ambulatory blood pressure in the transition from normo- to microalbuminuria. A longitudinal study in IDDM patients. Diabetes 1994; 43:1248-53.

151. Mangili R, Deferrari G, DiMario U, et al: Arterial hypertension and microalbuminuria in IDDM: the Italian Microalbuminuria Study. Diabetologia 1994; 37:1015-24.

152. Schultz CJ, Neil HAW, Dalton RN, et al: Blood pressure does not rise before the onset of microalbuminuria in children followed from diagnosis of type 1 diabetes. Diabetes Care 2001; 24:555-60.

153. Mathiesen ER, Ronn B, Jensen T, et al: Relationship between blood pressure and urinary albumin excretion in development of microalbuminuria. Diabetes 1990; 39:245-49.

154. Poulsen PL, Juhl B, Ebbehoj E, et al: Elevated ambulatory blood pressure in microalbuminuric IDDM patients is inversely associated with renal plasma flow. A compensatory mechanism? Diabetes Care 1997; 20:429-32.

155. Osterby R, Bangstad H-J, Nyberg G, et al: A quantitative ultrastructural study of juxtaglomerular arterioles in IDDM patients with micro- and normoalbuminuria. Diabetologia 1995; 38:1320-7.

156. Osterby R, Asplund J, Bangstad H-J, et al: Glomerular volume and the glomerular vascular pole area in patients with insulin-dependent diabetes mellitus. Virchows Arch 1997; 431:351-7.

157. Osterby R, Hartmann A, Bangstad H-J: Structural changes in renal arterioles in Type I diabetic patients Diabetologia 2002; 45:542-9.

158. Benhamou PY, Halimi S, De Gaudemaris R, et a;: Early disturbances of ambulatory blood pressure load in normotensive type I diabetic patients with microalbuminuria. Diabetes Care 1992; 15:1614-9.

159. Moore WV, Donaldson DL, Chonko AM, et al: Ambulatory blood pressure in type I diabetes mellitus. Comparison to presence of incipient nephropathy in adolescents and young adults. Diabetes 1992; 41:1035-41.

160. Lafferty AR, Werther GA, Clarke CF: Ambulatory blood pressure, microalbuminuria, amd autonomic neuropathy in adolescents with type 1 diabetes. Diabetes Care 2000; 23:533-8.

161. Lurbe E, Redon J, Kesani A, et al: Increase in nocturnal blood pressure and progression to microalbuminuria in type 1 diabetes. N Engl J Med 2002; 347:797-805.

162. Nielsen S, Schmitz A, Poulsen PL, et al: Albuminuria and 24-h ambulatory blood pressure in normoalbuminuric and microalbumnuric NIDDM patients. Diabetes Care 1995; 18:1434-41.

163. Rutter MK, McComb JM, Forster J, et al: Increased left ventricular mass index and nocturnal systolic blood pressure in patients with Type 2 diabetes mellitus and microalbuminuria. Diabet Med 2000; 17:321-5.

164. Hansen KW, Poulsen Christiansen JS, Mogensen CE: Determinants of 24-h blood pressure in IDDM patients. Diabetes Care 1995; 18:529-35.

165. Bodmer CW, Patrick AW, How TV, Williams G: Exaggerated sensitivity to NE-induced vasoconstriction in IDDM patients with microalbuminuria. Possible etiology and diagnostic implications. Diabetes 1992; 41:209-14.

166. Trevisan R, Bruttomesso D, Vedovato M, et al: Enhanced responsiveness of blood pressure to sodium intake and to angiotensin II is associated with insulin resistance in IDDM patients with microalbuminuria. Diabetes 1998; 47:1347-53.

167. Imanishi M, Yoshioka K, Okumura M, et al: Sodium sensitivity related to albuminuria appearing before hypertension in type 2 diabetic patients. Diabetes Care 2001; 24:111-6.

168. Chiarelli F, Catino M, Tumini S, et al: Increased Na+/Li+ countertransport activity may help to identify type 1 diabetic adolescents and young adults at risk for developing persistent microalbuminuria. Diabetes Care 1999; 22:1158-64.

169. Nannipieri M, Penno G, Rizzo L, et al: Transcapillary escape rate of albumin in type II diabetic patients. The relationship with microalbuminuria and hypertension. Diabetes Care 1997; 20:1019-26.

170. Krowlewski AS, Fogarty DG, Warram JH: Hypertension and nephropathy in diabetes mellitus: what is inherited and what is acquired? Diab Res Clin Pract 1998; 39(Suppl):S1-14.

171. Qiu C, Williams MA, Leisenring WM, et al: Family history of hypertension and type 2 diabetes in relation to preeclampsia risk. Hypertens 2003; 41:408-13.

172. Walker SP, Higgins JR, Brennecke SP: Ambulatory blood pressure monitoring in pregnancy. Obst Gynecol Surv 1998; 53:636-44.

173. Higgins JR, de Swiet M: Blood-pressure measurement and classification in pregnancy. Lancet 2001; 357:131-5

174. Flores L, Levy I, Aguilera E, et al: Usefulness of ambulatory blood pressure monitoring in pregnant women with type 1 diabetes. Diabetes Care 1999; 22:1507-11.

175. Cundy T, Slee F, Gamble G, Neale L: Hypertensive disorders of pregnancy in women with type 1 and type 2 diabetes. Diabet Med 2002; 19:482-9.

176. Hanson U, Persson B: Epidemiology of pregnancy-induced hypertension and preeclampsia in Type 1 (insulin-dependent) diabetic pregnancies in Sweden. Acta Obst Gynecol Scand 1998; 77:620-4.

177. Caritis S, Sibai B, Hauth J, et al: Predictors of preeclampsia in women at high risk. National Institute of Child Health and Human Development Network of Maternal-Fetal Medicine Units. Am J Obst Gynecol 1998; 179:946-51.

178. Sibai BM, Caritis S, Hauth J, et al: Risks of preeclampsia and adverse neonatal outcomes among women with pregestational diabetes mellitus. Am J Obst Gynecol 2000; 182:364-9.

179. Sowers JR, Saleh AA, Sokol RJ: Hyperinsulinemia and insulin resistance is associated with preeclampsia in African-Americans. Am J Hypertens 1995; 8:1-4.

180. Fuh MM, Yin CS, Pet D, et al: Resistance to insulin-mediated glucose uptake and hyperinsulinemia in women who had preeclampsia during pregnancy. Am J Hypertens 1995; 8:768-71.

181. Van Beek E, Peeters LLH: Pathogenesis of preeclampsia: a comprehensive model. Obst Gynecol Surv 1998; 53:233-9.

182. Roberts JM, Cooper DW: Pathogenesis and genetics of preeclampsia. Lancet 2001; 357:53-56.

183. Lachmeijer AMA, Dekker GA, Pals G, et al: Searching for preeclampsia genes: the current position. Eur J Obst Gynecol Reprod Biol 2002; 105:94-113.

184. Dekker G, Sibai B: Primary, secondary, and tertiary prevention of preeclampsia. Lancet 2001; 357:209-215.

185. Sibai BM: Prevention of preeclampsia: a big disappointment. Am J Obst Gynecol 1998; 179:1275-8.

186. Duley L, Henderson-Smart D, Knight M, King J: Antiplatelet drugs for prevention of pre-eclampsia and its consequences: systematic review. BMJ 2001; 322:329-33.

187. Chappell LC, Seed PT, Briley AL, et al: Effect of antioxidants on the occurrence of pre eclampsia in women at increased risk; a randomized trial. Lancet 1999; 354:810-816.

188. Luttun A, Carmeliet P: Soluble VEGF receptor Flt1: the elusive preeclampsia factor discovered? J Clin Invest 2003; 111:600-2.

189. Dicker D, Feldberg, Peleg, et al. Pregnancy complicated by diabetic nephropathy. J Perin Med 1986; 14: 299-306.

190. Biesenbach G, Stoger H, Zasgornik J. Influence of pregnancy on progression of diabetic nephropathy and subsequent requirement of renal replacement therapy in female type I diabetic patients with impaired renal function. Nephrol Dial Transplant 1992; 7: 105-109.

191. Kimmerle R, Zass R-P, Cupisti S, et al. Pregnancies in women with diabetic nephropathy: long-term outcome for mother and child. Diabetologia 1995; 38: 227-235.

192. Miodovnik M, Rosenn BM, Khoury JC, et al. Does pregnancy increase the risk for development and progression of diabetic nephropathy? Am J Obst Gynecol 1996:174:1180-91.

193. Reece EA, Leguizamon G, Homko C. Stringent controls in diabetic nephropathy associated with optimization of pregnancy outcomes. J Mat-Fetal Med 1998; 7:213-216.

194. Katz A, Davison J, Hayslet J, et al: Pregnancy in women with kidney disease. Kidney Intl 1980; 18:192-206

195. Hou SH, Orlowski J, Pahl M, et al: Pregnancy in women with end stage renal disease: treatment of anemia and preterm labor. Am J Kidney Dis 1993; 21:16-22.

196. Yankowitz J, Piraino B, Laifer A, et al. Use of erythropoieitin in pregnancies complicated by severe anemia of renal failure. Obst Gynecol. 1992; 80:485-488.

197. Braga J, Marques R, Branco A, et al. Maternal and perinatal implications of the use of human recombinant erythroitin. Acta Obst Gynecol Scand 1996; 75:449-453.

198. Balasoiu D, van Kessel KC, van Kats-Renaud HJ, et al: Granulocyte function in women with diabetes and asymptomatic bacteriuria. Diabetes Care 1997; 20:392-5.

199. Geerlings SE, Stolk RP, Camps MJL, et al: Risk factors for symptomatic urinary tract infection in women with diabetes. Diabetes Care 2000; 23:1737-41.

200. Geerlings SE, Stolk RP, Camps MJL, et al: Consequences of asymptomatic bacteriuria in women with diabetes mellitus. Arch Int Med 2001; 161:1421-7.

201. Geerlings SE, Meiland R, van Lith EC, et al: Adherance of type 1-fimbriated *Escherichia coli* to uroepithelial cells. More in diabetic women than in control subjects. Diabetes Care 2002; 25:1405-9.

202. Davison JM, Sprott MS, Selkon JB: The effect of covert bacteriuria in schoolgirls on renal function at 18 years and during pregnancy. Lancet 1984; 2:651-5.

203. Harding GKM, Zhanel GG, Nicolle LE, et al: Antimicrobial treatment in diabetic women with asymptomatic bacteriuria. N Engl J Med 2002; 347:1576-83.

204. Eskenazi B, Fenster L, Sidney S: A multivariate analysis of risk factors for preeclampsia. JAMA 1991; 266:237-41.

206. Muhlhauser I, Bender R, Bott U, et al: Cigarette smoking and progression of retinopathy and nephropathy in type 1 diabetes. Diab Med 1996; 13:536-43.

207. Remuzzi G: Effect of cigarette smoking on renal function and vascular endothelium. Contrib Nephrol 2000; 130:45-52.

208. Baggio B, Budakovic A, Dalla Vestra M, et al: Effects of cigarette smoking on glomerular structure and function in type 2 diabetic patients. J Am Soc Nephrol 2002; 13:2730-6.

209. Chuahiran T, Wesson DE: Cigarette smoking predicts faster progression of type 2 established diabetic nephropathy despite ACE inhibition. Am J Kidney Dis 2002; 39:376-82.

210. Yasin SY, Bey Doun SN. Hemodialysis in pregnancy. Obst Gynec Surv 1988; 43: 655-68.

211. Jakobi P, Ohel G, Szylman P, et al: Continuous ambulatory peritoneal dialysis as the primary approach in the management of severe renal insufficiency in pregnancy. Obst Gynecol 1992; 79:808-10.

212. Hou S: Frequency and outcome of pregnancy in women on dialysis. Am J Kidney Dis 1994; 23:60-63.

213. Okundaye I, Abrinko P, Hou S: Registry of pregnancy in dialysis patients. Am J Kidney Dis 1998; 31:766-773

214. Romao JE, Luders C, Kahhale S, et al: Pregnancy in women on chronic dialysis. A single-center experience with 17 cases. Nephron 1998; 78:416-422.
215. Bagon JA, Vernaeve H, De Muylder X, et al: Pregnancy and dialysis. Am J Kidney Dis 1998; 31:756-765
216. Chao A-S, Huang J-Y, Lien R, et al: Pregnancy in women who undergo long-term hemodialysis. Am J Obst Gynecol 2002; 187:152-6
217. Jones DC, Hayslett JP: Outcome of pregnancy in women with moderate or severe renal insufficiency. N Engl J Med 1996; 335:226-32.
218. Hou S: Pregnancy in chronic renal insufficiency and end-stage renal disease. Am J Kidney Dis 1999; 33:235-52.
219. Mogensen CE. Progression of nephropathy in long-term diabetics with proteinuria and effect of initial antihypertensive treatment. Scand J Clin Lab Invest 1976; 36: 383-7.
220. Parving H-H, Smidt UM, Friisberg B, et al: A prospective study of glomerular filtration rate and arterial blood pressure in insulin-dependent diabetics with diabetic nephropathy. Diabetologia 1981; 20:457-461.
221. Austin SM, Lieberman JS, Newton LD, et al: Slope of serial glomerular filtration rate and the progression of diabetic renal disease. J Am Soc Nephrol 1993; 3:1358-1370.
222. Alaveras AEG, Thomas SM, Sagriotis A, Viberti GC: Promoters of progression of diabetic nephropathy: the relative roles of blood glucose and blood pressure control. Nephrol Dial Transpl 1997; 12 (Suppl 2):71-4.
223. Hovind P, Rossing P, Tarnow L, et al: Progression of diabetic nephropathy. Kidney Intl 2001; 59:702-9.
224. Rossing K, Jacobsen P, Hommel E, et al: Pregnancy and progression of diabetic nephropathy. Diabetologia 2002; 45:36-41.
225. Chaturvedi N, Stephenson JM, Fuller JH, et al. The relationship between pregnancy and long-term maternal complications in the EURODIAB IDDM complications study. Diabet Med 1995; 12: 494-9.
226. Hemachandra A, Ellis D, Lloyd CE, Orchard TJ: The influence of pregnancy on IDDM complications. Diabetes Care 1995; 18:950-4.
227. Kaaja R, Sjoberg L, Hellstedt T, et al: Long-term effects of pregnancy on diabetic complications. Diabet Med 1996; 13: 165-9.
228. Kitzmiller JL: Sweet success with diabetes. The development of insulin therapy and glycemic control for pregnancy. Diab Care 1993; 16 (Suppl 3): 107-21.
229. Holley JL, Bernardini J, Quadri KHM, et al: Pregnancy outcomes in a prospective matched control study of pregnancy and renal disease. Clin Nephrol 1996; 45:77-82.
230. Biesenbach G, Grafinger P, Zasgornik J, Stoger H: Perinatal complications and three-year followup of infants of diabetic mothers with diabetic nephropathy stage IV. Renal Failure 2000; 22:573-80.
231. Cunningham FG, Cox SM, Harstad TW, et al: Chronic renal disease and pregnancy outcome. Am J Obst Gynecol 1990; 163:453-9.
232. Lindheimer MD, Katz AI: Pregnancy in the renal transplant patient. Am J Kidney Dis 1992; 19:173-6.
233. Abe S, Amagasaki Y, Kaniski K, et al: The influence of antecedent renal disease on pregnancy. Am J Obst Gynecol 1985; 153:508-14.
234. Jungers P, Houillier P, Chauveau D, et al: Pregnancy in women with reflux nephropathy. Kidney Intl 1996; 50:593-9.
235. Jungers P, Chauveau D, Choukroun G, et al: Pregnancy in women with impaired renal function. Clin Nephrol 1997; 47:281-8.
236. Jungers P, Chauveau D: Pregnancy in renal disease. Kidney Intl 1997; 52:871-85.

237. Packham DK: Aspects of renal disease and pregnancy. Kidney Intl 1993; 44(Suppl 42):S64-7.

238. Rizzoni G, Ehrich JH, Broyer M, Brunner FP: Successful pregnancies in women on renal replacement therapy: report from the EDTA Registry. Nephrol Dial Transplant 1992; 7:279-87.

239. Hou S: Pregnancy in women on dialysis, in Nissenson AR and Fine RN, ed, *Dialysis Therapy*, Third Edition, Hanley and Belfus, Phila., 2002, pp 519-522.

240. Greene MF, Hare JW, Krache M, et al: Prematurity among insulin-requiring diabetic gravid women. Am J Obst Gynec 1989; 161: 106-11.

241. Garner PR, D'Alton ME, Dudley DK, et al: Preeclampsia in diabetic pregnancies. Am J Obst Gynec 1990; 163: 505-8.

242. Lyall F, Greer IA: Pre-eclampsia: a multifaceted vascular disorder of pregnancy. J Hypertens 1994; 12:1339-45.

243. Ness RB, Roberts JM: Heterogenous causes constituting the single syndrome of preeclampsia: a hypothesis and its implications. Am J Obst Gynecol 1996; 175:1365-70.

244. Pridjian G, Puschett JB: Preeclampsia. Part 1: Clinical and pathophysiologic considerations. Part 2: Experimental and genetic considerations. Obst Gynecol Surv 2002; 57:598-640.

245. Lyall F, Greer IA, Boswell F, Fleming R: Suppression of serum vascular endothelial growth factor immunoreactivity in normal pregnancy and in pre-eclampsia. Br J Obst Gynaecol 1997; 104:223-8.

246. Livingston JC: Reductions of vascular endothelial growth factor and placental growth factor concentrations in severe preeclampsia. Am J Obst Gynecol 2000; 183:1554-7.

247. Morris NH, Eaton BM, Dekker G: Nitric oxide, the endothelium, pregnancy and pre-eclampsia. Br J Obst Gynecol 1996; 103:4-15.

248. Schobel HP, Fischer T, Heuszer, et al: Preeclampsia – a state of sympathetic overactivity. N Engl J Med 1996; 335:1480-5.

249. Greenwood JP, Scott EM, Walker JJ, et al: The magnitude of sympathetic hyperactivity in pregnancy-induced hypertension and preeclampsia. Am J Hypertens 2003; 16:194-9.

250. Claxton CR, Brands MW: Nitic oxide opposes glucose-induced hypertension by suppressing sympathetic activity. Hypertens 2003; 41:274-8.

251. Davidge ST: Oxidative stress and altered endothelial cell function in preeclampsia. Semin Reprod Endocrinol 1998; 16:65-73.

252. Roberts JM, Hubel CA: Is oxidative stress the link in the two-stage model of pre-eclampsia? Lancet 1999; 354:788-9.

253. Zusterzeel PLM, Wanten GJA, Peters WHM, et al; Neutrophil oxygen radical production in preeclampsia with HELLP syndrome. Eur J Obst Gynecol Reprod Biol 2001; 99:213-8.

254. Makino A, Skelton MM, Zou A-I, et al: Increased renal medullary oxidative stress produces hypertension. Hypertens 2002; 39(part 2):667-72.

255. Roberts JM, Pearson G, Cutler J, Lindheimer M: Summary of the NHLBI Worhng Group on Research on Hypertension During Pregnancy. Hypertens 2003; 41:437-45.

256. Conrad KP, Benyo DF: Placental cytokines and the pathogenesis of preeclampsia. Am J Reprod Immunol 1997; 37:240-9.

257. RedmanCW, Sacks GP, Sargent IL: Preeclampsia: an excessive maternal inflammatory response to pregnancy. Am J Obst Gynecol 1999; 180:499-506.

258. Chambers JC, Fusi L, Malik IS, et al: Association of maternal endothelial dysfunction with preeclampsia. JAMA 2001; 285:1607-12.

259. Mellembakken JR, Aukrust P, Olafsen MK, et al: Activation of leukocytes during the uteroplacental passage in preeclampsia. Hypertens 2002; 39:155-60.

260. Lafayette RA, Druzin M, Sibley R, et al: Nature of glomerular dysfunction in pre-eclampsia. Kidney Intl 1998; 54:1240-9.

261. Kincaid-Smith PS: The renal lesion of preeclampsia revisited. Am J Kidney Dis 1991; 17:144-8.

262. Nochy D, Heudes D, Glotz R, et al; Pre-eclampsia associated focal and segmental glomerulosclerosis and glomerular hypertrophy: a morphometric analysis. Clin Nephrol 1994; 42:9-17.

263. Naicker T, Randeree IGH, Moodley J, et al: Correlation between histological changes and loss of anionic charge of the glomerular basement membrane in early onset pre-eclampsia. Nephron 1997; 75:201-7.

264. Osicka TM, Houlihan CA, Chan JG, et al: Albuminuria in patients with type 1 diabetes is directly linked to changes in the lysosome-mediated degradation of albumin during renal passage. Diabetes 2000; 49:1579-84.

265. Brockelsby J, Hayman R, Ahmed A, et al: VEGF via VEGF receptor-1 (Flt-1) mimics preeclamptic plasma in inhibiting uterine blood vessel relaxation in pregnancy: implications in the pathogenesis of preeclampsia. Lab Invest 1999; 79:1101-11.

266. Vuorela P, Helske S, Hornig C, et al: Amniotic fluid-soluble vascular endothelial growth factor receptor-1 in preeclampsia. Obst Gynecol 2000; 95:353-7.

267. Zhou Y, McMaster M, Woo K, et al; Vascular endothelial growth factor ligands and receptors that regulate human cytotrophoblast survival are dysregulated in severe preeclampsia and hemolysis, elevated liver enzymes, and low platelet syndrome. Am J Pathol 2002; 160:1405-23.

268. Maynard SE, Min J-Y, Merchan J, et al: Excess placental soluble fms-like tyrosine kinase 1 (sFlt) may contribute to endothelial dysfunction, hypertension, and proteinuria in preeclampsia. J Clin Invest 2003; 111:649-58.

269. Ahmed A, Li XF, Dunk C, et al: Co-localization of vascular endothelial growth factor and its Flt-1 receptor in human placenta. Growth Factors 1995; 12:235-43.

270. Clark DE, Smith SK, Sharkey AM, Charnock-Jones DS: Localization of VEGF and expression of its receptors flt and KDR in human placenta throughout pregnancy. Hum Reprod 1996; 11:1090-8.

271. Clark DE, Smith SK, He Y, et al: A vascular endothelial growth factor antagonist is produced by the human placenta and released into the maternal circulation. Biol Reprod 1998; 59:1540-8.

272. Ostendorf T, Kunter U, Eitner F, et al: VEGF165 mediates glomerular endothelial repair.J Clin Invest 1999; 104:913-23.

273. Eremina V, Sood M, Haigh J, et al: Glomerular-specific alterations of VEGF-A expression lead to distinct congenital and acquired renal diseases. J Clin Invest 2003; 111:707-16.

274. Rey E, LeLorier J, Burgess E, et al: Report of the Canadian Hypertension Society Conference: 3. Pharmacologic treatment of hypertensive disorders in pregnancy. Can Med Assoc J 1997; 157:1245-54.

275. Brown MA, Hague WM, Higgins J, et al: The detection, investigation and mangement of hypertension in pregnancy: full consensus statement. Aust NZ J Obst Gynaecol 2000; 40:139-155.

276. National High Blood Pressure Education Program Working Group on High Blood Pressure in Pregnancy: Report of the National High Blood Pressure Education Program Working Group on High Blood Pressure in Pregnancy. Am J Obst Gynecol 2000; 183:S1-22.

277. Seely EW: Hypertension in pregnancy: a potential window into long-term cardiovascular risk in women. J Clin Endocrinol Metab 1999; 84:1858-61.

278. Novelli GP, Valensise H, Vasapollo B, et al: Left ventricular concentric geometry as a risk factor in gestational hypertension. Hypertens 2003; 41:469-75.

279. Joint National Committee: The sixth report of the Joint National Committee on detection, evaluation, and treatment of high blood pressure. Arch Int Med 1998; 57:2413-46.

280. Mosca L, Grundy SM, Judelson D, et al: Guide to preventive cardiology for women. AHA/ACC Scientific Statement: Consensus Panel Statement. Circ 1999; 99:2480-84.

281. Bakris GL, Williams M, Dworkin L, et al: Preserving renal function in adults with hypertension and diabetes: a consensus approach. Am J Kidney Dis 2000; 36:646-61.

282. American Diabetes Association: Position statement: standards of medical care for patients with diabetes mellitus. Diabetes Care 2003; 26(Suppl 1):S39-40.

283. Von Dadelszen P, Ornstein MP, Bull SB, et al: Fall in mean arterial pressure and fetal growth restriction in pregnancy hypertension: a meta-analysis. Lancet 2000; 355:87-92.

284. Sibai BM: Chronic hypertension in pregnancy. Obst Gynecol 2002; 100:369-77.

285. Lydakis C, Lip GYH, Beevers M, Beevers DG: Atenolol and fetal growth in pregnancies complicated by hypertension. Am J Hypertens 1999; 12:541-7.

286. Magee LA, Bull SB, Koren G, Logan A: The generalizability of trial data; a comparison of β-blocker trial participants with a prospective cohort of women taking β-blockers in pregnancy. Eur J Obst Gynecol Reprod Biol 2001; 94:205-210.

287. Easterling TR, Carr DB, Brateng D, et al: Treatment of hypertension in pregnancy: effect of atenolol on maternal disease, preterm delivery, and fetal growth. Obst Gynecol 2001; 98:427-33.

288. Easterling TR, Brateng D, Schmucker B, Brown Z, Millard SP: Prevention of preeclampsia: a randomized trial of atenolol in hyperdynamic patients before onset of hypertension. Obst Gynecol 1999; 93:725-33.

289. Salvesen DR, Higueras MT, Brudenell M, et al. Doppler velocimetry and fetal heart studies in nephropathic diabetics. Am J Obst Gynec 1992; 167: 1297-1303.

290. Ogburn PL Jr, Kitzmiller JL, Hare JW, et al. Pregnancy following renal transplantation in class T diabetes mellitus. JAMA 1986; 225: 911-5.

291. Armenti VT, McGrory CH, Cater J, et al. The national transplantation registry: comparison between pregnancy outcomes in diabetic cyclosporine-treated female kidney recipients and CyA-treated female pancreas-kidney recipients. Transpl Proc 1997; 29: 669-70.

292. Sturgiss SN, Davison JM: Perinatal outcome in renal allograft recipients: prognostic significance of hypertension and renal function before and during pregnancy. Obst Gynecol 1991; 78:573-7.

293. Armenti VT, Ahlswede KM, Ahlswede BA, et al: Variables affecting birthweight and graft survival in 197 pregnancies in cyclosporine-treated female kidney transplant recipients. Transplantation 1995; 59:476-9.

294. Davison JM: The effect of pregnancy on kidney function in renal allograft recipients. Kidney Int 1985; 27: 74-9.

295. Pirson Y, Van Lierde M, Ghysen J, et al: Retardation of fetal growth in patients receiving immunosuppressive therapy. N Engl J Med 1985; 313:328-31.

296. Pickrell MD, Sawers , Michael J: Pregnancy after renal transplantation: severe intrauterine growth retardation during treatment with cyclosporine A. Br Med J 1988; 296:828.

297. Salmela KT, Kyllonen LEJ, Holmberg C, Gronhagen-Riska C: Impaired renal function after pregnancy in renal transplant recipients. Transplantation 1993; 56:1372-5.

298. Queipo-Zaragoza JA, Vera-Donoso CD, Soldevila A, et al: Impact of pregnancy on kidney transplant. Transpl Proc 2003; 35:866-7.

299. Cararach V, Carmona F, Monleon FJ, Andreu J: Pregnancy after renal transplantation: 25 years experience in Spain. Br J Obst Gynecol 1993; 100:122-5.

300. Oz BB, Hackman , Einarson T, Koren G: Pregnancy outcome after cyclosporine therapy during pregnancy: a meta-analysis. Transplantation 2001; 71:1051-5.

301. Kainz A, Harabacz I, Cowlrick IS, et al: Review of the course and outcome of 100 pregnancies in 84 women treated with tacrolimus. Transplantation 2000; 70:1718-21.

302. Sturgiss SN, Davison JM: Effect of pregnancy on long-term function of renal allografts. Am J Kidney Dis 1992; 19:167-172.

303. Armenti VT, Ahlswede KM, Ahlswede BA, et al: National transplantation Pregnancy registry – outcomes of 154 pregnancies in cyclosporine-treated female kidney transplant recipients. Transplantation 1994; 57:502.

304. Di Paolo S, Monno R, Stallone G, et al: Placental imbalance of vasoactive factors does not affect pregnancy outcome in patients treated with cyclosporine A after transplantation. Am J Kidney Dis 2002; 39:776-83.

305. Pergola PE, Kancharia A, Riley DJ: Kidney transplantation during the first trimester of pregnancy: immunosuppression with mycophenolate mofetil, tacrolimus, and prednisone. Transplantation 2001; 71:994-7.

306. Eisenberg JA, Armenti VT, McGrovy CH, et al: National transplantation pregnancy registry (NTPR): use of muromonab-CD3 (OKT3) during pregnancy in female transplant recipients. Am Soc Transplant Phys 1997; 20:108.

307. Morris STW, McMurray JJV, Rodger RSC, et al: Endothelial function in renal transplant recipients maintained on cyclosporine. Kidney Intl 2000; 57:1100-6.

308. Armenti VT, Coscia LA, Dunn SR, et al: National Transplantation Pregnancy Registry: pregnancy outcomes in female kidney recipients treated with Neoral vs. Tacrolimus based regimens. Transplantation 2000; 69(Suppl):S322

309. Stanley CW, Gottlieb R, Zager R, et al: Developmental well-being in offspring of women receiving cyclosporine post-renal transplant. Transplant Proc 1999; 31:241-2.

310. Di Paolo S, Schena A, Morrone LF, et al: Immunologic evaluation of infants from cyclosporine treated kidney transplanted mothers during the first year of life. Analysis of lymphocyte subpopulations and immunoglobulin serum levels. Transplantation 2000; 69:2049-55.

311. Scott JR, Branch DW, Holman J: Autoimmune and pregnancy complications in the daughter of a kidney transplant patient. Transplantation 2002; 73:815-7.

312. Armenti VT, Moritz MJ, Coscia LA, Philips LZ: Parenthood after transplantation: what are the risks? Transplantation 2002; 73:677-8.

313. Neugarten J, Silbiger SR: The impact of gender on renal transplantation. Transplantation 1994; 58:1145-52.

314. Meier-Kriesche H-U, Ojo AO, Leavey SF, et al: Differences in etiology for graft loss in female renal transplant recipients. Transpl Proc 2001; 33:1288-90.

315. Tyden G, Bratterstrom C, Bjorkman U, et al: Pregnancy after combined pancreas-kidney transplantation. Diabetes 1989; 39(Suppl 1):43-5.

316. Skannal DG, Miodovnik M, Dungy-Poythress LJ, First MR. Successful pregnancy after combined renal-pancreas transplantation: a case report and literature review. Am J Perinatol 1996; 13: 383-7.

317. Van Winter JT, Ogburn PL Jr, Ramin KD, et al: Pregnancy after pancreatic-renal transplantation because of diabetes. Mayo Clinic Proc 1997; 72:1044-7.

318. Karaitis LK, Nankivell BJ, Lawrence S, et al. Successful obstetric outcome after simultaneous pancreas and kidney transplantation. Med J Aust 1999; 170:368-370.

319. McGrory CH, Groshek MA, Sollinger HW, et al: Pregnancy outcomes in female pancreas-kidney transplants. Transpl Proc 1999; 31:652-3.

320. Barrou BM, Gruessner AC, Sutherland DE, Gruessner RW. Pregnancy after pancreas transplantation in the cyclosporine era: report from the International Pancreas Transplant Registry. Transplantation 1998:65:524-7.

321. Biesenbach G, Margreiter R, Konigsrainer A, et al: Comparison of progression of macrovascular diseases after kidney or pancreas and kidney transplantation in diabetic patients with end-stage renal disease. Diabetologia 2000; 43:231-4.

322. First MR, Combs CA, Weiskittel P, Miodovnik M: Lack of effect of pregnancy on renal allograft survival or function. Transplantation 1995; 59: 472-6.

323. Tanabe K, Kobayashi C, Takahashi K, et al: Long-term renal function after pregnancy in renal transplant recipients. Transpl Proc 1997; 29:1567-8.

324. Wilson GA, Coscia LA, McGrory CH, et al: National Transplantation Pregnancy Registry: postpregnancy graft loss among female pancreas-kidney transplants. Transpl Proc 2001; 33:1667-9.

325. Mahanty HD, Cherikh WS, Chang GJ, et al: Influence of pretransplant pregnancy on survival of renal allografts from living donors. Transplantation 2001; 72:228-32.

326. Rebibou J-M, Chabod J, Alcalay D, et al: Flow cytometric evaluation of pregnancy-induced anti-HLA immunization and blood transfusion-induced reactivation. Transplantation 2002; 74:537-40.

327. Lindheimer MD, Katz AI: Pregnancy in the renal transplant patient. Am J Kidney Dis 1992; 19:173-6.

328. Jindal RM: Posttransplant diabetes mellitus: a review. Transplantation 1994; 58:1289-98.

329. Hjelmesaeth J, Midtvedt K, Jenssen T, Hartmann A: Insulin resistance after renal transplantation. Impact of immunosuppressive and antihypertensive therapy. Diabetes Care 2001; 24:2121-6.

EVOLUTION WORLDWIDE OF RENAL REPLACEMENT THERAPY IN DIABETES

Rudy Bilous

Audrey Collins Teaching Unit, Education Centre, James Cook University Hospital, Marton Road, MIDDLESBROUGH, TS4 3BW

INTRODUCTION

Since the last edition, the numbers of patients entering renal replacement therapy (RRT) with diabetic nephropathy as their primary disease continues to rise world-wide, although there are signs that the rate of increase has stabilised in the USA [1] and Japan [2]. Although short-term (1 year) mortality adjusted for age declined from 40.4 to 23.2 per 100 patient years in the decade 1986-96 in the USA, more recent data suggest that no further improvement has occurred since then [3]. Long-term survival of patients on RRT remains much less good for diabetic compared to non-diabetic recipients [3,4].

It must be remembered that much of the data summarised in this chapter are extracted from registers of patients who have been <u>accepted</u> onto RRT programmes. They are therefore an underestimate of the true prevalence of renal failure in diabetes as many patients will not survive until end-stage renal disease (ESRD). Secondly, some registers and country reports are less than comprehensive, with low ascertainment rates even in well-established European centres [5]. Finally, methods of reporting differ between registers. Historically, the USRDS data retrieval only began after patients had survived 90 days of RRT, but now it includes all (not just Medicare) ESRD patients from first treatment [1]. Data from Europe [5] and Japan [2] also relate to entry onto RRT.

Nonetheless, reported differences and contrasts in the incidence and outcome within and between countries raise intriguing questions about both the pathophysiology of diabetic nephropathy and optimum management of ESRD in diabetes. The following areas will be covered in turn:

1. Evolution of acceptance of diabetic patients onto RRT.
2. Impact of age, type of diabetes and ethnicity of subject population.
3. Mode and outcome of RRT used to treat diabetic patients.
4. Suggested management strategies.

EVOLUTION OF ACCEPTANCE OF DIABETIC PATIENTS ONTO RRT

The USRDS has shown a year on year increase in the incidence of new diabetic patients entering RRT to 44.2% of the total enrolled in 2000 (41,107 of 92,906 patients) [1]. This represents a rate of 146.3 per million population (pmp). The annual increase in incidence rates for diabetic ESRD fell from 14% in 1988-92 to 9% in 1992-96, and <7% in 1996-2000, but this rate was still higher than that recorded for major non-diabetic causes. Overall prevalence seems to be showing a decline in the annual rate of increase from 15% in 1988-92 to 11% in 1992-96 and <8.0% in 1996-2000; however, in 1982, diabetic patients would comprise only 3% (21pmp) patients on RRT in an average dialysis centre, whereas nationally the figures were 26.1% (188pmp) in 1991 and 40% (384pmp) in 2000 [1].

In Canada, the percentage of patients with diabetes commencing haemodialysis (HD) rose from 13% in 1981-5 to 27% in 1994-7. Moreover, the projected diabetes ESRD incidence for over 65 year olds is >250pmp in 2005, an increase of three-fold from 1995 [6].

In Japan the incidence of diabetes as a cause of RRT requiring haemodialysis (HD), (which represents 95% of all RRT), rose from 31.2% (60pmp) to 36.2% (84.7pmp) in 1998, and 36.5% (92pmp) in 2000 [2]. The prevalence in 1996 was 21.6% (209pmp) total population, which is more than double the figure for 1986 (10.5%). Taiwan was second only to the USA in the incidence of ESRD in 2000 (311pmp) and 31.7% (98.6pmp) had diabetes [7], but unlike Japan there was an almost 10% increase from 1998 (table 1). In contrast only 4.3% of patients in Shanghai were recorded as having diabetic ESRD in 1999.

In Australia and New Zealand the incidence of diabetic ESRD rose from 4 to 14 and 6 to 28pmp respectively over the decade from 1986 – 96 [9].

Table 1. Percent (PMP) of incident patients entering RRT with diabetes recorded as main cause of ESRD. Adapted from USRDS 2002 – Annual Data Report (reference 3).

	1998	1999	2000
Austria	30.0 (25.8)	31.3 (28.7)	32.7 (29.4)
Brunei	32.3 (62.0)	39.0 (69.4)	45.1 (94.7)
Canada	30.0 (41.4)	31.3 (45.7)	32.0 (45.8)
Catalunya	19.8 (26.7)	19.0 (28.5)	19.9 (28.5)
Czech Republic	31.0 (41.2)		33.0 (49.8)
Finland	33.6 (30.2)	31.9 (28.7)	31.4 (29.5)
Germany	33.0 (48.8)	34.6 (51.2)	36.2 (63.8)
Greece	21.6 (24.6)	21.5 (26.7)	25.5 (40.0)
Hungary	18.3 (23.2)	21.1 (26.0)	19.9 (25.7)
Japan	36.2 (84.7)	35.0 (87.2)	36.5 (92.0)
Netherlands	15.5 (14.6)	14.0 (13.7)	16.7 (15.5)
Norway	10.2 (9.2)	12.1 (10.8)	15.2 (13.5)
Sweden	23.0 (29.2)	21.7 (27.1)	25.1 (31.6)
Taiwan	28.7 (82.7)	29.8 (93.9)	31.7 (98.6)
USA	43.5 (136.2)	43.4 (141.1)	43.4 (146.3)

In Europe, recent data collection is much less complete than previously, and it is hard to draw firm conclusions across frontiers since 1992 [4,5]. However, the EDTA registry now collects data from regional and national registers and it is possible to detect some recent trends [5]. Comparative data extracted from the registers from Austria, Finland, French-Belgium, The Netherlands, Norway and Scotland showed an increase in diabetic ESRD from 9.5 to 23% of all incident patients from 1980-84 to 1996-99. There was a wide range between these areas in 1999 however with 31.3% (42.3pmp) in Austria; 31.9% (28.7pmp) in Finland; 12.1% (10.8pmp) in Norway and 14% (13.7pmp) in The Netherlands. These rates have been steadily increasing from 1998 to 2000 in

Austria and other central European countries such as Germany and the Czech Republic, but remaining more stable in Scandinavia and Northern Europe [5] (table 1).

Consistent with this observation is the UK Renal Registry for 2002, which covers approximately 72% of the adult population and reports an 18% (16.8pmp) incidence of diabetic ESRD, also stable for the last few years [10]. There was wide geographical variation however, diabetes accounts for around 30% (26.9pmp) of incident patients in Derby but only 10% (8.5pmp) in Gloucestershire, perhaps the reflecting the influence of the proportion of ethnic minorities.   Overall prevalence of diabetic ESRD was just over 10% (approximately 54.7pmp) [10].

In Germany, the total incidence and prevalence of patients entering RRT from all causes of renal failure was 156 and 713pmp in 1998, with diabetes representing 48 and 150pmp respectively [11]. Two years later, the incidence of diabetic ESRD was 36.2% (63.4pmp) [7]. In Catalunya in Spain, the incidence of patients with diabetes entering RRT rose from 8 to 19.8pmp from 1984-94 [12]. In Madrid there was a similar rise from 10 to 21pmp over the same period, rising to 32 pmp in 1998 [13]. In France the proportion of diabetic patients entering RRT in 1995-96 was 40% in Alsace but only 13.2% for the rest of the mainland [14].

In the Balkan countries in 2000 the prevalence of diabetic ESRD was 9.2% (41.4pmp) in Bosnia/Herzegovina [15] and approximately 10% (43.8pmp) in Croatia [16]. Absolute percentages are lower here because of the incidence of other specific diseases such as Balkan nephropathy. In Turkey the figures were 15.1% (54.1pmp) in 2000 [17].

Latin America demonstrates one of the difficulties in interpreting data from countries with vastly differing Gross National Product per person (GNP). Prevalent rates of RRT in 1997 varied from 20.7pmp (Bolivia, GNP $617 per capita) to 861pmp (Puerto Rico, GNP $26,977). However, there are striking differences in the proportion of diabetic patients (incidence 57% of 254pmp in Puerto Rico and 16.3% of 132pmp in Uruguay). The reasons for these differences are unclear but again may reflect ethnicity as the rates in Puerto Rico are very similar to those seen in Hispanic Americans [18,19].

The USRDS reports a range of incidence of diabetic ESRD internationally from 3.6% (0.5pmp) in Russia to 45.1% (94.7pmp) in Brunei (figure 1) [7].

The overall message is of a continuing and exponential growth in diabetic patients entering RRT in nearly all countries (table 1).

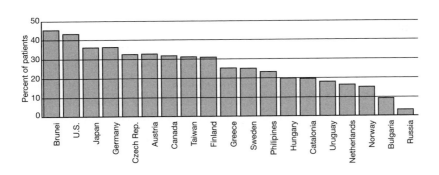

Fig. 1. Percentage of incident ESRD patients with diabetes recorded as cause. Range 3.6% (0.5pmp) in Russia to 45.1% (94.7pmp) in Brunei. Figure reproduced from USRDS Report 2002 with permission (reference 7).

IMPACT OF AGE, TYPE OF DIABETES AND ETHNICITY OF POPULATION

Part of the explanation for the increasing numbers of diabetic patients on RRT has been a relaxation of age limits for entry. Diabetes prevalence increases dramatically with age and one of the major risk factors for the development of nephropathy is duration of disease. Thus it is no surprise that as the average age of acceptance onto RRT for all causes of ESRD has increased from 45.8 years in 1977 to 57.4 years in 1992 in Europe, and the number of new patients commencing RRT over 65 years of age at acceptance increased from 9 to 37% of the total over the same period of time[4], that the proportion with diabetes has jumped dramatically. More recent data from 6 European centres showed an increase of 14 years in the mean age of incident RRT patients from 1980-1999 [5]. In Japan the mean age rose from 51.9 to 62.2 years over the period 1983-97 [2], and in the USA the increase in median age of incidence of ESRD was slightly less dramatic from approximately 62 years in 1988 to 64 years in 2000. In the USA, the median age of diabetic ESRD patients on haemodialysis (HD) was 63.9 years in 2000 [19]. Diabetes remains the commonest single cause of ESRD in those aged over 65 years entering RRT in the USA from 1990-2000 (41.6%) [1].

Although the cumulative incidence and rates of development of nephropathy are similar for both types of diabetes [20], a smaller proportion of patients with type 2 enter RRT, probably because of excess cardiovascular mortality prior to developing ESRD [21]. However as there are numerically many more patients with type 2 diabetes, and the treatments for cardiovascular disease become more effective, they represent a greater and growing proportion of the diabetic population on RRT (table 2). The reported figures are not totally reliable however, because the categorisation of patients by type of diabetes has been shown to be imprecise [22]. However the percentage of incident type 2 patients in 1999 in largely white Europid populations varies from 81% in Austria to 32% in Scotland (table 2) and are increasing by between 10 and 20% per annum in the EDTA registry area [23]. Using a carefully designed algorithm for the diagnosis of diabetes type, Cowie et al [24] found an increased probability of developing ESRD over a 10 year period of 5.82% in type 1 but only 0.5% in type 2 African American and Europid patients. However there was a suggestion of an increasing incidence in type 2 patients over the decade 1974-83. The proportion of diabetic patients with carefully defined type 2 diabetes on RRT varies from 50-90% in Europid populations world-wide [25]. The latest USRDS Report does not discriminate between diabetes type, but approximately 71% of 143,854 patients registered with diabetic ESRD from 1993-7 were recorded as type 2 (table 2) [26].

It is difficult to separate the impact of type of diabetes from ethnic factors. In Japan for example, >90% of patients on RRT have type 2 diabetes [27] but this is a reflection of the remarkably low incidence of type 1 nationally. Many ethnic groups have high prevalences of both type 2 diabetes and nephropathy [28], and countries with minorities with these characteristics will reflect an over preponderence in their RRT population.

Table 2. Worldwide incidence and prevalence of ESRD in patients with diabetes mellitus.

Country	Population studied	Year of observation	Prevalence per million pop.		Incidence per million pop.		Type 2 diabetes %	Ref.
			All causes	Diabetes	All causes	Diabetes		
USA	National	1997	1105	366	287	120	71	26
	Europid	1993-7			63%	40%	67	
	Native American				1.5%	65%	81	
	African American				30%	39%	75	
	Asians/ Pacific Islanders				3.2%	43%	80	
Japan	National	1994	1149	209	194	60	>90	27
Europe (EDTA)		1994	312	61	59	10		4
Australia	National	1993	427	33	65	10	64	25
	Europid		374	23	54	7	48	
	Aboriginal		1129	335	338	125	85	
New Zealand	National		406	58	65	20	79	25
	Europid	1993	311	16	37	4	55	
	Maori/ Pacific Islanders		648	273	166	91	83	
UK	National	2001	547	55	93	17	31	10
Austria	National	1999			128	40	81	5, 23
Finland	National	1999			91	29	50	5, 23
Netherlands	National	1999			80	13	56	5, 23
Scotland	National	1999			82	14	32	5,23

For example, in 1993 diabetic Aboriginal patients in Australia and Maori/Pacific Islanders in New Zealand receiving RRT were 85% and 83% type 2 respectively, compared to Europid populations of 48 and 55% in the same countries (table 2) [25]. The USRDS reports incidences of ESRD for the year 2000 for all causes of 996pmp for African Americans, 716 pmp for Native Americans, 455 pmp for Hispanics and 393pmp for Asian/Pacific Islanders, compared to 217pmp for Europids [19]. Analysis of incidence data from 1990-2000 has revealed that although Native Americans with diabetic ESRD represented just 2.3% of the total diabetic population receiving RRT, diabetes accounted for 69.1% of all those registered on the database. The figures for Asian/Pacific Islanders were similarly discrepant at 3.5 and 46.3%; whereas those for African Americans were 29.1 and 42.2%; and for Europids 62.6 and 43.6% respectively [19]. The annual incidence rates of HD for diabetic ESRD declined in Native Americans by 4.1% between 1996-2000, whereas there were increases of 4.2, 1.2, 3.0 and 7.7% for Hispanic, Asian/Pacific Islander, African American and Europid patients respectively [19]. Cowie et al [24] found an increased ratio of probability of developing ESRD in the 1980's of 1.62 and 3.93 for type 1 and type 2 diabetic African Americans respectively, when compared to Europids.

From 1992 –96 in Australia, diabetes was the primary cause of renal failure for 42% of Aboriginals compared to 18% of the overall incident ESRD population. The figures for New Zealand were 61% of Maori, and 49% Pacific Islanders compared to 36% nationally [9].

In the UK there has been a dramatic increase in ESRF in patients from Southern Asia (India, Pakistan, Bangladesh, Sri Lanka) and the West Indies, such that in 1991-2 these patients were accepted onto RRT at a rate of 239 and 220 pmp respectively [29], with diabetes as a major cause in both groups. Ethnicity is inadequately recorded in the latest UK Renal Registry Report, but the reported prevalence of diabetic ESRD in 2001 was 20%, double the national rate [10].

The reported risk of developing diabetic ESRD is up to fourteen-fold in South Asians compared to Europid patients in Leicester. Interestingly South Asian patients also have an increased risk of approximately five-fold for non-diabetic ESRD [28].

The reasons for the increased incidence of diabetes and its complications in ethnic minorities are not understood and are currently the source of intense controversy, particularly the low birth weight - thrifty phenotype hypothesis. Whatever the cause, the consequence will be rapidly increasing numbers of patients with diabetic ESRD world-wide for the foreseeable future [30].

MODE OF TREATMENT AND OUTCOME

There is a wide range of preferred RRT options for diabetic ESRD world-wide for reasons that are cultural/religious (eg. low transplantation rates in Japan) [2], financial (eg. higher rates of HD) in some European countries because of its link to government remuneration), and medical (eg. theoretical advantages of CAPD v. HD) [31]. No randomised control trials have ever been performed, perhaps for obvious reasons, thus it is hard to draw firm conclusions about preferred treatment.

A recent meta-analysis for all ESRD patients could not demonstrate a survival advantage for HD v PD. Unfortunately this analysis was not able to explore the effect of diabetes and dialysis modality on survival [32].

International comparisons of outcome must be made with caution because of differences in acceptance rates onto RRT, patient demographics, socio-economic factors, and national health care legislation. Nonetheless, with these provisos it is still useful to look at different practice and results world-wide.

In the USA in 2000, 16.3% of prevalent diabetic patients with ESRD had a functioning transplant (Tx), 77.5% were on HD and 6.3% were on a form of peritoneal dialysis (PD) [32]. In the UK in 2001, 28.6% had a functioning graft, 46% were on HD and 25.4% were on PD compared to 50.5%, 34.4% and 15.1% for non-diabetic patients [10]. In Europe in 1992 the percentage of prevalent RRT was 15% transplant, 68% HD and 32% PD with wide variations between countries [4]. For France and Scandinavia the proportions were 25% and 30% for Tx, 65% and 37% for HD, and <10% and 30% for PD respectively. More recent data from Catalunya report rates of 21.6, 72.8 and

5.5% for Tx, HD and PD with around 50% of those transplanted receiving a combined kidney and pancreas graft [12]. In Japan in 1996, 95% of diabetic patients were on HD and 5% on PD [2].

In most reported series, survival is best in those diabetic patients receiving a kidney transplant [3,12], but this almost certainly reflects a degree of patient selection.   In an attempt to overcome this bias, workers from the USA compared the survival of patients receiving a kidney during 1991-6, to those who had been accepted onto the transplant programme but who did not receive a graft in the same period. Survival was dramatically better for the transplanted patients, and diabetic subjects were particularly advantaged with an estimated increase in survival of 11 years [33]. Short term survival for diabetic patients has gradually increased in the USA over the decade until 1996 with a reduction of 45% from the death rate of 40.4 per 100 patient years recorded in 1986 [34]. Prevalent death rates in 1995 ranged from approximately 75 per 1000 patient years for 15-19 year olds to >300 per 1000 patient years for 60-64 year olds, and >400 per 1000 patient years for >70 year olds. These rates were highest for Europid patients [35].   For non-diabetic patients, the rates were approximately 40, 200, and >300 per 1000 patient for 15-19, 60-64, and >70 year olds respectively. Survival rates have not changed significantly since 1994 [3].

In the USA during 1993-5 for never transplanted patients aged 20-44 years, the death rate was approximately twice as high in diabetic compared to non-diabetic patients (160.7 v. 83.3 per thousand patient years), but this was five times the rate seen in diabetic subjects with a functioning transplant (31.4 per thousand patient years); and this in turn was almost three times the rate in non-diabetic transplant recipients over the same period (11.9 per thousand patient years). The major cause of death in these diabetic patients was cardiovascular disease (49% for never transplanted, 30% for functioning transplant v. 29% and 22% for non-diabetic patients respectively) [35]. The latest registry report confirms a 2.5 fold increase in death rate (approx 85 v 255 per 1000 patient years) for diabetic and cardiovascular disease patients >65 years of age with chronic kidney disease, compared to the age and CV disease matched background population. This ratio rises to almost four fold for those diabetic patients on dialysis. Interestingly these ratios are only slightly less for non-diabetic patients[3] (figure 2). Five year survival rates for diabetic patients are not given separately in these reports.

For the whole of Europe, the latest information on survival relates to >60 year olds on treatment from 1983-92 [4]. For diabetic patients, five year survival rates were 23% for 60-64 year olds and 18% for 70-74 year olds compared to 56% and 36% for non-diabetic ESRD respectively, but the proportion dying from cardiovascular causes was not very different between diabetic and non-diabetic >60 year olds (59 v. 55%) [4]. More recent reports from individual centres in Europe show a wide range of survival rates. In Spain the Catalunya Registry reports a five year survival of 30% for all diabetic patients entering RRT from1984-94 compared to 65% for those without diabetes [12], whilst in Madrid a 54% five year survival is reported in diabetic patients registered from1983-98[13]. However in Alsace, France, the two year survival in 84 patients with diabetic nephropathy admitted to the Dialysis Unit was only 32% [36]. The ERA-EDTA Registry has reported a combined 5 year survival from 6 national and regional registers for 1990-99 of 38%, 19% and 49% for type 1, type 2 and non-diabetic patients on HD respectively [5,23].

Diabetic patients in Southern Europe (Italy, Spain and Portugal) seem to do significantly better than those in the North, whatever the form of dialysis. A similar phenomenon has been reported for Hispanic compared to Europid diabetic patients in Texas [37] and for African American v. Europid patients in the USA as a whole [3]. The reasons are not entirely clear but may be a reflection of the lower incidence of ischaemic heart disease, perhaps secondary to dietary factors.

In Japan, 5 and 10 year survival for diabetic patients on HD from 1983 onwards was 47% and 21% respectively, compared to 71% and 53% for

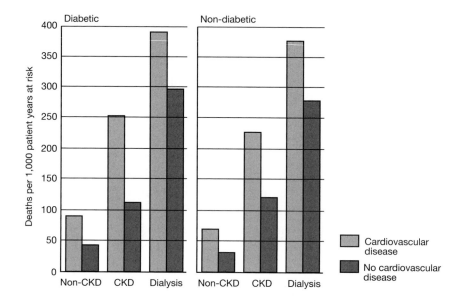

Fig. 2. All cause mortality in the general medicare and dialysis populations in diabetic and non-diabetic patients age 65 and over. Patients are categorised by the presence or absence of cardiovascular disease. They are also grouped according to presence of chronic kidney disease (CKD) or dialysis. Figure reproduced from the USRDS report 2002 with permission (reference 3).

patients with chronic glomerulonephritis [2]. Detailed causes of death are not provided, and the data are not age banded. Recent survival rates appear to have declined, perhaps as a result of accepting older and more ill patients onto RRT [38]. These survival rates on HD [39] remain better than for Europe and the USA [3] although the differences may be becoming smaller [38]. This might reflect longer and more effective dialysis in the Japanese patients and studies are currently ongoing to explore this proposition. Better survival in Japanese patients may also be explained by their lower risk of cardiovascular disease. Sudden cardiac death and myocardial infarction account for around 11% of deaths in 1996 in diabetic ESRD patients on HD in Japan, compared to 35% in the USA [2,3].

In all centres, survival is strongly influenced by pre-existing co-morbidity. Heart failure increases the relative risk of mortality by 45% for diabetic patients in all ethnic groups [2,3]. Because of the increased rate of cardiovascular death in diabetic patients on all modalities of RRT, many centres are advocating full vascular investigation prior to ESRD with coronary angiography in high risk subjects [40]. One centre has reported improved survival in patients who undergo coronary artery bypass grafting prior to renal transplantation [41].

SUGGESTED MANAGEMENT STRATEGIES

One of the key factors determining outcome of RRT for all patients is clinical status at entry. This is particularly true for diabetic patients in whom there is often considerable co-morbidity [19]. The guidelines for referral suggested by the kidney working group of the St Vincent Declaration include joint assessment by nephrologist and diabetologist once serum creatinine exceeds 200μmol/l [42]. In the UK, the Renal Association has suggested nephrology referral once serum creatinine exceeds 150μmol/l, although some have questioned the practicality of this guideline. Reports from a German centre and from Alsace suggest that in practice many patients are presenting in established renal failure [36,43]. In addition, specific treatments of proven worth such as angiotensin converting enzyme inhibitor drugs, and good blood pressure control were either absent or inadequate. Moreover, no mention is made in these reports of cholesterol lowering therapy, and despite the high prevalence of cardiovascular disease in the French patients, less than 10%

received a beta-blocker and only 25% were on treatment with aspirin [36]. A randomised trial of multiple risk factor intervention versus conventional therapy has been described by the Steno Hospital in Denmark in microalbuminuric type 2 patients, showing a significant reduction in numbers progressing to nephropathy after 7-8 years (RR 0.39; 95% CI 0.17 – 0.87; p = 0.003) [44]. A major priority for all of us looking after diabetic patients with renal complications is to improve our pre-ESRD care because only then are we likely to see no significant reductions in those needing RRT and improvements in survival.

CONCLUSIONS:

1. Incidence of diabetic ESRD is increasing world-wide, particularly in Southern Asian, Afro-Caribbean, Native American, Hispanic, Aboriginal and Pacific Islander populations. Rates in North American Europid subjects may be slowing down. The vast majority of this increase is of type 2 diabetes.

2. Acceptance of diabetic patients onto RRT is consequently increasing with a prevalence of around 384 pmp in the USA in 2000. European rates are much less than this but growing rapidly, particularly in Germany and Austria.

3. Survival on RRT is less good for diabetic patients who tend to have higher death rates from cardiovascular disease. Regional and ethnic variations in causes and rates of mortality need further study. Renal transplantation is the recommended option.

4. Early specialist referral and aggressive management of vascular risk factors and established arterial disease in the pre-ESRD patient is recommended.

REFERENCES

1. United States Renal Data System 2002 – Annual Data Report. Chapter 1. Incidence and Prevalence. pp 42-56. National Institutes of Health. Bethesola USA.
2. Shinzato T, Nakai S, Akiba T, et al. Report of the annual statistical survey of the Japanese Society for dialysis therapy in 1996. Kidney Int 1999; 55, 700-712.
3. United States Renal Data System 2002 – Annual Data Report. Chapter 9, Survival, Mortality and Causes of Death. pp 152-164. National Institutes of Health. Bethesola USA.
4. Valderrabano F, Berthoux F C, Jones E H P, Mehls O. Report on management of renal failure in Europe XXV, 1994. Endstage renal disease and dialysis report. Nephrol Dial Transplant 1996; 11: suppl 1:2-21
5. van Dijk P C W, Jager K J, deCharro F et al. Renal Replacement Therapy in Europe: the results of a collaborative effort by the ERA – EDTA registry and 6 National or Regional registries. Nephrol Dial Transplant 2001; 16, 1120-1129.

6.   Schaubel D E, Fenton S S A, Trends in mortality rates on hemodialysis in Canada 1981-1997. Kidney Int 2000; 57 suppl 74: s66-73.

7.   United States Renal Data System 2002 – Annual Data Report, chapter 13 International Comparisons pp 206-213. National Institues of Health. Bethesola USA.

8.   Guanyu W, Nan C, Giaqui Q, Shanyan L, Qinjun X, Dechang D, Nephrology, Dialysis and Transplantation in Shang-Hai, 1999. Nephrol Dial Transplant 2000: 15: 961-963.

9.   Disney APS Some trends in chronic renal replacement therapy in Australia and New Zealand, 1997. Nephrol Dial Transplant 1998; 13: 854-859.

10. UK Renal Registry Report 2002. UK Renal Registry, Bristol, UK.

11. Frei U. Schober-Halstenberg and the Quaisi-Niere Task Group. Annual Report of the German Renal Registry 1998. Nephrol Dial Transplant 1999; 1085-1090

12. Rodriguez J A, Cleries M, Vela E and Renal Registry Committee. Diabetic patients on renal replacement therapy: Analysis of Catalan Registry Data. Nephrol Dial Transplant 1997; 12: 2501-2509.

13. Perez-Garcia R, Rodriguez Beniteze P, Verde E, Valderrabano F. Increasing of renal replacement therapy (RRT) in diabetic patients in Madrid. Nephrol Dial Transplant 1999; 14: 2525-2527.

14. Cordonnier D G, Halimi S, Zaoui P. Health policies and epidemiology of diabetes among dialysed pateints in France. Nephrol Dial Transplant 1999: 2519.

15. Mesic E, Resic H, Halilbasic A, Komljenovic I, Vasilj M, Vucicevic L, Trnacevic S. Renal Replacement Therapy in Bosnia and Herzegovina: Report of the Society of Nephrology, Dialysis and Transplantation of Bosnia and Herzegovina and Nephrol Dial Transplant 2003 18 661-663.

16. Rutkowski B et al. Changing pattern of end-stage renal disease in Central and Eastern Europe. Nephrol Dial Transplant 2000; 15: 156-160.

17. Erek E, Suleymanlar G, Serdengecti K et al. Nephrology, Dialysis and Transplantation in Turkey. Nephrol Dial Transplant 2002; 17: 2087-2093.

18. Cean J F, Gonzalez-Martinez F, Schwedt E, et al. Renal Replacement Therapy in Latin America, Kidney Int 2000; 57 suppl 74: s55-59.

19. United States Renal Data System 2002 – Annual Data Report. Chapter 2, Patient Characteristics. pp 58-71. National Institutes of Health. Bethesola USA.

20. Hasslacher C, Ritz E, Wahl P, Michael C. Similar risks of nephrology in patients with type I and type II diabetes mellitus. Nephrol Dial Transplant 1989; 4: 859-863.

21. Adler A I, Stevens R J, Manley S E, Bilous R W, Cull CA, Holman R R, on behalf of the UKPDS Group. Development and progression of Nephropathy in type 2 diabetes: The United Kingdom Prospective Diabetes Study UKPDS (UKPDS 64). Kidney Int 2003; 63: 225-232.

22. Catalano C, Postorino M, Kelly P J et al. Diabetes mellitus and renal replacement therapy in Italy: prevalence, main characteristics and complications. Nephrol Dial Transplant 1995; 10788-96.

23. Briggs D, Personal Communication.

24. Cowie C C, Port F K, Wolfe R A, Savage P J, Moll P P, Hawthorne V M. Dispaities and incidence of diabetic endstage renal disease according to race and type of diabetes. N Engl J Med 1989; 321: 1074-1079.

25. Ritz E, Rychliki, Locatelli F, Halimi S, End-stage renal failure in type II diabetes: a medical catastrophe of World Wide dimensions. AMJ Kid Dis 1999; 34: 795-808.

26. United States Renal Data Sytem 1999 – Annual Data Report. II Incidence and prevalence. Am J Kid Dis 1999; 34: suppl 1: S40-50.

27. Valderrabano F, Berthoux F C, Jones E H P, Mehls O. Report on management of renal failure XXV, 1994. Endstage renal disease and dialysis report. Nephrol Dial Transplant 1996; 11: suppl 1: 2-21.

28. Buck K, Feehally J. Diabetes and renal failure in Indo-Asians in the UK – A paradigm for the study of disease susceptibilty. Nephrol Dial Transplant 1997; 12: 1555-1557.

29. Raleigh V S, Diabetes and hypertension in Britain's ethnic minorities: implications for the future of renal services. BMJ 1997; 314: 209-213.

30. Amos A F, McCarty D J, Zimmet P. The rising global burden of diabetes and its complications: Estimates and projections to the year 2010. Diabetic Medicine 1997; 14: suppl 5: S7-85.

31. Mazzuchi N, Fernandez-Caen J, Carbonell E. Criteria for selection of ESRD treatment modalities. Kidney Int 2000; 57 suppl 74: S136-43.

32. Ross S, Dong E, Gordon M, Connelly J, Kevasz M, Iyengar M, Mujais S K.Meta-analysis of outcome studies in end-stage renal disease. Kidney Int 2000; 57 suppl 74: S28-38.

33. United States Renal Data System 2002 – Annual Data Report. Chapter 3. Treatment Modalities pp72-81. National Institues of Health. Bethesola USA.

34. Wolfe R A, Ashby V B, Milford E L, Ojo A O, Ettenger R E, Agodoa L Y C, Held P J, Port F K. Comparison of mortality in all patients on dialysis, patients on dialysis awaiting transplantation and recipients of a first cadaveric transplant. N Engl J Med 1999; 341: 1725-30.

35. United States Renal Data System 1997 – Annual Report Data. VI Causes of death. Am J Kid Dis 1997; 30: suppl 1: S107-117.

36. Chantrel F, Enache I, Bouiller M, Kolb I, Kunz K, Petitjean P, Moulin B, Hannedouche T. Abysmal prognosis of patients with type 2 diabetes entering dialysis. Nephrol Dial Transplant 1999; 14: 129-136.

37. Medina R A, Pugh J A, Monterrosa A, Cornell J. Minority advantage in diabetic endstage renal disease survival on haemodialysis: due to different proportions of diabetic type? Am J Kid Dis 1996; 28: 226-234.

38. Akiba T, Nakai S, Shinzato T, Yamazaki C, Kitaoka T, Kubo K, Maeda K, Why has the gross mortality of dialysis patients increased in Japan? Kidney Int 2000; 57: suppl 74: S60-65.

39. Shinzato T, Nakai S, Akiba T et al. Survival in long term haemodialysis patients: results from the annual survey of the Japanese Society for Dialysis Therapy. Nephrol Dial Transplant 1997; 12: 884-888.

40. Manske CL, Thomas W, Wang Y, Wilson R F. Screening diabetic transplant candidates for coronary artery disease: identification of a low risk sub-group. Kidney Int 1993; 44: 617-621.

41. Manske C L, Wang Y, Rector T, Wilson R F, White C W. Coronary revascularisation in insulin dependent diabetic patients with chronic renal failure. Lancet 1992; 340: 998-1002.

42. Viberti G C, Mogensen C E, Passa P, Bilous R W, Mangili R. St Vincent Declaration, 1994: Guidelines for the prevention of diabetic renal failure. In, The kidney and hypertension in diabetes mellitus, second ed, Mogensen C E ed. Boston, Dordrecht, London: Kluwer Academic Publishers, 1994; pp 515-527.

43. Pommer W, Bressel F, Chen F, Molzahn M. There is room for improvement of pre-terminal care in diabetic patients with endstage renal failure – the epidemiological evidence in Germany. Nephrol Dial Transplant 1997; 12: 1318-1320.

44. Gaede P, Vedel P, Larsen N, Jensen G V H, Parvin g H-H, Pedersen O. Multi-factorial intervention and cardiovascular disease in patients with type 2 diabetes. N Engl J Med 2003; 348: 383-93.

38

HEMODIALYSIS AND CAPD IN TYPE 1 AND TYPE 2 DIABETIC PATIENTS WITH ENDSTAGE RENAL FAILURE

Ralf Dikow and Eberhard Ritz
Department Internal Medicine, Ruperto Carola University Heidelberg, Germany

Not too long ago type 2 diabetes was mostly considered a contraindication against renal replacement therapy (RRT). An impressive body of evidence has meanwhile accumulated upon which selection of therapeutic options in such patients can be based. Although diabetic patients, particularly type 2, continue to have a poorer outcome on RRT than non-diabetic patients, survival has become progressively better. Recent strategies to improve prognosis by appropriate timing of the start of treatment, by preventing cardiovascular complications in the predialytic stage, and by optimising glycemic control as well as lipid lowering are very promising indeed.

EPIDEMIOLOGY

As shown in table 1, in different countries the incidence of patients with type 2 diabetes requiring RRT has increased progressively during the last decade [1], according to the EDTA registry [2], the German experience [3, 4] and the US renal data system [5] and various national registries. From 1990-1999, the incidence of type 1 diabetic patients entering RRT ranged from 7.6 per million population (pmp) in Austria to 17.9 pmp in Denmark (compared to 7 pmp in Heidelberg 1998-2000; ref. 4) and of type 2 diabetes from 9.4 pmp in Denmark to 32.8 pmp in Austria (compared to 94 pmp in Heidelberg). The annual percent increase of type 2 diabetic patients entering RRT in different was +13.6% per year ranging from +10% in Austria to +20.9% in francophone Belgium [2]. Such rapid recent rise explains the markedly higher values in the recent local evaluation [4] compared to the data from earlier periods [2]. There is a substantial discrepancy between the incidence and the prevalence of diabetic patients (table 2). This is explained by the fact that survival of diabetic patients is considerably worse than in non-diabetic patients. This point is illustrated by the results of a prospective study on incident dialysis patients in Germany by Koch [6] as illustrated in figure 1. The 5 year survival of 5% in type 2 diabetic patients correspond to the survival in patients with metastasising gastrointestinal carcinoma. Survival rates in diabetic patients are much better in countries such as Japan [7] and this is presumably related to the lower rate of cardiovascular death in Japan. Nevertheless even in Germany survival of diabetic patients, mostly (90%) type 2, has improved in recent years [8].

Table 1. Incidence of patients admitted to renal replacement programs with diabetes as a co-morbid condition according to national registries (data are given as patients per million population (pmp) or percent).

Country	Year	New patients total (pmp)	Diabetes (% of total)	Diabetes (pmp)
Australia	(2000)	93.7	22	20.3
Catalunya	(2000)	146	19.8	28.9
Denmark	(2000)	67.5	15.8	28.8**
Germany	(2001)	73.3	36	26.4
Heidelberg*	(2001)	183	48.9	101***
New Zealand	(2000)	91.8	35	32.0
Poland	(2000)	67.5	15.8	10.6
Turkey	(2001)	89.7	25.3	22.7
United States	(2001)	317	42.8	136

*	according to ref. 4
**	type 1 diabetes 14.8 pmp, type 2 diabetes 14.0 pmp
***	type 1 diabetes 6 pmp, type 2 diabetes 92 pmp

It is obvious from Table 1, that in Europe the absolute rates of admission differ widely between different countries. A North-South gradient continues to persist. It is primarily admission for RRT of patients with type 2 diabetes as a co-morbid condition, which continues to increase. The diagnostic classification poses some problems [1]. Registry figures tend to underestimate the renal burden of diabetes. Diabetes was found in no less than 50% of patients admitted for renal replacement therapy in Heidelberg [4]. Clinical features of classical Kimmelstiel Wilson's disease were found only in 60%, however. Atypical presentation consistent with ischemic nephropathy accounted for 13% and known primary renal disease, e.g. polycystic disease, analgesic nephropathy, glomerulonephritis, with superimposed diabetes for 27% of the cases. Survival of the diabetic patient on hemodialysis is similar whether or not diabetic or non-diabetic renal disease accounts for endstage renal failure [6]. In our series, in 11% of the patients diabetes had not been diagnosed at the time of admission presumably because the patients had lost weight secondary to anorexia, thus self-correcting hyperglycemia. It is known that between 5 and 10% of patients [1] develop diabetes on dialysis de novo, presumably because they were pre-diabetic to begin with or because they had been a temporary reversal of hyperglycemia following weight loss from anorexia in the predialytic stage and recurrence after weight gain on dialysis. Gilbertson et al. [9] recently found that by the end of the first year of RRT close to two thirds of patients of RRT have recognized diabetes in the USA, further illustrating that registry data are confounded by diagnostic difficulties. It is also of interest that an increasing proportion of patients, 27% in the series of Schwenger [8], present as acute irreversible renal failure or acute on chronic renal failure, mostly after cardiac or septic complications with or without radiocontrast administration. The prognosis of patients admitted as acute renal failure is particularly poor [8, 10].

Late referral continues to be a problem [8, 11]. In Heidelberg the median interval between referral and start of dialysis was 17 weeks [8]. One year mortality was 37% in diabetics referred < 17 weeks and only 7.3% for those patients referred > 17 weeks. Patients referred late had even more insufficient control of risk factors (see table 2). They also had no vascular access as the main factor causing increased morbidity and mortality when patients had to be put on hemodialysis (HD) acutely. Insufficient control of risk factors is the more deplorable since cardiovascular death and particularly ischemic heart disease account for approximately 60% of deaths on hemodialysis in type 2 diabetic patients [2].

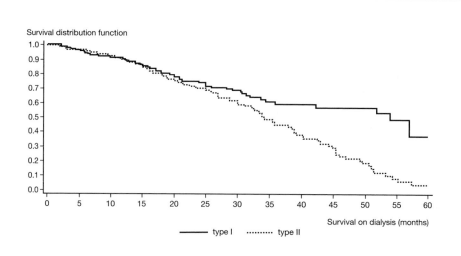

Fig. 1. Survival distribution function of 412 diabetic patients (181 type 1 and 231 type 2) with end-stage renal disease (after ref. 6).

Table 2. Status of diabetic patients at the time of admission to a renal unit (multicentric, nationwide retrospective study). 173 patients, 16 type 1 diabetes, 157 type 2 diabetes (ref. 88).

	Median (Range)
Measured C_{Cr} (ml/min)	29 (1-216)
Systolic BP (mmHg)	170 (120-260)
Diastolic BP (mmHg)	90 (60-180)
HbA1c (%)	7.9 (4.9-15.7)
No antihypertensive treatment	18%
ACE-inhibitor treatment	52%
Ophthalmological examination	30.6%
(within 12 months prior to admission)	

MANAGEMENT PROBLEMS ON HEMODIALYSIS

Vascular access

In the past it was felt that the known difficulty to create a functioning vascular access was mainly the result of venous run-off problems. Recently it has been recognised that inadequate arterial inflow is the major cause of fistula malfunction in diabetic patients because of sclerosis and calcification of the radial artery. Sclerosed arteries are unable to dilate and to remodel to accommodate an increase in blood flow from approximately 15 ml/min. to 500-1000 ml/min, as required for a functioning AV fistula [12]. The quality of the arterial wall, the diameter of the arterial lumen and the flow rate can be assessed by Doppler/duplex investigation, which has recently become an essential part of the preoperative diagnostic work-up. If the distal radial artery is severely sclerotic, one must usually establish a more proximal anastomosis. Use of native vessels is clearly the first choice and results of PTFE grafts are definitely inferior [13]. Surgeons who create a high elbow fistula achieve actual fistula survival rates, which are no longer different in diabetic and non-diabetic patients; such high fistulas are certainly justified in view of the limited life expectancy of diabetic patients on HD [14] (figure 2A and 2B). Atherosclerosis of the arteries of the palmar arch is frequent, and may lead to a "steal phenomenon" with finger gangrene [14]. If a PTFE graft is used monomelic neuropathy resulting from ischemia of the nerves may be seen [15].

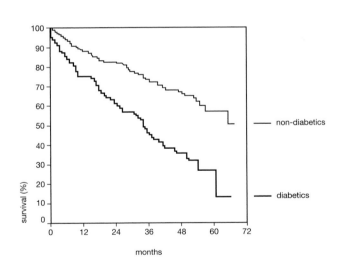

Fig. 2A Cumulative actuarial patient survival rates comparing non-diabetic and diabetic patients (after ref 14).

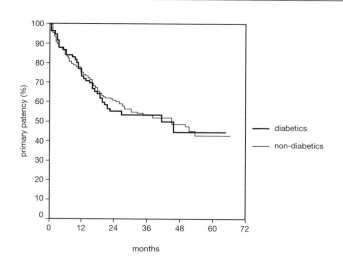

Fig. 2b. Actuarial primary fistula patency rates comparing non-diabetic and diabetic patients (after ref. 14).

The new DOQI guidelines recommend to prepare the patient for future kidney replacement therapy [dialysis and transplantation], and to create a vascular access once the estimated GFR has declined to <30 mL/min/1.73 m^2 (http://www.kidney.org/professionals/doqi/kdoqi/p8_cpm.htm).

Initiation of renal replacement therapy [RRT]

Most nephrologists agree that RRT should be started earlier in the diabetic than in the non-diabetic patient, approximately at a GFR of 15 ml/min. An even earlier start may be justified when hypervolemia and blood pressure become uncontrollable, when the patient is anorectic and cachectic and when the patient vomits as the combined result of uremia and diabetic gastroparesis. A new concept has been proposed by Lameire and collaborators, i.e. the integrated treatment program [16]. This is based on the reasoning that residual renal function is longer preserved on CAPD compared to HD. CAPD tends to become inefficient, however, when residual renal function is gone. There are no controlled data available to document better survival with this strategy, but observational data indeed look encouraging [16].

Hypertension

In advanced renal failure, blood pressure [BP] tends to be higher in diabetic compared to non-diabetic patients at any given level of GFR. Exchangable sodium is increased [17]; consequently, control of hypervolemia is the major challenge in the treatment of the hypertensive patient with diabetes. Blood pressure is characterised by a high amplitude because of reduced aortic compliance. This point is important because blood pressure amplitude or more direct indicators of aortic compliance such as pulse wave velocity, are powerful predictors of survival on RRT [18]. Pulse pressure and impaired elasticity of central arteries are major predictors of death in non-diabetic patients, and increased aortic stiffness contributes to higher all-cause and cardiovascular mortality in diabetic patients on HD [19].

BP on HD is characterised by an abnormal circadian profile with inadequate nighttime decrease or even an increase. This constellation in the type 2 diabetic is associated with poor cardiovascular prognosis [20]. In the patient on RRT it has been shown that BP levels in the lower normotensive range are associated with better survival [21]. Contraintuitively several recent epidemiological series showed that in the short run (2 years) low pre-dialysis BP values rather than high BP values are associated with higher mortality [22, 23]. There is agreement that this finding is the result of reverse causality, i.e. higher mortality in patients who suffer from cardiac disease. In any case because cardiac problems [24] are frequent in diabetic patients, circumspection and caution is required when fixing the target blood pressure, because hypotension, either orthostatic or during dialysis sessions [6] is associated with higher mortality. Over-aggressive lowering of blood pressure by volume subtraction must be avoided [25]. This is a particular risk in patients with low diastolic blood pressures as a result of reduced aortic compliance, because in this case coronary perfusion [which occurs during diastole] will be compromised [26].

The single most effective approach to control hypertension of the diabetic on HD is volume control by providing a low salt diet, determined ultrafiltration during dialysis sessions and selection of a lower dialysate Na^+-concentration [27, 28]. To avoid intradialytic hypotension, long dialysis sessions, omission of antihypertensive agents immediately before dialysis sessions, controlled ultrafiltration and correction of anemia by EPO therapy are helpful. Particularly impressive are recent observations that daily dialysis renders the majority of patients normotensive and abrogates the need of antihypertensive medication [29], although because of co-morbid conditions many diabetic patients don't qualify for this option.

Cardiovascular complications

Coronary heart disease, i.e. MI, AP, CABG, PTCA or pathology on coronary angiography is more frequent in diabetic (46.4%) than non-diabetic patients (32.2%) [30]. Obviously much of coronary pathology is acquired prior to dialysis. In preterminal diabetic compared to non-diabetic patients, the odds ratio for a new cardiovascular event was 5.3 [31] and progression, i.e. new events or worsening of existing pathology was seen in 20% of the patients over 23 months. In 433 Canadian patients, 116 of whom were diabetics, the latter had more frequently LVH, IHD and CHF [32] (table 3). No difference between diabetic and non-diabetic patients was found with respect to de novo appearance of progression of LVH and CHF. In contrast, the relative risk to develop IHD de novo, and in parallel CV mortality, were significantly higher in diabetic patients, suggesting accelerated atherogenesis. It is of note that although transplantation reduces the risk it does not completely abrogate it. Recently it was found, that the hazard ratio to develop an acute coronary syndrome after transplantation was still 0.38 and the rate of new events was 0.79% per patient year compared to 1.67 prior to transplantation [33]. In diabetic patients, advanced 3-vessel disease and severe coronary calcification are more frequent [34].

If the diabetic patient on dialysis develops an acute coronary syndrome, his chances of survival are very poor [35]. Fig. 3 shows survival after MI in dialysed patients and separately in dialysed diabetic patients. Unfortunately, up-to-date interventions including lysis, PTCA or CABG are not widely used in the high risk population of renal patients irrespective of the presence or absence of diabetes [36]. Although the impressive results of the DIGAMI study document benefit of intensified insulin and glucose treatment [37], this strategy is not widely adopted in dialysed diabetic patients despite the presence of insulin resistance even in non-diabetic renal patients [38]. The risk of an adverse cardiac outcome in IHD is amplified in the diabetic because of the coexistence of LVH [32], congestive heart failure [39], disturbed sympathetic function [40] and microvessel disease with arteriolar thickening and deficient capillarisation [41] as well as deranged cardiomyocyte metabolism [38].

Much new information has accrued with respect to intervention. There is no doubt that interventional management is superior to conservative management with betablockers [42], but it had remained controversial whether PTCA ($\pm$ stent) or coronary bypass is the preferred modality of treatment. Although prospective data are not available very compelling observational information in a large patient sample indicates that CABG is associated with higher inhospital death rates (12.5% vs. 5.4% in PTCA), but has the advantage of better longterm survival (56.9% vs. 52.9%) [43]. The must powerful predictors of cardiac death were old age and diabetes. The relative risk was 1.37 in diabetics. Table 4 compares the results of cardiac intervention in diabetic and non-diabetic dialysis patients [44]. Compared to PTCA without stent, PTCA + stent provided some benefit in non-diabetic, but not in diabetic patients. Similar to the results of the BARI study in non-renal patients [45] CABG was more beneficial in both non-diabetic and diabetic patients. It is important that this benefit was seen only when internal mammary grafts were used and not with saphenous bypass grafts.

Table 3 Cardiac findings in diabetic patients on dialysis (after ref. 32).

Baseline	Diabetic patients (n=116)	Non-diabetic patients (n=317)	p
concentric left ventricular hypertrophy	50%	38%	0.04
ischemic heart disease	32%	18%	0.003
cardiac failure	48%	24%	0.00001
Follow up	adjusted relative risk (diabetic/non-diabetic)		p
Ischemic heart disease	3.2		0.0002
Overall mortality	2.3		0.0001
Cardiovascular mortality	2.6		0.0001

Table 4. Comparison of cardiac intervention in diabetic and non diabetic dialysis patients (after ref. 44).

Compared to PTCA without stent	Relative risk of all-cause death	
	PTCA+Stent	Coronary artery bypass surgery
Non-diabetic	0.9 (0.86-0.97)	0.79 (0.7-0.85)
Diabetic	0.99* (0.91-1.08)	0.81** (0.75-0.86)

*   p= N.S.
**   p=0.0001

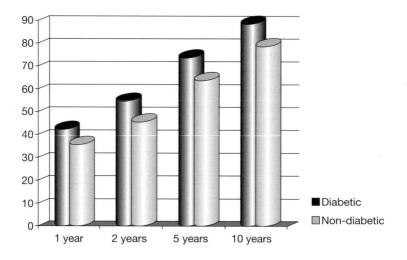

Fig. 3. Cardiac mortality after acute myocardial infarction in non-diabetic and diabetic dialysis patients (after ref. 35).

There is some discussion concerning the use of betablockers and statines. Norepinephrine is predictive of cardiac death in dialysis patients [46]. In dialysis patients with CHF, a prospective trial documented functional improvement by administration of carvedilol compared to placebo [47]. We had strongly advocated more liberal use of betablockers in patients with diabetes [48], based on the observation that only 3% of dialysed type 2 diabetic patients who died from cardiac causes were on betablockers, but no less than 13% of those who survived [6]. A benefit has meanwhile also been suggested by an observational study indicating that mortality was substantially less in dialysed patients (including diabetic patients) on betablockers [49].

Current recommendations suggest that LDL cholesterol should be lowered to values < 100 m g/dl in diabetic patients. Whether unique pathomechanisms operate in the atherogenesis in diabetics with ESRD, and whether statines are also indicated in this condition, is currently investigated in a prospective trial [50].

Several predictors of cardiac death have been identified in diabetic patients, i.e. a history of vascular disease, specifically myocardial infarction or angina pectoris [51], proliferative retinopathy and polyneuropathy (presumably inducing an imbalance of autonomic cardiac innervation) [6] and serum lipid levels [52]. The latter observation is remarkable because in non-diabetic patients on HD, an inverse relation between cholesterol and survival is seen presumably because low cholesterol is an index of malnutrition [53]. In prospective studies, strong predictors of CV death were smoking [54] as well as poor glycemic control prior to dialysis [55] or on HD [56].

The diabetic foot

Both neuropathic and ischemic foot problems are common in the uremic diabetic patient. In the 4D study, 16% of type 2 diabetic patients entering RRT had a history of amputation [49]. In the US, the rate of lower limb amputation in patients on RRT has risen progressively in recent years and is higher by a factor of 10 in the diabetic patient on RRT compared to the diabetic population at large [57]. The proportion of patients requiring amputation on dialysis is approximately 4% per year [58].

Glycemic control

The change of insulin requirements on HD is not uniform. Dialysis treatment partially reverses insulin resistance, so that insulin requirements often become less than before dialysis. In some patients, however, insulin requirements increase presumably because of reversal of anorexia and increased food consumption. It is most convenient to use dialysates that contain glucose, usually about 200 mg/dl, to allow administration of insulin at the usual times of the day with reduced risk of hypoglycemic or hyperglycemic episodes. Glucose containing dialysates cause also less hypotensive episodes [59].

Adequate control of glycemia is important because hyperglycemia causes thirst, high fluid intake and hypervolemia as well as an osmotic shift of water and K^+ from the intracellular to the extracellular space. The results are circulatory congestion and hyperkalemia. Diabetics with poor glucose control are also more susceptible to infection. Most important, however, is the finding that in type 2 diabetic patients mortality is increased with poor glycemic control before dialysis [55] and on RRT [56]. The actuarial survival was 31.7% when HbA1c was < 7.5% compared to 12.1% when it was > 7.5%. Assessment of glycemic control by using HbA1c is confounded by carbamylation of Hb, by altered red blood cell survival and by assay interference from uremia [60]. HbA1c values above 7.5% cause modest over-estimation of hyperglycemia in diabetic patients with ESRD. When EPO therapy is started, reticulocytes and young erythrocytes which had not had prolonged exposure to hyperglycemia enter the circulation and transiently cause artificial lowering of HbA1c.

There has been a recent trend to institute insulin treatment, including basal/bolus schedules, much earlier in type 2 diabetes with renal disease than used in the past. Insulin treatment is obligatory when patients have infections or undergo surgery. Insulin administration is also particularly useful to control malnutrition. Most sulfonylurea compounds (or their metabolites) with the exception of glimepirid and gliquidon, are excreted via the kidney and pose the risk of hypoglycemia. It is of interest that the newer glinides [61] and glitazones [62] do not cumulate in renal failure.

Anemia
Patients with diabetic nephropathy tend to have more severe anemia than non-diabetic patients. In a small series of type 1 diabetic patients [63] nearly 50% of the patients were anemic, compared to matched control patients with glomerulonephritis. More severe anemia in type 2 diabetic patients with more advanced renal disease compared to matched non-diabetic controls was also found by Ishimura [64] and by ourselves [4]. A multivariate analysis in a retrospective cohort found that diabetes increased the odds of anemia in renal disease [65]. Interestingly diabetic patients have a similar rise of EPO levels in response to hypoxia compared to healthy individuals [66], but inadequately low EPO concentrations in relation to the degree of anemia [67]. Interestingly a low EPO concentration is a predictor of more rapid loss of renal function [68]. There is some evidence that anemia is associated with more severe diabetic retinopathy [69] and that reversal of anemia causes regression of macula edema [70]. The role of anemia and its reversal by EPO in patients with peripheral artery disease is unclear. One retrospective study claimed an adverse effect [71], but the relative roles of improving oxygen supply vs. increasing viscosity and its adverse effect of microrheology have not been worked out. Anemia has also been claimed to either improve [72] or aggravate [73] insulin resistance, but confounding effects of EPO treatment on appetite and food intake have not been excluded. There are some intriguing suggestions that reversal of anemia reduces the rate of progression of renal disease [74, 75], but controlled evidence with sufficient biostatistical power is not available.

Current guidelines suggest work-up for anemia when Hb is < 12 g/dl in adult males and postmenopausal females and < 11g/dl in premenopausal females [76]. Two major studies currently investigate whether prevention of anemia by administration of EPO ameliorates cardiovascular surrogate markers and improves outcome. Currently expert groups recommend a target Hb of 12 g/dl.

Miscellaneous

One of the major unresolved problems in RRT of diabetic patients is malnutrition. It is usually the composite result of anorexia, chronic infections (diabetic foot), muscular wasting from polyneuropathy and impaired GI absorption because of gastroparesis. There is no "golden bullet solution" and the approach must be individualised.

On average, hyperparathyroidism is much less pronounced in diabetic compared to non-diabetic patients on HD [77]. This is in part explained by the shorter duration of uremia in diabetic patients because of more rapid progression, but there are also indications that glucose and insulin interfere with the parathyroid gland [78].

CONTINUOUS AMBULATORY PERITONEAL DIALYSIS (CAPD)

According the US Renal Data System [5] 7.1% of all patients with diabetes receiving renal replacement therapy are treated with PD, whilst 75.4% receive maintenance HD and 17.5% undergo transplantation. The proportion varies largely between countries, illustrating that selection of treatment modalities is strongly influenced by logistics and reimbursement policies and not only by medical considerations. There are very good a priori reasons to offer initially CAPD treatment to diabetic patients. In diabetic patients with ESRD, forearm vessels are often sclerosed, so that it is not possible to create a fistula [12]. The alternative of hemodialysis via intravenous catheters (instead of using av fistulas or grafts) is not ideal in the long run, because often blood flow is low and the risk of infection is high. Longterm dialysis via catheter was identified as one major predictor of poor patient survival on HD [79]. Furthermore, it has been stated that during the first two years of RRT in general survival is better for patients including diabetic patients treated with PD compared to HD [80] except the very elderly [81]. The survival advantage is no longer demonstrable beyond the second year, presumably because by then the residual renal function has decayed. It has been stated that PD has the advantage of providing slow and sustained ultrafiltration without rapid fluctuations of fluid volumes and electrolyte concentration, features, which are advantageous for blood pressure control and prevention of heart failure. These considerations have led to the interesting concept [16] of starting patients on PD and transferring them to HD when residual renal function has decayed. Recent analysis showed that unexpectedly mortality on PD is higher than on HD, including in diabetic patients [82], although this had not been a uniform experience [L. Tarnov, personal communication]. The issue is currently moot. In the past it was thought that CAPD offers the attractive alternative of administering insulin by injection into the CAPD fluid with the goal of providing insulin via the "physiological" portal route. Unfortunately this poses many practical problems: uncertainties of dosage, since insulin binds to the surfaces of dialysis bags and tubing and degradation by insulinases in the peritoneum [83]. Moreover, absorption from the peritoneal cavity shows large interindividual variations and there is no firm evidence that this mode of administration permits better control of glycemia or dyslipidemia [84]. This approach has meanwhile been almost universally abandoned.

Although protein is lost across the peritoneal membrane, more in diabetic than in non-diabetic patients, the main nutritional problem is gain of glucose and calories, because high glucose concentrations in the dialysate are necessary for osmotic removal of excess body fluid. The daily rate of glucose absorption is 100-150 g and a CAPD patient is exposed to 3-7 tons of fluids containing 50-175 kg glucose per year. The use of glucose-containing fluid has an interesting disadvantage, which has been recognised only recently [85]. Heat sterilisation of glucose under acid conditions creates highly reactive glucose degradation products [GDPs] such as methylglyoxal, glyoxal, formaldehyde, 3-deoxyglucosone and 3,4-dideoxyglucosone-3-ene [86]. GDPs are cytotoxic. They cause formation of advanced glycation endproducts (AGE) in the peritoneal cavity and are absorbed into the systemic circulation [87]. Even in non-diabetic patients on CAPD, deposits of AGE are found in the peritoneal membrane. AGE stimulate fibrogenesis and neoangiogenesis via VEGF. As a result peritoneal membrane characteristics deteriorate leading to inefficacy of CAPD. The capillary abnormalities in the peritoneal membrane resemble what is seen in retinal and renal capillaries and led to the snappy, but misleading term "local diabetes mellitus", which is seen even in non-diabetic patients. There is a strong move to avoid GDPs by heat sterilisation of 2 compartment bags. In prospective studies, CAPD fluid thus sterilised was much less toxic than conventional CAPD fluid despite high glucose concentrations [88].

STRATEGIES TO IMPROVE DIALYSIS OUTCOME

The key to improving dialysis outcome is more appropriate management of diabetic patients in the pre-dialysis phase to avoid the currently unsatisfactory cardiovascular state of patients at the time of referral to the nephrologist [4, 89]. It is of interest that the majority of type 2 diabetics (in contrast to the type 1 diabetics) is referred by general practitioners who tend to grossly underestimate the degree of renal dysfunction by paying attention only to serum creatinine concentration. This concentration is misleadingly low in these often malnourished cachectic patients. It has been strongly recommended to calculate the Cockroft Gault clearance (www.dopps.org) or to measure endogenous creatinine clearance. Further common problems are the failure to recognise coronary disease [particularly because IHD and MI are often silent] and to underestimate the importance of LVH.

These considerations and the necessity to create a useable vascular access in due time [12] require an interdisciplinary approach incorporating the nephrologist early into the treatment team.

A complementary strategy is to take type 2 diabetic patients out of dialysis programs and to transplant them. It has recently been recognised that for unknown reasons long duration of hemodialysis treatment interferes, for unknown reasons, with longterm graft outcome [90]. In view of the currently unacceptably high waiting times on the transplantation (TX) waiting list this increases the move to use life donor transplants from related or unrelated donors. Mortality after TX is higher in high risk individuals such as the elderly or the diabetic than in the average graft recipients. Nevertheless survival after TX is still better than survival in patients on the waiting list. The proportional benefit after TX is even greater in diabetics [91]. Whilst there is no doubt that pancreas/kidney transplantation is the method of choice for the type 1 diabetic which almost normalises survival [92] compared to life donor non-diabetic graft recipients, the remaining dilemma is TX in the type 2 diabetic. Most type 2 diabetics are of course excluded because of age and co-morbidity, but it has recently been shown that a surprisingly good outcome can be achieved in carefully selected type 2 diabetic patients when vascular disease [specifically coronary heart disease] has been excluded [93]. We strongly urge to consider transplantation in the younger hemodialysed type 2 diabetic who is free of vascular disease. The use of simultaneous pancreas/kidney transplantation in type 2 diabetic patients is currently under investigation. Further progress will hopefully come from steroid-free novel immunosuppressive treatments.

It has been a long way from the catastrophic early results of RRT in diabetic patients [94] until today's results had been achieved. The above considerations give reason for cautious optimism that further improvement can be achieved in the future.

REFERENCES

1. Ritz E, Rychlik I, Locatelli F, Halimi S: End-stage renal failure in type 2 diabetes: a medical catastrophe of worldwide dimensions. Am J Kidney Dis. 1999; 34: 795-808.
2. Jager KJ: Incidence and outcome of renal replacement therapy in patients with diabetes mellitus in a number of European countries. *In press* (*full quotation will be given in the galleys*).
3. Frei U, Schober-Halstenberg HJ: Nierenersatztherapie in Deutschland; Bericht 2000. Berlin 2001. www.quasi-niere.de.
4. Schwenger V, Mussig C, Hergesell O, Zeier M, Ritz E: Incidence and clinical characteristics of renal insufficiency in diabetic patients. Dtsch Med Wochenschr. 2001; 126: 1322-1326.
5. United States Renal Data System: *USRDS 2001 Annual Data Report*, Bethesda, The National Institute of Health, National Institute of Diabetes and Digestive and Kidney Diseases, 2001.
6. Koch M, Thomas B, Tschope W, Ritz E: Survival and predictors of death in dialysed diabetic patients. Diabetologia 1993; 36: 1113-1117.
7. Iseki K, Tozawa M, Iseki C, Takishita S, Ogawa Y: Demographic trends in the Okinawa Dialysis Study (OKIDS) registry (1971-2000). Kidney Int 2002; 61: 668-675.
8. Schwenger V, Hofmann A, Kalifeh N, Meyer T, Zeier M, Hörl WH, Ritz E: Uremic patients: late referral – early death. Dtsch Med Wochenschr. 2003 *in press*.
9. Gilbertson DT, Xue JL, Collins AJ: The increasing burden of diabetes in United States ESRD patients. J Am Soc Nephrol. 2002; 13: 646A.
10. Chantrel F, Enache I, Bouiller M, Kolb I, Kunz K, Petitjean P, Moulin B, Hannedouche T: Abysmal prognosis of patients with type 2 diabetes entering dialysis. Nephrol Dial Transplant. 1999;14: 129-136.
11. Jungers P: Late referral: loss of chance for the patient, loss of money for society. Nephrol Dial Transplant 2002;17: 371-375.
12. Konner K, Nonnast-Daniel B, Ritz E: The arterio-venous fistule. J Am Soc Nephrol. 2003 *in press*.
13. Wedgewood KR, Viggins PA, Guillou PJ: A prospective study of end-to-side versus side-to-side arteriovenous fistulas for hemodialysis. Brit J Surg. 1984; 71: 640-642.
14. Konner K: Primary vascular access in diabetic patients: an audit. Nephrol Dial Transplant. 2000; 15: 1317-1325.
15. Miles AM: Vacular steal syndrome and ischaemic monomelic neuropathy: two variants of upper limb ischaemia after haemodialysis vascular access surgery. Nephrol Dial Transplant. 1999; 14: 297-300.

16. Van Biesen W, Davies S, Lameire N: An integrated approach to end-stage renal disease. Nephrol Dial Transplant. 2001;16: Suppl 6: 7-9.

17. O'Hare JA, Ferriss JB, Brady D, Twomey B, O'Sullivan DJ: Exchangeable sodium and renin in hypertensive diabetic patients with and without nephropathy. Hypertension 1985; 7(suppl 2): II-43 – II-48.

18. Blacher J, Guerin AP, Pannier B, Marchais SJ, Safar ME, London GM: Impact of aortic stiffness on survival in end-stage renal disease. Circulation 1999; 99: 2434-2439.

19. Shoji T, Emoto M, Shinohara K, Kakiya R, Tsujimoto Y, Kishimoto M, Ishimura E, Tabata T, Nishizawa Y: Diabetes mellitus, aortic stiffness, and cardiovascular mortality in end-stage renal disease. J Am Soc Nephrol. 2001; 12: 2117-2124.

20. Nakano S, Fukuda M, Hotta F, Ito T, Ishii T, Kitazawa M, Nishizawa M, Kigoshi T, Uchida K: Reversed circadian blood pressure rhythm is associated with occurrences of both fatal and nonfatal vascular events in NIDDM subjects. Diabetes 1998; 47: 1501-1506.

21. Schomig M, Eisenhardt A, Ritz E: Controversy on optimal blood pressure on haemodialysis: normotensive blood pressure values are essential for survival. Nephrol Dial Transplant 2001;16: 469-474.

22. Zager PG, Nikolic J, Brown RH, Campbell MA, Hunt WC, Peterson D, Van Stone J, Levey A, Meyer KB, Klag MJ, Johnson HK, Clark E, Sadler JH, Teredesai P: "U" curve association of blood pressure and mortality in hemodialysis patients. Medical Directors of Dialysis Clinic, Inc. Kidney Int 1998; 54: 561-569.

23. Port FK, Hulbert-Shearon TE, Wolfe RA, Bloembergen WE, Golper TA, Agodoa LY, Young EW: Predialysis blood pressure and mortality risk in a national sample of maintenance hemodialysis patients. Am J Kidney Dis 1999; 33: 507-517.

24. Zoccali C: Cardiovascular risk in uraemic patients-is it fully explained by classical risk factors? Nephrol Dial Transplant. 2000; 15: 454-457.

25. Dikow R, Adamczak M, Henriquez DE, Ritz E: Strategies to decrease cardiovascular mortality in patients with end-stage renal disease. Kidney Int Suppl 2002; 80: 5-10.

26. Zoccali C: Arterial pressure components and cardiovascular risk in end-stage renal disease. Nephrol Dial Transplant 2003;18: 249-252.

27. Krautzig S, Janssen U, Koch KM, Granolleras C, Shaldon S: Dietary salt restriction and reduction of dialysate sodium to control hypertension in maintenance haemodialysis patients. Nephrol Dial Transplant 1998;13: 552-553.

28. Ozkahya M, Ok E, Cirit M, Aydin S, Akcicek F, Basci A, Dorhout Mees EJ. Regression of left ventricular hypertrophy in haemodialysis patients by ultrafiltration and reduced salt intake without antihypertensive drugs. Nephrol Dial Transplant 1998; 13: 1489-1493.

29. Kooistra MP, Vos J, Koomans HA, Vos PF. Daily home haemodialysis in The Netherlands: effects on metabolic control, haemodynamics, and quality of life. Nephrol Dial Transplant 1998; 13: 2853-2860.

30. Stack AG, Bloembergen WE: A cross-sectional study of the prevalence and clinical correlates of congestive heart failure among incident US dialysis patients. Am J Kidney Dis. 2001; 38: 992-1000.

31. Levin A, Djurdjev O, Barrett B, Burgess E, Carlisle E, Ethier J, Jinda K, Mendelssohn D, Tobe S, Singer J, Thompson C: Cardiovascular disease in patients with chronic kidney disease: getting to the heart of the matter. Am J Kidney Dis. 2001; 38: 1398-1407.

32. Foley RN, Culleton BF, Parfrey PS, Harnett JD, Kent GM, Murray DC, Barre PE: Cardiac disease in diabetic end-stage renal disease. Diabetologia 1997; 40: 1307-1312.

33. Hypolite IO, Bucci J, Hshieh P, Cruess D, Agodoa LY, Yuan CM, Taylor AJ, Abbott KC: Acute coronary syndromes after renal transplantation in patients with end-stage renal disease resulting from diabetes. Am J Transplantat 2002; 2: 274-281.

34. Raggi P, Boulay A, Chasan-Taber S, Amin N, Dillon M, Burke SK, Chertow GM: Cardiac calcification in adult hemodialysis patients. A link between end-stage renal disease and cardiovascular disease? J Am Coll Cardiol. 2002; 39: 695-701.

35. Herzog CA, Ma JZ, Collins AJ: Poor long-term survival after acute myocardial infarction among patients on long-term dialysis. New Engl J Med. 1998; 339: 799-805.

36. Shlipak MG, Heidenreich PA, Noguchi H, Chertow GM, Browner WS, McClellan MB: Association of renal insufficiency with treatment and outcomes after myocardial infarction in elderly patients. Ann Intern Med. 2002; 137: 555-562.

37. Malmberg K, Norhammer A, Wedel H, Ryden L: Glycometabolic state at admission: important risk marker of mortality in conventionally treated patients with diabetes mellitus and acute myocardial infarction. Circulation 1999; 99: 2626-2632.

38. Dikow R, Ritz E: Cardiovascular complications in the diabetic patient – an update in 2003. Nephrol Dial Transplant. 2003; *in press*.

39. Foley RN, Parfrey PS, Sarnak MJ: Epidemiology of cardiovascular disease in chronic renal disease. J Am Soc Nephrol. 1998; 9: S16-S23.

40. Standl, Schnell O: A new look at the heart in diabetes mellitus: from ailing to failing. Diabetologia 2000; 43: 1455-1469.

41. Amann K, Ritz E: Microvascular disease – the Cinderella of uraemic heart disease. Nephrol Dial Transplant. 2000; 15: 1493-1503.

42. Manske CL, Wang Y, Rector T, et al: Coronary revascularization in insulin-dependent diabetic patients with chronic renal failure. Lancet 1992; 340: 998-1002.

43. Herzog CA, Ma JZ, Collins AJ: Long-term outcome of dialysis patients in the United States with coronary revascularization procedures. Kidney Int. 1999; 56: 324-332.

44. Herzog CA, Ma JZ, Collins AJ: Comparative survival of dialysis patients in the United States after coronary angioplasty, coronary artery stenting, and coronary artery bypass surgery and impact of diabetes. Circulation 2002; 106: 2207-2211

45. Comparison of coronary bypass surgery with angioplasty in patients with multivessel disease. The Bypass Angioplasty Revascularization Investigation (BARI) Investigators. N Engl J Med 1996; 335: 217-25.

46. Zoccali C, Mallamaci F, Parlongo S, Cutrupi S, Benedetto FA, Tripepi G, Bonanno G, Rapisarda F, Fatuzzo P, Seminara G, Cataliotti A, Stancanelli B, Malatino LS, Cateliotti A: Plasma norepinephrine predicts survival and incident cardiovascular events in patients with end-stage renal disease. Circulation 2002; 105: 1354-1359.

47. Cice G, Ferrara L, Di Benedetto A, Russo PE, Marinelli G, Pavese F, Iacono A: Dilated cardiomyopathy in dialysis patients—beneficial effects of carvedilol: a double-blind, placebo-controlled trial. J Am Coll Cardiol 2001; 37: 407-411.

48. Zuanetti G, Maggioni AP, Keane W, Ritz E: Nephrologists neglect administration of betablockers to dialysed diabetic patients. Nephrol Dial Transplant. 1997; 12: 2497-2500.

49. Bragg JL, Mason NA, Maroni BJ, Held PJ, Young EW: Beta-adrenergic antagonist utilization among hemodialysis patients. Data from the DOPPS study. Lecture from the Annual Meeting of the American Society of Nephrology, Philadelphia 2002.

50. Wanner C, Krane V, Ruf G, März W, Ritz E: Rationale and design of a trial improving outcome of type 2 diabetics on hemodialysis. Kidney Int. 1999; 56: S222-S226.

51. Koch M, Kutkuhn B, Grabensee B, Ritz E: Apolipoprotein A, fibrinogen, age, and history of stroke are predictors of death in dialysed diabetic patients: a prospective study in 412 subjects. Nephrol Dial Transplant. 1997; 12: 2603-2611.

52. Tschöpe W, Koch M, Thomas B, Ritz E: Serum lipids predict cardiac death in diabetic patients on maintenance hemodialysis. Nephron 1992; 64: 354-358.

53. Chertow GM, Johansen KL, Lew N, Lazarus JM, Lowrie EG: Vintage, nutritional status, and survival in hemodialysis patients. Kidney Int 2000; 57: 1176-1181.

54. Foley RN, Herzog CA, Collins AJ: Smoking and cardiovascular outcomes in dialysis patients: The United States Renal Data System Wave 2 Study. Kidney Int 2003; 63:1462-1467.

55. Wu MS, Yu CC, Yang CW, Wu CH, Haung JY, Hong JJ, Fan Chiang CY, Huang CC, Leu ML: Poor pre-dialysis glycaemic control is a predictor of mortality in type II diabetic patients on maintenance haemodialysis. Nephrol Dial Transplant 1997; 12: 2105-2110.

56. Morioka T, Emoto M, Tabata T, Shoji T, Tahara H, Kishimoto H, Ishimura E, Nishizawa Y: Glycemic control is a predictor of survival for diabetic patients on hemodialysis. Diabetes Care 2001; 24: 909-913.

57. Eggers PW, Gohdes D, Pugh J: Nontraumatic lower extremity amputations in the Medicare end-stage renal disease population. Kidney Int. 1999; 56: 1524-1533.

58. Schömig M, Ritz E, Standl E, Allenberg J: The diabetic foot in the dialyzed patient. J Am Soc Nephrol. 2000; 11: 1153-1159.

59. Simic-Ogrizovic S, Backus G, Mayer A, Vienken J, Djukanovic L, Kleophas W: The influence of different glucose concentrations in haemodialysis solutions on metabolism and blood pressure stability in diabetic patients. Int J Artif Organs 2001; 24: 863-869.

60. Joy MS, Cefalu WT, Hogan SL, Nachman PH: Long-term glycemic control measurements in diabetic patients receiving hemodialysis. Am J Kidney Dis. 2002; 39: 297-307.

61. Hasslacher C: Safety and efficacy of repaglinide in type 2 diabetic patients with and without impaired renal function. Diabetes Care 2003; 26: 886-891.

62. Chapelsky MC, Thompson-Culkin K, Miller AK, Sack M, Blum R, Freed MI: Pharmacokinetics of rosiglitazone in patients with varying degrees of renal insufficiency. J Clin Pharmacol 2003 Mar;43(3):252-259.

63. Bosman DR, Winkler AS, Marsden JT, MacDougall IC, Watkins PJ: Anemia with erythropoietin deficiency occurs early in diabetic nephropathy. Diabetes Care 2001; 24: 495-499.

64. Ishimura E, Nishizawa Y, Okuno S et al. Diabetes mellitus increases the severity of anemia in non-dialyzed patients with renal failure. J Nephrol. 1998; 11: 83-86.

65. Kazmi WH, Kausz AT, Khan S et al. Anemia: an early complication of chronic renal insufficiency. Am J Kidney Dis. 2001; 38: 803-812.

66. Bosman DR, Osborne CA, Marsden JT et al. Erythropoietin response to hypoxia in patients with diabetic autonomic neuropathy and non-diabetic chronic renal failure. Diabetes Med. 2002; 19: 65-69.

67. Dikow R, Schwenger V, Schomig M, Ritz E: How should we manage anaemia in patients with diabetes? Nephrol Dial Transplant. 2002; 17: S67-S72.

68. Inomata S, Itoh H, Imai H: Serum levels of erythropoietin as a novel marker reflecting the severity of diabetic nephropathy. Nephron 1997; 75: 426-430.

69. Shorb SR: Anemia and diabetic retinopathy. Am J Ophthalmol. 1985; 100: 434-436.

70. Friedman EA, Brown CD, Berman DH: Erythropoietin in diabetic macular edema and renal insufficiency. Am J Kidney Dis. 1995; 26: 202-208.

71. Wakeen M, Zimmermann SW; Association between human recombinant EPO and peripheral vascular disease in diabetic patients receiving peritoneal dialysis. Am J Kidney Dis. 1998; 32: 488-493.

72. Spaia S, Pangalos M, Askepidis N et al. Effect of short-term rhu-EPO treatment on insulin resistance in hemodialysis patients. Nephron 2000; 84; 320-325.

73. Rigalleau V, Blanchetier V, Aparicio M et al. Erythropoietin can deteriorate glucose control in uremic non-insulin dependent diabetic patients. Diabet Met. 1998; 24: 62-65.

74. Jungers P, Choukronn G, Oualim Z et al. Beneficial influence of recombinant human erythropoietin therapy on the rate of progression of chronic renal failure in pre-dialyisis patients. Nephrol Dial Transplant. 2001, 16: 307-312.

75. Kuriyama S, Tomonari H, Yoshida H, et al: Reversal of anemia by erythropoietin therapy retards the progression of chronic renal failure, especially in non-diabetic renal patients. Nephron 1997; 77: 176-185.

76. EBPG. European Best Practise Guidelines for the Management of Anemia in Patients with Chronic Renal Failure. Nephrol Dial Transplant. 1999; 14 (suppl. 5): 1-5.

77. Inaba M, Okuno S, Nagasue K, Otoshi T, Kurioka Y, Maekawa K, Kumeda Y, Imanishi Y, Ishimura E, Ohta T, Morii H, Kim M, Nishizawa Y: Impaired secretion of parathyroid hormone is coherent to diabetic hemodialyzed patients. Am J Kidney Dis 2001; 38(4 Suppl 1): S139-42.

78. Sugimoto T, Ritter C, Morrissey J, Hayes C, Slatopolsky E: Effects of high concentrations of glucose on PTH secretion in parathyroid cells. Kidney Int 1990; 37: 1522-1527.

79. Sehgal AR, Leon JB, Siminoff LA, Singer ME, Bunosky LM, Cebul RD: Improving the quality of hemodialysis treatment: a community-based randomized controlled trial to overcome patient-specific barriers. JAMA 2002; 287: 1961-1967.

80. Heaf JG, Lokkegaard H, Madsen M: Initial survival advantage of peritoneal dialysis relative to haemodialysis. Nephrol Dial Transplant. 2002; 17: 112-117.

81. Winkelmayer WC, Glynn RJ, Mittleman MA, Levin R, Pliskin JS, Avorn J: Comparing mortality of elderly patients on hemodialysis versus peritoneal dialysis: a prospective score approach. J Am Soc Nephrol. 2002; 13: 2353-2362.

82. Ganesh SK, Hulbert-Shearon T, Port FK, Eagle K, Stack AG: Mortality Differences by Dialysis Modality among Incident ESRD Patients with and without Coronary Artery Disease. J Am Soc Nephrol 2003; 14: 415-424.

83. Khanna R, Oreopoulos DG: CAPD in patients with diabetes mellitus. In: Gokal R, ed. Continuous Ambulatory Peritoneal Dialysis. London: Churchill Livingstone. 1986; 12: 291-306.

84. Nevalainen PI, Lahtela JT, Mustonen J, Pasternak A: Subcutaneous and intraperitoneal insulin therapy in diabetic patients on CAPD. Peritoneal Dial Int. 1996; 16: S288-S291.

85. Wieslander AP: Cytotoxicity of peritoneal dialysis fluid – is it related to glucose breakdown products? Nephrol Dial Transplant. 1996; 11: 958-959.

86. Linden T, Cohen A, Deppisch R, Kjellstrand P, Wieslander A: 3,4-Dideoxyglucosone-3-ene (3,4-DGE): a cytotoxic glucose degradation product in fluids for peritoneal dialysis. Kidney Int. 2002; 62: 697.

87. Zeier M, Schwenger V, Deppisch R, Haug U, Weigel K, Bahner U, Wanner C, Schneider H, Henle T, Ritz E: Glucose degradation products in PD fluids: Do they disappear from the peritoneal cavity and enter the systemic circulation? Kidney Int 2003; 63: 298-305.

88. Rippe B, Simonsen O, Heimburger O, Christensson A, Haraldsson B, Stelin G, Weiss L, Nielsen FD, Bro S, Friedberg M, Wieslander A: Long-term clinical effects of a peritoneal dialysis fluid with less glucose degradation products. Kidney Int. 2001; 59: 348-357.

89. Keller C, Ritz E, Pommer W, Stein G, Frank J, Schwarzbeck A: Quality of treatment of renal failure in diabetics in Germany. Dtsch Med Wschr. 2000; 125: 240-244.

90. Mange KC, Joffe MM, Feldman HI: Effect of the use or nonuse of long-term dialysis on the subsequent survival of renal transplants from living donors. N Engl J Med 2001; 344: 726-31.

91. Wolfe RA, Ashby VB, Milford EL, Ojo AO, Ettenger RE, Agodoa LYC, Held PJ, Port FK: Comparison of mortality in all patients on dialysis, patients on dialysis awaiting transplantation, and recipients of a first cadaveric transplant. N Engl J Med. 1999; 341: 1725-1730.

92. Becker BN, Brazy PC, Becker YT, Odorico JS, Pintar TJ, Collins BH, Pirsch JD, Leverson GE, Heisey DM, Sollinger HW: Simutaneous pancreas-kidney transplantation reduces excess mortality in type 1 diabetic patients with end-stage renal disease. Kidney Int. 2000; 57: 2129-2135.

93. Mieghem AV, Fonck C, Coosemans W, Vandeleene B, Venrenterghem Y, Squifflet JP, Pirson Y: Outcome of cadaver kidney transplantation in 23 patients with type 2 diabetes mellitus. Nephrol Dial Transplant. 2001; 16: 1686-1691.

94. Ghavamian M, Gutch CG, Kopp KF, Kolff WJ: The sad truth about hemodialysis in diabetic patients. JAMA 1972; 222: 1386-1389.

39

KIDNEY AND PANCREAS TRANSPLANTS IN DIABETES

[1]Amy L. Friedman, [2]Eli A. Friedman,

[1]Department of Surgery, Yale University School of Medicine , and , [2]Department Medicine, Downstate Medical Center, Brooklyn, New York USA

Diabetes mellitus leads the causes of end-stage renal disease (ESRD) in the United States (US), Japan, and most nations in industrialized Europe. As tabulated in the latest US Renal Data System (USRDS) Report (2002), of 96,192 patients begun on therapy for ESRD during 2000, 41,772 (43.4%) had diabetes, an *incidence* rate of 145 per million population [1] (figure 1). Reflecting their relatively higher death rate compared to other causes of ESRD, the *prevalence* of US diabetic ESRD patients on December 31, 2000, was 34% (131,173 of 378,862 patients). Both glomerulonephritis and hypertensive renal disease rank below diabetes in frequency of diagnosis among new ESRD patients, substantiating the contention of Mauer and Chavers that "Diabetes is the most important cause of ESRD in the Western world [2]".

According to the 2002 National Diabetes Fact Sheet issued by the US Centers for Disease Control and Prevention [3], more than 16 million people in the US have diabetes – one third of whom are unaware of their disorder. Among US adults, the prevalence of diagnosed diabetes increased 49% from 1990 to 2000. During 2003 in the US, an estimated 798,000 people will have newly diagnosed diabetes while 187,000 people will die from diabetes. Depending on age, race, and gender, diabetes in 1996 ranked from 8th (White men 45 to 65 years) to 4th (Black women 45 years and over) leading cause of death [4]. Health care expenditures for diabetes in the US amount to a minimum of $100 billion and may be as high as $150 billion annually. The full impact of diabetic complications is unmeasured but in addition to the toll of ESRD includes 82,000 lower limb amputations, and 24,000 cases of blindness.

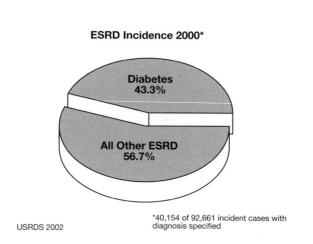

USRDS 2002

*40,154 of 92,661 incident cases with diagnosis specified

Figure 1. Extracted from the USRDS 2002 Annual Data Report [1] diabetes accounts for nearly half of all incident patients with ESRD. The great majority of new diabetic ESRD patients have type 2 diabetes.

OPTIONS FOR ESRD TREATMENT IN DIABETES

Diabetic ESRD patients are managed similarly to non-diabetic ESRD patients with two exceptions: 1) simultaneous pancreas and kidney transplantation is a diabetes-specific therapy and 2) opting for no treatment, meaning electing passive suicide, is the choice more often selected for and by diabetic than by nondiabetic individuals (Table 1). While the goal of uremia therapy is to permit an informed patient to select from a menu of available regimens, realities of program resources usually channel the diabetic ESRD patient to that treatment preferred by the supervising nephrologist. Illustrating this point, the first advocated option for newly treated ESRD is likely to be peritoneal dialysis performed as continuous ambulatory peritoneal dialysis (CAPD) in Toronto, home hemodialysis in Seattle, and a renal transplant in Minneapolis. No prospective, controlled trials of dialytic therapy — of any type — versus kidney transplantation have been reported or are likely to be initiated. Therefore, what follows reflects an acknowledged bias in interpreting the bias of others.

Table 1. OPTIONS IN UREMIA THERAPY FOR DIABETIC ESRD PATIENTS

1.	No Specific Uremia Intervention = Passive Suicide
2.	Peritoneal Dialysis
	Intermittent Peritoneal Dialysis (IPD)
	Continuous Ambulatory Peritoneal Dialysis (CAPD)
	Continuous Cyclic Peritoneal Dialysis (CCPD)
3.	Hemodialysis
	Facility Hemodialysis
	Home Hemodialysis
4.	Renal Transplantation
	Cadaver Donor Kidney
	Living Donor Kidney
5.	Pancreas plus Kidney Transplantation
	Type 1
	?Type 2

Confusion over diabetes type is frequent when evaluating diabetic ESRD patients. Underscoring the difficulty in determining diabetes type is the report that in Sweden, as many as 14% of cases originally diagnosed as non-insulin-dependent diabetes mellitus (type 2 diabetes) progressed to type 1 diabetes, while 10% of newly diagnosed diabetic individuals could not be classified [1]. Islet ß-cell dysfunction in type 2 diabetes, noted in 27.2% of 56,059 subjects, varies with the different genetic defects associated with characteristic patterns of altered insulin secretion that can be defined clinically [6]. Subjects with mild glucose intolerance and normal fasting glucose concentrations and normal glycosylated hemoglobin levels consistently manifest defective ß-cell function, a component of type 2 diabetes that is present before onset of overt hyperglycemia. The degree of hyperglycemia assessed by the level of hemoglobin A_{1c} (HbA$_{1c}$) is the best predictor of microvascular and macrovascular complications of diabetes [7]. At the other extreme, it is well established that some patients with type 1 diabetes maintain a measurable level of pancreatic ß-cell activity for many years after onset of their disease [8] sometimes thwarting the utility of C-peptide measurements to distinguish type 1 diabetes from type 2 diabetes [9].

Diabetes in America and Europe is overwhelmingly type 2, fewer than seven percent of diabetic Americans are insulinopenic, C-peptide negative persons who have type 1 diabetes. ESRD in diabetic persons reflects the demographics of diabetes *per se* [10] in that: 1. The incidence [11] is higher in women, blacks [12], Hispanics [13], and native Americans [14]. 2. The peak incidence of ESRD in diabetes occurs from the 5th to the 7th decade. Inferred from these relative attack rates, is the reality that blacks over the age of 65 face a seven times greater risk of diabetes-related renal failure than do whites. In the urban US, it is not surprising, therefore, that ESRD associated with diabetes is mainly a disease of poor, elderly blacks [15]. Vasculopathic complications of diabetes including the onset and severity of hypertension are at least as severe in type 2 diabetes as in type 1 diabetes [16]. In fact, recognition of the high prevalence of proteinuria and azotemia in carefully followed individuals with type 2 diabetes contradicts the view that type 2 diabetes only infrequently induces nephropathy [17]. Although there are differences between type 1 diabetes and type 2 diabetes in terms of genetic predisposition [18] and racial expression, clinical expression of the two disorders - particularly manifestations of nephropathy - are remarkably similar as a correlate of disease duration.

Careful observation of the course of nephropathy in type 1 and type 2 diabetes indicates strong similarities in rate of renal functional deterioration [19] and onset of comorbid complications Figure 2). Early nephromegaly, as well as both glomerular hyperfiltration and microalbuminuria, previously thought limited to type 1 diabetes, are now recognized as equally prevalent in type 2 diabetes [20]. Lack of precision in diabetes classification provokes confusing terms like "insulin requiring" to explain treatment with insulin in persons thought to have *resistant* type 2 diabetes. In fact, present criteria are unable to classify as many as one-half of diabetic persons as specifically type 1 or type 2 diabetes [21,22].

Consequently, literature reports of the outcome of ESRD therapy by diabetes type are few and imprecise.

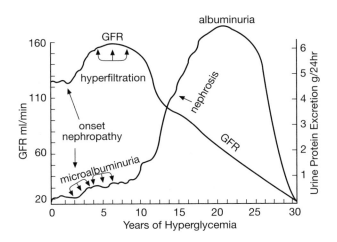

Figure 2.The natural history of kidney disease in diabetes begins with the pathophysiologic perturbations of increased glomerular filtration rate (GFR) termed hyperfiltration, and the excretion of small amounts of albumin termed microalbuminuria. Thereafter, proteinuria, nephrosis, azotemia, and ESRD follow in sequence. These stages are similar in type 1 and type 2 diabetes

CO-MORBID RISK FACTORS

Management of a diabetic person with progressive renal insufficiency is more difficult than in an age and gender matched non-diabetic person. The toll of coincident extrarenal disease — especially blindness, limb amputations, and cardiac disease — limits or preempts rehabilitation. For example, provision of a hemodialysis vascular access in a non-diabetic patient is minor surgery, whereas a diabetic patient, after even minimal surgery, risks major morbidity from infection or deranged glucose regulation. As a group, diabetic patients manifesting ESRD suffer a higher death rate due to cardiac decompensation, stroke, sepsis and pulmonary disease than do nondiabetic ESRD patients. Listed in Table 2 are the major co-morbid concerns in the management of diabetic ESRD patients. Diabetic retinopathy ranks at the top — with heart and lower limb disease — as major concerns in overall patient care. More than 95 per cent of diabetic individuals, in industrialized countries where advanced healthcare is readily available, who begin maintenance dialysis, or receive a renal allograft, have undergone laser treatment and/or vitrectomy surgery for retinopathy. Laser and/or vitreous surgery are best integrated as a component of comprehensive management (Figure 3) [23] Consultation — even in asymptomatic patients — with a collaborating cardiologist familiar with uremia in diabetic patients defines the timing of usually required heart evaluation. Coronary angiography (if indicated), will detect those for whom prophylactic coronary artery angioplasty or bypass surgery is likely to extend life. Similarly, the renal team should include a podiatrist who delivers regular surveillance of patients at risk of major lower extremity disease, thereby reducing the risk of amputations, a complication noted in about 20% who do not receive podiatric care. Autonomic neuropathy — expressed as gastropathy, cystopathy, and orthostatic hypotension — is a frequently overlooked, highly prevalent disorder impeding life quality in the diabetic with ESRD. Diabetic cystopathy, though common, is frequently unrecognized and confused with worsening diabetic nephropathy and is sometimes interpreted as allograft rejection in diabetic kidney transplant recipients (figure 4). In 22 diabetic patients who developed renal failure — 14 men and 8 women of mean age 38 years — an air cystogram detected cystopathy in 8 (36%) manifested as detrusor paralysis in 1 patient; severe malfunction in 5 patients (24%)); and mild impairment in 1 patient. Older male patients should be examined to exclude a prostatic component of obstruction. Encouragement to the patient adapting to a regimen of frequent voiding and self-application of manual external pressure above the pubiic symphysis (Crede Maneuver) plus administration of oral bethanechol usually permits resumption of spontaneous voiding. Finally, repeated self-catheterization of the bladder may be the only means to avoid an indwelling catheter when an atonic bladder is unresponsive to the above protocol.

Table 2. Diabetic complications which persist and/or progress during ESRD

1.	Retinopathy, glaucoma, cataracts.
2.	Coronary artery disease. Cardiomyopathy.
3.	Cerebrovascular disease.
4.	Peripheral vascular disease: limb amputation.
5.	Motor neuropathy. Sensory neuropathy.
6.	Autonomic dysfunction: diarrhea, dysfunction, hypotension.
7.	Myopathy.
8.	Depression.

Diabetic Nephropathy
Comprehensive Management

SPECIALIST	FREQUENCY
Cardiologist*	Annually to prn
Dentist*	Semiannually to prn
Endocrinologist	prn
Gastroenterologist	prn
Neurologist	prn
Nurse-Educator*	Monthly to prn
Nutritionist	prn
Ophthalmologist*	Semiannually or prn
Podiatrist*	Monthly

*essential

Figure 3.A large team is required to manage the myriad complications experienced by the typical diabetic ESRD patient.

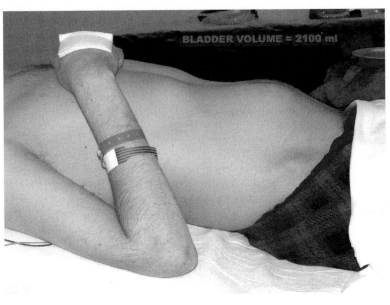

Courtesy of Dr Amy L Meguira, MD

Figure 4. Undiagnosed diabetic cystopathy may be confused for renal allograft rejection when unexplained azotemia is noted in a long-term diabetic patient. In the illustrated patient, 2,100 ml of urine was removed by a bladder catheter from a noncontracting bladder

731

Gastroparesis afflicts one-quarter to one-half of azotemic diabetic persons when initially evaluated for renal disease [24]. Other expressions of autonomic neuropathy — obstipation and explosive nighttime diarrhea — often coexists with gastroparesis [25]. Obstipation responds to daily doses of cascara, while diarrhea is treated with psyllium seed dietary supplements one to three times daily plus loperamide [26] in repetitive 2 mg. doses until symptoms abate or a total dose of 18 mg daily.

Cardiovascular Disease

Heart disease, the leading cause of death among patients with diabetes mellitus, is often advanced at the time of a candidate's initial consideration for transplantation and can certainly progress during the years a patient awaits organ availability on the cadaver waiting list. Khauli et. al. identified 38% of diabetic ESRD patients with coronary artery disease, in 1986, an era of far more conservative referral and exclusions of obese and/or aged transplant candidates than the current approach [27]. Failure to recognize critical heart disease may lead to loss of the allograft and the patient's demise. Presence of minimal pump dysfunction or angiographically demonstrable coronary artery lesions that are either asymptomatic or responsive to drugs, need not preclude transplantation so long as expectations are realistic and management fastidious. In fact, successful engraftment of a renal transplant may induce overall improvement in the diabetic recipient's cardiac function. Indeed, Abbott et. al. reported a lower risk of hospitalization for congestive heart failure after transplantation when compared to patients with ESRD due to diabetes on the renal transplant waiting list [28].

Determination of the specific individual's overall level of cardiac risk in advance of transplantation, a surgical procedure that may be associated with hemodynamic instability, hemorrhage, prolonged anesthesia, reoperation to address technical complications, hypertension and infection, is crucial as the patient and transplant team assess whether or not an organ transplant is a reasonable option. Should severe coronary artery disease be discovered, revascularization of the myocardium by coronary artery bypass or angioplasty becomes an absolute requirement in preparation for transplantation [29]. Khauli et. al. first reported the use of coronary angiography for detecting the presence and severity of coronary artery disease and left ventricular dysfunction in 48 diabetic patients scheduled for a kidney transplant. The benefit of pre-transplant myocardial revascularization was inferred from the uniform successful outcome in 23 diabetic patients, none of whom died. The remarkably good two-year patient and graft survival for living donor and cadaver donor recipients given "standard" immunosuppression with azathioprine and prednisone was 81% and 68%, and 61% and 32%, respectively.

We concur with Philipson et. al. who studied 60 diabetic patients being considered for a kidney transplant and advised that "patients with diabetes and end-stage renal disease who are at highest risk for cardiovascular events can be identified, and these patients probably should not undergo renal transplantation [30]." The basis for this position was an analysis of treatment outcome in which only seven patients had a negative thallium stress test, four of whom received a kidney transplant, without subsequent "cardiovascular events'. By contrast, of 53 diabetic patients with either a positive or non-diagnostic stress thallium tests, cardiac catheterization was employed to identify 26 patients with mild or no coronary disease or left ventricular dysfunction; 16 patients in this group received kidney transplants without cardiovascular incident. In a subset of ten patients with moderate heart disease, of whom 8 received renal transplants, two died of heart disease, while of thirteen patients with severe coronary artery disease or left ventricular malfunction, eight died before receiving a transplant, three from cardiovascular disease.

SELECTING UREMIA THERAPY (figure 5)

Depending on age, severity of co-morbid disorders, available local resources, and patient preference, the uremic diabetic patient may be managed according to different protocols. Diabetic ESRD patients select the no further treatment option, equivalent to passive suicide, more frequently than do nondiabetic patients [31]. Such a decision is understandable for blind, hemiparetic, bed-restricted limb amputees for whom life quality has been reduced to what is interpreted as unsatisfactory. On the other hand, attention to the total patient may restore a high quality of life that was unforeseen at the time of ESRD evaluation [32].

Unfortunately, in both Europe and the US, so called "preterminal care in diabetic patients with ESRD" is deficient in amount and quality [33] with inadequate attention to control of hypertension, hyperlipidemia or ophthalmologic intervention [34]. For the large majority — over 80% of diabetic persons who develop ESRD in the US — maintenance hemodialysis is the only renal replacement regimen that will be employed (figure 6).

Approximately 12% of diabetic persons with ESRD will be treated by peritoneal dialysis while the remaining 8% will receive a kidney transplant. To perform maintenance hemodialysis requires establishment of a vascular access to the circulation. Creation of what has become the *standard access* — an internal arteriovenous fistula in the wrist — is often more difficult in a diabetic than in a nondiabetic person because of advanced systemic atherosclerosis. For many diabetic patients with peripheral vascular calcification and/or atherosclerosis, creation of an access for hemodialysis necessitates resort to synthetic (PTFE) prosthetic vascular grafts.

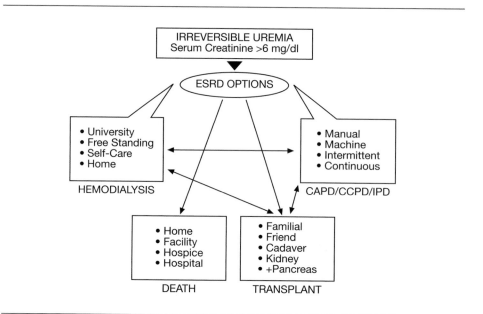

Figure 5. Selecting from a broad array of treatment options for the diabetic ESRD patient demands full presentation of what might be done including exploration of all available donor sources (intra and extrafamilial).

The typical hemodialysis regimen requires three weekly treatments lasting 4 to 5 hours each, during which extracorporeal blood flow must be maintained at 300 to 500 ml/min. Motivated patients trained to perform self-hemodialysis at home gain the longest survival and best rehabilitation afforded by any dialytic therapy for diabetic ESRD. When given hemodialysis at a facility, however, diabetic patients fare less well, receiving significantly less dialysis than nondiabetic patients due, in part, to hypotension and reduced access blood flow [35]. Maintenance hemodialysis does not restore vigor to diabetic patients as documented by Lowder et al., in 1986, who reported that of 232 diabetics on maintenance hemodialysis, only seven were employed, while 64.9 per cent were unable to conduct routine daily activities without assistance [36]. Approximately 50% of diabetic patients begun on maintenance hemodialysis die within two years of their first dialysis.

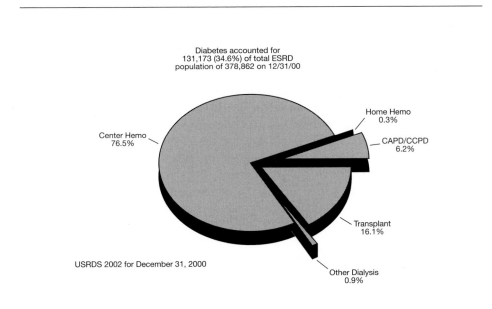

Diabetes accounted for
131,173 (34.6%) of total ESRD
population of 378,862 on 12/31/00

Home Hemo
0.3%

Center Hemo
76.5%

CAPD/CCPD
6.2%

Transplant
16.1%

USRDS 2002 for December 31, 2000

Other Dialysis
0.9%

Figure 6.Hemodialysis is the most widely applied ESRD therapy in diabetes. The option most likely to result in full rehabilitation, kidney transplantation, is utilized in fewer than 1 in 6 diabetic ESRD patients.

PERITONEAL DIALYSIS

In the US, peritoneal dialysis sustains the life of about 12% of diabetic ESRD patients. Continuous ambulatory peritoneal dialysis (CAPD) holds the advantages of freedom from a machine, performance at home, rapid training, minimal cardiovascular stress and avoidance of heparin [37]. To permit CAPD, an intraperitoneal catheter is implanted one or more days before CAPD is begun. Typically, CAPD requires exchange of 2 to 3 liters of sterile dialysate, containing insulin, antibiotics, and other drugs, 3 to 5 times daily. Mechanical cycling of dialysate, termed continuous cyclic peritoneal dialysis (CCPD) can be performed during sleep.

CAPD and CCPD pose the constant risk of peritonitis as well as a gradual decrease in peritoneal surface area. Some clinicians characterize CAPD as "a first choice treatment" for diabetic ESRD patients [38]. A less enthusiastic judgment of the worth of CAPD in diabetic patients was made by Rubin et al. in a largely black diabetic population treated with CAPD in Jackson, Mississippi [39]. Only 34% of patients remained on CAPD after two years, and at three years, only 18% continued on CAPD. According to the USRDS, survival of diabetic ESRD patients treated by CAPD is significantly less than on hemodialysis. A decision to select CAPD, therefore, must be individual-specific after weighing its benefits including freedom from a machine and electrical outlets, and ease of travel against the disadvantages of unremitting attention to fluid exchange, constant risk of peritonitis, and disappearing exchange surface. As concluded in a Lancet editorial: "Until the frequency of peritonitis is greatly reduced, most patients can expect to spend only a few years on CAPD before requiring a different form of treatment, usually haemodialysis [40]."

Evaluation of Transplant Candidacy
Armed with the knowledge that transplantation of a kidney and, perhaps, a pancreas, is the sole renal replacement therapy offering the uremic diabetic substantial likelihood of prolonged survival, the transplant team bears the onus of excluding only those candidates for whom the moderate technical demands of the transplant operation are anticipated to be excessively risky, or those individuals with comorbidities that are anticipated to be worsened substantially by the requisite use of pharmacologic immunosuppression. The consensus that offering access to the scarce pool of cadaveric organs to patients who are far older and sicker than the ideal, young candidates transplanted in earlier eras is now justifiable, has developed sequentially. With steadily improving outcomes, refinement of anti-rejection drug therapies, and the pioneering efforts of individual transplant groups who advocated on behalf of specific population segments (after the model of the Minnesota transplant team that first demonstrated that diabetes was not an insurmountable risk factor) [41], renal transplantation must now be weighed as an option in the management of every

Medicare covered ESRD patient. Accordingly, the transplant candidate is not approached with the expectation that indefinite longevity, full sight or independent ambulation must be anticipated in order to vindicate allocation of an organ to that individual. We continue to consider the presence of ongoing systemic infection that is likely to compromise short or immediate term survival of the patient or organ, the presence of malignancy that is likely to be progressive in the presence of immunosuppression, or the inability to comprehend or comply with the post-transplantation regimen of medication utilization or medical supervision needed to protect the engrafted organ or its host, as the principle contraindications to acceptance of a transplant candidate (Table 3).

Table 3. Evaluation of transplant candidacy for diabetic ESRD patients

Absolute Contraindications
Acute systemic infection (bacterial, fungal or viral)
Progressive malignancy
Likely survival < 2 years
Inability to comply with medications or medical advice
Inability to give informed consent

Relative Contraindications
Age > 70 years
Body Mass Index > 40
Unreconstructable Coronary Artery Disease
Incurable chronic infection (HIV, hepatitis C, hepatitis B)
Indolent malignancy (e.g., prostate cancer, multiple non-melanoma skin cancers)

Pancreas Transplantation

The largest data repository from which data regarding the outcome of pancreas transplantation may be gleaned is the International Pancreas Transplant Registry (IPTR), now reporting on >17,000 transplants of which 11,500 were performed in the U.S [42]. Solitary pancreas transplantation (PTA; pancreas transplant alone) represents only 5 % of reported cases with the lowest one year graft survival (78 %). Transplanting a cadaver donor pancreas in a recipient with a functioning renal allograft (PAK; pancreas after kidney) is the most popular strategy for candidates with a living kidney donor even though two separate operations are required and represented 13.2 % of cases. Superior pancreatic graft survival is reported for SPK (simultaneous cadaveric pancreas and kidney) over PAK recipients; 83 vs. 79 %, inter group differences such as 1) duration of pre-transplant maintenance dialysis 2) duration of state of immunosuppression prior to pancreas transplantation and 3) HLA identity or difference of renal and pancreatic donors probably contribute to this perhaps insignificant difference.

PANCREAS TRANSPLANT OPTIONS IN DIABETES: WHO?, WHEN?

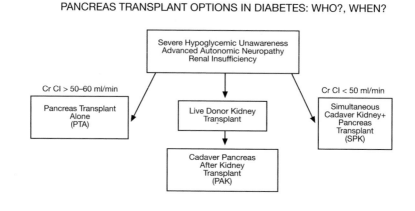

Figure 7.Assignment to a pancreas transplant alone is rarely indicated when the creatinine clearance is above 50 ml/min unless hypoglycemia is crippling. A combined pancreas and kidney transplant can permit full rehabilitation ("cure of diabetes") for a decade or longer.

Pancreatic duct management in the US is predominantly by enteric drainage (as opposed to bladder drainage) in SPK transplants (67 %) vs 51% for PAK and 42% for PTA, the type of duct drainage did not affect graft survival rates. Pancreatic allograft loss from rejection is declining in frequency, currently 4 %, 6 % and 8 % per year for SPK, PAK and PTA, respectively. Unfortunately, pancreas transplantation performed in patients with extensive extrarenal disease, has neither arrested nor reversed diabetic retinopathy, diabetic cardiomyopathy, or extensive peripheral vascular disease [43]. A comparison of survival of diabetic ESRD patients treated with a renal allograft or dialysis is given in figure 8.

Reports of beneficial effects on visual acuity and the need for additional posttransplant laser therapy are generated principally from patients with more mild disease [44]. The most remarkable result is that patient survival from all pancreas transplants in the US in the most recent era (1997 – 2001) is > 95% [41].

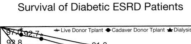

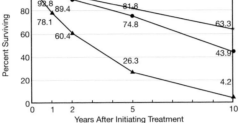

Figure 8. Extracted from the USRDS 2002 Annual Report[1], it is evident that diabetic ESRD patients given either a live donor or cadaver donor kidney transplant have much higher survival than those treated by dialysis (combined peritoneal and hemodialysis). Fewer than one in 10 diaabetic ESRD patients survive a decade.

Combined Pancreas Plus Kidney Transplantation

For many uremic individuals with type 1 diabetes, a combined kidney plus pancreas transplant has evolved as an important option because of its ability to offer superior glycemic control and improved quality of life. As both kidney graft survival and overall mortality are approximately equivalent following kidney alone versus dual organ transplantation alone at many centers, neither the survival of the patient nor the success of the kidney transplant need be jeopardized by the addition of a pancreas graft. Further on the positive side of the ledger, anecdotal reports indicate that recipients of combined pancreas and kidney transplants have greater stabilization of diabetic eye disease than do kidney recipients. On the other hand, a somber review of the surgical risk of 445 consecutive pancreas transplants from the pioneer University of Minnesota program noted that relaparotomy was required in 32% of recipients while perioperative mortality was 9% [45]. Based on a serious surgical complication rate of 35%, these workers advise that donors over 45 years old not be used while recipients over 45 years old be given a kidney graft alone.

It is true that recipients of combined pancreas plus kidney grafts experience greater morbidity, a reality that can be justified by the evidence that a pancreas graft will both prevent recurrent diabetic nephropathy, and may result in improvements in sensory/motor neuropathy. Newer immunosuppressive drug regimens are improving the outlook for pancreas transplantation. For example, matched-pair analysis of pancreas and kidney graft recipients immunosuppressed with tacrolimus plus prednisone had an 88% first year survival compared with 73% immunosuppressed with cyclosporine plus prednisone [46]. Switching from cyclosporine to tacrolimus with or without mycophenolate mofetil appeared to increase graft survival rates with a low rate of rejection episodes. Other reasonable strategies now include daclizumab induction combined with tacrolimus, mycophenolate mofetil and steroids [47], and thymoglobulin induction combined with tacrolimus and mycophenolate mofetil [48].

Following simultaneous pancreas kidney transplants, but not after a kidney transplant alone, hyperlipidemia reverts to normal, affording a hint of perhaps better cardiovascular outcomes as well. In those with normal or only mild renal disease, the decision to proffer an isolated pancreas transplant is more complex. Consistently, success rates for solitary pancreas transplants are lower than after combined simultaneous or dual sequential organ transplants. Suitable candidates for an isolated pancreas graft are those younger than 45 years suffering repeated bouts of disabling hypoglycemia or ketoacidosis unresponsive to other measures. More difficult to judge is whether or when individuals who have advancing diabetic complications with relatively intact renal function (creatinine clearance >60 mL/min) should be considered for an isolated pancreas transplant. An encouraging report from the Minnesota Transplant Team observed that a successful pancreas transplant after five or more years of euglycemia will reverse established pathologic changes of diabetic nephropathy including disappearance of nodular glomerular lesions [49]. At ten years, eight patients with type I diabetes and normal glycosylated hemoglobin values achieved with pancreas transplantation, progressive reduction in the median urinary albumin excretion rate, in the thickness of the glomerular and tubular basement membranes, and in the mesangial fractional volume – a remarkable accomplishment [50]. Pancreas transplantation is an important option in the treatment of type 1 diabetes so long as alternative strategies to provide equal glycemic control with less or no immunosuppression or less overall morbidity remain elusive.

Transplantation of Pancreatic Islets

The main attraction of pancreatic islet over whole organ pancreas transplantation as a diabetes cure is the potential technical simplicity and avoidance of the risks of a major surgical procedure by simple injection of a small volume suspension of islets. To date, however, clinical success, indicated not only by some signs of persistent islet function but by true insulin independence, has been achieved in only a small fraction of diabetic islet recipients. Nevertheless, enthusiasm for this attractive approach to ameliorating type 1 diabetes persists in many active investigators.

Pancreatic islets are durable. Insulin-producing islets can be isolated with a relatively simple and reproducible technique utilizing enzymatic digestion (trypsin) of the whole pancreas in rodent, canine and primate species. Human islets are also culled by mincing and enzyme digestion of normal pancreas glands obtained from cadaver donors [51], or resected for disease [52]. Freshly isolated islets can be safely transported across great distances meaning that the isolation laboratory need not be located at, or even in proximity, to the transplant center.

Heterotopic sites employed in rodent, dog and primate trials of islet implantation included: the peritoneum [53], thymus [54], testicle [55,56] spleen [57] kidney capsule [58], and liver [59] but only the last two are clinically practical; the liver is preferred. Underscoring the longevity of pancreatic islets is the use of intrahepatic autotransplanted islets from pancreas glands removed to treat chronic pancreatitis successfully preventing endocrine insufficiency [60]. Technically successful islet transplants may undergo progressive graft loss presumed associated with their ectopic location such as nutritional toxins, intestinal bacteria and endotoxins. Transplanted islets are also subject to recurrence of the same T-cell mediated autoimmune beta-cell destruction that originally caused the host's type 1 diabetes. Recipients of pancreatic segments from identical twins can experience rapidly recurrent diabetes without any evidence of rejection, strongly implicating such an autoimmune mechanism in the graft failure [61]. So called gentle immunosuppression may have protected one identical twin recipient of a simultaneous pancreas kidney graft from autoimmune mediated insulitis [62]. Exploratory attempts to use porcine islet xenotransplants provoked the worry that a porcine retrovirus may infect the human host resulting in an ongoing halt of further trials [63,64]. Analysis of the infectious risks to both individual patients and the whole human species is underway [65,66]. Strictly controlled, islet xenotransplantation may very well become a cost effective therapy for diabetes in the new millennium. Immunoisolation barriers and other imaginative approaches such as islet immunomodulation prior to transplantation through tissue culture, antibody application and even ultraviolet irradiation remain promising [67].

Most exciting has been the impressive recent experience with clinical human islet transplantation reported by the Edmonton, Alberta group [68]. Using a steroid immunosuppressive protocol including basliximab, sirolimus and tacrolimus, insulin independence beyond 1 year has been achieved with transplantation of a minimum of 9,000 islets/kg (this often requires sequential transplantation from islets procured from more than 1 pancreas) in 12 type 1 diabetics. This first clinical success has provoked renewed enthusiasm for an approach that is well tolerated and is distinctly less morbid than whole organ transplantation.

Pancreas Transplantation for Type 2 Diabetes
Until the past 7 to 8 years, pancreas transplantation in type 2 diabetic recipients was thought contraindicated because of their persistent secretion of insulin. The pathophysiologic problem in type 2 disease was attributed to insulin resistance rather than insulin lack. Furthermore, advanced age and obesity, usually present in type 2 diabetes, are associated with increased morbidity and mortality from all surgical procedures and specifically following pancreas transplantation [69]. Difficulty in obtaining adequate anatomic visualization, poor healing and peri-operative complications such as deep vein thrombosis raise the rate of technical complications in obese subjects. Exogenous obesity greater than 20% of normal weight, (a condition that includes most type 2 diabetic individuals) is reason to deny a pancreas transplant. Further apprehension over the wisdom of performing a pancreas transplant in type 2 recipients is the fear that exposure of donor beta cells to an environment of insulin resistance will promote their overstimulation and ultimate exhaustion meaning functional graft loss [70]. Thus, in view of the limited supply of suitable cadaver pancreas glands, limiting their grafting to type 1 diabetic recipients is understandable and consistent with the goal of maximizing duration of graft function.

At variance with the foregoing, after reviewing the outcome of inadvertent pancreas transplantation in type 2 diabetes, Sasaki et al report a fascinating experience with 13 intentional simultaneous pancreas-kidney transplants in recipients with elevated C-peptide levels establishing their diabetes as type 2

[70]. Graft survival in these type 2 diabetic recipients was an impressive 100 % with a mean follow-up of 46 months. Our experience with a single patient, also identified as having type 2 diabetes, following inadvertent pancreas transplantation has been similarly encouraging; the recipient lost a primary pancreas graft to venous thrombosis but is insulin independent 42 months after transplantation of a second pancreas. The IPTR experience reports 5% of pancreas transplants were performed for type 2 diabetes with graft survival rates equal to those in type 1 patients [71].

PATIENT SURVIVAL DURING TREATMENT OF ESRD

Prospective studies of renal transplantation compared with peritoneal or hemodialysis do not overcome limitations imposed by patient and physician refusal to permit random assignment to one treatment over another. As a generalization, younger patients with fewer complications are assigned to renal transplantation while residual older, sicker patients are treated by dialysis. Combined kidney/pancreas transplants are restricted (with rare exploratory exceptions) to those with type 1 diabetes who are younger than age 50. Reports from the European Dialysis and Transplant Association (EDTA) Registry, summarized by Brunner et al., demonstrate the singular and understandable effect of age on survival during treatment for ESRD "irrespective of treatment modality and of primary renal disease [72]." At 10 and 15 years after starting treatment, 58% and 52% respectively of patients who were 10 to 14 years old when begun on ESRD therapy were alive, compared to 28% and 16% who were alive at 10 and 15 years of those who were 45 to 54 years old when starting ESRD therapy. A similar effect of increasing age is noted in recipients of living related donor kidney transplants. In the early 1980s, kidney recipient survival was 92% at 5 years for patients younger than 15, 87% for the 15 to 44 year old cohort and 72% for those aged 45 or older.

Overall patient and graft survival following renal transplantation continue to slowly rise thanks to advances in overall medical care and, more specifically, to improved therapeutic windows associated with modern immunosuppressive agents such as sirolimus, mycophenolic acid and basiliximab. Graft survival for diabetic recipients of living donor kidneys is currently 95% and 89% at 1 and 3 years, versus 90% and 79% at 1 and 3 years after cadaver donor kidneys [73]. Early outcomes do not differ between diabetics and non-diabetics; collective graft survival rates of transplants performed between 1996 – 2001 in the U.S. are 90.2% for diabetics at 1 year, versus rates of 88.5 – 93.4% for patients with all other diagnoses. Long-term, however, diabetics have a lower survival rate, due principally to deaths from cardiovascular disease. Rajagopalan and colleagues observed equivalent graft survival between diabetics and non-diabetics ten years after kidney transplantation, though patient survival was 10% lower among diabetics [74]. Although the long-term prognosis is limited for diabetics, it is clear from groups like Hypolite et al. [75] reporting a decreased likelihood of hospitalization for acute coronary syndromes for diabetics after renal transplantation (0.79% per patient year) compared to those still on the waiting list (1.67% per patient year), that those diabetics who acquire kidney transplants have optimized their chances of survival.

Diabetes adds a severe restriction on life anticipation, imparting a threefold rise in risk of dying compared with either chronic glomerulonephritis or polycystic kidney disease. In England, diabetic and nondiabetic patients starting CAPD or hemodialysis in seven large renal units between 1983-1985 were monitored prospectively over four years. Of 610 new patients (median age 52 years, range 3-80 years) beginning CAPD and 329 patients (median age 48 years, range 5-77 years) starting hemodialysis, patient survival estimates at 4 years were 74% for hemodialysis and 62% for CAPD [76]. Survival on CAPD and maintenance hemodialysis is lower in the U.S. than in Europe. An explanation for diabetic dialysis patients' better survival in Europe is not evident, though the growing application of American practices of dialyzer reuse and shortened treatment hours have been incriminated as promoting fatal underdialysis [77].

The case for or against CAPD as a preferred therapy is still open. On the positive side, for example, is the report of Maiorca et al. who detailed an 8 year experience at a single center in Italy which offered "all treatments" for ESRD [78]. Survival at 5 years was equivalent for CAPD and hemodialysis patients but 98% of those started on hemodialysis continued hemodialysis while only 71% of CAPD treated patients remained on CAPD (p<0.01). Contending that survival on hemodialysis or CAPD is now equivalent, Burton and Walls determined life-expectancy using the Cox Proportional Hazards statistical methodology for unequal group analysis in 389 patients accepted for renal replacement therapy in Leicester between 1974 and 1985 [79]. There were no statistically significant differences between the relative risk of death for patients on CAPD (1.0), those on hemodialysis (1.30), and those who received a kidney transplant (1.09). CAPD, the authors concluded "is at least as effective as haemodialysis or transplantation in preserving life." For the present, substantiation of the superiority of one ESRD treatment over another is lacking whether for the total population of ESRD patients or for the subset with diabetic nephropathy (Table 3) [80].

CO-MORBIDITY INDEX FOR DIABETIC PATIENTS

To aid in grading the course of diabetic patients over the course of ESRD treatment we inventory the type and severity of common co-morbid problems. Numerical ranking of this inventory constitutes a co-morbid index (Table 4). As remarked above, comparison between treatments (hemodialysis versus CAPD [81] versus renal transplantation versus combined kidney and pancreas transplantation) demands that patient subsets be equivalent in severity of illness before application of the treatment modality under study.

Table 4. Morbidity in diabetic kidney transplant recipients

THE CO-MORBIDITY INDEX

1)	Persistent angina or myocardial infarction.
2)	Other cardiovascular problems, hypertension, congestive heart failure, cardiomyopathy.
3)	Respiratory disease.
4)	Autonomic neuropathy (gastroparesis, obstipation, diarrhea, cystopathy, orthostatic hypotension.
5)	Neurologic problems, cerebrovascular accident or stroke residual.
6)	Musculoskeletal disorders, including all varieties of renal bone disease.
7)	Infections including AIDS but excluding vascular access-site or peritonitis.
8)	Hepatitis, hepatic insufficiency, enzymatic pancreatic insufficiency.
9)	Hematologic problems other than anemia.
10)	Spinal abnormalities, lower back problems or arthritis.
11)	Vision impairment (minor to severe - decreased acuity to blindness) loss.
12)	Limb amputation (minor to severe - finger to lower extremity).

Mental or emotional illness (neurosis, depression, psychosis). To obtain a numerical Co-Morbidity Index for an individual patient, rate each variable from 0 to 3 (0 = absent, 1 = mild - of minor import to patient's life, 2 = moderate, 3 = severe). By proportional hazard analysis, relative significance of each variable isolated from the other 11.

Only limited data suggests an advantage other than well being for strict metabolic control once uremia has developed. On the other hand, it is reasonable to anticipate that all of the benefits to native kidneys of blood pressure and blood glucose control should be conferred on a renal transplant, retarding the recurrence of diabetic nephropathy in the kidney allograft. In a comparison of renal transplant biopsies taken 2.5 years post-transplant, 92% of recipients of a combined pancreas and renal transplant but only 35% of recipients with renal transplant alone had normal glomerular basement membrane thickness [82]. Glomerular mesangial volume expansion in the renal transplant, another early sign of recurrent diabetic nephropathy, is also retarded by the presence of a functioning pancreatic transplant. Anemia in azotemic diabetic patients adds to co-morbidity and is responsive to treatment with recombinant erythropoietin. Concern over a possible increase in severity of hypertension as red cell mass increases is based on an early finding that ambulatory maintenance hemodialysis patients evince such a change [83]. To expedite management of the myriad micro- and macrovascular complications that are manifested as azotemia increases, an orderly approach is advised. Subsequent selection of ESRD therapy for a diabetic individual whose kidneys are failing requires appreciation of the patient's family, social, and economic circumstances. Home hemodialysis, for example, is unworkable for a blind diabetic who lives alone. Deciding upon a kidney transplant requires knowledge of the patient's family structure, including its willingness to participate by donating a kidney. Without premeditation, the diabetic ESRD patient is subjected to repetitive, inconclusive studies instead of implementation of urgently required treatment (such as panretinal photocoagulation or arterial bypass surgery).

Autonomic Neuropathy
Throughout transplant surgery, and the day or two before oral feeding is resumed, metabolic control of plasma glucose concentration is best effected by frequent hourly (when needed) measurements of glucose and an intravenous infusion of 1-4 units per hour of regular insulin. Bethanechol, which may be given in combination with metoclopramide also improves gastric motility. Constipation, sometimes evolving into obstipation, is a frequent problem following transplantation. Effective stimulants to resume spontaneous defecation are early ambulation, stool softening agents, and suspension of cascara. Autonomic neuropathy may, at the other extreme, induce explosive and continuous liquid diarrhea enervating and dehydrating the post-operative diabetic patient. With the high incidence of clostridium difficile infection among hospitalized patients often exacerbating symptoms we find that loperamide given hourly in doses as high as 4 mg/hr almost always halts diarrhea.

A Life Plan [84] may elect "no treatment" when life extension is unacceptable. Illustrating this point, a blind, hemiparetic diabetic patient experiencing daily angina and nocturnal diarrhea, who is scheduled for bilateral lower limb amputation may chose death despite his family's plea that he start maintenance dialysis. Because azotemic diabetic patients typically are depressed, however, a rational decision to die must be distinguished from temporary despair over a current setback. Despondent diabetics, on occasion, respond to visits by rehabilitated dialysis patients or transplant recipients by reversing their decision to die. It is unwise to coerce acceptance of dialysis or a kidney transplant, when life has minimal (or even negative) value. Diabetic patients forced into uremia therapy by family or the health care team are often noncompliant to dietary and drug regimens, thereby expressing behavior culminating in passive suicide.

Pregnancy

Pregnancy, rare among ESRD patients on dialysis, make occur following successful transplantion. The National Transplantation Pregnancy Registry (NPTR) includes 31 female pancreas-kidney recipients who bore 45 pregnancies with an 80 % rate of live births; 53% of births occurred with Cesarean sections. While 75% of births were premature (less than 37 weeks of gestation), 57% of babies had low birth weight (< 2500 grams), and 53% of newborns had complications only 1/36 died. There is a substantial (8%) risk of a rejection episode during the pregnancy, and a 16% rate of graft loss within 2 years of delivery. Remarkably, all pancreatic allografts supported pregnancies without the development of hyperglycemia. Data for pregnancies among female kidney recipients are similar although specific outcomes for diabetic recipients are not available [85].

REHABILITATION (figure 9)

Inferences extracted from the study of rehabilitation in the diabetic ESRD patient are that: 1) Patients fare best when participating in their treatment regimen. 2) A functioning renal transplant permits markedly superior rehabilitation than that attained by either peritoneal dialysis or hemodialysis. Unfortunately, bias in assignment to a specific treatment may have prejudiced the favorable view of kidney transplants to the extent that statistical corrections (Cox Proportional Hazards technique) cannot compensate for group differences. Studies in which the mean age of transplant patients is a decade younger than the CAPD or hemodialysis groups are likely to discern better functional status in the younger group. Another variable affecting the magnitude of rehabilitation attained in diabetic and nondiabetic ESRD patients is the progressive increase in age of newly treated patients. In the US, for example, patients over the age of 69 years who comprised 27% of all dialysis patients in

1979, increased by 450% between 1974 and 1981, and will make up 60% of all dialysis patients by the year 2010. An ageing ESRD population has a declining rate of employment and increasingly prevalent comorbid complications. An extremely optimistic picture of rehabilitation during maintenance hemodialysis was projected by a state-wide longitudinal prospective study of 979 ESRD patients in Minnesota in which the Karnofsky scoring system [86] was employed to assess patient well being [87]. Initial Karnofsky scores showed that 50% of all patients were able to care for themselves when starting treatment. After two years of maintenance hemodialysis, a remarkable 78% of patients maintained or improved their functional status. Kidney transplant recipients, however, had higher initial Karnofsky scores than did those relegated to long-term dialysis. Selection for a kidney transplant gleaned the most functional patients leaving a residual population of less functional patients. Thereafter, comparisons of relative rehabilitation in transplant and dialysis groups are flawed by selection bias favoring kidney transplant recipients.

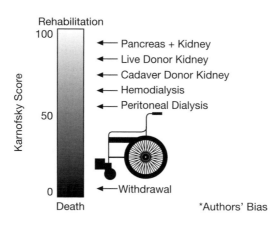

Figure 9. Relative rehabilitation is depicted as a Karnofsky Score. Clearly solid organ transplants (kidney and pancreas) permit the best recovery. How much of the superiority of transplantation is attributable to biased patient selection ("cherry picking") is undetermined.

The Minnesota description of well being on maintenance hemodialysis is highly atypical. Sustaining this point, for example, is the nationwide survey of maintenance hemodialysis patients, in which Gutman, Stead and Robinson measured functional assessment in 2,481 dialysis patients irrespective of location or type of dialysis [88]. Diabetic patients achieved very poor rehabilitation; only 23% of diabetic patients (versus 60% of nondiabetic patients) were capable of physical activity beyond caring for themselves. Lowder et al discerned the same very low level of rehabilitation [23]. More recent confirmation of this point was afforded by Ifudu et al. who documented pervasive failed rehabilitation in a multicenter studies of diabetic and non-diabetic [89], and elderly inner-city [90] hemodialysis patients. The inescapable conclusion of studies to date is that maintenance hemodialysis, in most instances, does not permit return to life's responsibilities for diabetic individuals.

Impotence

Whether caused by arterial insufficiency, mechanical disruption of the pelvic nerves during transplantation, the use of exacerbating antihypertensive medications and diabetic neuropathy, erectile dysfunction is common in diabetic ESRD patients and, in a minority of patients, may improve after a successful kidney transplant. Unless due to psychiatric cause, impotence in diabetes has a poor prognosis. Resort to a penile prosthesis, pre-coital intrapenile injections, intraurethral instillation of prostaglandins and, more recently, the use of Sildenafil, may be appropriate for rehabilitation when impotence persists.

Advanced glycosylated endproducts

In health, protein alteration resulting from a nonenzymatic reaction between ambient glucose and primary amino groups on proteins to form glycated residues called Amadori products is termed the Maillard reaction. After a series of dehydration and fragmentation reactions, Amadori products are transformed to stable covalent adducts called advanced glycosylation endproducts (AGEs). In diabetes, accelerated synthesis and tissue deposition of AGEs is proposed as a contributing mechanism in the pathogenesis of clinical complications [91]. Accumulation of AGEs in the human body is implicated in aging and in complications of renal failure [92] and diabetes [93]. AGEs are bound to a cell surface receptor (RAGE) inducing expression of vascular cell adhesion molecule-1 (VCAM-1), an endothelial cell surface cell-cell recognition protein that can prime diabetic vasculature for enhanced interaction with circulating monocytes thereby initiating vascular injury [94].

Glomerular hyperfiltration, characteristic of the clinically silent early phase of diabetic nephropathy may be induced by Amadori protein products — in rats, infusion of glycated serum proteins induces glomerular hyperfiltration [95]. Nitric oxide, produced by endothelial cells, the most powerful vasodilator influencing glomerular hemodynamics [96], has enhanced activity in early experimental diabetes [97]. Subsequently, AGEs, by quenching nitric oxide synthase activity, limit vasodilation and reduce glomerular filtration rate [98]. Clarification of the interaction of AGEs with nitric oxide may unravel the mystery of the biphasic course of diabetic glomerulopathy — sequential hyperfiltration followed by diminished glomerular filtration.

Pharmacologic prevention of AGE formation is an attractive means of preempting diabetic microvascular complications because it bypasses the necessity of having to attain euglycemia, an often unattainable goal. Pimagidine (aminoguanidine), interferes with non-enzymatic glycosylation [99] and reduces measured AGE levels leading to its investigation as a potential treatment. Pimagidine was selected because its structure is similar to "-hydrazinohistidine, a compound known to reduce diabetes-induced vascular leakage, while having opposite effects on histamine levels [100].

Pimagidine treatment in rats made diabetic with streptozotocin preempts complications viewed as surrogates for human diabetic complications. Representative examples from a large literature include: 1) Preventing development of cataracts in rats 90 days after being made "moderately diabetic" (<350 mg/dl plasma glucose); lens soluble and insoluble AGE fractions were inhibited by 56% and 75% by treatment with aminoguanidine 25 mg/kg body weight starting from the day of streptozotocin injection [101]. 2) Blocking AGE accumulation (measured by tissue fluorescence) in glomeruli and renal tubules in rats 32 weeks after induction of diabetes 32 weeks earlier; ponalrestat, an aldose reductase inhibitor, did not block AGE accumulation [102]. Treatment of streptozotocin-induced diabetic rats with pimagidine prevents glomerular basement membrane thickening typical of renal morphologic changes noted in this model of diabetic nephropathy [103]. 3) Reducing severity of experimental diabetic retinopathy as judged by a decrease in the number of acellular capillaries by 50% and complete prevention of arteriolar deposition of PAS-positive material and microthrombus formation after 26 weeks of induced diabetes in spontaneous hypertensive rats [104]. 4)

Ameliorating slowing of sciatic nerve conduction velocity dose dependently after treatment at three doses of 10, 25, and 50 mg/kg for 16 weeks [105]. Autonomic neuropathy (neuroaxonal dystrophy), however, was not prevented by treatment with pimagidine [106]. 5) Preventing development of the "stiff myocardium" that is a main component of diabetic cardiomyopathy [107]. 6) Preventing the diabetes-induced 24% impairment in maximal endothelium-dependent relaxation to acetylcholine for phenylephrine precontracted aortas by treatment for 2 months in a dose of 1 g/kg/day [108]. Blocking AGE formation to impede development of diabetic complications [109,110]. is an attractive strategy because of elimination of the necessity for euglycemia [111].

Pimagidine treatment significantly prevents NO activation and limits tissue accumulation of AGEs. Corbett et al. speculate that pimagidine inhibits interleukin-1 beta-induced nitrite formation (an oxidation product of NO) [112]. Uremia in diabetes is associated with both a high serum level of AGEs and accelerated macro and microvasculopathy. The renal clearance of AGE-peptides is 0.72 " 0.23 ml/min for normal subjects and 0.61 " 0.2 ml for diabetics with normal glomerular filtration (p value NS) [113]. Diabetic uremic patients accumulate advanced glycosylated end-products in "toxic" amounts that are not decreased to normal by hemodialysis or peritoneal dialysis [114] but fall sharply, to within the normal range, within 8 hours of restoration of half-normal glomerular filtration by renal transplantation [115]. It follows that the higher mortality of hemodialysis treated diabetic patients compared with those given a renal transplant may relate — in part — to persistent AGE toxicity.

Separate multicenter trials of aminoguanidine (Pimagidine) were conducted in adults with type I and type II diabetes and documented, fixed proteinuria of at least 500 mg/day, and a plasma creatinine concentration of <1.0 mg/dL (88 ?mol/L) in women or <1.3 mg/dL (115 ?mol/L) randomly assigned to treatment with aminoguanidine or placebo for four years. In the type 1 trial, reported in abstract, 56 sites enrolled 69 subjects randomized to receive 150 or 300 mg of aminoguanidine orally b.i.d. versus placebo with a mean treatment exposure of 2.5 years. Throughout the study, more than 90% of subjects in both treatment and placebo groups were concurrently treated with either an angiotensin converting enzyme inhibitor or receptor blocker. Compared with the placebo group, the aminoguanidine group evinced a significant (<0.05) reduction in doubling of serum creatinine concentration in those who had proteinuria >2g/24h. There was a nonsignificant "trend" toward slowing the creatinine rise in the entire group. Simultaneously, protection against diabetic retinopathy and a decrease in hyperlipidemia was noted in the treated group. Side effects in the aminoguanidine group included a transient flu-like syndrome, worsening anemia, and development of antinuclear autoantibodies (ANA) [116]. A similar study in 599 subjects with type 2 diabetes enrolled in 84 centers in Canada and the US was interrupted because of liver function abnormalities in the aminoguanidine treated group. Other adverse effects of aminoguanidine treatment included myocardial infarction, congestive heart failure, atrial fibrillation, anemia, ANA titre conversion, and upper GI symptoms [117,118].

Other agents
Although aminoguanidine inhibits initial stages of glycation in a hyperglycemic millieux, it only minimally blocks post-Amadori AGE formation. Other drugs, with promising activity against post-Amadori stages and/or effective breaking of crosslinks are underevaluation including desferrioxamine, D-penicillamine, pentoxifylline, pioglitazone, and metformin [119]. ALT-946, another thiazolidine derivative AGE inhibitor, is more potent than aminoguanidine in inhibiting AGE-protein cross-linking (both in vitro and in vivo) [120]. Compared with ALT-946 treated rats, albuminuria and AGE staining was twice as high in untreated diabetic rats, thereby providing a rationale for clinical trials in diabetic nephropathy [121].

At present, potential application of aminoguanidine (1827 Library of Medicine citations as of April 2003), related molecules, or AGE breakers remains a promise unfulfilled. Lessons learned from broad investigative experience with aminoguanidine center about the species differences between induced-diabetes in the rat, diabetes in the dog, and the human disease. While no further human trials of aminoguanidine have reached even the Phase 1 Trial stage, it is likely that AGEs will persist as a target for both prevention and amelioration of diabetic micro and macrovascular complications.

POST-TRANSPLANT DIABETES MELLITUS (PTDM)

Post-transplant diabetes mellitus (PTDM), a well-documented complication of tissue and organ transplantation was initially recognized in the steroid-azothioprine era with an incidence of 7-15% of patients [122,123]. More potent immunosuppressive drugs, especially the calcineurin inhibitors cyclosporine and tacrolimus, increased allograft survival and decreased the dose of corticosteroid drugs but were associated with a higher incidence of PTDM (cyclosporine 3-6% [124-127], tacrolimus 15-32% [128]). Maes et al. hypothesized that the calceneurin inhibitors are diabetogenic [129]. Data extracted from the USRDS show a cumulative incidence of PTDM at 3, 12 and 36 months of 9.1, 16 and 24% [130].

No clear understanding of the pathogenesis of PTDM is in hand. While steroid administration is linked to insulin resistance [131], both cyclosporine and tacrolimis may perturb carbohydrate metabolism by direct injury to pancreatic beta cell function resulting in diminished insulin synthesis or release [132-34], and decreased peripheral insulin sensitivity. Other, established risk factors for PTDM that may be additive to immunosuppressive drugs include race, older age, obesity, family history of diabetes, and certain HLA subtypes [135].

In the general population, both type 1 and type 2 diabetes are associated with extrarenal comorbid complications that shorten life. It has been suggested that PTDM is as prone to comorbid complications as non-transplant diabetes. In one study, renal allograft survival was significantly lower in PTDM patients at 12 years (48%) as compared with 70% in control patients, with no difference in patient survival [136]. By contrast, the larger USRDS study (vide supra), including over 11,000 patients who received a first kidney transplant between 1996-2000, PTDM was associated with increased graft failure (RR 1.63, 1.46-1.84, $p < 0.0001$), death-censored graft failure (RR 1.46, 1.25-1.70, p< 0.0001), and mortality (RR 1.87, 1.60-2.18, $p < 0.0001$). Friedman et al.'s pre-cyclosporine era study (vide supra) found a 67% 2-year patient survival in transplant recipients with PTDM, compared with 83% survival in control patients. The USRDS analysis of 7092 nondiabetic recipients of first-kidney transplants between 1996 and 1998 who were followed for 3 years demonstrated a heightened risk of death (risk ratio 1.87) in those with PTDM. Cardiovascular disease, primarily acute myocardial infarction, is also the leading cause of death in renal transplant recipients with intact graft function [137], and PTDM probably contributes to this through the known atherosclerosis-promoting actions of hyperglycemia and hyperinsulinemia [138]. In a 5-year follow-up study of 1347 renal transplant recipients with or without a functioning allograft, risk of death from ischemic heart disease was 20.8 times higher in transplanted diabetic patients, compared with a 6.4-fold higher risk in transplanted non-diabetic patients [139].

The UK Prospective Diabetes Study (UKPDS) demonstrated that macrovascular complications are strongly correlated with duration of diabetes and degree of hyperglycemia. A 1% decrease in glycosylated hemoglobin in the UKPDS significantly reduced the risk of myocardial infarction or death [140]. Whether the same benefit of intensified glucose regulation will accrue in PTDM has not been demonstrated. Awaiting definitive clinical trials, it seems prudent to emphasize careful blood glucose regulation in all diabetic renal transplant recipients. including those with PTDM, to forestall diabetic complications and death.

Post-Transplant Long-Term Management

Diabetic recipients of renal transplants spend more days during more frequent hospitalizations than do non-diabetic patients [141] for management of allograft failure, infections, peripheral vascular insufficiency or cardiac disease. Perturbations in plasma glucose levels due to changing doses of corticosteroids can usually be managed at home. Hospital admission is necessitated when extreme hypo or hyperglycemia becomes life threatening.

A comparison of present ESRD therapies for diabetes is given in table 5. Isolated restoration of normal renal function in a diabetic with ESRD does not reverse concomitant advanced extrarenal micro- and macrovasculopathy. Starting with the immediate post-transplant period, management of the diabetic renal transplant recipient is often complex demanding attention from diverse subspecialists. In many instances, determining a single pathogenetic mechanism after interpretation of renal scans, sonograms, biopsies, and tests of glomerular and tubular function is still largely an art based on experience. The complex clinical judgements often required to restore euglycemia, baseline renal graft function and to treat infection in the setting of profound immunosuppression are best accomplished under the direction of transplant professionals, whether surgeons or nephrologists, with collaborating consultants involved as needed. Overall, survival of diabetic patients with ESRD has been improving annually over the past decade whether treated by peritoneal dialysis, hemodialysis, or a kidney transplant (figure 10). Illustrating this point is the five year allograft function of 60.1% in diabetic cadaver kidney transplant recipients versus a five year allograft function of 60.3% of all recipients reported to the USRDS [1] This encouraging progress in therapy reflects multiple small advances in understanding of the pathogenesis of extrarenal micro- and macrovasculopathy in a previously inexorable disease, coupled with intensified regulation of hypertension and hyperglycemia. Identifying the perturbed biochemical reactions underlying the pathogenesis of diabetic vasculopathy C especially the adverse impact of accumulated advanced glycosylated end-products (AGEs) C raises the possibility of preempting end-organ damage without necessarily correcting hyperglycemia.

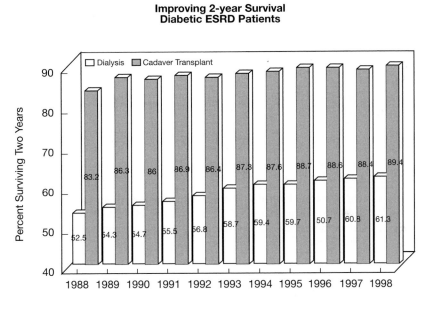

**Improving 2-year Survival
Diabetic ESRD Patients**

USRDS 2002

Figure 10. Two year survival of diabetic ESRD patients as reported in the USRDS Annual Data Report, 2002[1]. Reflecting incremental improvements in management, especially better attention to blood pressure regulation and metabolic control, survival of ESRD patients treated on hemodialysis or with a cadaver donor renal transplant have shown a progressive improvement in survival.

Table 5. Comparison of ESRD options for diabetic patients

FACTOR	PERITONEAL DIALYSIS	HEMODIALYSIS	KIDNEY TRANSPLANT
Extensive extrarenal disease	No limitation	No limitation except for hypotension	Excluded in substantive cardiovascular insufficiency
Geriatric patients	No limitation	No limitation	Arbitrary age exclusion as determined by program
Complete rehabilitation	Rare, if ever	Very few individuals	Common so long as graft functions
Death rate	Much higher than for nondiabetics	Much higher than for nondiabetics	About the same as nondiabetics
First year survival	About 75-80%	About 75-80%	>90%
Survival to second decade	Almost never	Fewer than 5%	About 1 in 5
Progression of complications	Usual and unremitting. Hyperglycemia and hyperlipidemia accentuated.	Usual and unremitting. May benefit from metabolic control.	Interdicted by functioning pancreas + kidney. Partially ameliorated by correction of azotemia.
Special advantage	Can be self-performed. Avoids swings in solute and intravascular volume level.	Can be self-performed. Efficient extraction of solute and water in hours.	Cures uremia. Freedom to travel. Neuropathy, retinopathy may improve
Disadvantage	Peritonitis. Hyperinsulenemia, hyperglycemia, hyperlipidemia. Long hours of treatment. More days hospitalized than either hemodialysis or transplant.	Blood access a hazard for clotting, hemorrhage and infection. Cyclical hypotension, weakness. Aluminum toxicity, amyloidosis.	Cosmetic disfigurement, hypertension, personal expense for cytotoxic drugs. Induced malignancy. HIV transmission.
Patient acceptance	Variable, usual compliance with passive tolerance for regimen.	Variable, often noncompliant with dietary, metabolic, or antihypertensive component of regimen.	Enthusiastic during periods of good renal allograft function. Exalted when pancreas proffers euglycemia.

Table 5. (cont.)

FACTOR	PERITONEAL DIALYSIS	HEMODIALYSIS	KIDNEY TRANSPLANT
Bias in comparison	Delivered as first choice by enthusiasts though emerging evidence indicates substantially higher mortality than for hemodialysis.	Treatment by default. Often complicated by inattention to progressive cardiac and peripheral vascular disease.	All kidney transplant programs preselect those patients with fewest complications. Exclusion of those older than 45 for pancreas + kidney simultaneous grafting obviously favorably predjudices outcome.
Relative cost	Most expensive over long run	Less expensive than kidney transplant in first year, subsequent years more expensive.	Pancreas + kidney engraftment most expensive uremia therapy for diabetic. After first year, kidney transplant — alone — lowest cost option.

REFERENCES

1. US. Renal Data System, USRDS 2002 Annual Data Report Atlas of End-Stage Disease in the United States, National Institutes of Health, National Institute of Diabetes and Digestive and Kidney Diseases. Bethesda, MD, 2002.
2. Mauer SM, Chavers BM. A comparison of kidney disease in type I and type II diabetes. Adv Exp Med Biol 1985; 189:299-303.
3. Centers for Disease Control and Prevention. Diabetes: Disabling, deadly, and on the rise 2002. National Diabetes Fact Sheet: National estimates and general information on diabetes in the United States. National Center for Chronic Disease Prevention and Health Promotion, Atlanta, GA, 2002.
4. National Center for Health Statistics. Health, United States, 1998. Hyattsville, Maryland: Public Health Service. 1999.
5. Blohme G, Nyström L, Arnqvist HG, et al. Male predominance of type 1 (insulin-dependent) diabetes in young adults: results from a 5-year prospective nationwide study of the 15-34 age group in Sweden. Diabetologia 1993; 35:56-62.
6. Polonsky KS. The ß-cell in diabetes: From molecular genetics to clinical research. Diabetes 1995;44:705-717.
7. Harris MI, Eastmen RC. Early detection of undiagnosed non-insulin-dependent diabetes mellitus. JAMA 1996;276:1261-1262.
8. Rossing P, Hougaard P, Parving HH. Risk Factors for Development of Incipient and Overt Diabetic Nephropathy in Type 1 Diabetic Patients: A 10-year prospective observational study. Diabetes Care 2002;25(5):859-64.

9. Wahren J, Johansson B-L, Wallberg-Henriksson H, Linde B, Fernqvist-Forbes E, Zierath JR. C-peptide revisited - new physiological effects and therapeutic implications. J Intern Med 1996;240:115-124.

10. Zimmet PZ. Kelly West Lecture 1991. Challenges in diabetes epidemiology — from West to the rest. Diabetes Care, 1992; 15:232-252.

11. Harris M, Hadden WC, Knowles WC, et al. Prevalence of diabetes and impaired glucose tolerance and plasma glucose levels in U.S. population aged 20-74 yr, Diabetes 1987; 36:523-534.

12. Stephens GW, Gillaspy JA, Clyne D, Mejia A, Pollak VE. Racial differences in the incidence of end-stage renal disease in Types I and II diabetes mellitus. Am J Kidney Dis 1990; 15:562-567.

13. Haffner SM, Hazuda HP, Stern MP, Patterson JK, Van-Heuven WA, Fong D. Effects of socioeconomic status on hyperglycemia and retinopathy levels in Mexican Americans with NIDDM. Diabetes Care (1989) 12:128-134.

14. National Diabetes Data Group. Diabetes in America. NIH Publication No. 85-1468, August 1985.

15. Council on Ethical and Judicial Affairs. Black-white disparities in health care. JAMA 1990; 163:2344-2346.

16. Melton L. J., Palumbo, P. J., and Chu, C.P. Incidence of diabetes mellitus by clinical type. Diabetes Care 1983; 6:75-86.

17. Ritz E, Stefanski A. Diabetic nephropathy in Type II diabetes. Am J Kidney Dis 1996;2:167-194.

18. Sheehy MJ. HLA and insulin-dependent diabetes. A protective perspective. Diabetes 1992; 41:123-129.

19. Biesenback G, Janko O, Zazgornik J. Similar rate of progression in the predialysis phase in type I and type II diabetes mellitus. Nephrol Dial Transplant 1994;9:1097-1102.

20. Wirta O, Pasternack A, Laippala P, Turjanmaa V. Glomerular filtration rate and kidney size after six years disease duration in non-insulin-dependent diabetic subjects. Clinical Nephrology 1996;45:10-17.

21. Abourizk NN, Dunn JC. Types of diabetes according to National Diabetes Data Group Classification. Limited applicability and need to revisit. Diabetes Care 1990 13:1120-1122.

22. Sims EAH, Calles-Escandon J. Classification of diabetes. A fresh look for the 1990s? Diabetes Care 1990 13:1123-1127

23. Berman DH, Friedman EA, Lundin AP. Aggressive ophthalmological management in diabetic ESRD: A study of 31 consecutively referred patients. Amer J Nephrol, 1992; 12:344-350.

24. Clark DW, Nowak TV. Diabetic gastroparesis. What to do when gastric emptying is delayed. Postgrad Med 1994; 95:195-198, 201-204.

25. Battle WM, Cohen JD, Snape WJ Jr. Disorders of colonic motility in patients with diabetes mellitus. Yale J Biol Med 1983;56:277-283.

26. Lux G. Disorders of gastrointestinal motility — diabetes mellitus. Leber Magen Darm 1989;19:84-93.

27. Khauli RB, Steinmuller DR, Novick AC, et al. 1986. A Critical Look at Survival of Diabetics with End-Stage Renal Disease: Transplantation Versus Dialysis Therapy. Transplantation 41:598-602.

28. Abbott KC, Hypolite IO, Hshieh P, et al. 2001. The impact of renal transplantation on the incidence of congestive heart failure in patients with end-stage renal disease due to diabetes. J Nephrol 2001; 14(5):369.

29. Braun WE, Phillips D, Vidt DG, et al. 1983. The Course of Coronary Artery Disease in Diabetics with and without Renal Allografts. Transplant Proc 15: 1114-1119.

30. Philipson JD, Carpenter BJ, Itzkoff J, Hakala TR, Rosenthal JT, Taylor RJ, Puschett JB. 1986. Evaluation of cardiovascular risk for renal transplantation in diabetic patients. Am J Med 81:630-634.

31. Meisel A. The Right to Die. New York: John Wiley and Sons; 1989; 122.

32. Kjellstrand CM. Practical aspects of stopping dialysis and cultural differences. in Ethical Problems in Dialysis and Transplantation. Eds Carl M. Kjellstrand and John B. Dossetor. Kluwer Academic Publishers, Dordrecht, 1992.

33. Pommer W, Bressel F, Chen F, Molzahn There is room for improvement of preterminal care in diabetic patients with end-stage renal failure — The epidemiological evidence in Germany. Nephrol Dial Transplant 1997;12:1318-1230.

34. Passa P Diabetic nephropathy in the NIDDM patient on the interface between diabetology and nephrology. What do we have to improve? Nephrol Dial Transplant 1997;12:1316-1317.

35. Cheigh J, Raghavan J, Sullivan J, Tapia L, Rubin A, Stenzel KH. Is insufficient dialysis a cause for high morbidity in diabetic patients? 1991; J Amer Soc Nephrol 317 (abstract).

36. Lowder, G. M., Perri, N. A., and Friedman, E. A. Demographics, diabetes type, and degree of rehabilitation in diabetic patients on maintenance hemodialysis in Brooklyn. J Diabetic Complications 1988; 2:218-226.

37. Lindblad, A. S., Nolph, K. D., Novak, J. W., and Friedman, E. A. A survey of the NIH CAPD Registry population with end-stage renal disease attributed to diabetic nephropathy. J Diabetic Complications 1988 2:227-232.

38. Legrain, M., Rottembourg, J., Bentchikou A. et al. Dialysis treatment of insulin dependent diabetic patients. Ten years experience. Clin Nephrol 1984;21:72-81.

39. Rubin J, Hsu H. Continuous ambulatory peritoneal dialysis: Ten years at one facility. Amer J Kidney Dis 1991;17:165-169.

40. Prevention of peritonitis in CAPD. Lancet 1991;337:22-23.

41. Sutherland DE. Gores PF. Farney AC. Wahoff DC. Matas AJ. Dunn DL. Gruessner RW. Najarian JS. 1993. Evolution of kidney, pancreas, and islet transplantation for patients with diabetes at the University of Minnesota. 40. an Journal of Surgery. 166(5):456-91.

42. Gruessner AC, Sutherland DE. 2001. Analysis of United States and non-US pancreas transplants reported to the United network for organ sharing (UNOS) and the international pancreas transplant registry (IPTR) as of October 2001. Clin Transplant:41-72, 2001.

43. Ramsay RC, Goetz FC, Sutherland DE, Mauer SM, Robison LL, Cantrill HL, Knobloch WH, Najarian JS. 1988. Progression of diabetic retinopathy after pancreas transplantation for insulin – dependent diabetes mellitus. N Engl J Med 318: 208-214.

44. Koznarova R, Saudek F, Sosna T, et al. 2000. Beneficial effect of pancreas and kidney transplantation on advanced diabetic retinopathy. Cell Transplant 9(6):903-8.

45. Gruessner RW, Sutherland DE, Troppmann C, Benedetti E, Hakim N, Dunn DL, Gruessner AC. 1997. The surgical risk of pancreas transplantation in the cyclosporine era: an overview. J Am Coll Surg 185: 128-144.

46. Gruessner RW. 1997. Tacrolimus in pancreas transplantation : a multicenter analysis. Tacrolimus Pancreas Transplant Study Group. Clin Transplant 11: 299-312.

47. Stratta RJ, Alloway RR, Hodge E, Lo A. 2002. A multicenter, open-label, comparative trial of two daclizumab dosing strategies vs. no antibody induction in combination with tacrolimus, mycophenolate mofetil, and steroids for the prevention of acute rejection in simultaneous kidney-pancreas transplant recipients: interim analysis. Clin Transplant 16(1):60-8.

48. Trofe J, Stratta RJ,, Egidi MF, et. Al. 2002. Thymoglobulin for induction or rejection therapy in pancreas allograft recipients: a single center experience. Clin Transplant 16 Supl 7:34-44.

49. Fioretto P, Steffes MW, Sutherland Der, Goetz FC, Mauer M. 1997. Successful pancreas transplantation alone reverses established lesions of diabetic nephropathy in man. J Am Soc Nephrol 8: 111A.

50. Fioretto P, Steffes MW, Sutherland DE, et al. 1998. Reversal of lesions of diabetic nephropathy after pancreas transplantation. N Engl J Med 339(2):115-7.

51. Marshak S, Leibowitz G, Bertuzzi F, Socci C, Kaiser N, Gross DJ, Cerasi E, Melloul D. 1999. Impaired beta-cell functions induced by chronic exposure of cultured human pancreatic islets to high glucose. Diabetes 48(6):1230-1236.

52. Rabkin JM, Leone JP, Sutherland DE, Ahman A, Reed M, Papalois BE, Wahoff DC. 1997. Transcontinental shipping of pancreatic islets for autotransplantation after total pancreatectomy. Pancreas 15(4):415-9.

53. Rabkin JM, Leone JP, Sutherland DE, Ahman A, Reed M, Papalois BE, Wahoff DC. 1997. Transcontinental shipping of pancreatic islets for autotransplantation after total pancreatectomy. Pancreas 15(4):415-9.

54. Sutherland DE. 1994. Intraperitoneal transplantation of microencapsulated canine islet allografts with short-term, low-dose cyclosporine for treatment of pancreatectomy – induced diabetes in doge. Transplantation Proceedings 26(2):804.

55. Tuch BE, Wright DC, Martin TE, Keogh GW, Deol HS, Simpson AM, Roach W, Pinto AN. 1999. Fetal pig endocrine cells develop when allografted into the thymus gland. Transplantation Proc 31(1-3):670-674.

56. Ar'Rajab A, Dawidson IJ, Harris RB, Sentementes JT. 1994. Immune privilege of the testis for islet xenotransplantation (rat to mouse). Transplant Proc 26(6):3446.

57. Gray DW. 1990. Islet isolation and transplantation techniques in the primate. Surgery, Gynecology and Obstetrics. 170(3):225-232.

58. Eow CK, Shimizu S, Gray DW, Morris PJ. 1994. Successful pancreatic islet autotransplantation to the renal subcapsule in the cynomolgus monkey. Transplantation 57(1):161-4.

59. Stevens RB, Lokeh A, Ansite JD< Field MJ, Gores PF, Sutherland De. 1994. Role of nitric oxide in the pathogenesis of early pancreatic islet dysfunction during rat and human intraportal islet transplantation. Transplantation proceedings 26(2):692.

60. Robertson GS, Dennison AR, Johnson PR et al. 1998. A review of pancreatic islet autotransplantation. Hepatogastroenterology 45: 226-235.

61. Sibley R, Sutherland Der, Goetz F, Michael AF. 1985. Recurrent diabetes mellitus in the pancreas iso- and allograft. A light and electron microscopic and immunohistochemical analysis of four cases. Lab Invest 53:132-144.

62. Benedetti E, Dunn T, Massad MG< Raofi V, Bartholomew A, Gruessner RW, Brecklin C. 1999. Successful living related simultaneous pancreas-kidney transplant between identical twins. Transplantation 67(6):915-8.

63. Butler D. 1999. FDA warns on primate xenotransplants. Nature 398:549.

64. Bach FH, Fineberg HV. 1998. Call for moratorium on xenotransplants Nature 391:326.

65. Weiss RA. 1999. Xenografts and retroviruses. Science 285:1221-1223.

66. Paradis K, Langford G, Long Z, Heneine W, Sandstrom P, Switzer WM, Chapman LE, Lockey C, Onions D, The XEN 111 Study Group and Otto E. 1999. Search for cross-species transmission of porcine endogenous retrovirus in patients treated with living pig tissue. Science 285:1236-1241.

67. Lau H, Reemstma K, Hardy MA. 1984, Prolongation of rat islet allograft survival by direct ultraviolet irradion of the graft. Science 223:607-609.

68. Ryan EA, Lakey JR, Paty BW, et al. 2002. Successful islet transplantation: continued insulin reserve provides long-term glycemic control. Diabetes 51(7):2148—57.

69. Odorico JS, Becker YT, Van der Werf W, Collins B, D'Alessandro AM, Knechtle SJ, Pirsch JD, Sollinger HW.   1997. Advances in pancreas transplantation: the University of Wisconsin experience. In Clinical Transplants 1997, Cecka and Terasaki, Eds. UCLA tissue typing laboratory, Los Angeles, California.

70. Sasaki TM, Gray RS, Ratner RE, Currier C, Aquino A, Barhyte DY, Light JA. 1998. Successful long-term kidney-pancreas transplants in diabetic patients with high C-peptide levels. Transplantation 65:1510-1512.

71. Gruessner AC, Sutherland DE. 2001. Analysis of United States and non-US pancreas transplants reported to the United network for organ sharing (UNOS) and the international pancreas transplant registry (IPTR) as of October 2001. Clin Transplant:41-72, 2001.

72. Brunner, F.P., Fassbinder, W., Broyer, M., Oules, R., Brynger, H., Rizzoni, G., Challah, S., Selwood, N. H., Dykes, S. R., and Wing, A.J.: Survival on renal replacement therapy: data from the EDTA Registry. Nephrol Dial Transplant 3:109-122, 1988.

73. Organ procurements and transplantation network kidney Kaplan-Meier graft survival rates for transplants performed: 1996-2001. based on OPTN data as of March 28, 2003. http://www.optn.org/latestData/rptStrat.asp.

74. Rajagopalan PR, Rogers J, Chavin C, et al. 2001. Cadaveric renal translantation in African-Americans in South Carolina. In Clinical Transplants 2001. Cecka and Terasaki, Eds. UCLA Immunogenetics Center, Los Angeles. Pp. 143-147.

75. Hypolite IO, Bucci J, Hshieh P, et. al. 2002. Acute coronary syndromes after renal transplantation in patients with end-stage renal disease resulting from diabetes. Amer J Transplant 2(3):274081.

76. Gokal, R., Jakubowski, C., King, J., Hunt, L., Bogle, S., Baillod, R., Marsh, F., Ogg, C., Oliver, D., Ward, M., et al.: Outcome in patients on continuous ambulatory peritoneal dialysis and haemodialysis: 4-year analysis of a prospective multicentre study. Lancet 2:1105-1109, 1988.

77. Friedman EA. <u>Death on Hemodialysis: Preventable or Inevitable?</u> 1994, Kluwer Academic Publishers, Dordrecht, The Netherlands.

78. Maiorca, R., Cancarini, G., Manili, L., Brunori, G., Camerini, C., Strada, A., and Feller, P.: CAPD is a first class treatment: results of an eight-year experience with a comparison of patient and method survival in CAPD and hemodialysis. Clin Nephrol 30 (Supp 1):S3-S7, 1988.

79. Burton, P. R., and Walls, J.: Selection-adjusted comparison of life-expectancy of patients on continuous ambulatory peritoneal dialysis, haemodialysis, and renal transplantation. Lancet 1:1115-1119, 1987.

80. Keshaviah P, Collins AJ, Ma JZ, Churchill DN, Thorpe KE. Survival comparison between hemodialysis and peritoneal dialysis based on matched doses of delivered therapy. J Am Soc Nephrol. 2002;13 Suppl 1:S48-52.

81. Miguel A, Garcia-Ramon R, Perez-Contreras J, Gomez-Roldan C, Alvarino J, Escobedo J, Garcia H, Lanuza M, Lopez-Menchero R, Olivares J, Tornero F, Albero D. Comorbidity and Mortality in Peritoneal Dialysis: A Comparative Study of Type 1 and 2 Diabetes versus Nondiabetic Patients. Nephron. 2002;90(3):290-6.

82. Wilczek HE, Jaremko G, Tyden G, Groth CG. Evolution of diabetic nephropathy in kidney grafts. Evidence that a simultaneously transplanted pancreas exerts a protective effect. Transplantation 1995;59:51-57.

83. Lebel M, Kingma I, Grose JH, Langlois S. Effect of recombinant human erythropoietin therapy on ambulatory blood pressure in normotensive and in untreated borderline hypertensive hemodialysis patients. Amer J Hypertension 1995;8:545-551.

84. White CA, Pilkey RM, Lam M, Holland DC. Pre-dialysis clinic attendance improves quality of life among hemodialysis patients. BMC Nephrol. 2002 5;3(1):3.

85. Armenti FT, Radomski JS, Moritz MJ, et al. 2001. Report from the National Transplantation Pregnancy Registry (NPTR): outcomes of pregnancy after transplantation. Clinical Transplants 2001, Cecka and Terasaki, eds. UCLA Immunogenetics Center, Los Angeles. Pp 97-105.

86. Karnofsky, D. A., and Burchenal, J. H.: The clinical evaluation of chemotherapeutic agents in cancer, in MacLeod CM (ed): Evaluation of Chemotherapeutic Agents. Columbia University Press, New York, 1949, pp 191-205.

87. Carlson, D. M., Johnson, W. J., and Kjellstrand, C. M.: Functional status of patients with end-stage renal disease. Mayo Clin Proc 62:338-344, 1987.

88. Gutman, R. A., Stead, W. W., and Robinson, R. R.: Physical activity and employment status of patients on maintenance dialysis. N Engl J Med 304:309-313, 1981.

89. Ifudu O, Paul H, Mayers JD, Cohen LS, Brezsynyak WF, Herman AI, Avram MM, Friedman EA. Pervasive failed rehabilitation in center-based maintenance hemodialysis patients. Am J Kidney Die 1994;23:394-400.

90. Ifudu O, Mayers J, Matthew J, Tan CC, Cambridge A, Friedman EA. Dismal rehabilitation in geriatric inner-city hemodialysis patients. JAMA 1994;271:29-33.

91. Brownlee M, Cerami A, Vlassara H. Advanced glycosylation end products in tissue and the biochemical basis of diabetic complications. N Engl J Med 1988;318:1315-1321.

92. Sell DR, Monnier VM. End stage renal disease and diabetes catalyze the formation of a pentose-derived crosslink from aging human collagen. J Clin Invest 1990;85:380-384.

93. Vlassara H, Bucala R, Striker L. Pathogenic effects of advanced glycosylation: biochemical, biological, and clinical implications for diabetes and aging. J Lab Invest 1994;70:138-151.

94. Schmidt AM, Hori O, Chen JX, Li JF, Crandall J, Zhang J, Cao R, Yan SD, Brett J, Stern D. Advanced glycation endproducts interacting with their endothelial receptor induce expression of vascular cell adhesion molecule-1 (VCAM-1) in cultured human endothelial cells and in mice. J Clin Invest 1995;96:1395-1403.

95. Sabbatini M. Sansone G, Uccello F, Giliberti A, Conte G, Andreucci VE. Early glycosylation products induce glomerular hyperfiltration in normal rats. Kidney Int 1992;42:875-881.

96. Moncado S, Palmer RMJ, Higgs EA. Nitric oxide: physiology, pathophysiology, and pharmacology. Pharmacological Reviews 1991;43:109-142.

97. Bank N, Aynedjian HS. Tole of EDRF (nitric oxide) in diabetic renal hyperfiltration. Kidney Int 1993;43:1306-1312.

98. Bucala R, Tracey KJ, Cerami A. Advanced glycosylation products quench nitric oxide and mediate defective endothelium-dependent vasodilation in experimental diabetes. J Clin Invest 1991;87:432-438.

99. Edelstein D, Brownlee M. Mechanistic studies of advanced glycosylation end product inhibition by aminoguanidine. Diabetes 1992;41:26-29.

100. Brownlee M, Vlassara H, Kooney T, Ulrich P, Cerami A. Aminoguanidine prevents diabetes-induced arterial wall protein cross-linking. Science 1986;232:1629-1632.

101. Swamy-Mruthinti S, Green K, Abraham EC: Inhibition of cataracts in moderately diabetic rats by aminoguanidine. Experimental Eye Research 62:505-510, 1996.

102. Soulis-Liparota T, Cooper ME, Dunlop M, Jerums G: The relative roles of advanced glycation, oxidation and aldose reductase inhibition in the development of experimental diabetic nephropathy in the Sprague-Dawley rat. Diabetologia 38:387-394, 1995.

103. Ellis EN, Good BH. Prevention of glomerular basement membrane thickening by aminoguanidine in experimental diabetes mellitus. Metabolism 1991;40:1016-1019.

104. Hammes HP, Brownlee M, Edelstein D, Saleck M, Martin S, Federlin K: Aminoguanidine inhibits the development of accelerated diabetic retinopathy in the spontaneous hypertensive rat. Diabetologia 37:32-35, 1994.

105. Miyauchi Y, Shikama H, Takasu T, Okamiya H, Umeda M, Hirasaki E, Ohhata I, Nakayama H, Hakagawa S: Slowing of peripheral motor nerve conduction was ameliorated by aminoguanidine in streptozotocin-induced diabetic rats. European J Endocrinology 134:467-473, 1996.

106. Schmidt RE, Dorsey DA, Beaudet LN, Reiser KM, Williamson JR, Tilton RG. Effect of aminoguanidine on the frequency of neuronal dystrophy in the superior mesenteric sympathetic autonomic ganglia of rats with streptozotocin-induced diabetes. Diabetes 1996;45:284-290.

107. Norton GR, Candy G, Woodiwiss AJ: Aminoguanidine prevents the decreased myocardial compliance produced by streptozotocin-induced diabetes mellitus in rats. Circulation 93:1905-1912, 1996.

108. Archibald V, Cotter MA, Keegan A, Cameron NE: Contraction and relaxation of aortas from diabetic rats: effects of chronic anti-oxidant and aminoguanidine treatments. Naunyn-Schmiedbergs Arch Pharm 353:584-591, 1996.

109. Brownlee M. 1989. Pharmacological modulation of the advanced glycosylation reaction. Prog Clin Biol Res, 304:235-248.11

110. Nicholls K, Mandel TE. 1989. Advanced glycosylation end-products in experimental murine diabetic nephropathy: effect of islet isografting and of aminoguanidine. Lab Invest, 60:486-491.

111. Lyons TJ, Dailie KE, Dyer DG, Dunn JA, Baynes JW. 1991. Decrease in skin collagen glycation with improved glycemic control in patients with insulin-dependent diabetes mellitus. J Clin Invest, 87:1910-1915.

112. Corbett JA, Tilton RG, Chang K, Hasan KS, Ido Y, Wang JL, Sweetland MA, Lancaster JR Jr., Williamson JR, McDaniel ML. Aminoguanidine, a novel inhibitor of nitric oxide formation, prevents diabetic vascular dysfunction. Diabetes 1992;4:552-556.

113. Vlassara H. Serum advanced glycosylation end products: a new class of uremic toxins? Blood Purif 1994;12:54-59.

114. Papanastasiou P, Grass L, Rodela H, Patrikarea A, Oreopoulos D, Diamandis EP. Immunological quantification of advanced glycosylation end-products in the serum of patients on hemodialysis or CAPD. Kidney Internat 1994;46:216-222.

115. Makita Z, Radoff S, Rayfield EJ, Yang Z, Skolnik E, Delaney V, Friedman EA, Cerami A, Vlassara H. 1991. Advanced glycosylation end products in patients with diabetic nephropathy. New Engl J Med 325:836-842.

116. Whittier F, Spinowitz B, Wuerth JP, Cartwright K. Pimagidine (PG) safety profile in patients with Type I diabetes mellitus (DM). H Am Soc Nephrol 1999;10:184A (abstract).

117. Freedman BI, Wuerth J-P, Cartwright K et al. Design and baseline characteristics for the aminoguanidine Clinicl Trial in Overt Type 2 Diabetic Nephropathy (ACTION II). Control Clin Trials 1999;20:453-410.

118. Alteon Inc. Pimagidine hydrochloride (aminoguanidine hydrochloride) Unpublished data.

119. Rahbar S, Natarajan R, Yerneji K, Scott S, Gonzales N, Nadler JL. Evidence that pioglitazone, metformin and pentoxifylline are inhibitors of glycation. Clin Chem Acta 2000;301:65-77.
120. Forbes, JM, Soulis, T, Thallas, V, et al. Renoprotective effects of a novel inhibitor of advanced glycation. Diabetologia 2001; 44:108.
121. Abdel-Rahman E, Bolton WK. Pimagedine: a novel therapy for diabetic nephropathy. Expert Opin Investig Drugs 2002;11(4):565-74.
122. Friedman EA, Shyh TP, Beyer MM, Manis T, Butt KM.New onset diabetes after transplantation in kidney transplant recipients. Am J Nephrol 1985;5(3):196-202.
123. Fryer JP, Granger DK, Leventhal JR, Gillingham K, Najarian JS, Matas AJ. Steroid related complications in the cyclosporine era. Clin Transplant 1994;8(3 Pt 1):224-229.
124. First MR, Gerber DA, Hariharan S, Kaufman DB, Shapiro R New onset diabetes after transplantation mellitus in kidney allograft recipients: incidence, risk factors, and management. Transplantation 2002 Feb 15;73(3):379-86.
125. Roth D, Milgrom M, Esquenazi V, Fuller L, Burke G, Miller J: Posttransplant hyperglycemia. Increased incidence in cyclosporine-treated renal allograft recipients. Transplantation 1989 Feb;47(2):278-81.
126. Cosio FG, Pesavento TE, Osei K, Henry ML, Ferguson RM: Post-transplant diabetes mellitus: increasing incidence in renal allograft recipients transplanted in recent years. Kidney Int 2001 Feb;59(2):732-7.
127. Sumrani NB, Delaney V, Ding ZK, Davis R, Daskalakis P, Friedman EA, Butt KM, Hong JH. Diabetes mellitus after renal transplantation in the cyclosporine era—an analysis of risk factors. Transplantation 1991 Feb;51(2):343-7.
128. Weir MR, Fink JC. Risk for new onset diabetes after transplantation mellitus with current immunosuppressive medications. Am J Kidney Dis 1999;34:1-13.
129. Maes BD, Kuypers D, Messiaen T, Evenepoel P, Mathieu C, Coosemans W, Pirenne J, Vanrenterghem YF: Posttransplantation diabetes mellitus in FK-506-treated renal transplant recipients: analysis of incidence and risk factors. Transplantation 200127;72(10):1655-61.
130. Kasiske BL, Snyder JJ, Gilbertson D, Matas AJ. Diabetes mellitus after kidney. transplantation in the United States. Am J Transplant 2003;3(2):178-85.
131. Hjelmesaeth J, Hartmann A, Kofstad J, Stenstrom J, Leivestad T, Egeland T, Fauchald P: Glucose intolerance after renal transplantation depends upon prednisolone dose and recipient age. Transplantation 1997 Oct 15;64(7):979-83.
132. Duijnhoven EM, Boots JM, Christiaans MH, Wolffenbuttel BH, Van Hooff JP.Influence of tacrolimus on glucose metabolism before and after renal transplantation: a prospective study. J Am Soc Nephrol 2001;12(3):583-8.
133. Filler G, Neuschulz I, Vollmer I, Amendt P, Hocher B: Tacrolimus reversibly reduces insulin secretion in paediatric renal transplant recipients. Nephrol Dial Transplant 2000;15:867.
134. Hathaway DK, Tolley EA, Blakely ML, Winsett RP, Gaber AO: Development of an index to predict new onset diabetes after transplantation mellitus. Clin Transplant 1993;7:330-338.Hathaway DK, Tolley EA, Blakely ML, Winsett RP, Gaber AO: Development of an index to predict new onset diabetes after transplantation mellitus. Clin Transplant 1993;7:330-338.
135. Silva F, Queiros J, Vargas G, Henriques A, Sarmento A, Guimaraes S.Risk factors for new onset diabetes after transplantation mellitus and impact of this complication after renal transplantation. Transplant Proc 2000;32:2609-2610.

136. Miles AM, Sumrani N, Horowitz R, Homel P, Maursky V, Markell MS, Distant DA, Hong JH, Sommer BG, Friedman EA. Diabetes mellitus after renal transplantation: as deleterious as non-transplant-associated diabetes? Transplantation 1998;65:380-384.

137. Ojo AO, Hanson JA, Wolfe RA, Leichtman AB, Agodoa LY, Port FK.Long-term survival in renal transplant recipients with graft function. Kidney Int 2000;57:307-313.

138. Schneider DJ, Nordt TK, Sobel BE. Attenuated fibrinolysis and accelerated atherogenesis in type II diabetes patients. Diabetes 1993;42:1-7.

139. Lindholm A, Albrechtsen D, Frodin L, Tufveson G, Persson NH, Lundgren G. Ischemic heart disease—major cause of death and graft loss after renal transplantation in Scandinavia. Transplantation 1995 ;60:451-457.

140. Stratton IM, Adler AI, Neil HA, Matthews DR, Manley SE, Cull CA, Hadden D, Turner RC, Holman RR. Association of glycaemia with macrovascular and microvascular complications of type 2 diabetes (UKPDS 35): prospective observational study. BMJ 2000;321:405-412.

141. Najarian JS, Sutherland DER, Simmons RL, et al. 1979. Ten year experience with renal transplantation in juvenile onset diabetics. Ann Surgery 190:487-500.

40

COMBINATION THERAPY FOR HYPERTENSION AND RENAL DISEASE IN DIABETES

[1]Peter D. Hart, and [2]George L. Bakris,

[1]*Department of Medicine, Cook County Hospital, Chicago, IL and* [2]*The Rush Hypertension Center, Department of Preventive Medicine, Rush-Presbyterian-St. Luke's Medical Center, Chicago, IL 60612.*

INTRODUCTION

Hypertension and diabetes are the leading cause of end stage renal disease (ESRD in the USA [1]. Clearly, cardiovascular disease accounts for more than half of the morbidity and mortality seen in people with diabetes, with hypertension being the strongest predictor of death from diabetic nephropathy [2].

In 1997, the sixth report of the Joint National Committee on detection, evaluation, and treatment of high blood pressure (JNC VI) recommends initiation of antihypertensive drug therapy in *all* people with diabetes and a blood pressure (BP) greater than 130/85 mmHg [3]. However, results of more recent studies support a lower blood pressure goal of <130/80 mmHg in patients with diabetes [4], a goal original put forth by the National Kidney Foundation in 2000 and now recommended by the American Diabetes Association and the JNC VII, Table 1. However, in spite of the recent advances in drug therapy and recommendations for preventive strategies, an analysis of the NHANES III data base demonstrated that only 11% of patients with type 2 diabetes and hypertension being treated for hypertension actually achieved the JNC VI goal BP of <130/85mmHg[5]. That compared to 27% of the general population having blood pressure to a goal of <140/90 mmHg [3].

Table 1- Recommended Goal BP and initial therapy in patients with Diabetes or kidney disease to reduce cardiovascular and retard progression of nephropathy.

What is the Goal BP and Initial therapy in Kidney Disease or Diabetes to Reduce CV Risk?

Group	Goal BP (mmHg)	Initial Therapy
• KDOQI (NKF) (2003)	<130/80	ACE Inhibitor/ARB*
• JNC VII? (2003)	<130/80	ACE Inhibitor/ARB*
• Am. Diabetes Assoc. (2003)	<130/80	ACE Inhibitor/ARB*
• Canadian HTN Soc. (2002)	<130/80	ACE Inhibitor/ARB
• Am. Diabetes Assoc. (2002)	<130/80	ACE Inhibitor/ARB
• Natl. Kidney Fdn.-CKD (2002)	≤130/80	ACE Inhibitor/ARB*
• Natl. Kidney Fdn. (2000)	≤130/80	ACE Inhibitor*
• British HTN Soc. (1999)	<140/80	ACE Inhibitor
• WHO/ISH (1999)	<130/85	ACE Inhibitor
• JVC VI (1997)	<130/85	ACE Inhibitor

* Indicates use with diuretic

In all clinical trial more than 80% of patients with diabetic nephropathy and hypertension require two or more antihypertensive medications to attain the JNC VI recommended blood pressure goal of 130/85 mmHg [3,6]. Clinical trials that randomized participants with either diabetes and Stage 2 or higher nephropathy, (GFR <80 ml/min), to two different levels of blood pressure control showed that to achieve the desired lower BP goal, an average of 3.2 different antihypertensive medications per day was required, (Figure 1). In these and other trials, it was common to add a medication whose antihypertensive action provides complementary, additive or synergistic antihypertensive effects through different mechanisms, i.e. a diuretic with a beta blocker, an angiotensin converting enzyme (ACE) inhibitor or angiotensin receptor blocker (ARB) with a diuretic or calcium antagonist [7,8].

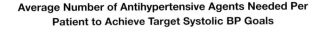

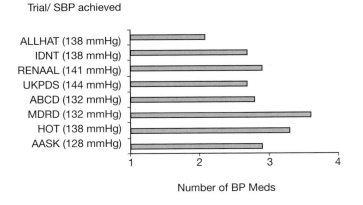

Figure 1- A summary of recent randomized trials showing the average number of antihypertensive agents needed per person to achieve blood pressure goals

Perhaps the most consist data on drug adherence demonstrate that simplification of a drug regimen significantly improves adherence. To further improve adherence and drug related side effects, fixed-dose combinations of antihypertensive drugs with complementary modes of action have been developed [8]. These medications combine a lower dose of two different antihypertensive drugs that, in a fixed dose combination, reduce arterial pressure to a greater degree than either agent alone thus, enhancing efficacy and tolerability. The evolution of fixed-dose combination antihypertensive therapy is summarized in a recent review [9] and in Table 2.

This review will focus on the available evidence from both animal models of hypertension and renal disease as well as clinical studies that examine the efficacy of different classes of antihypertensive medications, either alone or combined, to either retard or prevent development of diabetic renal disease. The discussion will concentrate on combination therapy with an ACE inhibitor, ARB, diuretic or calcium channel blocker (CCBs) as one of the components.

Table 2. Historical Evolution of Fixed Dose Combination

1960's
Ser-Ap-Es (reserpine-hydralazine-hydrochlorothiazide)
Methyldopa/thiazide diuretic

1970's
Thiazide/ Various[K+] Sparing Diuretic
Thiazide/Spironolactone
 Beta blocker/thiazide diuretic
Clonidine/thiazide diuretic

1980's
ACE inhibitor/thiazide diuretic

1990's
(Low dose) β- Blocker /thiazide diuretic
Calcium Channel Blocker/ACE inhibitor
Beta Blocker/Dihydropyridine Calcium Channel Blocker
Angiotensin II Receptor Blocker/Diuretic

RENAL MORPHOLOGY AND HEMODYNAMICS

Brief overviews of the renal hemodynamic and morphologic changes that occur in the diabetic kidney are presented (Figure 2). This is done in an effort to improve the understanding of how and why, at a comparable blood pressure level, combinations of various antihypertensive medications slow progression of diabetic nephropathy to a greater extent than either of the individual components.

Early changes observed in the diabetic kidney include an increase in efferent arteriolar tone and a loss of autoregulation [10-11]. These changes lead to an increase in intraglomerular capillary pressure, which results in cell stretch and activation of various autocrine and paracrine factors associated with tissue injury [11-12]. In addition, glomerular membrane permeability and endothelial injury is increased and microalbuminuria ensues, a risk factor for cardiovascular disease, in general and indicative of nephropathy in Type 1 diabetes [13-16]. The earliest morphologic change is mesangial matrix expansion and in some cases interstitial inflammation, the latter portends a poor renal prognosis [15-17]. The role of the renin angiotensin system (RAS) in diabetic nephropathy cannot be overemphasized. Blocking the RAS slows down the progression of established diabetic nephropathy in type I diabetes mellitus and inhibiting angiotensin II formation retards or impedes the progression from microalbuminuria to established diabetic nephropathy in people with type I diabetes mellitus [18-21]. The situation could be the same for type 2 diabetes mellitus as has been seen in numerous studies [22-25].

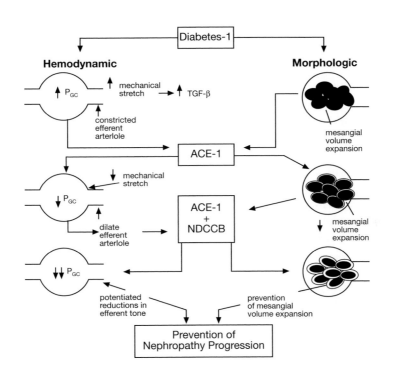

Figure 2- A representation of the renal hemodynamic and morphologic effects of ACE inhibitors (ACE-I) and nondihydropyridine calcium channel blockers (NDCCB), PGC- Intraglomerular capillary pressure
(***Adapted from Kilaru PK and Bakris GL. Calcium channel blockade and/or ACE inhibition in diabetic hypertensive nephropathy. IN Combination Drug Therapy for Hypertension . Opie LH and Messerli F, (eds). Lippincott-Raven Publ., Philadelphia, 1997, pp.123-138.)

INDIVIDUAL ANTIHYPERTENSIVE AGENTS

Experimental evidence demonstrates that reductions in intraglomerular capillary pressure, through either profound reductions in systemic arterial pressure or dilation of the efferent arteriole, slow progression of diabetic renal disease [4, 8, and 18]. Drugs that reduce efferent arteriolar tone and intraglomerular pressure include the ACE inhibitors, ARB and certain CCBs [4, 13, 18, and 26]. In clinical studies, however, only the ACE inhibitors and the ARBs demonstrate a consistent and persistent reduction in albuminuria and proteinuria as well as an attenuated progression in nephropathy associated with type 1 and type 2 diabetes [21-31].

Angiotensin converting enzyme inhibitors (ACEI)
Blood pressure reduction to within the goal recommended has been shown to slow progression of both diabetic and non-diabetic renal disease, but ACE inhibitors appear to preserve renal function to even greater extent than other agents do when achieved blood pressure <140/90 mmHg [21-33]. The benefit of ACE inhibitors on diabetic glomerulosclerosis is thought to result from attenuation of angiotensin II effects on blood pressure, glomerular hemodynamics, and tissue fibrosis indirectly through effects on TGF-beta [18-20]. Inhibition of angiotensin II occurs with ACE inhibitors and ARBs.

Angiotensin receptor blockers (ARBs):
ARBs are currently the best tolerated of all antihypertensive agents, with an apparent beneficial profile similar to ACE inhibitors yet with side effect profile similar to placebo [34]. Recent clinical trials show that ARBs, when appropriately dosed, have renoprotective and cardio-protective effects to a similar magnitude as ACE inhibitors [35-41]. Clinical trials have demonstrated that ARBs are safe and effective for the treatment for hypertension in patients with impaired renal function and produces renal hemodynamic effects akin to those seen with ACE inhibitors [22, 34-36]. Moreover, ARBs do not directly interfere with any enzymatic process in the renin angiotensin system (RAS). In contrast to ACE inhibitors, ARBs have no significant direct effect on angiotensin II production or bradykinin metabolism. This more targeted mechanism, may account for the excellent tolerability profiles observed with ARBs [37-39]. Two recent clinical trials involving more than 3200 people with nephropathy associated with type 2 diabetes solidifies the role of this class as renoprotective agents. The Irebesartan Diabetic Nephropathy Trial (IDNT) [40] and the Reduction of Endpoints in NIDDM with the AII Antagonist Losartan (RENAAL)[41] Both demonstrated a 16 to 20% risk reduction of renal disease

progression compared to placebo and 23% risk reduction for time dialysis or doubling of creatinine compared to amlodipine in the IDNT.

Calcium Channel Blockers (CCBs)

Antihypertensive agents that do not reduce intraglomerular pressure or reduce membrane permeability to albumin may not slow progression of nephropathy unless blood pressure is lowered well below that of agents that lower intraglomerular pressure [10, 13, 18]. Furthermore, dihydropyridine CCBs are well known not to protect against morphologic progression of renal disease [18, 42-44]. Studies using 24 hour blood pressure monitoring in a rat model of renal insufficiency were performed where animals were randomized to four different CCBs, two long acting dihydropyridines, amlodipine or felodipine, as well as the nondihydropyridine agents, verapamil and diltiazem [42]. In this and four other studies, given similar levels of blood pressure reduction, the nondihydropyridines prevented development of glomerulosclerosis and the rise in proteinuria [42-46]. Conversely, the dihydropyridines did not protect against development of renal injury or proteinuria at comparable blood pressure levels. A lack of morphologic protection and increase in proteinuria has also been noted in a salt-sensitive, DOCA-salt, rat model as well as the SHR model [47]. It should also be noted that in addition to dihydropyridine CCBs, prevention of mesangial expansion or glomerulosclerosis has never been shown for alpha-blockers in animal models of diabetes [18, 47-49]. This lack of benefit of alpha blockade was also seen clinically, in the Antihypertensive and lipid lowering treatment to prevent heart attack trial (ALLHAT), the alpha-blocker, doxazosin, was discontinued because of a higher incidence of congestive heart failure and less benefit in preventing ischemic heart disease compared with the diuretic chlorthalidone [50]. This was also true in the 15,000 diabetic participants in the study.

A lack of effect by dihydropyridine CCBs on albuminuria reduction in people with 300 mg per day or more of albuminuria is also seen clinically [30,31,40,44]. Agardh et al, showed that patients with type 2 diabetes and microalbuminuria randomized to either an ACE inhibitor (lisinopril) or CCB (nifedipine retard), the ACE inhibitor group had a significantly greater reduction in albumin excretion compared to the CCB group. Moreover, this occurred in spite of comparable reductions in blood pressure. In a separate study, an increase in protein excretion of as much as 50% has also been shown in Type II diabetic African-Americans with albuminuria randomized to isradipine.

The reason for this absence of effect on albuminuria by dihydropyridine CCBs relates to a lack of effect on glomerular membrane permeability, in spite of adequate blood pressure reduction to levels around 140/90mmHg[13,15,18,44]. Results from a recently completed two year randomized, prospective trial in 28 type 2 diabetic patients with nephropathy, demonstrates no alteration of glomerular membrane permeability or albuminuria with once-daily nifedipine whereas there was a clear reduction in membrane permeability and albuminuria with once-daily diltiazem [13]. Additionally, several long-term clinical trials have examined the effects of long acting dihydropyridine CCBs on both changes in albuminuria as well as progression of renal disease [51-55]. Two of these studies demonstrated that in patients with diabetic nephropathy the initial reduction in albuminuria seen with the dihydropyridine CCBs does not persist beyond the first year [52, 54]. Moreover, in one of these studies, the rate of decline in renal function in the group randomized to nifedipine was significantly faster than the group randomized to the ACE inhibitor [50]. In a separate study, Zucchelli et.al. followed patients with chronic renal disease, randomized to either nifedipine or an ACE inhibitor, for three years [53]. At study end, no significant differences in proteinuria or the slopes of glomerular filtration rate (GFR) declines were noted. However, in the third year, people randomized to nifedipine were more than five times more likely to start dialysis. Another study of patients with early diabetic nephropathy, randomized to either an ACE inhibitor or amlodipine and followed for three years, noted no difference between groups in reduction of microalbuminuria [54]. Lastly, a four -year randomized double-blinded trial in people with mild renal insufficiency and Type 1 diabetes showed that with comparable blood pressure control, there was no substantive reduction from baseline albuminuria and no worsening of left ventricular hypertrophy with a dihydropyridine CCB as compared to an ACE inhibitor [56].

It should be noted, however, that adverse renal outcomes with dihydropyridine CCBs have been documented only in people with albuminuria of >300 mg/d, not those with normo- or microalbuminuria [40, 44]. In the diabetic subgroup of the ALLHAT, however, cardiovascular events, especially stroke were reduced with this class of antihypertensive agents in the more than 15,000 diabetic patients seen in this trial. While albuminuria was not assessed in this trial, patients with advanced renal disease were excluded. Thus, this subclass of CCBs is safe in people with normal renal function even if they have diabetes.

In contrast to the dihydropyridine CCBs, three different meta-analyses note that nondihydropyridine CCBs reduce albuminuria and slow the decline in GFR among patients with established diabetic nephropathy [44, 57-59]. This observation is further supported by two long-term trials in patients with type 2 diabetic nephropathy. These studies demonstrated that long acting verapamil or diltiazem slowed progression of established diabetic renal disease to a degree similar to an ACE inhibitor [27, 60].

Many factors may contribute to the disparate effects of the different subclasses of CCBs on both surrogate end-points as well as progression of renal disease in those with macroalbuminuria. These differences are reviewed, in detail, elsewhere [44, 61]. It is clear, however, that blood pressure reduction is the ultimate goal that uniformly leads to preservation of renal function. Thus, when the achieved systolic blood pressure is below 120mmHg or dihydropyridine CCB, are combined with ACE inhibitors, no significant differences in renal protection is observed between the subclasses of CCBs in animal models studied [44, 62-64].

COMBINATION ANTIHYPERTENSIVE THERAPY

The majority of patients with diabetic nephropathy require two or more antihypertensive agents to effectively reduce blood pressure levels to recommended goal [4].   Thus, combination agents individually shown to reduce blood pressure and albuminuria as well as preserve renal function and morphology should be the preferred agents.

ACE inhibitor/ dihydropyridine CCB combinations
Few animal studies have evaluated the effects of an ACE inhibitor/CCB combination on various aspects of renal disease [44, 45, 65-68]. One of these studies showed that combination therapy with a fixed-dose of an ACE inhibitor, benazepril, and dihydropyridine CCB, amlodipine blunted the rise in albuminuria and prevented progression to glomerulosclerosis in contrast to amlodipine alone [63].   Similar results were also observed in a recent clinical study that examined changes in proteinuria and GFR with this combination [64]

ACE inhibitor/ nondihydropyridine CCB combinations
In contrast to ACE inhibitor/ dihydropyridine CCB combinations, animal studies that combine a nondihydropyridine CCB with an ACE inhibitor have demonstrated a potentiation of ACE inhibitor associated reductions in proteinuria [44, 65-67]. Two of these studies also showed relatively greater preservation of renal morphology [43, 45]. Moreover, the fixed-dose

combination of verapamil with trandolapril showed protection of glomerular morphology, in the absence of blood pressure control [45]. The additive antiproteinuric effects of the fixed-dose combination, verapamil plus trandolapril, has also been observed in randomized, multicenter, clinical trials of patients diabetic nephropathy with comparable blood pressure control [65].

Apart from the additive antiproteinuric effects of fixed-dose ACE inhibitor/ nondihydropyridine CCB combinations, clinical studies have also shown that fixed-dose combinations have less side effect profile than either agent alone [66,67,69]. Schneider, et al confirmed that in patients with type II diabetes and hypertension, this combination did not aggravate insulin resistance nor elevate lipid levels compared to patients who were treated with β-blockers and chlorthalidone [67].

The most common cause of death in people with diabetes and nephropathy is due to cardiovascular disease [70]. The following facts emerge from all the clinical trials that have evaluated CCBs for reduction of cardiovascular events: First, an average of 3 different antihypertensive agents is needed to achieve blood pressure goals. Second, in post-hoc analyses of clinical trials use of a CCB with an ACE inhibitor or ARB is associated with preservation of renal function and reduction in cardiovascular events [71-74]. Lastly, in patients with macroalbuminuria i.e. > 300 mg/day albuminuria, dihydropyridine CCBs does not reduce progression of nephropathy as well as an ARB, regardless of blood pressure reduction [40].

ACE inhibitor/ARB combinations
Decreased angiotensin II formation or action is beneficial in diabetic nephropathy because it reduces both systemic and glomerular hypertension, proteinuria and the tendency to form abnormal amounts of glomerular and interstitial matrix protein and decreases in aldosterone formation. Thus, a therapeutic goal in diabetic nephropathy might be to inhibit angiotensin II effects as completely as possible. ACE inhibitor therapy reduces but do not totally eliminate angiotensin II effects [75], however, combining an ACE inhibitor with an ARB blocks more than 90% of the effect [76]. The data, however, with such combinations is mixed in clinical outcome studies. The Candesartan and Lisinopril microalbuminuria (CALM) trial examined the effect of a combination of ACE inhibitor and ARB on microalbuminuria compared to either agent alone in patients with type 2 diabetes. The results showed that the ACEI/ARB combination led to a 50% reduction in urinary albumin: creatinine ratio compared to candesartan (24%) and lisinopril (39%) [77]. Of note, blood

pressure levels were lower with the combination therapy compared to the individual agents alone. Another study by Ruilope et al randomized 108 people with renal insufficiency to either an ARB alone, in two different doses, or these same doses in combination with a low dose ACE inhibitor. In this study the blood pressure lowering effects of the combination were significantly better with no significant adverse effects on measures of renal function including serum creatinine and potassium [78]. A recent study by the Steno Diabetes group also showed that use of high dose ACE inhibitor with high dose ARB also further reduces albuminuria; however, blood pressure was also further reduced [79]. Agarwal et al, however, showed that when maximum doses of ACE inhibitors are used, addition of an ARB did not lead to further blood pressure reduction or antiproteinuric effect [80]. Finally we have the results of the COOPERATE trial that demonstrated fewer renal outcomes such as ESRD and doubling of creatinine when the combination of an ACE inhibitor and an ARB were used in an Asian population of 240 people [81]. This study has many problems not the least of which it is underpowered for the primary endpoint. When these data are viewed in the context of the ValHeFT study in heart failure where mortality was not further reduced with an ACE inhibitor/ARB combination but there was a reduction in morbidity, it is unclear whether this combination is truly of benefit [82]. Thus, the role of combining an ACE inhibitor with an ARB remains unclear with regard to cardiovascular outcomes. It does appear to reduce proteinuria, however. Combining ACE inhibitors with drugs such as aldosterone receptor antagonists may provide far greater benefit with regard to both proteinuria reduction as well as cardiovascular outcomes [83-84], the data are pending.

CONCLUSIONS

Current recommendations from all guideline committees indicate that the goal blood pressure for those with diabetes or any type of kidney disease is <130/80 mmHg. The majority of patients with diabetic nephropathy require a minimum of two to three antihypertensive agents to achieve this goal, therefore combination therapy is highly recommended by guideline committees [3, 4, and 85]. In order to provide maximum cardiovascular and kidney protection the antihypertensive regimen should include a minimum of two agents notably ACE inhibitors or ARBs with a diuretic. Diuretics preferable to CCBs since they demonstrated a reduced incidence of heart failure development in the ALLHAT compared to diuretics. Given the difficulties with medication adherence in these patients, the advantages of fixed dose combinations are obvious. Use of initial fixed-dose combination therapy has been shown to achieve the blood pressure goal of <130/85 mmHg faster in patients with hypertension and diabetes that starting with conventional monotherapy. The results of the study of hypertension and the efficacy of Lotrel in Diabetes (SHIELD) trial demonstrate that in patients with type 2 diabetes, initiating treatment with a fixed dose combination resulted in higher percentage of patients achieving blood pressure goal compared to monotherapy with subsequent addition of diuretics [86]. In spite of this data, current available evidence is insufficient to assess whether fixed-dose antihypertensive therapy offers a distinct advantage to reduce renal and cardiovascular mortality compared to use of the individual components used separately. The first cardiovascular endpoint trial to test the hypothesis that starting with a combination without a diuretic of a fixed dose combination versus one without a diuretic is just underway. The results will be known in 2007. Until then combination therapy offers a viable alternative to improve adherence by reducing the number of pills taken, minimize drug-related side effects, and most importantly reducing the cost because of reimbursement in certain countries [87-89].

REFERENCES

1.   (www.usrds.gov;2002).
2.   Sievers ML, Bennett PH, Roumain J, Nelson RG; Effect of hypertension on   mortality in Pima Indians. Circulation 1999; 100(1): 33-40
3.   Joint National Committee on Detection, Evaluation, and Treatment of High Blood Pressure. The sixth report of the Joint National Committee on Detection, Evaluation, and Treatment of High Blood Pressure (JNC VI). Arch Intern Med 1997; 154:2413-2446
4.   Bakris GL, Williams M, Dworkin L, Elliot WJ, Epstein M, Toto R, Tuttle K, Douglas J, Hsueh W, Somer J: Preserving renal function in adults with hypertension and diabetes: A consensus approach. National Kidney Foundation Hypertension and Diabetes executive Committees working group. Am J Kidney Diseases 2000; 36(3): 646-661
5.   Coresh J, Wei GL, McQuillan G, Brancatil FL, Levey AS, Jones C and Klag MJ: Prevalence of high blood pressure and elevated serum creatinine level in the United States: findings from the third National Health and Nutrition Examination Survey (1988-1994). Arch.Intern.Med.2001; 161 (9): 1207-1216.
6.   Sheinfeld GR and Bakris GL. Benefits of combination angiotensin-converting enzyme inhibitor and calcium antagonist therapy for diabetic patients. Am J Hypertension 1999;12:80S-85S
7.   Waeber B, Brunner HR. Main objectives and new aspects of combination treatment of hypertension. J Hypertens 1995; 13 (Suppl):S15-S19.
8.   Epstein M and Bakris GL. Newer approaches to antihypertensive therapy using fixed dose combination therapy: Future perspectives. Arch Intern Med. 1996;156:1969-1978.
9.   Sica AD. Rationale for fixed-dose combinations in the treatment of Hypertension. Drugs. 2002; 62(3):443-462

10. Griffin KA, Picken MM and Bidani AK. Deleterious effects of calcium channel blockade on pressure transmission and glomerular injury in rat remnant kidneys. J Clin. Invest 1995; 96: 793-800.

11. Makrilakis K and Bakris GL. New therapeutic approaches to achieve the desired blood pressure goal. Cardiovasc Rev. & Reports 1997;18:10-16.

12. Bakris GL, Walsh MF, Sowers JR. Endothelium, mesangium interactions: Role of insulin-like growth factors . IN: Endocrinology of the Vasculature (Sowers JR, ed). Humana Press Inc. New Jersey, 1996, pp.341-356.

13. Smith AC, Toto R, Bakris GL Differential effects of calcium channel blockers on size selectivity of proteinuria in diabetic glomerulopathy. Kidney Int. 1998;54:889-896

14. Bakris GL. Microalbuminuria: Prognostic Implications. Curr Opin in Nephrol and Hypertens 1996;5(3):219-233.

15. Drumond MC , Kristal B , Myers BD , Deen WM Structural basis for reduced glomerular filtration capacity in nephrotic humans. J Clin Invest 1994 ;94(3):1187-1195

16. Garg JP and Bakris GL. Microalbuminuria: marker of vascular dysfunction, risk factor for cardiovascular disease. *Vasc.Med* 2002;7 (1):35-43.

17. Steffes MW, Osterby R, Chavers B, and Mauer SM. Mesangial expansion as a central mechanism for loss of kidney function in diabetic patients. Diabetes 1989;38:1077-1081.

18. Anderson S, Rennke HG, Brenner BM. Nifedipine versus fosinopril in uninephrectomized diabetic rats. Kidney Int 1992;41:891-897.

19. Parving H, Hommel E, Nielsen M, Giese J: Effect of captopril on blood pressure and kidney function in normotensive insulin dependent diabetics with nephropathy. Br Med J 1989;299:533-536.

20. Bakris GL, Slataper R, Vicknair N, Sadler R: ACE inhibitor mediated reductions in renal size and microalbuminuria in normotensive, diabetic subjects. J Diab Compl 1994;8:2-6.

21. Viberti G; Mogensen CE; Groop LC; Pauls JF. Effect of captopril on progression to clinical proteinuria in patients with insulin-dependent diabetes mellitus and microalbuminuria. European Microalbuminuria Captopril Study Group JAMA 1994;271(4):275-9.

22. Sica DA and Bakris GL. Type 2 diabetes: RENAAL and IDNT—the emergence of new treatment options. J.Clin.Hypertens.(Greenwich.) 2002;4 (1):52-57.

23. Parving HH, Lehnert H, Brochner-Mortensen J, Gomis R, Andersen S, and Arner P. The effect of irbesartan on the development of diabetic nephropathy in patients with type 2 diabetes. N.Engl.J.Med. 2001;345 (12):870-878.

24. Ravid M, Lang R, Rachmani R, Lishner M. Long-term renoprotective effect of angiotensin-converting enzyme inhibition in non-insulin-dependent diabetes mellitus. Arch Intern Med 1996;156:286-289

25. Sakamoto N: Effects of long-term enalapril treatment on persistent microalbuminuria in well- controlled hypertensive and normotensive NIDDM patients. Diabetes Care 1994;17:420-424

26. Nakamura M, Notoya M, Kohda Y, Yamashita J, Takashita Y, and Gemba M. Effects of efonidipine hydrochloride on renal arteriolar diameters in spontaneously hypertensive rats. Hypertens.Res. 2002;25 (5):751-755.

27. Bakris GL, Copley JB, Vicknair N, Sadler R, Leurgans S. Calcium channel blockers versus other antihypertensive therapies on progression of NIDDM associated nephropathy: Results of a six year study. Kidney Int. 1996;50:1641-1650.

28. Lebovitz HE, Wiegmann TB, Cnaan A: Renal protective effects of enalapril in hypertensive NIDDM: role of baseline albuminuria. Kidney Int Suppl 1994;45:S150-S155.

29. Lewis EJ, Hunsicker LG, Bain RP, Rohde RD for the Collaborative Study Group. The effect of angiotensin converting enzyme inhibition on diabetic nephropathy. N Engl J Med 1993;329:1456-1462.

30. Agardh CD, Garcia-Puig J, Charbonnel B, Angelkort B, Barnett AH. Greater reduction of urinary albumin excretion in hypertensive Type II diabetic patients with incipient nephropathy by lisinopril than by nifedipine. J Human Hypertens 1996;10:185-192.

31. Guasch A, Parham M, Zayas CF, Campbell O, Nzerue C, Macon E. Contrasting effects of calcium channel blockade versus converting enzyme inhibition on proteinuria in African Americans with non-insulin dependent diabetes mellitus and nephropathy. J Am Soc Nephrol 1997;8: 793-798.

32. Maschio G, Alberti D, Janin G, Locatelli F, Mann JEF, Motolese M, Ponticelli C, Ritz E, Zucchelli P, and the Angiotensin-Converting-Enzyme Inhibition in Progressive Renal Insufficiency Study Group. Effect of the angiotensin-converting-enzyme inhibitor benazepril on the progression of chronic renal insufficiency. N Engl J Med 1996;334:939-945

33. Venkart C, Ram S, Fierro G. The Benefits of Angiotensin II Receptor Blockers in patients with renal insufficiency of failure. Am J Ther.1998;5(2): 101-105

34. Bakris GL, Weber MA, Black HR, Weir MR. Clinical efficacy and safety profiles of AT1 receptor antagonists. Cardiovasc Reviews and Reports 1999;20:77-100

35. Pitt B, Segal R, Martinez FA, Meurers G, Cowley AJ, Thomas I, Deedwania PC, Ney DE, Snavely DB, Chang PI Randomised trial of losartan versus captopril in patients over 65 with heart failure. Lancet 1997;349:747-752

36. Dahlof B, Devereux RB, Kjeldsen SE, Julius S, Beevers G, Faire U, Fyhrquist E, Ibsen H, Kristiansson K, Lederballe-Pedersen O, Lindholm LH, Nieminen MS, Omvik P, Oparil S, and Wedel H. Cardiovascular morbidity and mortality in the Losartan Intervention For Endpoint reduction in hypertension study (LIFE): a randomised trial against atenolol. Lancet 2002;359 (9311):995-1003.

37. Kang PM, Landau AJ, Eberhardt RT, Frishman WH: Angiotensin II receptor antagonists: a new approach to blockade of the renin-angiotensin system. Am Heart J 1994;127:1388-1401

38. Goldberg AI, Dunlay MC, Sweet CS: safety and tolerability of Losartan potassium, an angiotensin II receptor antagonist, compared with hydrocholothiazide, atenolol, felodipine ER, and angiotensin –converting enzyme inhibitors for the treatment of systemic hypertension. Am J Cardiol 1995;75:793-795.

39. Dahlof B, Keller SE, Makris L, et al: Efficacy and tolerability of Losartan potassium and atenolol in patients with mild to moderate essential hypertension. Am J Hypertens 1995:8:578-583

40. Lewis EJ, Hunsicker LG, Clarke WR, Berl T, Pohl MA, Lewis JB, Ritz E, Atkins RC, Rohde R, and Raz I. Renoprotective effect of the angiotensin-receptor antagonist irbesartan in patients with nephropathy due to type 2 diabetes. N Engl J Med 2001; 345 (12): 851-860

41. Brenner BM, Cooper ME, de Zeeuw D, Keane WF, Mitch WE, Parving HH, Remuzzi G, Snapinn SM, Zhang Z, and Shahinfar S. Effects of losartan on renal and cardiovascular outcomes in patients with type 2 diabetes and nephropathy. N Engl J Med 2001; 345 (12): 861-869.

42. Griffin KA, Picken MM, Bakris GL, Bidani AK Class differences in the effects of calcium channel blockers in the rat remnant kidney model. Kidney Int 1999; 55(5):1849-1860.

43. Gaber L, Walton C, Brown S, Bakris, GL: Effects of different antihypertensive treatments on morphologic progression of diabetic nephropathy in uninephrectomized dogs. Kidney Int 1994;46:161-169

44. Koshy S and Bakris GL. Therapeutic approaches to achieve desired blood pressure goals: focus on calcium channel blockers. Cardiovasc.Drugs Ther. 14 (3):295-301, 2000.

45. Munter K, Hergenroder S, Jochims K, Kirchengast M. Individual and combined effects of verapamil or trandolapril on glomerular morphology and function in the stroke prone rat. J Am Soc Nephrol 1996;7:681-686.

46. Brown SA, Walton CL, Crawford P & Bakris GL. Long-term effects of different anti-hypertensive regimens on renal hemodynamics and proteinuria. Kidney Int 1993, 43:1210-1218.

47. Dworkin LD, Tolbert E, Recht PA, Hersch JC, Feiner H, Levin RI. Effects of amlodipine on glomerular filtration, growth and injury in experimental hypertension. Hypertension 1996; 27:245-250

48. Jyothirmayi GN, Alluru I, Reddi AS. Doxazosin prevents proteinuria and glomerular loss of heparan sulfate in diabetic rats. Hypertension 1996;27:1108-1114

49. Rachmani R, Levi Z, Slavachevsky I, Half-Onn E, Ravid M Effect of an alpha-adrenergic blocker, and ACE inhibitor and hydrochlorothiazide on blood pressure and on renal function in type 2 diabetic patients with hypertension and albuminuria. A randomized cross-over study. Nephron 1998;80(2):175-182

50. ALLHAT collaborative research group: Major cardiovascular events in hypertensive patients randomized to doxazosin vs. clorthalidone: the antihypertensive and lipid-lowering treatment to prevent heart attack trial (ALLHAT). JAMA 2000; 283: 2013-4

51. Abbott K, Smith AC, Bakris GL. Effects of dihydropyridine calcium antagonists on albuminuria in diabetic subjects. J. Clin Pharmacol. 1996;36:274-279.

52. Jerums G, Allen TJ, Campbell DJ, Cooper ME, Gilbert, RE, Hammond JJ, Raffaele J, and Tsalamandris C. Long-term comparison between perindopril and nifedipine in normotensive patients with type 1 diabetes and microalbuminuria. Am.J.Kidney Dis. 2001;37 (5):890-899.

53. Zucchelli P, Zuccala A, Borghi M, et. al., Long term comparison between captopril and nifedipine in the progression of renal insufficiency Kidney Int 1992 42:452-458.

54. Velussi M, Brocco E, Frigato F, Zolli M, Muollo B, Maioli M, Carraro A, Tonolo G, Fresu P, Cernigoi A, Fioretto P, Nosadini R. Effects of cilazapril and amlodipine on kidney function in hypertensive NIDDM patients. Diabetes 1996;45:216-222

55. Locatelli F, Carbarns IR, Maschio G, Mann JF, Ponticelli C, Ritz E, Alberti D, Motolese M, Janin G, Zucchelli P Long-term progression of chronic renal insufficiency in the AIPRI Extension Study. The Angiotensin-Converting-Enzyme Inhibition in Progressive Renal Insufficiency Study Group. Kidney Int Suppl, 1997;63:S63-S66

56. Tarnow L, Sato A, Ali S, Rossing P, Nielsen FS, Parving HH Effects of nisoldipine and lisinopril on left ventricular mass and function in diabetic nephropathy. Diabetes Care 1999;22(3):491-494

57. Gansevoort RT, Sluiter WJ, Hemmelder MH, de Zeeuw D, de Jong PE. Antiproteinuric effect of blood pressure lowering agents: a meta-analysis of comparative trials. Nephrol Dial Transplant 1995;10:1963-1974

58. Maki DD, Ma JZ, Louis TA, Kasiske BL: Effect of antihypertensive agents on the kidney. Arch Intern Med 1995 ;155:1073-1082.

59. Kloke HJ, Branten AJ, Huysmans FT, Wetzels JF Antihypertensive treatment of patients with proteinuric renal diseases: risks or benefits of calcium channel blockers? Kidney Int 1998;53(6):1559-1573

60. Bakris GL, Mangrum A, Copley JB, Vicknair N, Sadler R. Calcium channel or beta blockade on progression of diabetic renal disease in African-Americans. Hypertension 1997;29:744-750

61. Tarif N and Bakris GL Preservation of renal function: the spectrum of effects by calcium channel blockers. Nephrol Dial Transpl, 1997;12:2244-2250.

62. Bakris GL, Griffin KA, Picken MM, and Bidani AK. Combined effects of an angiotensin converting enzyme inhibitor and a calcium antagonist on renal injury. J Hypertension 1997;15:1181-1185

63. Wenzel RO, Helmchen U, Schoeppe W, Schwietzer G. Combination treatment of enalapril with nitrendipine in rats with renovascular hypertension. Hypertension 1994;23: 114-122.

64. Fogari R, Zoppi A, Mugellini A, Lusardi P, Destro M, Corradi L. Effect of benazepril plus amlodipine vs. benazepril alone on urinary albumin excretion in hypertensive patients with type II diabetes and microalbuminuria. Clin Drug Invest 1996:11:50-55.

65. Bakris GL, Weir MR, DeQuattro V, McMahon FG. Effects of an ACE inhibitor/calcium antagonist combination on proteinuria in diabetic nephropathy. Kidney Int.1998; 54:1283-1289

66. Holzgreve H. Safety profile of the combination of verapamil and trandolapril. J Hypertens. 1997;15(suppl 2): S51-S53.

67. Schneider M, Lerch M, Papiri M, Buechel P, Boehlen L, Shaw S, Risen W, Weidmann P. Metabolic neutrality of combined verapamil-trandolapril treatment in contrast to beta-blocker-low-dose chlorthalidone treatment in hypertensive type II diabetes. J Hypertens. 1996;14:669-677.

68. Herlitz H, Harris K, Risler T, Boner G, Bernheim J, Chanard J, and Aurell M. The effects of an ACE inhibitor and a calcium antagonist on the progression of renal disease: the Nephros Study. Nephrol.Dial.Transplant. 2001;16 (11):2158-2165.

69. Muijsers RBR, Curran MP, Perry CM. Fixed Combination Trandolapril/Verapamil Sustained-Release: A review of its use in essential hypertension. Drugs 2002;62:2539-2567.

70. Nelson RG, Knowler WC, Pettitt DJ, Bennett PH. Kidney diseases in diabetes. In Diabetes In America National Institutes of Health Pub. No.95-1468, 2nd edition, 1995, pp. 349-400

71. Hansson L, Zanchetti A, Carruthers SG, Dahlof B, Elmfeldt D, Julius S, Menard J, Rahn RK, Wedel H, Westerling S. Effects of intensive blood-pressure lowering and low dose aspirin in patients with hypertenstion: principal results of the Hypertension Optimal Treatment (HOT) randomised trial. HOT Study Group Lancet, 1998; 351: 1755-1762.

72. Staessen JA, Thijs L, Gasowski J, Cells H, Fagard RH. Treatment of isolated systolic hypertension in the elderly: further evidence from the systolic hypertension in Europe (Syst-Eur) trial. Am J Cardiol 1998; 82(9B):20R-22R.

73. Bakris GL, Matthew R. Weir MR, Shahnaz Shanifar S, Zhongxin Zhang Z, Janice Douglas J , David J. van Dijk DJ and Barry M. Brenner BM for the RENAAL Study Group Effects of Blood Pressure Level on Progression of Diabetic Nephropathy: Results from the RENAAL study Arch Intern Med, In Press

74. Pepine CJ, Handberg-Thurmond E, Marks RG, Conlon M, Cooper-DeHoff R, Volkers RP and Zellig P. Rationale and design of the International Verapamil SR/Trandolapril Study (INVEST): an Internet-based randomized trial in coronary artery disease patients with hypertension. J.Am.Coll.Cardiol. 1998;32 (5):1228-1237.

75. Nussberger J, Brunner DB, Waeber B, Brunner HR: Specific measurement of angiotensin metabolites and in vitro generated angiotensin II in plasma. Hypertension 1986;6:476-482.

76. Forclaz A, Maillard M, Nussberger J, Brunner HR, and Burnier M. Angiotensin II receptor blockade: is there truly a benefit of adding an ACE inhibitor? Hypertension 2003;41 (1):31-36.

77. Mogensen CE, Neldam S, Tikkanen I, et al; Randomised controlled trial of dual blockade of rennin-angiotensin system in patients with hypertension, microalbuminuria, and non-insulin dependent diabetes: the candesartan and lisinopril microalbuminuria (CALM) study. BMJ, 2000; 312(7274): 1440-1444

78. Ruilope LM, Aldigier JC, Ponticelli C, Oddou-Stock P, Botten F, Mann JF for the European Group for the Investigation of valsartan in chronic renal disease. Safety of the combination of valsartan and benazepril in patients with chronic renal disease. J Hypertens, 2000;18(1):89-95.

79. Garg J and Bakris GL. Angiotensin converting enzyme inhibitors or angiotensin receptor blockers in nephropathy from type 2 diabetes. Curr.Hypertens.Rep. 2002; 4 (3):185-190.

80. Agarwal R; Add-on Angiotensin receptor blockade with maximized ACE inhibition. Kidney Int; 2001;59(6):2282-2289

81. Nakao N, Yoshimura A, Morita H, Takada M, Kayano T, and Ideura T. Combination treatment of angiotensin-II receptor blocker and angiotensin-converting-enzyme inhibitor in non-diabetic renal disease (COOPERATE): a randomised controlled trial. Lancet 2003;361 (9352):117-124.

82. Cohn JN and Tognoni G. A randomized trial of the angiotensin-receptor blocker valsartan in chronic heart failure. N.Engl.J.Med. 2001;345 (23):1667-1675.

83. Pitt B, Williams G, Remme W, Martinez F, Lopez-Sendon J, Zannad F, Neaton J, Roniker B, Hurley S, Burns D, Bittman R, and Kleiman J. The EPHESUS trial: eplerenone in patients with heart failure due to systolic dysfunction complicating acute myocardial infarction. Eplerenone Post-AMI Heart Failure Efficacy and Survival Study. Cardiovasc.Drugs Ther. 2001;15 (1):79-87.

84. Pitt B, Zannad F, Remme WJ, Cody R, Castaigne A, Perez A, Palensky J, and Wittes J. The effect of spironolactone on morbidity and mortality in patients with severe heart failure. Randomized Aldactone Evaluation Study Investigators. N.Engl.J.Med. 1999;341 (10):709-717 1999.

85. Anonymous. Summary of Revisions for the 2003 Clinical Practice Recommendations. Diabetes Care 2003;26 (1 Suppl):S3.

86. Bakris GL and Weir MR on behalf of the SHIELD Trial Investigators Achieving Goal Blood Pressure in Patients with Type 2 Diabetes: Conventional versus Fixed-Dose Combination Approaches J Clinical Hypertens, In Press

87. Simeon G, Bakris G. Socioeconomic impact of diabetic nephropathy: can we improve the outcome? J Hypertens 1997;15 (Suppl 2):S77-S82.

88. Elliot WJ, Weir DR, Black HR. Cost-effectiveness of the new lower blood pressure goal of JNC VI for diabetic hypertensives. Arch Intern Med 2000, 167:1277-1283

89. Ifudu O: Benefits of combination antihypertensive therapy in progressive chronic renal failure. Am J Manag Care 1999; 5:429S-448S (suppl II)

41

MICROALBUMINURIA IN ESSENTIAL HYPERTENSION: CARDIOVASCULAR AND RENAL IMPLICATIONS

Vito M. Campese*, Roberto Bigazzi, and Stefano Bianchi
* *Division of Nephrology, University of Southern California, Los Angeles, USA, and Unita'*
Operativa di Nefrologia, Spedali Riuniti, Livorno, Italy

INTRODUCTION

The presence of microalbuminuria in patients with insulin-dependent (IDDM) and non-insulin-dependent diabetes mellitus (NIDDM) is a well recognized marker of generalized microvascular and glomerular damage, and, as such, it predicts progressive renal disease as well as cardiovascular morbidity and mortality [1-3]

A large body of evidence indicates that microalbuminuria in patients with essential hypertension is also predictive of cardiovascular and renal events. As such, measurement of urinary albumin excretion (UAE) is a useful tool to predict cardiovascular and renal disease in patients with essential hypertension.

MICROALBUMINURIA IN ESSENTIAL HYPERTENSION: INCIDENCE AND RELATIONSHIP WITH LEVELS OF BLOOD PRESSURE

The prevalence of microalbuminuria in patients with essential hypertension varies enormously among different studies with rates ranging between 5 and 37 percent [4-7]. In a study of 11 343 non-diabetic hypertensive patients with a mean age of 57 years, microalbuminuria was present in 32% of men and 28% of women (P < 0.05) and increased with age, and with severity and duration of hypertension [8].

Most studies have demonstrated a significant relationship between levels of blood pressure and UAE [9-12], but some studies have failed to confirm the existence of this relationship [13]. Knight et al have found that subjects with high-normal blood pressure manifest urine albumin excretion greater than individuals with normal or optimal blood pressure [14].

In general, a better correlation between levels of blood pressure and UAE is observed when continuous ambulatory measurements are used instead of occasional blood pressure readings in the office. Giaconi et al [15] found a significant correlation between day-time diastolic blood pressure and UAE, whereas Cerasola et al [16] observed a significant correlation between 24 hr systolic and diastolic blood pressure and UAE. Knight et al have found that high-normal blood pressure is significantly associated with microalbuminuria compared with optimal blood pressure [17].

In a study of 63 patients with essential hypertension and 21 healthy volunteers we observed a blunted or absent nocturnal dipping of blood pressure in hypertensive patients with microalbuminuria compared to patients with normal UAE and normotensive healthy individuals (Figure 1) [18]. Twenty-four hypertensive patients failed to show the normal night-time fall in blood pressure of at least 10/5 mm Hg and were defined 'non-dippers'; the remaining were defined as 'dippers'. The median UAE in non-dippers was significantly greater than dippers and normal subjects. A significant correlation between night-time systolic, night-time diastolic and 24-hour systolic blood pressure and UAE was present in hypertensive patients. This study indicates that essential hypertensive patients with microalbuminuria manifest reduced night-time blood pressure dipping and altered circadian blood pressure profile. The increase in UAE in non-dipper hypertensive patients suggests the presence of greater renal damage than in dippers. Others have shown an association between reduced nocturnal dipping of blood pressure and increased UAE in patients with essential hypertension, [19] and in patients with type 1 [20] or type 2 [21] diabetes mellitus. In patients with type 1 diabetes mellitus, an increase in systolic blood pressure during sleep precedes the development of microalbuminuria [22].

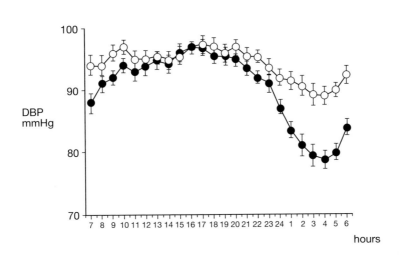

Figure 1. Mean hourly diastolic blood pressure (DBP) values in patients with essential hypertension with (open circle) and without (closed circles) microalbuminuria. [Adapted from Ref. 18].

MICROALBUMINURIA AND SERUM LIPIDS

Microalbuminuria and hyperlipidemia frequently coexist in patients with essential hypertension. We have observed that serum levels of lipoprotein (a), low-density lipoprotein (LDL) cholesterol, and triglycerides are higher whereas levels of HDL-cholesterol are lower in hypertensive patients with microalbuminuria compared with patients without microalbuminuria. (Figure 2). Using multiple regression analysis we observed that lipoprotein (a) and nocturnal blood pressure values were the variables best correlated with UAE [23].

Haffner et al [24] observed higher serum levels of triglycerides and lower HDL cholesterol in non diabetic subjects with microalbuminuria compared with subjects without microalbuminuria. Others observed a significant correlation between UAE and levels of triglycerides and apolipoprotein B [25,26].

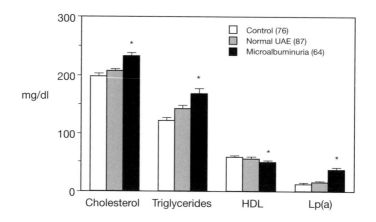

Figure 2. Serum levels of lipoproteins in 76 normotensive healthy subjects, 87 patients with essential hypertension and normal urinary albumin excretion (UAE) and 64 hypertensive patients with microalbuminuria. Values in patients with microalbuminuria were significantly (p<0.001 by ANOVA) greater than in hypertensive patients with normal UAE and normotensive healthy subjects.

The mechanisms for the association between microalbuminuria and serum lipid abnormalities are not clear. One possible explanation is that the urinary loss of protein causes the rise in serum levels of lipoproteins. This hypothesis is supported by evidence that urinary losses of large amounts of proteins lead to increased serum levels of total and LDL cholesterol [27,28] and lipoprotein(a) [29,30]. Some studies have indicated that in diabetic patients, loss of small amounts of albumin in the urine may cause substantial alterations of serum lipoproteins [31,32].

An alternative hypothesis is that hyperlipidemia causes renal damage and increased UAE. This hypothesis is supported by evidence that lipid abnormalities may contribute to the progression of renal disease [33] both in experimental nephropathy in animals [34] as well as in humans with diabetic [35] or with non-diabetic nephropathy [36]. Patients with familial type III hyperlipidemia manifest generalized atherosclerosis and glomerulosclerosis with massive foam cells accumulation within the glomeruli [37]. These patients may also manifest glomerulopathy characterized by intraglomerular lipoprotein thrombi even in the absence of generalized atheroschlerosis [38]. Recent studies have suggested that this form of lipoprotein glomerulopathy may be linked to variants in apoE molecule [39,40].

The mechanism(s) responsible for the deleterious effects of lipids on glomerular injury are not well established. The resemblance between glomerular mesangial cells and vascular smooth muscle cells and the important role played by the latter cells in the process of atherosclerosis suggests that accumulation of lipids in the mesangial cells may cause or accelerate glomerulosclerosis. In glomerulosclerotic glomeruli, lipids accumulate in mesangial cells and glomerular macrophages along with collagen, laminin and fibronectin. This process resembles that of atherosclerosis. Klahr et al [41] have suggested that mesangial cells exposed to increased amounts of lipoproteins incorporate lipids which, in turn, stimulate proliferation and deposition of excessive glomerular basement membrane matrix. This ultimately leads to progressive glomerulosclerosis. Experimental evidence suggests that elevated concentration of apoB-containing lipoproteins contributes to progression of renal injury [42]. LDL, VLDL and IDL promote the proliferation of human mesangial cells in vitro [43]. Chemokines, monocyte chemoattractant protein-1 (MCP-1) may play a pivotal role in mediating lipid-induced nephrotoxicity, whereas lovastatin, an HMG CoA-reductase inhibitor reduces the gene expression of this protein [44]. A high cholesterol diet up-regulates macrophage-colony stimulating factor (M-CSF), vascular adhesion molecules-1 (VCAM) and intracellular adhesion molecule-1 (ICAM) in glomerular mesangial cells from ExHC rats [45], suggesting that hypercholesterolemia may cause pro-inflammatory responses within the glomeruli, with activations chemotactic and adhesion molecules and recruitment of macrophages.

Agents that lower serum lipids ameliorate renal injury in experimental models of renal disease [46]. In subtotally nephrectomized rats, atorvastatin reduced TGF-ß1 expression, macrophage infiltration in glomeruli and tubulointerstitium, and this was associated with reduced urine protein excretion [47]. Statins appear to influence important intracellular pathways involved in inflammatory and fibrogenic processes involved in progressive renal injury [48]. Statins also reduce mesangial cell expression and production of chemokines such as MCP-1 and macrophage-colony stimulating factor (M-CSF), as well as vascular adhesion molecules-1 (VCAM) and intracellular adhesion molecule-1 (ICAM-1). Lovastatin inhibits activation of transcription nuclear factor-kB (NKF-kB), which plays a major role in gene expression involved in inflammatory response of mesangial cells.

MICROALBUMINURIA, INSULIN RESISTANCE AND HYPERINSULINEMIA IN ESSENTIAL HYPERTENSION

A substantial number of patients with essential hypertension manifest insulin resistance and hyperinsulinemia [49,50]. Hyperinsulinemia is considered a risk factor for atherosclerotic cardiovascular diseases [51].

Plasma insulin response to an oral glucose load was enhanced in hypertensive patients compared with control subjects [52]. A significant direct correlation was present between insulin area-under-the-curve and urinary albumin excretion rate. Using the euglycemic clamp technique, we observed a 35% reduction of peripheral glucose uptake stimulated by insulin in patients with essential hypertension and microalbuminuria [53]. This appeared to be secondary to a reduction of glycogen synthesis in skeletal muscle cells. A significant correlation between UAE and insulin resistance has been described in white patients with essential hypertension [54], and in young African-Americans [55]. Kuusisto et al [56] studied the impact of hyperinsulinemia and microalbuminuria, alone or in combination, on the incidence of cardiovascular events in 1069 elderly subjects followed for an average of 3.5 years. Forty-eight percent of males and 60.8% of females had hypertension. The incidence of fatal and non-fatal cardiovascular events was significantly greater in patients with than in those without microalbuminuria. By contrast, the incidence of cardiovascular events was only slightly, but not significantly increased in patients with higher serum insulin levels. The combined presence of microalbuminuria and hyperinsulinemia increased the probability of fatal and non-fatal cardiovascular events, even after adjusting for other risk factors, such as male sex, cigarette smoking, hypertension and serum cholesterol levels.

In all, the data supports microalbuminuria as a consistent correlate of iperinsulinemia and insulin resistance in normotensive and hypertensive individuals.

The significance of the association between hyperinsulinemia, insulin resistance and microalbuminuria in essential hypertension is uncertain. Microalbuminuria and insulin resistance have been observed in non-diabetic normotensive subjects with genetic predisposition for hypertension [57,58]. This suggests that microalbuminuria and insulin resistance could be both genetically determined and cosegregate with hypertension. Alternatively, insulin resistance and hyperinsulinemia could be causally related to microalbuminuria. Finally, enhanced plasma insulin response to glucose, insulin resistance and microalbuminuria could be a consequence of hypertension or one of its pathogenetic mechanisms.

Insulin could increase UAE directly or indirectly. Insulin could contribute to arteriosclerosis, renal damage and microalbuminuria through its effects on blood pressure, lipid metabolism, and throphic actions on vascular smooth muscle cells. Insulin infusion into femoral arteries induced intimal and medial proliferation and accumulation of cholesterol and fatty acids in animals [59]. In vitro, insulin stimulates the proliferation of smooth muscle cells and collagen deposition by growth-promoting factors [60]. Insulin may increase cholesterol and triglycerides synthesis and enhance LDL-receptor activity in arterial smooth muscle cells, fibroblasts and mononuclear cells [61,62].

An alternative hypothesis is that insulin alters glomerular hemodynamics and/or permeability directly or in association with catecholamines, angiotensin II, glucagone and sodium retention. Insulin contributes to salt-sensitivity of blood pressure by sodium retention [63], and activation of the sympathetic nervous system [64]. Salt-sensitive individuals manifest abnormal renal hemodynamic responses to high salt intake characterized by increased filtration fraction and intraglomerular pressure, and greater UAE than salt resistant patients [65].

Insulin may alter glomerular membrane permeability [66] and endothelial function [67,68].

Finally, both insulin resistance and microalbuminuria could be the result of alterations of the microcirculation caused by long standing hypertension. This explanation seems less likely, because hyperinsulinemia, insulin resistance and microalbuminuria may precede the appearance of high blood pressure and are not universally found in patients with established hypertension.

MICROALBUMINURIA AND ENDOTHELIAL FUNCTION

UAE is dependent upon the integrity of the glomerular basement membranes, but it may also be influenced by mechanical and humoral factors that may affect the permselectivity of the basement membranes as well as endothelial function. As such, microalbuminuria may reflect systemic dysfunction of the vascular endothelium, a structure intimately involved in permeability, hemostasis, fibrinolysis and blood pressure control. Pedrinelli et al [69] have shown greater concentration of Von Willebrand Factor antigen – a glycoprotein secreted in greater amount when the vascular endothelium is damaged – in hypertensive patients with microalbuminuria than in patients without and controls. Albumin transport is increased in rat aorta in the early phase of hypertension [70]. Cottone et al [71] have shown increased blood levels of endothelin-1, basic fibroblast growth factor, and platelet derived growth facto in hypertensive patients with microalbuminuria compared to those with normal UAE and suggested a cause-effect relationship between endothelial dysfunction and UAE.

Endothelial dysfunction pay expose hypertensive patients to increased cardiovascular risk.

MICROALBUMINURIA AND CARDIOVASCULAR DISEASE

It is now well recognized that an increase in UAE is associated with an increased incidence of cardiovascular disease and events, including left ventricular hypertrophy [72,73], increased thickness of the carotid artery, myocardial ischeamia [74,75], coronary heart disease [77], peripheral vascular disease [77] stroke [78], and hypertensive retinopathy [79].

In a group of patients with essential hypertension we observed [21] that those patients who displayed an increase in UAE, also manifested an increased thickness of the carotid artery (Fig 3), a recognized marker of atherosclerosis that correlates with the incidence of coronary heart disease. Other investigators have confirmed these findings [80].

In a study of 11 343 non-diabetic hypertensive patients, among patients with microalbuminuria, 31% had coronary artery disease, 24% had left ventricular hypertrophy, 6% had had a stroke, and 7% had peripheral vascular disease. In patients without MAU, these rates were 22%, 14%, 4%, and 5% respectively (P < 0.001). Further, in patients with coronary artery disease, left ventricular hypertrophy, stroke, and peripheral vascular disease, UAE was significantly greater than in patients who did not have these complications (P < 0.001) [8].

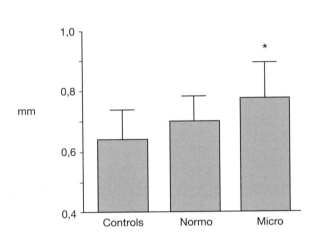

Figure 3. Thickness of the media-intima carotid artery in hypertensive patients with normal urinary albumin excretion (normo), patients with microalbuminuria (micro) and normotensive healthy subjects (control). The difference between patients with microalbuminuria and patients with normal urinary albumin excretion was significant (P<0.01). [From Ref. 80 with permission].

We have shown that hypertensive Individuals with microalbuminuria manifest an Increased prevalence of silent myocardial Ischemia [81].

In a prospective cohort study of 631 subjects aged 50 to 75 years (54% of these patients had impaired glucose tolerance or NIDDM), Jager et al [82] observed that microalbuminuria and peripheral arterial disease were both independent predictors of cardiovascular and all-cause mortality, especially among hypertensive subjects. In a prospective study of 2085 non-diabetic individuals, the relative risk of ischemic heart disease associated with microalbuminuria was 2.3 and was independent of other conventional atherosclerotic risk factors [83].

We performed a retrospective cohort analysis of 141 hypertensive individuals followed-up for approximately 7 years. Fifty-four patients had microalbuminuria and 87 had normal UAE. At baseline, the two groups had similar age, weight and blood pressure, but serum cholesterol, triglycerides, and uric acid were higher and HDL cholesterol lower in patients with microalbuminuria than those with normal UAE. During follow-up, 12 cardiovascular events occurred in the 54 patients with microalbuminuria and only 2 events in the 87 patients with normal UAE. Multiple regression analysis showed that UAE cholesterol and diastolic blood pressure were independent predictors of cardiovascular outcome [84].

In conclusion, the presence of microalbuminuria in patients with essential hypertension carries an increased risk of cardiovascular disease and events.

MICROALBUMINURIA AND NEPHROANGIOSCLEROSIS.

Data from the United States Renal Data System (USRDS) show that over the past decade, the incidence of renal failure as a consequence of essential hypertension has steadily increased. This phenomenon is particularly striking when one considers that substantial progress has been achieved in the treatment of established hypertension and in the prevention of other cardiovascular complications. Can we predict the patients at risk for developing renal failure due to hypertension, and more specifically is microalbuminuria such predictor?

Schmieder and his collaborators [85] followed a group of hypertensive subjects with normal renal function for 6 years and observed no correlation between baseline urinary protein excretion and worsening of renal function. Ruilope et al [86], on the other hand, followed a cohort of hypertensive subjects with and without microalbuminuria for 5 years. Hypertension in these patients was treated with diuretics and β-blockers alone or in combination. Patients with microalbuminuria at the time of baseline evaluation manifested a more rapid decline in renal function than patients without microalbuminuria.

In a retrospective analysis of 141 hypertensive individuals followed for approximately 7 years, we observed a greater decrease of creatinine clearance among hypertensive patients with microalbuminuria than patients with normal UAE (-12.1±2.77 vs. -7.1±0.88 ml/min; P<0.05) [84].

In a large population of non-diabetic subjects, Pinto-Sietsma et al observed an association between UAE and renal function characterized by an elevated creatinine clearance in the stages of slightly elevated albuminuria and a lower creatinine clearance in those individuals with higher UAE. This study suggests that screening for albuminuria may identify non-diabetic subjects who are at risk for developing renal functional loss [87].

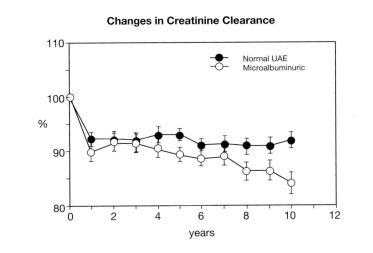

Figure 4 The line graphs show the changes in rate of clearance of creatinine over time for hypertensive patients with microalbuminuria (closed circles) and patients with normal urinary excretion of albumin (open circles). (From Ref. 84 with permission).

REFERENCES

1.   Messent JW, Elliot TG, Hill RG, Jarret RJ, Keen H, Viberti GC. Prognostic significance of microalbuminuria in insulin-dependent diabetes mellitus: a twenty-three-year follow-up study. Kidney Int 1992; 41: 836-839.

2. Mau Pedersen M, Christensen CK, Mogensen CE. Long-term (18 years) prognosis for normo-and microalbuminuric type 1 (insulin-dependent) diabetic patients. Diabetologia 1992; 35: A60.
3. Schmitz A, Vaeth M. Microalbuminuria: a major risk factor in non-insulin-dependent diabetes. A ten-year follow-up study of 503 patients. Diabet Med 1988; 5: 126-134.
4. Gerber LM, Shmukler C, Alderman MH. Differences in urinary albumin excretion rate between normotensive and hypertensive white and non white subjects. Arch Intern Med 1992;152: 373-377.
5. Bigazzi R, Bianchi S, Campese VM, Baldari G. Prevalence of microalbuminuria in a large population of patients with mild to moderate essential hypertension. Nephron 1992; 61: 94-97.
6. Redon J, Liao Y, Lozano JV, Miralles A, Baldo E. Factors related to the presence of microalbuminuria in essential hypertension. Am J Hypertens 1994; 7(9 Pt1): 801-807.
7. Jensen JS, Feldt-Rasmussen B, Borch-Johnson K, Clausen P, Appleyard M, Jensen G. Microalbuminuria and its relation to cardiovascular disease and risk factors. A population-based study of 1254 hypertensive individuals. J Human Hypertens 1997;11:727-732.
8. Agrawal B, Berger A, Wolf K, Luft FC. Microalbuminuria screening by reagent strip predicts cardiovascular risk in hypertension. J Hypertens 1996 Feb;14(2):223-8
9. Pedersen EB, Mogensen CE. Effect of antihypertensive treatment on urinary albumin excretion, glomerular filtration rate, and renal plasma flow in patients with essential hypertension. Scand J Clin Lab Invest 1976; 36: 231-237.
10. Parving HH, Jensen HE, Mogensen CE, Evrin PE. Increased urinary albumin excretion rate in benign essential hypertension. Lancet 1974; i: 1190-1192
11. James A, Fotherby MB, Potter JF. Screening tests for microalbuminuria in non-diabetic elderly subjects and their relation to blood pressure. Clin Sci 1995;88:185-190.
12. West JNW, Gosling P, Dimmitt SB, Littler WA. Non-diabetic microalbuminuria in clinical practice and its relationship to posture, exercise and blood pressure. Cli Sci 1991;81: 373-377.
13. Opsahl JA, Abraham PA, Halstenson CE, Keane WF. Correlation of office and ambulatory blood pressure measurements with urinary albumin and N-acetyl-beta-D-glucosaminidase excretions in essential hypertension. Am J Hypertens 1988;1: S117-S120.
14. Knight EL, Kramer HM, Curhan GC. High-normal blood pressure and microalbuminuria. Am J Kidney Dis 2003;41:588-595.
15. Giaconi S, Levanti C, Fommei E, Innocenti F, Seghieri G, Palla L, Palombo C, Ghione S. Microalbuminuria and casual and ambulatory blood pressure monitoring in normotensives and in patients with borderline and mild essential hypertension. Am J Hypertens 1989; 2:259-26.
16. Cerasola G, Cottone S, Mule G, Nardi E, Mangano MT, Andronico G, Contorno A, Li Vecchi M, Gaglione P, Renda F, Piazza G, Volpe V, Lisi A, Ferrara L, Panepinto N, Riccobene R. Microalbuminuria, renal dysfunction and cardiovascular complication in essential hypertension. J Hypertens 1996;14: 915-920
17. Knight EL, Kramer HM, Curhan GC. High-normal blood pressure and microalbuminuria. Am J Kidney Dis 2003;41:588-595.
18. Bianchi S, Bigazzi R, Baldari G, Sgherri GP, Campese VM. Diurnal variation of blood pressure and microalbuminuria in essential hypertension. Am J Hypertens 1994;7: 23-29.
19. Redon J, Liao Y, Lozano JV, Miralles A, Pasqual JM, Cooper RS. Ambulatory blood pressure and microalbuminuria in essential hypertension: role of circadian variability. J Hypertens 1994; 12: 947-953.

20. Berrut G, Hallab M, Bouhanick B, Chameau AM, Marre M, Fressinaud P. Value of ambulatory blood pressure monitoring in type I (insulin-dependent) diabetic patients with incipient diabetic nephropathy. Am J Hypertens 1994; 7: 222-227.

21. Equiluz-Bruck S, Schnack C, Kopp HP, Schernthaner G. Non dipping of nocturnal blood pressure is related to urinary albumin excretion rate in patients with type 2 diabetes mellitus. Am J Hypertens 1996; 9: 1139-1143.

22. Lurbe E, Redon J, Kesani A, et al: Increase in nocturnal blood pressure and progression to microalbuminuria in type 1 diabetes. New Engl J Med 2002;347:797-805.

23. Bigazzi R, Bianchi S, Nenci R, Baldari D, Baldari G, Campese VM. Increased thickness of the carotid artery in patients with essential hypertension and microalbuminuria. J Hum Hypertens 1995;9: 827-833.

24. Haffner SM, Stern MP, Gruber KK, Hazuda HP, Mitchell BD, Patterson JK. Microalbuminuria. A marker for increased cardiovascular risk factors in nondiabetic subjects? Arteriosclerosis 1990; 10: 727-31.

25. Nosadini R, Cipollina MR, Solini A, Sambataro M, Morocutti A, Doria A, Fioretto P, Brocco E, Muollo B, Frigato F. Close relationship between microalbuminuria and insulin resistance in essential hypertension and non-insulin dependent diabetes mellitus. J Am Soc Nephrol 1992; 3:S56-S63.

26. Mimran A, Ribstein J, DuCailar G. Is microalbuminuria a marker of early intrarenal vascular dysfunction in essential hypertension? Hypertension 1994; 23(part2): 1018-1021.

27. Kaysen GA. Hyperlipidemia of the nephrotic syndrome. Kidney Int 1991;3 (suppl 31): S8-S15.

28. Keane WF, Peter JV St, Kasiske BL. Is the aggressive management of hyperlipidemia in nephrotic syndrome mandatory?. Kidney Int 1992;42 (suppl 38): S134-S141.

29. Newmark SR, Anderson CF, Donadio JV, Ellefson RD. Lipoprotein profiles in adult nephrotics. Mayo Clin Proc 1975; 50: 359-366.

30. Thomas ME, Freestone AL, Persaud JW, Varghese Z, Moorhead JF. Raised lipoprotein(a) [Lp(a)] levels in proteinuric patients. J Am Soc Nephrol 1990; 1: 344A.

31. Jenkins AJ, Steel JS, Janus ED, Best JD. Increased plasma apoprotein(a) levels in IDDM patients with microalbuminuria. Diabetes 1991; 40: 787-790.

32. Kapelrud H, Bangstad HJ, Dahl-Jorgensen K, Berg K, Hanssen KF. Serum Lp(a) lipoprotein concentrations in insulin dependent diabetic patients with microalbuminuria. Brit Med J 1991; 303: 675-678.

33. Keane WF. Lipids and the kidney. Kidney Int 1994; 46: 910-920.

34. Keane WF, Kasiske BL, O'Donnel MP, Kim Y. Hypertension, hyperlipidemia and renal damage. Am J Kidney Dis 1993; 21 (suppl 2): 43-50.

35. Mulec H, Johnson SA, Bjorck S. Relationship between serum cholesterol and diabetic nephropathy. Lancet 1990; i:1537-1538.

36. Tolins JP, Stone BG, Raij L. Interactions of hypercholesterolemia and hypertension in initiation of glomerular injury. Kidney Int 1992; 41:1254-1261.

37. Amatruda JM, Margolis S, Hutchins GM: Type III hyperlipoproteinemia with mesangial foam cells in renal glomeruli. Arch Pathol 1974;98:51-54.

38. Saito T, Sato H, Kudo K, Oikawa S, Shibata T, Hara Y, Yoshinaga K, Sakaguchi H. Lipoprotein glomerulopathy: Glomerular lipoprotein thrombui in a patient with hyperlipoportinemia. Am J Kidney Dis 1989;13:148-153.

39. Oikawa S, Suzuki N, Sakuma E, Saito T, Namai K, Kotake H, Fujii Y, Toyota T. Abnormal lipoprotein and apolipoprotein pattern in lipoprotein glomerulopathy. Am J Kidney Dis 1991;18:553-558.

40. Saito T, Oikawa S, Sato H, Sato T, Ito S, Sasaki J. Lipoprotein glomerulopathy: significance of lipoprotein and ultrastructural features. Kidney Int 1999;55:(Suppl 71):S-37-S41.

41. Klahr S, Schreiner G, Ichikawa I.   The progression of renal disease. New Engl J Med 1988; 318: 1657-1666.

42. Attman PO, Alaupovic P, Samuelsson O. Lipoprotein abnormalities as a risk factor for progressive nondiabetic renal disease. Kidney Int 1999;56(Suppl 71):S-14-S17.

43. Nishida Y, Oda H, Yorioka N. Effect of lipoproteins on mesangial cell proliferation. Kidney Int 1999;56(Suppl 71):S-51-S-53.

44. Park YS, Guijarro C, Kim Y, Massy ZA, Kasiske BL, Keane WF, O'Donnell MP. Lovastatin reduces glomerular pacrophage influx and expression of monocyte chemoattractant protein-1 mRNA in nephrotic rats. Am J Kidney Dis 1998;31:190-194.

45. Hattori M, Nikolic-Paterson DJ, Miyazaki K, Isbel NM, Lan HY, Atkins RC, Kawaguchi H, Ito K. Mechanisms of glomerular macrophage infiltration in lipid-induced renal injury. Kidney Int 1999;55(Suppl 71)S-47-S50.

46. Keane WF, Mulcahy WS, Kasiske BL, Kim Y, O'Donnell MP. Hyperlipidemia and progressive renal disease. Kidney Int 1991; 39 (Suppl 31): S41-S48.

47. Jandeleit-Dahm K, Cao Z, Cox AJ, Kelly DJ, Gilbert RE, Cooper ME. Role of hyperlipidemia in progressive renal disease: focus on diabetic nephropathy. Kidney Int 1999;56(Suppl 71):S-31-S-36.

48. Oda H, Keane WF. Recent advances in statins and the kidney. Kidney Int 1999;56(Suppl 71):S-2-S-5.

49. Ferrannini E, Buzzigoli G, Bonadonna R, Giorico MA, Oleggini M, Graziadei L, Pedrinelli R, Brandi L, Bevilacqua S. Insulin resistence in essential hypertension. N Eng J Med 1987; 317: 350-357.

50. Swislocki AL, Hoffman BB, Reaven GM. Insulin resistance, glucose intolerance and hyperinsulinemia in patients with hypertension. Am J Hypertens 1989; 2: 419-423

51. Fuller JH, Shipley MJ, Rose G, Jarret RJ, Keen H. Coronary heart disease risk and impaired glucose tolerance: The Whitehall Study. Lancet 1980; i: 1373-1376.

52. Bianchi S, Bigazzi R, Valtriani C, Chiapponi I, Sgherri G, Baldari G, Natali A, Ferrannini E Campese VM. Elevated serum insulin levels in patients with essential hypertension and microalbuminuria. Hypertension 1994;23: 681-687.

53. Bianchi S, Bigazzi R, Quinones Galvan A, Muscelli E, Baldari G, Pecori N, Ciociaro D, Ferranini E, Natali A. Insulin resistance in microalbuminuric hypertension: sites and mechanism. Hypertension 1995; 26: 789-795.

54. Doria A, Fioretto P, Avogaro A, Carraro A, Morocutti A, Trevisan R, Frigato F, Crepaldi G, Viberti GC, Nosadini R. Insulin resistance is associated with high sodium-lithium countertransport in essential hypertension. Am J Physiol 1991;261: 684-691.

55. Falkner B, Kushner H, Levison S, Canessa M. Albuminuria in association with insulin and sodium-lithium countertransport in young african americans with borderline hypertension. Hypertension 1995;25: 1315-1321.

56. Kuusisto J, Mykkanen L, Pyorealea K, Laakso M. Hyperinsulinemic microalbuminuria. A new risk indicator for coronary heart disease. Circulation 1995; 9: 831-837.

57. Ferrari P, Weidmann P, Shaw S, Giachino D, Riesen W, Alleman Y, Heynen G. Altered insulin sensitivity, hyperinsulinemia, and dyslipidemia in individuals with a hypertensive parent. Am J Med 1991;91:589-596.

58. Grunfeld B, Balzareti M, Romo M, Gimenez M, Gutman R. Hyperinsulinemia in normotensive offspring of hypertensive parents. Hypertension 1994; 231 (Suppl 1): I12-I15.

59. Cruz AB, Amatuzio DS, Grande F, Hay LJ. Effect of intraarterial insulin on tissue cholesterol and fatty acids in alloxan diabetic dogs. Circ Res 1961; 9: 39-43

60. Capron L, Jarnet J, Kazandjian S, Housset E. Growth promoting effects of diabetes and insulin on arteries. Diabetes 1988; 35: 973-978.

61. Oppenheumer MJ Sundquist K, Bierman EL. Down-regulation of high-density lipoprotein receptor in human fibroblats by insulin and IGF-I. Diabetes 1989; 38: 117-122.

62. Krone W, Greten H. Evidence for post-transcriptional regulation by insulin of 3 Hydroxy-3-methylglutaryl coenzyme A reductase and sterol synthesis in human mononuclear leucocytes. Diabetologia1984; 26:366-369.

63. DeFronzo RA, Cooke CR, Andres R, Faloona GR, David PJ. The effect of insulin on renal handling of sodium, potassium, calcium, and phosphate in man. J Clin Invest 1975; 55: 845-855.

64. Christensen NJ, Gundersen HJG, Hegedus L, Jacobsen F, Mogensen CE, Osterby R, Vittinghus E. Acute effects of insulin on plasma noradrenaline and the cardiovascular system. Metabolism 1980; 29: 1138-1145.

65. Bigazzi R, Bianchi S, Baldari D, Sgherri G, Baldari G, Campese VM. Microalbuminuria in salt-sensitive patients: a marker for renal and cardiovascular risk factors. Hypertension 1994; 23: 195-199.

66. Hilsted J, Christensen NJ. Dual effect of insulin on plasma volume and transcapillary albumin transport. Diabetologia 1992; 35: 99-103.

67. Elliot TG, Cockcroft JR, Groop PH, Viberti GC, Ritter JM. Inhibition of nitric oxide synthesis in forearm vasculature of insulin-dependent diabetic patients: blunted vasocontriction in patients with microalbuminuria. Clin Sci 1993; 83: 687-693.

68. Stehouwer CDA, Nauta JJP, Zeldenrust GC, Hackeng WHL, Donker AJM, den Ottolander GJH. Urinary albumin excretion, cardiovascular disease, and endothelial dysfunction in non-insulin dependent diabetes mellitus. Lancet 1992; 340: 319-323.

69. Pedrinelli R Giampietro O, Carmassi F, et al: Microalbuminuria and endothelial dysfunction in essential hypertension. Lancet 1994;344:14-18.

70. Tedgui A, Merval R, Esposito. Albumin transport characteristics of rat aorta in early phase of hypertension. Clin Res 1995;71:932-942.

71. Cottone S, Vadala' A, Mangano MT, et al. Endothelium-derived factors in microalbuminuric and normoalbuminuric essential hypertensives. Am J Hypertens 2000;13:172-176.

72. Redon J, Gomez-Sanchez MA, Baldo E, Casal MC, Fernandez ML, Miralles A, Gomez-Pajuelo C, Rodicio JL, Ruilope LM. Microalbuminuria is correlated with left ventricular hypertrophy in male hypertensive patients. J Hypertens 1991; 9 (Suppl.6): S148-S149.

73. Pedrinelli R, Bello VD, Catapano G, Talarico L, Materazzi F, Santoro G, Giusti C, Mosca F, Melillo E, Ferrari M. Microalbuminuria is a marker of left ventricular hypertrophy but not hyperinsulinemia in non diabetic atherosclerotic patients. Arteriosclerosis and Thrombosis 1993; 13: 900-906.

74. Agewall S, Persson B, Samuelsson O, Ljungman S, Herlitz H, Fageberg B. Microalbuminuria in treated hypertensive men at high risk of coronary disease. The Risk Factor Intervention Study Group. J Hypertens 1993;11: 461-469.

75. Horton RC, Gosling P, Reeves CN, Payne M, Nagle RE. Microalbumin excretion in patients with positive exercise electrocardiogram tests. Eur Heart J 1994; 15: 1353-1355.

76. Kuusisto J, Mykkanen L, Pyorealea K, Laakso M. Hyperinsulinemic microalbuminuria. A new risk indicator for coronary heart disease. Circulation 1995; 9: 831-837.

799

77. Yudkin JS, Forrest RD, Jackson CA. Microalbuminuria as predictor of vascular disease in non-diabetic subjects. Islington Diabetes Survey. Lancet 1988; ii: 530-533.
78. Damsgaard EL, Froland A, Jorgensen OD, Mogensen CE. Prognostic value of urinary albumin excretion rate and other risk factors in elderly diabetic patients and non-diabetic control subjects surviving the first 5 years after assessment. Diabetologia 1993;36:1030-1036.
79. Cerasola G, Cottone S, D'Ignoto G, Grasso L, Mangano MT, Carapelle E, Nardi E, Andronico G, Fulantelli MA, Marcellino T, Seddio G. Micro-albuminuria as a predictor of cardiovascular damage in essential hypertension. J Hypertens 1989; 7(suppl 6) : S332-S333.
80. Mykkanen L, Zaccaro DJ, O'Leary D, Howard G, Robbins DC, Haffner SM. Microalbuminuria and carotid artery intima-media thickness in nondiabetic and NIDDM subjects. Stroke 1997;28:1710-1716.
81. Bianchi S, Bigazzi R, Campese VM. Silent ischemia is more prevalent among hypertensive patients with microalbuminuria and salt sensitivity. J Hum Hypertens 2003;17:13-20.
82. Jager A, Kostense PJ, Ruhe' HG, Heine RJ, Nijpels G, Dekker JM, Bouter LM, Stehouwer CDA. Microalbuminuria and peripheral arterial disease are independent predictors of cardiovascular and all-cause mortality, especially among hypertensive subjects. Five-year follow-up of the Hoorn study. Arterioscler Thromb Vasc Biol 1999;19:617-624.
83. Borch-Johnsen K, Feldt-Rasmussen B, Strandgaard S, Scroll M, Jensen JS. Urinary albumin excretion: an independent predictor of ischemic heart disease. Arterioscler Thromb Vasc Biol 1999;19:1992-1997
84. Bigazzi R, Bianchi S, Baldari G, Campese VM. Microalbuminuria predicts cardiovascular and renal insufficiency in patients with hypertension. J Hypertens 1998; 16: 1325-1333.
85. Schmieder RE, Veelken R, Gatzka CD, Ruddel H, Schachinger H. Predictors for hypertensive nephropathy: results of a 6-year follow-up study in essential hypertension. J Hypertens 1994; 13: 357-365.
86. Ruilope LM, Campo C, Rodriguez-Artalejo F, Lahera V, Garcia Robles R, Rodicio JL. Blood pressure and renal function: therapeutic implications. J Hypertens 1996; 14: 1259-1263.
87. Pinto-Sietsma SJ, Janssen WMT, Hillege HL, navis G, De Zeeuw D, De Jong PE. Urinary albumin excretion is associated with renal functional abnormalities in a nondiabetic population. J Am Soc Nephrol 2000; 11:1882-1888.

42

A COMPARISON OF PROGRESSION IN DIABETIC AND NON-DIABETIC RENAL DISEASE: SIMILARITY OF PROGRESSION PROMOTERS

Gerjan Navis[1,2], Peter T. Luik[1], Dick De Zeeuw[2,1,] Paul E De Jong[1].

Department of Internal Medicine, Division of Nephrology[1] and Department of Clinical Pharmacology[2], University Medical Center, Groningen, The Netherlands.

The prevention of progressive renal function loss remains the major challenge for nephrologists today. Traditionally the progressive nature of renal function loss was attributed to the underlying disease, with a major role for hypertension [1]. The hypothesis, however, that common mechanisms account for progressive renal function loss in many different renal conditions regardless the nature of initial renal damage [2] was fueled by several observations. These include the linear renal function deterioration that occurs in many patients regardless their initial renal disease [3], as well as the similarity in histopathological abnormalities in end-stage kidneys with different underlying diseases. Systemic [4] and glomerular [5] hypertension, proteinuria [6] and lipid abnormalities [7] are assumed to be common mediators in the pathogenesis of focal segmental glomerulosclerosis, the alleged final common pathway of progressive renal disease [8]. Here we will briefly review current knowledge on progressive renal function loss in human diabetic and non-diabetic renal disease and on the response to intervention treatment. We will focus on clinical evidence regarding the hypothesis that common mechanisms underlie progressive renal function loss in diabetic and non-diabetic renal disease; this will help to devise future prevention strategies.

NATURAL HISTORY

The initiation and progression of renal damage.

In IDDM the natural history of nephropathy is well-characterized, as, contrary to non-diabetic renal disease and partly NIDDM, most patients come to medical attention years before renal abnormalities develop. It is still not understood why some 30 to 40 per cent of diabetic patients develop nephropathy whereas others don't; familial clustering, however, since long suggests genetically determined susceptibility [9;10] and indeed, for NIDDM genetic factors presdisposing to nephropathy were recently identified [11]. In diabetic patients that develop nephropathy, a typical, biphasic clinical course of renal function occurs, with elevated GFR in the early stages, followed by micro-albuminuria [12;13]. The elevated GFR presumably reflects glomerular hypertension, due to afferent arteriolar dysfunction with increased transmission of systemic pressure to glomerular capillaries. The ensuing glomerular capillary damage and protein leakage are important mechanisms in initiation and perpetuation of renal damage in these patients [14]. These functional abnormalities are accompanied by renal and glomerular enlargement [15]. The transition from normoalbuminuria to microalbuminuria is associated with a slight increase in systemic blood pressure [16]. When micro-albuminuria progresses to overt proteinuria, usually in association with a further rise in arterial blood pressure, glomerular filtration rate decreases, and gradual progression to end-stage renal failure occurs, albeit with large interindividual differences in progression rate [12]. In NIDDM the sequence of events in development of nephropathy is somewhat more complicated to unravel, as patients present at a later stage, often have pre-existent hypertension, and moreover renal abnormalities are already present in a considerable proportion of the patients by the time diabetes is diagnosed. Yet, recent data support a bifasic course of GFR in NIDDM as well [13]. Moreover, data in a cohort of NIDDM patients normotensive at diagnosis support the concordance of albuminuria and a rise in blood pressure during follow-up in this population as well [17].

In non-diabetic renal disease the factors that initiate renal damage are heterogeneous, and can include primarily glomerular or vascular, or tubulo-interstitial damage. Little is known about possible factors preceding the development of non-diabetic renal disease, as by the time patients come to medical attention overt renal damage is usually present. Patients with hypertension may be an exception. Remarkably, microalbuminuria [18] as well as glomerular hyperfiltration [19], two hallmarks of incipient diabetic nephropathy, occur in subsets of patients with essential hypertension. In the general population an association between high-normal blood pressure and albuminuria was observed as well [20]. Interestingly, in the general population we observed a biphasic relationship between albuminuria and creatinine clearance with a striking similarity to the pattern in diabetes, with an association between hyperfiltration and micro-albuminuria or high high-normal albumin excretion and hypofiltration becoming more prevalent among those with microalbuminuria [21]. Whereas in non-diabetic populations the prognostic value of microalbuminuria and glomerular hyperfiltration for long term renal function are not yet established, nevertheless, these data suggest that the sequence of events in diabetic and nephropathy also occurs in at least some forms of non-diabetic renal damage.

The contribution of factors specific for the underlying disease as determinants of progression rate relative to common factors is not equivocal - and probably not uniform -across different renal conditions. In diabetes, the impact of glycemic control on renal prognosis in IDDM and NIDDM represents a clear-cut diagnosis-specific renal risk factor [22;23]. In non-diabetic patients, studies on the role of the underlying disorder provide conflicting data, with no effect of underlying disease on progression rate in some studies [3;24], whereas other studies found a faster progression rate in glomerulonephritis and diabetic nephropathy than in chronic pyelonephritis, analgesic nephropathy or hypertensive nephrosclerosis [6;25-30]. In most studies, polycystic kidney disease is associated with a faster progression rate as well [27;30-33] although not uniformly so [6;19]. Taken together, the nature of the underlying disease appears not to be indifferent to the rate of long-term renal function loss. Of note, in conditions where the primary cause of damage can be reliably eliminated (such as obstructive uropathy, analgesic abuse, or primary hypertension) the course of renal function is more favorable than in conditions where the initiating factors cannot (or not reliably) be annihilated (e.g diabetic nephropathy, glomerulonephritis, or polycystic kidney disease). This suggests that either primary causes still exert effect, or that they trigger the alleged common perpetuating factors to a greater extent than other conditions.

Whereas in nephropathy due to IDDM, linear progression appears to be the rule [34], in non-diabetic renal disease [6;31] or NIDDM [35], considerable subpopulations [up to 20-25% of the patients] may have stable renal function or non-linear progression. Such a heterogeneity in patient populations might partly explain the difficulties in reproducing clear-cut renoprotective effects obtained by specific treatment modalities in experimental animals, in particular for nondiabetic renal disease [6;36].

Common progression promoters

In diabetic as well as non-diabetic populations [3] considerable interindividual variability is apparent in the rate of renal function loss for any given disease. Many studies investigated the determinants of this variability (see also Table 1), evaluating the clinical relevance of common progression promoters identified in experimental renal disease, such as systemic and glomerular hypertension, proteinuria, lipid abnormalities, obesity, low grade inflammation and smoking.

In the interpretation of these studies, however, the close interaction of these factors as to their effects on long-term renal function [2] should be kept in mind. As a consequence, their respective contributions are often hard to dissect.

In both diabetic [37;38] and non-diabetic renal disease [6;32;33;39] the severity of proteinuria is a predictive factor for progression rate. Interestingly, Wight [32] showed that differences in progression rate between most renal conditions were no longer apparent after correction for proteinuria (with the sole exception of polycystic kidney disease). Moreover, the association between proteinuria and progression not only occurs in conditions where proteinuria might reflect activity of the primary glomerular disorder, such as diabetic nephropathy and glomerulonephritis, but also in chronic pyelonephritis [6].

Taken together, this evidence strongly suggests that, once a certain renal disorder is present, the severity of proteinuria rather than the underlying disorder per se predicts renal outcome. The case of polycystic kidney disease however, illustrates that disease-specific mechanisms may predominate over common mechanisms in some conditions [40;41].

Importantly, the reduction of proteinuria at onset of antihypertensive therapy predicts the subsequent course of renal function, in both non-diabetic [42] and diabetic [43] proteinuric renal patients. Remarkably, this is independent of the way the reduction of proteinuria was achieved [i.e. drug therapy or low protein diet [33;44] or class of drug [42]]. For therapeutic purposes, importantly, this allows early identification of patients who need more aggressive renoprotective intervention. The pathophysiological basis of the prognostic impact of antiproteinuric response is likely to be twofold. First, the reduction in proteinuria identifies subjects with less severe renal structural damage – as suggested by retrospective data in man [45], and by prospective data in experimental proteinuria [46].

Table 1. Clinical characteristics of progressive renal function loss in diabetic and non-diabetic renal disease

	Diabetic nephropathy	*Non-diabetic nephropathy*
Natural history		
Course of renal hemodynamics	Typically biphasic	Possibly biphasic in some conditions
Renal function loss	Invariably progressive	Progressive in many patients.
predictors of progression	Diabetes control Proteinuria Blood pressure Cholesterol DD genotype ACE gene *Obesity [NIDDM]?* Smoking Low-grade inflammation?	Underlying disease Proteinuria Blood pressure Cholesterol DD genotype ACE gene Obesity Smoking Low-grade inflammation?
Prevention of progressive renal function loss		
Protein restriction	Probably effective	Effective
Antihypertensive therapy	Effective	Effective; benefit proportional to severity of proteinuria.
Predictors	Initial antiproteinuric effect	Initial antiproteinuric effect
Renoprotection	Initial renal hemodynamic effect	Initial renal hemodynamic effect
Response to specific renoprotective drugs		
ACE inhibitors/ AT1 blockers	Reduce proteinuria Reduce progression rate Independent from blood pressure effect	Reduce proteinuria Reduce progression rate Independent from blood pressure effect
Non-ACE inhibitor antihypertensives	Reduce proteinuria in a strongly pressure-dependent fashion	Slight, pressure-dependent effect on proteinuria

Although difficult to substantiate prospectively in man, these data would implicate that renoprotective efficacy could be optimized by starting as early as possible in the course of the disease, which can be considered in line with the data in diabetic subjects – where ACE inhibition has been shown to be effective not only in the treatment, but also in the prevention of progression towards nephropathy [47]. Second, a poor antiproteinuric response leads to a higher residual proteinuria, which in turn further aggravates renal damage. In addition to the early antiproteinuric response, also the early response of glomerular filtration to antihypertensive therapy predicts the subsequent course of renal function in diabetic as well as non-diabetic patients [42] with a more favorable course in subjects with a slight initial drop in filtration - presumably reflecting a drop in filtration pressure . Again, this predictive effect does not depend on the mode of intervention, as it occurs irrespective of the class of drug (i.e ACEi or beta-blocker) and also applies to the early response to low protein diet [44].

As to hypertension, in IDDM the development of hypertension is closely associated with transition from normoalbuminuria to microalbuminuria [16] and subsequently with further progression to overt proteinuria and progressive renal function loss [48-50]. In NIDDM, the timecourse is less extensively documented, and presumably more diverse, as almost half of the patients is hypertensive at the time of diagnosis [51], yet blood pressure was found as a major risk factor for the progression to diabetic nephropathy [17;52]. In non-diabetic renal disease also, high blood pressure is usually associated with a poor renal outcome [24;27;32;33], and moreover, the antihypertensive response to treatment is associated with reduction of the rate of renal function loss [4]. Blood pressure was a strong predictor for end stage renal failure in the large MRFIT cohort [53]. Yet, somewhat surprisingly, several studies in renal patients failed to demonstrate that blood pressure was an independent determinant of progression rate [6;26;27]. In these studies, however, proteinuria and blood pressure were closely related and a predominant effect of proteinuria might obscure the role of a co-linear factor such as blood pressure.

Lipid profile is increasingly recognized as relevant to progression rate. An elevated serum cholesterol is associated with a faster progression rate in IDDM [54;55], NIDDM [17] and non-diabetic renal diseases [42;56]. There is no definitive proof however, that this reflects an independent effect of lipids - as patients with more severe hyperlipidemia also tend to be the ones with the more severe proteinuria [57].

Morbid obesity - usually associated with impaired glucose tolerance, insulin resistance or overt diabetes - is a well-known cause for so-called obesity-related glomerulopathy, a proteinuric condition with glomerular enlargement and eventually glomerulosclerosis [58]. Recent data support a role for less extreme obesity as a risk enhancer in primary renal conditions as well, i.e, IgA nephropathy [59], after unilateral nephrectomy [60] and in renal transplant patients [61], albeit not uniformly so [62]. Elevated filtration pressure is likely to be involved as a mechanism, as suggested by the elevated GFR and filtration fraction in morbidly obese subjects and in obese hypertensives [63;64]. This may promote proteinuria – as suggested by the beneficial effects of weight reduction on proteinuria in both non-diabetic and diabetic subjects [65]. Remarkably the association between higher BMI and elevated filtration fraction is already present in moderately overweight subjects [66], suggesting that on a population basis the impact of excess body weight on renal risk may be larger than recognized. Considering the diabetes-like renal abnormalities in obesity and the alleged role of insulin resistance, one might expect BMI to be a prominent renal risk factor in diabetes as well – at least in NIDDM. However, data are not uniform. Whereas Ravid et al found that higher BMI predicted faster progression towards albuminuria [17] – Lee at al reported a negative association between overweight and renal failure in NIDDM [52] – a discrepancy that may partly be explained by competing cardiovascular and renal risks. In IDDM - where overweight is less prevalent - the role of BMI as a renal risk factor has not been well-defined – and is likely to be more complex considering the interactions between glycemic control and body weight.

Association studies suggested that low-grade inflammation might be associated with progressive renal function loss in diabetic [67;68] as well as non-diabetic renal disease [69] and in the general population. A post-hoc analysis of the MDRD-study, however, reported that higher CRP (and leptin) was not an independent risk factor for the progression of non-diabetic kidney disease [70]. Further prospective studies are needed in this respect.

Smoking is increasingly recognized as a renal risk factor, as reviewed recently [71]. In type I [72] and type II diabetes mellitus [73] smoking accelerates the rate of progression from microalbuminuria to macroalbuminuria and rate of progressive renal function loss. Prospective data in IDDM, however, could not confirm this [74]. In non-diabetic subjects, smoking was associated with renal risk as well [75], in hypertensive renal damage [76-78], as well as renal transplant recipients. [79] Moreover, smoking is associated with albuminuria and a biphasic renal function pattern in the general population [80].

The recent developments in genetics provide a basis to unravel the genetic factors underlying in the interindividual difference in the progression of renal diseases. So far, most data are available on the insertion/deletion polymorphism of the ACE-gene, which was found to be a determinant of the rate of renal function loss in patients with nondiabetic [81] as well as diabetic nephropathy [82-84] with an increased rate of renal function loss in patients homozygous for the D-allele. However, the results from different studies are far from uniform, which should not come as a surprise for the role of a common genetic variant in a multifactorial condition like progressive renal function loss. Rather, this prompts to identify the conditions that allow this genetic variant to exert a pathophysiologically relevant effect. In this respect, it may be significant that a large prospective study in type I diabetes mellitus, found the D-allele to be a risk factor for progression of diabetic nephropathy especially when glycemic control was poor [85] suggesting gene-environment interaction with glycemic status. These data are in line with our observations on angI responses in uncomplicated IDDM, that also showed interaction between ACE-genotype and glycemic control [86]. Moreover, interaction with sodium status was observed, which is in line with prior observations in non-diabetic subjects, where high sodium intake elicited differences in the responses of blood pressure and proteinuria to ACEi between the different genotypes [87]. The interaction between ACE genotype and sodium intake was confirmed in a prospective study on angI responses in healthy volunteers [88]. Data on the clinical impact of ACE genotype on the antiproteinuric response to ACE inhibition are so far conflicting in non-diabetic as well as diabetic patients and suggest impact of interaction with other factors, such as sodium status, and gender. [87;89;90]. [91;92]. Further studies will have to elucidate the nature of these interactions.

RESPONSE TO RENOPROTECTIVE TREATMENT

As a matter of clinical common sense, renoprotective treatment should, first, aim at eliminating primary damaging factors. This may halt progression in some patients with specific disorders, such as obstructive uropathy [6] and analgesic nephropathy [93]. In diabetes, strict metabolic control can reverse early hyperfiltration, and retard the progression of renal function loss [22].

Progressive renal function loss in the large proportion of patients in whom the initial cause of renal damage is no longer present [3], however, prompted the development of additional treatment strategies aimed at intervention with factors thought to be involved in the alleged final common pathway for progressive renal function loss; i.e, systemic and glomerular pressure, proteinuria and lipid abnormalities.

Intervention studies have focussed on reduction of blood pressure and reduction of protein intake. Reduction of blood pressure has proven a cornerstone of renoprotective intervention in non-diabetic and diabetic renal disease [4;24;57]. Restriction of dietary protein intake has elicited extensive discussions as to its efficacy and feasibility - but all in all it appears that a well-kept low protein diet indeed retards the rate of renal function loss on non-diabetic and diabetic renal patients [94;95]. Increasing evidence supports the role of reduction of proteinuria as a mechanism of renoprotection, in diabetic and non-diabetic renal disease. As already mentioned above, the reduction in proteinuria at onset of treatment predicts subsequent renoprotective efficacy in non-diabetic as well as diabetic subjects. Moreover, drug regimens that reduce proteinuria more effectively invariably provide more effective long-term renoprotection.

The question whether RAS-blockade, by virtue of its specific renal effects, offers better renoprotection than other antihypertensives has long been subject of debate. Experimental data long since supported the assumption of specific renoprotective effects of RAS-blockade, [96] and in man renoprotective effects beyond reduction of blood pressure were supported by studies in normotensive diabetic patients where ACE inhibition was able to reverse microalbuminuria [97] and to prevent progression to overt proteinuria [98;99]. Moreover, in both diabetic and non-diabetic patients ACE inhibitors can reduce proteinuria [100;100;101], progression rate [102] and the risk to reach end stage renal failure or death [57] Nevertheless, the interpretation as to specific renal effects was hampered by the slightly more effective blood pressure reduction by the ACE-inhibitor regimens [57;103].

The results of several recent large clinical trials now allow the conclusion that indeed RAS-blockade has specific renoprotective effects in addition to its effects on blood pressure. This applies to both ACE-inhibition and AT1-blockade, and has been demonstrated in diabetic as well as non-diabetic renal damage [104-107]. Across these different studies, the better renoprotective effect is consistently explained by the better antiproteinuric efficacy of the RAS-blockers.

Several important insights have been gained from the large intervention trials of the last decade. First, importantly, in non-diabetic patients the long-term benefit of lower blood pressure (whether or not achieved with ACE inhibitors) on renal function was more pronounced in proteinuric patients [108-111]. Thus, like diabetic patients [in whom proteinuria is the hallmark of renal involvement], proteinuric patients with non-diabetic renal disease display greater renal sensitivity to the effect of elevated systemic blood pressure than their non-proteinuric counterparts. Whether this similarity simply reflects the long-term benefits of reduction of proteinuria secondary to the lower blood pressure, or whether proteinuria is a marker (or even a mediator) of the susceptibility of the glomerular vascular bed to hypertensive damage is as yet unknown. Second, the specific benefit of RAS-blockade over other modes of antihypertensive therapy appears to be proportional to the severity of proteinuria across non-diabetic and diabetic populations [112-114] [104] Finally, recent studies have shown that dual blockade of the RAS reduces proteinuria and progression rate more effectively than monotherapy with ACE inhibitor or AT1 blockade [115-117].

Individual differences in the response to renoprotective intervention.

In spite of the major improvements in renoprotective treatment, nevertheless in many patients the response to antihypertensive and antiproteinuric intervention is suboptimal, with residual proteinuria, and consequently ongoing renal function loss. In fact, the interindividual differences in responsiveness to antiproteinuric intervention by far exceed the differences in efficacy between different regimens – which is in line with a well-designed analysis in essential hypertension [118] This notion – which is often overlooked – underlines the importance of unravelling the mechanisms underlying individual differences in responsiveness to therapy. By applying different treatment schedules in the same patients, we could demonstrate that responsiveness to antiproteinuric intervention is indeed an individual characteristic – both in non-diabetic and diabetic nephropathy. The individual differences were not altered by increasing the dose of the ACE inhibitor, by increasing the dose of the AT1 blocker, or by switching from one class to the other – or even by switching to NSAID [119]. The difference between good and poor responders persisted when the mean response for the group was unaltered, but, remarkably, also when the mean response for the group was enhanced by dose increase or dietary sodium restriction. In other words, manoeuvres that enhance therapy response at group level do not make the poor responders catch up with the good responders –

neither in diabetic, nor in non-diabetic proteinuric patients [120]. Thus, in order to improve renoprotective efficacy in poor responders, other modes of intervention, and combined intervention in different pathophysiological pathways will be have to be explored [121].

CONCLUSIONS AND IMPLICATIONS FOR RENOPROTECTIVE TREATMENT

Promoters for progression in patients with diabetic and non-diabetic nephropathy display striking similarities. Moreover, predictors for efficacy of long-term renoprotective therapy are similar as well. This supports the hypothesis that common mechanisms underlie progressive renal function loss in diabetic and many non-diabetic renal patients, with the possible exception of specific diagnostic categories, such as polycystic kidneys [34], where disease-specific mechanisms may be the main determinants of progression. The similarities are most readily apparent for patients with proteinuria, supporting the assumption that proteinuria is pivotal in the alleged common mechanisms [8].

Several implications for renoprotective treatment can be derived from the current evidence. First, to provide renoprotection in proteinuric patients (with or without diabetes) target blood pressure should be lower than in non-proteinuric patients. For diabetic patients the need for a low target blood pressure has already gained general acceptance [122]. For non-diabetic proteinuric patients, data from the MDRD study demonstrated that the lowest mean arterial pressure attained ($\leq$92 mmHg, corresponding to 125/75 mmHg) provided improved renoprotection, without signs of a J-shape pattern[123]. From a renal perspective, therefore, target mean arterial blood pressure in proteinuric patients may have to be even lower than 90 mmHg. For such an aggressive approach to be feasible, short-term titration criteria predictive for long-term renoprotection are indispensable - but fortunately, reduction of proteinuria is a consistent predictor for long term outcome, in diabetic as well as non-diabetic patients. The latter suggests that specific titration for reduction of proteinuria may allow to further improve renoprotective efficacy in diabetic as well as non-diabetic patients, and it is recommended that future studies explore the renoprotective potential of specific titration for proteinuria reduction.

Studies including hard end-points have demonstrated that regimens based on RAS-blockade provide better reduction of proteinuria and consequently renoprotection – and recent data indicate that dual blockade of the RAS may even be more effective. Nevertheless, therapeutic benefit is still suboptimal in a substantial proportion of the patients – and exploration of regimens combining blockade in different pathophysiological pathways may provide a strategy to further improve the efficacy of long-term renoprotection.

REFERENCES

1   Ellis A. Natural history of Bright's disease; clinical, histological and experimental observations. The vicious circle in Bright's disease. Lancet 1942; i:72-76.

2   Klahr S, Schreiner G, Ichikawa I. The progression of renal disease. N Engl J Med 1988; 318(25):1657-1666.

3   Mitch WE, Walser M, Buffington GA, Lemann J, Jr. A simple method of estimating progression of chronic renal failure. Lancet 1976; 2(7999):1326-1328.

4   Alvestrand A, Gutierrez A, Bucht H, Bergstrom J. Reduction of blood pressure retards the progression of chronic renal failure in man. Nephrol Dial Transplant 1988; 3(5):624-631.

5   Brenner BM, Meyer TW, Hostetter TH. Dietary protein intake and the progressive nature of kidney disease: the role of hemodynamically mediated glomerular injury in the pathogenesis of progressive glomerular sclerosis in aging, renal ablation, and intrinsic renal disease. N Engl J Med 1982; 307(11):652-659.

6   Williams PS, Fass G, Bone JM. Renal pathology and proteinuria determine progression in untreated mild/moderate chronic renal failure. Q J Med 1988; 67(252):343-354.

7   Keane WF, Kasiske BL, O'Donnell MP, Kim Y. The role of altered lipid metabolism in the progression of renal disease: experimental evidence. Am J Kidney Dis 1991; 17(5 Suppl 1):38-42.

8   Remuzzi G, Bertani T. Is glomerulosclerosis a consequence of altered glomerular permeability to macromolecules? (editorial). Kidney Int 1990; 38(3):384-394.

9   Seaquist ER, Goetz FC, Rich S, Barbosa J. Familial clustering of diabetic kidney disease. Evidence for genetic susceptibility to diabetic nephropathy (see comments). N Engl J Med 1989; 320(18):1161-1165.

10   Tarnow L. Genetic pattern in diabetic nephropathy. Nephrol Dial Transplant 1996; 11(3):410-412.

11   Vardarli I, Baier LJ, Hanson RL, Akkoyun I, Fischer C, Rohmeiss P et al. Gene for susceptibility to diabetic nephropathy in type 2 diabetes maps to 18q22.3-23. Kidney Int 2002; 62(6):2176-2183.

12   Mogensen CE. Natural history and potential prevention of diabetic nephropathy in insulin-dependent and non-insulin-dependent diabetic patients. In: El Nahas A, Mallick NP, Anderson S, editors. Prevention of progressive chronic renal failure. Oxford, 1993: 278-279.

13   Vora JP, Dolben J, Dean JD, Thomas D, Williams JD, Owens DR et al. Renal hemodynamics in newly presenting non-insulin dependent diabetes mellitus. Kidney Int 1992; 41(4):829-835.

14   Parving HH, Kastrup H, Smidt UM, Andersen AR, Feldt-Rasmussen B, Christiansen JS. Impaired autoregulation of glomerular filtration rate in type 1 (insulin-dependent) diabetic patients with nephropathy. Diabetologia 1984; 27(6):547-552.

15   Feldt-Rasmussen B, Hegedus L, Mathiesen ER, Deckert T. Kidney volume in type 1 (insulin-dependent) diabetic patients with normal or increased urinary albumin excretion: effect of long-term improved metabolic control. Scand J Clin Lab Invest 1991; 51(1):31-36.

16   Poulsen PL, Hansen KW, Mogensen CE. Ambulatory blood pressure in the transition from normo- to microalbuminuria: a longitudinal study in IDDM. Diabetes 1994; 43(10):1248-1253.

17   Ravid M, Brosh D, Ravid-Safran D, Levy Z, Rachmani R. Main risk factors for nephropathy in type 2 diabetes mellitus are plasma cholesterol levels, mean blood pressure, and hyperglycemia. Arch Intern Med 1998; 158(9):998-1004.

18   Parving HH, Mogensen CE, Jensen HA, Evrin PE. Increased urinary albumin-excretion rate in benign essential hypertension. Lancet 1974; 1(7868):1190-1192.

19   du CG, Ribstein J, Mimran A. Glomerular hyperfiltration and left ventricular mass in mild never- treated essential hypertension. J Hypertens Suppl 1991; 9(6):S158-S159.

20   Knight EL, Kramer HM, Curhan GC. High-normal blood pressure and microalbuminuria. Am J Kidney Dis 2003; 41(3):588-595.

21   Pinto-Sietsma SJ, Janssen WM, Hillege HL, Navis G, de Zeeuw D, de Jong PE. Urinary albumin excretion is associated with renal functional abnormalities in a nondiabetic population. J Am Soc Nephrol 2000; 11(10):1882-1888.

22   Effect of intensive therapy on the development and progression of diabetic nephropathy in the Diabetes Control and Complications Trial. The Diabetes Control and Complications (DCCT) Research Group. Kidney Int 1995; 47(6):1703-1720.

23   Stratton IM, Adler AI, Neil HA, Matthews DR, Manley SE, Cull CA et al. Association of glycaemia with macrovascular and microvascular complications of type 2 diabetes (UKPDS 35): prospective observational study. BMJ 2000; 321(7258):405-412.

24   Brazy PC, Fitzwilliam JF. Progressive renal disease: role of race and antihypertensive medications. Kidney Int 1990; 37(4):1113-1119.

25   Ahlem J. Incidence of human chronic renal insufficiency. A study of the incidence and pattern of renal insufficiency in adults during 1966-71 in Gotheburg. Acta Med Scand 1975; supp 582:1-50.

26   Stenvinkel P, Alvestrand A, Bergstrom J. Factors influencing progression in patients with chronic renal failure. J Intern Med 1989; 226(3):183-188.

27   Locatelli F, Marcelli D, Comelli M, Alberti D, Graziani G, Buccianti G et al. Proteinuria and blood pressure as causal components of progression to end-stage renal failure. Northern Italian Cooperative Study Group. Nephrol Dial Transplant 1996; 11(3):461-467.

28   Rutherford WE, Blondin J, Miller JP, Greenwalt AS, Vavra JD. Chronic progressive renal disease: rate of change of serum creatinine concentration. Kidney Int 1977; 11(1):62-70.

29   Hannedouche T, Chauveau P, Fehrat A, Albouze G, Jungers P. Effect of moderate protein restriction on the rate of progression of chronic renal failure. Kidney Int Suppl 1989; 27:S91-S95.

30   Rosman JB, Langer K, Brandl M, Piers-Becht TP, van der Hem GK, ter Wee PM et al. Protein-restricted diets in chronic renal failure: a four year follow- up shows limited indications. Kidney Int Suppl 1989; 27:S96-102.

31   Bergstrom J, Alvestrand A, Bucht H, Gutierrez A, Stenvinkel P. Is chronic renal disease always progressive? Contrib Nephrol 1989; 75:60-67.

32   Wight JP, Salzano S, Brown CB, el Nahas AM. Natural history of chronic renal failure: a reappraisal. Nephrol Dial Transplant 1992; 7(5):379-383.

33   Oldrizzi L, Rugiu C, Valvo E, Lupo A, Loschiavo C, Gammaro L et al. Progression of renal failure in patients with renal disease of diverse etiology on protein-restricted diet. Kidney Int 1985; 27(3):553-557.

34   Jones RH, Hayakawa H, Mackay JD, Parsons V, Watkins PJ. Progression of diabetic nephropathy. Lancet 1979; 1(8126):1105-1106.

35   Gall MA, Nielsen FS, Smidt UM, Parving HH. The course of kidney function in type 2 (non-insulin-dependent) diabetic patients with diabetic nephropathy. Diabetologia 1993; 36(10):1071-1078.

36   Levey AS. Measurement of renal function in chronic renal disease. Kidney Int 1990; 38(1):167-184.

37   Keane WF, Brenner BM, de Zeeuw D, Grunfeld JP, McGill J, Mitch WE et al. The risk of developing end-stage renal disease in patients with type 2 diabetes and nephropathy: The RENAAL Study. Kidney Int 2003; 63(4):1499-1507.

38   Ruggenenti P, Gambara V, Perna A, Bertani T, Remuzzi G. The nephropathy of non-insulin-dependent diabetes: predictors of outcome relative to diverse patterns of renal injury. J Am Soc Nephrol 1998; 9(12):2336-2343.

39   Ruggenenti P, Perna A, Mosconi L, Pisoni R, Remuzzi G. Urinary protein excretion rate is the best independent predictor of ESRF in non-diabetic proteinuric chronic nephropathies. "Gruppo Italiano di Studi Epidemiologici in Nefrologia" (GISEN). Kidney Int 1998; 53(5):1209-1216.

40   Woo D. Apoptosis and loss of renal tissue in polycystic kidney diseases. N Engl J Med 1995; 333(1):18-25.

41   Grantham JJ. Polycystic kidney disease—there goes the neighborhood. N Engl J Med 1995; 333(1):56-57.

42   Apperloo AJ, de Zeeuw D, de Jong PE. A short-term antihypertensive treatment-induced fall in glomerular filtration rate predicts long-term stability of renal function. Kidney Int 1997; 51(3):793-797.

43   Rossing P, Hommel E, Smidt UM, Parving HH. Reduction in albuminuria predicts diminished progression in diabetic nephropathy. Kidney Int Suppl 1994; 45:S145-S149.

44   el Nahas AM, Masters-Thomas A, Brady SA, Farrington K, Wilkinson V, Hilson AJ et al. Selective effect of low protein diets in chronic renal diseases. Br Med J (Clin Res Ed) 1984; 289(6455):1337-1341.

45   Lufft V, Kliem V, Hamkens A, Bleck JS, Eisenberger U, Petersen R et al. Antiproteinuric efficacy of fosinopril after renal transplantation is determined by the extent of vascular and tubulointerstitial damage. Clin Transplant 1998; 12(5):409-415.

46   Kramer AB, Laverman GD, van Goor H, Navis GJ. Interindividual differences in antiproteinuric response to ACEi in established adriamycin nephrosis are predicted by pre-treatment renal damage. J Pathol 2003; in press.

47   Ravid M, Brosh D, Levi Z, Bar-Dayan Y, Ravid D, Rachmani R. Use of enalapril to attenuate decline in renal function in normotensive, normoalbuminuric patients with type 2 diabetes mellitus. A randomized, controlled trial. Ann Intern Med 1998; 128(12 Pt 1):982-988.

48   Hasslacher C, Ritz E, Terpstra J, Gallasch G, Kunowski G, Rall C. Natural history of nephropathy in type I diabetes. Relationship to metabolic control and blood pressure. Hypertension 1985; 7(6 Pt 2):II74-II78.

49   Mogensen CE, Christensen CK. Blood pressure changes and renal function in incipient and overt diabetic nephropathy. Hypertension 1985; 7(6 Pt 2):II64-II73.

50   Rossing P, Hommel E, Smidt UM, Parving HH. Impact of arterial blood pressure and albuminuria on the progression of diabetic nephropathy in IDDM patients. Diabetes 1993; 42(5):715-719.

51   Hypertension in Diabetes Study (HDS): I. Prevalence of hypertension in newly presenting type 2 diabetic patients and the association with risk factors for cardiovascular and diabetic complications. J Hypertens 1993; 11(3):309-317.

52   Lee ET, Lee VS, Lu M, Lee JS, Russell D, Yeh J. Incidence of renal failure in NIDDM. The Oklahoma Indian Diabetes Study. Diabetes 1994; 43(4):572-579.

53   Klag MJ, Whelton PK, Randall BL, Neaton JD, Brancati FL, Ford CE et al. Blood pressure and end-stage renal disease in men. N Engl J Med 1996; 334(1):13-18.

54   Krolewski AS, Warram JH, Christlieb AR. Hypercholesterolemia—a determinant of renal function loss and deaths in IDDM patients with nephropathy. Kidney Int Suppl 1994; 45:S125-S131.

55   Mulec H, Johnsen SA, Wiklund O, Bjorck S. Cholesterol: a renal risk factor in diabetic nephropathy? Am J Kidney Dis 1993; 22(1):196-201.

56   Yang WQ, Song NG, Ying SS, Liang HQ, Zhang YJ, Wei MJ et al. Serum lipid concentrations correlate with the progression of chronic renal failure. Clin Lab Sci 1999; 12(2):104-108.

57   Maschio G, Alberti D, Janin G, Locatelli F, Mann JF, Motolese M et al. Effect of the angiotensin-converting-enzyme inhibitor benazepril on the progression of chronic renal insufficiency. The Angiotensin-Converting- Enzyme Inhibition in Progressive Renal Insufficiency Study Group. N Engl J Med 1996; 334(15):939-945.

58   Kambham N, Markowitz GS, Valeri AM, Lin J, D'Agati VD. Obesity-related glomerulopathy: an emerging epidemic. Kidney Int 2001; 59(4):1498-1509.

59   Bonnet F, Deprele C, Sassolas A, Moulin P, Alamartine E, Berthezene F et al. Excessive body weight as a new independent risk factor for clinical and pathological progression in primary IgA nephritis. Am J Kidney Dis 2001; 37(4):720-727.

60   Praga M, Hernandez E, Herrero JC, Morales E, Revilla Y, Diaz-Gonzalez R et al. Influence of obesity on the appearance of proteinuria and renal insufficiency after unilateral nephrectomy. Kidney Int 2000; 58(5):2111-2118.

61   Meier-Kriesche HU, Arndorfer JA, Kaplan B. The impact of body mass index on renal transplant outcomes: a significant independent risk factor for graft failure and patient death. Transplantation 2002; 73(1):70-74.

62   Johnson DW, Isbel NM, Brown AM, Kay TD, Franzen K, Hawley CM et al. The effect of obesity on renal transplant outcomes. Transplantation 2002; 74(5):675-681.

63   Ribstein J, du CG, Mimran A. Combined renal effects of overweight and hypertension. Hypertension 1995; 26(4):610-615.

64   Reisin E, Messerli FG, Ventura HO, Frohlich ED. Renal haemodynamic studies in obesity hypertension. J Hypertens 1987; 5(4):397-400.

65   Morales E, Valero MA, Leon M, Hernandez E, Praga M. Beneficial effects of weight loss in overweight patients with chronic proteinuric nephropathies. Am J Kidney Dis 2003; 41(2):319-327.

66   Bosma RJ, Homan van der Heide JJ, Oosterop EJ, de Jong PE, Navis G. Association between a higher body mass index and an unfavorable renal hemodynamic profile in healthy non-obese subjects. J Am Soc Nephrol 2002; 13:628A.

67   Weiss MF, Rodby RA, Justice AC, Hricik DE. Free pentosidine and neopterin as markers of progression rate in diabetic nephropathy. Collaborative Study Group. Kidney Int 1998; 54(1):193-202.

68   Myrup B, de Maat M, Rossing P, Gram J, Kluft C, Jespersen J. Elevated fibrinogen and the relation to acute phase response in diabetic nephropathy. Thromb Res 1996; 81(4):485-490.

69   Panichi V, Migliori M, De Pietro S, Taccola D, Bianchi AM, Norpoth M et al. C reactive protein in patients with chronic renal diseases. Ren Fail 2001; 23(3-4):551-562.

70   Sarnak MJ, Poindexter A, Wang SR, Beck GJ, Kusek JW, Marcovina SM et al. Serum C-reactive protein and leptin as predictors of kidney disease progression in the Modification of Diet in Renal Disease Study. Kidney Int 2002; 62(6):2208-2215.

71   Orth SR. Smoking and the kidney. J Am Soc Nephrol 2002; 13(6):1663-1672.

72   Telmer S, Christiansen JS, Andersen AR, Nerup J, Deckert T. Smoking habits and prevalence of clinical diabetic microangiopathy in insulin-dependent diabetics. Acta Med Scand 1984; 215(1):63-68.

73   Chuahirun T, Wesson DE. Cigarette smoking predicts faster progression of type 2 established diabetic nephropathy despite ACE inhibition. Am J Kidney Dis 2002; 39(2):376-382.

74   Hovind P, Rossing P, Tarnow L, Parving HH. Smoking and progression of diabetic nephropathy in type 1 diabetes. Diabetes Care 2003; 26(3):911-916.

75   Orth SR, Stockmann A, Conradt C, Ritz E, Ferro M, Kreusser W et al. Smoking as a risk factor for end-stage renal failure in men with primary renal disease. Kidney Int 1998; 54(3):926-931.

76   Regalado M, Yang S, Wesson DE. Cigarette smoking is associated with augmented progression of renal insufficiency in severe essential hypertension. Am J Kidney Dis 2000; 35(4):687-694.

77   Horner D, Fliser D, Klimm HP, Ritz E. Albuminuria in normotensive and hypertensive individuals attending offices of general practitioners. J Hypertens 1996; 14(5):655-660.

78   Mimran A, Ribstein J, DuCailar G, Halimi JM. Albuminuria in normals and essential hypertension. J Diabetes Complications 1994; 8(3):150-156.

79   Sung RS, Althoen M, Howell TA, Ojo AO, Merion RM. Excess risk of renal allograft loss associated with cigarette smoking. Transplantation 2001; 71(12):1752-1757.

80   Pinto-Sietsma SJ, Mulder J, Janssen WM, Hillege HL, de Zeeuw D, de Jong PE. Smoking is related to albuminuria and abnormal renal function in nondiabetic persons. Ann Intern Med 2000; 133(8):585-591.

81   van Essen GG, Rensma PL, de Zeeuw D, Sluiter WJ, Scheffer H, Apperloo AJ et al. Association between angiotensin-converting-enzyme gene polymorphism and failure of renoprotective therapy. Lancet 1996; 347(8994):94-95.

82   Fujisawa T, Ikegami H, Kawaguchi Y, Hamada Y, Ueda H, Shintani M et al. Meta-analysis of association of insertion/deletion polymorphism of angiotensin I-converting enzyme gene with diabetic nephropathy and retinopathy. Diabetologia 1998; 41(1):47-53.

83   Parving HH, Jacobsen P, Tarnow L, Rossing P, Lecerf L, Poirier O et al. Effect of deletion polymorphism of angiotensin converting enzyme gene on progression of diabetic nephropathy during inhibition of angiotensin converting enzyme: observational follow up study (see comments). BMJ 1996; 313(7057):591-594.

84   de Azevedo MJ, Dalmaz CA, Caramori ML, Pecis M, Esteves JF, Maia AL et al. ACE and PC-1 gene polymorphisms in normoalbuminuric Type 1 diabetic patients: a 10-year prospective study. J Diabetes Complications 2002; 16(4):255-262.

85   Hadjadj S, Belloum R, Bouhanick B, Gallois Y, Guilloteau G, Chatellier G et al. Prognostic value of angiotensin-I converting enzyme I/D polymorphism for nephropathy in type 1 diabetes mellitus: a prospective study. J Am Soc Nephrol 2001; 12(3):541-549.

86   Luik PT, Kerstens MN, Beusekamp BJ, Dullaart RP, de Jong PE, Hoogenberg K et al. Glycemic control determines renal and systemic pressor sensitivity to angiotensins in uncomplicated type I diabetic patients. J Am Soc Nephrol 2001; 12:150A.

87   van der Kleij FG, Schmidt A, Navis GJ, Haas M, Yilmaz N, de Jong PE et al. Angiotensin converting enzyme insertion/deletion polymorphism and short- term renal response to ACE inhibition: role of sodium status. Kidney Int Suppl 1997; 63:S23-S26.

88   van der Kleij FG, de Jong PE, Henning RH, de Zeeuw D, Navis G. Enhanced Responses of Blood Pressure, Renal Function, and Aldosterone to Angiotensin I in the DD Genotype Are Blunted by Low Sodium Intake. J Am Soc Nephrol 2002; 13(4):1025-1033.

89   Penno G, Chaturvedi N, Talmud PJ, Cotroneo P, Manto A, Nannipieri M et al. Effect of angiotensin-converting enzyme (ACE) gene polymorphism on progression of renal disease and the influence of ACE inhibition in IDDM patients: findings from the EUCLID Randomized Controlled Trial. EURODIAB Controlled Trial of Lisinopril in IDDM. Diabetes 1998; 47(9):1507-1511.

90   Jacobsen P, Rossing K, Rossing P, Tarnow L, Mallet C, Poirier O et al. Angiotensin converting enzyme gene polymorphism and ACE inhibition in diabetic nephropathy. Kidney Int 1998; 53(4):1002-1006.

91   Perna A, Ruggenenti P, Testa A, Spoto B, Benini R, Misefari V et al. ACE genotype and ACE inhibitors induced renoprotection in chronic proteinuric nephropathies1. Kidney Int 2000; 57(1):274-281.

92   Yoshida H, Mitarai T, Kawamura T, Kitajima T, Miyazaki Y, Nagasawa R et al. Role of the deletion of polymorphism of the angiotensin converting enzyme gene in the progression and therapeutic responsiveness of IgA nephropathy. J Clin Invest 1995; 96(5):2162-2169.

93   Hauser AC, Derfler K, Balcke P. Progression of renal insufficiency in analgesic nephropathy: impact of continuous drug abuse. J Clin Epidemiol 1991; 44(1):53-56.

94   Pedrini MT, Levey AS, Lau J, Chalmers TC, Wang PH. The effect of dietary protein restriction on the progression of diabetic and nondiabetic renal diseases: a meta-analysis. Ann Intern Med 1996; 124(7):627-632.

95   Levey AS, Adler S, Caggiula AW, England BK, Greene T, Hunsicker LG et al. Effects of dietary protein restriction on the progression of advanced renal disease in the Modification of Diet in Renal Disease Study. Am J Kidney Dis 1996; 27(5):652-663.

96   Zatz R, Meyer TW, Rennke HG, Brenner BM. Predominance of hemodynamic rather than metabolic factors in the pathogenesis of diabetic glomerulopathy. Proc Natl Acad Sci U S A 1985; 82(17):5963-5967.

97   Rudberg S, Aperia A, Freyschuss U, Persson B. Enalapril reduces microalbuminuria in young normotensive type 1 (insulin-dependent) diabetic patients irrespective of its hypotensive effect. Diabetologia 1990; 33(8):470-476.

98   Mathiesen ER, Hommel E, Giese J, Parving HH. Efficacy of captopril in postponing nephropathy in normotensive insulin dependent diabetic patients with microalbuminuria. BMJ 1991; 303(6794):81-87.

817

99   Kvetny J, Gregersen G, Pedersen RS. Randomized placebo-controlled trial of perindopril in normotensive, normoalbuminuric patients with type 1 diabetes mellitus. QJM 2001; 94(2):89-94.

100   Heeg JE, de Jong PE, van der Hem GK, de Zeeuw D. Efficacy and variability of the antiproteinuric effect of ACE inhibition by lisinopril. Kidney Int 1989; 36(2):272-279.

101   Bjorck S, Nyberg G, Mulec H, Granerus G, Herlitz H, Aurell M. Beneficial effects of angiotensin converting enzyme inhibition on renal function in patients with diabetic nephropathy. Br Med J (Clin Res Ed) 1986; 293(6545):471-474.

102   Bjorck S, Mulec H, Johnsen SA, Norden G, Aurell M. Renal protective effect of enalapril in diabetic nephropathy. BMJ 1992; 304(6823):339-343.

103   Giatras I, Lau J, Levey AS. Effect of angiotensin-converting enzyme inhibitors on the progression of nondiabetic renal disease: a meta-analysis of randomized trials. Angiotensin-Converting-Enzyme Inhibition and Progressive Renal Disease Study Group. Ann Intern Med 1997; 127(5):337-345.

104   Jafar TH, Schmid CH, Landa M, Giatras I, Toto R, Remuzzi G et al. Angiotensin-converting enzyme inhibitors and progression of nondiabetic renal disease. A meta-analysis of patient-level data. Ann Intern Med 2001; 135(2):73-87.

105   Lewis EJ, Hunsicker LG, Clarke WR, Berl T, Pohl MA, Lewis JB et al. Renoprotective effect of the angiotensin-receptor antagonist irbesartan in patients with nephropathy due to type 2 diabetes. N Engl J Med 2001; 345(12):851-860.

106   Brenner BM, Cooper ME, de Zeeuw D, Keane WF, Mitch WE, Parving HH et al. Effects of losartan on renal and cardiovascular outcomes in patients with type 2 diabetes and nephropathy. N Engl J Med 2001; 345(12):861-869.

107   Wright JT, Jr., Bakris G, Greene T, Agodoa LY, Appel LJ, Charleston J et al. Effect of blood pressure lowering and antihypertensive drug class on progression of hypertensive kidney disease: results from the AASK trial. JAMA 2002; 288(19):2421-2431.

108   Jafar TH, Stark PC, Schmid CH, Landa M, Maschio G, Marcantoni C et al. Proteinuria as a modifiable risk factor for the progression of non- diabetic renal disease. Kidney Int 2001; 60(3):1131-1140.

109   Klahr S, Levey AS, Beck GJ, Caggiula AW, Hunsicker L, Kusek JW et al. The effects of dietary protein restriction and blood-pressure control on the progression of chronic renal disease. Modification of Diet in Renal Disease Study Group. N Engl J Med 1994; 330(13):877-884.

110   Lewis EJ, Hunsicker LG, Bain RP, Rohde RD. The effect of angiotensin-converting-enzyme inhibition on diabetic nephropathy. The Collaborative Study Group. N Engl J Med 1993; 329(20):1456-1462.

111   Peterson JC, Adler S, Burkart JM, Greene T, Hebert LA, Hunsicker LG et al. Blood pressure control, proteinuria, and the progression of renal disease. The Modification of Diet in Renal Disease Study. Ann Intern Med 1995; 123(10):754-762.

112   Navis G, de Zeeuw D, de Jong PE. ACE-inhibitors: panacea for progressive renal disease. Lancet 1997; 349(9069):1852-1853.

113   Ruggenenti P, Perna A, Gherardi G, Garini G, Zoccali C, Salvadori M et al. Renoprotective properties of ACE-inhibition in non-diabetic nephropathies with non-nephrotic proteinuria. Lancet 1999; 354(9176):359-364.

114   Randomised placebo-controlled trial of effect of ramipril on decline in glomerular filtration rate and risk of terminal renal failure in proteinuric, non-diabetic nephropathy. The GISEN Group (Gruppo Italiano di Studi Epidemiologici in Nefrologia). Lancet 1997; 349(9069):1857-1863.

115 Laverman GD, Navis G, Henning RH, de Jong PE, de Zeeuw D. Dual renin-angiotensin system blockade at optimal doses for proteinuria. Kidney Int 2002; 62(3):1020-1025.

116 Mogensen CE, Neldam S, Tikkanen I, Oren S, Viskoper R, Watts RW et al. Randomised controlled trial of dual blockade of renin-angiotensin system in patients with hypertension, microalbuminuria, and non-insulin dependent diabetes: the candesartan and lisinopril microalbuminuria (CALM) study. BMJ 2000; 321(7274):1440-1444.

117 Nakao N, Yoshimura A, Morita H, Takada M, Kayano T, Ideura T. Combination treatment of angiotensin-II receptor blocker and angiotensin-converting-enzyme inhibitor in non-diabetic renal disease (COOPERATE): a randomised controlled trial. Lancet 2003; 361(9352):117-124.

118 Dickerson JE, Hingorani AD, Ashby MJ, Palmer CR, Brown MJ. Optimisation of antihypertensive treatment by crossover rotation of four major classes. Lancet 1999; 353(9169):2008-2013.

119 Bos H, Andersen S, Rossing P, de Zeeuw D, Parving HH, de Jong PE et al. Role of patient factors in therapy resistance to antiproteinuric intervention in nondiabetic and diabetic nephropathy. Kidney Int 2000; 57 Suppl 75:S32-S37.

120 Laverman GD, Zeeuw DD, Navis G. Between-patient differences in the renal response to renin-angiotensin system intervention: clue to optimising renoprotective therapy? J Renin Angiotensin Aldosterone Syst 2002; 3(4):205-213.

121 Ruggenenti P, Brenner BM, Remuzzi G. Remission achieved in chronic nephropathy by a multidrug approach targeted at urinary protein excretion. Nephron 2001; 88(3):254-259.

122 Mogensen CE, Keane WF, Bennett PH, Jerums G, Parving HH, Passa P et al. Prevention of diabetic renal disease with special reference to microalbuminuria (see comments). Lancet 1995; 346(8982):1080-1084.

123 Lazarus JM, Bourgoignie JJ, Buckalew VM, Greene T, Levey AS, Milas NC et al. Achievement and safety of a low blood pressure goal in chronic renal disease. The Modification of Diet in Renal Disease Study Group.

43

SCIENTIFIC BASIS FOR NEW GUIDELINES FOR THE TREATMENT OF HYPERTENSION IN TYPE 2 DIABETES

[1] Klavs Würgler Hansen, [2] Per Løgstrup Poulsen and [2] Carl Erik Mogensen

1) Medical dept., Silkeborg Centralsygehus, Silkeborg, Denmark, and 2) Medical Dept. M, Aarhus Kommunehospital, Aarhus, Denmark

INTRODUCTION

In 1993 the American Diabetes Association (ADA) stated that antihypertensive treatment should be started in diabetes if blood pressure exceeded 140/90 mmHg, with the goal of reduction to less than 130/85 mmHg [1]. Exactly the same target values was proposed in the latest (sixth) edition of JNC (1997) and WHO/ISH (1999) and nearly the same (<130/80 mmHg) by the 2003 position paper from ADA and the 2003 version of the European society of hypertension [2-4]. The 1993 strategy for antihypertensive treatment in diabetic patients was based on 1) extrapolation from the very large intervention studies in non-diabetic patients 2) knowledge from epidemiological studies in (largely) type 2 diabetic patients but without evidence from prospective studies in type 2 diabetic patients. Between 1993 and 2003 a number of large important intervention studies in type 2 diabetes have been published.

THE BASIS FOR GUIDELINES BEFORE 1993

The major epidemiological studies available in 1993 were the Framingham and MRFIT diabetic cohorts. In the very large MRFIT cohort the cardiovascular mortality was increased by a factor 2 to 4 (depending on number of additional risk factors) in diabetic patients and a clear association with systolic blood pressure was demonstrated with no threshold value [5].

It is less clear why a goal of < 130/85 mmHg was chosen in 1993. Probably this was based on the general assumption that the goal should be lower in diabetic patients because of diabetes per se is an important cardiovascular risk factor. The exact value 130/85 mmHg may be a consequence of the JNC stratification of a normal (<140/90 mmHg) blood pressure into high normal (140-130/90-85 mmHg), normal (130-120/85-80 mmHg) and optimal (<120/80mmHg) blood pressure. From a definition point of view diabetic patients should at least obtain a blood pressure, which could be designated as normal i.e. < 130/85 mmHg.

THE BASIS FOR GUIDELINES IN 2003

The major studies in type 2 diabetic patients are listed in table 1 and can be separated in 1) placebo controlled studies 2) trials looking for the optimal blood pressure goal 3) trials comparing different antihypertensive drugs 4) trials exploring the effect of ACE-inhibitors/AT1 blockers in normo- or microalbuminuric patients or patients with overt nefropathy. 5) trials with the combination of ACE-inhibitors and AT1 blockers. Some studies serves two purposes.

PLACEBO CONTROLLED STUDIES IN HYPERTENSIVE TYPE 2 DIABETIC PATIENTS

Both the SHEP [6]and Syst-Eur [7] trials were placebo controlled studies in isolated systolic hypertensive patients with a secondary publication of the results from the diabetic subpopulation (about 10 % diabetic patients). The SHEP study was based on thiazide diuretics and Syst-Eur on a calcium channel blocker (nitrendipin), with the option of supplementation with ACE inhibitors or diuretics. In both studies the incidence of CVD events in the placebo arm was about the double in diabetic patients compared with non-diabetic patients. The relative risk reduction for cardiovascular events in the SHEP study was similar (about 30 %) in both diabetic and non-diabetic patients. The active antihypertensive treated diabetic patients in the SHEP study had their risk for CVD events reduced to a level comparable with untreated (placebo) patients without diabetes. In contrast the Syst-Eur trial showed a very high relativ risk reduction (about 70 %) in diabetic patients compared with non-diabetic patients

(30 %). As a consequence the risk for CVD events in hypertensive diabetic patients in the Syst-Eur trial, was reduced to the level for antihypertensive treated patients without diabetes.

Table 1. Important trials with antihypertensive drugs in type 2 diabetic patients in the period 1993-2002

Placebo controlled studies in isolated systolic hypertension
1) SHEP (1996) [6]
2) Syst-Eur (1999) [7]

Trials exploring the optimal blood pressure goal
3) UKPDS:38 (1998) [8]
4) HOT (1998) [9]
5) ABCD (2000+2002) [11,12]

Trials exploring the optimal drug
6) UKPDS:39 (beta blockers vs ACE-inhibitors) (1998) [13]
7) FACET (dihydropyridin calcium antagonists vs ACE-inhibitors) (1998) [15]
8) ABCD (dihydropyridin calcium antagonists vs ACE-inhibitors) (1998) [16]
9) CAPPP (betablockers/diuretics vs ACE-inhibitors) (1999) [14]
10) STOP-2 (betablockers/diuretics vs ACE-inhibitors vs dihydropyridin calcium antagonists) (2000) [22]
11) NORDIL (betablockers/diuretic vs non dihydropyridin calciumantagonist) (2000) [21]
12) IDNT (AT blockers+convent. vs dihydropyridin calciumantagonist + convent.)(2001)[17]
13) LIFE (betablocker vs ACE inhibitor) (2001) [23]
14) MARVAL (AT1 blockers vs dihydropyridin calcium antagonist) (2002) [32]
15) ALLHAT (thiazide vs dihydropyridin calcium antagonist vs ACE inhibitors) (2002) [19]

Trials exploring the effects of ACE-inhibitors in normoalbuminuric patients
14) Ravid (1998)[24]
15) HOPE (2000) [28]

Trials exploring the effects of ACE-inhibitors or AT1 blockers in microalbuminuric patients
15) Ravid (1993) [25]
16) Steno Type 2 study (1999,2003) [26,27]
17) HOPE (2000) [28]
18) IRMA II (2001) [31]
19) MARVAL (2002)[32]

Trials exploring the effects of combination of ACE inhibitors and AT1 blockers
19) CALM (2001) [33]

Trials exploring the effects of AT1 blockers in diabetic nephropathy
20) RENAAL (2001)[18]
21) IDNT (2001).[17]

Table 2: Acronyms

MRFIT: Multiple risk factor intervention trial
SHEP: The systolic hypertension in the elderly program
Syst-Eur: The systolic hypertension in europe trial
UKPDS: United Kingdom prospective diabetes study
HOT: The hypertension optimal treatment
ABCD: Appropiate blood pressure control in diabetes
FACET: The fosinopril versus amlodipine cardiovascular events randomized trial
CAPPP: The captopril prevention project
STOP: The swedish trial in old patients with hypertension
NORDIL: The nordic diltiazem study
HOPE: Heart outcomes prevention evaluation
RENAAL: Reduction end points in NIDDM with the angiotensin II antagonist losartan
IDNT: Irbesartan type II diabetic nephropathy trial
IRMA: Irbesartan type II diabetes with microalbuminuria trial
CALM: Candesartan and lisinopril microalbuminuria study
MARVAL: The microalbuminuria reduction with valsartan study
PROGRESS: The perindopril protection against recurrent stroke study
LIFE: The losartan intervention for endpoint reduction in hypertension study
ALLHAT: The antihypertensive and lipid-lowering treatment to prevent heart attack trial
DETAIL: Diabetics exposed to telmisartan and enalapril
ONTARGET: The ongoing telmisartan alone and in combination with ramipril global end point trial

---

This promising results of the Syst-Eur study should be evaluated on the background that this was a placebo controlled study i.e. the study drug (nitrendipine) is clearly much more efficient (in both diabetic and non-diabetic patients) than placebo for prevention of complications related to hypertension. It should be noted that 43 % of the patients receiving nitrendipine also received an ACE-inhibitor.

OPTIMAL BLOOD PRESSURE GOAL

The tight blood pressure control part of the UKPDS study [8] showed a significant reduction of any diabetes related end point, macrovascular disease (except myocardial infarction), diabetes related death and of retinal complications. The baseline blood pressure was 160/94 mmHg and the aim in the tight blood pressure control arm was < 150/85 mmHg (achieved 144/82 mmHg) and the aim in the less tight control arm was < 180/105 mmHg (achieved 154/87 mmHg). In the tight control group 29 % needed 3 or more antihypertensive drugs.

In the HOT study [9] baseline blood pressure (measured automatically with the Visomat OZ, oscillometric device) was 173/105 mmHg and in the diabetic subgroup the frequency of major CVD events was gradually decreased with lower diastolic target blood pressure without evidence of a J curve phenomenon. The frequence of major CVD events in the group with target <80 mmHg (achieved 144/81mmHg) was 11.9/1000 patients/year, which was significantly lower than the event rate (24.4/1000 patients/year) in the group with target < 90 mmHg (achieved 148/85 mmHg). The usual interpretation is an effect of reduction of blood pressure per se in the diabetic subpopulation (not seen in the total study population). However in the < 80 mmHg group, the number of diabetic patients treated with ACE inhibitors in addition to the main drug felodipine is unknown and it could be argued that part of the observed beneficial effect possibly should be ascribed to a drug effect in addition to a mere blood pressure lowering effect. It should be noted that despite an attempt to reach the target < 80 mmHg, the achieved blood pressure for more than half the patients in this group was > 80 mmHg leaving the question open whether the protocol target (< 80 mmHg) or the achieved target (< 85 mmHg) should be the goal for guidelines. In addition it should be mentioned as a caveat that the HOT study did not use ordinary auscultatory blood pressure measurements but an automatic device which in a subsequently published validation study [10] was shown to underestimate the diastolic blood pressure significantly by 0.9 mmHg and underestimated the systolic blood pressure by 6.4 mmHg. If these differences, as stated, were independent of the level of blood pressure, it could be argued that the true targets were a diastolic blood pressure of < 81, <86 and < 91 mmHg respectively and that the achieved blood pressure in the group with target < 81 mmHg was 150/82 mmHg.

In the part of the ABCD study enrolling hypertensive patients [11] (n=470) no difference in the primary end point (creatine clearance) was reported with intensive antihypertensive treatment (achieved BP 132/78 mmHg) as compared with moderate treatment (achieved BP 138/86 mmHg). All cause mortality (not a prespecified end point) was lower in the intensive treatment arm (5,5 %) versus the moderate treatment arm (10,7 %). In the part of the ABCD study encompassing normotensive patients [12] (n=480), intensive antihypertensive therapy (achieved BP 128/75 mmHg) reduced the progression rates from normo-to microalbuminuria and overt nephropathy, reduced progression of retinopathy, and reduced the incidence of cerebrovascular disease as compared with moderate therapy (achieved BP 137/81 mmHg)

OPTIMAL DRUG

In UKPDS a beta-blocker [13] was compared with an ACE-inhibitor with no difference in the outcome. A larger proportion of patients on beta-blockers (35 %) than on ACE-inhibitors (22 %) terminated treatment due to possible side effects. In the beta-blocker group weight gain was significantly higher throughout the study (3.4 versus 1.6 kg) and HBA_{1c} significantly higher for the first four years (7.5 versus 7.0 %).

In the CAPPP study [14] analysis of the diabetic subpopulation showed large risk reduction (66%) for myocardial infarction in the captopril versus the conventional (thiazide, beta-blocker) group. Even total mortality was lower in captopril treated patients.

Although some methodological problems exist, two studies (FACET,ABCD) comparing dihydropyridine calcium antagonists with ACE-inhibitors both reported increased frequency of cardiovascular disease in the calcium antagonist group [15,16]. This has raised some concern as to the safety of dihydropyridine calciumantagonist in diabetes. However in the IDNT study amlodipine performed similar to placebo, but inferior to AT1-blockers [17]. In the RENAAL study the impressive result of AT1-blockers was achieved despite frequent (60%) co-medication with dihydropyridine calcium antagonist[18]. Furthermore the ALLHAT study did not report any differences in the primary end point (fatal and non-fatal myocardial infarction) between amlodipine, lisinopril and chlorthalidone [19,20].

In the NORDIL study no difference was noted for a combined cardiovascular end point between diltiazem and conventional drugs (thiazide or beta-blockers) [21].

In the STOP-2 study no difference for the primary end point (fatal CV disease) was seen, when conventional drugs (diuretics/beta-blockers) were compared with ACE-inhibitors or dihydropyridine calcium antagonists. Myocardial infarction was significant less frequent in the ACE-inhibitor group than in the dihydropyridine calcium antagonist group [22].

In the LIFE study inclusion criteria was hypertension and ECG determined left ventricular hypertrophy [23]. Total mortality during 5 years treatment was significantly lower (11 %)) in AT1-blocker group than in the beta-blocker group (17 %). The results was even more impressing for patients with untreated hypertension at baseline. The favourable results of blocking the renin-angiotensin system with an AT1-blocker (losartan) in the LIFE study as compared to beta-blockage (atenolol) contrast the results from the UKPDS using an ACE-inhibitor and an identical beta-blocker [13]. This puzzling controversy may be caused by the inherent difference between AT1-blockers and ACE-inhibitors or the presence of left ventricular hypertrophy. Also the patients were older and the blood pressure higher at baseline in the LIFE study (table 3). The frequency of combined AT1-blocker and thiazide treatment was high (60 %) in the LIFE study.

Table 3. Comparison of the LIFE and UKPDS studies

	Left ventricular hypertrophy (ECG)	Atenolol compared with:	Add. treatment with diuretics	Age (yrs)	BP baseline	Achieved BP (A arm)	Achieved BP (L- and C- arm Respectively)	Total mortality (pr 1000/yr A-arm)	Total mortality (pr 1000/yr L and C-arm respectively)
LIFE	100%	L	Approx. 46% (thiazide)	67	177/96	148/79	146/79	37.2	22.5
UKPDS	?%	C	Approx. 30% (frusemide)	56	159/94	143/81	144/83	20.8	23.8

A= atenolol; C= captopril; L=losartan

In the ALLHAT study thiazide diuretic (chorthalidone) reduced systolic blood pressure 2 mmHg more than lisinopril throughout the study period [19]. This may explain why thiazide prevented aggregate cardiovascular event points slightly more efficient than lisinopril (19.9 events/100 person/6year versus 20.8 events/100 persons/6year). Thiazide also prevented symptoms of heart failure more than lisinopril. From the nature of the study design lisinopril could not be combined with diuretics, while the well accepted combination with beta-blockers was possible for the thiazide arm. The overall medication in patients who needed more than one drug was somewhat artificial (including open label atenolol, reserpine, clonidine and hydralazine). One third of the participants were black. Data of HbA1c and urinary albumin excretion are lacking [20]. ALLHAT also included an alpha-blocker arm (doxazosin), which was discontinued prematurely due to increased frequency of heart failure.

ACE-INHIBITORS IN NORMOALBUMINURIC, NORMOTENSIVE PATIENTS

In a six year follow-up study by Ravid et al. enalapril 10mg reduced the risk for progression to microalbuminuria from 19% to 7 % and the age dependent decline in creatinine clearance was attenuated [24].

ACE-INHIBITORS IN MICROALBUMINURIC PATIENTS

Ravid has shown a reduction of the frequency of diabetic nephropathy by ACE-inhibitor treatment in normotensive lean microalbuminuric type 2 diabetic patients [25]. With a multiple intervention approach, including ACE inhibitor treatment irrespective of blood pressure the same was shown in the Steno type 2 study. The baseline blood pressure was about 147/86 mmHg and the achieved blood pressure was 136/78 mmHg in the intensive treated group compared with 144/81 mmHg in the group receiving standard care [26]. In a recent 7.8 year follow-up the frequency of nephropathy was reduced by 61 % in the intensive treated group [27].

In the HOPE study [28] diabetic patients without heart failure were included if 1) they had established CVD *or* 2) possess one risk factor which could be smoking, hypertension, dyslipedemia or microalbuminuria. The main end point was a combination of cardiovascular mortality, myocardial infarction or stroke. This composite end point was clearly reduced in the diabetic patients with previous cardiovascular event or with microalbuminuria whereas no significant effect was seen for diabetic patients without previous cardiovascular events or without microalbuminuria. Since the inclusion criteria are multiple and not mutually exclusive, it is impossible to draw any conclusions with respect to effect on the main composite end point in microalbuminuric type 2 diabetic patients without previous cardiovascular event (if any) or without hypertension.

The effect of ACE-inhibition in diabetic patients was not independent of blood pressure, but much more prominent in patients with the highest baseline systolic blood pressure (Gerstein HC, lecture 30/9 99, EASD meeting, Brussels). At the final visit office systolic BP was 140 mmHg in ramipril patients and 143 mmHg in placebo patients. In the HOPE study ramipril/placebo was administered in the evening. A small substudy using ambulatory BP monitoring reports much larger BP differences during the night than measured in the office [29]. Systolic night BP after one year was reduced by 17 mmHg in ramipril patients and by 8 mmHg in placebo patients. Reduction of night blood pressure is of particular importance for prevention of cardiovascular events [30]. Thus the blood pressure independent effect of ramipril is questionable.

In IRMAII the freqency of progression to urinary albumin excretion > 200 microg/min was reduced from 15 % (placebo) to 5 % (irbesartan 300mg) in a dose dependent manner [31]. In the MARVAL study valsartan lowered urinary albumin excretion more than amlodipine [32].

DUAL BLOCKADE

The principle of dual blockage is discussed in chapter 30. In the CALM study a further reduction of systolic BP from about 147 to 136 mmHg was accomplished by combining ongoing treatment with lisinopril or candesartan [33].

AT1-BLOCKERS IN DIABETIC NEPHROPATHY

IDNT and RENAAL showed relative risk reduction of 32 % and 16 % respectively for development of the primary end point (mortality or end stage kidney disease or doubling of se-creatinine) when an AT1-blocker was added to ongoing conventional treatment [17,18]. In the RENAAL study it could be calculated that end stage renal failure was postponed by two years. An average of four different drug classes was necessary in the IDNT study.

SUMMARY

Trials published in 1993-2002 has underscored the paramount importance of tight blood pressure control, which can reduce both macro-and microvascular complications. The actual goal for diastolic blood pressure should be < 80 mmHg or < 85 based on the interpretation of the HOT study. Unfortunately this study had diastolic blood pressure as intervention and target value, however the main clinical problem in type 2 diabetic patients is isolated systolic hypertension comprising about 2/3 of the hypertensive population [34]. The achieved blood pressure in most studies is far above 130 mmHg (fig 1) and recommendations to obtain a systolic blood pressure < 130 mmHg is still not evidence based, but relies on epidemiological results.

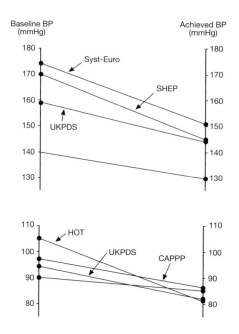

Fig. 1. Baseline and achieved blood pressure in five large intervention trials in hypertensive type 2 diabetic patients: The Syst-Eur and SHEP trials included patients with isolated systolic hypertension. The CAPPP and HOT studies were based on diastolic hypertension. The levels for intervention (> 140/90 mmHg) and goal (<130/85 mmHg) proposed by most international guidelines are presented for comparison (heavy black lines)

In the UKPDS study any diabetes related event and myocardial infarction both declined with lower systolic blood pressure (11-12 % reduction for a 10 mmHg reduction of blood pressure) without any threshold value [35]. Thus the principle of "the lower the better" is reinforced by the UKPDS study, but results from epidemiological studies are less important than results from intervention studies as basis for treatment guidelines. On top of the practical problems of achieving a goal of < 130 systolic in type 2 diabetic patients is the problem of "white coat hypertension" or "isolated clinic hypertension".

This problem is particular important for the older population with systolic hypertension. In the Syst-Eur trial the systolic day-time average blood pressure was 20 mmHg lower than the systolic clinic blood pressure [30].

Analysis of a subpopulation of the Syst-Eur population in which ambulatory blood pressure was performed demonstrated (in the placebo group) a much clearer association between cardiovascular events and ambulatory blood pressure (mainly night value) than clinic blood pressure [30].

For this reason it is at the moment not evidence based to recommend a reduction of systolic blood pressure to < 130 mmHg in all type 2 diabetic patients. The actual guidelines from several international and national institutions are shown in table 4 [2-4,36-38].

The possible effects of ACE-inhibitors and AT1- blockers "beyond the reduction of blood pressure" has been much debated. Must studies claiming a blood pressure independent effect have compared with placebo. Even minor reductions of blood pressure is considered important in diabetic patients. Some large scale studies comparing ACE- inhibitors with other drugs have failed to proof any difference in the primary end point (UKPDS, ALLHAT, STOP-2).

The fact that most type 2 diabetic patients needs several antihypertensive drugs to reach the goal renders the question about drug priority less important. There is strong evidence for choosing ACE-inhibitors in patients with congestive heart disease, and in patients with normal left ventricular function but microalbuminuria or a previous cardiovascular event (HOPE). Similar strong evidence supports the preference for AT1-blockers in patients with microalbuminuria, diabetic nephropathy or left ventricular hypertrophy (RENAAL, IDNT, IRMA II, MARVAL, LIFE).

It is noteworthy that most studies demonstrating favourable effects of ACE-inhibitors/AT1-blockers have combined with thiazide diuretics in a large proportion of the patients. This also applies to the PROGRESS study (containing 13 % diabetic patients) [39]. The combination of low dose thiazide and ACE-inhibitors/AT1-blockers is suggested as a primary step [38,40]. With some reservation for the ALLHAT study, the present data suggest that dihydropyridine calcium antagonist should not be used as monotherapy (FACET, ABCD, to some extent STOP-2) because other drugs are more efficient, at least when renal complications are present (IDNT). Dihydropyridine calcium antagonists are useful secondary line drugs when combined with blockade of the renin-angiotensin system (FACET, RENAAL).

Table 4: Present (2003) international and national guidelines for antihypertensive treatment in type 2 diabetes. All guidelines recommend intensive BP reduction for patients with nephropathy. goal < 130-120/80-75 mmHg

Institution or Society	Intervention	Goal
WHO/ISH 1999 [4] JNC VI 1997[3]	BP > 140/90 (consider intervention if high normal BP i.e. 140-130/90-85)	BP< 130/85
ADA 2003 [2]	BP > 140/90	BP< 130/80
BHS 1999 [36]	BP > 140/90	BP < 140/80
European Policy Group 1999 [37]	BP > 140/90	BP< 140/85
National Kidney Foundation and Diabetes Executive Committees Working Group 2000[38]	BP> 130/85	BP< 130/80
European Society of Hypertension-European Society of Cardiology 2003	BP> 130/85	BP< 130/80

The head to head comparison of ACE-inhibitors versus AT1-Blockers and the effect of their combination are the objective for important ongoing studies (DETAIL, CALM II, ONTARGET) [41-43]. Also the question about the optimal dose of these drugs is unsolved. The frequency of cardiovascular events in type 2 diabetes is still very high, in particular in those with nephropathy. The role for spironolactone [44], new aldosterone antagonist and vasopeptidase inhibitors needs to be explored.

REFERENCES

1   Consensus Statement. Treatment of hypertension in diabetes. Diabetes Care 1993; 16: 1394-1397
2   American Diabetes Association. Standards of medical care for patients with diabetes mellitus. Diabetes Care 2003; 26: Suppl.1:S33-S51.
3   The Joint National Commitee on Detection, Evaluation, and Treatment of High Blood Pressure. The sixth report of the joint national committee on detection, evaluation, and treatment of high bloood pressure. Arch Intern Med 1997; 157: 2413-2446
4   1999 Guidelines for the management of hypertension: Meromandum from a World Health Organization/International Society of Hypertension meeting. Guidelines sub-committee. J Hypertens 1999; 17:151-183
5   Stamler J,Vaccaro O, Neaton JD, Wentworth D for the multiple risk factor intervention trial research group. Diabetes, other risk factors, and cardivascular mortality for men screened in the multiple risk factor intervention trial. Diabetes Care 1993; 16: 434-44
6   Curb JD, Pressel SL, Cutler JA, Savage PJ, Applegate WB et al for the Systolic Hypertension in the Elderly Programme Cooperative Research Group. JAMA 1996; 23: 1886-1892
7   Tuomilehto J, Rastenyte D, Birkenhäger WH, Thijs L, Antikainen R, Bulpitt CJ, Fletcher AE, Forette F, Goldhaber A, Palatini P, Sarti C, Fagard R for the systolic hypertension in europe trial investigators. Effects of calcium-channel blockade in older patients with diabetes and systolic hypertension. N Eng J Med 1999; 340: 677-684
8   UK Prospective Diabetes Study Group. Tight blood pressure control and risk of macrovascular and microvascular complications in type 2 diabetes: UKPDS 38. BMJ 1998; 317: 703-713
9   Hansson L, Zanchetti A, Carruthers SG, Dahlöf B, Julius S, Ménard J, Rahn KH, Wedel H, Westerlin S. Effects of intensive blood -pressure lowering and low-dose aspirin in patients with hypertension: principal results of the Hypertension Optimal Treatment (HOT) randomised study. Lancet 1998; 13: 1755-1762
10   Lithell H, Berglund L. Validation of an oscillometric blood pressure measuring device: A substudy of the HOT study. Blood Pressure 1998; 7: 149-152
11   Estacio RO, Jeffers BW, Gifford N, Schrier RW. Effect of blood pressure control on diabetic microvascular complications in patients with hypertension and type 2 diabetes. Diabetes Care 2000; 23 (suppl 2): B54-B64
12   Schrier RW, Estacio R, Esler A, Mehler P. Effects of agressive blood pressure control in normotensive type 2 diabetic patients on albuminuria, retinopathy and strokes. Kidney Int 2002; 61: 1086-1097

13   UK prospective Diabetes Study Group. Efficacy of atenolol and captopril in reducing risk of macrovascular and microvascular complications in type 2 diabetes: UKPDS 39. BMJ 1998; 317: 713-720

14   Hansson L,Lindholm LH, Niskanen L, Lanke J,Hedner T, Niklason A, Luomanmäki K, Dahlöf B, de Faire U, Mörlin C, Karlberg BE, Wester PO, Björck JE. Effect of angiotensin-converting-enzyme inhibition compared with conventional therapy on cardiovascular morbidity and mortality in hypertension: the Captopril Prevention Project (CAPPP) randomised trial. Lancet 1999;353:611-616.

15   Tatti P, Pahor M, Byington RP, Mauro PD, Guarisco R, Strollo G, Strollo F. Outcome results of the fosinopril versus amlodipine cardiovascular events randomised trial (FACET) in patients with hypertension and NIDDM. Diabetes Care 1998; 21: 597-603

16   Estacio RO, Jeffers BW, Hiatt WR, Biggerstaff SL, Gifford N, Schrier RW. The effect of nisoldipine as compared with enalapril on cardiovascular outcomes in patients with non-insulin-dependent diabetes and hypertension. N Eng J Med 1998; 338: 645-653

17   Lewis EJ, Hunsicker LG, Clarke WR, Berl T, Pohl MA et al. Renoprotective effect of the angiotensin-receptor antagonist irbesartan in patients with nephropathy due to type 2 diabetes. N Eng J Med 2001; 345: 851-860

18   Brenner BM, Cooper MA, De Zeeuw D, Keane WF, Mitch WE et al. Effects of losartan on renal and cardiovascular outcomes in patients with type 2 diabetes and nefropathy. N Eng J Med 2001; 345: 861-869

19   The ALLHAT officiers and coordinators for the ALLHAT collaborative research group. Major outcomes in high-risk hypertensive patients randomized to angiotensin-converting enzyme inhibitor or calcium channel blocker vs diuretic. JAMA 2002; 288: 2981-2997

20   Barzilay JI, Jones CL, Davis BR, Basile JN, Goff DC, Ciocon JO, Sweeney ME, Randall OS. Baseline characteristics of the diabetic participants in the antihypertensive and lipid-lowerin treatment to prevent heart attack trial (ALLHAT). Diabetes Care 2001; 24: 654-658

21   Hansson L, Hedner T, Lund-Johansen P, Kjeldsen SE, Lindholm LH, Syvertsen JO, Lanke J, de Faire U, Dahlöf B, Karlberg BE. Randomised trial of effects of calcium antagonists compared with diuretics and beta-blockers on cardiovascular morbidity and mortality in hypertension: the Nordic Diltiazem (NORDIL) study. Lancet 2000; 356:359-365

22   Lindholm LH, Hansson L, Ekbom T, Dahlöf B, Lanke J, Linjer E, Scherstén B, Wester P-O, Hedner T, de Faire U. Comparison of antihypertensive treatments in preventing cardiovascular events in elderly diabetic patients: results from the swedish trial in old patients with hypertension. J Hypertens 2000; 18: 1671-1675

23   Lindholm LH, Ibsen H, Dahlöf B, Devereux RB, Beevers G et al. Cardiovascular morbidity and mortality in patients with diabetes in the losartan intervention for endpoint reduction in hypertension study (LIFE): a randomised trial against atenolol. Lancet 2002; 359: 1004-10.

24   Ravid M, Brosh D, Levi Z, Bar-Dayan Y, Rovid D, Rachmani R. Use of enalapril to attenuate decline in renal function in normotensive, normoalbuminuric patients with type 2 diabetes mellitus. Ann Int Med 1998; 128: 982-988

25   Ravid M, Savin H, Jutrin I, Bental T, Katz B, Lishner M. Long-term stabilizing effects of angiotensin-converting enzyme inhibition on plasma creatinine and on proteinuria in normotensive type II diabetic patients. Ann Intern Med 1993; 118: 577-581

26   Gæde P, Vedel P, Parving H-H, Pedersen O. Intensified multifactorial intervention in patients with type 2 diabetes and microalbuminuria: the Steno type 2 randomised study. Lancet; 353: 617-622

27   Gæde P, Vedel P, Larsen N, Jensen GV, Parving HH, Pedersen OB. Multifactorial intervention and cardiovascular disease in patients with type 2 diabetes. N Eng J Med 2003; 348; 383-393

28   Heart outcomes Prevention Evaluation (HOPE) study investigators. Effects of ramipril in cardiovascular and microvascular outcomes in people with diabetes mellitus: results of the HOPE and MICRO-HOPE substudy. Lancet 2000; 355: 253-59

29   Svensson P, de Faire U, Sleight P, Yusuf S, Östergren J. Comparative effects of ramipril on ambulatory and office blood pressures. Hypertens 2001; 38: e28-e32

30   Staessen JA, Thijs L, Fagard R, O´Brien ET, Clement D, Leeuw PW, Mancia G, Nachev C, Palatini P, Parati G, Tuomilehto J, Webster J for the Systolic Hypertension in Europe Trial Investigators. Predicting cardiocasvular risk using conventional vs ambulatory blood pressure in older patients with systolic hypertension. JAMA 1999; 282: 539-546

31   Parving H-H, Lehnert H, Bröchner-Mortensen J, Gomis, Andersen S, Arner P. The effect of irbesartan on the development of diabetic nephropathy in patients with type 2 diabetes. N Eng J Med 2001; 345: 870-878.

32   Viberti CG, Wheeldon NM. Microalbuminuria reduction with valsartan in patients with type 2 diabetes mellitus. Circulation 2002; 106: 672-678.

33   Mogensen CE, Neldam S, Tikkanen I, Oren S, Viskoper R, Watts RW, Cooper ME. Randomised controlled trial of dual blockade of renin-angiotensin system in patients with hypertension, microalbuminuria, and non-insulin dependent diabetes: the candesartan and lisinopril microalbuminuria (CALM) study. BMJ 2000; 321: 1440-44

34   Tarnow L, Rossing P, Gall M-A, Nielsen FS, Parving H-H. Prevalence of arterial hypertension in diabetic patients before and after the JNC-V. Diabetes Care 1994; 17: 1247-1251

35   Adler AI, Stratton IM, Neil HAW, Yudkin JS, Matthews DR, Cull CA, Wright AD, Turnaer RC, Holman RR. Association of systolic blood pressure with macrovascular and microvascular complications of type 2 diabetes (UKPDS 36): prospective observational study. BMJ 2000; 321; 412-419

36   Ramsay LE, Williams B, Johnston GD, MacGregor GA, Poston L, Potter L, Poulter NR, Russel G for the British Hypertension Society. Guidelines for the management of hypertension: report of the third working party of the British Hypertension Society. J Hum Hypertens 1999; 13: 569-592

37   European Diabetes Policy Group 1999. A desktop guide to type 2 diabetes mellitus. Diabetic Med 1999; 16: 716-730

38   Bakris GL, Williams M, Dworkin L, Elliott WJ, Epstein M, Toto R, Tuttle K, Douglas J, Hsueh W, Sowers J. Preserving renal function in adults with hypertension and diabetes: A consensus approach. Am J Kidney Dis 2000; 36: 646-61

39   PROGRESS collaborative group. Randomised trial of a perindopril-based blood pressurre-lowering regimen among 6105 individuals with previous stroke or transient ischemic attack. Lancet 2001; 358: 1033-1041

40   Williams B. Drug treatment for hypertension (editorial). BMJ 2003; 326; 61-62

41   Rippin J, Bain SC, Barnett AH. Rationale and design of diabetics exposed to telmisartan and enalapril (DETAIL) study. J Diabetes Complications 2002; 16: 195-200

42   Andersen NH, Knudsen ST, Poulsen PL, Poulsen SH, Helleberg K, Eiskjær H, Hansen KW, Bek T, Mogensen CE. Dual blockade with candesartan cilexetil and lisinopril in hypertensive patients with diabetes mellitus. Journal of the renin angiotensin aldosterone system (in press 2003)

43 Yusuf S. From the HOPE to the TARGET and the TRANSCEND studies: challenges in improving prognosis. Am J Cardiol 2002; 89(2A): 18A-25A

44 Sato A, Hayashi K, Naruse M, Saruta T. Effectiveness of aldosterone blockade in patients with diabetic nephropathy. Hypertens 2003; 41: 64-68

44

REGULATORY CONSIDERATIONS IN THE DEVELOPMENT OF THERAPIES FOR DIABETIC NEPHROPATHY AND RELATED CONDITIONS

Alexander Fleming
President and CEO, Kinexum LLC, Ridge Street, Harper's Ferry, WV, USA

INTRODUCTION

The importance of regulation in the drug development process is well appreciated, but the principles and practices of the major regulatory agencies overseeing therapeutic development are much less understood even by well-informed academicians. This chapter is intended to provide a better understanding of the regulatory framework and processes that are pertinent to therapeutic development in general and the advancement of therapies for diabetic nephropathy and related conditions in particular.

RECENT DEVELOPMENTS IN THERAPEUTIC REGULATION

The modern history of therapeutic evaluation and regulation and pertinent, more recent global developments are discussed in this book's previous edition. While some differences persist in the philosophies and approaches of the three major regulatory regions (Europe, Japan and the United States), convergence continues towards a single set of global standards. The International Conference on Harmonisation of Technical Requirements for the Registration of Pharmaceuticals for Human Use (ICH) [1] has continued to produce harmonized guidances for the pharmaceutical industry. Most recently the Food and Drug Administration and the counterpart European and Japanese authorities have adopted the ICH guidances for the "Common Technical Document." This outlines a single format and guide to content for registration submissions acceptable to all three authorities. While unnoticed by the public, the adoption of the CTD represents another very significant step towards global convergence in the pharmaceutical world. Full texts of all these and other ICH documents can be found at the FDA website.** While ICH is intended to provide guidance for pharmaceutical developers, many of these ICH products are discourses on scientific principles and practices for all involved or interested in the development of therapies.

THE EVOLVED MODERN PRINCIPLES OF THERAPEUTIC EVALUATION

The ICH movement and other efforts have led to the concept that good scientific principles and practices of pharmaceutical evaluation should be understood and utilized by all those involved in the development of therapies.[2] Reviews of principles for designing clinical trials and evaluating their data abound [3,45]. Others are more directly applied to the regulatory context [6,7,8]. Some of these regulatory principles are summarised below:

BENEFIT/RISK RELATIONSHIP

The final regulatory decision about whether or not to sanction the availability of a therapy is based on the perceived balance of benefits and risks that the therapy affords for the population of patients for whom it is intended. The availability of other therapies, the expected course of not treating the condition and other considerations will influence the amount of risks that can be accepted for the benefits provided. Ultimately a licensing decision for a therapy relies on the knowledge and judgment of experts in and outside of government. Collectively, these experts must provide an understanding of all the relevant scientific, clinical, ethical, legal, and administrative issues that are involved.

EFFECTIVENESS

The estimate of a therapy's effectiveness, i.e. ability to produce health benefits in the intended patient or user population, is determined by all experience in

---

** http://www.fda.gov/cder

which relevant biologic responses to the therapy and, sometimes, related therapies are measured. The range of data afforded by this experience form a hierarchy of value ranging from that provided by the most rigorously controlled study to the single anecdotal report. Effectiveness is an overall conclusion to be distinguished from efficacy, which characterizes the positive results of single experiments (ranging from in vitro studies to large clinical trials). Regulatory authorities may state, a priori, minimally acceptable outcomes necessary for claiming effectiveness, but this is a preliminary estimate based on assumptions about the quality of the data and safety outcomes, which cannot be confirmed until all studies have been completed and analyzed.

Circumstances can alter the magnitude of response or the response itself that regulators will ultimately accept as adequate to show effectiveness. An important attribute of a regulatory authority is to abide by its commitments to accept specified outcomes as indicative of effectiveness. This imperative must be balanced by the equally important need to take into account important scientific developments that may occur over the considerable amount of time involved in developing a therapy.

Not uncommonly, therapeutic development and regulatory approval must rely on outcomes that predict clinical benefits, i.e. surrogate endpoints, instead of the demonstration of direct clinical benefits themselves. In many cases, use of surrogate endpoints may be the only practical means by which therapies for chronic diseases and conditions can be developed. Blood glucose and cholesterol levels are well know examples of surrogates by which many therapies for diabetes and hyperlipidemia were developed and more recently have been confirmed as producing clinical benefits. The selection of surrogates should reflect an expert consensus, but this approach is not infallible. Probably the best know example of a surrogate that was used to justify marketing approval and was later discredited is from the development of agents for suppression of ventricular arrhythmias. The Cardiac Arrhythmia Suppression Trial (CAST) [9] evaluated the survival benefit conferred by treatment with one of three agents. These therapies were approved on the basis of efficacy in reducing frequency of ventricular arrhythmias following myocardial infarction. Instead of the anticipated reduction of cardiac deaths, CAST revealed that all three therapies were associated with an excess of total mortality compared to placebo. This experience does not invalidate the surrogate approach. It only shows the value of confirming clinical benefit for therapies that were approved on the basis of surrogate outcomes. When viewed from a broad perspective, the benefits to patients that have resulted from the use of surrogates in therapeutic development far exceed the harm that this approach has caused.

Because surrogate outcomes reflect human judgments based on the best available information at a point in time, additional data may alter the estimated value of a surrogate and thereby change the acceptability of the surrogate as a primary efficacy outcome. In effect, an authority might reject a previously accepted surrogate outcome that has been discredited, or it might accept a surrogate measure as a primary outcome that has since been validated.

SAFETY

In no case is therapeutic safety absolute. A safety profile can be estimated only for the dose, disease, and population in which it has been tested. The safety risks predicted by preclinical and clinical experience that can be accepted to justify further human exposure—investigational or as approved clinical use—depend on the severity of the disease itself, availability of therapeutic alternatives, and ultimately the benefit that the treatment affords. In general, an adequate definition of a therapy's safety profile requires far greater numbers of patients and duration of treatment than is required to define effectiveness. Given the extent and duration of investigation that is reasonable to require of developers before a therapy can be approved for its indicated use, only relatively frequently occurring adverse reactions can be detected prior to marketing (typically no lower than a 0.05% incidence) [10]. Detection during marketed use of rare but serious toxicities such as major organ failure can alter a therapy's benefit to risk relationship enough to warrant restrictions on the use of the therapy or even withdrawal of its marketing approval.

Ongoing evaluation of a new therapy's safety beyond the date of its marketing approval is therefore essential. In some cases, large controlled trials are required, as a condition for approval, to be performed in the post approval period. Such studies are most likely to be required when unresolved safety issues persist and the therapy is intended for chronic use in large populations. Large post approval studies may also be used to demonstrate major benefits, such as positive effects on survival, which could not practically be shown in pre-approval studies. Reporting by health providers and patients of toxicity associated with therapies is a very important source of information for further refining the estimates of their safety profiles. Such reports must be carefully compiled and evaluated by the marketer and regulatory authority alike, especially during the first years of marketing but for an indefinite time beyond this initial period as well. Finally, epidemiological approaches can also be used to better define issues of safety and effectiveness.

ANIMAL TESTING

Despite the increasing importance of in vitro methodologies, animal testing is the primary means of evaluating the desired and toxic effects of a potential human therapy prior to introduction of the therapeutic agent into humans. Ethical understandings dictate that some evidence of a therapy's efficacy as well as safety be obtained prior to exposing humans to a new compound. Wholly satisfactory animal models for evaluating safety and efficacy rarely exist. For some therapies, such as vaccines and antidepressants, indirect surrogate measures in animals or even in vitro approaches are all that can be used to predict clinical benefit prior to human exposure. Animal models may over predict as much as under predict clinical benefits of treatments for humans. The development of therapies for diabetes has frequently been associated with seemingly appropriate animal models that strongly suggested human efficacy, which nonetheless could not be confirmed in human trials.

For general toxicology evaluation, larger animals such as dogs and non-human primates tend to better approximate human intermediary and drug metabolism than small animals. Large animals are less feasibly used for providing the large numbers of animals required for examining multiple doses and gender differences. On the other hand, the much shorter life span and faster metabolism of small animals provide a means of simulating life long exposure to a candidate therapy. Small animals such as mice and rats may therefore provide better or at least complementary models for exploring long term toxicity including carcinogenicity. Because of considerable size and metabolic differences among experimental animals and humans, it is important to relate toxic effects across species to exposure, i.e., the amount of the therapeutic agent that animals from each species "sees" over time. This exposure to the therapeutic agent is generally expressed as the blood concentration of the agent integrated over a given period of time.

The significance for humans of a therapy's toxic effects in animals requires interpretation in every case. Known differences in drug metabolism or sensitivity between the test animal and humans may help to allay concerns about the potential for toxicity in humans. However, some findings in animals even at very large multiples of the anticipated human exposure cannot be dismissed. It must be understood that high exposures to a therapy are used in animals, in part, to compensate for the relatively short duration of exposure that can be obtained in animals compared to chronic use in humans. On the other hand, for a multitude of reasons, the absence of a toxic effect in animals does not exclude the possibility of the toxic effect in humans. Experimental animals are generally more uniform genetically, are studies under highly controlled conditions, and results are very unlikely to have any value in predicting rare, idiosyncratic toxicity in humans.

The practice of providing animal toxicology data in the official physician product information though common is of dubious value because of the inability of most physicians to interpret such data. Ultimately, all that matters are human safety data, but these may not become available until years of human use have elapsed. Some long term issues like carcinogenicity are almost never systematically addressed with human data. Animal toxicology data should be seen as only supplementary to data from human experience. The role of animal toxicology testing is primarily for protecting the safety of subjects and patients involved in pre-approval clinical investigation. By and large, the data from controlled clinical trials are the basis of determining a therapy's benefit to risk relationship and forming the body of information aimed at guiding patients and physicians in its safe and appropriate use when the therapy is first approved.

THE LEARN AND CONFIRM PARADIGM

Ethical and scientific considerations require that therapeutic development proceed carefully through a series of measured steps within the well know four phases of therapeutic investigation. Earliest investigation is spent in understanding how the healthy human body handles and tolerates the therapeutic agent. Subsequent studies start to show what the agent does to the body. At this point, hypotheses begin to form (or sharpen, if preclinical data had initiated them) about how the agent could be used to provide health benefits. A hypothesis that a therapy could provide a heath benefit warranting regulatory approval is provided by at least one and usually several small to medium sized, well controlled clinical studies. This hypothesis is confirmed with one and usually two more large studies that not only confirm efficacy (effectiveness) but provide enough patients to estimate the safety profile for the therapy's intended use. On the basis of the totality of data from all these clinical and preclinical studies, the regulatory authority with the help of experts determines if the therapy's benefit to risk relationship is acceptable. Thus, therapeutic development proceeds through cycles of learning and confirming—starting when or frequently before a therapy is identified and proceeding into and through the period of marketed use. The learn and confirm concept [11] expresses the epistemological basis of therapeutic development. That is, knowledge about a therapy is gained by repetitively advancing hypotheses and systematically testing them. In the fullness of time, knowledge about the benefits and risks of a therapy asymptotically approaches but never reaches complete understanding.

The FDA, by its interpretation of its legally defined authority, has set a fairly rigorous standard for demonstration of effectiveness. To warrant marketing approval, the FDA in most cases has required that at least two well controlled studies show differences in primary efficacy outcomes that are statistically significant (generally defined as $p<.05$). The Agency has more recently shown a willingness to accept a single, well-designed large trial with a treatment effect on the primary outcome, which is highly statistically significant. In effect, the significance level of such a trial should reach the equivalent composite significance of two independent trials each with significance at the $p=.05$ level, i.e., a significance level of $p<.0025$.*** In

---

*** Biostatistical significance does not directly equate to clinical meaningfulness. A highly statistically significant effect can theoretically be reached with a treatment effect that is not clinically meaningful, especially if large numbers of patients are studied. However, when the primary efficacy outcome(s) and the biostatistical plan for the registration grade studies have been prospectively stated by the sponsor and agreed to by the FDA, an outcome with a significance level of $p<.05$ is implicitly understood if not explicitly stated to indicate a clinically meaningful effect. Frequently, the sponsor, with the FDA's concurrence, will state the magnitude of a clinically meaningful effect *a priori*. The study is then sized to provide a stated probability that the study will, at a stated p value, be able to reject the null hypothesis (i.e. exclude that the demonstrated treatment effect is less than that considered to be clinically meaningful).

general, however, two trials (each with somewhat different designs) are to be preferred over a single trial. Two trials reduce the possibility of an unperceived systematic error or bias in the design or interpretation of a single study leading to an incorrect conclusion. The FDA has also accepted single studies to justify new drug approvals under other conditions. These include when a survival benefit has been clearly demonstrated, when no other therapy is available for a life threatening disorder, and when the disorder affects a very small population.

REGULATORY FLEXIBILITY

Therapeutic regulatory authorities must continue to balance their two major responsibilities: to facilitate the development of therapies that are desperately needed and to protect the public from unsafe, ineffective, or inadequately labeled therapies. The dictum, primum non nocere, is not tenable in this context. Nearly everyone recognizes that no therapy, approved or under investigation, is without risks. To strike a reasonable balance between these imperatives, regulators have to approve therapies before the risks are definitively established. To require such information prior to approval would, at a minimum, deprive patients of needed therapy for a period of time. In many cases, this requirement would deter therapeutic developers from ever seeking new therapies for chronic diseases. As part of an overall approach to managing risks, regulators are more and more taking into account the actual medical practice and other conditions under which a new therapy will be used. For example, the regulators must ask how consistently will patients be adequately monitored for toxicity known to be caused by the therapy. The concern of regulators about a therapy's significant toxicity will not be diminished by the availability of a highly effective monitoring test if the test is unlikely to be regularly used in everyday practice. Thus, regulators must weigh a number of considerations on a case-by-case basis as to just what body of evidence is required prior to proceeding with a given study and, finally, what is needed for marketing approval. A particularly difficult problem is to weigh modest therapeutic benefit for many or most patients against a severe risk for a very few patients.

PERSISTING DIFFERENCES IN APPROACHES TO THERAPEUTIC EVALUATION

While ICH and other initiatives have achieved considerable agreement among the major regulatory authorities and therapeutic developers about the principles with which they evaluate therapies, significant differences exist in how the regulatory authorities execute their responsibilities. Other important differences between European and US regulatory approaches are summarized in table 1.

Table 1 Selected Differences in Pharmaceutical Regulation between the European Union and the United States

Aspect	United States	Europe
Typical level of ethical review	Institutional	Community or region
Level of review	Raw data	Reports and summaries
Standard control group	Placebo	Active treatment
Size of regulatory authority	Very large	Small
Basis of authority	Federal	Multinational and transnational
Economic considerations	Excluded from licensing process	Reflected in the kinds of studies that are required for licensing
Emphasis used in assuring data integrity	Verification that reported data match data in source documents	Evaluation of all systems and procedures involved in recording and handling data
Public access to data and basis of decision making	Limited only to proprietary information	Limited to expert and regulatory summaries

Examples are provided of typical differences in perspective and/or practice between Europe and the United States. Exceptions to these typical characterisations abound. Europe itself is not monolithic in its regulation and development of therapies.

REGULATORY SITUATION FOR DIABETES THERAPIES

Therapeutic development for diabetes therapies and related conditions has exploded in the post-DCCT era. The FDA's approach to regulation of therapies for diabetes drugs has also evolved [12]. While some significant compounds have been put into use for oral therapy of type 2 diabetes and recombinant insulin and insulin analogs provide some attractive features, a true therapeutic breakthrough has not occurred during this time [13]. Results of the Diabetes Control and Complications Trial (DCCT) and the United Kingdom Prevention of Diabetes Study (UKPDS) have stimulated greater awareness of the value of improving glycemic control and, to some extent, some success in achieving better glycemic control among type 1 and 2 patients. However, the average patient's glycemic control is far from acceptable. Diabetes complications will therefore continue to be a major cause of morbidity and mortality, and treatments for diabetic complications will be much needed for the foreseeable future.

For obvious reasons, development of therapies for diabetic complications is inherently more difficult than that for treatments of glycemic and other metabolic abnormalities of diabetes. Extraordinary amounts of time and resources have been invested in aldose reductase inhibitors, primarily as treatments for peripheral neuropathy but also for nephropathy and retinopathy. Convincing clinical benefits have yet to be shown for compounds in this therapeutic class [14,15]. Until recently, only one therapy for a diabetic complication of any kind was approved by the FDA.

Captopril (CapotenTM , Bristol-Myers Squibb Co.), an angiotensin converting enzyme inhibitor (ACEI) originally approved for treatment of hypertension was approved in early 1994 by the FDA for treatment of diabetic nephropathy [16]. The approval was based largely on results of a double-blind, placebo-controlled clinical trial that involved 409 patients at 30 centers in the United States and Canada. Captopril treatment was associated with a 50 percent reduction in the combined risk of death or of kidney failure requiring dialysis or a transplant compared to placebo. The trial was conducted in patients with type 1 diabetes who had proteinuria (24 hour urinary excretion >500 mg) and retinopathy. Subsequent trials have since demonstrated a benefit of captopril on progression to overt proteinuria in patients with 20-200 microgram/min. Thus, ACEI therapy has become standard therapy for patients with proteinuria of any degree in type 1 and 2 patients even though the original lower limit for proteinuria of 500 mg has not been modified in Captopril's approved indication. Moreover, ACEI therapy has become an attractive choice for treating hypertension uncomplicated by proteinuria in patients with diabetes largely because of the anticipation that this therapy will forestall the development of renal dysfunction as well as provide some other benefits [17].

846

Though ACEI has become a standard of care in the treatment nephropathy in patients with type 2 diabetes, clinical outcome data from trials involving type 2 patients have not been available. Three trials have recently been reported, which demonstrate that angiotensin receptor blockers (ARB) slow progression of nephropathy in type 2 patients [18,19,20]. All three studies showed a substantial reduction in the rate of progression of diabetic nephropathy in a combined total of over 3500 randomized patients treated with ARBs. These trials were the basis of regulatory approval of Avapro® (Bristol Myers Squibb, irbesartan) and Cozaar® (Merck & Co., losartan) for treatment indications in type 2 patients. Importantly, the use of ACEI was not allowed in either of these three studies. An additive effect of ACE inhibition and angiotensin II receptor blockade in reducing proteinuria has since been reported for patients with type 1 diabetes [21].

ACEI efficacy in reducing the progression of diabetic nephropathy is substantial, but not fully effective in forestalling this complication. Complementary therapeutic approaches should be pursued to fully avert the development of nephropathy. Because ACEI and now ARB have become standard therapies, the development of new therapies will be more challenging. The therapeutic window for subsequent treatments is considerably smaller since no nephropathy trial can be ethically conducted without ACEI therapy. For example, captopril therapy itself might fall short of producing statistically significant treatment effects in the same trials on which approval was based if a comparably effective background therapy had been used by most of the patients in the trial.

The other major obstacle for development of additional therapies aimed at preventing nephropathy is the strong secular trend in risk factor reduction for this complication. Improved glycemic and blood lipid control, decreased smoking, earlier detection and treatment of microalbuminuria all serve to lower the rate of progression to renal dysfunction and ESRD. Thus, the absolute treatment effect being pursued in the development of new therapies continues to shrink. It should be recognized, however, that a substantial number of patients will progress to disabling nephropathy despite the use of captopril therapy and all other currently recognized interventions. Captopril itself is not risk free. This therapy is recognized to cause anaphylactic-like reactions, angioedema, neutropenia/agranulocytosis, and increased proteinuria with occasional nephrotic syndrome. For all these reasons, additional anti-nephropathic therapies, particularly those that can be used preventatively in a general population, are very much needed.

AMINOGUANIDINE: A CASE STUDY OF THERAPEUTIC DEVELOPMENT

The understanding led by Cerami, Brownlee and others that chronic exposure to high glucose concentration results in chemical modification of proteins has resulted in a major therapeutic target for preventing and treating diabetic complications. Cerami's sentinel work in this area also resulted in the identification of glycated hemoglobin (hemoglobin A1c) as a diagnostic tool of immense importance not only to clinical therapeutics but to the development of therapies for glycemic control [22].

Aminoguanidine (Pimagedine, Alteon) is the first anti-glycation compound to be evaluated in clinical trials. Pimagedine has been shown to inhibit the formation of glycation end products (AGEs), which are strongly implicated in the development of micro- and macrovascular complications. Although the protective effects of pimagedine appear to be predominantly mediated by a reduction in pathologic glycation [23], this compound also functions as an inhibitor of nitric oxide synthase and oxidative stress, which are potential contributing factors to the development of tissue damage in diabetic patients [24] In animal models of diabetes and diabetic complications, treatment with pimagedine resulted in the prevention or reduction of retinopathy [25,26], and the amelioration of albuminuria [27]. Pimagedine also prolonged the survival of diabetic rats made azotemic by renal ablation, suggesting that it has protective effects even in cases of existing renal damage [28] Moreover, Pimagedine has demonstrated potential benefits against macroangiopathy, including anti-atherogenic effects in cholesterol-fed rabbits [29] and reduced infarct volume in a rat model of focal cerebral ischemia [30].

In a double-blind, placebo-controlled, 28-day trial, circulating hemoglobin advanced glycation end-products (AGE) levels were reduced significantly (by approximately 28%) in patients receiving an average dose of 1200 mg/day Pimagedine in contrast to no significant change in those receiving placebo [31]. To assess the efficacy of Pimagedine in diabetic patients with microvascular complications, three pivotal clinical trials have been initiated in North America. ACTION I (A Clinical Trial In Overt Nephropathy) was conducted in 690 patients with type 1 diabetes [32]. The results of ACTION I suggest that Pimagedine could provide important benefits to patients with early diabetic nephropathy. The treatment effect on time to doubling in serum creatinine, the pre-defined primary outcome measure, did not reach statistical significance. However, the study does provide other evidence that this therapy improves renal function. Reduction in proteinuria is the most compelling finding. Many experts may accept the treatment effect on proteinuria itself as a reflection of a significant clinical benefit. Statistically significant reductions in LDL cholesterol, and triglycerides, as well as lowered diastolic blood pressure were also seen. In addition, the data indicated favorable outcomes in measures of renal function, including creatinine clearance and filtration rate, as well as in the inhibition of the progression of retinopathy.

ACTION II was conducted in 599 patients with type 2 diabetes. However, an external monitoring committee recommended the discontinuation of this trial because of an insufficient risk/benefit ratio based upon data currently available at that time [33]. A third multicenter trial of patients with early diabetic nephropathy was undertaken in Europe, but was canceled due to slow enrollment and difficulty maintaining a placebo group. Finally, enrollment is also in progress for a trial of Pimagedine in type 1 and type 2 diabetic patients with end stage renal disease.

The development of Pimagedine therapy illustrates many of the principles expressed in the first part of this chapter. For example, the developers of this therapy evaluated the preclinical data and other considerations prior to making a decision about which therapeutic applications should be targeted. This therapy could conceivably be of value for a wide variety of conditions including aging itself. Pimagedine's developers decided that the condition for which the projected benefit to risk relationship was most acceptable is the prevention of progression from overt, but mild diabetic nephropathy to end stage renal failure. From the preclinical data, Pimagedine therapy could be seen to have some real and theoretical risks that would not be as well tolerated for conditions for which patients were at less risk from the disease itself. The choice of the patient population was influenced by other important considerations including the event rate for primary outcomes and the biology of the disease and the intervention itself. These considerations would determine the size and duration of the trial.

The designs of the major Pimagedine nephropathy studies reflected considerable confidence in this therapeutic approach. These sizable, very long, and costly studies were designed to definitively (as much as is possible to do prior to marketing) demonstrate the benefit risk relationship of the therapy. The developers had clear direction for designing the study. They drew on the model of the captopril study, which had been used to successfully win a nephropathy indication for that drug. Disappointingly, the primary outcome results fell just short of achieving statistical significance in ACTION I. Why? The relatively small effect on general renal function and progression to end-stage renal disease is clearly related to the originally unanticipated, almost universal use of captopril therapy by patients in this trial. This illustrates a hazard for any long-term trial. The imposition of a new standard background therapy during the course of a trial, just as occurred in this case, decreases the absolute magnitude of efficacy that can be achieved in the trial. Use of a background therapy undermines the biostatistical power of a trial to demonstrate a treatment effect of the new therapy. The data suggest that Pimagedine, as monotherapy would have about the same effects on renal function and proteinuria as captopril. Similarly, captopril would likely be shown to have marginal efficacy if it were re-examined as add-on therapy to background Pimagedine treatment.

The Pimagedine situation presents some regulatory quandaries. The ACTION I trial failed to obtain statistical significance in the primary outcome, but an over all reading of the trial results as well as the circumstances of the trial would suggest to most experts that the therapy is efficacious. However, the FDA expects that the primary outcome will be convincingly affected by the new therapy in order to approve it. Picking other outcomes in a non pre-specified way after the trial is completed is considered an exploratory approach that requires subsequent confirmation. The other major problem for Pimagedine is that the second trial, ACTION II, was intended to confirm the results of ACTION I.

The two studies together would meet the FDA's "well controlled trials" requirement. Though in retrospect the lack of positive outcomes in ACTION II can be explained (patients had more advance disease and the presence of other co-morbidities), this leaves Pimagedine with at most one positive study. What are the sponsor and the FDA to do with results that fall short after a very large investment and good faith effort to provide a therapy that is much needed? One possible approach is discussed in the following section.

Until now, the clinical discussion of Pimagedine has been confined to therapeutic efficacy. Demonstrating effectiveness is only half the challenge for the developers of Pimagedine or any other therapy. To receive regulatory approval, the risks of the therapy have to be defined and the relationship of these risks to the benefits provided by the therapy has to be acceptable. Significant toxicity has been associated with Pimagedine therapy in ACTION I.

The most notable observation was of crescentic glomerulonephritis associated with high anti-neutrophil cytoplasmic antibodies in three patients treated with the high dose of Pimagedine. No such cases were seen in the lower dose group, and the low dose treatment appears to provide benefits comparable to those achieved in the high dose group. Furthermore, what would appear to be a reliable monitoring procedure has been identified for discontinuing therapy before this syndrome can develop. A transient flu-like syndrome and mild anemia were also associated with therapy [34]. Because of the much-increased danger from macrovascular complications faced by patients with overt nephropathy who progress to end stage renal disease, these risks from Pimagedine therapy may yet be acceptable.

Some account must also be made of the fact that captopril itself is not without its own risks and cannot be used by every patient who is at high risk for developing end stage renal disease. Ultimately, it is the responsibility of the review scientists at the FDA and other regulatory authorities to weigh these considerations and determine whether the therapy should be approved or not and what additional information will be required in either case.

SURROGATES FOR DIABETIC NEPHROPATHY

As discussed above, regulatory authorities should appropriately modify requirements for therapeutic approval as scientific understanding evolves. These and other considerations ought to be taken into account in adjusting the requirements for therapies aimed at prevention and treatment of diabetic nephropathy. One possible approach is the use of well-accepted surrogate outcomes. Proteinuria is the leading candidate for this role in the case of Pimagedine and other therapies for nephropathy. In the original captopril trial, protein excretion was reduced by 30% in the first 3 months of captopril therapy, this reduction was maintained for the rest of the trial, and the effect on proteinuria correlated with the primary efficacy outcomes. A large body of evidence now supports the view that excreted protein itself is a tubular toxin [35]. Some experts now regard proteinuria as not only a reflection of dysfunction for all glomerulopathies, but as one of the common etiologic pathways on which all these diseases converge [36-41]. In streptozotocin-induced diabetic rats, the albuminuric-lowering effects of both pimagidine and ACEI have recently been associated with normalisation of glomerular protein kinase C. These data suggest that despite entirely different mechanisms of action, the renoprotective effects of these agents likewise converge at a common biochemical pathway [42]. Reduction of protein excretion regardless of cause could thereby be justified as a therapeutic objective [43]. By extension, protein excretion could be accepted as a reasonable surrogate if not outright clinical outcome on which a nephropathy indication could be based. The FDA has also implemented a provision for, in effect, provisionally approving a life saving therapy on the basis of one or more surrogate outcomes. As a condition of approval, the sponsor is obligated to finish or conduct a study in the post-approval period, which confirms the therapy's clinical benefit.

While the case for the predictive value of proteinuria continues to build, those with a more conservative perspective will still insist that developers of new therapies be required to show effects on the same kind of outcomes like time to doubling of serum creatinine and progression to end stage renal disease (ESRD). This is likely to be the expectation of regulatory authorities for the foreseeable future.

CONCLUSIONS

Of diabetic microvascular complications, nephropathy is the most important in terms of mortality and economic impact. Diabetic nephropathy is the most common cause of end stage renal disease and dialysis dependency in the industrialized world. The importance of this disorder and the rapidly expanding knowledge about its pathophysiology warrant the attention that it has been shown in this book and numerous other efforts. Clearly, much remains to be accomplished. The concerted efforts of patients, clinicians, academicians, therapeutic developers, regulators, and politicians are necessary to achieve effective preventions and treatments within the next decade.

REFERENCES

1. J. Showalter, International Conference on Harmonization. The Journal of Biology & Business 1(2): 90-93.

2. G.A.Fleming, Beyond Drug Evaluation: The Science of Drug Evaluation, Molecular Medicine 2:5, 1996.

3. S.J.Pocock. Clinical trials: a Practical Approach. John Wiley, New York, 1983.

4. L.M. Friedman, C.D. Furberg, D.L. DeMets. Fundamentals of Clinical Trials. Second Edition. PSG, Boston, 1985.

5. A. H. Zwinderman , T. F. Cleophas. In Statistics Applied to Clinical Trials. Kluwer Academic Publishers, Dordrecht, May 2002

6. R. Temple. A regulatory authority's opinion about surrogate endpoints. In Nimmo WS, Tucker GT, eds. Clinical Measurement in Drug Evaluation. Vol. 3, p. 21. Chichester: John Wiley and Sons, Ltd, 1995.

7. R. Temple. Difficulties in evaluating positive control trials. Proceedings of the American Statistical Association, Biopharmaceutical Section, 1983.

8. F. A. Rozovsky, R. K. Adams. In Clinical Trials and Human Research: A Practical Guide to Regulatory Compliance, Jossey-Bass (Wiley Company), New York, May 2003,

9. The Cardiac Arrhythmia Suppression Trial Investigators. Effect of the anti-arrhythmic moricizine on survival after myocardial infarction. New England Journal of Medicine. 327: 227-233, 1992.

10. FDA Guideline for Industry. The Extent of Population Exposure to Assess Clinical Safety: For Drugs Intended for Longterm Treatment of Non-Life-Threatening Conditions (ICH E1). 1995. http://www.fda.gov/cder/guidance/iche1a.pdf

11. L. B. Sheiner. Learning versus confirming in clinical drug development. J Clin Pharm Ther, 61(3):275-291, 1997

12. G.A. Fleming. American Heart Journal 138: S338-S345, 1999

13. G.A. Fleming, S. Jhee, R. Coniff, H. Riordan, M. Murphy, N. Kurtz, N.Cutler. In Optimizing Therapeutic Development in Diabetes. Greenwich Medica Media, London, pp. 47-60, 1999.

14. The Sorbinil Retinopathy Trial Research Group: A randomized trial of sorbinil, an aldose reductase inhibitor in diabetic retinopathy, Arch Ophthalmol 108:1234-1244, 1990.

15. M. Foppiano, G. Lombardo, Worldwide pharmacovigilance systems and tolrestat withdrawal. Lancet 349: 399-400, 1997

16. E.J. Lewis, L.G. Hunsicker, R.P. Bain, & R.D. Rohde, for the Collaborative Study Group. The effect of angiotensin-converting-enzyme inhibition on diabetic nephropathy. New England Journal of Medicine 329(20):1456-1462, 1993.

17. Heart Outcomes Prevention Evaluation (HOPE) Study Investigator. Effects of ramipril on cardiovascular and microvascular outcomes in people with diabetes mellitus: results of the HOPE study and MICRO-HOPE substudy Lancet 355, 253-259, 2000.

18. E. J. Lewis, L. G. Hunsicker, W. R. Clarke, T. Berl, M. A. Pohl, J. B. Lewis, E. Ritz, R. C. Atkins, R. Roh, I. de Raz. Renoprotective effect of the angiotensin-receptor antagonist irbesartan in patients with nephropathy due to type 2 diabetes. N.Engl.J.Med. 345:851-860, 2001

19. B.M. Brenner, M. E. Cooper, D. de Zeeuw, W.F. Keane, W.E. Mitch, H.H. Parving, G. Remuzzi, S.M. Snapinn, Z. Zhang, S. Shahinfar. Effects of losartan on renal and cardiovascular outcomes in patients with type 2 diabetes and nephropathy N.Engl.J.Med. 345:861-869, 2001

20. H. H. Parving, H. Lehnert, J, R. Brochner-Mortensen, Gomis, S. Andersen, P. Arner. The effect of irbesartan on the development of diabetic nephropathy in patients with type 2 diabetes. N.Engl.J.Med. 345:870-878, 2001

21. P. Jacobsen, S. Andersen, B.R. Jensen. H.H. Parving. Additive Effect of ACE Inhibition and Angiotensin II Receptor Blockade in Type I Diabetic Patients with Diabetic Nephropathy. J Am Soc Nephrol 14(4):992-9, 2003

22. A. Fleming, S,Jhee, R. Coniff, H,Riordan, M. Murphy, N. Kurtz, N. Cutler. In Optimizing Therapeutic Development in Diabetes. Greenwich Medica Media, London, pp. ix-x, 1999.

23. T. Soulis-Liparota, M, Cooper, D. Papazoglou, B. Clarke, G. Jerums. Retardation by aminouanidine of development of albuminuria, mesangial expansion, and tissue fluorescense in streptozotocin-induced diabetic rat. Diabetes; 40(10):328-1334, 2000

24. C.W. Yang, C.C.Yu, Y.C. Ko, C.C. Huang. Aminoguanidine reduces glomerular inducible nitric oxide synthase (iNOS) and transforming growth factor-beta 1 (TGF beta) mRNA expression and diminshes glomerulosclerosis in NZB/W F1 mice. Clin Exp Immunol 113(2): 258-264, 1998

25. H.P.Hammes, M. Brownlee, D. Edelstein, M. Saleck, S. Martin, K. Federlin. Aminoguanidine inhibits the development of accelerated diabetic retinopathy in the spontaneous hypertensive rat. Diabetologia 1994; 37(1):32-35.

26. H.P. Hammes, D. Strodter , A. Weiss, R.G. Bretzel, K. Federlin, M. Brownlee. Secondary intervention with aminoguanidine retards the progression of diabetic retinopathy in the rat model. Diabetologia 1995; 38(6): 656-660.

27. D. Edelstein, M. Brownlee,. Aminoguanidine ameliorates albuminuria in diabetic hypertensive rats. Diabetologia 1992; 35(1): 96-97.

28. E.A. Friedman, D.A. Distant, J.F. Fleishhacker, T.A. Boyd, K. Cartwright. Aminoguanidine prolongs survival in azotemic-induced diabetic rats. AM J Kidney Dis 1997; 30(2): 253-259.

29. S. Panagiotopoulos, R.C. O'Brien, R. Bucala, M.E. Cooper, G. Jerums.. Aminoguanidine has an anti-atherogenic effect in the cholesterol-fed rabbit. Atherosclerosis 1998; 136(1): 125-131.

30. G.A. Zimmerman, M. Meistrell 3rd, O. Bloom, K.M.Cockroft, M. Bianchi, D. Risucci, J. Broome, P. Farmer, A. Cerami, H. Vlassara, et al. Neurotoxicity of advanced glycation endproducts during focal stroke and neuroprotective effects of aminoguanidine. Proc Natl Acad Sci USA 1994; 92(9): 3744-3748.

31. Makita Z, Vlassara H, Rayfield E, Cartwright K, Friedman E, Rodby R, Cerami A, Bucala R, Hemoglobin-AGE: a circulating marker of advanced glycosylation. Science 1992: 258(5082): 651-653.

32. G. Appel, K. Bolton , B. Freedman, J-P. Wuerth, K. Cartwright. Pimagedine (PG) Lowers Total Urinary Protein (TUP) and Slows Progression of Overt Diabetic Nephropathy in Patients with Type 1 Diabetes Mellitus. Abstract: American Society of Nephropathy Annual Meeting [A0786] 1999.

33. Script No.2320. Side Effects with Alteon's pimagedine. March 25, 1998, p. 24.

34. F. Whittier, B. Spinowitz, J-P. Wuerth, K. Cartwright. Pimagedine safety profile in patients with type I diabetes mellitus. Abstract: American Society of Nephropathy Annual Meeting [A0941] 1999.

35. M.E. Thomas, N.J. Brunskill, K.P. Harris, E Bailey, J.H. Pringle, P.N. Furness, J. Walls Proteinuria induces tubular cell turnover: A potential mechanism for tubular atrophy. Kidney International: 55(3):890-8. 1999.

36. The GISEN Group (Gruppo Italiano di Studi Epidemiologici in Nefrologia. Randomised placebo-controlled trial of effect of ramipril on decline in glomerular filtration rate and risk of terminal renal failure in proteinuric, non-diabetic nephropathy Lancet 349: 1857-63, 1997.

37. P.L. Kimmel, G.J. Mishkin, W.O. Umana. Captopril and renal survival in patients with human immunodeficiency virus nephropathy. American Journal Of Kidney Diseases 28: 202-8, 1996.

38. S.Wakai, K. Nitta, K. Honda, S. Horita, H Kobayashi, K.Uchida, W.Yumura, H. Nihei. Relationship between glomerular epithelial cell injury and proteinuria in IgA nephropathy. Nippon Jinzo Gakkai Shi 40(5):315-21, 1998.

39. F. Locatelli, D. Marcelli, M. Comelli, D. Alberti, G. Graziani, G. Buccianti, B. Redaelli, A. Giangrande. roteinuria and blood pressure as causal components of progression to end-stage renal failure. Northern Italian Cooperative Study Group. Nephrology Dialysis Transplant, 11(3):461-7, 1996.

40. G. Remuzzi. Renoprotective Effect of ACE Inhibitors: Dissecting the Molecular Clues and Expanding the Blood Pressure Goal. American Journal of Kidney Diseases 34: 951-954. 1999

41. K. Sharma, B.O. Eltayeb, T.A. McGowan, et al. Captopril induced reduction of serum levels of transforming growth factor-ß1 correlates with long-term renoprotection in insulin-dependent diabetic patients. American Jounal of Kidney Disease 34:818-823, 1999

42. T.M. Osicka, Y. Yu, S Panagiotopoulos, et al. Prevention of albuminuria by aminoguanidine or ramipril in streptozoticin-induced diabetic rats is associated with the normalization of glomerular protein kinase C. Diabetes 49: 87-93, 2000.

43. W.F. Keane, G. Eknoyan. Proteinuria, Albuminuria, Risk, Assessment, Detection, Elimination (PARADE): A Position Paper of the National Kidney Foundation American Journal of Kidney Diseases 33: 1004-1010, 1999.

45

DIABETES, HYPERTENSION, AND KIDNEY DISEASE IN THE PIMA INDIANS.

William C Knowler[1], Robert G Nelson[1], David J Pettitt[2]
[1]National Institute of Diabetes and Digestive and Kidney Diseases, Phoenix, Arizona, USA
[2]Sansum Medical Research Institute, Santa Barbara, California, USA

INTRODUCTION

Hypertension and kidney disease are well-known concomitants of both type 1 and type 2 diabetes mellitus. Hypertension, kidney disease, and diabetes are associated with each other, but the associations vary between populations, and the causal interpretations, especially regarding hypertension and diabetic nephropathy, are controversial. The complications of diabetes have been studied extensively among the Pima Indians of Arizona, U.S.A. In this chapter, we describe the epidemiology of diabetic kidney disease and its relationship with hypertension in the Pima Indians.

THE PIMA INDIAN DIABETES STUDY

The Pima Indians have the world's highest reported incidence and prevalence of diabetes [1]. Since 1965, this population has participated in a longitudinal epidemiologic study of diabetes and its complications [2]. At each examination, conducted at about two-year intervals, an oral glucose tolerance test was performed and classified according to the World Health Organization criteria [3]. Throughout the study, urine samples with at least a trace of protein on dipstick were assayed for total protein, and the urine protein-to-creatinine ratio was used as an estimate of the protein excretion rate [4]. Since 1982, the urine samples were assayed for albumin, and a urine albumin-to-creatinine ratio was used as an estimate of the urinary albumin excretion rate [5]. Blood pressure was measured at each examination with the subject at rest in the supine position [6].

Kidney function was studied in more detail in a subset of nondiabetic and diabetic Pima Indians. These studies include serial measurements of glomerular filtration rate (GFR), renal plasma flow, albumin and IgG excretion, and glomerular capillary permeability to dextran particles of different sizes [7].

The prevalence of diabetes in Pima Indians is almost 13 times as high as in the mostly white population of Rochester, Minnesota [1]. Diabetes occurs in over one-third of Pima Indians aged 35-44 years and in over 60% of those ≥45 years old [2]. Many cases develop before the age of 25 years. Pima Indians develop only type 2 diabetes [8, 9], and they differ from other populations in that the disease develops at younger ages [1, 2]. Diabetic complications also develop at rates similar to those of other populations. In contrast to populations in which type 2 diabetes usually develops later in life, many Pima Indians have diabetes of sufficient duration for nephropathy to develop.

THE COURSE OF DIABETIC NEPHROPATHY IN PIMA INDIANS

The onset of type 2 diabetes in Pima Indians is characterized, on average, by a rise in GFR and a modest size-selective abnormality of the glomerular capillary wall [10, 11]. Abnormally elevated albuminuria is another characteristic early sign of diabetic nephropathy. In a cross-sectional study of albuminuria in Pima Indians ≥15 years of age, abnormal albuminuria was defined by a urine albumin-to-creatinine ratio ≥ 30 mg/g [5]. Abnormal albuminuria is subdivided by ratios ≥ 30 mg/g and < 300 mg/g, called microalbuminuria, and ratios ≥ 300 mg/g, called macroalbuminuria. Abnormal albuminuria was found in 8% of those with normal glucose tolerance, 15% of those with impaired glucose tolerance, and 47% of those with diabetes [5]. The prevalence was also related to the duration of diabetes, varying from 29% within five years of diagnosis to 86% after 20 years of diabetes. The high prevalence in diabetes and the relationship with diabetes duration indicate that albuminuria is a complication of diabetes, but there is also a substantial prevalence in those with normal or impaired glucose tolerance, indicating that diabetes is not the sole cause of abnormal albuminuria in this population. Abnormal albuminuria is often followed by more serious kidney disease. Among diabetic Pimas, the degree of albuminuria over the range of values < 300 mg/g predicts the subsequent incidence of overt nephropathy, defined by a protein-to-creatinine ratio ≥1.0 g/g [12].

Among diabetic Pima Indians, the incidence rate of elevated albuminuria (≥30 mg/g) is similar to that previously reported in type 1 diabetes [13]. The incidence of overt diabetic nephropathy, defined by urine protein/creatinine ≥1.0g/g, is shown in figure 1. Incidence rates increased with duration of diabetes, at least until 25 years. Beyond 25 years of diabetes, the incidence rate appears to have stabilized or declined, although the trend with time is uncertain because the standard errors of the rates are high at long durations due to limited observations. Thus it remains uncertain whether beyond a certain duration of diabetes, Pima Indians pass a period of susceptibility to development of nephropathy, as reported after 15-20 years of type 1 diabetes [14, 15].

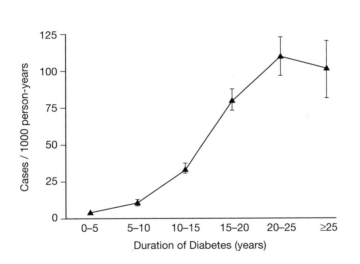

Fig. 1. Incidence rates of overt nephropathy (urine protein-to-creatinine ratio ≥1.0 g/g) by duration of diabetes in Pima Indians. The rates ± standard errors are shown. Adapted from Kunzelman et al [4].

GFR was measured in Pimas with diabetes of ≥5 years duration with normal albuminuria (n=20) or with macroalbuminuria (n=34) [16]. At baseline, those with macroalbuminuria had, on average, lower GFR and higher blood pressure. During 48 months of follow-up of 30 of those with macroalbuminuria, the GFR declined by an average of 9 ml/min per year, higher than the rate of decline reported for similar patients with type 1 diabetes. The slope of GFR over time was highly correlated with the increase in urinary albumin or IgG clearance. Dextran sieving studies suggested that the progressive decline in GFR is caused by a decline in average density of glomerular pores, which is accompanied by a widening of the pore size distribution and increased transglomerular passage of plasma proteins.

Figure 2 summarizes the degree of albuminuria, expressed as an albumin-to-creatinine ratio, in five groups of subjects followed for up to four years [7]. On average, those with impaired glucose tolerance, newly diagnosed diabetes, or longstanding diabetes with normoalbuminuria (by definition) had normal urine albumin excretion at baseline. There was little change, on average, during follow-up of those in the first two groups. The degree of albuminuria tended to increase, however, in all three groups with long-standing diabetes, whether they had normo-, micro-, or macro-albuminuria at baseline. During this time, GFR increased in persons with impaired glucose tolerance or newly diagnosed diabetes, was relatively stable in those with longstanding diabetes with normo- or micro-albuminuria, and declined in those with macro-albuminuria at baseline (figure 2). The major predictor of declining GFR was the degree of albuminuria. By contrast, baseline GFR did not predict change in GFR or in albuminuria. Thus the degree of elevation in albumin excretion is the major predictor of worsening diabetic nephropathy.

In diabetic persons, the onset of clinical proteinuria, defined by the urinary excretion of at least 500 mg protein per day, heralds a progressive decline of kidney function that often leads to end-stage renal disease (ESRD) [17]. Figure 3 shows the cumulative incidence of ESRD as a function of the duration of proteinuria in Pima Indians and, using similar definitions of proteinuria, in whites with type 1 [15] or type 2 diabetes [18]. Coronary heart disease is a frequent cause of death in older persons with diabetes, and proteinuria may, in part, account for the lower incidence of ESRD in whites with type 2 diabetes. Due to the relatively young age at onset of diabetes in Pima Indians and their lower death rate from coronary heart disease [19], the cumulative incidence of ESRD in this population more closely resembles that of whites with type 1 diabetes than those with type 2 diabetes.

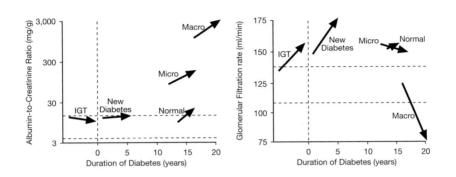

Fig. 2. Changes in median urinary albumin-to-creatinine ratio (left) and mean glomerular filtration rate (right) from baseline to the end of follow-up in persons with impaired glucose tolerance (IGT), newly diagnosed diabetes, and longstanding diabetes according to baseline albuminuria. Each arrow connects the value at the baseline examination and the value at the end of follow-up. The vertical dashed line indicates the time of diagnosis of diabetes, and the horizontal dotted lines the 25th through 75th percentiles of values in subjects with normal glucose tolerance. Adapted from Nelson et al. [7].

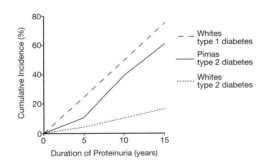

Fig. 3. Cumulative incidence of end stage renal disease by duration of proteinuria. Adapted from Nelson et al. [17], Krolewski et al. [15], and Humphrey et al. [18].

When expressed as a function of duration of diabetes, the cumulative incidence of ESRD is also nearly identical in the Pimas with type 2 diabetes and the whites with type 1 diabetes [20]. Other studies comparing persons with type 1 diabetes or type 2 diabetes in the same populations have concluded that the duration-specific risk of ESRD is similar in the two types of diabetes [17, 21].

The incidence of ESRD is also very high among other American Indians [reviewed in 22], but diabetes is apparently not responsible for as great a proportion of cases of ESRD in some of the other American Indian tribes. The degree of albuminuria was higher in Pima Indians than in several other American Indian tribes, even when controlled for differences in age, sex, fasting plasma glucose, blood pressure, and fibrinogen [23].

The greater degree of albuminuria in Pima Indians compared with the other American Indian tribes [23], the increased risk of diabetic nephropathy in Pima Indians whose parents have hypertension [24], and the familial aggregation of diabetic nephropathy in this [25] and other populations suggest that susceptibility to diabetic nephropathy may be genetically transmitted, as reviewed in Chapter 8. A genetic segregation analysis suggested that the family aggregation results from a major genetic effect on the prevalence of diabetic nephropathy conditional on the duration of diabetes [26]. Further evidence for genetic susceptibility to diabetic nephropathy comes from a genetic linkage study in which 98 diabetic sibling pairs affected with nephropathy were included in a genome-wide scan. A DNA marker on chromosome 7q was tentatively linked to nephropathy (single marker LOD = 2.73, multipoint LOD = 2.04), suggesting that a genetic element in the region of this marker influences susceptibility to diabetic nephropathy [27]. A parametric linkage analysis, using the segregation model [26] to incorporate data from diabetic siblings without nephropathy, suggested an additional locus on chromosome 18q (multipoint LOD = 1.49) [28]. Other factors, including duration of diabetes, blood pressure, level of glycemia, and pharmacologic treatment of diabetes are associated with the development of kidney disease in Pima Indians [4, 17, 20]. Risk of diabetic nephropathy is also higher in offspring exposed to diabetes in utero [29] or who were in the lowest or highest extremes of the birth weight distribution [30]; these exposures are also risk factors for diabetes itself [31]. There was no evidence that hantavirus infection, which has been implicated in kidney disease in other populations, is involved in diabetic nephropathy in the Pimas [32]. Nearly all of the excess mortality associated with diabetes in this population occurs in persons with clinically detectable proteinuria, and the age-sex-adjusted death rate in diabetic subjects without proteinuria is no greater than the rate in nondiabetic subjects [33]. Thus, proteinuria is a marker not only for diabetic kidney disease, but identifies those with diabetes who are at increased risk for a number of macro- and microvascular complications and for death. Similar findings reported in persons with type 1 diabetes suggest a common underlying cause for albuminuria and the other associated diabetic complications, both renal and extrarenal [34].

Autopsy studies indicate that intercapillary glomerular sclerosis, typical of diabetic nephropathy in other ethnic groups, is the predominant kidney disease in the Pimas [35], although other glomerular lesions were found in some nondiabetic Pimas [36]. In kidney biopsies from 51 diabetic Pima Indians, total glomerular volume and mesangial volume were positively correlated with stage of diabetic nephropathy. Moreover, clinical nephropathy was associated with thickening of the glomerular basement membrane and a lower number of podocytes per glomerulus [37]. In a 4-year follow-up of 16 diabetic persons with microalbuminuria, lower podocyte number per glomerulus predicted increasing urinary albumin excretion, suggesting that podocyte injury plays an important role in the development and progression of diabetic nephropathy [38]. A 35 percent reduction in the number of podocytes per glomerulus in 12 diabetic patients with microalbuminuria who had two kidney biopsies separated by 4 years provides further evidence that podocyte loss characterizes the early course of diabetic glomerular injury [39]. Ensuing alterations in the remaining podocyte foot processes may contribute to the progressive loss of glomerular size selectivity that occurs in diabetic patients with macroalbuminuria [40].

RELATIONSHIP OF BLOOD PRESSURE TO DIABETES AND KIDNEY DISEASE

The relationships of blood pressure to glucose tolerance, hyperinsulinemia, and insulin resistance have been examined in many populations. A difficulty in examining these relationships is that many drugs used in treating high blood pressure may also affect insulin resistance or glycemia. Thus, correlations of these variables are difficult to interpret if studies include subjects taking antihypertensive drugs; yet if such subjects are excluded, the associations might be underestimated because of exclusion of those with the most severe hypertension. One approach is to divide blood pressure into two categories, hypertension or not, and include those treated with antihypertensive drugs as hypertensive regardless of their measured blood pressure. Even this approach may not be satisfactory, however, as many diabetic patients are treated with antihypertensive drugs for cardio- or renoprotection rather than because of hypertension, a practice likely to increase in the future in view of evidence of benefit [41-45].

Blood pressure (or hypertension) is related to glucose tolerance in Pima Indians. The age-sex-adjusted prevalence rates of hypertension (systolic blood pressure ≥160 mm Hg, diastolic blood pressure ≥ 95 mm Hg, or receiving antihypertensive drugs) among those with normal glucose tolerance, impaired glucose tolerance, or diabetes were 7%, 13%, and 20%, respectively, an almost three-fold difference [6]. Similarly, as continuous variables, blood pressure and two-hour plasma glucose concentrations were correlated among subjects who were not treated with either antihypertensive or hypoglycemic drugs. This relationship, also observed in other populations, may be explained by hyperinsulinemia, as serum insulin concentrations tend to be higher in persons with impaired glucose tolerance and in some persons with diabetes than in those with normal glucose tolerance. Yet in the Pimas blood pressure has a much stronger correlation with plasma glucose than with serum insulin concentrations, and the partial correlation of blood pressure with fasting insulin, controlled for age, sex, BMI, and glucose, is practically zero [6]. Thus the relationship, at least among the Pimas, is primarily with glucose, and the correlation with insulin may be secondary.

In addition to studies of blood pressure and serum insulin concentrations, the correlation of blood pressure with insulin resistance was assessed by the euglycemic clamp. In a study of three racial groups, among nondiabetic, normotensive subjects not taking any medicines, blood pressure and insulin resistance were correlated only among whites, but not among blacks or Pima Indians [46]. While this study confirmed previous reports of a correlation of blood pressure with insulin resistance in whites, it suggests that such a relationship is race-specific, and hence does not indicate that insulin resistance is an important or consistent cause of hypertension.

Although blood pressure and plasma glucose concentrations are correlated and the prevalence of hypertension is related to 2-hr glucose, even among nondiabetic subjects, hyperglycemia is not the only factor of importance for blood pressure in diabetes. Among adult Pima Indians, urinary albumin-to-creatinine ratios were higher with progressively worse glucose tolerance or longer duration of diabetes, and among diabetic patients were higher in those treated with insulin [47]. Regardless of the degree of hyperglycemia and duration of diabetes, those with hypertension had greater albuminuria. The associations of each of these variables with albuminuria were highly significant, but the causal directions underlying them have not been determined. The relationship of insulin treatment with albuminuria is similar to that of insulin treatment with many complications of diabetes [4 , 5, 19, 48-50] and might reflect more severe diabetes (i.e. those with greater hyperglycemia or more complications have a greater need for insulin treatment).

Blood pressure and kidney disease are clearly related, although the causes of this relationship are not clear and are debated extensively, with some arguing that the elevated blood pressure in diabetes is only secondary to diabetic nephropathy [34, 51], and others that elevated blood pressure is due to a genetic predisposition that contributes to the development of diabetic nephropathy [52, 53]. In the Pima Indians, higher blood pressure *before* the onset of diabetes confers a greater risk of kidney disease *after* diabetes develops (figure 4) [54], and among the diabetic subjects with normo- or micro-albuminuria, higher blood pressure predicts increasing urinary albumin excretion rates [7]. On the other hand, higher blood pressure does not predict ESRD in diabetic Pima Indians who already have proteinuria [17]. This suggests that blood pressure may contribute to the initiation of diabetic nephropathy [54], but less to its progression once proteinuria has developed [17]. The higher pre-diabetic blood pressure in those destined to have elevated albuminuria after the onset of diabetes may be an early manifestation of an underlying susceptibility to kidney disease which develops only in the presence of diabetes. This susceptibility factor for nephropathy may also be a risk factor for diabetes [54].

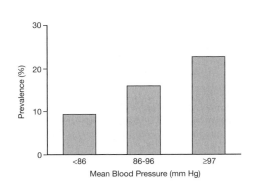

Fig. 4. Prevalence of elevated albuminuria (urine albumin-to-creatinine ratio ≥100 mg/g) after the diagnosis of diabetes by prediabetic blood pressure. Adapted from Nelson et al. [54].

CONCLUSIONS

Hypertension and kidney disease are common complications of diabetes in the Pima Indians, as they are in other populations, and persons with these conditions have a particularly bad prognosis. Almost all of the excess mortality in diabetic Pimas is associated with nephropathy. The higher prevalence of abnormal albumin excretion in diabetic subjects who had higher blood pressures before the onset of diabetes suggests that the hypertension of diabetes is not entirely secondary to diabetic nephropathy, but that higher blood pressure contributes to this complication.

REFERENCES

1. Knowler WC, Bennett PH, Hamman RF, Miller M: Diabetes incidence and prevalence in Pima Indians: a 19-fold greater incidence than in Rochester, Minnesota. Am J Epidemiol 108:497-505, 1978.
2. Knowler WC, Pettitt DJ, Saad MF, Bennett PH: Diabetes mellitus in the Pima Indians: incidence, risk factors, and pathogenesis. Diabetes/Metabolism Reviews 6:1-27, 1990.
3. Diabetes mellitus: report of a WHO study group. WHO Technical Report Series 727. Geneva, World Health Organization, 1985.
4. Kunzelman CL, Knowler WC, Pettitt DJ, Bennett PH: Incidence of nephropathy in type 2 diabetes mellitus in the Pima Indians. Kidney Int 35:681-687, 1989.
5. Nelson RG, Kunzelman CL, Pettitt DJ, Saad MF, Bennett PH, Knowler WC: Albuminuria in Type 2 (non-insulin-dependent) diabetes mellitus and impaired glucose tolerance in Pima Indians. Diabetologia 32:870-876, 1989.
6. Saad MF, Knowler WC, Pettitt DJ, Nelson RG, Mott DM, Bennett PH: Insulin and hypertension: relationship to obesity and glucose intolerance in Pima Indians. Diabetes 39:1430-1435, 1990.
7. Nelson RG, Bennett PH, Beck GJ, Tan M, Knowler WC, Mitch WE, Hirschman GH, Myers BD, for the Diabetic Renal Disease Study: Development and progression of renal disease in Pima Indians with non-insulin-dependent diabetes mellitus. N Engl J Med 335:1636-1642, 1996.
8. Knowler WC, Bennett PH, Bottazzo GF, Doniach D: Islet cell antibodies and diabetes mellitus in Pima Indians. Diabetologia 17:161-164, 1979.
9. Dabelea D, Palmer JP, Bennett PH, Pettitt DJ, Knowler WC: Absence of glutamic acid decarboxylase antibodies in Pima Indian children with diabetes mellitus (letter). Diabetologia 42:1265-1266, 1999.
10. Myers BD, Nelson RG, Williams GW, Bennett PH, Hardy SA, Berg RL, Loon N, Knowler WC, Mitch WE: Glomerular function in Pima Indians with non-insulin-dependent diabetes mellitus of recent onset. J Clin Invest 88:524-530, 1991.
11. Nelson RG, Tan M, Beck GJ, Bennett PH, Knowler WC, Mitch WE, Blouch K, Myers BD: Changing glomerular filtration with progression from impaired glucose tolerance to Type II diabetes mellitus. Diabetologia 42:90-93, 1999.

12. Nelson RG, Knowler WC, Pettitt DJ, Saad MF, Charles MA, Bennett PH: Assessment of risk of overt nephropathy in diabetic patients from albumin excretion in untimed urine specimens. Arch Int Med 151:1761-1765, 1991.

13. Nelson RG, Knowler WC, Pettitt DJ, Hanson RL, Bennett PH: Incidence and determinants of elevated urinary albumin excretion in Pima Indians with NIDDM. Diabetes Care 18:182-187, 1995.

14. Andersen AR, Christiansen JS, Andersen JK, Kreiner S, Deckert T: Diabetic nephropathy in Type 1 (insulin-dependent) diabetes: an epidemiological study. Diabetologia 25:496-501, 1983.

15. Krolewski AS, Warram JH, Cristlieb AR, Busick EJ, Kahn C: The changing natural history of nephropathy in Type 1 diabetes. Am J Med 78:785-793, 1985.

16. Myers BD, Nelson RG, Tan M, Beck GJ, Bennett PH, Knowler WC, Blouch K, Mitch WE: Progression of overt nephropathy in non-insulin-dependent diabetes. Kidney Int 47:1781-1789, 1995.

17. Nelson RG, Knowler WC, McCance DR, Sievers ML, Pettitt DJ, Charles MA, Hanson RL, Liu QZ, Bennett PH: Determinants of end-stage renal disease in Pima Indians with type 2 (non-insulin-dependent) diabetes mellitus and proteinuria. Diabetologia 36:1087-1093, 1993.

18. Humphrey LL, Ballard DJ, Frohnert PP, Chu C-P, O'Fallon WM, Palumbo PJ: Chronic renal failure in non-insulin-dependent diabetes mellitus: a population-based study in Rochester, Minnesota. Ann Intern Med 111:788-796, 1989.

19. Nelson RG, Sievers ML, Knowler WC, Swinburn BA, Pettitt DJ, Saad MF, Garrison R, Liebow IM, Howard BV, Bennett PH: Low incidence of fatal coronary heart disease in Pima Indians despite high prevalence of non-insulin-dependent diabetes. Circulation 81:987-995, 1990.

20. Nelson RG, Newman JM, Knowler WC, Sievers ML, Kunzelman CL, Pettitt DJ, Moffett CD, Teutsch SM, Bennett PH: Incidence of end-stage renal disease in Type 2 (non-insulin-dependent) diabetes mellitus in Pima Indians. Diabetologia 31:730-736, 1988.

21. Hasslacher C, Ritz E, Wahl P, Michael C: Similar risks of nephropathy in patients with type I and type II diabetes mellitus. Nephrol Dial Transplant 4:859-863, 1989.

22. Nelson RG, Knowler WC, Pettitt DJ, Saad MF, Bennett PH: Diabetic kidney disease in Pima Indians. Diabetes Care 16:335-341, 1993.

23. Robbins DC, Knowler WC, Lee ET, Yeh J, Go OT, Welty T, Fabsitz R, Howard BV: Regional differences in albuminuria among American Indians: an epidemic of renal disease. Kidney Int 49:557-563, 1996.

24. Nelson RG, Pettitt DJ, de Courten MP, Hanson RL, Knowler WC, Bennett PH: Parental hypertension and proteinuria in Pima Indians with NIDDM. Diabetologia 39:433-438, 1996.

25. Pettitt DJ, Saad MF, Bennett PH, Nelson RG, Knowler WC: Familial predisposition to renal disease in two generations of Pima Indians with Type 2 (non-insulin-dependent) diabetes mellitus. Diabetologia 33:438-443, 1990.

26. Imperatore G, Knowler WC, Pettitt DJ, Kobes S, Bennett PH, Hanson RL: Segregation analysis of diabetic nephropathy in Pima Indians. Diabetes 49:1049-1056, 2000.

27. Imperatore G, Hanson RL, Pettitt DJ, Kobes S, Bennett PH, Knowler WC, and the Pima Diabetes Genes Group: Sib-pair linkage analysis for susceptibility genes for microvascular complications among Pima Indians with type 2 diabetes mellitus. Diabetes 47: 821-830, 1998.

28. Imperatore G, Knowler WC, Nelson RG, Hanson RL: Genetics of diabetic nephropathy in the Pima Indians. Current Diabetes Reports 1: 275-281, 2001.

29. Nelson RG, Morgenstern H, Bennett PH: Intrauterine diabetes exposure and the risk of renal disease in diabetic Pima Indians. Diabetes 47: 1489-1493, 1998.

30. Nelson RG, Morgenstern H, Bennett PH: Birth weight and renal disease in Pima Indians with type 2 diabetes mellitus. Am J Epidemiol 148: 650-656, 1998.

31. Dabelea D, Hanson RL, Bennett PH, Roumain J, Knowler WC, Pettitt DJ: Increasing prevalence of type II diabetes in American Indian children. Diabetologia 41: 904-910, 1998.

32. de Courten MP, Ksiazek TG, Rollin PE, Kahn AS, Daily PJ, Knowler WC: Seroprevalence study of hantavirus antibodies in Pima Indians with renal disease. J Infectious Dis 171:762-763, 1995.

33. Nelson RG, Pettitt DJ, Carraher MJ, Baird HR, Knowler WC: Effect of proteinuria on mortality in NIDDM. Diabetes 37:1499-1504, 1988.

34. Deckert T, Feldt-Rasmussen B, Borch-Johnsen K, Jensen T, Kofoed-Enevoldsen A: Albuminuria reflects widespread vascular damage. The Steno hypothesis. Diabetologia 32:219-226, 1989.

35. Kamenetzky SA, Bennett PH, Dippe SE, Miller M, LeCompte PM: A clinical and histologic study of diabetic nephropathy in the Pima Indians. Diabetes 23:61-68, 1974.

36. Schmidt K, Pesce C, Liu Q, Nelson RG, Bennett PH, Karnitschnig H, Striker LJ, Striker GE: Large glomerular size in Pima Indians: lack of change with diabetic nephropathy. J Am Soc Nephrol 3:229-235, 1992.

37. Pagtalunan ME, Miller PL, Jumping-Eagle S, Nelson RG, Myers BD, Rennke HG, Coplon NS, Sun L, Meyer TW: Podocyte loss and progressive glomerular injury in type II diabetes. J Clin Invest 99: 342-348, 1997.

38. Meyer TW, Bennett PH, Nelson RG: Podocyte number predicts long-trem urinary albumin excretion in Pima Indians with type II diabetes and microalbuminuria. Diabetologia 42: 1341-1344, 1999.

39. Lemley KV, Abdullah I, Myers BD, Meyer TW, Blouch K, Smith WE, Bennett PH, Nelson RG: Evolution of incipient nephropathy in type 2 diabetes mellitus. Kidney Int 58:1228-1237, 2000.

40. Lemley KV, Blouch K, Abdullah I, Boothroyd DB, Bennett PH, Myers BD, Nelson RG: Glomerular permselectivity at the onset of nephropathy in type 2 diabetes mellitus. J Am Soc Nephrol 11:2095-2105, 2000.

41. UK Prospective Diabetes Study (UKPDS) Group: Efficacy of atenolol and captopril in reducing risk of macrovascular and microvascular compliations in type 2 diabetes: UKPDS 39. Br Med J 317: 713-720, 1998.

42. Heart Outcomes Prevention Evaluation (HOPE) Study Investigators: Effects of remipril on cariovascular and microvascular outcomes in people with diabetes mellitus: results of the HOPE study and MICRO-HOPE substudy. Lancet 355: 253-259, 2000.

43. Lewis EJ, Hunsicker LG, Clarke WR, Berl T, Pohl MA, Lewis JB, Ritz E, Atkins RC, Rohde R, Raz I, for the Collaborative Study Group: Renoprotective effect of the angiotensin-receptor antagonist irbesartan in patients with nephropathy due to type 2 diabetes. N Engl J Med 345:851-860, 2001.

44. Brenner BM, Cooper ME, de Zeeuw D, Keane WF, Mitch WE, Parving H-H, Remuzzi G, Sapinn SM, Zhang Z, Shahinfar S, for the RENAAL Study Investigators: Effects of losartan on renal and cardiovascular outcomes in patients with type 2 diabetes and nephropathy. N Engl J Med 345:861-869, 2001.

45. Parving H-H, Lehnert H, Bröchner-Mortensen, Bomis R, Andersen S, Arner P, for the Irbesartan in Patients with Type 2 Diabetes and Microalbuminuria Study Group: The effect of irbesartan on the development of diabetic nephropathy in patients with type 2 diabetes. N Engl J Med 345: 870-878, 2001.

46. Saad MF, Lillioja S, Nyomba BL, Castillo C, Ferraro R, DeGregoria M, Ravussin E, Knowler WC, Bennett PH, Howard BV, Bogardus C: Racial differences in the relation between blood pressure and insulin resistance. N Engl J Med 324:733-739, 1991.

47. Knowler WC, Nelson RG, Pettitt DJ: Diabetes, hypertension, and kidney disease in the Pima Indians compared with other populations. In Mogensen CE, ed: The Kidney and Hypertension in Diabetes Mellitus, 2nd ed., Kluwer Academic Publishers, Boston, 1994, pp. 53-62.48. Knowler WC, Bennett PH, Ballintine EJ: Increased incidence of retinopathy in diabetics with elevated blood pressure: a six-year followup study in Pima Indians. N Eng J Med 302:645-650, 1980.

49. Liu QZ, Knowler WC, Nelson RG, Saad MF, Charles MA, Liebow IM, Bennett PH, Pettitt DJ: Insulin treatment, endogenous insulin concentration, and ECG abnormalities in diabetic Pima Indians: cross-sectional and prospective analyses. Diabetes 41:1141-1150, 1992.

50. Nagi DK, Pettitt DJ, Bennett PH, Klein R, Knowler WC: Diabetic retinopathy assessed by fundus photography in Pima Indians with impaired glucose tolerance and non-insulin-dependent diabetes mellitus. Diabetic Med 14: 449-456, 1997.

51. Mathiesen ER, Rønn B, Jensen T, Storm B, Deckert T: Relationship between blood pressure and urinary albumin excretion in development of microalbuminuria. Diabetes 39:245-249, 1990.

52. Viberti CG, Keen H, Wiseman MJ: Raised arterial pressure in parents of proteinuric insulin-dependent diabetics. Br Med J 295:551-517, 1987.

53. Krolewski AS, Canessa M, Warram JH, Laffel LMB, Christlieb AR, Knowler WC, Rand LI: Predisposition to hypertension and susceptibility to renal disease in insulin-dependent diabetes mellitus. N Engl J Med 318:140-145, 1988.

54. Nelson RG, Pettitt DJ, Baird HR, Charles MA, Liu QZ, Bennett PH, Knowler WC: Prediabetic blood pressure predicts urinary albumin excretion after the onset of type 2 (non-insulin-dependent) diabetes mellitus in Pima Indians. Diabetologia 36:998-1001, 1993.

55. McCance DR, Hanson RL, Pettitt DJ, Jacobsson LTH, Bennett PH, Bishop DT, Knowler WC: Diabetic nephropathy: a risk factor for diabetes in offspring. Diabetologia 38:221-226, 1995.

46

THE DEVELOPMENT AND PROGRESSION OF CLINICAL NEPHROPATHY IN WHITE PATIENTS WITH TYPE 2 DIABETES

Amanda I. Adler

Diabetes Trials Unit, Oxford Centre for Diabetes and Endocrinology, Churchill Hospital, Headington, Oxford OX3 7LJ, UK

Nephropathy is one of the most characteristic complications of diabetes. Individuals without diabetes are twice as likely to identify renal disease, compared to cardiovascular disease, as a complication of diabetes [1]. Diabetic renal disease, described since the second century A.D. [2], burdens patients and health care systems to the extent that US government officials have referred to the "enormity of the problem of diabetic renal failure" [3]. The proportion of patients with end stage renal disease (ESRD) who also have diabetes varies from approximately 25% in the UK and Canada to over 40% in the US [4] [5] [6] making diabetic nephropathy the main reason for renal replacement therapy [4].

Although type 2 diabetes accounts for the overwhelming majority of all diabetes mellitus, the clinical course of nephropathy in type 2 diabetes is less well described than it is in type 1 diabetes [7]. Fortunately, prospective studies are accumulating including those of early stage nephropathy [8] [9] [10, 11] [12], later stage nephropathy [13] and studies addressing from early to late nephropathy including from the diagnosis of diabetes [14] [15]. Because of ethnic differences in the incidence of nephropathy in type 2 diabetes [16, 17], this chapter will concentrate on populations comprised largely, or entirely, of white Caucasians. It will also concentrate on clinical trials and cohort studies, either prospective studies or retrospective, of moderate to large size. This chapter will attempt to summarize estimates of the rate of development and worsening of nephropathy over time, that is, incidence rates rather than prevalence.

Varying definitions, and somewhat confusing nomenclature, used in studies of diabetic nephropathy lead to challenges when comparing results. Moreover, categorization systems have changed over time. Previously, five stages defined disease, including early hypertrophy/hyperfunction, glomerular lesions without clinical disease, incipient diabetic nephropathy defined by low levels of proteinuria, persistent proteinuria and declining renal function, and, finally, end-stage renal disease [18] [19]. Recent epidemiologic studies of renal disease incorporate the classification of chronic kidney disease (CKD) based on five stages of progression, itself based on glomerular filtration rate [20] [21].

This chapter uses the clinical stages based on the older classification, i.e. (degrees of) proteinuria, because of the strong association between albuminuria and subsequent nephropathy [22], elevation in creatinine, and end-stage renal disease.

RATES OF PROGRESSION OF NEPHROPATHY

Using data collected in Rochester, Minnesota, epidemiologists recorded the progression of nephropathy among 1301 residents with type 2 diabetes [14]. Subjects diagnosed with diabetes from 1945 to 1969 were followed to 1982 for the onset of "persistent proteinuria" defined as a urine protein value of greater than 40 mg/dl on two random spot urine sample obtained during routine medical care. Excluding the 8.2% of subjects who had persistent proteinuria diagnosed before or within 6 months after diagnosis of diabetes, diabetic individuals developed persistent proteinuria at a rate of 1.5% per year and chronic renal failure at a rate of 0.13% per year [23]. Persistent proteinuria was a strong (hazard ratio 12.1) and independent risk factor for the development of chronic renal failure. Despite the high relative risk, the absolute risk was modest. Patients with persistent proteinuria were unlikely to develop chronic renal failure; the cumulative incidence was 16.8% 15 following the diagnosis of persistent proteinuria. The median duration of persistent proteinuria in the Rochester cohort was 7 years compared to 9.7

872

years in the UK Prospective Diabetes Study UKPDS [15] [23], acknowledging differences in the definitions used between the two studies.

In a different part of the Midwestern United States, Southern Wisconsin, investigators followed a population-based, predominantly white cohort of individuals with type 2 diabetes for the emergence of "gross proteinuria", defined as spot urine protein concentration of $\geq$ 30 mg/l. Investigators observed that 33% of patients not taking insulin (n=418) developed gross proteinuria in 10 years, compared with 40% of patients taking insulin (n=376) [11]. The study used a semi-quantitative determination of urine protein using a reagent stick.

In Denmark, Gall and co-workers followed 191 patients with type 2 diabetes for the development of "incipient diabetic nephropathy" defined as persistent microalbuminuria of 30 – 299 mg/24 hours in two out of three 24 hour urine collections [8]. Among patients normoalbuminuric at the start of the observation period, 23% develop incipient diabetic nephropathy in five years.

In Finland, 108 patients with type 2 diabetes and normal albumin excretion. In the nine-years of follow-up, 34% progressed to microalbuminuria or worse renal function. Approximately 24% of patients developed microalbuminuria alone. However, some one in five patients died during follow-up, and true incidence rates were not reported [9].

By comparison, Ravid and his colleagues followed patients with type 2 in Israel aged 40 to 60 years for the development of microalbuminuria defined as urinary protein excretion of 30 – 300 mg/24 hours. Patients were followed for a mean of 7.8 years during which time 19% of patients had developed microalbuminuria.

Among the 5147 diabetic men participating in the Multiple Risk Factor Intervention Trial (MRFIT) study, some 83% of whom were white, the age-adjusted incidence of ESRD was 199.8 per 100,000 person years, or approximately 0.2% per year. Hence, while diabetes itself was associated with a nine-fold increased in risk over men with diabetes for the development of ESRD due to any cause, the absolute rate of ESRD remained low.

Compared to the MRFIT study, UK Prospective Diabetes Study, UKPDS, was of a similar size, duration, and proportion of white participants, but also measured the spectrum of diabetic nephropathy. The UKPDS was a randomized, non-blinded clinical trial that investigated the effects of intensive policies for the control of blood glucose and blood pressure on the complications of type 2 diabetes in newly diagnosed subjects, 82% of whom were white [15]. Because of the size of the study (5102, of whom 5097 had measures of urinary albumin measurements), and relatively long follow-up (median 10.4 years), the study provided an opportunity to observe the (treated) natural history of nephropathy. Subjects were excluded from the UKPDS if the plasma creatinine concentration was >175 mmol/L among other exclusions [24] [25] [26] [27].

Stages of nephropathy were defined based on urinary albumin concentration measured annually from a morning spot urine and plasma creatinine. Subjects were designated as having "no nephropathy" in the absence of microalbuminuria or worse renal function. Patients were designated as being in the stage of microalbuminuria if the urine albumin was in the range of 50 to 299 mg/L [28] [24] on two consecutive annual visits with a plasma creatinine was < 175 µmol/L. A patient was also deemed microalbuminuric if a urinary albumin in the range of microalbuminuria was followed in the next year by worse nephropathy or death from renal or cardiovascular causes. Patients were designated as being in the stage of macroalbuminuria if their urine albumin was ≥ 300 mg/L at two consecutive annual visits with a plasma creatinine was < 175 mmol/L, or if a urinary albumin value in the macroalbuminuric range was followed in the next year by worse renal function or death from renal or cardiovascular causes. Patients were designated as being in the stage of elevated plasma creatinine or renal replacement therapy if their plasma creatinine was ≥175 µmol/L on two consecutive annual visits, or if a creatinine ≥175 µmol/L was followed the next year by renal dialysis, renal transplant, or death.

The annual rates of transition from stage to stage of nephropathy and to death are shown in Figure 1. Patients progressed through *each stage* from no nephropathy to elevated plasma creatinine or renal replacement therapy at 2 –3 % per year. Individuals had a lower probability of skipping stages in a given year.

Annual death rates increased with increasing nephropathy (Figure 1). Patients with elevated plasma creatinine, but without renal replacement therapy, had an annual death rate of 18.9% (95% confidence interval, CI, 13.3% - 24.6%). For patients with macroalbuminuria, the annual death rate of 4.6% (3.5%-5.7%) exceeded the rate of progression to worse nephropathy (CI, 2.3%, 1.5% - 3.0%). Relative to patients in the stage of no nephropathy, those with microalbuminuria, macroalbuminuria, or an elevated plasma creatinine or renal replacement therapy had a 2.2 fold, 3.4 fold, and 13.9 fold increased risk of death, respectively.

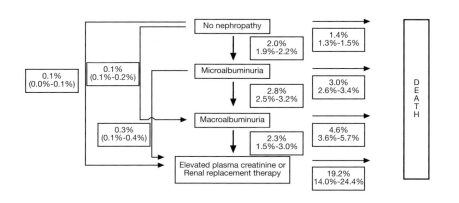

Fig.1. Annual transition rates with 95% confidence intervals through the stages of nephropathy and to death from any cause

The most common cause of death at all stages of nephropathy was cardiovascular disease, including deaths from stroke, myocardial infarction, sudden death and peripheral vascular disease, with a trend for increasing risk of cardiovascular death with increasing nephropathy (p<0.0001). The annual death rate due to cardiovascular disease was 0.7% for subjects in the no nephropathy stage, 2.0% for those with microalbuminuria, and 3.5% for those with macroalbuminuria and 12.1% for those with elevated plasma creatinine or renal replacement therapy. Correspondingly, the proportion of all deaths due to cardiovascular disease increased with each stage of increasing albuminuria being 51% of deaths in no nephropathy stage, 66% of deaths in those with microalbuminuria, and 75% of deaths in those with macroalbuminuria.

Reflecting the rising mortality rate with increasing nephropathy, the proportion of patients alive at ten years following onset of a given stage of nephropathy fell with increasing nephropathy. Of patients with no nephropathy at diagnosis of diabetes, 87.1% were alive after ten years falling to 8.5% for those ten years following the onset of elevated plasma creatinine or renal replacement therapy [15].

The Heart Outcomes and Prevention Evaluation Study (HOPE), also a randomized clinical controlled trial, provided prospective observations on the progression of renal disease in type 2 diabetes. The trial demonstrated, in patients at high risk for cardiovascular disease including 3498 individuals with diabetes, the success of ramipril in reducing risk for cardiovascular, as well as renal, disease [29]. The study also identified that microalbuminuria increased the risk for subsequent cardiovascular disease [30], as well as for the risk of greater degrees of albuminuria [12]. Specifically, investigators observed that 34% of diabetic patients developed new microalbuminuria defined as a urine albumin-creatinine ratio of ≥2 mg/mmol over the course of the median 4.5 year follow-up. Investigators defined "clinical proteinuria" as a urine albumin excretion greater than or equal to 300 mg/d or urine protein was ≥ 500 mg/d or the albumin creatinine ratio was >36 mg/mmol. Of patients with microalbuminuria at baseline, 23% developed clinical proteinuria compared to only 1.5% of those without microalbuminuria, evidencing the importance of extant albuminuria to the progression of diabetes renal disease, as well as the low overall incidence of clinical proteinuria among patients without microalbuminuria. The greater the urinary albumin/creatinine at the beginning of the study, the greater the risk of developing clinical proteinuria. It is of note that levels of albuminuria below that traditionally defined as microalbuminuria were also associated with an increased risk of nephropathy [12].

DISCUSSION

Incidence rates of albuminuria and more advanced nephropathy help us to understand the natural history of disease, as well as providing information to health care workers, modelers, clinical trialists, economists, health planners and insurers. Studies of the development and progression of nephropathy in type 2 diabetes show that patients with diabetes are at overwhelmingly greater risk for nephropathy than are patients without, as are patients with an existing degree of albuminuria. The rate of progression is fairly constant through the stages of nephropathy; hence, individuals are likely to develop microalbuminuria but less likely to develop greater degrees of nephropathy. The modest rates of progression to ESRD means that subjects with microalbuminuria are not necessarily destined for worse renal function. Indeed, ESRD remains a relatively rare complication of diabetes, yet also one that significantly burdens those who do develop it. Because a high proportion of patients with diabetes die from cardiovascular disease, a risk increased by the presence of early nephropathy, the low rate of ESRD is due in part to the competing risk of death.

In theory, then, the rate of ESRD could rise given a drop in the prevalence of factors that increase the risk of cardiovascular death, but not the risk of ESRD to the same extent. Based on UKPDS observations, subjects with macroalbuminuria and elevated plasma creatinine have a greater probability of dying in any year than of requiring renal replacement therapy. If a therapy decreased the risk of MI without decreasing progressive albuminuria, this relationship could change. On a related note, if the age of diagnosis of type 2 diabetes continues to fall [31], the burden of advanced renal disease will likely worsen, in part because younger patients with ESRD live longer than older patients [32].

In general, patients in the UKPDS were less likely to develop microalbuminuria and then macroalbuminuria than patients in Denmark or Israel. Investigators in the HOPE studied predicted that 50% of study participants, in whom duration of diabetes was not specifically reported, would develop microalbuminuria by 10 years [12]; by comparison half that percentage would be expected to develop microalbuminuria based on UKPDS observations [15].

Not all renal disease in patients with type 2 diabetes stems necessarily from diabetes [33] [13], although diabetes accounts for the vast majority. Unless the proportion of non-diabetic nephropathy present in type 2 diabetes differs markedly between cohorts, this would not account for differences in rates.

The rates of development and progression of albuminuria and worse nephropathy reported do not take into account factors that accelerate, or retard, progression. Risk factors which have been shown to have independent (i.e. controlling for the presence potential confounders) associations with the development of albuminuria in type 2 diabetes in at least one prospective study include age, male sex, glycemia, the presence of retinopathy or cardiovascular disease, systolic and diastolic blood pressure, smoking cigarettes, urine albumin excretion, body mass index, duration of diabetes, digoxin use, and dyslipidemia [10] [9] [8, 11, 14]. The rates observed in the reviewed studies are most generalizable to populations with similar characteristics and definitions of disease.

Nor do the above-mentioned rates of progression of nephropathy in type 2 diabetes take into account therapies that have been shown to reduce the occurrence and progression [24, 34, 35] [12]. Since these therapies are recently reported, as well as gaining in popularity [36], the progression of nephropathy may slow in future. That microalbuminuria itself is a risk factor for greater degrees of albuminuria, renal failure, and death, particularly from cardiovascular disease and including congestive heart failure, has been repeatedly observed [30, 37, 38] [39] [22] [40] [41] [42] and was first observed by Mogensen [43]. The implication is that agents that retard the early progression of nephropathy, i.e. the primary prevention of microalbuminuria, have the potential to influence not only the development of renal failure, but of cardiovascular disease as well.

Future studies would improve on existing knowledge were they larger or longer. This would provide more precise estimates of the rate of infrequent events such as ESRD. Longer studies might also identify changes in annual rates of progression over time, and test the hypothesis that there is a group of individuals who lack susceptibility to diabetic nephropathy [44]. Future studies could model the risk for nephropathy and cardiovascular disease using continuous, rather than categorical values of urine albumin-creatinine value, in order to gain information and understanding, just as HOPE study investigators estimated an approximate 6% increase in risk in cardiovascular disease for every 0.4 mg/mmol increase in albumin creatinine ratio [30]. Once reliable data on rates exist, then the magnitude of the potential benefit from effective interventions can be estimated.

REFERENCES

1. UK Diabetes, Diabetes in the UK - the missing million. 2000, Diabetes UK: London.
2. Tattersal, R., The History of Diabetic Nephropathy, in Diabetic Nephropathy, C. Mogensen, Editor. 2000, Aventis Pharma: Bridgewater.
3. Teutsch, S., J. Newman, and P. Eggers, The problem of diabetic renal failure in the United States: An overview. American Journal of Kidney Diseases, 1989. 8: p. 11-13.

4.   Ansell, D. and T. Feest The Second Annual Report ; The UK Renal Registry. 1999, The UK Renal Registry, Southmead Hospital: Bristol.

5.   Schaubel, D., et al., End-stage renal disease in Canada: prevalence projections to 2005. Canadian Medical Association Journal, 1999. 160: p. 1557-63.

6.   US Renal Data System, Excerpts from the USRDS Annual Data Report. American Journal of Kidney Disease, 2000. 36: p. S1-S239.

7.   Parving, H.H., Initiation and progression of diabetic nephropathy. New England Journal of Medicine, 1996. 335: p. 1682-3.

8.   Gall, A.M., et al., Risk factors for development of incipient and overt diabetic nephropathy in patients with non-insulin dependent diabetes mellitus: prospective, observational study. BMJ, 1997. 314: p. 783-788.

9.   Forsblom, C., et al., Predictors of progression from normoalbuminuria to microalbuminuria in NIDDM. Diabetes Care, 1998. 21: p. 1932-8.

10. Ravid, M., et al., Main risk factors for nephropathy in type 2 diabetes mellitus are plasma cholesterol levels, mean blood pressure, and hyperglycemia. Archive Internal Medicine, 1998. 158: p. 998-1004.

11. Klein, R., et al., Ten-Year incidence of gross proteinuria in people with diabetes. Diabetes, 1995. 44: p. 916-923.

12. Mann, J., et al., Development of Renal Disease in People at High Cardiovascular Risk: Results of the HOPE Randomized Study. J Am Soc Nephrol, 2003. 14: p. 641-7.

13. Brancati, F., et al., Risk of end-stage renal disease in diabetes mellitus: a prospective cohort study of men screened for MRFIT. Multiple Risk Factor Intervention Trial. JAMA, 1997. 278: p. 2069-74.

14. Ballard, D.J., et al., Epidemiology of persistent proteinuria in type II diabetes mellitus; Population-based study in Rochester, Minnesota. Diabetes, 1988. 37: p. 405-12.

15. Adler, A., et al., Development and progression of nephropathy in type 2 diabetes: The United Kingdom Prospective Diabetes Study (UKPDS 64). Kidney Int, 2003. 63: p. 225-232.

16. Lopes, A.A.S. and F.K. Port, Differences in the patterns of age-specific balck/white comparisons between end-stage renal disease attributed and not attributed to diabetes. American Journal of Kidney Diseases, 1995. 25: p. 714-721.

17. Karter, A., et al., Ethnic disparities in diabetic complications in an insured population. JAMA, 2002. 287: p. 2519-27.

18. Mogensen, C., C. Christensen, and E. Vittinghus, The stages in diabetic renal disease with emphasis on the stage of incipient diabetic nephropathy. Diabetes, 1983. 12: p. 7-10.

19. Pugh, J., The Epidemiology of Diabetic Nephropathy. Diabetes/Metabolism Reviews, 1989. 5: p. 531-546.

20. Coresh, J., et al., Prevalence of chronic kidney disease and decreased kidney function in the adult US population: Third National Health and Nutrition Examination Survey. Am J Kidney Dis, 2003. 41: p. 1-12.

21. Foundation, N.K., K/DOQI clinical practice guidelines for chronic kidney disease: evaluation, classification, and stratification. Am J Kidney Dis, 2002. 39(Suppl 1): p. S1-S266.

22. Parving, H.-H., et al., Does microalbuminuria predict diabetic nephropathy? Diabetes Care, 2002. 25: p. 406-7.

23. Humphrey, L.L., et al., Chronic renal failure in non-insulin-dependent diabetes mellitus. Annals of Internal Medicine, 1989. 111: p. 788-796.

24. UKPDS Group, Intensive blood-glucose control with sulphonylureas or insulin compared with conventional treatment and risk of complications in patients with type 2 diabetes (UKPDS 33). Lancet, 1998. 352: p. 837-53.

25. UKPDS Group, Effect of intensive blood-glucose control with metformin on complications in overweight patients with type 2 diabetes (UKPDS 34). Lancet, 1998. 352: p. 854-865.

26. UKPDS Group, Tight blood pressure control and risk of macrovascular and microvascular complications in type 2 diabetes (UKPDS 38). British Medical Journal, 1998. 317: p. 703-713.

27. UKPDS Group, Efficacy of atenolol and captopril in reducing risk of macrovascular and microvascular complications in type 2 diabetes (UKPDS 39). British Medical Journal, 1998. 317: p. 713-720.

28. UKPDS Group, UK Prospective Diabetes Study X. Urinary albumin excretion over 3 years in diet-treated Type 2 (non-insulin-dependent diabetic patients, and association with hypertension, hyperglycaemia and hypertriglyceridaemia. Diabetologia, 1993. 36: p. 1021-1029.

29. Gerstein, H., et al., Rationale and design of a large study to evaluate the renal and cardiovascular effects of an ACE inhibitor and vitamin E in high-risk patients with diabetes. The MICRO-HOPE Study. Diabetes Care, 1996. 19: p. 1225-8.

30. Gerstein, H., et al., Albuminuria and risk of cardiovascular events, death, and heart failure in diabetic and nondiabetic individuals. JAMA, 2001. 286: p. 421-6.

31. Fagot-Campagna, A., et al., Type 2 diabetes among North American children and adolescents: an epidemiologic review and a public health perspective. Journal of Pediatrics, 2000: p. 664-72.

32. Fleischmann, E., et al., Influence of excess weight on mortality and hospital stay in 1346 hemodialysis patients. Kidney Int., 1999. 55: p. 1560-7.

33. Kasinath, M., et al., Nondiabetic renal disease in patinets with diabetes mellitus. American Journal of Medicine, 1983. 75: p. 613-617.

34. Parving, H.H., et al., The effect of irbesartan on the development of diabetic nephropathy in patients with type 2 diabetes. New England Journal of Medicine, 2001. 345: p. 870-878.

35. Brenner, B.M., et al., Effects of Losartan on renal and cardiovascular outcomes in patients with type 2 diabetes and nephropathy. New England Journal of Medicine, 2001. 345: p. 861-869.

36. EUROASPIRE I and II Group, Clinical reality of coronary prevention guidelines: a comparison of EUROASPIRE I and II in nine countries. EUROASPIRE I and II Group. European Action on Secondary Prevention by Intervention to Reduce Events. Lancet, 2001. 357: p. 972-3.

37. Stephenson, J.M., et al., Proteinuria and mortality in diabetes: the WHO Multinational Study of Vascular Disease in Diabetes. Diabetic Medicine, 1995. 12: p. 149-155.

38. Mattock, M., et al., Prospective study of microalbuminuria as predictor of mortality in NIDDM. Diabetes, 1992. 41: p. 736-41.

39. Vaur, L., et al., Development of Congestive Heart Failure in Type 2 Diabetic Patients With Microalbuminuria or Proteinuria: Observations from the DIABHYCAR (type 2 DIABetes, Hypertension, CArdiovascular Events and Ramipril) study. Diabetes Care, 2003. 26: p. 855-860.

40. Gall, M.-A., et al., Albuminuria and poor glycemic control predict mortality in NIDDM. Diabetes, 1995. 44: p. 1303-09.

41.   Dinneen, S. and H. Gerstein, The association between microalbuminuria and mortality in non-insulin dependent diabetes mellitus: a systematic overview of the literature. Arch Intern Med, 1997. 157: p. 1413-18.

42.   Baigent, C., K. Burbury, and D. Wheeler, Premature cardiovascular disease in chronic renal failure. Lancet, 2000. 356: p. 147-52.

43.   Mogensen, C., Microalbuminuria predicts clinical proteinuria and early mortality in maturity-onset diabetes (Abstr.). Diabetologia, 1983. 181.

44.   Breyer, J., Diabetic Nephropathy, in Primer on Kidney Diseases, A. Greenberg, Editor. 1998, Academic Press: San Diego. p. 215-219.

MICROALBUMINURIA, BLOOD PRESSURE AND DIABETIC RENAL DISEASE: ORIGIN AND DEVELOPMENT OF IDEAS

Carl Erik Mogensen

Medical Department M, Diabetes and Endocrinology, Aarhus Kommunehospital, Aarhus University Hospital, Aarhus, Denmark
(Modified from Diabetologia, 1999; 42: 263-285, with permission – And based upon the Claude Bernard Lecture, Helsinki, 1998)

INTRODUCTION

Microalbuminuria and diabetic renal disease are closely linked [1-14] and are associated with hyperglycemia, increasing, blood pressure and often antecedent hyperfiltration [1, 2]. Microalbuminuria usually indicates the beginning of diabetic nephropathy as opposed to overt nephropathy characterized by clinical proteinuria and most often reduced GFR according to generally defined standards [14-15] but it has even broader implications because it is also often found in cardiovacsular disease [9] and in essential hypertension as first described by Parving et al. [16]. This indicates that microalbuminuria is involved in early renal and vascular disorders, which can predict advancing renal disease as well as the progression of cardiovascular disease [17]. This concept of exact prediction however is becoming increasingly complex because many patients are treated with anti-hypertensive drugs and other types of interventions when microalbuminuria is diagnosed; such measures often return albumin excretion to normal [18-19]. Further in population-based studies microalbuminuria is not uncommon, especially in elderly people where it is also strongly related to cardiovascular disease and mortality, as in both in Type 1 (insulin-dependent) and Type 2 (non-insulin-dependent) diabetes mellitus [20-29]. Whether it should be considered as a part of the metabolic syndrome is still doubtful as it relates more specifically to high blood pressure and glucose intolerance rather than to dyslipedimia and obesity [30]. In diabetic pregnancy, an increase of microalbuminuria predicts complications [31].

Thus microalbuminuria can be considered as an early sign of damage not only of the kidney but also generally the cardiovascular system [9, 17, 28, 32]. For intervention strategies to prevent or reverse the abnormality, also with perspectives of hard end-points, it is crucial to define and recognize pathogenetic risk factors involved in the aetiology of disease [33-41]. It is, however, equally important to consider early signs of disease and microalbuminuria indicates detectable renal structural damage [42-48], but structural lesions are also found in normoalbuminuria before development of microalbuminuria as related to long-term metabolic derangement [45]. Changes are also found in muscle capillaries [49].

Table 1. Studies related to nephromegaly, hyperfiltration and microalbuminuria

Phenomenon	Nephromegaly	Hyperfiltration	Immune-measurement of albumin meaurement	Microalbuminuria Type 1 diabetes
Early observation	Paris 1849 C. Bernard [63]	Belgium/Italy Switzerland [347-49]	Upsala [99]	London, Aarhus [100, 355-56]
Subsequent studies and observations	Several pathologists (but not carefully documented)	Denmark [350-51]	London, RIA [354]	Follow-up: London, Copenhagen, Aarhus [73, 115, 116]
Newer studies	Aarhus 1973 [67, 68], Copenhagen 1991 [346]	Boston [70], Stockholm [71], London [352]	Aarhus [355-357]	Many studies [360-62]
Confirmed and/ or clinically significant	Munich 1998 [69] Predictive of renal disease - not clinically used.	Minneapolis [353] Clinical assessment may be problematic	Rapid procedures Aarhus [102-104] Widely used [112,328]	Important guidelines [358, 362]. Cyclosporine results in renal damage [363]

If we can diagnose and intervene with effective strategies at an even earlier stage, e. g. at hyperfiltration [45, 50-56] or guided by provocation tests [57, 58] or with very early risk factors, such as poor glycemic control we might be able to further improve prognosis [45].

Very early risk factors to be considered could be pre-natal, such as genetic elements, birth-weight and familial predisposition to renal and vascular disease. The interrelation of risk factors seems to some extent, however, to have confused the medical community for years. This also applies to the pathogenetic importance of hyperglycaemia per se, not only because of poor recognition of hyperglycaemia before the glycated haemoglobin-era, but also the failure to recognize that the two important risk factors, e.g. high blood pressure and increased blood glucose concentrations, must be considered together. These are fundamental risk factors for cardiovascular disease also, and in diabetes and hyperlipidaemia with effective antilipid intervention they could be of equal or even greater importance [59] Considered together, the long-term occurrence over the years of high blood glucose and high blood pressure is highly indicative of the development of renal disease, other microvascular lesions and also macrovascular disease. Conversely, low blood pressure may be protective, even with long-standing diabetes and poor glycaemic control [60]. A similar pattern with respect to cardiovascular disease is observed in non-diabetic populations [61].

Another confounding issue has been the seemingly independent development of retinopathy and renal disease in some situations. Some studies have failed to recognize that morphological diagnosis of renal disease (based upon biopsies) is often lacking in epidemiological studies, in contrast to visible retinopathy, although clinically meaningful microvascular eye and renal disease usually develop in a very concordant fashion, at least in type 1 diabetes [62].

This review discusses how pertinent concepts of diabetic renal disease have developed over the years (tables 1-4) based upon my personal systematic review of the literature and attempt to try to reach some conclusions [63]. It also focuses on earlier diagnosis based on exact measures such as ambulatory blood pressure, provocation tests and precise monitoring of glomular filtration rate (GFR) as well as other renal function tests to define the earliest possible stage predictive of incipient or overt disease (Tables 5-6). Several new theoretical concepts are mentioned briefly (Table 7) and new important intervention is reviewed (Tables 8-10).

Table 2. Glomerulopathy, epidemiology, metabolic syndrome, and significance of near-normal glycemia.

Phenomenon	Glomerulo-pathy and proteinuria	Epidemiology of microalbuminuria and mortality, incl. T2DM	The metabolic syndrome	Significance of long-term glycemic control
Early observation	Kimmelstiel and Wilson, 1936 [364]	London, Epidemiology [100] Aarhus, Mortality [123-124]	Sweden 1923 [162] England 1939 [163-64] France 1949 [165] Italy 1965 [166]	Keiding 1952 [369] Providing the concept Pirart 1978 [84]
Subsequent studies	Several pathologists, e.g. Gellman [365]	Aarhus [128] Fredericia [20] London [27]	Ferranini [32] Reaven [367] Hoorn Study [30]	Scandinavia [370] Gothenburg [371] Kumamoto [40]
Newer studies	Aarhus/ Minneapolis (Morphometry) [47] Japan [137]	Mortality data firmly confirmed [125]	Concept used by many investigators, but correlation not too close [368].	DCCT [41] Oslo/Aarhus [48] Copenhagen [15] UKPDS [138]
Confirmed and/or clinically significant	Several reviews [45, 366]	Used now in all epidemiological and large trials [141, 160]	Still somewhat ill defined [30,167]. One element requires screening for the other risks [368].	Several guidelines (widely accepted, but AHT may be equally important)

NEPHROMEGALY AND HYPERFILTRATION

The origin of ideas often goes much further back than investigators in the research field acknowledge. Thus, nephromegaly had been observed more than a century before it was rediscovered. Claude Bernard [64], with quite another purpose in mind, observed pronounced nephromegaly in a patient with newly diagnosed diabetes who was in the care of M. Rayer in a Parisian Hospital in the 1840s and was examined after a sudden and unexpected death. The pronounced nephromegaly seen in the post mortem examination corresponds closely with new observations. Between 1848 and 1974 nephromegaly was not recognized clinically, although it seemed to be a common finding among pathologists. It was described in textbooks in France even before Claude Bernard [65]. Newer observations indicated considerable renal enlargement in experimental diabetes [66]. Nephromegaly was proposed as an index of long-term glycaemic control and could thus theoretically be used to document a possible relation between hyperglycaemia and later overt nephropathy [67-68].

This concept was recently expanded by the observation that diabetic patients with considerable nephromegaly were at greater risk of developing overt renal disease [69].

Table 3 The concept of renoprotection

Phenomenon	Protection by AHT. Incipient nephropathy (type 1)	Protection by AHT. Overt nephropathy (type 1)	Protection by AHT in microalbuminuria (Type 2)	ACE-I and renal protection
Early observation	Aarhus 1985 [216-17] Copenhagen [222] Melbourne [224] Paris [221]	Aarhus, 1976-1982 [234, 237] Copenhagen [238-40] Gothenburg [217]	Melbourne [321]	Aarhus [218,373] Paris [221] Copenhagen [222] Melbourne [224, 321]
Newer studies	Aarhus [199] Italy [372]	Many studies [241, 288]	Several studies (Table 8)	UKPDS (probably similar effect with beta-blockers) [139-140]
Confirmed and clinically significant	Several guidelines	Several guidelines [323-28]	Clinically used and Multifactorial intervention important [158]	Maybe more effective than ordinary AHT

AHT, antihypertensive treatment

887

The functional abnormality, to some extent concomitant with nephromegaly, is hyperfiltration and intrarenal hypertension, which was proposed to be of key pathogenetic relevance by Brenner and a key concept in nephrology [70].

Studies in diabetes indicate that hyperfiltration is of considerable importance [45, 56] as evidenced by several follow-up studies, most convincingly by Dahlquist et al. [71], however, microalbuminuria may be a stronger predictor [6]. Some studies have failed to document correlations possibly because of too broad inclusion criteria, e.g. patients with newly diagnosed diabetes before insulin treatment [56]. These patients are known to have pronounced hyperfiltration that can be reversed with treatment [72]. The predictive role of hyperfiltration could be difficult to study now, because there is a more intensified control in diabetes, both before and after the development of microalbuminuria. Even so, hyperfiltration, associated with microalbuminuria and slightly raised blood pressure [73], is likely to be strongly predictive of renal disease, perhaps to some extent because hyperfiltration in parallel to nephromegaly is related to poor metabolic control [68, 74]. In contrast to microalbuminuria, hyperfiltration and nephromegaly are, however, not included in the clinical evaluation of patients, partly because their presence under routine circumstances can be difficult to ascertain, as the procedures involved are technically demanding in the clinic.

Regarding mechanisms, atrial natriuretic peptide could be involved both in hyperfiltration [74] and microalbuminuria [75, 76]. The genesis of hyperfiltration is, however, likely to be multifactorial, possibly involving the renin-angiotensin system [76].

Interestingly, low creatinine clearance (not real GFR) has been reported in long-term normoalbuminuric female patients without information about S-creatinine (earlier reported to be normal). This observation can also be explained by more antihypertensive treatment, returning UAE to normal or to inaccurate urine collection (normal S-creatinine). Obviously, more structural lesions could be found [77].

We see no reason to measure GFR in such individuals but follow S-creatinine. In my view, renal biopsies have no place in the clinical management [2].

It has been suggested that there is a discrepancy between the development of renal disease and retinopathy so retinopathy, especially the background retinopathy is much more common than nephropathy. It has not been taken into consideration that the diagnoses of retinopathy is most often now based on retinal photographs, that is morphology. By contrast renal disease is diagnosed by the occurrence of microalbuminuria or proteinuria and only rarely through renal biopsies. With more exact morphological diagnosis the prevalence of the two microvascular lesions could be very similar. Actually, as shown by the Melbourne group, development of clinically important renal disease is strongly associated with the occurrence of retinopathy [62].

Thus, the basis for considering susceptibility factors distinct from the development of renal disease and retinopathy could be weakly founded. In Type 2 diabetes the appearance of retinopathy might be seen later but it usually correlates with that of glomerulopathy, and patients with retinopathy carrry a worse prognosis.

Nevertheless, it is still surprising and so far unexplained that some Type 2 patients have pronounced proteinuria, but not retinopathy, according to standard evaluation [78].

Table 4. Pathophysiological and genetic studies

Phenomenon	Complications, genetically determined?	Provocation tests (e.g. exercise)	24 h-amb. BP in diabetes	Dextran Ficoll and polyvinyl clearance
Early observation	Siperstein 1973 [82]	Karlefors [169]	Rubler 1982 [183]	Uppsala [203]
Subsequent observations	Deckert [83] Aarhus [42]	Aarhus [171-72]	Aarhus [184]	Düsseldorf [204] Aarhus [3, 72] Liège [205]
Newer studies	London [374] Boston [375] Copenhagen [86] France [376]	Only few studies [173]	Several studies [185-95]	Copenhagen [206, 209] San Francisco [207-208]
Clinical significance	Complications metabolically determined and modulated by hypertension [2]	Not used, but may be relevant in treatment trials [199, 377]	Of great value and should be used more clinically	Groningen [378] Not used any longer [3]

Table 5 *(continues on next page)*

STAGES IN THE DEVELOPMENT OF RENAL CHANGES AND LESIONS IN DIABETES MELLITUS (TYPE 1)

	Stage	Chronology	Main Structural changes or lesions	Glomerular filtration rate	Dextran clearance (% of GFR)
1	Acute renal hypertrophy-hyperfunction	Present at diagnosis of diabetes (reversible with good control)	Increased kidney size. Increased glomerular size	Increased by 20-50%	Normal
2	Normo-albuminuria (UAE<20 µg/min)	Almost all patients normo-albuminuric in first 5 years	On renal biopsy, increased BM thickness in some patients.	Increased by 20-50%	Normal
3	Incipient diabetic nephropathy, UAE 20-200 µg/min	Typically after 6-15 years (in ~35% of patients)	Further BM-thickening and mesangial expansion, arrestable with AHT[d] *	Still supra-normal values, predicted to decline with development of proteinuria	Normal
4	Proteinuria, clinical overt diabetic nephropathy	After 15-25 years (in ~35% of patients)	Clear and pronounced abnormalities *	Decline ~10 ml/min/year with clear proteinuria[c]	Abnormal to high mol dextrans (non-specific and only with low GFR) [2]
5	End-stage renal failure	Final outcome, after 25-30 years or more	Glomerular closure and advanced glomerulopathy*	<10 ml/min	Not studied

BM = Basement membrane; UAE = Urinary albumin excretion rate; AHT = Antihypertensive treatment.

[a]The best clinical marker of early renal involvement; [b]Mostly ACE-inhibition + diuretics;
[c]Without antihypertensive treatment
The classification was conceived and presented on ideas presented in ref. 2, and updated – Based on studies 1983-98 (refs. 2 and 14) . [d] Rudberg and Østerby et al [48]
Arteriolar hyalinosis and * increased interstitium

Table 5 *(continued)*

STAGES IN THE DEVELOPMENT OF RENAL CHANGES AND LESIONS IN DIABETES MELLITUS (TYPE 1)

	Albumin excretion Baseline UAE[a]	Exercise-induced UAE	Blood pressure	Reversible by strict insulin treatment	Arrestable or reversible by AHT
1	May be increased, but reversible	Increased, but reversible	Normal	Yes	No hypertension present. Microcirculatory changes modifiable
2	Normal by definition (12-20 µg/min may be abnormal)	Maybe abnormal after a few years	Normal (BP as in background population) Increase by 1 mmHg/year	Hyperfiltration reduced	Filtration fraction and UAE may be reduced [308]
3	Increase: ~20%/year (of glomerular origin)	Abnormal aggravation of baseline UAE, related to BP-increase	Incipient increase, ~3 mmHg/year (if untreated)	Microalbuminuria stabilized, GFR also stable (if HbA$_{1c}$ is reduced). Structural damage slower	Microalbuminuria reduced. Prevention of fall in GFR Arrestable by AHT[d]
4	Progressive clinical proteinuria[c] of glomerular origin	Pronounced increase in BP	High BP, increase by ~5 mmHg/year (if untreated)	Higher fall in GFR with poor control	Progression reduced (aiming at 130/80 mmHg)
5	Often some decline due to decreasing GFR	Not studied	High (if untreated)	No	No

BM = Basement membrane; UAE = Urinary albumin excretion rate; AHT = Antihypertensive treatment.

[a]The best clinical marker of early renal involvement; [b]Mostly ACE-inhibition + diuretics;
[c]Without antihypertensive treatment
The classification was conceived and presented on ideas presented in ref. 2, and updated – Based on studies 1983-98 (refs. 2 and 14) . [d] Rudberg and Østerby et al. [48].

Table 6. The endpoints: GFR-decline rate related to intermediary end-points in diabetic patients

Intermediary end-points	GFR-decline (young type 1 diabetic patients)	GFR-decline (middle-aged type 2 diabetic patients)
Microalbuminuria[a] (20-200 μg/min)	Decline in GFR[a] only seen with progression to proteinuria	Decline rate of GFR[a] usually not noteably different from normoalbuminuria
Proteinuria[b] (macroalbuminuria, >200 μg/min)	Clear decline in GFR[b] (Reduced by antihypertensive treatment)	Clear decline in GFR[c]. High mortality with increasing proteinuria
Blood pressure[b]	Controversy exists but a clear risk factor with co-existing abnormal albuminuria	Clear risk factor especially with co-existing abnormal albuminuria

Related to future mortality and ESRD with increasing power ([a]) ([b]) ([c])
ESRD, end-stage renal disease.

Table 7. Newer therapeutic concepts

	Aldose-reductose inhibition	Selective growth factor inhibition	Protein-kinase-C inhibition	Angiotensin II receptor blockade(*)	ACE-inhibition
Theoretical, basis, reference	Mau Pedersen [51]	Flyvbjerg, Ziaydeh [379-80]	King et al. [381]	Willem-heimer [382]	Schalkwijk [383] Friedman [384]]
Human studies	Mau Pedersen [51,52]	Few, Mau Pedersen [50]	Trials may be in progress	Many studies conducted and in progress [144-155]	In progress (So far not promising)
Clinically used	No	No	No	Widely used	No

(*) Dual blockade may be useful [146-47, 249-50].

GENETIC OR FAMILIAL FACTORS

Another key issue is that more than one risk factor must be present for the development of apparent clinical disease [79]. Thus isolated hyperglycaemia might not suffice to develop overt renal disease, whereas two co-existing risk factors namely, hyperglycaemia and high blood pressure are highly predictive as underscored in the UK prospective diabetes study [80, 81]. Conversely the development of microalbuminuria is usually accompanied by the development of increased blood pressure. Therefore, there should be recognition of both risk factors. In long-term studies, in diabetic patients without clinically meaningful microvascular lesions, blood pressure is lower than in the general population, which again supports the prerequisite of at least two risk factors in the genesis of renal disease [60].

Interestingly, clinical management was hampered for many years by the studies of Siperstein et al. [82] suggesting that morphological lesions can be present at or before the clinical diagnosis of diabetes. This would lend some support to genetic factors being decisive for the development of microvascular disease. A tempting, but dangerous conclusion would then be that the development of microvascular lesions is not responsive to better metabolic control but related to genetic "destiny" rather than to treatment failure [83]. These concepts were incorrect, at least for the kidney, as substantiated by the fundamental studies by Osterby who showed that structural lesions develop after diabetes has been present for some years [42-48]. In this context, muscle basement membrane might be less suited to measurement [49].

In his long-term follow-up studies, Pirart showed that glycaemic control was important for microvascular lesions and neuropathy [84]. Several European intervention studies confirm the correlation between hyperglycaemia and the development of renal disease [85]. It was not, however, until the Diabetes Control and Complications Trial (DCCT) [41] was completed that this was widely accepted in the United States, an attitude, which in retrospect, in many places could have had a deleterious effect on clinical management before 1993. This could also apply to the management of Type 2 diabetic patients, in whom metabolic control quite often is not perfect, but this will clearly change after publication of the UK Prospective Diabetes Study [80]. This landmark study also highlighted hypertension as an even more important risk factor.

Studies on genetic predisposition should be considered in the context of several risk factors [15, 79]. Interestingly, certain angiotensin-converting enzyme (ACE) genotypes have been shown initially but not subsequently to affect progression [86, 87], although data are diverse and might not relate to all populations [79, 87, 88]. In Type 2 diabetes there seems to be no such effect in Caucasians [86]. Familial predisposition to hypertension, also seen in affected patients, could still be important in a concordant, yet multifactorial, fashion [89,

90] and blood pressure should be treated once the patients become hypertensive. Recent work also suggests some racial and familial clustering of renal disease in black patients [91] but often such patient-material is small and familial clustering of environmental factors is just as likely [92].

An ambitious project has been proposed [93], possibly linking the very rare Finnish type of congenital nephrotic syndrome gene to diabetic nephropathy. The nephrin molecule is thought to be of utmost relevance. A multicenter project has been supported by a 15 million USD grant in 1999 from the Novo Nordisk Foundation to unravel over 10 years the mechanisms of diabetic vascular disease. Karl Tryggvason is the main investigator and co-founder of the company, BioStratum (www.Biostratum.com). However, so far, by May 2003, not a single relevant publication has appeared from the group – but interestingly negative data from another center in Finland [94].

BIRTH WEIGHT, CV-DISEASE AND MICROALBUMINURIA

It has been suggested that low birth weight could be predictive of cardiovascular renal disease in diabetes and in the general population [95-98]. Abnormally high birth weight could also be a problem. Small kidneys could relate to fewer glomeruli and an increase in the pressure gradient in existing tissue. This concept was not, however, supported by Danish studies on the relations between birth weight, renal and glomerular size [95, 96]. Also in population-based studies we failed to find any correlation between microalbuminuria or raised albumin secretion and birth weight. Nor was there any correlation between blood pressure and birth weight [25].

Therefore, in the Western world, it seems inconceivable that low birth weight could be an important determinant of essential hypertension or associated renal disease, in particular, because hypertension is highly prevalent in the Western population and found in perhaps 15-20 % of elderly people. Hypertension is more closely related to actual increased body mass index or abdominal adiposity. A relation between low birth weight and the much later development of diabetes and some element of cardiovascular disease might however exist in the present situations in many poor countries, but this may be of less relevance to the management of patients in the Western world [97, 98]. (See chapter by Jones and Nyengaard).

IMMUNE-BASED MEASUREMENT OF ALBUMINURIA IN LOW CONCENTRATIONS

Progress in medical research is often driven by new methodology and procedures, e.g. by more sensitive techniques. This was the case with the study of early development and early treatment of diabetes associated renal disease. The first study from 1961 describing measurements of albumin in normal urine was quite elaborate requiring pre-concentration of urinary albumin [99]. This completely changed after the introduction of radioimmuno-assays for albumin that often even required dilution of urine samples and led to the term microalbuminuria [100]. The introduction of such methods was important in the study of the early diabetes-associated renal impairment in cross-sectional and longitudinal studies. Radioimmuno-assays were, however, still laborious and time-consuming for clinical use and therefore it was an important step forward when immuno-turbidimetry and other immune precipitation tests were developed; this allowed processing of multiple samples of urine at high speed for use in clinical practice [12]. It was a major step forward in the clinical management of patients with diabetes [100-101] and also those with essenial hypertension [16-19].

Clinical management has benefited further from the introduction of effective and quick bedside and dipstick tests for measurement of albumin. The introduction of the Micral 1 and Micral 2 tests, which are not quantitative was of major benefit [102, 103], with the Micral 2 test being very efficient and easy to use in the clinic [103].

In our clinical laboratory a very good quantitative correlation has been obtained through the measurement of the albumin creatinine ratio by the DCA-2000 apparatus compared with measurement by immuno-turbidimetry [104], a new major technical step forward.

Thereby it is possible to rapidly measure not only HbA1C but also albumin and creatinine [104], an ideal situation for small clinics where large-scale measurements of these compounds are not always necessary.

We have thus experienced huge progress in our laboratory techniques from the initial extremely laborious methods in the early 1960s [99] to the very quick and efficient bedside tests of the 1990s [104], as well as excellent laboratory measurements using albumin creatinine ratios [105-114].

MICROALBUMINURIA IN TYPE 1 DIABETES

Three independent groups have consistently shown that microalbuminuria predicts overt renal disease in type 1 diabetes [73, 115, 116]. Consequently, it is now wide-spread clinical practice to screen for microalbuminuria, especially as it has subsequently been shown that intervention is effective (as described later). New follow-up studies of initial cohorts have also shown that micro-albuminuria is strongly predictive of mortality [117]. In a recent study with shorter follow-ups, on a very large number of patients, the same phenomenon was observed [118]. In this study the observation of the deleterious effects of albuminuria was also, however, based on patients with clinical proteinuria, excluded in previous studies because of their well-known poor outcome.

The recent follow-up study from the DCCT [119] clearly confirms the initial observation in Europe [73, 115, 116]. 31% of microalbuminuric patients developed proteinuria after further 4 years of conventional insulin treatment.

In patients with long-standing diabetes and late microalbuminuria it can be assumed that microalbuminuria increases relatively slowly [120]. Therefore these patients perhaps have a somewhat different and more benign prognosis. Such interpretations could, however, still be problematic because we are not dealing with distinct entities but rather we should regard the degree of albuminuria as a continuous variable (normo-micro-macro). New follow-up studies have indeed confirmed that microalbuminuria is a very strong predictor even with long diabetes duration [117, 121-122].

MICROALBUMINURIA IN TYPE 2 DIABETES

In a follow-up study first communicated in 1983 [123] it was shown that microalbuminuria in Type 2 diabetes is strongly predictive of an increased mortality risk [124]. This observation has since been confirmed in numerous studies [125]. Other factors could be associated with poor prognosis such as long-term hyperglycaemia and high blood pressure.

Microalbuminuria seems though to be the strongest overall predictor of mortality in accordance with studies in non-diabetic population-based studies. Interestingly, poor metabolic control has recently been shown to predict microalbuminuria [126,127] and could also be a risk factor for its progression, whereas high blood pressure is probably more important later on [128-135]. Poor glycaemic control correlates with typical diabetic glomerular lesions [136]. More so-called "unspecific" lesions can also be observed but non-diabetic microalbuminuric controls are lacking, which is problematic. Indeed there might be some misclassification of patients in such studies because albuminuria usually decreases with antihypertensive treatment. The "unspecific" lesions can also be considered as characteristic lesions in elderly type 2 diabetic patients, again making exact classification problematic, not necessarily in daily ordinary pathology practice but in scientific work, which is to be tested by other investigators.

Other studies have shown abnormalities in microalbuminuric type 2 diabetic patients in Japan [137]. Among the many risk factors analysed hyperglycaemia and hypertension seem to be of particular importance, as documented in initial studies on the relevance of higher albumin excretion rates in relation to other risk factors [8-10, 118-124]. Thus again there is a requirement for two risks; hyperglycaemia and high blood pressure factors usually combine to produce important clinical disease. Since microalbuminuria in Type 2 diabetes is a better predictor of cardiovascular than of microvascular disease other macrovascular disease factors must be taken into consideration.

Long-term glycaemic control as in the Kumamoto study [40] and the UK prospective diabetes study [138-141] has, however, proven rather efficient especially when combined with long-term antihypertensive treatment [140]. Detailed accounts of microalbuminuria in the UK study [141] have recently confirmed original data [123, 124].

DIFFERENCES BETWEEN TYPE 1 AND TYPE 2 DIABETES

More and more evidence suggests that the course of renal abnormalities is rather similar in Type 1 and Type 2 diabetes. Obviously, there are exceptions because patients with Type 2 diabetes tend to be elderly and obese. This means that hypertension is seen much earlier in Type 2 diabetes with subsequent renal damage.

Another important point is that Type 2 diabetes can remain undiagnosed for many years and therefore some patients will have renal and retinal as well as cardiovascular damage at the clinical diagnosis [29]. Risk factors for the development of renal disease include poor metabolic control and high, or increasing, blood pressure for both types. With microalbuminuria again glycaemic control and high blood pressure are important risk factors that can be controlled. In overt renal disease, there is a clear-cut correlation between blood pressure and decline in glomular filtration rate. There is also a correlation in Type 1 diabetes between glycaemic control and a decline in GFR but this is less clear in Type 2 diabetes where there seems to be no correlation between rate of decline of GFR and HbA$_{1C}$ [128].

Treatment modalities seem to be the same as confirmed by the UK prospective diabetes study [138-140]. An important point is that many patients with Type 2 diabetes have cardiovascular and cerebrovascular disease and they suffer premature mortality. Certainly, the course can be modulated by early anti-hypertensive treatment in type 2 diabetics [2], as shown in several trials (Table 8) [142-161], and also by lipid lowering [59].

MICROALBUMINURIA IN POPULATION BASED STUDIES

Microalbumininuria is present in 5-10% in elderly populations [20, 27] and usually relates to hypertension but also to other risk markers of cardiovascular disease, such as abdominal obesity, hypertension and hyperuricaemia. The relation between microalbuminuria and early mortality in population-based studies was first documented 10-15 years ago [20, 27]. Accordingly microalbuminuria should be included in epidemiological studies with focus on cardiovascular and metabolic diseases. In essential hypertension, microalbuminuria is often diagnosed and predictive of cardiovascular and also of progressive renal disease [170].

This is relevant to "Syndrome X" or the metablic syndrome where similar observations were made decades ago by Kylin in 1923, Himsworth in the 1930s, Vague in the 1940s, and Avogaro and Crepaldi in 1965 [162-166]. It is, however, still perhaps a too vaguely defined entity [167], which often most strongly relates to simple obesity. In contrast microalbuminuria is more related to high blood pressure and diabetes as shown in the Hoorn Study [30] and should not be included in the so-called"syndrome". The HOPE Study [142] documented that ACE-I in patients with risk factors is effective especially in those with microalbuminuria.

Table 8. New studies in T2DM, based upon microalbuminuria.

Study	Treatment	No. of patients	Duration of study	Effect on Micro-alb./alb.	Effect on BP	Additional effect parameter
HOPE, 2000 [142, 202]	Ram 10 mg at night vs. Pl	1140 micro (many T2DM)	4.5 yrs	Yes	Yes	Combined CV-outcome: Positive
ABCD, 2000 (Hypertensive pts) [143]	Nis vs. Enal	470	5 yrs	Yes	Yes	Creatinine Clearance Stable
Juliana Chan et al, 2000 [144]	Nif vs. Enal	102	5 yrs	Better with Enal	Yes	Renal function better with Enal in macro.
Lacourcière et al, 2000 [145]	Los vs. Enal	92	1 yr	Yes	Yes	Similar effect on GFR and albuminuria
CALM, 2000 [146, 147]	Can vs. Lis	199	24 W	Yes	Yes	Better effect with dual blockade on BP
Fernan-déz, 2001 [148]	Vera vs. Tran	103	6 M	Yes	Yes	Combination possible
Parving, 2001 [149, 385]	Irb vs. Pl	590	2 yrs	Yes	Yes	Dose-response-curve - (BP-independent?)
Sasso, 2002 [150]	Irb vs. pl	124	17 W	Yes	Yes	No correlation between M and BP-fall
Viberti, 2002 [151]	Val vs. Am	332	24 W	Yes (better with Val)	Yes	No correlation between M and BP-fall
Schrier, 2002 (Normotensive pts) [152]	Intensive vs. Moderate BP lowering	480	5 yrs	Yes	Yes	Less retinopathy and less incidence of stroke with intensive treatment
PREMIER, 2003 [153]	Per plus Inda (Preterax) vs. Enal	481	1 yr	Yes	Yes	Better effect with Preterax
Detail, 2005 [154]	Tel vs. Enal	252	5 yrs	Ongoing	Ongoing	GFR changes and strong end-points
Life, 2002 [155]	Los vs. At	Micros?	4.7 yrs	Possibly	No	Effect on mortality in diabetics
Epstein, 2003 [156,157]	Epl and ACE-I	215		Yes	Yes	Good effect also of combination
Steno II (Gaede), 2003 [158, 159]	Optimized Multifact. incl. lipid-lowering	120	8 yrs	Yes	Yes	GFR falls with progression to proteinuria - otherwise stable. Effect on CV disease.
DIAB-HYCAR 2003 [160]	Ram 1.25 mg vs. pl	3627	4 yrs	Minor	Minor	No effect on any important end-points (contrast to HOPE).

Am: Amlodipine; At: Atenolol; Can: Candesartan; Enal: Enalapril; Epl: Eplenerone; Inda: Indapamide; Irb: Irbesartan; Lis: Lisinopril; Los: Losartan; Nif: Nifedipine; Nis: Nisoldipine; Per: Perindopril; Pl: Placebo; Ram: Ramipril; Tel: Telmisartan; Tran: Trandolapril; V: Verapamil.

(The Allhat study did not include microalbuminuria [161])

The Fredericia Study is a Danish population-based study remarkable by including two generations. The first generation is a sub-group from a population-based study, which took place in the municipality of Fredericia, Denmark around 1981. The parent generation consisted of 228 subjects with diabetes and 223 control subjects to known diabetic subjects. The offspring generation was re-examined by Hauerslev et al [168] and a significant relation between microalbuminuria in the parental generation and hypertension in the offspring both of type 2 diabetic population and the non-diabetic population was found. The offspring generation was examined again in 1997-98, and the results showed a preserved diurnal blood pressure profile and normal blood pressure level in non-diabetic offspring of type 2 diabetic subjects [168], though the offspring was characterised by features of the metabolic syndrome.

PROVOCATION TESTS TO DETECT EARLY ABNORMALITIES IN RENAL FUNCTION

It was shown several years ago by Karlefors [169] that exercise induces a clear-cut increase in blood pressure, in particular, in diabetic patients with renal complications and blood pressure values in the upper normal range. We used this concept to describe and detect nascent changes in renal function prior to microalbuminuria and in certain patients quite a pronounced increase in albuminuria occurred during exercise, especially in those with preexisting microalbuminuria [170-73]. Increases in albuminuria are associated with raised blood pressure during exercise, an association that is quite strong. It is, however, not clear whether this test is predictive of advancing renal disease.

Although the idea seems quite attractive, clear-cut follow-up studies have not been conducted. Therefore, in the clinical situation multiple baseline measurements are preferred to precisely define the degree of early renal involvement. To this end we measure the albumin creatinine ratio at each visit to the clinic [12]. It has also been proposed that tests that block tubular reabsorption, e. g. by lysine or other dibasic amino-acids be used but again these are too complicated for clinical use [174-175] although, important physiological information on the nature of renal involvement in diabetes has thereby been obtained. By apparent complete blockade of tubular reabsorption, albumin excretion rises from 5 to approximately 300 µg/min, thus providing an estimate of transglomerular passage of albumin [57, 175]. In addition, other provocation factors have been examined [176-180].

24-H AMBULATORY BLOOD PRESSURE MEASUREMENTS

Ambulatory blood pressure measurements were first developed in the 1960s by Sokolow's and Pickering's groups [181-82] and used in the 1980s by Rubler in diabetic patients [183]. The technique used was initially quite difficult and demanding not only for the patient but also the physician. With the introduction of more user-friendly equipment, such as the SpaceLabs apparatus, it is now common clinical practice to take ambulatory blood pressure measurements in situations where there is uncertainty as to the precise level of blood pressure, both before and during treatment [184-202]. An important confounding issue to be avoided is the situation-induced "white-coat" hypertension, which is just as common in diabetic as in non-diabetic patients [197-199]. This is also extremely important in clinical trials because fewer patients could be required to document treatment effects [202]. More sophisticated questions might be answered by ambulatory blood pressure measurements. These include:

1. the effect of smoking which seems to increase blood pressure in diabetic patients in contrast to the paradoxical reduction in ambulatory blood pressure in non-diabetic patients [189];
2. the lower blood pressure in healthy women which is now well established but this conceivably protective biological feature is lost in diabetic patients [189-191];
3. the significance of a lack of nocturnal blood pressure "dips" in diabetic patients about which there are still some doubts [193].
4. possible increase in night BP by strict metabolic control which proved difficult to confirm [201].

In people with normoalbuminuria we have not found any major differences between those with and without diabetes and the phenomenon of dipping has been quite variable and not applicable in clinical settings. It has, however, been reported that Type 1 diabetic patients on intensive insulin therapy to some extent lack nocturnal dipping which is not present in large series of patients [201].

It is important to record ambulatory blood pressure when describing the antihypertensive effect of drugs, e.g. angiotensin-converting enzyme inhibitors. Thus, it is sometimes not possible, with the use of clinically based blood pressure, to detect a reduction in blood pressure that can only be unveiled during ambulatory blood pressure recordings. If it were not for these it could be argued that the inhibitors are renoprotective, even without any detectable effect on blood pressure. Thus by taking the ambulatory blood pressure we observed some blood pressure reduction in such patients, even in trials with relatively few patients. Again, this illustrates the danger of limiting the concept of renoprotection, by excluding the beneficial effect of blood pressure reduction. Multiple blood pressure measurements with the most exact procedures are therefore essential, also in the HOPE-study where reduced night blood pressure was observed [202]. In this study, medication was given at bed-time.

DEXTRAN AND POLYMER CLEARANCE

Dextran clearance was introduced to describe the glomerular permeability to a large range of molecular sizes [203-205] and the principle was used early in diabetic patients [204]. When we introduced this technique in our laboratory for diabetic patients [3, 72] we observed no change in dextran clearance in patients with neither newly diagnosed diabetes nor long-standing diabetes when correcting for prevailing glomular filtration rate [72], since these patients are often hyperfiltering. In patients with microalbuminuria, Deckert et al. [206], in contrast to other studies [207], also failed to find any changes. We were, however, able to see changes in patients with advanced clinical proteinuria but only by long-term collection of urine after dextran infusion and use of very high-molecular weight dextran [3].

Thus in patients with advanced proteinuria only small permeability defects could be described, which could be a paradox because these patients were clearly proteinuric or even nephrotic. Possibly the dextran molecule is not suitable for this purpose, perhaps because it uncoils during the glomerular filtration process and charged dextrans possibly aggregate suggesting a sporiously low clearance. The introduction of ficoll - a molecule with more fixed structure - could or could not provide new information on glomerular permeability to large molecules. Still, in the clinical situation, it is much easier and more practical (and better) to use endogenous plasma proteins as markers.

Newer studies, however, documented only limited change in ficoll clearance in proteinuric type 1 diabetic patients. As earlier described blocking the RAS reduced proteinuria, but had only a limited or a borderline effect on high molecular polymer clearance [208, 209].

RENAL AND OTHER ORGAN PROTECTION

To define risk markers for progressive renal as well as cardiovascular disease is clearly of interest academically but not necessarily of clinical importance as intervention might not always be possible. Theoretically, intervention should certainly be possible considering the two major risk factors, high blood pressure and hyperglycaemia. Renal protection, defined as any measure to prevent progression of renal impairment, could therefore include control of blood pressure and hyperglycaemia, based on observational risk factor studies, as poor glycaemic control is a major risk factor for progression from normo- to microalbuminuria [210]. In patients with microalbuminuria, glycaemic intervention is not, however, always clinically feasible, although highly desirable [15, 210-12]. The background could well be that patients with microalbuminuria previously have had poor metabolic control which could be inherently difficult to treat. In overt nephropathy, poor metabolic control is certainly associated with rapid progression [15]. Therefore during the entire course of renal involvement in diabetes good metabolic control is a main issue, likewise for the prevention of retinopathy, as well as cardiovascular disease, both in type 1 and type 2 diabetes. Table 7 describes the relation between intermediary end-points and the decline in glomular filtration rate. This is a dramatic change in concepts over the last 40 years as it has previously been argued that hypertension was "essential" to maintain sufficient organ (including renal) perfusion and survival [35].

EARLY ANTI-HYPERTENSION TREATMENT TO PREVENT PROGRESSION IN RENAL DISEASE IN MICROALBUMINURIC PATIENTS

In this context it is important to consider blood pressure as a continuous variable. This important concept was introduced by Pickering in his controversy with Platt [214]. It cannot be argued that there is a clearly defined level representing high blood pressure unless long-term studies are conducted to observe correlation between blood pressure and development of cardiovascular and renal lesions [215]. This applies to both Type 1 and Type 2 diabetes and the general population. Certainly, diabetic patients are more susceptible to renal damage than non-diabetic people or patients with essential hypertension, as related to blood pressure [18].

This was the basis for our early intervention study in which microalbuminuric Type 1 diabetic patients with so-called "normal" blood pressure were enrolled in a clinical trial with a self-controlled approach [213, 216-17]. In this study it was documented that antihypertensive treatment with beta-blockers could lead to regression of microalbuminuria.

Further studies along this line showed that antihypertensive combination treatment in such patients is associated with declining albuminuria and slow progression (no decline in GFR) in early diabetic renal disease [218-220]. At present most diabetic patients need combination therapy. The benefit of this new concept was clearly confirmed using angiotensin-converting enzyme inhibitors in the treatment of patients with microalbuminuria [221].

Numerous studies [222-228] have confirmed the effect of these inhibitors in type 1 diabetes leading to regression of microalbuminuria, as documented in a recent meta-analysis [229]. Interestingly, this effect is also seen in very early renal involvement in diabetes, such as in patients with early microalbuminuria [199] between 20 and 70 µg per min. In this 2-year controlled clinical trial the progression expected was seen in the untreated control group with a mean annual increase rate between 15 and 20 %. With treatment using ACE-inhibition, there was a clear-cut reduction in albuminuria as seen in earlier studies in which the subjects had a higher degree of microalbuminuria. Therefore treatment could be effective quite early, just after the development of microalbuminuria as now advocated by recent guidelines [230]. In one study [199], the specific renal impact of ACE-inhibition was clearly documented. A fall in albuminuria correlated with a fall in filtration fraction. The long-term aim is, however, not regression of microalbuminuria per se, although this might be a reliable surrogate marker, but to prevent a decline in GFR. This requires long-term studies over 6-8 years. Indeed, Mathiesen and co-workers [223] were able to show that the effect of ACE-inhibition is long lasting. Importantly, patients with clinical proteinuria had well-preserved GFR after a pause in treatment but only when ACE-inhibitors had been given over the previous 8 years. Without antihypertensive treatment, there was a clear-cut decline in GFR in those developing proteinuria.

This is the first study to document a long-term preservation of GFR in Type 1 diabetes [223] as seen in Type 2 diabetes [226, 227]. Table 8 shows an outline of 10 controlled studies in microalbuminuric type 1 diabetic patients [228-29]. Data include studies of 2 years duration or longer. Generally, microalbuminuria is reduced, but important new studies also indicate preservation of GFR and glomerular structure.

RENAL PROTECTION IN TYPE 1 DIABETES WITH OVERT NEPHROPATHY

There has been some discussion about the definition of renal protection in diabetes and in other renal diseases. In my view, a key point is that renal protection should mean that GFR (and renal structure) is better preserved by treatment, irrespective of its modality. It has been proposed that "renal protection" should be defined as a kind of treatment that preserves GFR, on top of the effect of blood pressure reduction. In my mind this definition is too narrow. Any kind of treatment that prevents a fall in GFR or reduces fall rates in GFR should be termed reno-protective. In many studies BP is not carefully recorded. A broader and weaker definition would be "reduction in proteinuria" since this is most often associated with the prevention of decline in GFR.

Initially, we studied early renal involvement in diabetes describing the now well-known phenomenon of hyperfiltration [1, 72, 231]. Subsequently it was found pertinent to study the natural course of renal function changes in diabetic patients, especially in those with microalbuminuria and clinical proteinuria [233-36]. It became clear that a rise in blood pressure was associated with a fall per period of time in GFR in proteinuric patients and therefore anti-hypertensive trials were initiated with a self-controlled design. This was essential to gain optimal sensitivity in new conceptually studies due to the limited number of patients [237].

It soon became clear that antihypertensive treatment with beta-blockers and diuretics and sometimes vasodilators was quite effective in preserving GFR [237-41] and in improving renal prognosis and survival [242-44]. These seem to be the first studies to document reno-protection (using the above definition) by antihypertensive treatment in diabetes specifically, and in fact, in renal disease in general. Later studies were conducted in other centres, in particular in Sweden [245] in patients with overt diabetic renal disease. All results suggested that the fall rate in GFR could be reduced by about 50 per cent from $10 \text{ ml} \cdot \text{min}^{-1} \cdot \text{year}^{-1}$ to $5 \text{ ml} \cdot \text{min}^{-1} \cdot \text{year}^{-1}$ or even more by more effective antihypertensive treatment and better glycemic control [15,241]. To some extent, this effect seems to be independent of the type of antihypertensive treatment and depends rather more on blood pressure reduction per se although

905

there still may be some disagreement [15, 246, 247]. The largest study so far conducted in overt renal disease in patients with Type 1 diabetes was the Collaborative Study in the United States [248]. Again this showed antihypertensive treatment to be effective in Type 1 diabetes. The study compared the use of ACE-inhibitors with other agents to control blood pressure. With a lower and more satisfactory degree of blood pressure attained during treatment, the effect with ACE-inhibitors and other agents was the same (Lewis, personal communication). In contrast with higher blood pressure the ACE-inhibitors seemed to be more efficient, although a strict cut-off has never been defined. Importantly, in this study the ACE-i-group obtained a significantly lower BP than the control group, a problem observed in several such trials. Such BP-differences may be crucial for observed renoprotection. In other studies it was found that the blood pressure level was important for the determination of the rate of decline in GFR and also some effect was observed by HbA1C as seen in other studies [15]. In non-diabetic renal disease blocking the RAS is also an important treatment strategy [249-51], including dual blockade [250-251].

In my mind, it is clearly not productive to exclude, by definition, antihypertensive treatment as a reno-protective measure. I would prefer that all measures, which protect against a decline in GFR be included in the definition both in diabetes and in other renal diseases. It is clear that antihypertensive treatment is important, however, in most renal diseases as suggested by long-term studies in 1982 [237], subsequently confirmed a decade later [248], also for cardiovascular disease.

GLYCAEMIC CONTROL AND GLYCAEMIC MEASURES

It would seem plausible that diabetic lesions in the kidney and in the eyes, specific for diabetes, are caused by the diabetic state, especially hyperglycaemia. For many years, there was doubt however about this association, mainly because of difficulties in documenting long-term glycaemic control. The large-scale observational study conducted by Pirart and co-workers, however, showed a clear correlation between glycaemic control and the development of microvascular and neurological complications [84]. Intervention studies conducted in Scandinavia and elsewhere supported these observations [15], which were later confirmed by the DCCT as to the development of microvascular and possibly also macrovascular lesions. This formed the basis of the concept of glucotoxicity [41]. Nyberg et al. were the first to observe fairly stable GFR in patients with well-controlled metabolism [252]. They showed that the decline in the rate of GFR correlated with HbA1C and strong evidence for an earlier effect was obtained in the DCCT [41]. Thereafter, optimal glycaemic control became the elusive gold standard for care in Type 1 diabetes. Most experts would very much support this view, also for Type 2 diabetes, when intervention studies related to microvascular disease are positive [40] and there is also a clear correlation between glycaemic control and the development of complications in observational studies [210, 241].

Over the past 25 years, we have observed a radical change in the management of patients, driven by new methods, such as home monitoring of blood glucose, insulin pumps, insulin pens, along with better monitoring of glycaemia, as well as better documentation of complications as measured by retinal photographs and microalbuminuria. Although insulin pumps were introduced around 1980 [253] and stimulated our hope for a practical way to achieve near-normoglycaemia [254-62]. For many reasons they are used only to a limited extent.

Pancreas transplantation, a more radical approach towards euglycaemia, was proposed even earlier and was also thought to have great promise [263-265]. The idea and its considerable impracticality have been critically evaluated recently [266]. A new longterm study [267] suggested that the glomerular lesions in diabetic nephropathy could heal not after 5 but after 10 years of normoglycaemia often by isolated pancreas transplantation. It should be noted that three of the eight patients in fact initially had normoalbuminuria, which in our experience is associated with limited lesions and a benign course, and by definition such patients do not have diabetic nephropathy. Four patients had microalbuminuria and only one proteinuria that is only one with overt nephropathy. Only open, nonsclerosed glomeruli were evaluated and no information on change in number of occluded glomeruli is available. Also analysis of interstitial expansion or vascular lesions would have been important considering necessary long-term treatment with Cyclosporin A. Biopsies were not taken from two patients at the follow-up because they had developed end-stage renal disease, so they were hardly normal from any point of view. The follow-up rate of the very initial total cohort (at year zero) is not recorded. A fall in GFR (from 108 to 74 ml/min) was noted in patients that were followed for 10 years, also hardly a sign of regression.

It would be important to see this study confirmed but for practical reasons this is not to be expected. The study could have problematic implications if it were to create overoptimistic views on the usefulness of pancreas transplantations. Also it is noteworthy that pancreas transplantation does not always lead to a complete return to normal metabolism [268].

ANGIOTENSIN-CONVERTING ENZYME-INHIBITORS AND ARBs

Angiotensin-converting enzyme-inhibitors are antihypertensive agents which in several experimental studies [269], and also in human studies in diabetes [219, 221-24], had a specific effect on renal function indicating reduction of trans-glomerular pressure. Thereby, a reduction in albuminuria has been shown by ACE-inhibitors; likewise, the rate of decline of GFR and even its arrest was seen in patients with microalbuminuria [223]. Therefore, the use of ACE-inhibitors has become a standard initial choice in early and late antihypertensive treatment of diabetic patients, but quite often combination therapy is required, also in clinical trials [222-23]. It is still debatable whether, with exactly the same effects on blood pressure, differences still remain between ACE-inhibitors and other anti-hypertensive agents.

According to the LIFE study an Angiotensin Receptor Blocker (ARB) is to be preferred compared to a beta-blocker in type 2 diabetes [155]. However, antihypertensive combination treatment is increasingly recommended [270-72].

Years ago, it was suggested that antihypertensive treatment could impair renal circulation and thus be deleterious [35]. The small reduction in GFR along with reduced proteinuria is likely to be indicative of a beneficial effect [15]. Based on many studies, we now know that low blood pressure obtained by treatment or spontaneously is protective against the development of more advanced glomerulopathy and decline in GFR. Renal vascular stenosis in diabetic patients very rarely poses clinical problems and needs usually not be screened for before treatment [273]. Interestingly, a famous case report documented only few diabetic lesions in a post-stenotic kidney [274].

THE CONCEPT OF ANTIHYPERTENSIVE COMBINATION THERAPY IN DIABETES

Quite often in clinical practice antihypertensive combination therapy has to be used. This is not surprising considering the complex nature of high blood pressure in diabetes. With particular regard to renal involvement it could be advantageous to use ACE-inhibitors because of their effect on glomerular pressure [269, 275]. Indeed, there could also be an additional effect on growth factors and cytokines by ACE-inhibition. Nevertheless, early on there may also be general hyperfusion related partly to cardiac involvement [276] that could be reduced by the use of beta-blockers. This concept of general vascular hyperperfusion in the genesis of vascular complications was proposed by Parving et al. [277]. In many Type 1 and Type 2 diabetic patients there are signs of sodium retention and therefore diuretic treatment could be beneficial.

Following these lines we have used a combination of beta-blockers and ACE-inhibitors [218-220] with diuretics as a basis therapy. This kind of treatment was effective in reducing albuminuria and persistent studies have shown long-term preservation of GFR in patients with early renal disease [220]. Therefore, this concept of treatment could prove important, also in the early management with only limited blood pressure increase. Very few side-effects are seen with early combination therapy where moderate doses can be used. Combinations including thiazides and beta-blockers are often used also in non-diabetics with some risk of developing glucose intolerance or diabetes with beta-blockers [278] but the proven relative benefits should be taken into consideration [279].

Newer studies suggest excellent antihypertensive effect in type 2 diabetes with microalbuminuria by combining an ACE-inhibitor with an angiotensin receptor-blocker [146]. This combination was also used in several other studies [147] as well as in non-diabetic renal disease [250-51].

RENAL INVOLVEMENT AND TREATMENT IN PATIENTS WITH TYPE 2 DIABETES, MICROALBUMINURIA AND PROTEINURIA

Patients in this category have a poor prognosis with a rapid decline in GFR, correlated with blood pressure, but not HbA1C [15, 280]. The prognosis is also poor because many patients develop cardiovascular disease, which is the most common cause for the observed considerable increase in mortality. Black people have a considerable higher risk for disease progression compared to white people [281]. Some controversy has arisen recently regarding calcium channel blockers in diabetes [282, 283], but they are often used in combination therapy, with blockers of the RAS as basis [158]. Table 8 summarizes major trials in type 2 diabetes published since year 2000 [142-61] – also summarized elsewhere.

It should be noted that the review by Brenner does not include information on microalbuminuria, which may indeed be an important concept in the prevention and amelioration of clinical diabetic renal disease and mortality, probably much more so early on in the disease [284]. For instance in the RENAAL and the IDNT studies [285-287] the effect on rate of progression in renal disease was significant but not pronounced and there was no effect on mortality. (Table 9)

In this recent review, Brenner discussed the development of mechanims as well as treatment and course of renal disease was reviewed including notes on diabetic renal disease. However, with overt proteinuria in diabetic patients, it is very difficult or impossible to accomplish remission. Nevertheless, it should also be emphasised that a number of European studies clearly showed a positive effect of antihypertensive treatment in overt diabetic renal disease in type 1 diabetes, irrespective of treatment modality [288].

In my mind, however, it is clear that early treatment, including screening of patients with microalbuminuria and well-preserved GFR would still be essential along with early antihypertensive treatment in general and better glycaemic control. So far treatment with the receptor blocker Losartan has been effective in normoalbuminuric and microalbuminuric essential hypertensive patients [289].

Table 9. AII AT1 receptor blocker (ARB) diabetic antihypertensive trials, RENAAL and IDNT [refs 285-87].

RENAAL TRIAL

- 1513 type 2 diabetic hypertensives with macroproteinuria and creatinine 1.9 mg/dl
- 3.1 yrs of follow-up
- Losartan vs. placebo, plus non-ACE antihypertensive therapy
- 16% risk reduction of composite end-point (p=0.024)
- The first clinical trial to show a reduction in ESRD incidence (28%) compared with a given traditional approach (p=0.002).

IDNT TRIAL

- 1715 type 2 diabetic hypertensives with macroproteinuria and creatinine 1.7 mg/dl
- 2.8 yrs follow-up
- Irbesartan vs. Amlodipine vs. placebo, plus non-ACE antihypertensive therapy
- 23% risk reduction of composite end-point with irbesartan compared with amlodipine (p=0.003) and 20% risk reduction of composite end-point with irbesartan compared with placebo (p=0.024).

THE ("FIXED") NATURAL HISTORY OF DIABETIC RENAL DISEASE, A SOUND CONCEPT?

The term "the natural history of diabetic renal disease" has been widely used [290] but it may no longer be appropriate, simply because we have and use many measures to change the course of renal disease in diabetic patients. The natural history can be a term used to describe the normal course in diabetic patients in purely observational studies. It is, however, now clear that the course of renal disease strongly relates to glycaemic control with HbA1c below 7,0 % microalbuminuria might not develop at all. Also when microalbuminuria is present there could be an effect of improved glycaemic control although this is difficult since control is often hard to achieve in these patients. In overt renal disease several observational studies in Type 1 diabetes have shown that the rate of decline in renal function is correlated with HbA1C, which excludes the term "natural history" and obviously only applies to poorly treated patients. In the case of normal blood pressure the rate of decline in GFR is actually low and long-term studies have shown that survivors of long duration quite frequently have lower than normal blood pressure [60].

RENAL BIOPSIES IN DIABETIC PATIENTS

Renal biopsies, originally introduced many years ago by Brun and Iversen [291], have been used in several diabetic nephropathy research projects with very remarkable results [42, 292-293]. However, in clinical practise costly renal biopsies in diabetic patients practically never changes clinical treatments. Also as a prognostic tool, biopsies are hardly interesting from a clinical point of view.

However, beneficial effect of antihypertensive treatment has been documented in a research project [48]. Non-diabetic lesions may be present in about 10 per cent of cases of type 2 diabetes [294-296] or even in zero percent [297], and clinical consequences are uncertain or non-existing. Indication may vary and diabetic renal disease as evidenced by microalbuminuria or proteinuria is hardly a reason for biopsy. Calculation of cost/benefit is missing.

ALTERNATIVES TO MICROALBUMINURIA?

Microalbuminuria has emerged as a very powerful clinical predictor of overt renal and cardiovascular disease. This was recently confirmed in the post DCCT-study [298] and the HOPE-study [142, 299]. Although the correlation to structural changes may not be perfect, especially in type 2 patients, microalbuminuria certainly predicts clinical proteinuria in both types of diabetes, and in type 2 diabetes, also cardiovascular mortality. The power of microalbuminuria is strengthened by continous follow-up in the diabetes clinic. It should be mentioned that ACE-inhibition and other antihypertensive agents may normalize microalbuminuria so evaluation of the actual clinical situation should be done after discontinuation of therapy for one or two months. Early treatment has also proven to improve prognosis. However, it would be useful to have alternatives to microalbuminuria, especially in evaluation of the long-term fate of patients, but so far this has not been possible [300-301].

New technologies have also failed to replace microalbuminuria or to add accurate predictions of the disease. Identification of genes has so far been clinically too unreliable and in some studies no association is found. Other substances to be measured in urine and blood have not added any new developments. It has been proposed that extra-cellular-matrix molecules or products of glycation could be of importance, but this needs still to be confirmed. Measurements of cellular function in skin and lympocytes are interesting research tools as also discussed elsewhere in this volume, but not useful enough in clinical evaluation. Also new imaging technologies, such as eg. Positron-emission tomography and magnetic resonance imaging have not been useful although further studies may be required [300].

It has been proposed that increasing serum prorenin preceeds the unset of microalbuminuria, a highly interesting area that needs further investigation [302-303]. However, the overlap between non-progressors and progressors is too large, and it is too demanding to evaluate serum prorenin in the diabetes clinic. However, the observation is very interesting, also because dual blockade of the renal angiotensin system seems to be useful in clinical practise (See chapter by Andersen NH).

It can thus be concluded that there are no alternatives in the present situation. Microalbuminuria quite accurately predicts renal disease, especially with careful follow-up and measurements of albumin excretion rate in the clinics.

Some American investigators are however, inclined to use much more invasive techniques such as renal biopsies [300, 304]. It was once asked: "Can the insulin-dependent diabetic patients be managed without kidney biopsy?"

CARDIOVASCULAR AND CEREBROVASCULAR ALONG WITH RENAL END-POINTS

Cardio- and also cerebro-vascular diseases are major causes of death in both Type 1 and Type 2 diabetes, especially when the kidney is affected. Although the concept of controlled clinical or therapeutic trial has evolved over the past 50 years [305, 306], only a few large trials have been conducted in diabetes, the first being the UGDP (University Group Diabetes Program) [307], which is now, after the UKPDS [138], mainly of historical interest. No real large-scale controlled trials were done when introducing sulphonylureas [308], biguanides or insulin but this has changed now [138]. Therefore there has been an increasing interest in cerebrovascular and cardiovascular end-points, especially in Type 2 diabetes with respect to effective modulation, mainly with antihypertensive treatment strategies, which show a beneficial effect (Table 8).

META-ANALYSIS IN DIABETES

The meta-analysis approach was originally worked out in the physical and mathematical sciences [305, 306] but was soon used in medical studies to combine, for instance, data from trials and from observational cohorts, e.g. on the correlation between hard endpoints such as mortality compared with risk factors such as blood pressure. Indeed studies with observations in many subjects have documented a clear linear correlation between hard end-points and blood pressure down to normal values.

Parving et al. did a modified meta-analysis of many small trials in the evaluation of progression of renal disease in Type 1 diabetic patients treated with ACE-inhibitors and non-ACE-inhibitors and found very similar progression rates during treatment [15, 240]. The analysis was before the Ed Lewis Study [248]. Most trials with microalbuminuric patients in Type 1 diabetes are of limited size and therefore it would be valuable to do meta-analysis also on such patients as done by Chaturvedi along with our group and others [229]. The beneficial effects on regression of microalbuminuria were better documented in this meta-analysis than in individual studies of homogeneous Type 1 diabetic patients. Table 10 shows results of a number of studies [322].

Table 10 (Continues on next page)
Controlled Studies of IDDM Microalbuminuric patients (duration of study ≥2y)

Study	Drugs	Baseline	Mean age: y	Mean BP	Duration of study, yrs
European Captopril Study (1994) [228]	Cap/Pla	46/46	32	124/77	2
North American Captopril Study (1995) [316]	Cap/Pla	70/73	33	120/77	2
EUCLID (1997) [317]	Lis/Pla	32/37	33	122/80	2
PRIMA (1997) [318]	Ram/Ram/Pla 1,25/5,0/-	18/19	-	?	2
Italian Microalbuminuria (1998) [319]	Lis/Nif/Pla	33/26/34	37	129/83	3
Mathiesen, Steno (1999) [223]	Cap+diu/Con	21/23	~29	126/77	8
ATLANTIS Paul O'Hare [320]	Ram/Ram/Pla 1,25/5,0/-	44/44/46	40	132/76	2
Melbourne DNSG [321]	Per/Nif/Pla	13/10/10	~30	132/77	2½
Padua/Aarhus (Low grade micro) (1998) [199, 322]	Lis/Pla	32/28	41	124/83 131/81	2
Rudberg (1999) [48]	Ena/Met/Ref	7/6/9	~19	125/81	~3
Europe 9/North Am. 1	Mostly ACE-I	All 727 pts	19-40	127/79	2,8

Cap = Captopril, Lis = Lisinopril, Ram = Ramipril, Per = Perindopril, Ena = Enalapril, Meto = Metoprolol, Nif = Nifidipine, Con = Control group, Pla = Placebo, Ref: Reference group, DD: Diabetes duration

Table 10 (Continued)
Controlled Studies of IDDM Microalbuminuric patients (duration of study ≥2y)

Study	DD. y	Mean or median UAE µg/min	Effect on UAE of drug	Effect on BP	Effect of GFR	Note
European Captopril Study (1994) [228]	17	55	↓	↓	No	European arm
North Am. Captopril Study (1995) [316]	18	62	↓	↓	Creatinine cl. stable	North American arm
EUCLID (1997) [317]	13	~42	↓	↓?	?	Little/No effect on normo
PRIMA (1997) [318]	24	61	No	No	No	HbA1C = 7.4
Italian Microalb. (1998) [319]	18	71	Lis ↓↓/Nif↓	L↓↓/Nif↓	S-crea: No	Effect with Nif
Mathiesen, Steno (1999) [223]	18	93	↓	?	Stable with Cap+Diu Diu	**Preservation of GFR by ACE-I**
ATLANTIS Paul O'Hare (1998) [320]	20	53	Ram 1,25+ 5 mg↓	↓	No	Not dose dependent HbA1C=11.0
Melbourne DNSG [321]	16	62	Per↓/Nif-	Tendency Per/Nif↓	No	No effect with Nif
Padua/Aarhus (Low grade micro) (1998) [199,322]	13,5 15,1	36 (range 20-70)	↓	↓(24h)	No	Effect in low micro related to FF
Rudberg (1999) [48]	11	~31	E↓/M↓/ref.-	No	No	**Preservation of structure by Ena/Met**
Europe 9/North Am. 1	16,7		Mainly ACE-I ↓	Mostly ↓		

Cap = Captopril, Lis = Lisinopril, Ram = Ramipril, Per = Perindopril, Ena = Enalapril, Meto = Metoprolol, Nif = Nifidipine, Con = Control group, Pla = Placebo, Ref: Reference group, DD: Diabetes duration

There are people who support the Petonian approach and believe that meta-analysis can be important even with non-homogeneity [309]. This has been questioned suggesting that meta-analysis does not always give the correct answer, especially if the question is not correctly formulated and patient material not homogeneous [310-315].

GUIDELINES BASED ON PATHOPHYSIOLOGICAL AND CLINICAL TRIALS

The World Health Organisation - International Society of Hypertension (WHO-ISH) Liaison Committee on hypertension was established in the mid-1970s and has subsequently produced several guidelines. New guidelines have recently appeared also related to hypertension in diabetes and related questions [230, 323-329]. Several of these new guidelines have a similar approach just as the JNC 7 Report published in JAMA, May 2003 [390]. There is a clear emphasis on early and effective antihypertensive treatment in patients with diabetes suggesting a lower threshold for the start of the treatment and also a lower blood pressure goal during treatment (~ 130/80 mmHg). Angiotensin-converting enzyme-inhibitors or ARBs are often preferred as initial agents but combination therapy is most often warranted including diuretics.

CONCLUDING REMARKS

This review describes observations in a number of areas related to diabetic renal disease and related topics. Over the past 30 years there has been a great change in the management of the patients with long-term diabetes as originally described by Lundbæk [330], based on the results of physiological and patho-physiological studies followed by clinical trials which have been quickly implemented into clinical practice and incorporated in revised guidelines. Not all ideas have proved successful although, at least so far, they may have provided important insight into the nature of the disease [82, 83, 94, 95, 120, 172, 206-208, 266-267, 300, 307, 331-340, 387-389]. Some erroneous concepts have, however, led to setbacks slowing down the introduction of effective treatment in patients. Further studies are needed to establish if glitazones directly reduce BP [340].

These concepts include a few very preliminary studies, which suggested complications are predominantly genetically determined and therefore not readily modifiable. Considering complications to be generated primarily by a combination of glycaemic and haemodynamic factors (especially high blood pressure) – and not clearly genetically determined makes the treatment option much more attractive to the clinician [301, 341].

The role of low protein diet is not discussed but Anitschkow and co-workers in St. Petersburg originally explored the potential nephrotoxic effect of dietary proteins in 1913 [342]. This subsequently gave rise to the cholesterol research since the rabbits fed were not only exposed to a high protein but also a high fat diet. The protein contents of the diabetic diet are still discussed [343, 344] but the diet in general and the cholesterol issue in diabetes, appeared later to be much more important [59, 329, 345, 386].

Acknowledgements. This review is dedicated to laboratory assistant Merete Moller, who over the years helped my co-workers and me in an extraordinary way to conduct studies described herein. I am also most grateful to Anna Honoré for careful secretarial work.

REFERENCES

1.   Mogensen CE (1989) Hyperfiltration, hypertension, and diabetic nephropathy in IDDM patients. (Based on the Golgi Lecture 1988, EASD meeting, Paris). Diabetes Nutrition & Metabolism 2: 227-244
2.   Mogensen CE (2003). Microalbuminuria and hypertension with focus on type 1 and type 2 diabetes. (Based upon the Anders Jahre lecture, Oslo Oct, 2002). Journal of Internal Medicine., 253: In press.
3.   Mogensen CE, Christensen CK, Vittinghus E (1983) The stages in diabetic renal disease. With emphasis on the stage of incipient diabetic nephropathy. Diabetes 32: 64-78
4.   Mogensen CE, Chachati A, Christensen CK et al. (1985-6) Microalbuminuria: an early marker of renal involvement in diabetes. Uremia Investigation 9: 85-95
5.   Mogensen CE (1987) Microalbuminuria as a predictor of clinical diabetic nephropathy. Kidney Int 31: 673-689
6.   Mogensen CE (1990) Prediction of Clinical Diabetic Nephropathy in IDDM patients. Alternatives to microalbuminuria? Diabetes 37: 761-767
7.   Mogensen CE (2003). New treatment guidelines for a patient with diabetes and hypertension. J Hypertens, 21(s1): S25-30.
8.   Mogensen CE, Hansen KW, Osterby R, Damsgaard EM (1992) Blood pressure elevation versus abnormal albuminuria in the genesis and prediction of renal disease in diabetes. Diabetes Care 15:1192-1204
9.   Mogensen CE, Damsgaard EM, Froland A (1992) GFR-loss and cardiovascular damage in diabetes: A key role for abnormal albuminuria. Acta Diabetol 29: 201-213

10. Mogensen CE, Damsgaard EM, Froland A, Nielsen S, de Fine Olivarius N, Schmitz A (1992) Microalbuminuria in non-insulin-dependent diabetes. Clin Nephrol [Suppl 1138:S28-S39

11. Mogensen CE, Christensen CK, Christensen PD (1993) The abnormal albuminuria syndrome in diabetes. Microalbuminuria: Key to the complications. In: Belfiore F, Bergman RN, Molinatti GM (eds) Current Topics in Diabetes Research. Front Diabetes. Karger, Basel, pp 86-121

12. Mogensen CE, Poulsen PL, Heinsvig EM (1993) Abnormal albuminuria in the monitoring of early renal changes in diabetes. In: Mogensen CE, Standl E (eds) Concepts for the Ideal Diabetes Clinic. Diabetes Forum Series, Volume IV Walter de Gruyter, Berlin, New York, pp 289-313

13. Mogensen CE (2000) Diabetic nephopathy: Natural history and management. In: Ei Nahas (ed) Mechanisms and clinical management of progressive renal failure. Oxford University Press, Oxford, pp 211-240

14. Mogensen CE (1998) Preventing end-stage renal disease. Diabetic Medicine, 15: S51-S56

15. Keane WF, Brenner BM, DeZeeuw D, Grunfeld JP, McGill J, Mitch WE, Ribeiro AB, Shahinfar S, Simpson RL, Snapinn SM, Toto R for the RENAAL Study Investigators (2003). The risk of developing end-stage renal disease in patients with type 2 diabetes and nephropathy: The RENAAL study. Kidn Int., 63: 1499-1507.

16. Parving H-H, Jensen HF-, Mogensen CE, Evrin PE (1974) Increased urinary albumin excretion rate in benign essential hypertension. Lancet 1: 1190-1192

17. Garg J, Bakris GL (2002). Microalbuminuria: marker of vascular dysfunction, risk factor for cardiovascular disease. Vascular Med, 7: 35-43.

18. Pedersen EB, Mogensen CE (1976). Effect of antihypertensive treatment on urinary albumin excretion, glomerular filtration rate and renal plasma flow in patients with essential hypertension. Scand J Clin Lab Invest, 36: 231-37.

19. Volpe M, Cosentino F, Ruilope LM (2003). Is it time to measure microalbuminuria in hypertension? J Hypertens, In press.

20. Damsgaard EM, Mogensen CE (1986) Microalbuminuria in elderly hyperglycaemic patients and controls. Diabetic Medicine 3: 430-435

21. De Jong P, Hillege HL, Pinto-Sietsma SJ, de Zeeuw D (2003). Screening for microalbuminuria in the general population: a tool to detect subjects at risk for progressive renal failure in an early phase? Nephrol Dial Transplant, 18: 10-13.

22. Damsgaard EM, Froland A, Jorgensen OD, Mogensen CE (1993) Prognostic value of urinary albumin excretion rate and other risk factors in elderly diabetic patients and non-diabetic control subjects surviving the first 5 years after assessment. Diabetologia 36: 1030-1036

23. Damsgaard EM, Froland A, Jorgensen OD, Mogensen CE (1990) Microalbuminuria as predictor of increased mortality in elderly people. BMJ 300: 297-300

24. Vestbo E, Damsgaard EG, Mogensen CE (1997) The relationship between microalbuminuria in first generation diabetic and non-diabetic subjects and microalbuminuria and hypertension in the second generation (a population based study). Nephrol Dial Transplant 12 [Suppl 2]: 32-36

25. Vestbo E, Damsgaard EM, Froland A, Mogensen CE (1996) Birth weight and cardiovascular risk factors in an epidemiological study. Diabetologia 39: 1598-1602

26. Vestbo E, Damsgaard EM, Froland A, Mogensen CE (1995) Urinary albumin excretion in a population based cohort. Diabet Med 12: 488-493

27. Yudkin JS, Forrest RD, Jackson CA (1988) Microalbumuminuria as predictor of vascular disease in non-diabetic subjects. Lancet ii:530-533

28. Mølgaard H, Christensen PD, Hermansen K, Sørensen KE, Christensen CK, Mogensen CE (1994). Early recognition of sympathovagal dysfunction in microalbuminuria. Importance for cardiac mortality in diabetes? Diabetologia, 37:788-796.

29. Olivarius de FN, Andreasen AH, Keiding N, Mogensen CE (1993) Epidemiology of renal involvement in newly-diagnosed middle-aged and elderly diabetic patients. Cross-sectional data from the population-based study "Diabetes care in General Practice", Denmark. Diabetologia 36: 1007-1016

30. Jager A, Kostense PJ, Nijpels G, Heine RJ, Bouter LM, Stehouwer CDA (1998) Microalbuminria is strongly associated with NIDDM and hypertension but not with the insulin resistance syndrome: the Hoorn Study. Diabetologia 41: 694-700

31. Ekbom P and the Copenhagen Pre-eclampsia in Diabetic Pregnancy Study Group (1999). Pre-pregnancy microalbuminuria predicts pre-eclampsia in insulin-dependent diabetes mellitus, The Lancet, 353: 377

32. Ferrannini E (1993) The metabolic syndrome. In: Mogensen CE (ed) Target organ damage in the mature hypertensive. Science Press, London, pp 2.31-2.49

33. Mogensen CE, Hansen KW, Mau Pedersen M, Christensen CK (1991) Renal factors influencing blood pressure threshold and choice of treatment for hypertension in IDDM. Diabetes Care 14: 13-26

34. Mogensen CE, Mau Pedersen M, Hansen KW, Christensen CK (1992) Microalbuminuria and the organ-damage concept in antihypertensive therapy for patients with insulin-dependent diabetes mellitus. Journal of Hypertension 10:S43-S51

35. Mogensen CE (1995) Diabetic Renal Disease: The Quest for Normotension - and Beyond. Diabetic Medicine 12: 756-769

36. Mogensen CE. Prevention and management of diabetic nephropathy. In Wilcox CS (ed.) Part III, Diabetic Nephropathy, Prepress Projects Ltd, UK., 2003 pp. 313-325

37. Mogensen CE (1990) Prevention and treatment of renal disease in insulin-dependent diabetes mellitus. Semin Nephrol:260-273

38. Mogensen CE (1994) Renoprotective role of ACE inhibitors in diabetic nephropathy. Brit Heart J 72 (l):38-45

39. Mogensen CE (1994) Systemic blood pressure and glomerular leakage with particular reference to diabetes and hypertension. J Intern Med 235: 297-316

40. Shichiri M, Kishikawa H, Ohkubo Y, Wake N (2000). Long-term results of the Kumamoto study on optimal diabetes control in type 2 diabetic patients. Diabetes Care, 23(S2): B21-29.

41. The Diabetes Control and Complications Trial Research Group (1993) The effect of intensive treatment of diabetes on the development and progression of long-term complications in insulin-dependent diabetes mellitus. New England Journal of Medicine 329: 977-986

42. Osterby RH (1965) A quantitative estimate of the peripheral glomerular basement membrane in recent juvenile diabetes. Diabetologia 1: 97-100

43. Osterby R (1971) Course of Diabetic Glomerulopathy. Acta Diabet Latina 8 (l):179-191

44. Osterby R (1972) Morphometric studies of the peripheral glomerular basement membrane in early juvenile diabetes. Development of initial basement membrane thickening. Diabetologia 8: 84-92

45. Berg UB, Torbjornsdotter TB, Jaremko G, Thalme B (1998) Kidney morphological changes in relation to long-term renal function and metabolic control in adolescents with IDDM. Diabetologia 41:1047-1056

46. Osterby R (1990) Basement membrane morphology in diabetes mellitus. In: Ellenberg & Rifkin's Diabetes Mellitus, theory and practice, 4th ed., Elsevier, N. Y., Amsterdam, London, pp 220-233

47. Osterby R (1996) Lessons from kidney biopsies. Diabetes Metabol Rev 12:151-174

48. Rudberg S, Østerby R, Bangstad H-J, Dahlquiest G, Persson B (1999). Effect of angiotensin converting enzyme inhibitor or beta blocker on glomerular structural changes in young microalbuminuric patients with type 1 (insulin-dependent) diabetes mellitus. Diabetologia, 42: 589-595.

49. Williamson JR, Vogler NJ, Kilo C (1971) Structural abnormalities in muscle capillary basement membrane in diabetes mellitus. Acta Diabet Latina 8 [Suppl l]: 1 17-134

50. Mau Pedersen M, Christensen SE, Christiansen JS, Pedersen EB, Mogensen CE, Orskov H (1990) Acute effects of the somatostatin analogue on kidney function in Type 1 diabetic patients. Diabetic Med 7: 304-309

51. Mau Pedersen M, Christiansen JS, Mogensen CE (1991) Reduction of glomerular hyperfiltration in normoalbuminuric IDDM patients by 6 months of aldose reductase inhibition. Diabetes 40: 527-531

52. Mau Pedersen M, Mogensen CE, Christiansen JS (1995) Reduction of glomerular hyperfunction during short-term aldose reductase inhibition in normoalbuminuric, insulin-dependent diabetic patients. Endocrinology and Metabolism 2: 55-56

53. Mau Pedersen M, Mogensen CE, Schonau Jorgensen F, Moller B, Lykke G, Pedersen 0 (1989) Renal effects of limitation of high dietary protein in normoalbuminuric insulin-dependent diabetic patients. Kidney Int 36 [Suppl 271:S115-S121

54. Mau Pedersen M, Winther E, Mogensen CE (1990) Reducing protein in the diabetic diet. Diabetes Metab 16:454-459

55. Mogensen CE (1986) Early glomerular hyperfiltration in insulin-dependent diabetics and late nephropathy. Scand J Clin Lab Invest 46: 201-206

56. Mogensen CE (1994) Glomerular hyperfiltration in human diabetes. Diabetes Care 17: 770-775

57. Mogensen CE, Solling K, Vittinghus E (1981) Studies on mechanisms of proteinuria using aminoacid-induced inhibition of tubular reabsorption in normal and diabetic man. Contr Nephrol 26: 50-65

58. Mogensen CE, Christensen CK, Christensen NJ, Gundersen HJG, Jacobsen FK, Pedersen EB, Vittinghus E (1981) Renal protein handling in normal, hypertensive and diabetic man. Contr Nephrol 24: 139-152

59. Heart Protection Study Collaborative Group (2002). MRC/BHF heart protection study of cholesterol lowering simvastatin in 20,536 high risk individuals: a randomised placebo-controlled trial. Lancet 360: 7-22.

60. Borch-Johnsen K, Nissen H, Salling N, Henriksen E, Kreiner S, Deckert T, Nerup J (1987). The natural history of insulin-dependent diabetes mellitus in Denmark. 1. Long-term survival with and without late diabetic complications. Diabetic Med 4: 211-16.

61. Vasan RS, Larson MG, Leip EP, Evans JC, O'Donnell CJ, Kannel WB, Levy D (2001). Impact of high-normal blood pressure on the risk of cardiovascular disease. N Engl J Med, 345: 1291-7.

62. Mogensen CE, Vigstrup J, Ehlers N (1985) Microalbuminuria predicts proliferative diabetic retinopathy. Lancet II:1512-1513

63. Petticrew M (2003) Why certain systematic reviews reach uncertain conclusions. BMJ, 326: 756-8.

64. Bernard C (1849) Compte Rendu de la Société du Biologie. Paris. Vol. 1: 80-81

65.   Rayer P (1839-41) Traité des maladies des Reins et des altérations de la sécrétion urinaire, etudiées en elles-mêmes et dans leurs rapports avec les maladies des uretèthres, de la vessie, de la prostate, de l'urèthre, etc. Libraire de l'Académie Royale de médicine, Paris

66.   Ross J, Goldmann JK (1971) Effect of streptozotocin-induced diabetes on kidney weight and compensatory hypertrophy in the rat. Endocrinology. 88: 1079-1082

67.   Mogensen CE, Andersen MJF (1973) Increased kidney size and glomerular filtration rate in early juvenile diabetes. Diabetes 22: 706-712

68.   Mogensen CE, Andersen MJF (1975) Increased kidney size and glomerular filtration rate in untreated juvenile diabetics. Normalization by insulin treatment. Diabetologia ll: 221-224

69.   Baumgartl HJ, Banholzer P, Sigl G, Haslbeck M, Standl E (1998) On the prognosis of IDDM patients with large kidneys. The role of large kidneys for the development of diabetic nephropathy. Nephrol Dial Transplant 13: 630-634

70.   Hostetter TH, Rennke HG, Brenner BM (1982) The case for intrarenal hypertension in the initiation and progression of diabetic and other glomerulopathies. Am J Med 72: 375-380

71.   Dahlquist G, Stattin EL, Rudberg S (2001). Urinary albumin excretion rate and glomerular filtration rate in the prediction of diabetic nephropathy: a long-term follow-up study of childhood onset type 1 diabetic patients. Nephrol Dial Transplant 16: 1382-86.

72.   Mogensen CE (1971) Kidney function and glomerular permeability in early juvenile diabetes. Scand J Clin Lab Invest 28: 79-90

73.   Mogensen CE, Christensen CK (1984) Predicting diabetic nephropathy in insulin-dependent patients. N Engl J Med 311: 89-93

74.   Mau Pedersen M, Christiansen JS, Pedersen EB, Mogensen CE (1992) Determinants of intra-individual variation in kidney function in normoalbuminuric insulin-dependent diabetic patients: importance of atrial natriuretic peptide and glycaemic control. Clinical Science 83: 445-451

75.   Eiskjær H, Mogensen CE, Schmitz A, Pedersen EB (1991) Enhanced urinary excretion of albumin and β-2 microglobulin in essential hypertension induced by atrial natriuretic peptide. Scand J Clin Lab Invest 51: 359-366

76.   Hollenberg NK, Price DA, Fisher NDL, Lansang MC, Perkins B, Gordon MS, Williams GH, Laffel LMB (2003). Glomerular hemodynamics and the renin-angiotensin system in patients with type 1 diabetes mellitus. Kidn Int, 63: 172-78.

77.   Camamori ML, Fioretto P, Mauer M (2003). Low glomerular filtration rate in normoalbuminuric type 1 diabetic patients. An indicator of more advanced glomerular lesions. Diabetes, 52: 1036-40.

78.   Christensen PK, Larsen S, Horn T, Olsen S, Parving HH (2000). Causes of albuminuria in patients with type 2 diabetes without diabetic retinopathy. Kidney Int. 58: 1719-31

79.   Mogensen CE (2003). Genetics and diabetic renal disease. Still a black hole. [editorial]. Diabetes Care, 26: 1631-32.

80.   Mogensen CE (1998) Combined high blood pressure and glucose in type 2 diabetes: double jeopardy (editorial). BMJ 317: 693-694

81.   American Diabetes Association (2003) Implications of the United Kingdom Prospective Diabetes study Diabetes Care 26, Suppl. 1 S28- S32

82.   Siperstein MD, Unger RH, Madison LL (1968) Studies of muscle Capillary Basement Membranes in Normal Subjects, Diabetic and Prediabetic Patients. J Clin Invest 47: 1973-1999

83.   Deckert T, Poulsen JE (1981) Diabetic nephropathy: fault or destiny? Diabetologia 21: 178-183

84. Pirart J (1978) Diabetes mellitus and its degenerative complications: a prospective study of 4,400 patients observed between 1947 and 1973. Diabetes Care 1: 168-188

85. Feldt-Rasmussen B, Mathiesen ER, Jensen T, Lauritzen T, Deckert T (1991) Effect of improved metabolic control on loss of kidney function in type 1 (insulin-dependent) diabetic patients: an update of the Steno studies. Diabetologia 34: 164-170

86. Tarnov L, Gluud C, Parving H-H (1998) Diabetic nephropathy and the insertion/deletion polymorphism of the angiotensin-converting enzyme gene. Nephrology Dialysis Transplantation 13: 410-412

87. Andersen S, Tarnow L, Cambien F et al. (2003). Long-term renoprotective effects of losartan in diabetic nephropathy: interaction with ACE-insertion/deletion genotype? Diabetes Care, 26: 1501-06.

88. Björck S, Blohmé G, Sylvén C, Mulec H (1997) Deletion insertion polymorphism of the angiotensin converting enzyme gene and progression of diabetic nephropathy. Nephrology Dialysis Transplantation 12: 67-70

89. Fagerudd JA, Tarnow L, Jacobsen P et al. (1998) Predisposition to essential hypertension and development of diabetic nephropathy in IDDM patients. Diabetes 47: 439-444

90. Rudberg S, Stattin E-L, Dahlquist G (1998) Familial and perinatal risk factors for micro- and macroalbuminuria in young IDDM patients. Diabetes 47:1121-1126

91. Cowie CC, Port F, Wolfe R, Savage PJ, Moll PP, Hawthorne VM (1989) Disparities in incidence of diabetic end-stage renal disease according to race and type of diabetes. N Engl J Med 321: 1074-1079

92. Borch-Johnsen K, Norgaard K, Hommel E, Mathiesen ER, Jensen JS, Deckert T, Parving H-H (1992) Is diabetic nephropathy an inherited complication? Kidney Int 41: 719-722

93. Tryggvason K. (1999). Unraveling the mechanisms of glomerular ultrafiltration: Nephrin, a key component of the slit diaphragm. J Am Soc Nephrol 10: 2440-45.

94. Petterson-Fernholm K, Forsblom C, Perola M, Groop P-H for the FinnDiane Study Group (2003). Polymorphisms in the nephrin gene and diabetic nephropathy in type 1 diabetic patients. Kidney Int, 63: 1205-1210.

95. Jacobsen P, Rossing P, Tarnow L, Hovind P, Parving HH (2003). Birth weight – a risk factor for progression in diabetic nephropathy? J Int Med, 253: 343-50.

96. Nyengaard JR, Bendtsen TF, Mogensen CE (1996) Low birth weight - is it associated with few and small glomeruli in normal persons and NIDDM (non-insulin-dependent diabetes mellitus) patients? Diabetologia 39: 1634-1637

97. Ravelli ACJ, van der Meulen JHP, Michels RPJ, Osmond C, Barker DJP, Hales CN, Bleker OP (1998) Glucose tolerance in adults after prenatal exposure to famine. Lancet 351:173-177

98. Yudkin JS, Stanner S (1998) Prenatal exposure to famine and health in later life. Lancet 351: 1361-1362

99. Bergaard l, Risinger G (1961) Quantitative immunochemical determination of albumin in normal human urine. Acta Soc Med Upsaliensis 66: 217-222

100. Keen H, Chlouverakis C (1964) Urinary albumin excretion and diabetes mellitus. Lancet ii: 1 155

101. Keen H, Chlouverakis C, Fuller J, Jarret RS (1969) The concomitants of raised blood sugar: studies in newly-detected hyperglycaemics. II. Urinary albumin excretion, blood pressure and their relation to blood sugar levels. Guy's Hospital Reports 118: 247-254

102. Poulsen PL, Mogensen CE (1995) Evaluation of a new semiquantitative stix for microalbuminuria. Diabetes Care 18: 732-733

103. Mogensen CE, Viberti GC, Peheim E et al. (1997) Multicenter evaluation of the Micral-test II test strip, an immunologic rapid test for the detection of microalbuminuria. Diabetes Care 20:1642-1646

104. Poulsen PL, Mogensen CE (1998) Clinical evaluation of a test for immediate and quantitative determination of urinary albumin-to-creatinine ratio. Diabetes Care 21: 97-98

105. Poulsen PL (1998). Office tests for microalbuminuria. In Mogensen CE (ed.) The Kidney and Hypertension in Diabetes mellitus, Kluwer Academic Publ., 1998, pp. 181-91.

106. Houlihan CA, Tsalamandris C, Akdeniz A, Jerums G (2002). Albumin to creatinine ratio: A screening test with limitations. Am J Kidney Dis, 39: 1183-89.

107. Mattix HJ, Hsu CY, Shaykevich S, Curhan G (2002). Use of albumin/creatinine ratio to detect microalbuminuria: Implications of sex and race. J Am Soc Nephrol, 13: 1034-39.

108. Claudi T, Cooper JG (2001). Comparison of urinary albumin excretion rate in overnight urine and albumin creatinine ratio in spot urine in diabetic patients in general practice. Scand J Prim Health Care, 19: 247-48.

109. Lum G (2000). How effective are screening tests for microalbuminuria in random urine specimens? Annals of Clinical & Laboratory Science, 30: 406-11.

110. Collins ACG, Vincent J, Newall RG, Mitchell KM, Viberti GC (2001). An aid to the early detection and management of diabetic nephropathy: assessment of a new point of care microalbuminuria system in the diabetic clinic. Diabet Med, 18: 928-32.

111. Croal BL, Mutch WJ, Clark BM, Dickie A, Church J, Noble D, Ross IS. The clinical application of a urine albumin: creatinine ratio point-of-care device. Clinical Chimica Acta, 2001; 15-21

112. Sacks DB, Bruns DE, Goldstein DE, Maclaren NK, McDonald JM, Parrott M (2002). Guidelines and recommendations for laboratory analysis in the diagnosis and management of diabetes mellitus. Clinica Chemistry 48: 436-72.

113. Mogensen CE. Microalbuminuria: concepts and definition. In Mogensen CE (ed.) Diabetic nephropathy in type 2 diabetes. Science Press, London, 2002, pp. 1-11.

114. Poulsen PL. Microalbuminuria: techniques of measurement and monitoring . The concept of early intervention. In Mogensen CE (ed.) Diabetic nephropathy in type 2 diabetes. Science Press, London, 2002, pp. 11-23.

115. Parving H-H, Oxenboll B, Svendsen PA, Christiansen JS, Andersen AR (1982) Early detection of patients at risk of developing diabetic nephropathy. A prospective study of urinary albumin excretion. Acta Endocrinol (Copenhagen) 100:550-555

116. Viberti GC, Hill RD, Jarret RJ, Argyropoulos A, Mahmud U, Keen H (1982) Microalbuminuria as a predictor of clinical nephropathy in insulin-dependent diabetes mellitus. Lancet I:1430-1432

117. Poulsen PL, Hjollund E, Nielsen MN, Knudsen ST, Andersen NH, Hansen KW, Mogensen CE. (2002) Microalbuminuria is the single most powerful predictor of 25-year mortality in type 1 diabetes. [Abstract]. Diabetologia, 45(S2): A76

118. Rossing P, Hougaard P, Borch-Johnsen K, Parving HH (1996). Risk factors for mortality in IDDM patients, a 10 years observational follow-up study. BMJ 313, 779-84.

119. The Diabetes Control and Complications Trial/Epidemiology of Diabetes Interventions and Compliations Research Group (2000). Retinopathy and nephropathy in patients with type 1 diabetes four years after a trial of intensive therapy. N Engl J Med, 342: 381-89.

120. Forsblom CM, Groop P-H, Ekstrand A, Groop LC (1992) Predictive value of microalbuminuria in patients with insulin-dependent diabetes of long duration. BMJ 305: 1051-1053

121. Arun CS, Stoddart J, Mackin P, Marshall SM (2003). Significance of microalbuminuria in long duration type 1 diabetes. Diabetes Care, In press.
122. Allen KV, Walker JD (2002). The prognostic significance of abnormal urinary albumin excretion in long-duration type 1 diabetes [Abstract]. Diabetes, 51(S2): A713
123. Mogensen CE (1983) Microalbuminuria in maturity onset, primarily type 2 (non-insulin-dependent) diabetes, predicts clinical proteinuria and early mortality. Diabetologia 26: 181 (Abstract)
124. Mogensen CE (1984) Microalbuminuria predicts clinical proteinuria and early mortality in maturity-onset diabetes. N Engl J Med 310: 356-360
125. Dinneen S, Gerstein HC (1997) The association of microalbuminuria and mortality in non-insulin-dependent diabetes mellitus. A systematic overview of the literature. Arch Intern Med 157:1413-1418
126. Tanaka Y, Atsumi Y, Matsuoka K, Onuma T, Tohjima T, Kawamori R (1998) Role of glycemic control and blood pressure in the development and progression of nephropathy in elderly Japanese NIDDM Patients. Diabetes Care 21:116-120
127. Forsblom CM, Groop P-H, Ekstrand A et al. (1998) Predictors of progression from normoalbuminuria to microalbuminuria in NIDDM. Diabetes Care 21:1932-1938
128. Schmitz A (1997) Microalbuminuria, blood pressure, metabolic control, and renal involvement. Longitudinal studies in white non-insulin-dependent diabetic patients. American Journal of Hypertension 10: 189S-197S
129. Schmitz A, Vaeth M, Mogensen CE (1994) Systolic blood pressure relates to the rate of progression of albuminuria in NIDDM. Diabetologia 37:1251-1258
130. Nielsen S, Schmitz A, Rehling M, Mogensen CE (1997) The clinical course of renal function in NIDDM patients with normo- and microalbuminuria. J Intern Med 241: 133-141
131. Nielsen S, Schmitz A, Rehling M, Mogensen CE (1993) Systolic blood pressure determines the rate of decline of glomerular filtration rate in Type 2 (non-insulin-dependent) diabetes mellitus. Diabetes Care 16: 1427-1432
132. Nielsen S, Schmitz A, Poulsen PL, Hansen KW, Mogensen CE (1995) Albuminuria and 24-h ambulatory blood pressure in normoalbuminuric and microalbuminuric NIDDM patients: a longitudinal study. Diabetes Care 18: 1434-1441
133. Nielsen S, Schmitz A, Derkx FHM, Mogensen CE (1995) Prorenin and renal function in NIDDM patients with normo- and microalbuminuria. J Intern Med 238: 499-505
134. Nielsen S, Schmitz A, Bacher T, Rehling M, Ingerslev J, Mogensen CE (1999). Transcapillary escape rate and albuminuria in Type II diabetes. Effects of short-term treatment with low-molecular weight heparin. Diabetologia, 42:60-67.
135. Nielsen S, Schmitz A, Knudsen RE, Dollerup J, Mogensen CE (1994) Enalapril versus bendroflumethiazide in type 2 diabetes complicated by hypertension. Q J Med 87: 747-754
136. Fioretto P, Stehouwer CDA, Mauer M et al. (1998) Heterogeneous nature of microalbuminuria in NIDDM: Studies of endothelial function and renal structure. Diabetologia 41: 233-236
137. Inomata S, Osawa Y, Itoh M (1987) Analysis of urinary proteins in diabetes mellitus - with reference to the relationship between microalbuminuria and diabetic renal lesions. J Jpn Diabetes Soc 30: 429-436
138. UKPDS 33 (1998) An intensive blood glucose control policy with sulphonylureas or insulin reduces the risk of diabetic complications in patients with Type 2 diabetes. Lancet 352:837-853

139. Turner R, Holman R, Stratton 1 et al. for United Kingdom Prospective Diabetes Study Group (1998) Tight blood pressure control and risk of macrovascular and microvascular complications in type 2 diabetes: United Kingdom prospective diabetes study 38. BMJ 317: 703-713

140. Holman R, Turner R, Stratton I et al. for United Kingdom Prospective Diabetes Study Group (1998). Efficacy of atenolol and captopril in reducing risk of macrovascular and microvascular complications in type 2 diabetes: United Kingdom prospective diabetes study 39. BMJ 317: 713-720

141. Adler AI, Stevens RJ, Manley SE, Bilous RW, Cull CA, Holman RR on behalf of the UKPDS group (2002). Development and progression of nephropathy in type diabetes: observations and modelling from the United Kingdom Prospective Diabetes Study. Kidney Int, 63: 225-32.

142. Heart Outcomes Prevention Evaluation (HOPE) Study Investigators (2000). Effects of ramipril on cardiovascular and microvascular outcomes in people with diabetes mellitus: results of the HOPE study and MICRO-HOPE substudy. *Lancet*, 355: 253-59.

143. Estacio RO, Jeffers BW, Gifford N, Schrier RW (2000). Effect of blood pressure control on diabetic microvascular complications in patients with hypertension and type 2 diabetes. *Diabetes Care*, 23(S2): B54-64.

144. Chan JCN, Ko GTC, Leung DHY, Cheung RC, Cheung MY, So WY (2000). Long-term effects of angiotensin-converting enzyme inhibition and metabolic control in hypertensive type 2 diabetic patients. *Kidney Int.*, 58: 590-600.

145. Lacourcière Y, Bélanger A, Godin C (2000). Long-term comparison of losartan and enalapril on kidney function in hypertensive type 2 diabetics with early nephropathy. *Kidney Int.*, 58: 762-69.

146. Mogensen CE, Neldam S, Tikkanen I, Oren S, Viskoper R, Watts RW, Cooper ME for the CALM study group (2000). Randomised controlled trial of dual blockade of renin-angiotensin system in patients with hypertension, microalbuminuria, and non-insulin dependent diabetes: the candesartan and lisinopril microalbuminuria (CALM) study. *BMJ*, 321: 1440-4.

147. Andersen NH, Mogensen CE (2002). Angiotensin converting enzyme inhibitors and angiotensin II receptor blockers: Evidence for and against the combination in the treatment of hypertension and proteinuria. *Current Hypertension Reports*, 4: 394-402.

148. Fernandez R, Puig JG, Rodriguez-Perez JC, Garrido J, Redon J on behalf of the TRAVEND Study Group (2001). Effect of two antihypertensive combinations on metabolic control in type 2 diabetic hypertensive patients with albuminuria: a randomised, double-blind study. *Journal of Human Hypertension*, 15: 849-56.

149. Parving HH, Lehnert H, Brochner-Mortensen J, Gomis R, Andersen S, Arner P for the Irbesartan in Patients with Type 2 Diabetes and Microalbuminuria Study Group (2001). The effect of irbesartan on the development of diabetic nephropathy in patients with type 2 diabetes. *N Engl J Med* 345: 870-8.

150. Sasso FC, Carbonara O, Persico M, Iafusco D, Salvatore T, D'Ambrosio R (2002). Irbesartan reduces the albumin excretion rate in microalbuminuric type 2 diabetic patients independently of hypertension. *Diabetes Care*, 25: 1909-13.

151. Viberti GC, Wheeldon NM, for the MicroAlbuminuria Reduction With VALsartan (MARVAL) study investigators (2002). Microalbuminuria reduction with valsartan in patients with type 2 diabetes mellitus. A blood pressure – independent effect. *Circulation*, 106: 672-78.

152. Schrier RW, Estacio RO, Esler A, Mehler P (2002). Effects of aggressive blood pressure control in normotensive type 2 diabetic patients on albuminuria, retinopathy and strokes. *Kidney Int*. 61: 1086-97.

153. Mogensen CE, Viberti GC, Halimi S, Ritz E, Ruilope L, Jermendy G (2003). Effect of low-dose perinodopril/indapamide on albuminuria in diabetes. PREterax in albuMInuria regression- PREMIER. *Hypertension*, 41: 1063-71.

154. Rippin J, Bain SC, Barnett AH. Rationale and design of diabetics exposed to telmisartan and enalapril (DETAIL) study (2002). *Journal of Diabetes and its Complications*, 16: 195-200.

155. Lindholm LH, Ibsen H, Dahlof B, Devereux RB, Beevers G, De Fair U (2002). Cardiovascular morbidity and mortality in patients with diabetes in the Losartan Intervention For Endpoint reduction in hypertension study (LIFE): a randomised trial against atenolol. *Lancet,* 359: 1004-10.

156. Epstein M, Buckalew V, Martinez F (2002). Antiproteinuric efficacy of epleronone, enalapril and epleronone/enalapril combination therapy in diabetic hypertensives with microalbuminuria [Abstract]. *Am J Hypertens*, 15: 24A.

157. Sato A, Hayashi K, Naruse M, Saruta T (2003). Effectiveness of aldosterone blockade in patients with diabetic nephropathy. *Hypertension,* 41: 64-68.

158. Gaede P, Vedel P, Larsen N, Jensen G, Parving HH, Pedersen O (2003). The Steno-2 study: intensified multifactorial intervention reduces the risk of cardiovascular disease in patients with type 2 diabetes and microalbuminuria. *New Engl J Med,* 348: 383-93

159. Gaede P, Beck M, Vedel P, Pedersen O (2001). Limited impact of lifestyle education in patients with type 2 diabetes mellitus and microalbuminuria: results from a randomized intervention study. *Diabetic Med,* 18: 104-8.

160. Marre M, Lievre M, Chatellier G for the DIABHYCAR study group (2002). Low-dose ramipril (1.25 mg/day) does not decrease cardiovascular events in type 2 diabetes patients with microalbuminuria/proteinuria: the DIABHYCAR (Type 2 DIAbetes, HYpertension, CArdivascular, Events and Ramipril Study [Abstract]. Diabetes, 51(S2): A171

161. The ALLHAT Officers and Coordinators for the ALLHAT Collaborative Research Group (2002). Major outcome in high-risk hypertensive patients randomized to angiotensin-converting enzyme inhibitor or calcium channel blocker vs. diuretic. The Antihypertensive and lipid-lowering treatment to prevent heart attack trial (ALLHAT). *JAMA,* 288: 2981-97.

162. Kylin E (1923) Studien über das Hypertonie-Hyperglykamie-Hyperurikaemie Syndrom. Zentralblatt fair Innere Medizin 7:105-112

163. Himsworth HP (1939) Mechanisms of diabetes mellitus (Goulstonian Lecture). Lancet 2: 1-6, 65-68, 118-122, 171-175

164. Himsworth HP (1949). The syndrome of diabetes mellitus and its causes. Lancet, March 19, 1949: 465-472

165. Vague J (1949) Le diabéte de la femme androide. Presse Med. Paris 57: 835-837

166. Avogaro P, Creapaldi G (1965) Essential hypertension, hyperlipemia, obesity and diabetes. European Association for the Study of Diabetes. Diabetologia 1: 137 (Abstract)

167. Jarrett RJ (1992) In defence of insulin: a critique of syndrome X. Lancet 340: 469-471

168. Hauerslev CF, Vestbo, E, Frøland A, Mogensen CE, Damsgaard EM. (2000). Normal blood pressure and preserved diurnal variation in offspring of type 2 diabetic patients characterised by the features of the Metabolic Syndrome. Diabetes Care, 23:283-89.

169. Karlefors T (1966) Circulatory studies during exercise with particular reference to diabetes. Acta Med Scand 180 [Suppl 4491]:1-87

170. Christensen CK (1991) The pre-proteinuric phase of diabetic nephropathy. Dan Med Bull 38:145-159

171. Vittinghus E, Mogensen CE (1981) Albumin excretion and renal hemodynamic response to physical exercise in normal and diabetic man. Scand J Clin Lab Invest 41: 627-632

172. Vittinghus E, Mogensen CE (1982) Graded exercise and protein excretion in diabetic man and the effect of insulin treatment. Kidney Int 21: 725-729

173. Mogensen CE, Vittinghus E (1975) Urinary albumin excretion during exercise in juvenile diabetes. A provocative test for early abnormalities. Scand J Clin Lab Invest 35: 295-300

174. Mogensen CE, Solling K (1977) Studies on renal tubular protein reabsorption: Partial and near complete inhibition by certain amino acids. Scand J Clin Lab Invest 37: 477-486

175. Mogensen CE, Vittinghus E, Solling K (1975) Increased urinary albumin, light chain, and beta-2-microglobulin excretion after intravenous arginine administration in normal man. Lancet II:581-583

176. Mogensen CE, Christensen NJ, Gundersen HJG (1978) The acute effect of insulin on renal haemodynamics and protein excretion in diabetics. Diabetologia 15: 153-157

177. Parving H-H, Christiansen JS, Noer I, Tronier B, Mogensen CE (1980) The effect of glucagon infusion on kidney function in short-term insulin-dependent juvenile diabetics. Diabetologia 19: 350-354

178. Parving H-H, Noer 1, Kehlet H, Mogensen CE. Svendsen PAa, Heding L (1977) The effect of short-term glucogen infusion on kidney function in normal man. Diabetologia 13: 323-325

179. Parving H-H, Noer 1, Mogensen CE, Svendsen PA (1978) Kidney function in normal man during short-term growth hormone infusion. Acta Endocrinol (Copenhagen) 89: 796-800

180. Mogensen CE, Vittinghus E, Solling K (1979) Abnormal albumin excretion after two provocative renal test in diabetes: Physical exercise and lysine injection. Kidney Int 16: 385-393

181. Hinman AT, Engel BT, Bickford AF (1962) Portable blood pressure recorder. Accuracy and preliminary use in evalutating intradaily variations in pressure. Am Heart J 63: 663—668

182. Richardson DW, Honour AJ, Fenton GW, Stott FH and Pickering GW (1964) Variation in arterial pressure throughout the day and night. Clin Sci 26: 445-460

183. Rubler S, Abenavoli T, Greenblatt HA, Dixon JF, Cieslik CJ (1982) Ambulatory blood pressure monitoring in diabetic males: A method for detecting blood pressure elevations undisclosed by conventional methods. Clin Cardiol 5: 447-454

184. Hansen KW, Christensen CK, Andersen PH, Mau Pedersen M, Christiansen JS, Mogensen CE (1992) Ambulatory blood pressure in microalbuminuric type 1 diabetic patients. Kidney Int 41: 847-854

185. Hansen KW, Klein F, Christensen PD et al. (1994) Effects of captopril on ambulatory blood pressure, renal and cardiac function in microalbuminuric type 1 diabetic patients. Diabetes Metab 20: 485-493

186. Hansen KW, Mau Pedersen M, Christensen CK, Christiansen JS, Mogensen CE (1992) Normoalbuminuria ensures no reduction of renal function in Type 1 (insulin-dependent) diabetic patients. J Intern Med 232: 161-167

187. Hansen KW, Mau Pedersen M, Christiansen JS, Mogensen CE (1993) Acute renal effects of angiotensin converting enzyme inhibition in microalbuminuric type 1 diabetic patients. Acta Diabetol 30: 149-153

188. Hansen KW, Mau Pedersen M, Christiansen JS, Mogensen CE (1993) Diurnal blood pressure variations in normoalbuminuric type 1 diabetic patients. J Intern Med 234: 175-180

189. Hansen KW, Mau Pedersen M, Christiansen JS, Mogensen CE (1994) Night blood pressure and cigarette smoking; disparate association in healthy subjects and diabetic patients. Blood Pressure 3: 381-388

190. Hansen KW, Mau Pedersen M, Marshall SM, Christiansen JS, Mogensen CE (1992) Circadian variation of blood pressure in patients with diabetic nephropathy. Diabetologia 35: 1074-1079

191. Hansen KW, Poulsen PL, Christiansen JS, Mogensen CE (1995) Determinants of 24-h blood pressure in IDDM patients. Diabetes Care 18: 529-535

192. Hansen KW, Poulsen PL, Mogensen CE (1994) Ambulatory blood pressure and abnormal albuminuria in type 1 diabetic patients. Kidney Int 45 [Suppl 45]:S134-S140

193. Hansen KW, Sorensen K, Christensen PD, Pedersen EB, Christiansen JS, Mogensen CE (1995) Night blood pressure: Relation to organ lesions in microalbuminuric type 1 diabetic patients. Diabet Med 12: 42-45

194. Poulsen PL, Hansen KW, Mogensen CE (1994) Ambulatory blood pressure in the transition from normo- to microalbuminuria. A longitudinal study in IDDM patients. Diabetes 43: 1248-1253

195. Poulsen PL, Ebbehoj E, Hansen KW, Mogensen CE (1997) 24-h blood pressure and autonomic function is related to albumin excretion within the normoalbuminuric range in IDDM patients. Diabetologia 40: 718-725

196. Poulsen PL, Bek T, Ebbehoj E, Hansen KW, Mogensen CE (1998) 24-h ambulatory blood pressure and retinopathy in normoalbuminuric IDDM patients. Diabetologia 41: 105-110

197. Poulsen PL, Ebbehoj E, Nosadini R, Fioretto P, Deferrai D, Crepaldi D, Mogensen CE (2001). Early ACE-i intervention in microalbuminuric patients with type 1 diabetes: Effects on albumin excretion, 24h ambulatory blood pressure and renal function. Diabetes and Metab., 27: 123-28.

198. Poulsen PL, Juhl B, Ebbehoj E, Klein F, Christiansen C, Mogensen CE (1997) Elevated ambulatory blood pressure in microalbuminuric IDDM patients is inversely associated with renal plasma flow. A compensatory mechanism? Diabetes Care 20: 429-432

199. Poulsen PL, Ebbehoj E, Mogensen CE (2001). Lisinopril reduces albuminuria during exercise in low-grade microalbuminuric type 1 diabetic patients: A double blind randomised study. J Intern Med, 249: 433-440.

200. Poulsen PL, Ebbehoj E, Hansen KW, Mogensen CE (1998) Effects of smoking on 24-h ambulatory blood pressure and autonomic function in normoalbuminuric insulin-dependent diabetes mellitus patients. Am J Hypertens 11: 1093-1099

201. Poulsen PL, Hansen KW, Ebbehøj E, Knudsen ST, Mogensen CE (2000). No deleterious effects of tight blood glocuse control on 24-h ambulatory blood pressure in normoalbuminuric insulin dependent diabetes mellitus patients. J Clin Endocrinol Metab, 85: 155-58.

202. Svensson P, de Faire U, Sleight P, Yusuf S, Ostergren J (2001). Comparative effects of ramipril on ambulatory and office blood pressures: a HOPE substudy. Hypertension, 38: E28-32.

203. Wallenius G (1954) Renal clearance of dextran as a measure of glomerular permeability. Acta Soc Med Upsaliensis [Suppl 4]

204. Lins H, Jahnke K, Scholtan W (1959) Ober die Permeabilität makromolekularer Stoffe. In: Oberdisse K, Jahnke K (eds) Die Niere bei diabetischen und anderen Nephropathien in Diabetes Mellitus. Proceedings of the Ill. Congress of the International Diabetes Federation. Georg Thieme Verlag, Stuttgart, pp 203-206

205. Lambert PP, Gassée JP, Askenasi R (1968) La perméabilité du rein aux macromolecules physiopathologie de la protéinurie. In: Lambert PP (ed) Acquisitions récentes de physiopathologie rénale. Editions Desoer S. A., Liège, Belgique, pp 181-214

206. Deckert T, Kofoed-Enevoldsen A, Vidal P, Norgaard K, Andreasen HB, Feldt-Rasmussen B (1993) Size- and charge selectivity of glomerular filtration in type 1 (insulin-dependent) diabetic patients with and without albuminuria. Diabetologia 36: 244-251

207. Myers BD, Nelson RG, Williams GW et al. (1991) Glomerular function in Pima Indians with noninsulin-dependent diabetes mellitus of recent onset. J Clin Invest 88: 524-530

208. Morelli E, Loon N, Meyer T, Peters W, Myers BD (1990) Effects of converting-enzyme inhibition on barrier function in diabetic glomerulopathy. Diabetes 39: 76-82

209. Andersen S, Blouch K, Bialek J, Deckert M, Parving HH, Myers BD (2000). Glomerular permselectivity in early stages of overt diabetic nephropathy. Kidn Int, 58: 2129-37.

210. Gaster B, Hirsch IB (1998) The effects of improved glycemic control on complications in type 2 diabetes. Archives of Internal Medicine 158: 134-140

211. Krolewski AS, Laffel LMB, Krolewski M, Quinn M, Warram JH (1995) Glycosylated hemoglobin and the risk of microalbuminuria in patients with insulin-dependent diabetes mellitus. N Engl J Med 332:1251-1255

212. Microalbuminuria Collaborative Study Group, UK (1995) Intensive therapy and progression to clinical albuminuria in patients with insulin dependent diabetes mellitus and microalbuminuria. BMJ 311: 973-977

213. Christensen CK, Mogensen CE (1985) The course of incipient diabetic nephropathy: Studies of albumin excretion and blood pressure. Diabetic Medicine 2: 97-102

214. Swales JD (1985). Platt versus Pickering: An episode of recent medical history. Keynes Press.

215. Viberti GC (2003). Pharmaceutical approaches to the management of hypertension in diabetes mellitus. In Mogensen CE (ed). Hypertension and Diabetes, vol. 3. Lippincott Williams and Wilkins, , London. In press.

216. Christensen CK, Mogensen CE (1985) Effect of antihypertensive treatment on progression of disease in incipient diabetic nephropathy. Hypertension 7:II-109-II-113

217. Christensen CK, Mogensen CE (1987) Antihypertensive treatment: long-term reversal of progression of albuminuria in incipient diabetic nephropathy. A longitudinal study of renal function. J Diabetes Complications 1: 45-52

218. Mau Pedersen M, Christensen CK, Hansen KW, Christiansen JS, Mogensen CE (1991) ACE-inhibition and renoprotection in early diabetic nephropathy. Response to enalapril acutely and in long-term combination wtih conventional antihypertensive treatment. Clin Invest Med 14: 642-651

219. Mau Pedersen M, Hansen KW, Schmitz A, Sorensen K, Christensen CK, Mogensen CE (1992) Effects of ACE inhibition supplementary to beta blockers and diuretics in early diabetic nephropathy. Kidney Int 41: 883-890

220. Mogensen CE, Pedersen M.M, Ebbehoj E, Poulsen PL, Schmitz A (1997) Combination therapy in hypertension-associated diabetic renal disease. International Journal of Clinical Practice [Suppl] 90: 52-58

221. Marre M, Chatellier G, Leblanc H, Guyenne T-T, Ménard J, Passa PH (1988) Prevention of diabetic nephropathy with Enalapril in normotensive diabetics with microalbuminuria. BMJ 297:1092-1095

222. Mathiesen ER, Hommel E, Giese J, Parving H-H (1991) Efficacy of captopril in postponing nephropathy in normotensive insulin-dependent diabetic patients with microalbuminuria. BMJ 303: 81-87

223. Mathiesen ER, Hommel E, Hansen HP, Smidt UM, Parving H-H. (1999) Randomised controlled trial of long term efficacy of captopril on preservation of kidney function in normtensive patients with insulin dependent diabetes and microalbuminuria. BMJ, 319; 24-25.

224. Melbourne Diabetic Nephropathy Study Group (1991) Comparison between perindopril and nifedipine in hypertensive and normotensive diabetic patients with microalbuminuria. BMJ 302:210-216

225. Barnes DJ, Cooper M, Gans DJ, Laffel L, Mogensen CE, Viberti GC (1996) Microalbuminuria Captopril Study Group. Captopril reduces the risk of nephropathy in insulin-dependent diabetic patients with microalbuminuria. Diabetologia 39: 587-593

226. Ravid M, Brosh D, Levi Z, Bar-Dayan Y, Ravid D, Rachmani R (1998). Use of enalapril to attenuate decline in renal function in normotensive, normoalbuminuric patients with type 2 diabetes mellitus. Ann Intern Med, 128: 982-988.

227. Ravid M, Brosh D, Levi Z, Bar-Dayan Y, Ravid D, Rachmani R (1998) Use of enalapril to attenuate decline in renal function in normotensive patients with type 2 diabetes mellitus. A randomized controlled trial. Ann Intern Med 128: 982-988

228. Viberti GC, Mogensen CE, Groop L, Pauls JF for the European Microalbuminuria Captopril Study Group (1994) Effect of captopril on progression to clinical proteinuria in patients with insulin-dependent diabetes mellitus and microalbuminuria. JAMA 271: 275-279

229. The ACE-inhibitors in Diabetic Nephropathy Trialist Group (2001). Should all patients with type 1 diabetes mellitus and microalbuminuria receive angiotensin-converting enzyme inhibitors? A meta-analysis of individual patient data. Ann Intern Med, 134: 370-79.

230. American Diabetes Ass (2003). Diabetic Nephropathy. Diabetes Care, 26(S1): S94-98.

231. Mogensen CE (1971) Glomerular filtration rate and renal plasma flow in short-term and long-term juvenile diabetes Scand J Clin Lab Invest 28: 91-100

232. Mogensen CE (1971) Maximum tubular reabsorption capacity for glucose and renal hemodynamics during rapid hypertonic glucose infusion in normal and diabetic man. Scand J Clin Lab Invest 28: 101-109

233. Mogensen CE (1976) Progression of nephropathy in longterm diabetes with proteinuria and effect of initial hypertensive treatment. Scand J Clin Lab Invest 36: 383-388

234. Mogensen CE (1976) High blood pressure as a factor in the progression of diabetic nephropathy. Acta Med Scand [Suppl 602]:29-32

235. Mogensen CE, Hansen KW, Mau Pedersen M, Christensen CK (1991) Renal factors influencing blood pressure threshold and choice of treatment for hypertension in IDDM. Diabetes Care 14[Suppl 4]:13-26

236. Mogensen CE (1997) How to protect the kidney in diabetic patients: with special reference to IDDM. Diabetes 46 [Suppl 2]S104-Slll

237. Mogensen CE (1982) Long-term antihypertensive treatment inhibiting progression of diabetic nephropathy. BMJ 285:685-688

238. Parving H-H, Smidt UM, Andersen AR, Svendsen PAA (1983) Early aggressive antihypertensive treatment reduces rate of decline in kidney function in diabetic nephropathy. Lancet 1:1175-1179

239. Parving H-H, Andersen AR, Schmidt UM, Hommel E, Mathiesen ER, Svendsen PAA (1987) Effect of antihypertensive treatment on kidney function in diabetic nephropathy. BMJ 294:1443-1447

240. Parving H-H, Jacobsen P, Rossing K, Smidt UM, Hommel E, Rossing P (1996) Benefits of long-term antihypertensive treatment on prognosis in diabetic nephropathy. Kidney Int 49:1778-1782

241. Hovind P, Rossing P, Tarnow L, Smidt UM, Parving HH (2001). Progression of diabetic nephropathy. Kidney Int, 59: 702-9.

242. Andersen S, Jacobsen P, Tarnow L, Rossing P, Juhl TR, Parving HH (2003). Time course of the antiproteinuric and antihypertensive effect of losartan in diabetic nephropathy. Nephrol Dial Transplant, 18: 293-97.

243. Parving H-H, Hommel E (1989) Prognosis in diabetic nephropathy. BMJ 299:230-233

244. Mathiesen ER, Borch-Johnsen K, Jensen DV, Deckert T (1989) Improved survival in patients with diabetic nephropathy. Diabetologia 32: 884-886

245. Björck S, Mulec H, Johnsen SA, Nordén G, Aurell M (1992) Renal protective effect of enalapril in diabetic nephropathy. BMJ 304: 339-343

246. Kurtz TW (2003). False claims of blood pressure – independent protection by blockade of the renin angiotensin aldosterone system? [Editorial]. Hypertension, 41: 193-96.

247. Weir MR, Dworkin LD (1998) Antihypertensive drugs, dietary salt, and renal protection: How low should you go and with which therapy? Am J Kidney Dis 32(l):1-22

248. Lewis E, Hunsicker L, Bain R, Rhode R (1993) The effect of angiotensin-converting enzyme inhibition on diabetic nephropathy. N Engl J Med 329:1456-1462

249. Ruggenenti P, Perna A, Gherardi G, Gaspari F, Benini R, Remuzzi G on behalf of the Gruppo Italiano di Studi Epidemiologici in Nefrologia (GISEN) (1998) Renal function and requirement for dialysis in chronic nephropathy patients on long-term ramipril: REIN follow-up trial. Lancet 352:1252-1256

250. Nakao N, Yoshimura A, Morita H, Takada M, Kayano T, Ideura T (2003). Combination treatment of angiotensin II receptor blocker and angiotensin-converting enzyme inhibitor in non-diabetic renal disease (COOPERATE): a randomised controlled trial. Lancet, 361: 117-24.

251. Campbell R, Sangalli F, Perticucci E, Aros C, Viscarrra C, Perna A, Remuzzi A, Bertocchi F, Fagiani L, Remuzzi G, Ruggenenti P (2003). Effects of combined ACE-inhibitor and angiotensin II antagonist treatment in human chronic nephropathies. Kidney Int, 63: 1094-1103.

252. Nyberg G, Blohmé G, Nordén G (1987) Impact of metabolic control in progression of clinical diabetic nephropathy. Diabetologia 30: 82-86

253. Pickup JC, Keen H, Parsons JA, Alberti KGMM (1978) Continuous subcutaneous insulin infusion: an approach to achieving normoglycaemia. BMJ 1: 204-207

254. Christensen CK, Christiansen JS, Christensen T, Hermansen K, Mogensen CE (1986) The effect of six months continuous subcutaneous insulin infusion on kidney function and size in insulin-dependent diabetics. Diabetic Medicine 3:29-32

255. Moller A, Rasmussen L, Ledet T, Christiansen JS, Christensen CK, Mogensen CE, Hermansen K (1986) Lipoprotein changes during CSII treatment in IDDM patients Scand J Clin Lab Invest 46: 471-475

256. Thuesen L, Christiansen JS, Sorensen KE et al. (1986) Exercise capacity and cardiac function in type 1 diabetic patients treated with continuous subcutaneous insulin infusion. A controlled study. Scand J Clin Lab Invest 46: 779-784

257. Hermansen K, Moller A, Christensen CK et al. (1987) Diurnal plasma profiles of metabolise and hormone concentration in insulin-dependent diabetic patients during conventional insulin treatment and continuous subcutaneous insulin infusion. A controlled study. Acta Endocrinol (Copenhagen) 114: 433-439

258. Mogensen CE (1988) Therapeutic interventions in nephropathy of IDDM. Diabetes Care 11 [Suppl 1]:10-15

259. Jakobsen J, Christiansen JS, Christensen CK, Hermansen K, Schmitz A, Mogensen CE (1988) Autonomic and somatosensory nerve function after two years of continuous subcutaneous insulin infusion in type 1 diabetes. Diabetes 37: 452-455

260. Hermansen K, Schmitz 0, Boye N, Christensen CK, Christiansen JS, Alberti KGMM, Orskov H, Mogensen CE (1988) Glucagon responses to intravenous arginine and oral glucose in insulin-dependent diabetic patients during six months conventional or continous subcutaneous insulin infusion. Metabolism 37: 640-644

261. Schmitz A, Christiansen JS, Christensen CK, Hermansen K, Mogensen CE (1989) Effect of pump versus pen treatment on glycemic control and kidney-function in longterm uncomplicated insulin-dependent diabetes-mellitus (IDDM). Dan Med Bull 36:176-178

262. Mogensen CE, Hansen KW (1990) Preventing or postponing renal disease in insulin-dependent diabetes by glycemic and nonglycemic intervention. In: Klinkmann H, Smeby LC (eds) Terminal Renal Failure: Therapeutic Problems, Possibilities, and Potentials. Contrib Nephrol, Karger, Basel78:73-101

263. Kelly WD, Lillehei RC, Merkel FK, Idezuki Y, Goetz FC (1967) Allotransplantation of the pancreas and duodenum along with the kidney in diabetic nephropathy. Surgery 61: 827

264. Dubernard JM, Traeger J, Neyra P, Touraine JL, Tranchant D, Blanc-Brunat N (1978) A new method of preparation of segmental pancreatic grafts for transplantation. Trials in dogs and in man. Surgery 84: 633

265. Sutherland DER, Gruessner RW, Dunn DL, Matas AJ, Humar A, Kandaswamy R, Mauer SM, Kennedy WR, Goetz FC, Robertson RP, Gruessner AC, Najarian JS (2001). Lessons from more than 1,000 pancreas transplants at a single institution. Ann Surg, 233: 463-501.

266. Manske CL (1999) Risks and benefits of kidney and pancreas transplantation for diabetic patients. Diabetes Care, 22 (S2): B114-120

267. Fioretto P, Steffes MW, Sutherland DER, Goetz FC, Mauer M (1998) Reversal of lesions of diabetic nephropathy after pancreas transplantation. N Engl J Med 339: 69-75

268. Nyberg G, Hoidaas H, Brekke IB, Hartmann A, Nordén G, Olausson M, Osterby R (1996) Glomerular ultrastructure in kidneys transplanted simultaneously with a segmental pancreas to patients with type 1 diabetes. Nephrol Dial Transplant ll: 1029-1033

269. Zatz R, Dunn BR, Meyer TW, Anderson S, Rennke HG, Brenner BM (1986) Prevention of diabetic glomerulopathy by pharmacological amelioration of glomerular capillary hypertension. J Clin Invest 77: 1925-1930

270. Solomon CG (2003). Reducing cardiovascular risk in type 2 diabetes. [Editorial]. New Engl J Med, 348: 457-9.

271. Frohlich ED (2003). Treating hypertension – what are we to believe? [Editorial]. New Engl J Med, 348: 639-41.

272. August P (2003). Initial treatment of hypertension. New Engl J Med, 348: 610-7.

273. Mogensen CE (2003). New treatment guidelines for a patient with diabetes and hypertension. J Hypertens, 21(S1): S25-30.

274. Berkman J, Rifkin H. (1973) Unilateral nodular diabetic glomeruloschlerosis (Kimmelsteil-Wilson). Report of a case. Metabolism Clin Exp 22; 715-722.

275. Mogensen CE (1992) Angiotensin converting enzyme inhibitors and diabetic nephropathy. Their effects on proteinuria may be independent of their effects on blood pressure. Editorial. BMJ 304: 327-328

276. Thuesen L, Christiansen JS, Falstie-Jensen N, Christensen CK, Hermansen K, Mogensen CE, Henningsen P (1985) Increased myocardial contractility in short-term type 1 diabetic patients: an echocardiographic study. Diabetologia 28:822-826

277. Parving H-H, Viberti GC, Keen H, Christiansen JS, Lassen NA (1983) Haemodynamic factors in the genesis of diabetic microangiopathy. Metabolism 32: 943-949
278. Dunder K, Lind L, Zethelius B, Berglund L, Lithell H. Increase in blood glucose concentration during antihypertensive treatment as a predictor of myocardial infarction: population based cohort study. BMJ, 326: 681-4.
279. Gress TW, Nieto FJ, Shahar E, Wofford MR, Brancati FL for the Atherosclerosis Risk in Communities Study (2000). Hypertension and antihypertensive therapy as risk factors for type 2 diabetes mellitus. NEJM, 342: 905-11.
280. Gall M-A, Borch-Johnsen K, Hougaard P, Nielsen FS, Parving H-H (1995) Albuminuria and poor glycemic control predicts mortality in NIDDM. Diabetes 44: 1303-1309
281. Krop JS, Coresh J, Chambless LE, Shahar E, Watson RL, Szklo M, Brancati FL (1999). A community-based study of explanatory factors for the excess risk for early renal function decline in blacks vs. whites with diabetes. Arch Intern Med, 159: 1777-83.
282. Abernethy DR, Schwartz JB (1999). Calcium antagonist drugs. New Engl J Med, 341: 1447-57.
283. Mogensen CE (1999) Drug treatment for hypertensive patients in special situations: Diabetes and hypertension. Clin Exp Hypertens, 21(5-6): 895-906.
284. Brenner BM (2002). Remission of renal disease: recounting the challenge, acquiring the goal. J Clin Invest, 110: 1753-58.
285. Brenner BM, Cooper ME, de Zeeuw D, Keane WF, Mitch WE, Parving HH et al for the Reduction of Endpoints in NIDDM with the Angiotensin II Antagonist Losartan (Renaal) Study Renaal Investigators: Effects of losartan on renal and cardiovascular outcomes in patients with type 2 diabetes and nephropathy. *New Engl J Med*, 2001; 345: 861-70.
286. Lewis EJ, Hunsicker LG, Clarke WR, Berl T, Pohl MA, Lewis JB et al. Renoprotective effect of the angiotensin.receptor antagonist irbesartan in patients with nephropathy due to type 2 diabetes. *N Engl J Med*, 2001; 345: 851-61
287. Ritz E, Dikow R. Angiotensin receptor antagonists in patients with nephropathy due to type 2 diabetes. *Ann Med.*, 2002; 34: 507-13.
288. Parving HH. (2001). Diabetic nephropathy: Prevention and treatment. Kidn Int., 60: 2041-55.
289. Nielsen S, Dollerup J, Nielsen B, Jensen HA, Mogensen CE (1997) Losartan reduces albuminuria in patients with essential hypertension. An enalapril controlled 3 months study. Nephrol Dial Transplant 12:19-23
290. Krolewski AS, Warram JH, Christlieb AR, Busick EJ, Kahn CR (1985) The changing natural history of nephropathy in type 1 diabetes. Am J Med 78: 785-794.
291. Brun C, Gormsen H, Hilden T, Iversen P, Raaschou F (1953). Diabetic nepropathy. Kidney biopsy and renal function tests. Am J Med, 15: 187-97.
292. Ditscherlein G. Nierenveränderungen bei Diabetikern. VEB Gustav Fischer Verlag Jena, 1969
293. Mauer SM, Steffes MW, Ellis EN, Sutherland DER, Brown DM, Goetz FC (1984) Structural functional relationships in diabetic nephropathy. J Clin Invest 74: 1143-1155
294. Schwartz MM, Lewis EJ, Leonard-Martin T, Lewis JB, Batlle D and the Collaborative Study Group (1998). Renal pathology patterns in type 2 diabetes mellitus: relationship with retinopathy. Nephrol Dial Transplant, 13: 2547-2552.
295. Olsen S, Mogensen CE (1996) How often is Type 2 diabetes mellitus complicated with non-diabetic renal disease? A material of renal biopsies and an analysis of the literature. Diabetologia 39: 1638-1645
296. Olsen S. The renal structural damage in patients with type 2 diabetes. In Mogensen CE (ed.) Diabetic Nephropathy in type 2 diabetes. Science Press, 2002, pp. 31-41.

297. Osterby R, Tapia J, Nyberg G (2001). Renal structures in type 2 diabetic patients with elevated albumin excretion rate. APMIS, 109: 751-61.

298. The Diabetes Control and Complications Trial/Epidemiology of Diabetes Interventions and Complications Research Group. (2000). Retinopathy and nephropathy in patients with type 1 diabetes four years after a trial of intensive therapy. N Engl J Med, 342: 381-9.

299. The Heart Outcomes Prevention Evaluation Study Investigators (2000) Effects of an angiotensin-converting-enzyme inhibitor, ramipril, on death from cardiovascular causes, myocardial infarction and stroke in high-risk patients. New Engl J Med, 342:145-53.

300. Caramori ML, Mauer M, Fioretto P (2000). The need for early predictors of diabetic nephropathy risk: is albumin excretion rate sufficient? Diabetes, 49: 1399-408.

301. Mogensen, Cooper (2003). Diabetic Renal disease: From recent studies to improved clinical practice. Diabetic Med, In press.

302. Luetscher JA, Kraemer FB, Wilson DM, Schwartz HC, Bryer-Ash M (1985). Increased plasma inactive renin in diabetes mellitus. N Engl J Med, 312

303. Deinum J, Rønn B, Mathiesen E, Derkx FHM, Hop WCJ, Shalekamp MADH (1999). Increase in serum prorenin precedes onset of microalbuminuria in patients with insulin-dependent diabetes mellitus. Diabetologia, 42: 1006-1010.

304. Fioretto P, Steffes MW, Mauer M (1994) Glomerular structure in nonproteinuric IDDM patients with various levels of albuminuria. Diabetes 43:1358-1364

305. The controlled therapeutic trial [editorial] (1948) BMJ 2: 791-792

306. Chalmers I (1998) Unbiased, relevant and reliable assessments in health care. BMJ 317:1167-1168

307. University Group Diabetes Program (1970) A study of the effects of hypoglycemic agents on vascular complications in patients with adult-onset diabetes. Diabetes 19 [Suppl 2]: 747-830

308. Creutzfeldt W (1994) The discovery of the oral treatment of diabetes mellitus with sulphonylureas. In: Mogensen CE, Standl E (eds) Research methodologies in Human Diabetes, part 1. Walter de Gruyter, Berlin, New York, pp 11-20

309. Peto R, Collins R, Gray R (1995) Large-scale randomized evidence: large, simple trials and overviews of trials. J Clin Epidemiol 48(1): 23-40

310. Thomson SG (1994) Why sources of heterogeneity in metaanalysis should be investigated. BMJ 309: 1351-1355

311. Feinstein AR (1995) Meta-analysis: statistical alchemy for the 21st century. J Clin Epidemiol 48: 71-79

312. Spitzer WO (1995) The challenge of meta-analysis (Editor's Keynote Address). J Clin Epidemiol 48:1-4

313. Victor N (1995) The challenge of meta-analysis: Discussion. Indications and contra-indications for meta-analysis. J Clin Epidemiol 48: 5-8

314. Sharp SJ, Thomson SG, Altman DG (1996) The relation between treatment benefit and underlying risk in metaanalysis. BMJ 313: 1550-1551

315. Lelorier J, Geneviève G, Benhaddad A, Lapierre J, Derderian F (1997) Discrepancies between meta-analyses and subsequent large randomized controlled trials. New Engl J Med 337: 536-542

316. Laffel LMB, McGill JB, Gans DJ on behalf of the North American Microalbuminuria Study Group. (1995). The beneficial effect of angiotensin-converting-enzyme inhibition with captopril on diabetic nephropathy in normotensive IDDM patients with microalbuminuria. Am Journ Med, 99: 497-504.

317. The Euclid Study Group. (1997). Randomised placebo-controlled trial of lisinopril in normotensive patients with insulin-dependent diabetes and normoalbuminuria or microalbuminuria. Lancet, 349: 1787-92.

318. Bojestig M, Karlberg B, Lindstrom T, Nystrom FH (2001). Reduction of ACE activity is insufficient to decrease microalbuminuria in normotensive patients with type 1 diabetes. Diabetes Care, 24: 919-24.

319. Crepaldi G, Carta Q, Deferrari G, Mangili R, Navalesi R, Santeusanio F, Spalluto A, Vanasia A, Villa GM, Nosadini R for the Italian Microalbuminuria Study Group in IDDM (1998). Diabetes Care, 21:104-110.

320. O'Hare JP, Bilbous R, Mitchell T, O'Callaghan CJ, Viberti GC (2000). Low-dose ramipril reduces microalbuminuria in type 1 diabetic patients without hypertension: results of a randomised controlled trial. Diabetes, 23: 1823-9.

321. Jerums G on behalf of the Melbourne Diabetic Nephropathy Study Group, Melbourne, Australia (1998). Ace inhibition vs. calcium-channel blockade in normotensive type 1 and type 2 diabetic patients with microalbuminuria. Nephrology Dial Trans, 13: 1065-66.

322. Poulsen PL (2003). ACE-inhibitor intervention in type 1 diabetes with low grade microalbuminuria. JRAAS, 4: 17-26.

323. Scottish Intercollegiate Guidelines Network. Management of Diabetes. A national clinical guideline. Nov. 2001.

324. 2003 European Society of Hypertension-European Society of Cardiology Guidelines for the Management of Arterial Hypertension. J Hypertension, In press, 2003.

325. Mooradian AD (2003). Cardiovascular disease in type 2 diabetes. Current Management Guidelines. Arch Int Med, 163: 33-40.

326. Onuigbo M, Weir MR (2003). Evidence-based treatment of hypertension in patients with diabetes mellitus. Diabetes, Obesity and Metabolism, 5: 13-26.

327. American Diabetes Association (2003) Treatment of hypertension in adults with diabetes. Diabetes Care 26(S1):S80-83.

328. American Diabetes Association (2003) Evidence-based nutrition principles and recommendations for the treatment and prevention of diabetes and related compliations. Diabetes Care 26 (S1):S51-62

329. WHO, Geneva 2003. WHO Technical report series 916. Diet, nutrition and the prevention of chronic diseases.

330. Lundbæk K (1953). Long-term diabetes. The clinical picture in diabetes mellitus of 15-25 years duration with a follow-up of a regional series of cases. Munksgaard, Copenhagen and Lange, Maxwell & Springer Ltd.

331. McCarty MF (1998) A central role for protein kinase C overactivity in diabetic glomerulosclerosis: implications for prevention with antioxidants, fish oil, and ACE inhibitors. Medical Hypotheses, 50: 155-65.

332. Wahren J and Johansson BL (1998). Ernst-Friedrich-Pfeiffer Memorial Lecture. New aspects of C-peptide physiology. Horm Metab Res, 30: A2-5

333. Oates J, Mylari BL (1999). Aldose reductase inhibitors: therapeutic implications for diabetic complications. Exp. Opin Invest Drugs, 8: 2095-2119.

334. Gambaro O, Kinalska I, Oksa A, Pont'Uch P, Hertlova M, Olsovsky J, Manitus J, Fedele D, Czekalski S, Perusicova J, Skrha J, Taton J, Grezeszak W, Crepaldi G (2002). Oral sulodexide reduces albuminuria in microalbuminuric and macroalbuminuric type 1 and type 2 diabetic patients: The Di.N.A.S. Randomized trial. J Am Soc Nephrol, 13: 1615-25.

335. Drummond K, Mauer M, for the International Diabetic Study Group (2002). The early natural history of nephropathy in type 1 diabetes. II Early renal structural changes in type 1 diabetes. Diabetes, 51: 1580-87.

336. Ebihara S, Nakamura T, Shimada N, Koide H (1998). Increased plasma metalloproteinase-9 concentrations precede development of microalbuminuria in non-insulin-dependent diabetes mellitus. Am J Kidney Dis, 32: 544-50.

337. Tikkanen T, Tikkanen I, Rockell MD et al. (1998). Dual inhibition of neutral endopeptidase and angiotensi-converting enzyme in rats with hypertension and diabetes mellitus. Hypertension, 32: 778-85.

338. Turner AJ, Murphy LJ (1996). Molecular pharmacology of endothelin converting enzyme. Biochem Pharmacol 51: 91-102.

339. Khalifah RG, Baynes JW, Hudson BG (1999). Amadorins: novel post-Amadori inhibitors of advanced glyaction reactions. Biochem Biophys Res. Commun, 257: 251-8.

340. Bakris G, Viberti GC, Weston WM, Heise M, Porter LE, Freed MI (2003). Rosiglitazone reduces urinary albumin excretion in type 2 diabetes. J Human Hypertension, 17: 7-12.

341. Cooper ME (1998) Pathogenesis, prevention and treatment of diabetic nephropathy. Lancet 352: 213-219

342. Anitschkow N, Chalatow S (1913) Uber experim. Cholesterinsteatose, Zentralbl. falg Pathol u. pathol Anst Bd 24: 379-403.

343. Pijls L, de Vries H, van Eijk JTM, Donker AJM (2002). Protein restriction, glomerular filtration rate and albuminuria in patients with type 2 diabetes mellitus: a randomized trial. Eur J Clin Nutr, 56: 1200-7.

344. Hansen HP, Tauber-Lassen E, Jensen BR, Parving HH (2002). Effect of dietary protein restriction on prognosis in patients with diabetic nephropathy. Kidney Int., 62: 220-8.

345. Sever PS, Dahlöf B, Poulter NR, Wedel H, Beevers G, Caulfield M, Collins R, Kjeldsen SE, Kristinsson A, McInnes GT, Mehlsen J, Nieminen M, O'Brien E, Östergren J for the ASCOT Investigators (2003). Prevention of coronary and stroke events with atorvastatin in hypertensive patients who have average or lower-than-average cholesterol concentrations in the Anglo-Scandinavian Cardiac Outcomes Trial – Lipid Lowering Arm (ASCOT-LLA): a multicentre randomised controlled trial. Lancet, 361: 1149-58.

346. Feldt-Rasmussen B, Hegedüs L, Mathiesen ER, Deckert T (1991). Kidney volume in type 1 (insulin-dependent) diabetic patients with normal or increased urinary albumin excretion: effect of long-term improved metabolic control. Scand J Clin Lab Invest, 51: 31-36

347. Cambier P (1934) Application de la théorie de Rehberg a l'etude clinique des affections rénales et du diabete. Annales Médicine 35: 273-299

348. Fiaschi E, Grassi B, Andres G (1952). La funzione renal nel diabete mellito. Rassegna di Fisiopatologia Clinica & Terapeutica 24: 373-410

349. Stadler G, Schmid R, Wolff MV (1960) Funktionelle Mikroangiopathie der Nieren beim behandelten Diabetes mellitus im Kindesalter. Dtsch Med Wochenschr 85: 346

350. Ditzel J, Schwartz M (1967) Abnormally increased glomerular filtration rate in short-term insulin-treated diabetic subjects. Diabetes 16: 264

351. Mogensen CE (1972) Glomerular filtration rate and renal plasma flow in long-term juvenile diabetics without proteinuria. BMJ 4: 257-259

352. Yip WJ, Jones LS, Wiseman JM, Hill C, Viberti GC (1996) Glomerular hyperfiltration in the prediction of nephropathy in IDDM. Diabetes 45:1729-1733

353. Mauer M, Drummond K for the International Diabetic Nephropathy Study Group (2002). The early natural history of nephropathy in type 1 diabetes. I Study design and baseline charachteristics of the study participants. Diabetes, 51: 1572-79.

354. Keen H, Chlouverakis C (1963) An immunoassay method for urinary albumin at low concentrations. Lancet ii: 913

355. Miles DW, Mogensen CE, Gundersen HJG (1970) Radioimmunoassay for urinary albumin using a single antibody. Scand J Clin Lab Invest 26: 5-11

356. Mogensen CE (1971) Urinary albumin excretion in early and long-term juvenile diabetes. Scand J Clin Lab Invest 28: 183-193

357. Mogensen CE (1988) Management of diabetic renal involvement and disease. Lancet I:867-870

358. Mogensen CE (1995) Management of early nephropathy in diabetic patients. Ann Rev Med 46: 79-93

359. Mogensen CE, Keane WF, Bennett PH et al. (1995) Prevention of diabetic renal disease with special reference to microalbuminuria. Lancet 346:1080-1084

360. Mogensen CE, Vestbo E, Poulsen PL et al. (1995) Microalbuminuria and potential confounders. A review and some observations on variability of urinary albumin excretion. Diabetes Care 18:572-581

361. Mogensen CE, Poulsen PL (1994) Epidemiology of microalbuminuria in diabetes and in the background population. Curr Opin Nephrol Hypertens 3: 248-256

362. Borch-Johnsen K, Wenzel H Viberti GC, Mogensen CE (1993) Is screening and intervention for microalbuminuria worthwhile in patients with insulin dependent diabetes? BMJ 306:1722-1725

363. Parving H-H, Tarnow L, Nielsen FS, Rossing P, Mandrup-Poulsen T, Osterby R, Nerup J (1999). Cyclosporine nephrotoxicity in type 1 diabetic patients. A 7-year follow-up study. Diabetes Care, 22: 478-83.

364. Kimmelstiel P, Wilson C (1936) Intercapillary lesions in the glomeruli of the kidney. Am J Pathol 12: 83-95

365. Gellman DD, Pirani C, Soothill JF, Muehrcke RC, Kark RM (1959) Diabetic nephropathy: a clinical and pathological study based on renal biopsies. Medicine 38: 321

366. Thomsen CAA (1965) The Kidney in Diabetes Mellitus. A Clinical and Histological Investigation Based on Renal Biopsy Material. Munksgaard, Copenhagen

367. Reaven GM (2002). Metabolic syndrome. Pathophysiology and Implications for Management of Cardiovascular Disease. Circulation, 106: 286-88.

368. Reaven GM (2003). Importance of identifying the overweigth patient who will benefit the most be losing weight. Ann Intern Med, 138: 420-23.

369. Keiding NR, Root HF, Marble A (1952) Importance of control of diabetes in prevention of vascular complications. JAMA 150:964-969

370. Wang PH, Lau J, Chalmers TC (1993) Meta-analysis of effects of intensive blood-glucose control on late complications of type 1 diabetes. Lancet 341: 1306-1309

371. Mulec H, Blohmé G, Grande B, Björck S (1998) The effect of metabolic control on rate of decline in renal function in insulin-dependent diabetes mellitus with overt diabetic nephropathy. Nephrol Dial Transplant 13: 651-655

372. Crepaldi G, Carta Q, Deferrari G et al. and The Italian Microalbuminuria Study Group in IDDM (1998) Effects of lisinopril and nifedipine on the progression to overt albuminuria in IDDM patients with incipient nephropathy and normal blood pressure. Diabetes Care 21: 104-110

373. Mau Pedersen M, Schmitz A, Pedersen EB, Danielsen H, Christiansen JS (1988) Acute and long-term renal effects of angiotensin converting enzyme inhibition in normotensive, normoalbuminuric insulin-dependent diabetic patients. Diabetic Med 5: 562-569

374. Viberti GC, Keen H, Wiseman MJ (1987) Raised arterial pressure in parents of proteinuric insulin-dependent diabetics. BMJ 295: 515-517

375. Doria A, Warram JH, Krolewski AS (1995) Genetic susceptibility to nephropathy in insulin-dependent diabetes: from epidemiology to molecular genetics. Diabetes Metab Rev 11: 287-314

376. Marre M (1999) Genetics and the predictions of complications in type 1 diabetes. Diabetes Care, 22: B53-B58

377. Tuominen JA, Ebeling P, Koivisto VA (1998) Long-term lisinopril therapy reduces exercise-induced albuminuria in normoalbuminuric normotensive IDDM patients. Diabetes Care 21: 1345-1348

378. Hemmelder MH, de Jong P, de Zeeuw D (1998). A comparison of analytic procedures for measurement of fractional dextran clearances. J Lab Clin Med, 132:390-403.

379. Flyvbjerg A, Hill C, Logan A (1999). Pathophysiological role of growth factors in diabetic kidney disease: Focus on innovative therapy. Trends in Endocrinology and Metabolism, 10: 267-272.

380. Wolf G, Ziyadeh FN (1999). Molecular mechanisms of diabetic renal hypertrophy. Kidney Int, 56: 393-405.

381. King GL, Ishii H, Koya D (1997). Diabetic vascular dysfunction: A model of excessive activation of protein kinase C. Kidney Int., 52:S77-S85.

382. Willenheimer R, Dahlöf B, Rydberg E, Erhard L (1999). AT_1-receptor blockers in hypertension and heart failure: clinical experience and future directions. European Heart Journal, 20: 997-1008.

383. Schalkwijk CG, Chaturvedi N, Twaafhoven H, van Hinsbergh VWM, Stehouwer CDA and the EUCLID Study Group (2002). Amadori-albumin correlates with microvascular complications and precedes nephropathy in type 1 diabetic patients. Eur J Clin Inv., 32: 500-506.

384. Friedman EA (1999). Advanced glycation end-products in diabetic nephropathy. Nephrol Dial Transplant, 14 (s3): 1-9.

385. Rossing K, Christensen PK, Andersen S, Hovind P, Hansen HP, Parving HH (2003). Comparative effects of Irbesartan on ambulatory and office blood pressure. A substudy of ambulatory blood pressure from the irbesartan in patients with type 2 diabetes and microalbuminuric study. Diabetes Care, 26: 569-74.

386. WHO/FAO (2003): www. who.int/hpr/nutrition/expertconsultationge.htm

387. Mogensen CE. The early detection of renal impairment in diabetes mellitus. The case for microalbuminuria and other biomakers. In Trull AK et al (eds.) Biomarkers of Disease. An evidence-based approach. Cambridge University Press, Cambridge, UK, pp. 76-95.

388. Mogensen CE (2002). Microalbuminuria in perspectives. In EA Friedman and FA L'Esperance, Jr (eds). Diabetic renal-retinal syndrome. Kluwer Academic Publ., Netherlands, pp. 106-120.

389. Knudsen ST, Bek T, Poulsen PL, Hove MN, Rehling M, Mogensen CE (2003). Effects of losartan on diabetic maculopathy in type 2 diabetic patients. A randomized, double-masked study. J Int Medicine, In press.

390. Chobanian AV, Bakris GL, Black HR, Cushman WC, Green LA, Izzo JL, Materson BJ, Oparil S, Wrigth Jr JT, Roccella EJ and the National High Blood Pressure Education Program Coordinating Committee (2003). The seventh report of the Joint National Committee on Prevention, Detection, Evaluation, and Treatment of high blood pressure. The JNC 7 Report. JAMA, 289: 2560-72.

INDEX